Howell-Jolly bodies—postsplenectomy

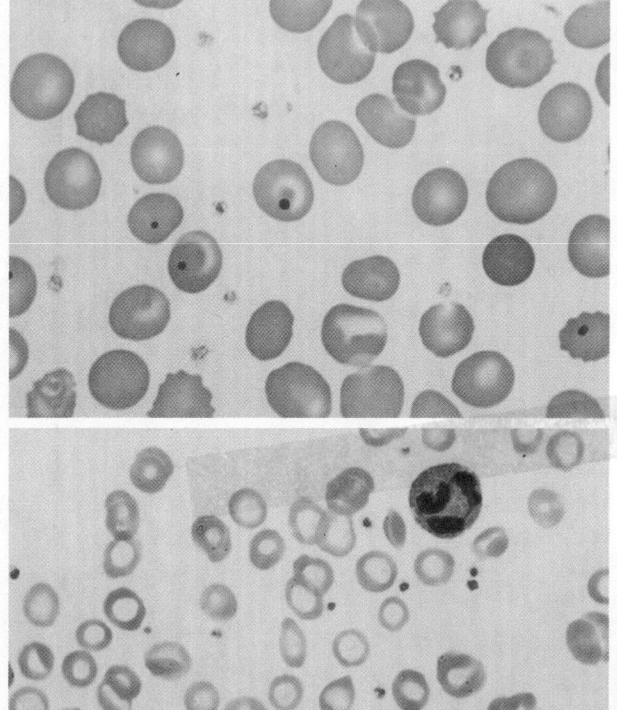

Microcytic hypochromic erythrocytes
in iron deficiency anemia

Ovalocytes in hereditary ovalocytosis

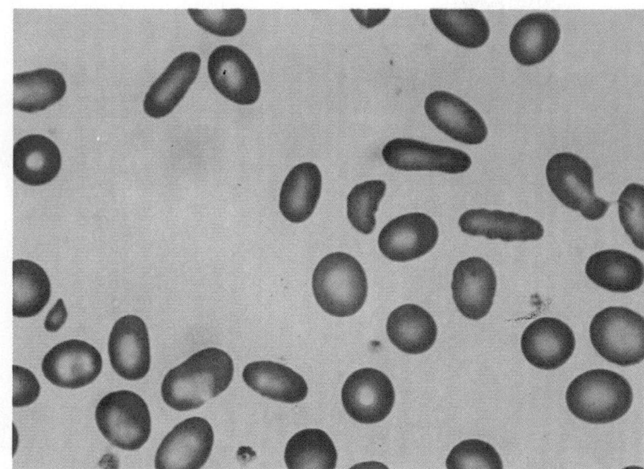

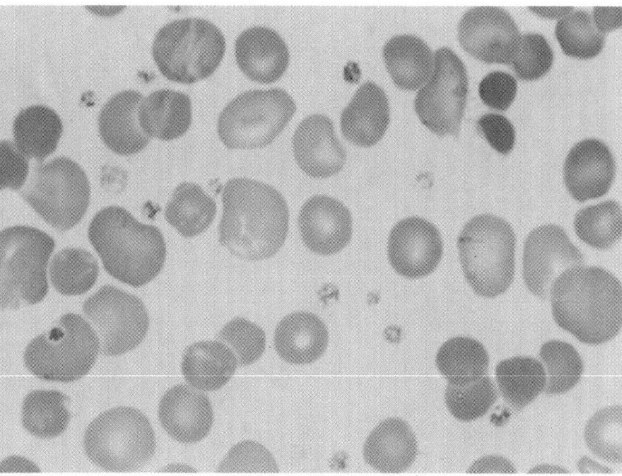

Polychromasia in peripheral blood in hemolytic anemia

Macrocytes and thrombocytopenia in pernicious anemia

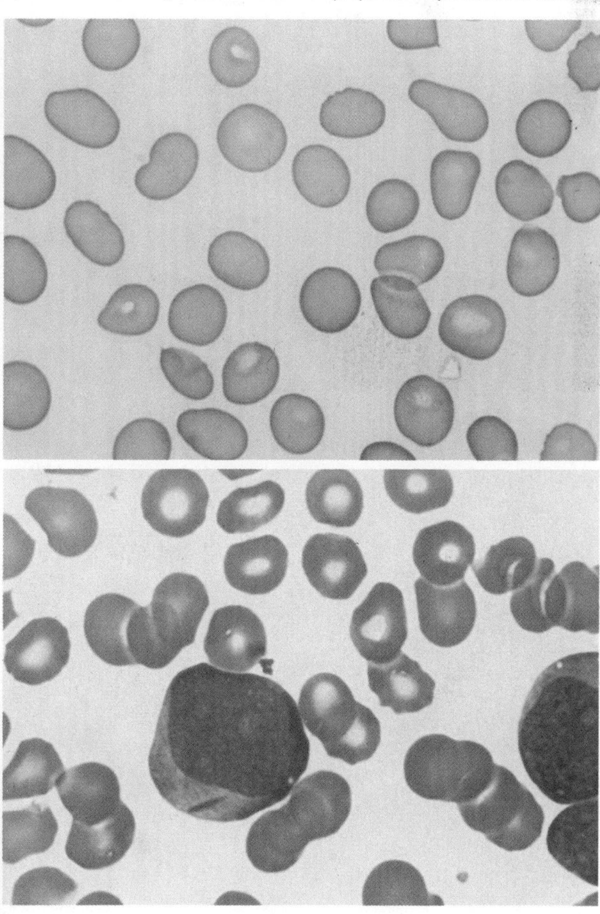

Myeloblast showing Auer rod

All × 1250

UNIVERSITY OF ROCHESTER LIBRARIES
3 9087 00474567 7

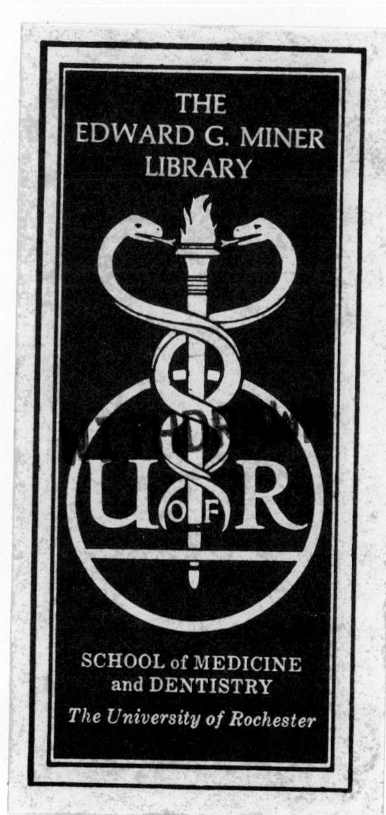
THE
EDWARD G. MINER
LIBRARY
U OF R
SCHOOL of MEDICINE
and DENTISTRY
The University of Rochester

AUTHORS

Chemistry

T. A. HYDE
M.D., M.R.C.Path., F.R.C.P.(C)

Pathologist, Hotel-Dieu of St. Joseph Hospital, Windsor, Ontario; Adjunct Professor in Clinical Chemistry, University of Windsor, Windsor, Ontario

LESLIE D. MELLOR
F.C.S.L.T., F.I.M.L.S.

Member, Canadian Society of Clinical Chemists; Chief Technologist, Department of Biochemistry, Women's College Hospital, Toronto, Ontario

Microbiology

STANLEY S. RAPHAEL

FRANK SPENCER
Ph.D.

Associate Professor, Department of Anthropology, Queens College of the City University of New York, Flushing, New York

Immunohematology and Hematology

MARTIN J. INWOOD
B.Sc., M.D., F.R.C.P.(C), F.I.M.L.S., L.C.S.L.T.

Chief, Divisions of Laboratory and Clinical Hematology, St. Joseph's Hospital, London, Ontario; Associate Professor, Department of Medicine, University of Western Ontario, London, Ontario

SAM THOMSON
B.A., F.I.M.L.S., A.R.T.

Chief Technologist, Division of Hematology and Blood Bank, St. Joseph's Hospital, London, Ontario; Lecturer in Advanced Medical Technology Program, Fanshawe College of Applied Arts and Technology, London, Ontario; Technical Director, Medical Services Laboratory, London, Ontario

NEVILLE J. BRYANT
A.R.T., F.A.C.B.S.

Serological Services Ltd. Toronto, Ontario

Histotechnology

STANLEY S. RAPHAEL

Lynch's MEDICAL LABORATORY TECHNOLOGY

Fourth Edition

Senior Author

STANLEY S. RAPHAEL

M.B., F.R.C.P.(C), F.R.C.Path.

Pathologist, Hotel-Dieu of St. Joseph Hospital, Windsor, Ontario

1983

W. B. Saunders Company

Philadelphia • London • Toronto • Mexico City • Rio de Janeiro • Sydney • Tokyo

W. B. Saunders Company: West Washington Square
Philadelphia, PA 19105

1 St. Anne's Road
Eastbourne, East Sussex BN21 3UN, England

1 Goldthorne Avenue
Toronto, Ontario M8Z 5T9, Canada

Apartado 26370—Cedro 512
Mexico 4, D.F., Mexico

Rua Coronel Cabrita, 8
Sao Cristovao Caixa Postal 21176
Rio de Janeiro, Brazil

9 Waltham Street
Artarmon, N.S.W. 2064, Australia

Ichibancho, Central Bldg., 22-1 Ichibancho
Chiyoda-Ku, Tokyo 102, Japan

Library of Congress Cataloging in Publication Data

Lynch, Matthew J.

Lynch's Medical laboratory technology.

1. Medical technology. I. Raphael, Stanley S. II. Title. III. Title: Medical laboratory technology. [DNLM: 1. Medical laboratory technology. 2. Technology, Medical. QY 25 L987m]

RB37.L9 1983 616.07′5 82–42570

ISBN 0–7216–7465–8

Listed here is the latest translated edition of this book, together with the language of the translation and the publisher:

Spanish (*2nd edition*)—Nueva Editorial Interamericana, Mexico

Front cover illustrations:
Top right—Ammonium urate crystals in urine.
Bottom right—Culture of *Sporothrix schenckii.*
Middle—ABO grouping: tube technique. Positive, top tube; negative, bottom tube.
Bottom left—Bone marrow in idiopathic thrombocytopenic purpura.
Top left—Liver section stained with aldehyde fuchsin to show HBsAg.

Lynch's Medical Laboratory Technology ISBN 0-7216-7465-8

Last digit is the print number: 9 8 7 6 5 4 3 2 1

A shy person does not learn, nor should
a short-tempered person teach.

Ethics of the Fathers, first century A.D.

PREFACE TO THE FOURTH EDITION

This fourth edition of *Lynch's Medical Laboratory Technology* is primarily intended and has been completely revised for use by students preparing for the M.T. (ASCP) or the R.T. (Canada). The authors have focused on the subjects delineated in the syllabi for these examinations and have emphasized preferred methodology, deleting alternative and less advantageous approaches. In doing so, we have achieved considerable economy in size. Between the first and third edition, the length of the book had doubled in 13 years, and although the subject has grown remarkably, a further increase of 50% would have increased the size of the book to more than 2000 pages, thus limiting its use to one of reference. This has never been our aim, which remains to produce a practical technical book that would answer successfully not only the question "how" but also "why."

Readers of previous editions will notice the extensive changes in each section, many parts of which have been completely rewritten, but we trust it retains the "clarity and concinnity" of which the late Dr. Lynch was such a master.

Many entirely new topics have been broached, and deeper explorations of established methodologies have been made, despite our self-imposed limitations of space. These include enzymatic methods for cholesterol and triglyceride estimation, sources of error in blood gas analysis, therapeutic drug monitoring, discussion of glycosylated hemoglobin and high-density lipoprotein cholesterol, and reviews of new methodologies for amylase and uric acid studies. In additon to an introduction to automation in bacteriology, there is an amplified section on preventive maintenance of laboratory apparatus, a revised section on spectrophotometer checking, and an updated section on automated biochemical instrumentation. There is also a broader consideration of anaerobic infections and a look at the basic chemistry of common bacteriological biochemical tests.

The authors would like to express their gratitude to colleagues who have impaired enlightenment and assistance. Dr. Jan Schwarz of the University of Cincinnati, Ohio, kindly reviewed the chapter on Mycology. Dr. P. Blaskovic of the Virology Laboratory of the Ontario Public Health Laboratory provided many of the illustrations in the chapter on Virology, and Dr. D. Yong of the Public Health Laboratory, Windsor, Ontario also gave his assistance in this matter. Mrs. Merilyn Donaghue, R.T., P. Harris, A.R.T., K. Leigh, A.R.T., Larry Stockwell, R.T., Ms. Miriam van Egmond, R.T., and Wayne Frenette, M.T. (ASCP) SI assisted in their areas of expertise. Mrs. Margaret Peto, once again with unfailing efficiency, saved the senior author from becoming completely overwhelmed in the mountain of paper from which this volume is distilled. Mr. Baxter Venable of Saunders provided us with the initial impetus and the benefit of his knowledge of our reader market to commence the revision. His encouragement was never further than the nearest telephone. Other members of the staff at Saunders showed much consideration and patience, and the senior author would particularly like to thank Mr. Alan Sorkowitz.

Sadly Mr. Culling died since the publication of the last edition. The authorship has been joined by Neville Bryant, who has made a valuable and erudite contribution to a close cooperative effort.

STANLEY S. RAPHAEL

CONTENTS

1

AN INTRODUCTION TO MEDICAL LABORATORY SCIENCE

It appears fitting to commence with a consideration of the physiology and the anatomy of the cell, which, in the final analysis, is the site of all the reactions with which we are concerned in laboratory medicine. In the recent past, with the electron microscope and advances in molecular biology, it has become possible to relate very accurately the structure of the cell to its function.

An average mammalian cell is some 15 to 20 μm (micrometer = 10^{-6} meter, formerly μ) in diameter and has a volume of 3000 to 6000 fL (femtoliters = 10^{-15} liter, formerly μ^3). Within the confines of this tiny space is a completely automated, computerized factory of an elegance and complexity that surpasses the imagination. By combining cell fractionation studies of the biochemists with electron microscopy, which gives a resolution of 1 nm to 0.5 nm (nanometer = $meter^{-9}$, formerly 10 Å), i.e., some 200 to 400 times the resolving power of the light microscope, many of the secrets of the cell have been laid bare.

ANATOMY OF THE CELL

Each cell is bounded by a cell membrane through which substances (metabolites, anabolites, and secretions) may pass in either direction under biological control. Some particles do not obey the usual thermodynamic rules in crossing the membrane but are facilitated in passing in one direction or the other by enzyme action. Within the cell cytoplasm there is *endoplasmic reticulum*, which is a complicated membranous structure on which *ribosomes* are located. The latter are small "jigs" that manufacture protein under nuclear control (see below). Numerous mitochondria are also present, and within these respiration occurs—that is, the oxidation of carbon and hydrogen components to CO_2 and H_2O with the production of energy. The energy is used in the performance of cellular functions.

Other intracellular structures include *lysosomes*, which are small formations containing varied enzymes capable of hydrolyzing most major groups of organic compounds, and the *Golgi complex*, in which the products of the cell (mucus and so forth) are assembled before secretion. Other subcellular bodies are present but will not be described here.

Each cell has a nucleus bounded by a nuclear membrane. The nucleus controls the metabolism and anabolism of the cell and also carries with it either the genetic information to reproduce itself or, in the case of a specialized gonadal cell, part of the information to reproduce a new individual. Within the nucleus are structures called *nucleoli*, which play an important role in the transmission of information from the nucleus to the cytoplasm (see below). The red blood cell, unlike most human cells, loses its nucleus in development and does not reproduce itself, but its substance is recycled by the body in the manufacture of new cells.

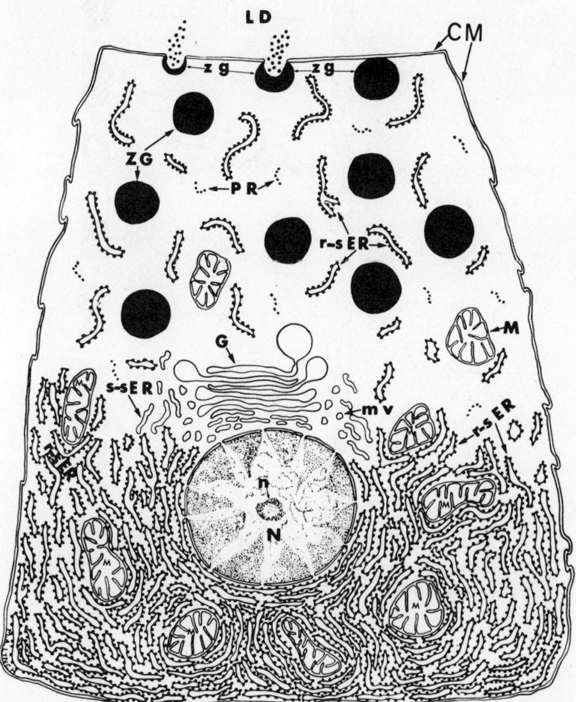

Figure 1–1 Pancreatic acinar cell. *LD*, lumen of ductule; *ZG*, zymogen granules; *zg*, same in process of secretion; *PR*, polyribosomes; *r-s ER, rough-surfaced endoplasmic reticulum, very abundant in basal (lower) part of cell, where it has long been referred to as ergastoplasm; G*, Golgi complex; *mv*, microvesicles; *M*, mitochondrion; *s-s ER*, smooth-surfaced endoplasmic reticulum; *N*, nucleus; *n*, nucleolus; *CM*, cell membrane.

The Nucleus

Every cell nucleus in the body contains 46 chromosomes, consisting of 44 autosomes ("self" chromosomes) and two sex chromosomes (2X in female and XY in male). On these chromosomes are carried all the inherited characteristics that govern the activity of every cell in the body. Each cell receives the same total legacy of inherited characteristics, yet, obviously, cells differ in appearance and functions throughout the body; most are specialized to some degree, and some are highly specialized. These differences, which underlie cell differentiation and specialization, are brought about by expression of some inherited characteristics and repression of others. The basis of all such expression lies in proteins, both structural and enzymatic, and when we say that a cell is highly specialized, we mean that it is producing and using enzymes that are either not produced by other cells or produced by them in different quantities and mixtures.

The chromosomes consist very largely of DNA (deoxyribonucleic acid).

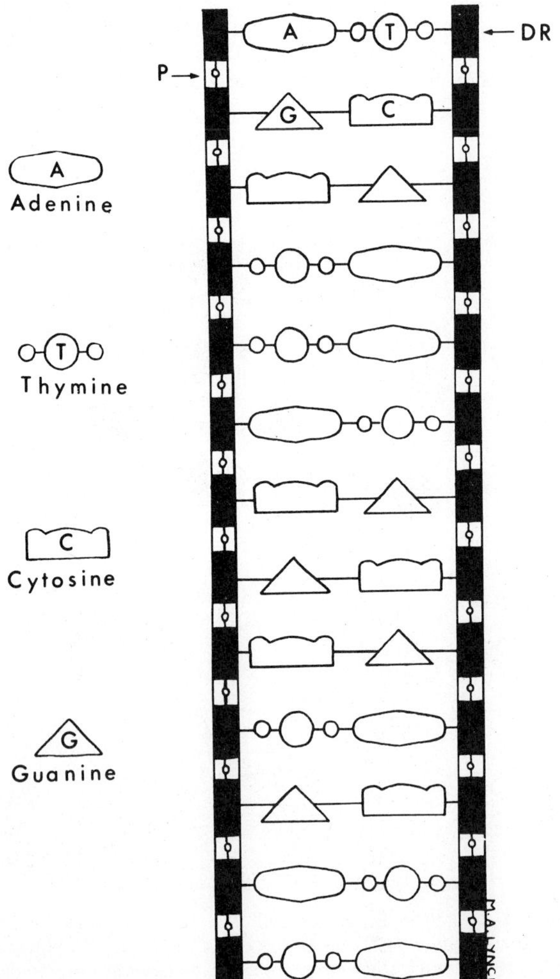

Figure 1–2 Portion of the double-stranded DNA molecule. *P*, phosphoric acid residues; *DR*, deoxyribose. Note the order of base pairing.

THE CHEMISTRY OF NUCLEIC ACIDS

The DNA molecule is composed of polymerized nucleotides, each of which is made up of phosphoric acid, the pentose deoxyribose, and a base. There are four bases: two purines, adenine and guanine, and two pyrimidines, thymine and cytosine. These organic bases, each in combination with a molecule of deoxyribose and of phosphoric acid, are the structural units—nucleotides—of DNA. The four nucleotides are named after their bases: adenylic, guanylic, thymidylic, and cytidylic acids.

The other type of nucleic acid in the cell, i.e., ribonucleic acid (RNA), has, with two exceptions, the same components in its makeup. The two exceptions are: (1) RNA has ribose instead of deoxyribose, and (2) it has the pyrimidine uracil instead of thymine. Thus the four nucleotides of RNA (ribonucleotides) are adenylic, guanylic, uridylic, and cytidylic acids. As will be seen from the structural formula of adenylic acid and from Figure 1–2, the bases are always linked to the pentose. Suitable hydrolysis of DNA or RNA liberates the nucleotides; further hydrolysis splits off the phosphoric acid from these and yields compounds consisting of base and pentose. These are known as nucleosides, which are also named after the constituent base: adenosine, guanosine, thymidine, uridine, and cytidine.

Organic Base	Corresponding Nucleotide*	Corresponding Nucleoside*
Adenine	adenylic acid	adenosine
Guanine	guanylic acid	guanosine
Thymine	thymidylic acid	thymidine
Uracil	uridylic acid	uridine
Cytosine	cytidylic acid	cytidine

*DNA derivatives may be differentiated by using the prefix "deoxy."

The DNA Helix

In 1953 Watson and Crick proposed their now famous concept and model of the chromosomal DNA structure. This represents the DNA molecule as a double-stranded structure, each strand parallel to its fellow but twisted or coiled about a common median longitudinal axis, i.e., in helical fashion, like two sides of a spiral staircase. A rope ladder also provides a good analogy. Let us first consider this hanging straight and vertically, its sides parallel and its rungs horizontal (Fig. 1–2). Each side rail of the ladder is made up of repeating units composed of phosphoric acid (P) joined to deoxyribose (DR). Each rung is attached on either side to a deoxyribose. Furthermore, each rung is formed of two pieces, spliced in the middle by a hydrogen bond. These "half rungs" all consist of one of the four bases, which are so arranged that if half of one rung is adenine, the other half of that rung *must* be thymine, and if one half is guanine, the other half *must* be cytosine. This natural law is known as the *Law, or Rule, of Base Pairing.*

If the rope ladder thus assembled is held fixed at its upper end and is then twisted around its long (vertical) axis until 10 rungs are present in one full twist or spiral, the result is a replica of the Watson-Crick model of DNA.

Duplication (Replication) of DNA Strands

The vast bulk of our knowledge of DNA, RNA, protein synthesis, and so forth, has come from study of lower forms of life, especially *Escherichia coli*. *E. coli* has but a single chromosome about 1 mm in length (when unfolded). This chromosome is double-stranded, as described before, and is calculated to contain six million nucleotides, which are chemically identical to those in higher forms of life; its molecular weight is about two billion.

As in all chromosomes, the two strands of DNA in *E. coli* are wound helically about a common axis, with 10 base pairs in every complete turn, i.e., every 3.4 nm of length. Under good conditions *E. coli* divides about every 20 minutes. Therefore, in this time it has to duplicate the six million nucleotides. Inexplicably, during this process the chromosome appears to form a closed circle; i.e., the two ends of each strand are joined. For each strand to duplicate itself it must very quickly unwind and separate from its fellow strand by cleavage of the H bonds uniting the base pairs between the strands. As it does this, a complementary base takes its place opposite each of the bases of the existing chromatid (single strand of DNA). In this manner a mirror-image chromatid is formed and joined by H bonds to the complementary bases of the parent chromatid. The rule of base pairing ensures that the daughter chromatid will be an exact copy of the strand that separated, which it (daughter) now replaces. Of course, the strand that separated (actually both parent strands separate in the same instant) also replicates for itself an exact copy of its original partner. Thus, when the *E. coli* divides into two, each of the "offspring" receives one chromosome in which one DNA strand is an old, or parent, strand and the other strand is new but is an exact copy of the second parent strand, which went to the other offspring. This is known as "semiconservative duplication" of DNA. Reference to Figure 1–3 will help clarify the mental picture of the process.

The speed with which this complicated feat is carried out is truly bewildering. In the case of *E. coli*'s dividing every 20 minutes, some 300,000 turns of the DNA molecule must unwind and duplicate in 20 minutes or less, i.e., 15,000 turns, and 150,000 pairs of nucleotides incorporated every minute!

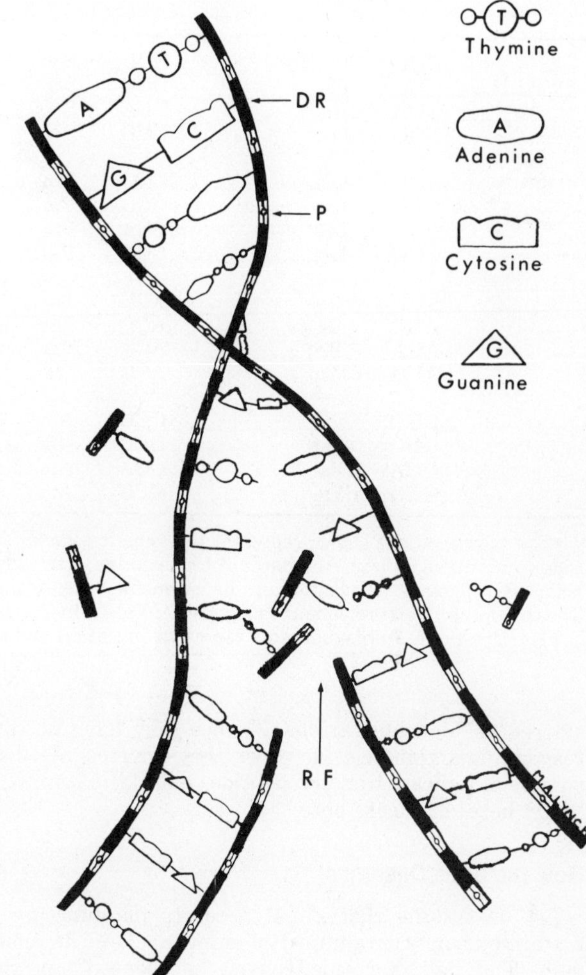

Figure 1–3 DNA replication. *DR*, deoxyribose; *P*, phosphoric acid residue; *RF*, replicating fork. See text for details.

THE GENETIC CODE

Besides proposing a model of DNA, Watson and Crick advanced the idea of a three-letter code. Using three-letter words from a four-letter alphabet, a total of 64 words (4 × 4 × 4) is possible. In the case of DNA, the letters of the code are the four bases, adenine, guanine, cytosine, and thymine, and the code words are the various combinations possible with any three of these four bases. The Watson-Crick proposal, then, was that all our genetic inheritance is encoded in the base sequences on each strand of our 46 chromosomes; that each three-base code word represents an amino acid; and that each of the many hundreds (prehaps more than 1000) of enzymes is encoded in a certain length of DNA strand having a total number of bases equal to at least three times the total number of amino acids in the enzyme molecule. Furthermore, the concept envisaged the sequence of bases spelling out the sequence of amino acids in the enzyme. All of this was subsequently proved.

Degeneracy of the DNA Code

From Watson and Crick's original proposal in 1953 the question naturally arose, "Why 64 code words for 20 amino acids?" Soon after the code was broken, it became apparent that several amino acids are represented by more than one code word, i.e., by more than one sequence of three bases. In the language of cryptography this meant that the code is degenerate.

The degeneracy is not uniform. Some amino acids such as serine have six codons (UCU, UCG, UCA, ACG, AGU, AGC), whereas others such as histidine have only two (CAU, CAC). The third base in the codon is more susceptible to degeneracy than the other two; for example, all alanine codons begin with GC. Strangely enough, in such a liberal coding of 64 codons for 20 amino acids, some amino acids do not have code words, and these amino acids have to be built subsequent to precursor formation; e.g., hydroxyproline is formed from proline. Three codons—UAG, UAA, and UGA—are con-

TABLE 1–1 RNA Codon Assignments*

UUU	Phe	UCU	Ser	UGU	Cys	UAU	Tyr
UUC	Phe	UCC	Ser	UGC	Cys	UAC	Tyr
UUA	Leu	UCA	Ser	UGA	†	UAA	†
UUG	Leu	UCG	Ser	UGG	Trp	UAG	†
CUU	Leu	CCU	Pro	CGU	Arg	CAU	His
CUC	Leu	CCC	Pro	CGC	Arg	CAC	His
CUA	Leu	CCA	Pro	CGA	Arg	CAA	Gln
CUG	Leu	CCG	Pro	CGG	Arg	CAG	Gln
AUU	Ile	ACU	Thr	AGU	Ser	AAU	Asn
AUC	Ile	ACC	Thr	AGC	Ser	AAC	Asn
AUA	Ile	ACA	Thr	AGA	Arg	AAA	Lys
AUG	Met	ACG	Thr	AGG	Arg	AAG	Lys
GUU	Val	GCU	Ala	GGU	Gly	GAU	Asp
GUC	Val	GCC	Ala	GGC	Gly	GAC	Asp
GUA	Val	GCA	Ala	GGA	Gly	GAA	Glu
GUG	Val	GCG	Ala	GGG	Gly	GAG	Glu

*The trinucleotides shown represent the genetic code as it is carried by m-RNA to the ribosomes. The amino acids that have a code word are as follows: Ala:alanine; Arg:arginine; Asn:asparagine; Asp:aspartic acid; Cys:cysteine; Gln:glutamine; Glu:glutamic acid; Gly:glycine; His:histidine; Ile:isoleucine; Leu:leucine; Met:methionine; Phe:phenylalanine; Pro:proline; Ser:serine; Thr:threonine; Trp:tryptophan; Tyr:tyrosine; Val:valine.

†The three code words marked † represent initiation and termination instructions.

sidered as "nonsense triplets," since they have no corresponding amino acid. However, they are recognized as signals to indicate that polypeptide chain formation will "start here" or "cease here."

How the Code Operates

Let us assume that a cell needs to manufacture a certain enzyme containing 120 amino acids in its molecule. The need for this enzyme is "sensed" by the *regulatory* gene for that enzyme. The regulatory gene then unbinds itself from the *operator* gene for the enzyme. Freeing of the operator gene permits the *structural* gene for that particular enzyme to go into action. These various controlling genes are all on the same chromosome but are spatially separated from each other. *Repression*, i.e., inhibition of synthesis of the particular enzyme caused by the binding of the regulatory gene to the operator gene, could be effected by folding of the molecule in such a way that genes spatially removed from each other could be superimposed and therefore occluded or rendered inactive. This fits with the observation that inactive portions of chromosomes are short and tightly coiled, i.e., heteropyknotic.

Since our hypothetical enzyme has 120 amino acids, the minimum length of the gene controlling its synthesis, i.e., its structural gene, must be 360 bases or 122.4 nm. Once free, this structural gene proceeds to make a complementary, single-strand copy of itself with the aid of an enzyme. The rules of base pairing obtain, but since this enzyme catalyzes the synthesis of m-RNA (messenger RNA) with DNA as the template, ribose is the pentose used and uracil is incorporated instead of thymine; i.e., uracil forms opposite adenine. The m-RNA in eukaryotic cells (including human cells) appears largely produced by the cell nucleoli.

This process by which a gene, represented by a certain number and sequence of bases on one DNA strand, is copied or transcribed into a strand of m-RNA is known as heterocatalytic RNA synthesis. It is to be distinguished from the autocatalytic replication of DNA in preparation for cell division and is more generally called *transcription*. The m-RNA will carry a chain of complementary bases from the nuclear DNA. Each set of three bases carrying genetic information from the nucleus encoding the message for one amino acid is called a *codon*. In our example there will be 120 codons.

The resultant 122.4 nm-long strand is a copy of the code on the DNA gene and is known as m-RNA. It is carried out into the cytoplasm, presumably by simple diffusion in the fluid moving through the nuclear pores. Once it is in the cytoplasm, free ribosomes attach themselves to it and, with the assistance of specific amino acid–carrying t-RNA (transfer RNA) molecules, translate its code into the enzyme protein—or at least into its constituent subunit peptide chains. This process is known as *translation*.

The t-RNA has two active areas on its molecule: a zone that accepts a specific amino acid and an area that carries an *anticodon* that is complementary to the codon carried by the matching messenger m-RNA.

The process of protein synthesis may be better appreciated by reference to Figure 1–4.

Further Considerations

We have seen that *E. coli* has some three million base pairs in its single chromosome. These may represent up to about 1000 genes. Viruses may have from less than 100 to several hundred genes. Each human cell probably has a million or more genes. We may ask, "Why so many?"

The answer may lie in some knowledge of information theory. This is closely related to current computer function and rests on a binary digit system, that is, a "yes" or "no" response. The data necessary to make a correct

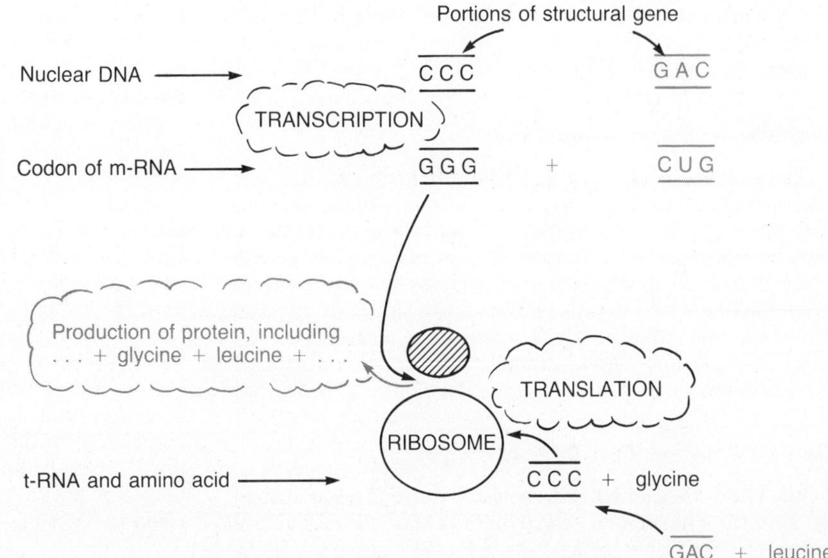

Figure 1–4 Steps in protein synthesis. *A*, adenine; *C*, cystosine; *G*, guanine; *U*, uracil.

decision from a certain number of choices can be calculated.

For two choices—need one decision to segregate the correct choice.

For four choices—two decisions are necessary; one discards two wrong choices and the next discards the remaining incorrect choice.

For eight choices—need three decisions; the first discards four bad choices, the second discards two of the remaining four, and the third discards the remaining incorrect choice.

For 16 choices—

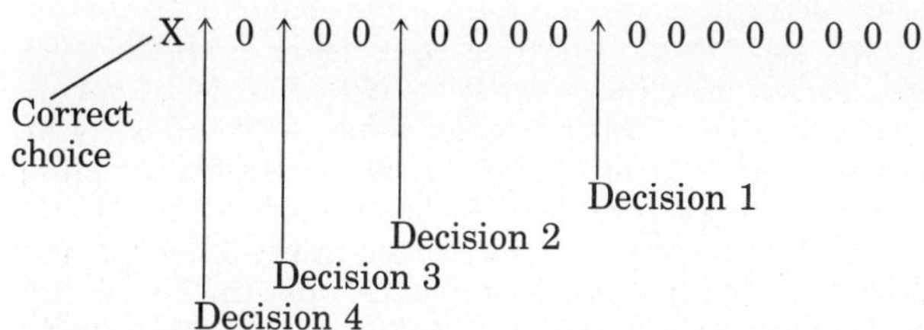

Thus, expressed mathematically, the correct choice of X possibilities requires $\log_2 X$ decisions.

A DNA molecule of M.W. 1,000,000 contains about 4000 nucleotide units. Since each nucleotide may be one of four, each nucleotide holds $\log_2 4 = 2$ pieces of information. The entire molecule contains 8000 pieces of information (4000 nucleotides × 2), which is not a great deal. When one considers that a cell must make its enzymes, protein, secretion, and so on, the mind can only reel at the amount of information stored in a sperm or an ovum, which between them must program the construction of a separate individual of many billion differentiated yet orchestrated cells! Even the lowly *E. coli* replicates itself perfectly every 20 minutes under good conditions, as well as building its own protein and maintaining its milieu in the interim. It has been said that even such a cell has 1000 times the information of a single volume of the *Encyclopaedia Britannica*.

Gene Control. Each cell probably requires more than 100 enzymes to carry out its functions, and some cell types may require far more. The sum of all the different enzymes in all the different cell types of the body may be well over 1000. Each of these is represented by a certain length of one or both DNA strands of one of the 46 chromosomes. Such a functional unit of the DNA strand, when spoken of as a code, is known as a *cistron*; in genetics it has long been referred to as the gene.

Each enzyme is controlled not by one but by at least two or three genes. The structural gene is that part of the DNA strand bearing the code that determines the actual constitution and quality of the protein to be made. It is not autonomous, but is controlled by its regulator gene, which decides when and for how long the structural gene shall work. Evidence suggests that the regulator gene may not exert this control directly on the structural gene or operon but through a third gene, the operator. The regulator gene appears to respond to concentrations of substances that are either substrates or products of the enzyme made by the operon or structural gene under its (regulator gene's) control. Thus, rising concentrations of substrate(s) cause the regulator gene to induce production of the enzyme by removing its repression of the operator so that the structural gene is allowed to "switch on." Conversely, as the products of the enzyme's action rise in concentration, the whole process is reversed by the regulator gene's repressing or "switching off" the structural gene by means of the operator gene. Obviously, in such a system control is very sensitively balanced by the relative concentrations of substrate and product.

Cell Division. Apparently cell division also is controlled by a mechanism broadly similar to that outlined. A regulatory gene for DNA replication exists. This seems to be under control of stimuli originating in the cell membrane. When activated, this gene directs the synthesis of an "initiator" substance that starts the replication process in motion. This takes place very shortly after a cell has divided. At a variably later date, other stimuli and genes set in motion the train of events leading to actual cell division.

Universality of the Genetic Code

Evidence to date suggests that all forms of life use the same basic DNA-RNA code. Minor variations and differences have been found, and certainly many more will be documented. Because of the universality of the code, it has become possible to perform feats of genetic engineering such as the production of human growth hormone and insulin by *E. coli.* This is achieved by inserting the necessary human gene into the bacterial chromosome.

Genetic Code and Cell Differentiation

We know that each cell receives the full inheritance of genetic characters. Experiments on the fertilized ovum of lower species and on the early generations of cells arising from it have shown that these are totipotent. After a few divisions, however, specialization begins to appear and the cells are multipotent rather than totipotent. The most plausible explanation for this limitation of capabilities is that certain genes have been suppressed. As the embryo continues to develop, more genes are suppressed and others are expressed in the different cell lines.

The genetic control in malignant cells is obviously slackened to some extent, and perhaps this is most dramatically shown by the inappropriate ectopic production of hormones by malignant cells. This would suggest strongly that the normal suppressive mechanism has ceased to function and that some genes that are normally suppressed in benign cells are expressed in their malignant counterparts. Examples of this phenomenon are the production of adrenocorticotrophic hormone in some cases of oat-cell carcinoma, and the production of insulin by connective tissue tumors of the thorax, retroperitoneum, or abdomen.

PROKARYOTIC AND EUKARYOTIC CELLS

Apart from references to *E. coli,* the cell to which we have directed major attention in this chapter has been the animal cell. Although there are features in common among all living cells and much fundamental knowledge has been obtained from the bacterium *E. coli,* there are essential differences between bacterial and animal cells.

Monera, which encompass the bacteria and blue-green algae, belong to the prokaryotic group. The nuclear DNA in these cells is not enclosed in a nuclear membrane, is a tightly coiled double helix, and is not adherent to any nuclear protein (histone). The ribosomes are smaller than those in eukaryotic cells. The latter also have an extensive endoplasmic reticulum, which is absent in prokaryotic cells, and they have specialized structures such as mitochondria and Golgi apparatus. The DNA of the nucleus of eukaryotic cells is divided into chromosomes, which undergo mitosis during cell division. Apart from *Mycoplasma*, the prokaryotic cells are typified by rigid cell walls, consisting of repeating mucopeptide units cross-linked by peptide chains. The differences between prokaryotic and eukaryotic cells are summarized in Table 1–2.

HUMAN CHROMOSOMES

As noted above, each human somatic cell contains 46 chromosomes, but these cannot be visualized in the interphase, which is the resting period between mitotic division. The *gametes* (sperm and ovum), which fuse to form the zygote, each contain 23 chromosomes; the zygote, which develops into the fetus and ultimately another individual, has the full complement of 46.

The chromosomes, as described above, consist of chains of DNA that carry the genetic code in *genes*. The latter are lengths of DNA that classically were considered as giving instructions for a particular inherited characteristic. With the solution of the method of transmission of genetic information these are also known as *cistrons*. They are transcribed by m-RNA to be translated in the cytoplasm. Each gene is present in a precisely determined position on a particular chromosome known as a *locus*. Contrasting genetic characteristics are carried on chromosomes in the same loci and are known as *alleles*. Naturally, only one allele can be found at any particular locus, but in the corresponding chromosome, the other allele may be present.

The 46 chromosomes are made from 23 homologous pairs. One of each pair is inherited from the father and

TABLE 1–2 Prokaryotic and Eukaryotic Cells

Cell Structure	Prokaryotic (e.g., *E. coli*)	Eukaryotic (e.g., liver cell)
Nucleus	Double helix of DNA without surrounding membrane. Acts as single chromosome. No histone present	DNA divided into chromosomes within nuclear membrane. Closely related to histones. Divides by mitosis
Wall	Rigid wall of repeating units of mucopeptide	Very thin flexible coat of acid mucopolysaccharide
Respiration	Occurs in membrane	Occurs in specialized structures, such as mitochondria
Intracellular membranes	None apparent	Complex endoplasmic reticulum
Ribosomes	Small and distributed in cytoplasm	Larger and may be attached to endoplasmic reticulum

the other from the mother; so in the same loci, there may be different or similar alleles. Twenty-two pairs of chromosomes are *autosomes* and are similar to one another, whether inherited from the mother or father; whereas the other pair are the sex chromosomes, which are dissimilar. These are called X and Y chromosomes. The entire chromosome make-up in any individual is his *karyotype*. A human male has 44 autosomes as well as an X and a Y chromosome, and a human female has 44 autosomes and two X chromosomes (XX). The normal human karyotype differs from that of any other species in terms of the number of chromosomes and their length and shape, as well as in the arrangement and coding of genes.

MITOSIS

Some description has been given above of the replication of chromosomal DNA that occurs at mitosis when the cell divides in the course of ordinary growth or replacement.

At the time of mitosis, the nuclear membrane vanishes and a structure called a *centriole* divides. The resulting two forms migrate to each end of the cell. The chromosomes replicate themselves, doubling the DNA content of the cell, and then each appears as two parallel strands *(chromatids)* joined at one point (the *centromere*). They then migrate to an equatorial plane and are connected from the centromeres to the centrioles by strands of protein known as a *spindle*. The centromere then divides, and each chromatid moves toward a centriole as if pulled by the spindle. The cytoplasm begins to divide and finally splits completely, leaving each group of chromatids, now chromosomes within new nuclear membranes, in one of the newly formed cells. These cells have the same 23 pairs of chromosomes and the same genes as the parent cell.

MEIOSIS

Each gamete, as stated above, carries 23 chromosomes: 22 autosomes and one sex chromosome. Each sperm will carry 22 + X or 22 + Y, and each ovum will carry 22 + X. To form a gamete, a specialized cell undergoes *reduction division*, in which the number of chromosomes in the parent cell is halved from the *diploid* number (46) to the haploid number (23). The details of meiotic division will not be delineated in detail, but it is important to realize that each pair of chromosomes is divided. During the course of division, genes on original maternal or paternal chromosomes may be exchanged, although they will occupy similar loci. The new chromosomes are not merely replicas of the original material in paternal or maternal chromosomes but mixtures of genes. This process is called genetic interchange, crossing over, or recombination, and it is a most exquisite and elegant method of altering genetic patterns carried by chromosomes and thus producing an almost incalculable number of differing combinations of characteristics. However, if gene loci are

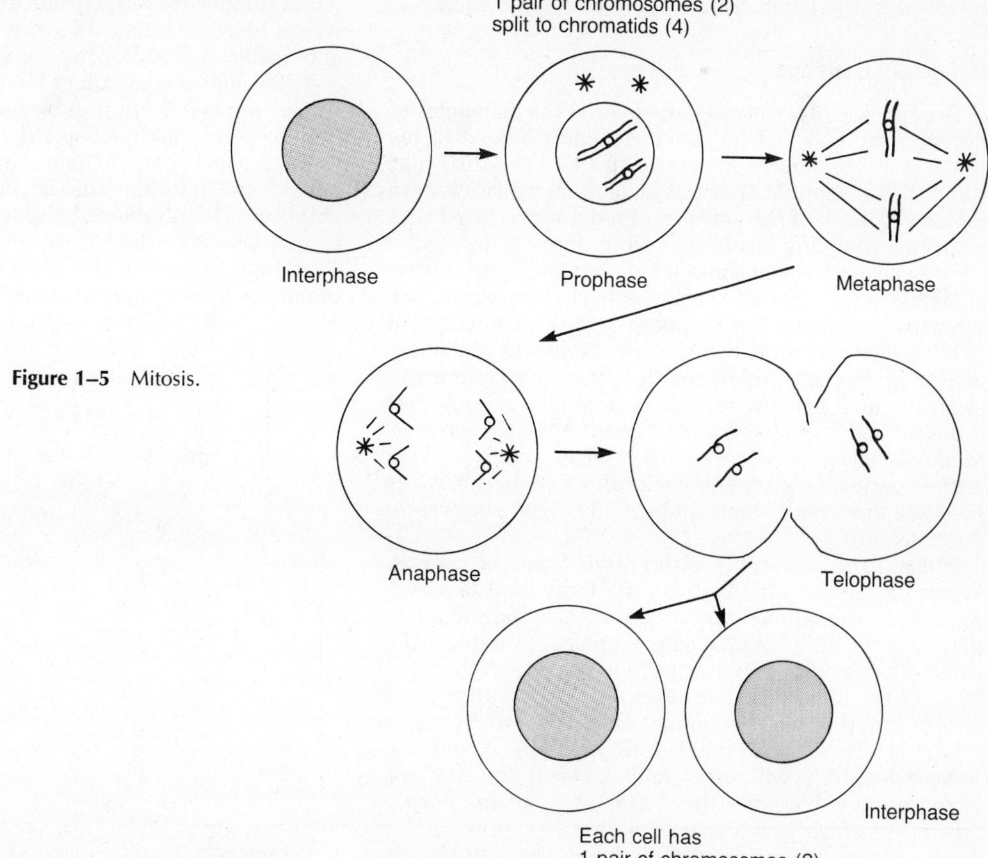

Figure 1–5 Mitosis.

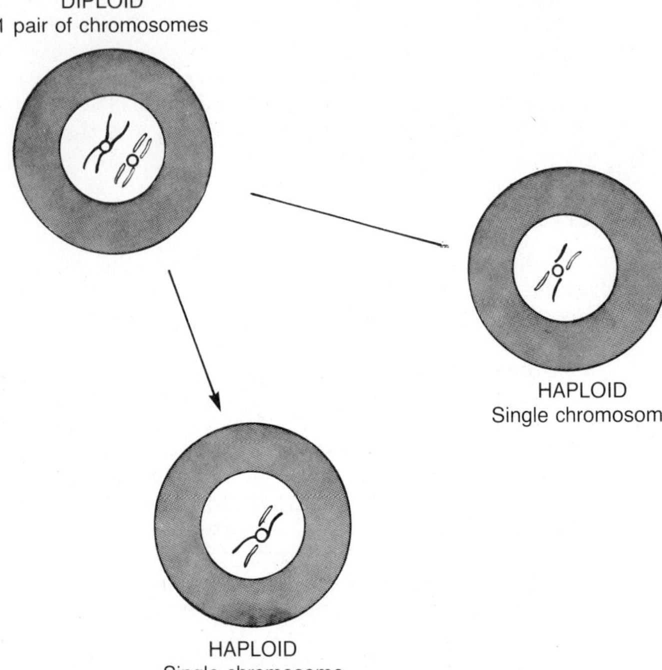

Figure 1–6 Meiosis with genetic interchange.

close together, they are less likely to be separated and are inherited together; i.e., they are *linked*. If, on the other hand, they are on different chromosomes, in different loci, they are likely to undergo *independent assortment* in the gametes and to the new generation.

Mendelian Genetics

The monk Gregor Mendel discovered the principles of heredity in 1865, but his work lay undiscovered in his lifetime and was not appreciated until 1900. Until that time, it was thought that physical characteristics were a blend of those of the parents. Mendel appreciated that continual blending would lead to uniformity, but experience and experiment showed him continual variability.

Mendel's laws stated that genetic characteristics are inherited as a unit and reappear or remain unchanged in subsequent generations; that two members of a single gene pair are not present in the same gamete but are separate and present in different gametes; and that different genes independently assort among gametes. Mendel's work was with garden peas and was done without any knowledge of molecular genetics, but his laws are universally applicable to all species that reproduce sexually.

Alleles are essentially alternative forms of a gene. When the alleles are identical, the individual is *homozygous*. If the alleles are different, the individual is *heterozygous*. In a heterozygote, if one gene produces the same effect as if the subject were homozygous, the gene is said to be *dominant*. For example, the gene that gives rise to group A blood is dominant to that which yields group O. Thus, both the heterozygote (AO) and the homozygote (AA) will have group A blood. The *genotype* of these individuals is either AO or AA, but the *phenotype* is A, which is the character that is expressed. An allele that is expressed only in a homozygous subject is a *recessive* gene, and in the example given previously is the gene carrying blood group O. Thus a patient who has the genotype OO will have group O blood. If both alleles are expressed, then the genes are *codominant*. An example with blood group analogies is the individual whose blood is group AB, in which case both heterozygote genes, A and B, are asserted.

Autosomal chromosomes have already been described. *Autosomal genes* are present on these chromosomes and may be inherited by offspring regardless of their sex. If the autosomal gene is dominant, it will be apparent in one of the parents and in half (statistically) of the children. The unaffected children will not transmit the characteristic to their children. If the gene is recessive, it will not appear in the parents but will appear in one of four of their children (statistically) regardless of sex.

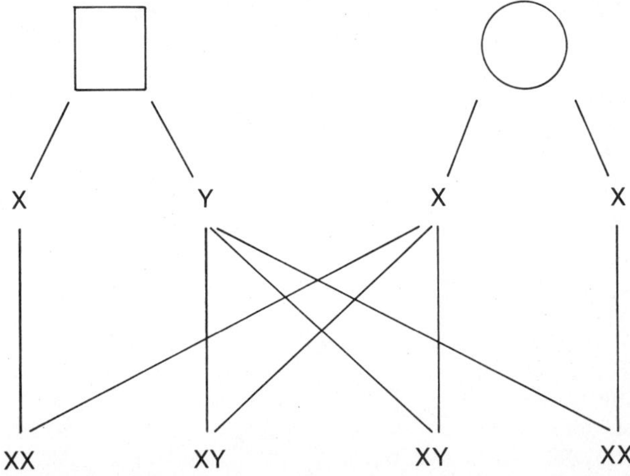

Figure 1–7 Possible results of mating for alleles X and Y.

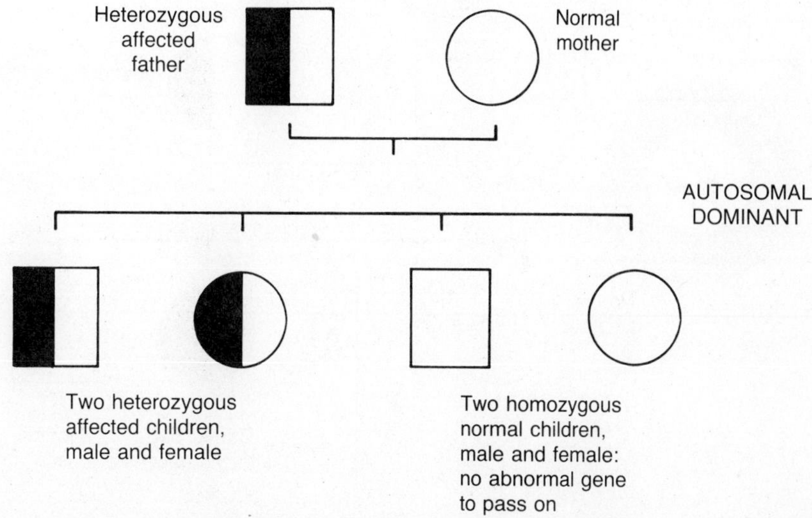

Figure 1–8 Results of mating with autosomal dominant and autosomal recessive genes.

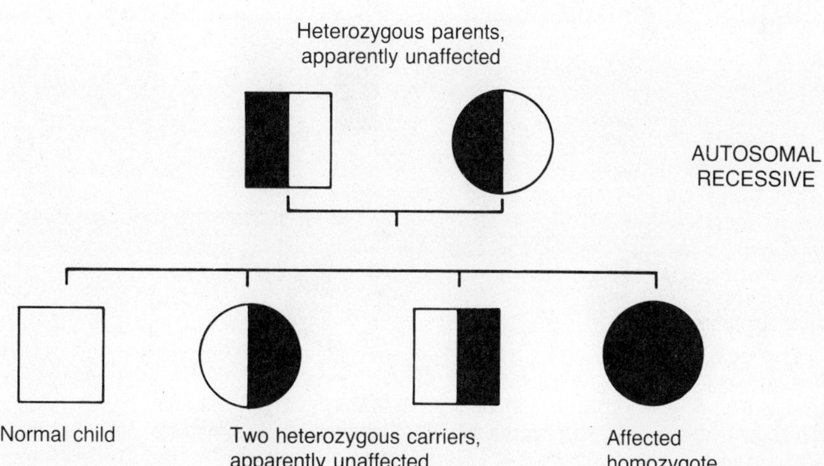

Two of the children will be heterozygous carriers without expression of the gene, and one will be a homozygous normal individual. The heterozygous carriers may pass the defect to their children if they marry other heterozygous carriers. Cystic fibrosis is a common disease that is inherited as an autosomal recessive trait.

X-Linked Inheritance

The term *X-linked inheritance* is applied when the gene is carried on the X chromosome. The male sex chromosome has apparently few gene loci. In the male, with the genotype XY, abnormal genes on the X chromosome will have no balancing alleles and will be expressed even if they are recessive. Thus, *X-linked recessive* disease (with the gene inherited from the mother) will always be expressed in the male, such as in hemophilia. The abnormal gene is transmitted from the affected male to all his daughters (and then to half of their sons) but not to his sons. *X-linked dominant* traits are transmissible to all the daughters of affected males but not to sons. The daughters will show the trait and will transmit it to half of their children regardless of sex. The female has the genotype XX, but in each cell, only one X is active. The other X chromosome is seen as a small nuclear condensation (the Barr body) and is not active. Which of the X chromosomes is functional appears to be the result of random chance. This phenomenon is known as the *Lyon hypothesis* and it has far-reaching consequences on the individual. Even in X-linked dominant disease, in which women would be expected to be at least as severely affected as men, experience has shown this condition to take a milder form in them. This follows from the fact that some proportion of the recessive, or normal, X chromosomes are expressed in some cells and mitigate the effects of abnormal X chromosomes expressed in other cells. If, during development, many cells express the normal gene, the disease or disorder will be very mild.

Cytogenetics

Much of the detailed methodology used in the demonstration of chromosomes is given in the third edition

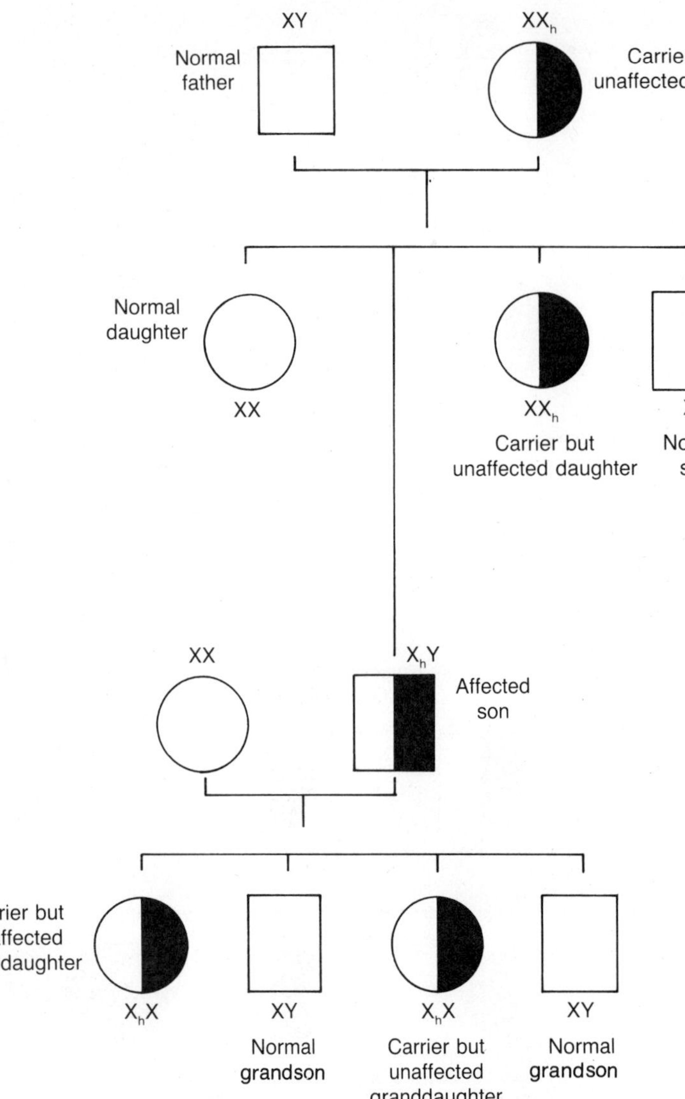

Figure 1–9 Pedigree of X-linked recessive disease (X_h, hemophilia).

of this book, and here only the general outlines will be described, since it is probably preferable to have cytogenetic diagnosis done in a specialized center.

Barr bodies can be demonstrated in cells from the buccal mucosa scraped from the inside of the cheek with a metal spatula. The cells are smeared on an albuminized slide and fixed in 95% ethanol. After at least 30 min fixation, the slides are taken through descending concentrations of alcohol to distilled water. They are then stained in 0.5% cresyl echt violet aqueous solution for 6 to 8 min. The slides are then dehydrated, cleared in xylene, and mounted. Barr bodies are seen as small condensations on the inner aspect of the nuclear membrane, and they are found in 20 to 80% of the cells of females. In normal males, less than 1 or 2% of the cells are positive.

Although much information may be gained by examination for Barr bodies or sex chromatin, much more is available from a complete cell karyotype. This may be obtained by culturing peripheral blood cells. In essence, a few drops of peripheral blood taken under aseptic conditions are added to a culture medium that includes phytohemagglutinin. The latter agglutinates red blood cells and promotes mitosis in lymphocytes. After a determined period, colchicine or a similar substance is added to the culture. Colchicine arrests mitosis at a phase in which the chromosomes are arranged at the equator of the cell. After the addition of colchicine, the cell is subjected to a hypotonic solution that causes it to swell and that disperses the chromosomes. The cells are then smeared on a slide, fixed, and stained.

For this purpose, several commercial kits are available. By using Gibco chromosome medium with phytohemaglutinin, it is convenient to add the blood to the medium and send the cell culture with all deliberate speed to a reference center, where the cells are cultured for 70 h at 37°C.

The chromosomes, or more accurately the centromeres, are displayed on the stained slides, and photomicrographs are made. The structures are cut out from enlarged photographs and arranged in pairs according to size. They are identified and numbered from 1 to 22 and X and Y. The completed karyotype is then examined for any abnormality.

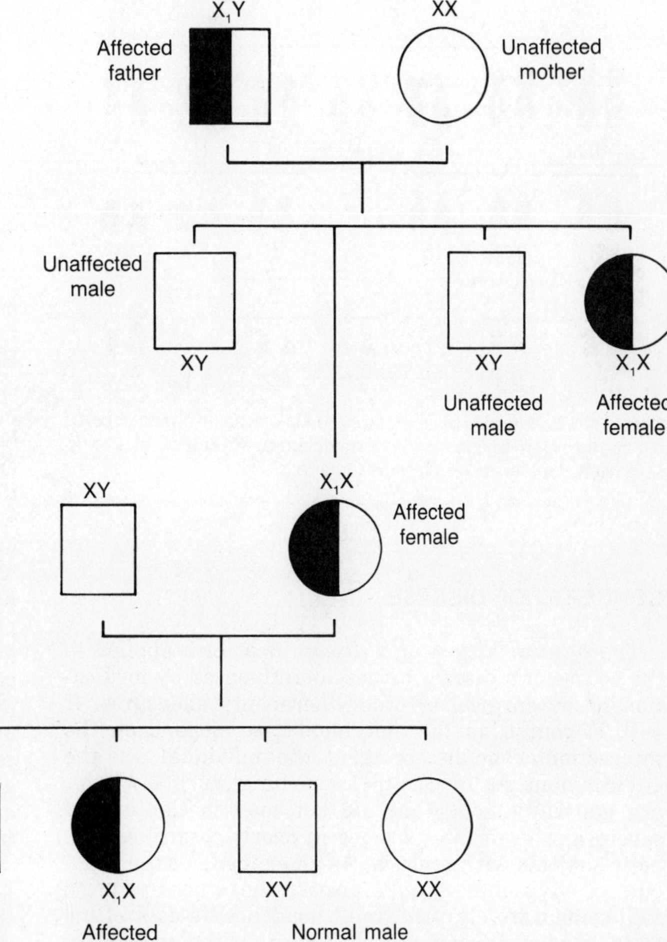

Figure 1–10 Pedigree of X-linked dominant trait (X_1).

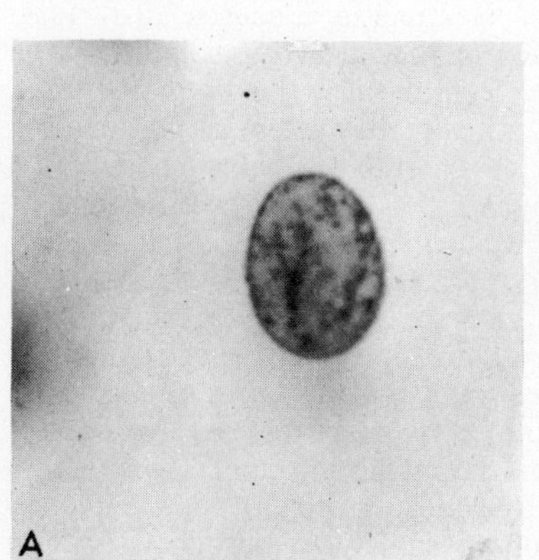

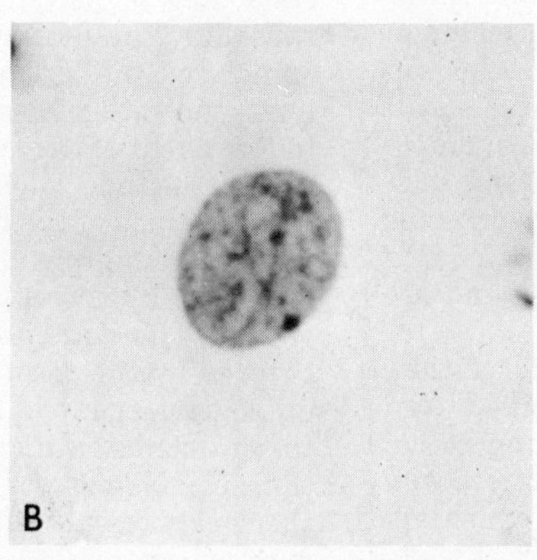

Figure 1–11 Interphase appearance of the sex chromatins. Interphase nuclei from normal showing sex chromatin mass attached to nuclear membrane in female cell *(B)* but not in a male cell *(A)*. (Courtesy of Dr. M. L. Barr, University of Western Ontario.)

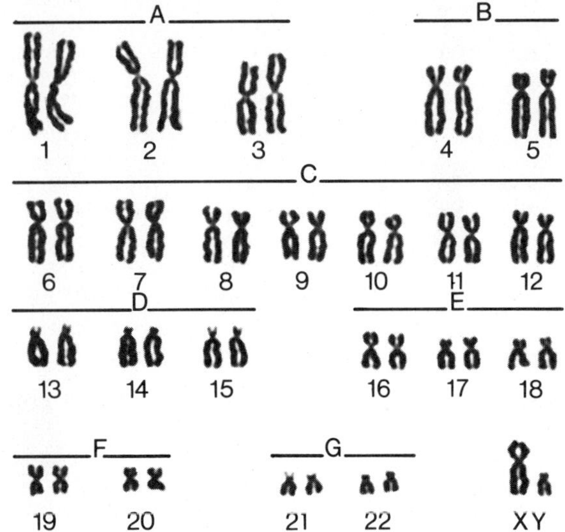

Figure 1–12 Normal male metaphase karyotype arranged according to the Denver system of nomenclature. (Courtesy of Dr. F. Sergovich, University of Western Ontario.)

CONCEPTS OF DISEASE

The *natural history of a disease* is a term applied to the course of a disease process uninfluenced by medication or by surgical or other therapeutic measures. It will, of course, in the individual case, depend on the interaction of the disease agent, the individual, and the environment. As an example, some fungi, such as *Mucor*, are generally nonpathogenic but may instigate very severe and even fatal disease in poorly controlled diabetic subjects with acidosis. As an example of the influence of environment, some diseases have been reduced to a comparatively very small incidence by controlling or improving environmental factors. In the case of tuberculosis, for example, in the United States in 1930 there were 101 cases reported per 100,000 population, whereas in 1978 there were only 12 cases per 100,000 population. Much of this improvement has come from the improvement in living standards during the intervening years. The provision of clean drinking water in the Western world has virtually eliminated cholera, while in less well developed areas the disease is still endemic and occasionally epidemic. A topical example of the influence of environment is the increased incidence of one type of cancer in persons exposed to asbestos (mesothelioma) and an even greater incidence of this cancer in persons who are exposed to asbestos and are cigarette smokers.

The *etiology* of disease is its cause or the derivation. In infections, etiological agents are well identified (e.g., *N. meningitidis* is the etiological agent of meningococcal meningitis). In other diseases, etiology may be less well defined. Such an example is atherosclerosis, which appears to be related to diet, smoking, sedentary habits, hypertension, and so forth. In some diseases, etiology is unknown, as it is with many types of cancer, although etiological factors are increasingly being brought to light.

Generally it is customary to consider etiological agents under the following headings:

1. Congenital
2. Inherited or familial
3. Traumatic
4. Inflammatory
5. Neoplastic
6. Metabolic
7. Nutritional
8. Vascular
9. Iatrogenic and drug induced
10. Physical agents, chemicals, x-rays, light, etc.
11. Autoimmune
12. Others (e.g., psychogenic or idiopathic)

The term *congenital disease* implies an abnormality present at birth that may or may not be manifest at that time and that is not genetic but acquired *in utero*. Examples are congenital syphilis, congenital heart disease, and so forth. Inherited or familial disease is genetically determined and may be present at birth or become apparent in later life. There are numerous examples, of which cystic fibrosis of the pancreas (autosomal recessive) and hemophilia (X-linked recessive) were referred to previously. Huntington's chorea is an autosomal dominant disease. Tyrosinemia is an autosomal recessive disease common in a French-Canadian population. Tay-Sachs disease has a similar hereditary pattern and occurs largely in Ashkenazi Jews. Some genetic disease is not carried from the parents but is caused by a change in the structure of DNA for that particular individual. Such a change is called *mutation*, and the affected individual is a *mutant*. Many mutations are lethal, and the zygote does not survive long in gestation. Achondroplastic dwarfism is carried as an autosomal dominant trait, but many cases occur as mutants.

Traumatic disease needs little description, but even here, there is a relationship between the individual and the agent. For example, in elderly people, fracture of the femur is much commoner than in younger people. The former are more likely to fall, their protective reflexes are slower, and their bones are more brittle. Inflammatory disease may be caused by bacteria, viruses, chlamydiae, fungi, or parasites and may be acute, subacute, or chronic. Neoplastic diseases are those caused by the formation of new growths, which may be benign or malignant. Benign growths do not spread from the site of origin, yet they have a metabolism independent of the general metabolism of the body. Such tumors include leiomyomas of the uterus (fibroids), fibroadenomas of the breast, lipomas, and so forth. Malignant tumors grow and metastasize to other locations in the body by direct spread or via lymphatics or blood vessels. There are numerous types, and all are generally covered by the term *cancer*. In some types of cancer an etiological agent is known or suspected; e.g., cancer of the bronchus is much commoner in cigarette smokers than in nonsmokers, and mesothelioma (a tumor of the chest cavity or peritoneal cavity) is closely associated with asbestos inhalation. Neoplastic disease is common, and in 1978, 20.6% of all deaths were caused by cancer.

Metabolic diseases include those related to intrinsic abnormalities of metabolism, as for example gout, in which there is a derangement of purine metabolism and crystals of uric acid are deposited in the tissues, especially in periarticular structures. In another metabolic disorder, phenylketonuria, the amino acid phenylalanine cannot be metabolized normally because of the deficiency of an enzyme, phenylalanine hydroxylase. The phenylalanine is abnormally metabolized to phenylpypyruvic acid because of the enzyme deficiency. The level of phenylalanine in the blood is elevated, and this has an effect on the development of the brain. If the deficiency is not treated, the child will become severely mentally retarded. As well as being of metabolic etiology, the disease is also inherited and is carried by an autosomal recessive gene.

Nutritional disease is of fairly self-evident nature and includes disease due to lack of adequate nutriments. This may result from simple insufficiency in the diet (as in starvation and vitamin deficiency) but may also occur secondary to malabsorption by the small bowel (as in sprue) or small-bowel inadequacy (following extensive small-bowel resection) or even in pregnancy, when additional demands by the fetus for such substances as folic acid are not met from the diet and the patient develops a deficiency macrocytic anemia.

Vascular diseases are common and are generally caused by atherosclerosis, in which the lumen of the vessel is reduced because of deposition of lipid and other materials on the inner arterial wall while an outer layer of the artery loses its elasticity, becomes fibrotic, and shows calcium deposition. These phenomena lead to reduction of blood flow to the part of the body served by the particular vessel. The reduction of blood flow is known as *ischemia*. A common example of this is coronary atherosclerosis, in which ischemia of the cardiac muscle may give rise to pain, especially on exertion, when the demand of the heart muscle for oxygen is greater. This particular ischemic symptom is known as angina pectoris, or angina of effort. If the blood supply is completely obstructed by a clot within the vessel lumen, the affected organ (or part of the organ) will show an *infarct*, which is a dead area resulting from the anoxemia. Myocardial infarction is often found to be due to obstruction of one or more coronary vessels by a blood clot, and stroke is the result of a similar type of obstruction involving the cerebral vessels. This group of vascular diseases is responsible for the majority of deaths in the advanced industrial societies.

Drug-induced disease is an adverse effect of a drug, and the spectrum of disease so caused is very large. Streptomycin may specifically damage the eighth cranial nerve, occasioning nerve deafness. A number of drugs, including primaquine (an antimalarial), sulfa compounds, phenacetin, and others, may cause hemolytic episodes in sensitive subjects. These are persons with deficiency of glucose-6-phosphate dehydrogenase in their red blood cells. The abnormal gene is carried on the X chromosome, and the disease is X linked. In sensitive patients (and in others as a result of high dosage), chloramphenicol may produce aplastic anemia. Penicillin may cause skin rashes, and many other drugs by a multiplicity of pathogenic pathways may cause adverse effects. The term *iatrogenic disease* is applied when the physician's action is responsible for the disease state. Many iatrogenic diseases are, of course, drug induced, but others include conditions such as stitch abscess, ischemic changes in the hand due to tight cast application after forearm facture, and so forth.

Chemicals and x-rays may cause disease. The latter were often implicated in the past for skin cancer, and, even now, if x-ray therapy is to be given, precautions must be taken to avoid damage to sensitive tissues such as bone marrow. A number of chemicals may cause dermatitis and other, more serious diseases. For example, vinyl chloride has been associated with the appearance of a vascular cancer of the liver (angiosarcoma).

Autoimmune disease is an extension of allergic disease. In the latter, as for example in hay fever, the patient reacts in a pathological fashion to the presentation of a foreign protein (usually pollen). In autoimmune disease, the patient reacts in an abnormal immune manner to his own tissues or to their components. Such disease includes some thyroid diseases, disseminated lupus erythematosus, some hemolytic anemias, and so forth. A further discussion involving this group of diseases will be found in a subsequent chapter.

The area of psychogenic disease does not impinge directly on the laboratory, but a physicochemical basis for some of these conditions, such as schizophrenia, is being actively investigated. Other diseases, such as peptic ulcer, thyrotoxicosis, and ulcerative colitis, may have a psychogenic etiological component.

Despite incredible medical advances, especially in the last 50 years, the etiology of some disease remains unknown or idiopathic. As mentioned previously, many cancers are in this category. A number of common skin diseases and nervous diseases have obscure etiologies, and throughout the discipline of pathology there remain groups of diseases with an unclear origin.

CHAPTER 1—REVIEW QUESTIONS

1. Give the essential differences between prokaryotic and eukaryotic cells.
2. Define the following terms:
   - genes
   - cistrons
   - alleles
   - autosomes
   - chromatids
   - meiosis
   - homozygous
   - phenotype
   - Lyon hypothesis
   - Barr bodies
   - autosomal dominant
   - mutation
3. Draw a family tree in which there is an X-linked recessive disease, to show the method of inheritance.
4. Give two examples of congenital disease and two of familial disease. What is the difference between congenital and familial disease?

BASIC PRINCIPLES OF LABORATORY WORK

LABORATORY SAFETY

Medical laboratory technology is a practical profession, and in addition to applying their skills to the many procedures of modern laboratory practice, technologists must also be constantly aware of the sources of accidents and potential hazards and the most effective counteraction to minimize injury and material damage.

The potential hazards of laboratory work are:

1. Fire and explosion from flammable solvents.
2. Poisonous, corrosive, and caustic reagents.
3. Burns and scalds, including electrical burns and electrical shock.
4. Lacerations from broken glass apparatus, microtome knives, and so forth.
5. Bacterial, viral, or parasitic infection.
6. Animal bites.
7. Radiation hazards.

Fire and Explosion

Flammable solvents—alcohols, ether, toluene, and xylene—are used in every department of the laboratory. The vapors of alcohols and especially ether are not only flammable but in certain circumstances explosive. The following precautions are recommended.

Quantities of solvents on the bench in bottles should be kept to the smallest volumes compatible with working needs.

Bulk quantities of solvents should be kept in a special storage room that is cool, well ventilated, and fireproof, if possible; that is equipped with foam-type fire extinguishers and away from all possible contact with naked flames or electrical sparks. Any tools used to open drum-stored solvents should be made of nonferrous metals such as bronze.

Before opening a bottle of any flammable solvent, one should check to see that there are no Bunsen burners alight within 6 feet. Ether should not be used in any room where there is a Bunsen flame, because its heavy vapor can travel along the bench or floor for a considerable distance. If practical, a well-ventilated fume hood should be used for any work with this solvent.

Flammable solvents should not be used in confined spaces where vapors may accumulate to form explosive mixtures with air.

Solutions containing flammable solvents must never be heated by Bunsen burners; explosion-proof boiling water baths, electrical hot plates, or heating mantles should be used, and any vapors should be condensed or carried off in the forced draught of a ventilating hood. These precautions are not necessary when the volume of fluid is very small.

If a solvent fire does occur in the laboratory, the following actions are indicated.

For a small fire involving a beaker or other container, cover with a larger vessel, smother with a wet cloth, or use a carbon dioxide foam-type fire extinguisher.

For a fire involving spilled solvent that covers a portion of the bench or floor, warn colleagues in the immediate vicinity, and use a foam-type extinguisher. If the fire is not brought under control almost immediately, evacuate the room, and without taking unnecessary risks, endeavor to prevent spread of the fire with extinguishers. If the laboratory is located in a hospital, alert the hospital fire fighting organization. If there is any real or potential danger to patients or staff, it is safer to contact the city or town fire department. In many hospitals the triggering of the hospital fire alarm system automatically sends a call to the local fire department. All laboratory personnel must know the location of fire extinguishers and alarms and be acquainted with the hospital's fire fighting organization.

Do not look for gas leaks by the use of a naked flame. This practice is always to be condemned, especially in small rooms and confined spaces. Commercially bottled gases contain added evil-smelling compounds to call attention to leaks. Locating a gas leak should be the responsibility of the hospital engineer or plumber.

Since modern electrically heated water baths are made of stainless steel, short circuits as a result of corrosion are highly unlikely. Nevertheless, it is preferable to use distilled rather than tap water for refilling water baths as the level drops owing to evaporation, adding about 5 milliliters per gallon of one of the proprietary anticorrosion and antifungal concentrates.

Poisonous, Corrosive, and Caustic Reagents

Although the technologist is usually aware that strong mineral acids and bases are dangerous substances, it is essential that a proper respect for their corrosive and poisonous nature be emphasized repeatedly. Familiarity still tends to breed contempt, and only the development of good technique as an automatic habit provides proper safeguards. In addition, many of the toxic substances in the laboratory (methyl alcohol, cyanides, and carbon tetrachloride) are unfamiliar to the student, who must be made aware of their poisonous effects.

The correct precautions in their handling should be included in the teaching of any procedure involving their use.

Strong Mineral Acids

These acids are sulfuric, hydrochloric, nitric, and perchloric. (Strong organic acids—acetic.)

These substances are rapidly destructive of body tissues, both externally and internally. The most common accidents are acid contamination of the hands, acid splashes in or near the eyes, and acid burns to the mouth from attempts to pipette directly from the bottle. (This last procedure should never be permitted.) Acid burns are slow to heal and frequently leave permanent scars. The following precautions are indicated: When pouring strong acids, making dilutions thereof, wear rubber gloves. Ideally, a rubber apron and goggles should also be worn, though these precautions are essential only when large amounts of acid (e.g., in carboys) are being handled or when even the smallest splash is very dangerous (e.g., with perchloric acid). Even when pouring from small bottles of strong acid, one must prevent splashing by *slow* pouring and by the use of bottles with pouring lips and plastic funnels. In any event, keep the face well away from the bottle when pouring acid.

The best solution to the problem of transferring strong acids from large containers is to use one of the various types of plastic pumps now available. These are made with a variety of screw caps and stoppers to fit most kinds of container. The use of plastic has also been extended to the packaging of reagents in cubic polyethylene containers fitted with an integral dispensing spout and tap. Strongly acid laboratory-made reagents can be safely dispensed from a suitable automatic or semiautomatic pipetting device.

The dilution of acids (especially sulfuric acid) with water produces heat. If a large amount of this acid is mixed with a small amount of water, enough heat can be produced to give an almost explosive reaction. Therefore, when diluting:

Always add acid to water.

Always pour very slowly, with frequent mixing.

If necessary, cool the diluted acid before adding any more strong acid.

Use a thin-walled Pyrex container—the heat may crack a thick-walled vessel.

Carefully wipe up any spillage on the outside of bottles or on the bench.

If the spillage of a concentrated acid, a concentrated base, or a flammable or toxic solvent exceeds the volume that can be safely wiped up with absorbent tissue or similar material, the preferred method is to use one of the commercially available neutralizing/absorbent powders; these are available for the safe cleanup of acids, bases, and solvents. The manufacturer's directions should be learned by the laboratory staff *before* the need arises.

Strong Bases

Both in the solid form (sodium hydroxide, potassium hydroxide) and in concentrated solution (sodium hydroxide, potassium hydroxide, ammonium hydroxide), the common bases can cause severe tissue damage, especially to the delicate membranes lining the mouth and esophagus. Dissolving solid sodium and potassium hydroxides in water generates a great deal of heat (this is the heating method used in the Clinitest tablet) and may be sufficient to crack a thick-walled glass vessel such as a graduate. Solutions of strong bases should be made with the same precautions as are used for strong acids. When sodium or potassium hydroxide is used in pellet form, constant stirring is essential to prevent "caking" of the pellets with the resultant localized overheating.

Ammonia is also dangerous because of its irritant vapor. This can cause damage to eyes and lungs, and strong ammonia solutions should be poured or transferred under the hood and never pipetted by mouth.

Strong Oxidants

These include strong solutions of hydrogen peroxide and perchloric acid and such solids as ferric nitrate, potassium dichromate, and chromic acid. These are dangerous to skin and eyes and also when brought into contact with oxidizable substances. The general precautions listed in the following section for poisons apply here as well.

Poisonous Compounds

This category includes all of the foregoing, to which the listed special precautions apply, plus compounds that have no marked effects on skin but are dangerous if taken internally, e.g., methyl alcohol, cyanides, ferrocyanide and ferricyanide, arsenical compounds, mercurial compounds, oxalates, nitroprussides, zinc compounds, lead compounds, barium compounds, elemental iodine, acrylamide, aromatic amines, and hydrocarbons. These substances may be ingested by:

1. Transfer to the technologist's hands and thence to mouth, food, and so forth.
2. Careless pipetting of solutions. *(No mouth pipetting should be performed.)*
3. Contamination of food, pipes, cigarettes, or pipettes laid on the bench. (Food should never be eaten in any laboratory.)

The precautions are obvious. It should be emphasized that proper labeling of all containers in a laboratory is essential, and this is particularly important with solutions of poisonous compounds.

Toxic Vapors

In some cases the level of ventilation in a laboratory may be adequate or tolerable for ordinary purposes but insufficient for the proper removal of toxic vapors. Ideally, any process that may produce a toxic vapor should be done under the hood, but this precaution is often overlooked. Students are not always aware that the vapors of acetone, chloroform, ether, formaldehyde, carbon tetrachloride, and methanol can be just as dangerous as the more obviously poisonous bromine. Procedures involving evaporation of these solvents in volumes greater than about 10 mL should be done under the hood or with a condenser. The use of the hood is the method of choice, since with condensed solvents the problem of disposal still remains. Large volumes of flammable or toxic liquids should not be poured down the sink; they must either be discarded in small amounts over a period of time or stored for qualified commercial disposal.

The toxic effects of the vapors of such solvents as carbon tetrachloride may be cumulative; that is, exposure to small concentrations at intervals over an extended period may finally result in a degree of toxic effect equal to exposure to a large concentration. Even if small quantities are being used, adequate ventilation must be maintained.

A source of a toxic vapor that is often overlooked is metallic mercury. All mercury spillage should be gathered up immediately with one of the various types of mercury collectors; merely sweeping the globules off the bench on to the laboratory floor is to be condemned. Under no circumstances should metallic mercury be dried in the hot air oven or discarded down laboratory sinks, where it may form amalgams with common metals, causing weakening and perforation of plumbing. The salvage of large quantities of mercury is best done by commercial experts using distillation.

In the past, sodium azide (NaN_3) was widely used as a preservative in some laboratory reagents, but it is less extensively used now. If the material is discarded in the sink, it may combine with lead or copper in the pipes to form explosive metal azides. Therefore if sodium azide ever needs to be discarded through the laboratory plumbing, only small quantities should be released at any one time, accompanied by much flushing water.

Burns and Scalds

Burns are caused by hot, dry objects—glassware or metal apparatus—and scalds by hot fluids and vapors. Excessive exposure to ultraviolet or infrared radiation can also cause burns.

A laboratory worker should not handle any glassware with bare hands unless he knows it is not hot or until he checks it first. It is essential that the correct equipment for the safe handling of hot apparatus be available—asbestos gloves, beaker and crucible tongs, test tube holders, and so forth. Electric hot plates and heating mantles should be placed so that accidental contact of hands or arms with the hot surfaces is minimized.

Scalds are usually the result of the boiling over of liquids, splashes, breakage of containers of hot liquid, or contact with steam. For example, heating the lower portion of the fluid in a test tube rapidly will often cause the violent expulsion of the contents and scalds to face and hands. Heating liquids in thick-walled glass containers and pouring hot liquids into cold containers can cause fracture of the glass and spillage of hot fluid. Thin-walled flasks may crack from direct contact with heat of a burner; a hot plate or asbestos mantle heater should be used. Round-bottomed flasks are much safer than the Erlenmeyer type for heating because of the lower stresses in the glass. Violent boiling of liquids with splashing can often be minimized by the use of quartz chips added to the container *before* heating is started. These are known commercially as "smooth boiling granules." They prevent superheating of the liquid.

Electrical Burns and Electrical Shock

The commonest causes of electrical shock in a laboratory are:

1. Using electrical apparatus or equipment with wet hands or while standing on a wet floor. The hospital or electrical engineer should fit a ground fault circuit interrupter (GFCI) to instruments that are at risk of causing electrical shock. The GFCI is a mechanism that disconnects the electrical supply as soon as a current imbalance is detected within the serving wires. Autopsy saws, for example, which may be used under potentially dangerous conditions, should always be fitted with a GFCI.
2. Faulty or overloaded wiring.
3. Attempting to service electrically powered apparatus without first disconnecting it. It should be remembered that, even when it is disconnected, any apparatus containing large condensers (also called capacitances) can store enough electrical energy to give a dangerous shock. Many instruments incorporate such large condensers to minimize line voltage variations.
4. Breakage of flask or beaker on an electrical hot plate, allowing water to short-circuit the power supply and possibly making the outer shell of the hot plate "live." In any case of such breakage, always disconnect the appliance before attempting to clean up the spilled fluid.

The safety precautions follow from the nature of the risk.

Never touch electrical apparatus with wet hands.

Do not overload electrical circuits by the use of multiple socket adapters.

Do not use metal tools, e.g., screwdrivers, inside "live" equipment. (See No. 4 above.)

Do not circumvent automatic power cut-off switches by the use of "jumpers."

Do not substitute fuses of higher rating than that specified by the manufacturer.

Keep cooling air intake filters clean and replace them according to schedule.

Disconnect electrical apparatus before servicing: merely switching them off is not enough.

Some types of circuit boards, in microprocessor-controlled instruments (which carry logic chips), can be ruined by static sparks. Be aware of the correct grounding methods.

There is a growing trend by manufacturers to provide sets of spare parts and circuit boards to permit in-laboratory service of instruments. This trend has been facilitated by the use of microprocessor control of automated equipment, with the concomitant ability to include self-diagnostic systems. This has the advantage that essential analytical services can be more easily maintained, but there is a strong obligation on the technologist to master thoroughly the instruction manuals and to carry out the work with careful attention to basic electrical safety rules as outlined above.

Most cases of electrical shock in a laboratory are

minor—painful but not dangerous. But if the accidental contact is strong (e.g., with wet hands), the shock can be severe enough to cause loss of consciousness. In such a case, remember, when removing the person from contact, to use some insulating cover on the hands, e.g., a lab coat, or pull the person away with a broom handle; otherwise, the rescuer may join the victim. Medical attention must be obtained immediately, and, if indicated, artificial respiration should be begun. The simplest method to learn and use is the "mouth-to-mouth" system.

Glass-Handling Accidents

Injuries resulting from cuts or lacerations from broken glass are the most common laboratory accidents, and it is essential that the chance of injury be minimized by correct handling and treatment of glassware.

Most of the necessary precautions in handling glassware are obvious, since they are just as appropriate for delicate objects of any nature. The precautions listed are those that are particularly applicable to laboratory glassware:

Remember that glass gives no warning of fracture; metal and wooden objects bend before breaking, as a rule.

Never use excessive force when assembling glass apparatus or inserting tubing in stoppers: always protect the hand with a cloth or heavy glove. Glass tubing should be moistened with distilled water before being inserted into rubber bungs. The introduction of Teflon stopcocks and stoppers for some types of burettes, separating funnels, and other apparatus prevents "freezing" during use, but the apparatus should be disassembled for cleaning immediately afterward; otherwise the Teflon tends to become locked into tubulures. If this occurs, place the apparatus in the deepfreeze overnight; the Teflon stopcock or stopper can be easily removed the next day.

The forces in a centrifuge impose great strains on centrifuge tubes, and if these have flaws or are cracked, they will fracture at quite moderate speeds. Centrifuge tubes of all sizes should fit the metal buckets reasonably well (it is risky to put a small tube into a large bucket), and the presence and condition of the rubber cushions in the bottom of the buckets should be checked. For high speeds (above 3000 rpm) round-bottomed tubes are stronger than the conical type, and at very high speeds plastic tubes may be necessary.

Improper storage of glass items in cupboards can lead to breakage. Items such as condensers, which are both fragile and awkward to store, should be kept on racks or in boxes. Items such as graduates and volumetric flasks, which are easily knocked over, must be arranged in the cupboard in such a way that any one item can be removed without risk of disturbing the remainder. Glassware should never be piled up in a cupboard.

Bacterial, Viral, or Parasitic Infection

The degree of risk to the technologist working with bacteriological material is related to the nature of the microorganism and to the standard technique. Some bacteria (e.g., the *Brucella*) and some viruses are so highly infective that even with optimum technique there is possibly still some risk, and extra precautions such as immunization may be indicated. But in most cases the adoption of good technique is more than adequate for safety.

Mailing Laboratory Samples

If material is to be sent by mail to reference laboratories, it must be packed with due regard to the current postal regulations. In the United States, information may be obtained from the National Standards Committee for Clinical Laboratory Standards, 771 East Lancaster Ave., Villanova, Pa. 19085, and their publication "Standard Procedures for the Handling and Transport of Diagnostic Medical Specimens and Etiologic Agents," TSH-5. For microbiological specimens, instructions are also available from the Biohazards Control Officer, Centers for Disease Control, Atlanta, Ga. 30333. The CDC publishes a guide to United States regulations on the topic.

In Canada, the information on parcel wrapping for medical materials is to be found in the Canada Postal Guide, Section 21.53, which is available in the post office. In case of difficulty, or for inquiries involving international regulations, the post office should be consulted.

Regarding viable microbiological specimens, in the U.S., federal regulations will allow the mailing of less than 50 mL of specimen securely closed in a watertight specimen container with sufficient absorbent material around it to absorb the entire contents in case of breakage. This is all to be enclosed in an outer shipping container of cardboard, wood, or corrugated fiber board bearing an "Etiologic Agents/Biomedical Material" red and white label (such labels are commercially available).

Infectious Hepatitis

In recent years, a new and serious hazard to laboratory personnel has arisen. Although the causes are only partially understood, the incidence of morbidity and even death from infectious hepatitis among hospital personnel, particularly those involved with renal dialysis units, has become a matter of concern. The commercial producers of lyophilized control sera test their products by the best available methods for the presence of the hepatitis-associated antigen, but they cannot yet guarantee its complete absence. The following precautions should be carefully noted. (See also pp. 19, 480, Chaps. 2 and 24.)

1. Any patient suspected or known to have hepatitis B should be identified as a high-risk case, and all blood samples should be taken, handled, and processed with strict precautions, using gloves and gowns when necessary. All samples must be specially identified with a suitable label, e.g., a red label.
2. *There should be no mouth pipetting of sera;* the availability of precise, rapid, hand-operated pipettors with capacities from 1 to 1000 microliters and from 1 to 5 milliliters makes mouth pipetting unnecessary.
3. Where large numbers of sera are being separated from centrifuged clots, poured into automatic analyzer cups or tubes, and subdivided into aliquots for further procedures, the handlers should wear, as a minimum, disposable plastic gloves and disposable aprons, and the

bench top should be covered with an absorbent paper sheet that is changed and incinerated daily. If the sera being handled are known to contain samples from hepatitis patients, the personnel should wear disposable paper masks; the centrifugation of sera produces finely dispersed aerosols that provide a high-risk source of infection. All blood "spills" must be cleaned up and disinfected immediately.

4. Effective provision must be made for disposal of used syringes and needles, preferably by incineration, or by readily accessible autoclaves.

5. All working areas must have adequate ventilation and "elbow room."

6. The work load must not be excessive; haste and pressure are incompatible with good handling techniques. *The importance of this factor is often underrated.*

7. If an automated process is available for tests done in large numbers, the associated reduction in serum handling is in itself a justification for automation.

8. The collection of patients' sera in order to prepare a control pool is not advised.

9. Centrifuges used for blood samples will soon accumulate a deposit of dried blood and serum on their inner surfaces unless it is removed with a strong detergent solution followed by thorough cleaning with a disinfectant. Finally, the inner surface should be given a *thin* layer of silicone grease to reduce adhesion of further contamination.

10. In large clinical laboratory departments, specimen receipt and handling should be done in separate rooms with effective ventilation for centrifuges.

11. The safety of laboratory personnel must be the active concern of a suitably qualified person with the power to institute safety procedures, train laboratory personnel in their application, and supervise the enforcement of specified procedures and with the responsibility to alert personnel to possible sources of infection through continually updated information about cases of hepatitis in both staff and patients. If any worker has any hand infection or open wound, he or she must not be allowed to handle blood specimens. If a worker sustains a cut or needle puncture during venipuncture or subsequent handling, this must be reported to the appropriate authority and advice obtained and given regarding the recognition of hepatitis.

12. Now that an effective vaccine against hepatitis B is available (although currently expensive), it will probably become advisable to immunize laboratory personnel, particularly those at increased risk, i.e., those who have frequent contact with blood from infective patients.

Suitable solutions for disinfection are described below (pp. 19 and 24).

Animal Handling

The correct techniques for handling laboratory animals are best taught by direct practical instruction.

It is essential that even minor scratches received from animals be treated properly; and if the animal has been inoculated with pathological material, the nature of this treatment may entail special measures to protect the technologist against the consequences of bites. Thus, even minor injuries *must* be reported immediately and proper treatment instituted.

Radiation Hazards

(See under Radioisotopes, p. 95.)

Further Recommendations

For a most complete and detailed discussion of laboratory safety, the handbook "Safety in Pathology Laboratories," produced by a working party of the Central Pathology Committee, Department of Health and Social Security, Alexander Fleming House, Elephant and Castle, London SE1 6BY, England, should be studied. The publication "CSLT Guidelines for Laboratory Safety," by A. R. Shearer, obtainable from Head Office, Canadian Society for Laboratory Technologists, P. O. Box 830, Hamilton, Ontario L8N 3N8, Canada, sets out practical rules for laboratory safety in a convenient form for ready reference. "Laboratory Safety at the Center for Disease Control" is obtainable from the CDC, Atlanta, Ga. 30333, as DHEW Publication No. CDC 76-8118. "Safety in the Clinical Laboratory" is a useful, well-illustrated manual.The authors are Henry, Olitzky, Lee, Walker, and Beattie, and it is published (1976) by Bio-Science Enterprises, Van Nuys, Calif. 91405.

LABORATORY GLASSWARE AND PLASTIC

Cleaning and Preparation of Glassware

Bacteriological Use

Choice of Detergent. There is a wide variety of detergents available for cleaning glassware, but the one chosen should satisfy the following criteria: (1) capable of softening the local water supply; (2) possesses the ability to remove organic material rapidly at a temperature of 60°C; (3) leaves glassware with a neutral pH following normal rinsing; (4) glassware should be free of antimicrobial factors following rinsing. To test for the absence of antimicrobial factors on glassware, three treated and three untreated bottles containing liquid culture media should be inoculated with a standard inoculum of a suitable test organism. Following overnight incubation, all six bottles should yield approximately identical viable counts.

Special attention must be given to new glassware, because resistant spores from packing material may be present. A convenient method is to boil the glassware in a detergent solution, thereby causing lysis of the organisms. Cool and wash thoroughly in tap water and then in distilled water. Dry in the hot air oven. Sterilize by autoclaving at 15 lb for 20 minutes.

Decontamination and Cleaning of Bacteriologically Dirty Glassware. During a normal working day in a microbiology department, a variety of glassware and apparatus becomes contaminated (including tube cultures), all of which has to be decontaminated before being sent to the washing-up area of the laboratory. Hence, following the completion of a procedure, all contaminated material or glassware should be placed in 3% Lysol or a similar disinfectant. This not only slowly destroys the organisms but also protects the laboratory worker, since the organisms, if they are beneath a fluid surface, are less likely to get into the atmosphere or onto environmental surfaces. When dealing with material suspected of containing *Mycobacterium tuberculosis, Bacillus anthracis,* or deep fungi, special care must be exercised, since these organisms are particularly resistant to decontamination and may infect those working in the laboratory. In the case of tubercle bacilli it is advisable to use 1% sodium hypochlorite rather than Lysol. This former reagent is also effective against hepatitis B virus. Some laboratory workers use a 5% solution for this purpose, and there are laboratories in which sodium hypochlorite is used for all routine decontamination. Commercial "Javex" is a 12% concentration of hypochlorite.

Two per cent glutaraldehyde is also a recommended decontaminant similar in activity and usefulness to hypochlorite and with the additional advantage of not being corrosive to metals.

Rubber gloves should be worn when handling these solutions. The effectiveness of the disinfection process depends on the thoroughness with which it is carried out.

Following this preliminary decontamination process, all glassware and other material for disposal should be autoclaved.

Obviously it is not possible to define an effective routine for the cleaning of dirty glassware that will be applicable to all situations. However, the following will suffice as an example of a procedure capable of yielding clean glassware:

1. Following autoclaving, the contents of bottles, tubes, flasks, and so forth, are drained of waste, and then the receptacles are placed in wire baskets.
2. Ideally these baskets should fit a commercial washing-up machine. But assuming such a machine is not available, these baskets are placed into a deep boiling sink with suitable detergent and boiled for 20 to 30 minutes.
3. Glassware is allowed to drain. Each bottle is then individually rinsed, then interior and exterior surfaces are scoured with an appropriate brush, rinsed, and stacked into another basket.
4. The basket is then transferred to a rinsing sink.
5. Following draining, the basket is transferred to still another sink, containing distilled water. After a draining period, the basket is placed in a hot air oven for drying.
6. After drying, the glassware is inspected. Dirty glassware is recycled; chipped and cracked glassware is rejected.

Disposable Plastic Equipment. By far the most common types of plastic encountered in the routine laboratory are the polypropylenes and polystyrenes. The polystyrenes are the cheapest and can be produced glass-clear; hence they have found wide application as disposable items in the microbiology laboratory. Such plastic equipment can be purchased presterilized from the manufacturer and is supplied in numerous forms, including Petri dishes, test tubes, syringes, precision pipettes, microtiter plates, microbiology diagnostic strips (e.g., Micro-ID; Fig. 14–11*B*), and so forth. The use of such equipment obviates the necessity for initial sterilization, and subsequent decontamination processing is much simpler.

Hematological Use

Glassware for hematological use must be free from detergent, because a minute concentration will lyse red cells. It is therefore inadvisable to use the method employed for bacteriological glassware, because it is difficult to remove the last traces of detergent. For general glassware, i.e., tubes, bottles, and so forth, wash thoroughly in tap water using a brush to remove obstinate dirt, place in dichromate cleaning fluid for 12 to 24 hours, and wash thoroughly in tap water and then in distilled water. Allow to drain and then dry in the hot air oven.

Microscope Slides. The degree to which the so-called precleaned microscope slide merits that description has improved, and pretreatment with dichromate is unnecessary. Rinsing in 70% ethyl or isopropyl alcohol followed by drying with a clean, soft cloth is adequate preparation for routine use.

Blood Pipettes. With the aid of a suction pump, draw through the pipette first tap water, then distilled water, and then acetone. Finally, let air flow through the pipette until it is dry.

Pipettes containing blood clots can be cleaned by first passing a pliable probe, e.g., nylon bristle, through the tip of the pipette and then using suction on the mouthpiece. Obstinate clots adhering to the wall of the pipette are removed by placing it in a 10% solution of potassium hydroxide for 12 to 24 hours.

To clean Wintrobe hematocrit tubes, pass a capillary pipette attached to a suction pump to the bottom of the tube and then immerse the tube in cold tap water. Distilled water is drawn through the tube in the same manner, followed by acetone. Dry by allowing air to flow through the tube or by placing in a warm (not hot) oven.

Biochemical Use

Glassware for biochemical use must not only look clean, it must be free from all forms of contaminating substances and, therefore, needs special attention. Tubes for general use may be cleaned in the following way: Soak for two to four hours in a weak solution—about 2% v/v—of a good "stripping" detergent* initially prepared in hot water. Rinse thoroughly in tap water, soak in 5% v/v hydrochloric acid solution, rinse again well in tap water, then with distilled water. Drain in the inverted position in a metal basket and dry in the hot air oven.

Glassware to be used for estimations of metal ions, i.e., sodium, potassium, calcium, lead, copper, zinc, and mercury, must, after being cleaned as described, be placed in 20% nitric acid for 12 to 24 hours, rinsed in three to four changes of distilled water, and then dried in the hot air oven.

Biochemical Pipettes. These must be placed in a jar containing dilute detergent immediately after use so that serum, blood, and chemical solutions do not dry in them. If an automatic pipette washer is available, the pipettes are placed in the pipette carrier, tip uppermost, and the carrier is then placed in the washer. The water supply is then regulated so that the washer fills and empties approximately 12 to 15 times per hour. After

*Conrad 70, Harleco, Philadelphia, Pa. 19143.

two hours, the carrier is removed and the pipettes are allowed to drain for 10 minutes. They are then placed in a container of distilled water, preferably hot. After the pipettes have filled with water, the carrier is raised above the level of the water and the pipettes are allowed to drain. This process is repeated twice more, a total of three changes of distilled water. The carriage is placed on the draining board for 10 minutes to allow the pipettes to drain thoroughly. They are then placed in a hot air oven at about 90°C until they are dry (about 1 hour).

Pipettes Containing Blood Clots. These are placed in 10% potassium hydroxide overnight before routine washing.

Greasy Pipettes. These should be placed in a "stripping" detergent solution for 12 to 24 hours. When a pipette washer is not available, pipettes may be washed by drawing tap water through them, followed by distilled water. The outside of the pipette is then wiped with a clean, soft cloth. They may be placed in the hot air oven at 90°C until they are dry.

Special Cleaning Methods

Permanganate Stains. These stains may be removed by steeping the article with a solution of 1% w/v ferrous sulfate in 25% v/v sulfuric acid or in 50% v/v hydrochloric acid.

Silver Nitrate Stains. To remove silver nitrate stains, steep the article overnight in concentrated ammonium hydroxide or place it in an iodine solution for 1 hour and then in a sodium thiosulfate solution for another hour.

Stopcock Grease. Stopcock grease may be removed by washing with organic solvents. Another grease solvent is a solution made by dissolving 100 g potassium hydroxide in 100 mL water, cooling, and adding 900 mL commercial grade 70% ethyl alcohol. This solution should not be used for very delicate glassware.

Resinous Matter. Soak the article in a mixture of five parts acetone, two parts commercial ether, and one part benzene. (Care! Flammable!) Leave for 30 minutes.

Hardened Blood Clots. Soak in a 5% solution of potassium hydroxide for minimum time necessary to dissolve the clot. Delicate apparatus may have to be treated with a warm solution of commercial pepsin or papain.

Brown Stains on Cell-Counting Pipettes. These can be removed by a short immersion in a commercial liquid bleach.

After use of any of the aforementioned methods, the articles should be very well rinsed in running tap water before proceeding with the usual cleaning routine.

USE OF PLASTIC APPARATUS IN BIOCHEMICAL LABORATORY WORK

Funnels, Graduates, Beakers. These are available in several types of plastic—polyethylene, polypropylene, and polycarbonate—and for many laboratory uses their survival time is far greater than that of glass versions. For reagent bottles, polypropylene is the best choice because of its almost complete inertness to most reagents. (The most important exception is fluorimetry; some plastics contain traces of highly fluorescent substances, and use of plastic ware in any stage of a fluorimetric analysis should be carefully checked.) The tall glass graduate's life is often short because of the ease with which it tips; if the transparent polycarbonate type is substituted, check for its resistance to solvents (see Table 2–1). For less critical measurements, such as 24-hour urine sample volumes, a large (2 liter) polyethylene graduate is quite suitable and almost indestructible. Plastic filter funnels have the disadvantage of retaining some stains permanently, but their low cost permits frequent replacement.

TABLE 2–1 PROPERTIES OF COMMON LABORATORY PLASTICS*

Plastic	Resistance to Heat	Resistance to Organic Solvents
Polyethylene	Low	Good
Polypropylene	Medium	Good
Polystyrene	Low	Poor
Polycarbonate	Medium	Poor
Nylon	Good	Good
Teflon	Excellent	Excellent
Polyvinyl chloride (tubing)	Low	Fair except to hydrocarbons

*Polyethylene, polystyrene, and polyvinyl chloride are not autoclavable; polypropylene, teflon, and polycarbonate are autoclavable.

Volumetric Flasks. The greater strength of the polypropylene volumetric flask has to be weighed against the difficulty of detecting improper cleaning or of seeing undissolved material. The glass flask is more resistant to solvents and heat.

Capped or Stoppered Tubes. We have found the plastic tube of about 12- to 15-mL capacity with a snap-on or push-fit closure very suitable when preparing dilutions for use with the atomic-absorption spectrophotometer or with determinations in which contamination is a critical problem, such as with plasma ammonia and serum iron. It is difficult to prepare glassware that is reliably free from trace elements on a routine basis; in our experience, the plastic tube is chemically clean. It is necessary to check each batch by filling with the diluent to be used, keeping overnight in the 56°C water bath, and then checking for such contamination as iron, calcium, and magnesium. This is done conveniently by processing the diluent as if it were a sample.

Micro Pipettes. Pipetting of serum by mouth suction, even using an extension rubber tube, should be eliminated. The main danger in this process is that of contracting hepatitis. Hand-operated, piston-type pipettors with disposable plastic tips in capacities from 1 to 1000 microliters are available from various sources. In the small- to medium-sized laboratory, in which a variety of procedures are done manually (phosphorus, cholesterol, microbilirubin, enzymes, total protein) using sample volumes in the 50- to 200-microliter range, these pipettors provide a sample and precise method for sample measurement. The coefficient of variation of the measurement is about 2 to 3% in routine use; better performance can be obtained after some practice. When unusually good precision in dilution is essential, as in serum calcium determination by atomic absorption spectrophotometry, the difference in viscosity between serum samples and aqueous standards introduces an error. One model of pipettor, which is designed for wash-out of the measured volume rather than expulsion by an extra movement of the piston, gives better results in this instance.

For many purposes the types of pipettors using glass capillaries rather than plastic tips are preferable.

Checking of Accuracy and Precision of Pipettes

"To Contain" (TC) Pipettes. These include hemoglobin pipettes and ultramicro pipettes. They can be checked by drawing in clean, dry mercury to the calibration mark, discharging it into a preweighed bottle, and reweighing. The contained volume is derived from the expression.

$$\frac{\text{Weight of mercury in pipette}}{\text{Weight of 1 mL mercury at the temperature of calibration (this is shown below).}}$$

Mercury Weight: Volume: Temperature Relationship

Temperature °C	Weight of 1 mL of Mercury
16	13.556 g
18	13.551 g
20	13.546 g
22	13.541 g
24	13.536 g

"To Deliver" (TD) Pipettes. These can be checked by delivering distilled water at the stated calibration temperature of the pipette and in the standard manner—emptying by gravity flow, no blowing out of last drop, pipette held close to the vertical with the tip against the inner surface of the vessel—into preweighed stoppered bottles. For most purposes the weight of 1 mL water can be taken as 1 gram: the weight of the fluid delivered in grams = capacity in mL.

"To Deliver with Blow Out" Pipettes. The calibration of blow out pipettes is similar to that used for "To Deliver" pipettes, except that the drop remaining in the tip after delivery is blown out once into the receiving vessel. This type of pipette has an etched ring near the mouthpiece.

"Between Two Marks" Pipettes. Checking of these pipettes is effected by weighing the water delivered between the two marks into a preweighed bottle.

The accuracy and precision of piston-type hand pipettors can be checked in a similar manner. Prepare 20 capped, numbered cups of the type used for continuous flow automatic analyzers. Record their individual weights. Using the technique specified for the pipette being tested, deliver repeated aliquots of water into the weighted cups, and cap. Reweigh. The weight differences will give the volumes delivered, and a mean value and standard deviation can be calculated by the method on p. 44. In our experience, a good quality piston-type pipettor should have a coefficient of variation

$$\left(\frac{\text{Standard deviation}}{\text{Mean value}} \times 100\right) \text{ of } 0.5\% \text{ or less}$$

The most accurate method for checking the calibrations of pipettes involves the use of a solution of a radioactively labeled compound. The ratio of the counts per minute of a dilution of that solution to the counts of the original solution provides a sensitive measure of the true dilution ratio and hence the accuracy of the pipette. This is not, however, a method for the average routine laboratory. A similar technique involving dilution of a dye and comparison of the absorbances of the dilution and the original dye solution requires a degree of photometric accuracy beyond that of the average routine laboratory spectrophotometer.

The matching of tube-type spectrophotometer cuvettes should be checked by filling each with a weakly acid solution of potassium dichromate that has an absorbance against a water blank of about 0.400 at 420 nm and reading the absorbance of each cuvette. The coefficient of variation of the readings should not exceed 0.5%.

OTHER FACTORS INFLUENCING ANALYTIC RESULTS

Preservatives for Laboratory Specimens

When specimens are to be sent to another laboratory or to a commercial laboratory, the types of samples required and their preservation and handling will be specified by the intended recipient. The large commercial bioassay organizations issue detailed handbooks with this and much other information. Within the hospital or other institution some specimens require special treatment to prevent deterioration before analysis, and the following notes apply to this situation.

Blood Glucose. The blood should be collected in a tube containing lithium iodoacetate, commercially available in the vacuum-tube systems. This preservative permits holding all of the blood samples from a glucose tolerance curve for simultaneous analysis or for checking unexpected results.

Serum Acid Phosphatase. This enzyme is extremely unstable. If the assay cannot be run immediately, add 10 mg disodium citrate for each milliliter of serum and freeze. In our experience, freezing alone does not always preserve elevated levels of acid phosphatase.

Plasma and Serum for Insulin, Renin. The separation and freezing of serum or plasma must be done quickly; for renin, a refrigerated centrifuge is desirable. Some workers avoid freezing of serum samples for insulin assay.

Blood for Acid-Base Determinations (pH, pCO_2, and so on). See p. 193.

Cerebrospinal Fluid. Immediate processing for both chemical and microbiological analyses is imperative. CSF glucose can be preserved as for blood glucose, previously mentioned.

Tissues and Cytological Samples. See pp. 760 and 787.

24-Hour Urine Collections

For glucose, collect with 10 mL of 10% w/v thymol in isopropanol.

For inorganic constituents—calcium, phosphate, sodium, and potassium—collect with 5 mL of concentrated hydrochloric acid.

For creatinine, and uric acid, refrigerate.

For quantitative porphyrins, collect with 5 g sodium carbonate.

For *d*-aminolevulinic acid, collect with 10 mL concentrated hydrochloric acid.
For urobilinogen and porphobilinogen, collect with 5 g sodium carbonate plus a layer of petroleum spirit (petroleum ether).
For steroids, refrigeration is preferable, since there is no risk of introducing chemical interference.
For catecholamines and VMA (3-methoxy-4-hydroxymandelic acid), collect with 10 mL concentrated hydrochloric acid.
For amylase, refrigerate.

When there is a conflict between the suggested preservatives—for example, if calcium and uric acid are to be assayed on the same collection and the added acid would precipitate the uric acid—make the collection with 10 mL of 10% w/v thymol in isopropanol, and, after mixing, acidify an aliquot of 10 mL with one drop of concentrated hydrochloric acid for the calcium estimation, or use refrigeration. Do not use the thymol-in-isopropanol preservative in collections for catecholamines.

The accurate collection of 24-hour urine specimens is facilitated if the laboratory provides suitable bottles with the correct preservative when indicated and a sheet of exact instructions. The use of the 24-hour creatinine excretion as an index of completeness of collection is to be regarded only as a guide to gross loss of urine. Any 24-hour output of less than 500 to 600 mL from an adult should be viewed with suspicion, as well as any collections that exactly fill the supplied bottle. If the bottle contains strong acid as a preservative, it should be clearly marked with a very large "DANGER—CORROSIVE" label; the possible inability of the patient, who is often entrusted by a busy nursing staff with the collection, to appreciate the danger of serious burns should not be overlooked.

Stability of Serum Constituents

It is recommended laboratory practice to store the unused portion of serum samples to permit repeat of doubtful or unusual results. Generally speaking, such repeat analyses will be requested or deemed necessary within two or three days of the original result, and, for the majority of serum constituents routinely assayed, freezing at $-10°C$ will preserve them adequately. Storing at refrigerator temperature (about 2 to 4°C) may lead to errors due to evaporation. Serum samples used for glucose analyses will be stable for at least 24 hours if taken with lithium iodoacetate as the preservative.

Stored sera should not be kept in corked tubes: this will give serious errors in calcium determinations. There are definite advantages in using plastic tubes with polyethylene stoppers for plasma and serum storage. Frozen plasma and serum samples must be well mixed by repeated inversion—not by vortexing—before analysis, since definite layering of the protein content occurs. Freezing of the plasma or serum samples also effectively inhibits bacterial growth that may produce erroneous results in automatic analyzers.

Drug Interference With Laboratory Tests

The concomitant increasing use of more sensitive methods of assay and the almost daily introduction of new drugs may confront the technologist with the possibility of erroneous laboratory results with little or no information about the probable causes. When this is suspected, the following measures to demonstrate that interference has made a result unreliable are suggested:

1. Repeat the assay to confirm the unusual or unexpected finding.
2. Repeat the determination, if possible, by a method using a different chemical or physical principle. An unusual blood urea nitrogen result by an automated diacetyl monoxime method should be checked by an enzymatic method using urease and the Berthelot reaction. A serum protein value by the biuret reaction can be checked with a refractometer.
3. With nonurgent tests, if medically possible, the patient should be taken off the drug and the test should be repeated.
4. Any suspicion that a test result may have been influenced by drug interference (or, for that matter, interference from any source, such as intravenous solutions or excessive amounts of heparin) should be brought to the attention of supervisory personnel to permit appropriate action.

As a general rule, any technique that enhances sensitivity without retaining specificity is liable to interference. One of the drawbacks to some fluorimetric methods is the associated interference caused by the widespread occurrence of highly fluorescent compounds in biological fluids and many drugs. In contrast, the high degree of specificity of atomic absorption and gas-liquid chromatographic techniques permits full use of their high sensitivity. A good source of assistance with this problem is the encyclopedic compilation of Caraway and Kammeyer (1972).

The published data on interferences is continually being extended. A detailed bibliography of drug interference with laboratory tests is given in a special issue of *Clinical Chemistry* (Young et al., 1975).

STERILIZATION AND THE LABORATORY

Inhibition and Killing of Microorganisms

1. Diagnostic microbiology endeavors to promote the growth and subsequent identification of pathogenic organisms in vitro, and considerations of hygiene and laboratory management require methods for the expeditious destruction of organisms once the diagnostic process is complete.
2. Aseptic methods are employed in surgical and other invasive procedures, and here some method of killing ambient organisms on instruments must be employed to achieve asepsis.
3. The laboratory is involved in the control of asepsis in the operating room.
4. The maintenance or achievement of sterility in culture media is naturally a function of the laboratory. Should the media be contaminated before inoculation with suspect material, identification of possible pathogens from the patient may be hindered.

For these four types of activity, different sterilization methods may be employed. Two groups of agents can be used to achieve sterilization:

Group I—Chemical Agents: (a) disinfectants, (b) antiseptics, (c) chemotherapeutics, and (d) gases and vapors.

Group II—Physical Agents: (a) moist heat, (b) dry heat, (c) visible and ultraviolet radiation, (d) atomic radiation, (e) ultrasonics, (f) mechanical filtration.

Some Definitions

The agents in groups I and II have specific modes of interference affecting an organism's natural equilibrium by means of essential enzyme activity, which results in either reversible or irreversible cellular changes. Thus it is important to appreciate that some agents kill, whereas others simply inhibit growth and multiplication.

Those agents producing reversible injury, namely, stasis or inhibition, are called bacteriostatic, and as such they do not manifest an immediately lethal action. Those agents causing irreversible injury, culminating in the rapid death of a cell, are termed bactericidal.

Sterilization is an absolute term indicating the total inactivation, i.e., destruction or removal, of all forms of microbial life in terms of their ability to reproduce (this includes the most resistant spores). The term does not necessarily imply the destruction of an organism's constitutive enzymes, the by-products of its metabolism, toxins, and so forth. By virtue of this fact, the term frequently is applied incorrectly to a situation characteristic of disinfection.

Disinfection is a term used to describe the activity of a chemical agent, such as a reduction in population numbers. It usually involves killing the organism, but without necessarily achieving sterility. There are, however, particular situations, such as those involving only nonsporing organisms, in which the entire population is destroyed. Here disinfection can be regarded as synonymous with sterilization. In practice, those disinfectants possessing the ability to kill important pathogens frequently are employed to render certain objects safe for use, e.g., a clinical thermometer.

The terms *disinfectant* and *antiseptic* are not synonymous; in fact, they define two distinct types of agents. Disinfectants are those substances which are toxic and capable of destroying microorganisms (including pathogens), but not necessarily resistant spores. By virtue of their properties, disinfectants are suitable only for those applications involving inanimate objects. By contrast, those chemical agents less toxic for mammalian tissue, yet capable of killing microorganisms, are known as antiseptics, and generally such agents act more slowly than disinfectants. By virtue of their low toxicity, antiseptics can be applied to skin surfaces and mucous membranes. Some antimicrobial chemicals possessing a low or differential toxicity frequently are employed as chemotherapeutics in the treatment of infectious diseases.

Chemical Disinfection

A Brief Consideration of Mode of Action. Chemical agents can affect normal cell function in a variety of ways, i.e., disruption of cell wall or membrane, injury to nuclear region, or enzyme inhibition.

Under certain conditions some agents may initiate precipitation of cell protein from the colloidal state, whereas others may be more specific and disrupt the cell membrane. Likewise, there are those agents that interfere with essential cell enzymes by removal of the free sulfhydryl groups or by antagonizing specific enzymatic reactions.

Factors Influencing Disinfection. The modus operandi of an organism's death naturally will vary according to the method employed, but despite this, the effect is the same: essential cellular proteins are degraded, causing a disturbance in metabolic activity, with the net result being that the cell's ability to develop and reproduce is obviated. The killing of bacteria by any means, physical or chemical, is influenced by a variety of factors: time, temperature, concentration, nature of the medium, and nature of the organism.

The killing rate of a chemical agent largely depends on its concentration and temperature, the rate usually increasing as the temperature is raised. For instance, a culture of *Salmonella paratyphi* is destroyed by exposure to 0.01% mercuric chloride for 2½ minutes at 31°C, and 36 minutes at 14°C. Under normal conditions most nonsporing microorganisms are susceptible to physical and chemical agents. However, the rate of death in a spore-bearing population differs. On exposure to chemical agents, population numbers are rapidly depleted for a short time; thereafter, destruction proceeds at a much slower rate.

As indicated, the concentration of a chemical disinfectant is an important factor influencing the killing rate. The higher the concentration of the germicide, the greater the rate of killing will be. With some agents, and in particular with the phenolic group of compounds, activity falls off very rapidly with dilution. Therefore it is important to appreciate that with a lowering of concentration there is a risk of reducing the agent's effectiveness to the point of little or no bactericidal action; indeed, there is the possibility that growth of the organism may be stimulated.

The activity of most germicides is reduced by the presence of organic matter, particularly that of protein, as found in body fluids. Hence, extraneous organic matter will combine with a disinfectant, reducing its effective concentration.

A bacterial culture always contains organisms of varying grades of resistance to disinfection, in which the most susceptible are the first to succumb, followed by those of greater resistance at successive intervals, until finally the most resistant members of the population are destroyed. It has been found that young cultures are extremely susceptible to disinfecting agents (for example, the time required to kill 99.9% of a 8-hour *E. coli* culture is 10 minutes), whereas old cultures tend to have a much higher resistance (for example, the time required to kill 99.9% of a 17-hour *E. coli* culture is approximately 27 minutes).

Spores are exceptionally resistant to the majority of disinfectants. Similarly, acid-fast bacilli and capsulated organisms are more difficult to destroy than noncapsulated organisms.

Evaluation of Disinfectants. The efficiency of a disinfectant is assessed by measuring the rate of kill against a range of organisms under specified conditions. The majority of methods employ phenol as a standard reference, so that a *phenol coefficient* (PC) is frequently quoted for disinfectants. The phenol coefficient is a figure comparing the dilutions of phenol and of another agent possessing equivalent killing power for a specific test organism.

A Consideration of Chemical Agents

Soaps and Detergents. These are surface agents. With the soaps, fatty acids adsorb to the cell membrane and the cation to the surrounding water. The cell membrane undergoes considerable strain and is subsequently disrupted. Detergents act in a similar manner. Compounds such as benzalkonium chloride (Zephiran) and cetrimonium bromide (Cetavlon) are useful cleansing agents and have considerable bacteriostatic and lesser bactericidal properties. They have been used widely for cleansing contaminated hospital areas. It should be noted that they are quite ineffective against *Ps. aeruginosa.* pHisoHex is a commercial compound containing a detergent and a chlorine-phenol antiseptic and is commonly used for cleaning skin.

Ethyl Alcohol. This agent produces denaturation of bacterial protein and is frequently employed as a skin disinfectant. The most effective disinfection occurs with a concentration between 50 and 70%—although any concentration between 70 and 95% will destroy approximately 90% of the normal resident skin flora in 2 minutes.

Phenols and Cresols. In the correct concentrations these compounds have highly bactericidal properties. They denature bacterial protein. Lysol is the most widely used of the cresols, and generally a 2 to 3% concentration is employed. These compounds are not greatly inactivated by the presence of organic matter, and they have little or no effect against spores.

Oxidizing Agents. Agents such as halogens, ozone, and hydrogen peroxide are either bacteriostatic or bactericidal. Their mode of action is either inhibition or destruction of $-SH$ or $-NH_2$ groups essential to many enzyme or coenzyme reactions. Halogens such as iodine and chlorine are effective as disinfectants because of their oxidative effects. The skin may be cleansed temporarily with such agents, but care should be taken not to use iodine or mercury solutions on sensitive (allergic) subjects. Iodine has long been used as a bactericidal agent, especially in the form of a tincture in 70% alcohol. Unfortunately this substance is allergenic to some and an irritant to many. A compound of iodine with polyvinyl pyrrolidone (Betadine) remains bactericidal but does not have the adverse effects of tincture of iodine.

One per cent sodium hypochlorite is very useful for the disposal of contaminated slides and swabs, including those with *M. tuberculosis.* It is also effective against hepatitis B virus. Bench tops are beneficially cleaned with this substance, and in case of spills, the offending area is covered with a 5% solution of hypochlorite for at least an hour before mopping up.

Salts and Organic Compounds of Heavy Metals. These have limited laboratory application. Mercury bichlorate in a concentration of 1:2000 to 1:5000 is used rarely as a hand disinfectant. Sodium ethylmercurithiosalicylate (Merthiolate) is used in 1:10,000 concentration for the preservation of sera. *Glutaraldehyde* as a 2% aqueous solution is a very effective disinfectant, especially since it does not corrode metal (unlike hypochlorite), and is effective against hepatitis B virus. Centrifuges can be treated with this substance.

Quaternary Ammonium Compounds. These are mixtures of high molecular alkyl, demethyl, benzyl ammonium chlorides and similar compounds. They have limited laboratory application but are employed widely in the food and dairy industries to sterilize equipment.

Glycerol. This chemical in a 50% solution kills bacteria, but not viruses, and thus finds a special application in the preservation of some vaccines; it is also used in preservation of agglutination sera.

Gases. Ethylene oxide is a colorless, odorless, poisonous, inflammable, and explosive gas, which if diluted with some inert substance such as carbon dioxide is an efficient sterilizer of surgical instruments, especially plastic materials which cannot be heat sterilized. The gas is also particularly useful in sterilizing apparatus such as heart-lung machines and respirators. It kills both vegetative organisms and spores in eight hours.

Beta-propiolactone is nonflammable and can be used as a liquid or gas, but it is toxic and an irritant.

Formaldehyde is an irritant water-soluble gas lethal to all kinds of vegetative microbes and spores. Bacterial cultures and suspensions usually are killed and fixed by the addition of formaldehyde to a concentration of 0.04 to 1.0%. Gaseous disinfection using formaldehyde frequently is employed for certain articles that cannot be wetted completely with solutions or that are damaged by wetting. The atmosphere must have a high relative humidity, over 60%, and a temperature of at least 18°C. The gas is liberated by heating or spraying formalin. When cold formalin is sprayed, an equal volume of ethanol is added to prevent polymerization. The best method is to boil formalin diluted with sufficient water to produce an adequate atmospheric humidity. Small articles, such as instruments, are disinfected by exposure to formaldehyde gas for at least three hours under air-tight conditions.

A Consideration of Physical Agents

Sterilization by Dry Heat. Sterilization by dry heat has limited application. The higher temperatures and prolonged exposure times required are often deleterious to many materials.

Incineration. A flame is an effective sterilizer and the simplest of methods. Naked flame heat often is employed in sterilizing platinum or Nichrome wire loops for inoculating or subculturing cultures. In flaming, large amounts of material should not be left on the loop, since this causes "spluttering" and dissemination of infective particles. To avoid this problem it is helpful to use a flame hood over the Bunsen burner, or to insert the loop into the lower part of the flame and slowly raise it into the hot zone of the flame. A small jar of Lysol containing a pad of lint can be used to rid the loop of excess material before flaming. The Bacti-Cinerator (Fig. 2–1) is an electrically heated apparatus that completely avoids the risks of aerosols. Contaminated material that is no longer required, such as paper, swabs, surgical dressings, animal cadavers, and so forth, is best disposed of by incineration.

Hot Air Oven. By this method, the process of heat transfer to the objects is by convection, radiation, and conduction. Hence, time must be allowed (1) for heat penetration, to bring all objects in the oven to the required temperature, (2) for the objects to be held at a

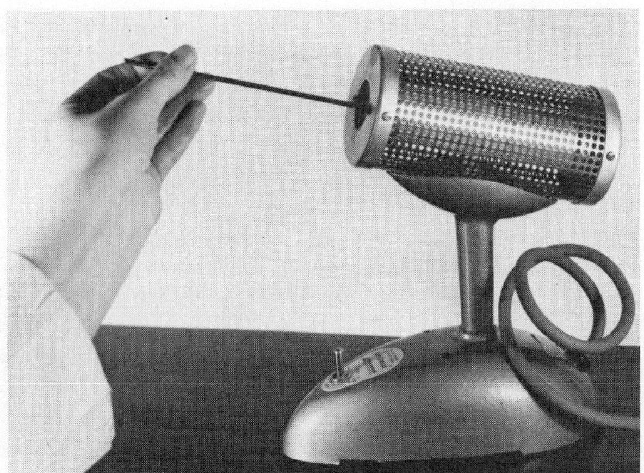

Figure 2–1 Bacti-Cinerator (Sherwood Medical Instruments, St. Louis, Mo. 63103). An electrically heated apparatus for the sterilization of bacterial loops that avoids the hazards of aerosols from a spluttering loop in the gas Bunsen burner.

standard temperature to kill organisms, and (3) for the oven to cool before opening. The entire process takes several hours, considerably longer than the moist heat process.

A temperature of 100°C dry heat for 1 hour will destroy nonsporing organisms; fungal spores required 115°C for 1 hour, and for the majority of bacterial spores a temperature of 160°C for 1 hour is required. It should be remembered that the hot air oven is unsuitable for material containing rubber or for apparatus with rubber bungs, washers, or stoppers. Likewise, apparatus made with both metal and glass will be ruined in a hot air oven because of the unequal expansion between glass and metal or the melting of the solder or cement. The oven is unsuitable for liquids or media. The oven is ideal for dry glassware, including assembled all-glass syringes.

Wrapping of the glassware before sterilization facilitates subsequent storage without chance of contamination. Remember that effective sterilization requires heating for 1 hour at 160°C; the temperature must be maintained for the entire period. After the hour has elapsed, the oven door should not be opened immediately, since a rapid change in temperature may cause cracking of glassware, and currents of air circulating into the oven may introduce contaminating organisms.

Sterilization by Moist Heat. By comparison with dry heat, the moist heat process of sterilization (particularly moist steam under pressure) has proved to be the most reliable and universally applicable method of sterilization. Moist heat is the most efficient lethal agent, sterilizing at a lower temperature and in a shorter time. Steam is a particularly effective lethal agent, since it penetrates all exposed surfaces of the treated material; further, in the process of steam's condensing on the cooler surfaces, heat is transferred by giving up its latent heat of vaporization, and this continues until a temperature equilibrium is reached.

Microbial death results from the coagulation and denaturation of structural proteins and cellular enzymes, which occurs more radily in the hydrated than in the dry state.

Boiling. Boiling is not usually adequate for routine bacteriology or surgery, since spore-bearing organisms are not killed by this method.

Steam Sterilization (Tyndallization). Exposure to steam at 100°C for 90 minutes will usually ensure sterility of material known not to contain spores, but surer methods are available. One variant of this method of steaming is known as tyndallization, or intermittent sterilization, in which the apparatus or medium to be sterilized is exposed to a temperature of 100°C for 30 minutes on three successive days. The principle is that spores fructify and subsequently are destroyed by additional heat. The germination of surviving spores is fostered by incubation at 37°C between periods of heating. The method finds its main application in sterilizing media containing sugars which may be degradated at higher temperatures.

Autoclave. The technical procedures in autoclaving are best learned by practice. The principle is that water under pressure boils at progressively higher temperatures. It is essential that the system utilize saturated steam; otherwise, the process becomes virtually a dry heat treatment, for which different time-temperature relationships exist. The implication here is that superheated steam (steam reheated) must be avoided. Also, it is essential in operating an autoclave that the residual air be completely exhausted and displaced. Those autoclaves operating on a downward displacement method (in which steam enters the chamber at the top, thus forcing air out at the bottom) require longer exposure times than those generally quoted. Using the downward displacement method, 25 minutes at 121°C (i.e., 15 lb/sq in) is adequate. With high-vacuum autocalves an effective time-pressure sterilizing formula is 15 lb/sq in for 15 minutes. The method is suitable for rubber-assembled apparatus and syringes that contain metal. It is unsuitable for many sugar-containing media, but is appropriate for those containing dextrose.

Filtration. The principle of filtration is that of "straining off" bacteria that are larger than the pores of the filter. Even viruses can be eliminated this way. Filters are of several types and grades.

Seitz Filters. Disposable asbestos filter pads, obtainable in various sizes, are made to fit into the standard Seitz filter apparatus or alternatively into special syringes. Two porosities are available: fine and extra fine, designated Type serum 1 and Type serum 3, respectively.

Membrane Filters. Millipore filters are porous membranes composed of pure and biologically inert cellulose, Teflon, polyvinyl chloride, and other substances with a remarkable array of filter characteristics for many medical and other purposes. Membrane filters with uniform pores are available. Those of filter size 0.22 μm are sufficient to provide a bacteriologically sterile filtrate.

Other Physical Methods of Sterilization. Occasionally, for instruments such as scalpel blades, scissors, or forceps, sterilization may be achieved by wetting with alcohol and then flaming it off. This procedure should be repeated several times to assure sterility. Its advantage is that it is rapid, but carbonization and the loss of cutting edge occur.

Other methods of sterilization include the use of ultraviolet light, but this has restricted application. Ultraviolet light is thought to be absorbed by bacterial

DNA, causing lethal mutation. Irradiation is being used for the sterilization of surgical packs. Both beta and gamma rays are effective. X-rays cause ionization, with the production of ions in the cells resulting in undesirable chemical combinations. Genetic changes also occur.

Supersonic and ultrasonic waves (9000 cycles per second and upward) may be used to rupture and disintegrate cells. It is thought that the bacteria are buffered and destroyed by minute gas bubbles forming in the suspension as a result of the sound waves.

Quality Control of Sterilization

Ideally, whichever method is chosen, it should be suitably controlled to ensure that the treatment has been adequate. However, not all the methods cited have an easy or convenient means of quality control. Obviously, when a new chemical agent for general disinfection is instituted, it should be evaluated according to the principles indicated (see p. 23) against those organisms usually encountered in the particular working situation.

Most hospital sterilization is done by autoclave or by ethylene oxide. A most convenient way to monitor sterility is by the use of a biological system that uses spores of *B. stearothermophilus* to test the adequacy of autoclaving and spores of *B. subtilis var. niger, globigii* for the adequacy of sterilization by ethylene oxide. The spores are impregnated in a paper strip together with a crushable ampule of modified trypticase soy broth with bromcresyl purple pH indicator* in a flexible plastic vial color coded to indicate the type of spore strip within.

The vial is placed strategically among the articles to be sterilized in the autoclave or gas sterilizer, and the materials are then sterilized. The vial is subsequently removed, and the ampule of medium is crushed within the plastic vial, allowing the medium to flood the spore strip. The vial is then incubated (at 56°C for the *B. stearothermophilus* and at 37 to 40°C for the *B. subtilis*) for 24 hours. Should the medium change from purple to yellow, the sterilization has been inadequate, since fructification of the spores has occurred. Small water bath incubators designed especially for the vials are obtainable, and these, along with prepared log books for performance entries, make the task of monitoring very easy.

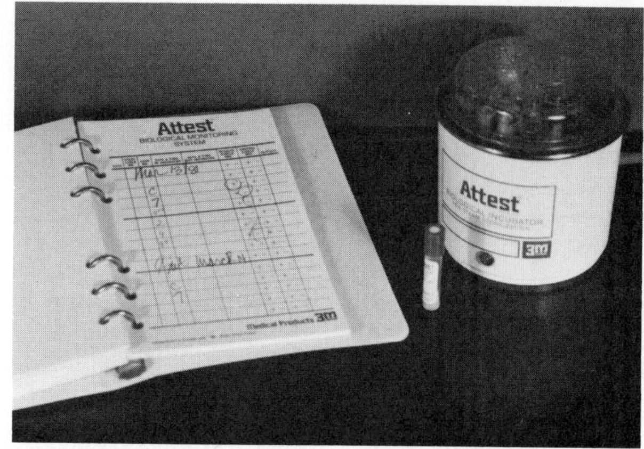

Figure 2–2 The Attest biological monitoring system (3M Company). Within a flexible vial there is a paper strip impregnated with *B. stearothermophilis* spores and a crushable glass ampoule containing broth and bromocresol purple indicator. The vial, seen between the recording book and the incubator in the illustration, is placed within a package to be sterilized. After the sterilization process, the ampoule of broth is crushed and the vial is placed in a plastic holder in a special incubator at 56°C. Bacterial growth is indicated when the medium changes from purple to yellow. A 48-hr incubation period is necessary to exclude the possibility of inadequate sterilization.

COLLECTION OF BLOOD SAMPLES

Venipuncture (Fig. 2–3)

Most blood samples are obtained by venipuncture. It is the easiest and most convenient method of obtaining an adequate volume of blood suitable for a variety of tests. The sample can be divided and treated as the prescribed investigations demand; thus, some may be mixed with anticoagulant to provide plasma or whole blood; some may be allowed to clot to provide serum (fluid part of blood less fibrinogen); clotting time may be accurately determined, smears made, blood cultures taken, and so on. For the busy laboratory it offers the fastest method of collecting samples from a large number of patients, allowing accurate dilution to be carried out with more leisure in the laboratory. It reduces the amount and variety of apparatus to be carried to the hospital wards. By providing sufficient blood it allows various tests to be repeated in case of accident or error or for the all-important checking of a doubtful result. It frequently allows the performance of additional tests that may be suggested by the results of those already ordered or that may occur to the clinician or laboratory physician as afterthoughts. It reduces the possibility of error resulting from dilution with tissue juices or constriction of skin vessels by cold or emotion that may occur in taking blood by finger puncture. Venipuncture should be undertaken only by experienced operators who have the patience and skill necessary to avoid causing discomfort to the patient.

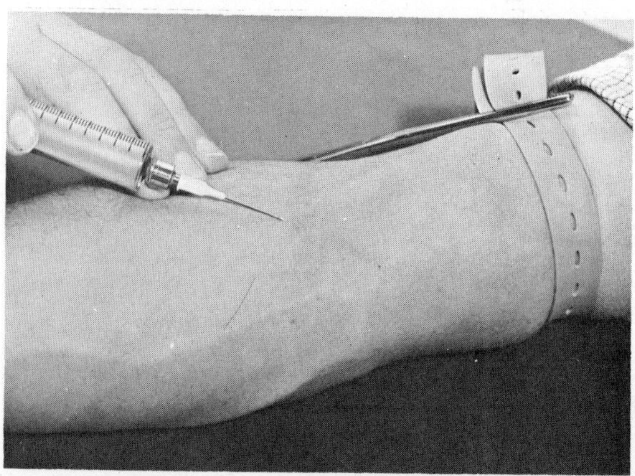

Figure 2–3 Performing a venipuncture.

*Attest system, Medical Products Division, 3M Co., St. Paul, Minn. 55101 and London, Ont. N6A 4T1.

Venipuncture is usually performed on the antecubital vein. This is easily located or palpated in most people (except the obese) and is usually prominent in manual workers, especially on the side of handedness. In many cases when the vein is not easily located it may be made to stand out by the patient's closing and opening his or her fist, or by massage, or both. A hot towel over the area may be helpful. Occasionally, the veins on the back of the hand may have to be used, but special care and experience are needed to prevent hematoma formation around these loose and poorly supported vessels. Venipuncture via the scalp, external jugular, subclavian, or femoral vessels demands the services of an experienced physician.

Once the vein is located, a check should be made to ensure that all the sample tubes and equipment required are in convenient readiness and accurately labeled (patient's name, room number, and nature of specimen written *legibly* on a suitable label). Many hospitals now use a preprinted label containing all the necessary patient data, and this system is highly recommended. The use of numerical codes to identify the patient is warranted. Blood may be taken with either a conventional syringe and needle or a commercially available evacuated tube with attached needle.*

The latter method has the advantage of:

1. A prepackaged sterile unit that requires no prior preparation.
2. A wide range of tube size and contained anticoagulant.
3. A safer method of taking blood, since the samples are taken directly into labeled tube.
4. The avoidance of syringe breakage.
5. No preparation of anticoagulants and containers.
6. Because the evacuated tubes are sterile, the prevention of possible bacterial contamination should there be any flowback of blood from tube to patient.

The technique for obtaining blood is essentially the same, whether conventional syringes or commercial evacuated tube systems are used. The syringe technique is described here.

A dry, sterile syringe of suitable size is assembled with aseptic care and a medium-length (shaft 2 to 4 cm), sterile, sharp, short-beveled needle of 20 to 21 gauge is securely fitted to the syringe nozzle, the sterile needle container remaining as protection over the needle shaft. The patient is then placed in a comfortable posture in which he or she can hold the selected arm comfortably and without fatigue. Avoid attempting to take blood from a sitting patient whose arm is unsupported. Place a chair alongside the bed, table, or bench being used by an ambulatory or outpatient so that the selected arm can be rested along the edge of the table or bed. Prepare the arm by swabbing the antecubital fossa with 70% ethanol or other suitable skin disinfectant. Apply a soft rubber tourniquet (Surgical white-rubber Penrose drain tubing is suitable or, alternatively, tourniquets can be purchased commercially) at a point about 6 cm above the bend of the elbow. This must not be applied too tightly as it will then constrict the artery as well as the veins. As a rough guide, it is sufficiently tight when its deep aspect sinks about 1 to 2 mm below the surrounding skin level. It should be secured by a "half bow" so that a gentle tug on the protruding end will release it.

Remove the protecting cap from the needle and hold the syringe so that the bevel of the needle is upward. Grasp the back of the patient's arm at the elbow and draw the skin slightly taut over the vein. Holding the needle so that its shaft parallels the course of the vein, pierce the skin along one edge of the vein. Advance the point of the needle 0.5 to 1 cm into the subcutaneous tissues and then pierce the vein wall. The blood may begin to enter the syringe spontaneously; if not, gently withdraw the piston at a rate equal to the flow of blood. The experienced and confident technologist may release the tourniquet now, and it is advisable to do so, since some hemoconcentration will develop after 1 minute of stasis. As soon as sufficient blood has entered the syringe, the tourniquet is released. Then (but not until the tourniquet has been released) the needle is quickly withdrawn and a ball of sterile cotton is applied to the puncture site, the patient being instructed to press on this. Flexing the elbow to hold the swab must be avoided.

The needle is removed from the syringe and the blood *gently* emptied into the appropriate containers. The containers are stoppered and those containing anticoagulant are inverted several times (not shaken). It is important not to eject the blood through the needle, not to use excessive force generally, and not to cause frothing in the tubes, since any of these is likely to lead to hemolysis.

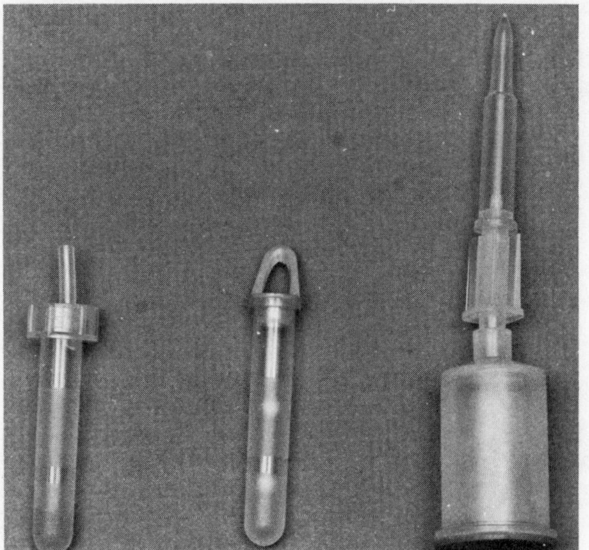

Figure 2–4 Tubes suitable for capillary blood sample collection. From left to right: Microtainer—Blood is collected through the attached capillary tube into anticoagulant: Microtainer—Once blood is collected, the capillary is removed, the plastic cap inserted, and the sample mixed. The sample can then be treated like a venous sample; Unopette—Blood is collected through the capillary directly into diluting fluid. Only those analyses for which the diluting fluid is suitable can be performed. A variety of different diluting fluids are available. (Tubes manufactured by Becton-Dickinson and Co., Rutherford, N.J. 07070.)

*Vacutainer, Becton-Dickinson and Co., Rutherford, N.J. 07070 and Mississauga, Ont. L5J 2M8.

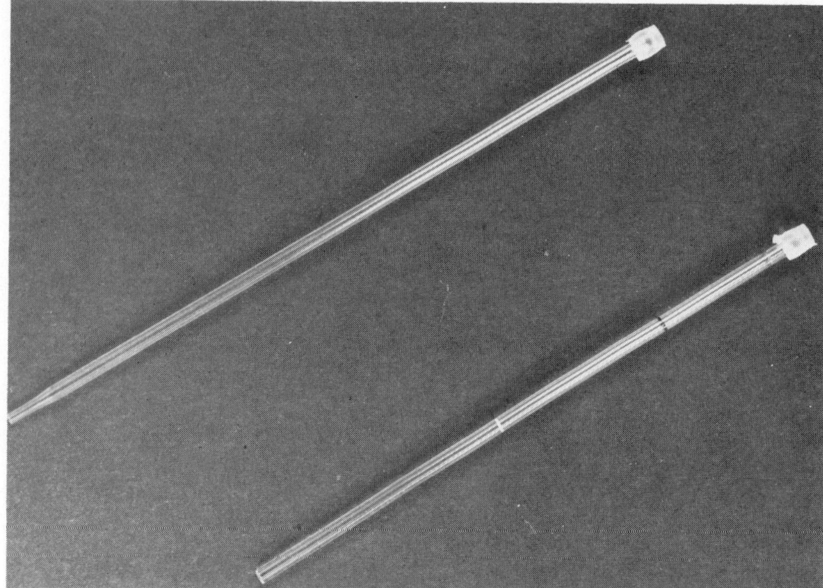

Figure 2–5 Capillary blood collection tubes. *Top,* Natelson microsample pipette; *bottom,* Miale prothrombin pipette.

Skin Puncture Technique—Micro Blood Samples

Skin puncture is frequently used when only small quantities of blood are required, e.g., for hemoglobin, for white cell and red cell counts, for blood smears, and for micro estimations in biochemistry. It is used when venipuncture is impractical, e.g., in infants and cases of extensive burns. A wide variety of collection tubes is available or may be made by the laboratory (Figs. 2–4 to 2–6). After filling they are sealed with a plastic stopper and can be centrifuged to obtain either serum or, in the case of a heparinized tube, plasma.

There are three usual sites for the puncture technique, the lobe of the ear, the pad of a finger, or (in infants) the heel. See Figure 4–17 for the recommended sites in taking blood samples from neonates. Whichever site is chosen, one must first make sure that it is warm so as to guarantee dilated skin vessels and thus a free flow of blood. If this is not the case, then the blood obtained will be small in amount and significantly different from venous blood because of either concentration by stasis, dilution with tissue fluid (squeezing), or both. Circulation may be improved in the lobe of the ear by rubbing with a piece of cotton. In the case of the hands or heels, immersion in water at 40°C for 5 minutes, followed by quick and vigorous drying with a warm towel, will produce the desired improvement in blood flow. Applying Infrarub,* a vasodilator cream, to the heel approximately 10 minutes before puncture also improves the availability and flow of blood. After preparation of the area with a suitable skin disinfectant, allow the skin to dry and then, using a sterile disposable lancet, make a 2- to 3-mm puncture. Allow the drops of blood to well up freely and naturally and do not squeeze with more than a gentle pressure, since this will dilute the blood with tissue fluid (lymph).

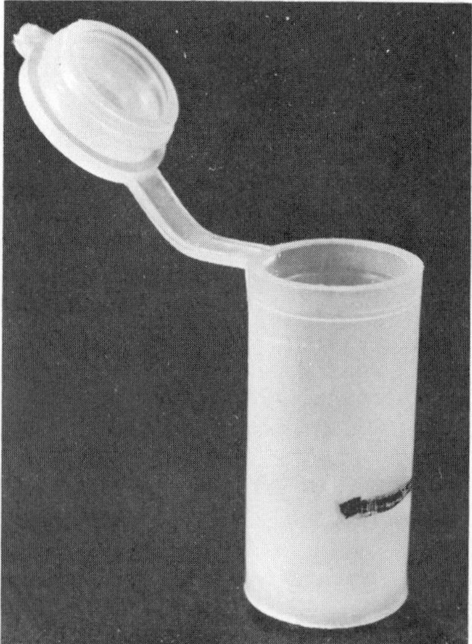

Figure 2–6 Plastic cup with lid suitable for microsamples. An appropriate amount of EDTA is added to the cup and blood is collected to the line. The cap is then shut and the sample mixed. (Manufactured by Cole Palmer Co., Chicago, Ill. 60648.)

Blood obtained by skin puncture is mostly capillary blood and differs slightly from venous blood, though in many cases the precise differences are not accurately established or agreed upon. Generally, capillary blood contains more glucose (10 to 20 mg more per dL) and more leukocytes (up to 1000 per μL) and has a higher red cell count and hemoglobin value (5%) and a lower platelet count (because platelets are lost by adherence to injured tissues). Also, the fragility of red cells obtained from capillary blood is less than that of venous erythrocytes (because of the lower pH of the latter).

One of the complications of heel puncture in infants in calcaneal osteomyelitis. To avoid this complication, heel punctures should (1) be performed on the most medial or lateral portions of the plantar surface of the heel, where the distance from skin to calcaneus is greatest; (2) be no deeper than 3 mm; (3) not be per-

*Whitehall Laboratories, Mississauga, Ont.

formed on the posterior curvature of the heel; and (4) not be performed through a previous puncture site.

Prevention of Hemolysis

1. Make sure the syringe and needle are dry. Plastic disposable apparatus is preferred.
2. Gentleness is the watchword. Avoid rough handling of blood at any stage.
3. Do not eject the blood from the syringe through the needle. Remove the needle first.
4. Avoid frothing by ejecting blood gently down the side of the tube.
5. Mix with anticoagulant by gentle inversion, not by shaking.
6. When obtaining blood by skin puncture, make sure the skin is dry before pricking and wipe off the first drop or two of blood. A thin coating of sterile petroleum jelly on the skin of the heel will promote good droplet formation and prevent spreading. Collection of heel-prick blood in a heparinized plastic tube or siliconized glass tube will obviate hemolysis.
7. If examination is to be delayed beyond 1 to 3 hours, do not allow the sample to stand unsealed or at room temperature. Stopper and store in a refrigerator at 4 to 10°C unless cold agglutinins are present, in which case it may be necessary to store blood in tubes in water bath at 37°C.
8. Do not freeze, because the red cells will hemolyze on thawing.
9. Make sure that all solutions with which blood is to be mixed or diluted are correctly prepared and are isotonic. Hypotonic solutions will lead to hemolysis.

Nosocomial Anemia

The increasing reliance on laboratory tests can result in considerable quantities of blood being withdrawn from patients. This is particularly true in a large hospital in which the laboratory may be fragmented into different departments scattered throughout the hospital. Therefore, some effort must be made to minimize the amount of blood withdrawn from patients. This can be done as follows:

1. The physician should not request unnecessary laboratory investigations.
2. Microcollection techniques should be used when possible.
3. The laboratory should perform as many laboratory tests on each sample as possible. This can be accomplished by having a central specimen reception area in the laboratory where all samples can be separated and the necessary amounts of serum, plasma, or blood sent to the relevant departments.
4. Small sample collection tubes (4 mL size) should be used.
5. Instruments that require only small volumes of blood should be used.

Anticoagulants

In most hematological and many biochemical examinations, unclotted blood is required. For this, a number of anticoagulants are available. The majority of these act by making calcium unavailable to the clotting mechanism, either by precipitating it as a salt (oxalates) or by binding it in a nonionized form (citrate and EDTA). Heparin acts as an antithrombin, i.e., it neutralizes thrombin. Finally, unclotted (fluid) blood may be obtained by removal of the fibrin as it forms (defibrination). The use of siliconized glassware does not prevent coagulation; it merely delays it by preventing activation of factor XII (Hageman) and the adhesion of platelets to wettable surface—i.e., it delays thromboplastin generation. The use of siliconized glassware or plasticware is essential in the investigation of certain clotting defects. The laboratory can either prepare anticoagulant tubes or, more conveniently, use the evacuated tube systems currently available.

Potassium Oxalate. Potassium oxalate alone is used frequently as an anticoagulant in biochemistry; 0.01 mL of a 30% solution is used for each 1.0 mL of blood required. It is placed in tubes and dried as already described.

Sodium Citrate. Trisodium citrate is the salt of choice. A 3.8% (w/v) solution is isotonic and is used in the proportion of one part citrate solution to four parts of blood in the Westergren ESR method, and one part citrate to nine parts blood in investigation of clotting mechanisms.

ACD (Acid Citrate Dextrose). The solution is used as an anticoagulant in blood transfusion, and may be used with advantage in the hematology laboratory to preserve red cell antigens when these are to be investigated. See p. 584 for the various solutions that are available.

EDTA. This is the dipotassium or disodium salt of ethylenediaminetetraacetic acid (EDTA). By chelation it prevents calcium from ionizing and is thus a very strong anticoagulant in the proportion of 1 to 2 mg per 1 mL of blood. The dipotassium salt is preferable, as it is the more soluble; but even with this the sample must be mixed well by inversion. EDTA has many advantages in hematology; e.g., white and red cell counts and hematocrit can be done even after the blood has stood for many hours. Likewise, good smears with well-preserved leukocyte and erythrocyte morphology can be obtained after 3 to 4 hours standing. Since EDTA tends to prevent surface adhesion and clumping of platelets, sufficiently accurate counts of these elements are possible in EDTA-treated blood many hours after withdrawal of the specimen. For routine laboratory use (5-mL samples of blood), 0.1 mL of 10% aqueous solution of potassium EDTA is dispensed in tubes and evaporated to dryness. It is the anticoagulant of choice for routine hematology. Anticoagulated samples may be stored overnight at 4°C without deterioration. Spontaneous agglutination of platelets can occur, causing spurious low platelet counts. This can be detected by examination of a peripheral blood film.

Fluoride. Fluoride combines with calcium and also acts as a powerful enzyme poison; hence it is used not only as an anticoagulant but also as a preservative, especially for blood (and CSF) glucose estimation when there is likely to be more than 1/2 to 1 hour's delay between the taking of the specimen and the actual analysis. 10 mg of sodium fluoride per 1 mL of blood is the usual concentration used.

Heparin. This is an excellent (and natural) anticoagulant, but it is more expensive than the artificial ones. It is the best anticoagulant to use (dry) when absolute minimal hemolysis is desired (e.g., for electrolyte determination and for red cell fragility determination). It is inadvisable to use it if it is desired to stain smears with Wright's or Leishman's stain, since it causes a diffuse blue coloration. It may be used in a concentration of 0.1 mg per 1 mL blood. Purified heparin usually contains at least 100 IU per mg, but the manufacturer's specifications should be consulted before any sample is used. Once the desired volume of the available preparation has been arrived at, it may be placed in tubes and evaporated to dryness at 37 to 56°C. Frequently, it is used as the solution; a drop is drawn into the syringe, the barrel of which is then moistened with it, and any excess is expelled.

Heparin, a complex acidic mucopolysaccharide, is available as the sodium, calcium, or ammonium salt. The latter is preferable for electrolyte determinations. It is worth remembering also that commercial heparin contains phosphate so that its use in inorganic phosphate estimations gives slightly higher values (approximately 0.2 mg per dL).

Defibrination. This is accomplished in a 50- or 100-mL Erlenmeyer flask, by using glass beads or a central glass rod or sealed tube to one end of which 0.5- cm lengths of fine (0.5 mm) glass rod or capillary tube have been fused. The upper end of the rod is held in the neck of the flask by a holed stopper. The blood (10 to 30 mL) is delivered into the flask immediately after withdrawal. The flask is held by its neck and rotated in a figure-8 motion for 5 to 10 minutes, by which time all the fibrin will have adhered to the beads or "hedgehog" end of the rod. The latter gives a better defibrinated sample with good WBC and RBC morphology, excellent for buffy coat preparation, and it gives a high serum yield. A simple method of defibrinating blood consists of using an applicator stick to one end of which three or four paper clips have been attached. This is easily twirled in the blood sample until all the fibrin has adhered to the clips.

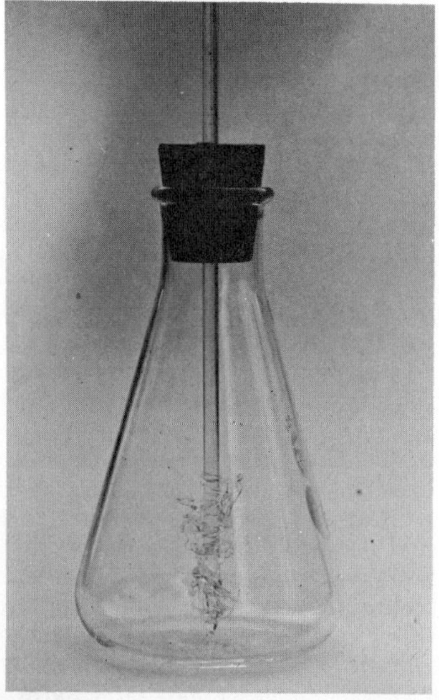

Figure 2–7 Apparatus for defibrinating blood.

Preparation of Siliconized Glassware. Use of siliconized glassware prevents or greatly reduces loss of platelets. The carefully cleaned and dried glassware is coated with a suitable dilution of a water-soluble silicone concentrate by immersion in the solution for 5 seconds or longer. Following this, the glassware is rinsed well with water and then dried (room temperature for 24 hours or, preferably, in a hot air oven at 100°C for 10 minutes).

THE MICROSCOPE

INTRODUCTION

The detailed examination of an object, whether by the unaided eye or with the help of a microscope, is basically dependent upon two factors: (i) contrast, and (ii) adequate lighting. Many examples of the problem of lack of contrast can be provided: the difficulty of seeing the traditional black cat in a cellar, a white house on the snow-covered prairie, or an unstained cell under the microscope using bright, direct light. Adequate lighting is essential for observation, a fact brought home to us at dusk when trying to read street signs while driving in a strange city, or when trying to examine a stained preparation of mixed bacteria under the oil-immersion (× 100) objective without the top lens of the condenser

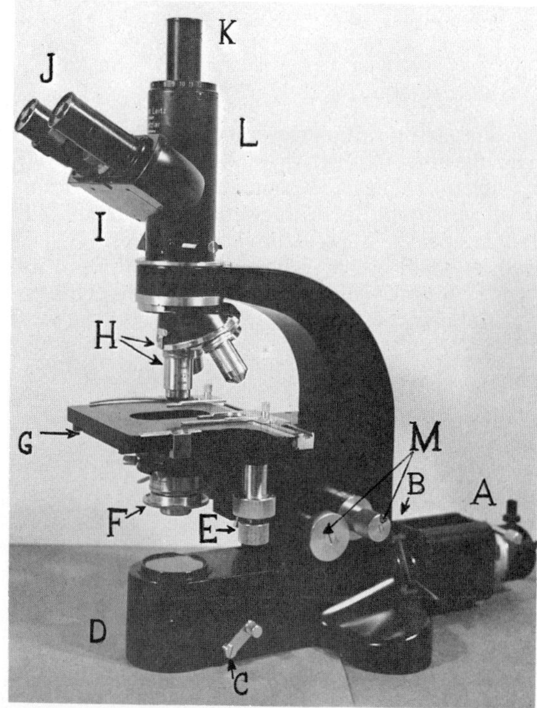

Figure 2–8 Binocular microscope. *A*, Lamp housing; *B*, filament-focusing lens and filters; *C*, collimator lens; *D*, housing of 45° angled mirror; *E*, coaxial mechanical stage controls; *F*, substage condenser and iris diaphragm; *G*, mechanical stage; *H*, revolving nosepiece and objectives; *I*, binocular prism housing; *J*, adjustable (for interocular distance) eyepieces; *K*, camera and projector tube; *L*, body tube; *M*, coarse and fine focusing knobs.

in position. One further factor involved is that, given adequate lighting of and contrast in the structures to be examined, it must be possible to separate them from each other. This is called *resolution*, and the ability of the eye or lens system to resolve such detail is expressed either as the minimum distance apart (when still resolvable) or as the number of lines to the inch that can be seen as separate and distinct. The unaided normal human eye can resolve (separate) objects 150 microns (μm) apart at a distance of 10 inches. If the object is illuminated properly with adequate contrast, then magnification of the image (with an adequate lens system) will greatly increase the resolution obtainable, the theoretical limit being approximately one-half the wavelength of the light employed. It can be seen, therefore, that the maximum visual resolution possible will be about 220 nm* with blue light, about 100 to 150 nm with ultraviolet light (using a photographic plate), and, theoretically, about 0.0005 nm using electrons (which at 50,000 volts have a wavelength of 0.001 nm). With the present type of electron microscope it is limited to about 0.02 to 0.03 nm owing to defects in the lenses that have not yet been corrected.

It therefore should be appreciated that only a properly prepared and stained specimen, which is critically illuminated and examined, with an adequately corrected and properly adjusted lens system, will give adequate resolution of the image. Furthermore, it should be realized that improperly adjusted microscopes or poorly prepared specimens can produce optical artifacts in the image that appear to be part of the object being examined.

The microscope is an expensive piece of laboratory equipment that is extremely sensitive and yet, if used intelligently, will give years of flawless performance. It is therefore worth spending some time to understand how it works and how to use it properly. If all microscopists had to buy their first microscope themselves, they would surely give them a great deal more care and attention, keeping them clean, dust-free, and properly adjusted. *Dust, dirt,* and *dried immersion oil* left on lenses are the greatest enemies of good resolution and should be scrupulously avoided.

Light

Light may be considered as a vibration in the ether (ether being a hypothetical substance filling the whole of space). It has been shown to have a constant speed of 186,000 miles per second (its precise speed is 2.9977×10^{10} cm per second), which is recognized as one of the most universal of the constants of nature.

However, when light passes through an *optically dense medium,* such as glass, it is slowed down or *retarded.* The degree of retardation will depend on the optical density of the material through which the light passes. This optical density usually is called the *refractive index* (RI) of a material and is expressed as *the ratio of the velocity of light in the air to the velocity of light in the unknown medium.* This can be measured quite simply with a refractometer. The RI of glass is approximately 1.5, depending upon the type of glass; the RI of water is 1.33; glycerin, 1.46; benzene, 1.5; and a diamond, 2.417.

The Lens

The lens is the basic component of a microscope, and its *aberrations* or faults place most of the limits on the microscope. An understanding of these aberrations is essential in the selection, evaluation, and use of the microscope.

The name *lens* refers to a piece of glass or other such transparent material that is usually circular and that has its faces ground and polished in such a manner that rays of light passing through it either converge (come together) or diverge (separate). Lenses that cause the light rays to converge and form images are called *positive lenses*; those that cause the rays to diverge and that do not form images are called *negative lenses.* These lenses can be easily identified, since positive lenses are thicker in the center, while negative lenses are thicker at the periphery.

Refraction

To understand the elementary optics of the microscope, it is necessary to know how and why a lens works.

The refraction or bending of light rays as they pass through a lens is caused by: (1) the shape of the lens and (2) the RI of the lens material (usually glass). As we pointed out, light rays are retarded while passing through an optically dense medium such as glass. Furthermore, if a light ray enters or leaves a glass surface at an angle to that surface, it will be bent or refracted. This phenomenon can be better understood if the light ray is thought of as having width; then, as the ray enters at an angle only one side will be slowed down, since the other side will be traveling at its original speed. This will produce a bend resembling a column of soldiers performing a right or left wheel (Fig. 2–9 illustrates this point). Another important concept in optics is that although a light ray usually leaves a lens on the opposite side from which it entered, it may on occasion leave on the same side. If we take an ordinary bull's-eye lens (as Fig. 2–10), we will see that a light ray entering the exact center of the lens will not be refracted (ray N) because both sides enter simultaneously; however, a similar ray (i) entering at a slight angle is refracted away from ray N. Ray (ii), entering at a greater angle, is refracted even more, in fact, along the surface of the lens; this is known as the *critical angle,* because exceeding this angle, as ray (iii) does, will result in the light's being refracted back into the lens. This is known as *total internal reflection,* and it explains how a prism works (Fig. 2–10).

Focus

If a positive lens is interposed between the sun and a piece of paper in such a position that the image of the sun is small and sharp, the paper will burn. The word *focus* originally meant burning place, and the distance from the paper at which the lens forms the sharpest image of the sun is its principal focus—for example, 4 inches or 6 inches—and this is what is meant by a lens with a 4-inch or 6-inch focus. In addition to a principal

*1 mm = 1000 μm; 1 μm = 1000 nm; 1 nm = 10 Å = 10^{-9} m.

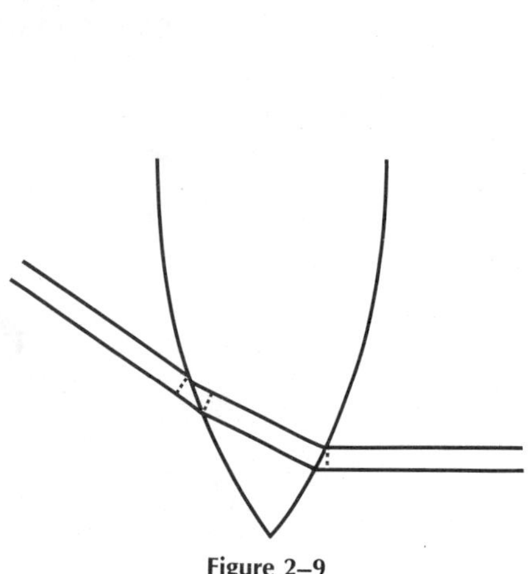

Figure 2–9

Figure 2–10

Figures 2–9 and 2–10 Refraction. For explanation, see text (p. 31).

focus, positive lenses also have *conjugate foci,* that is, they will form a sharp image on a screen at a distance that is dependent upon the distance of the object (from the lens); movement of the object either closer to or farther away from the lens will result in having to move the screen either farther away from or closer to the lens in order to maintain a sharp image (see Fig. 2–11). This is how we focus a projector when we move the lens back and forth between the object (slide) and the screen. As shown in Figure 2–11, bringing the object closer to the lenses causes the image to be more distant and therefore magnified. There is a direct relationship between the two, since the magnification will equal $\frac{\text{screen distance from the lens}}{\text{object distance from the lens}}$, e.g., $\frac{48}{6}$ ft = × 8 magnification and $\frac{160}{4}$ mm = × 40, these being the appropriate distances and magnification of the high dry objective lens of a microscope. In this latter case, however, there is no screen, because moving an object very close to a lens will cause the image (no matter where the screen is placed) to disappear (to infinity ∞). Another movement of the object even closer to the lens causes the image to reappear on the same side as the object. This is called a *virtual image* and can be seen by the eye (through the lens) but cannot be focused on a screen. It is this image that we see when looking through the microscope.

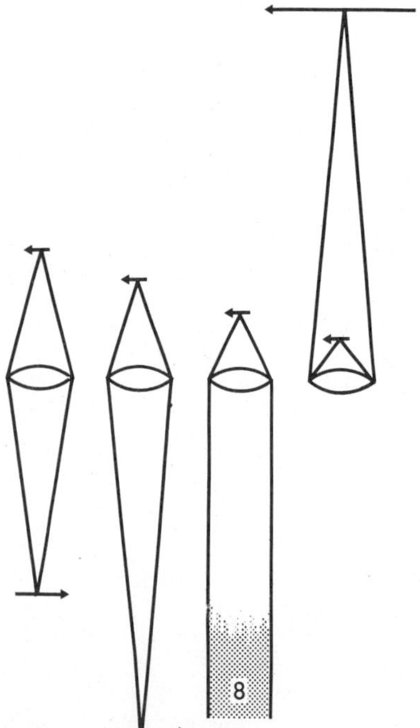

Figure 2–11 Focus. See explanation in text.

Faults or Aberrations of a Lens

Although there are several inherent faults in a lens, only two will be considered here, since a grasp of these, and of how they may be corrected, will serve as a key to understanding the others.

Spherical Aberration. This defect in a lens results from the curvature of the lens surface. The angle at which light rays, from any point in the object, will strike (and leave) the lens will differ at each part of the lens, and therefore they will be refracted to a greater or lesser degree (see Fig. 2–12). Those at the periphery will be refracted to the greatest degree, and those near the center to the least. This aberration cannot be corrected completely, but a fair degree of correction is achieved by adding a negative lens to the original lens. The negative lens is made of a different glass with a greater relative refractive index (for example, crown glass and

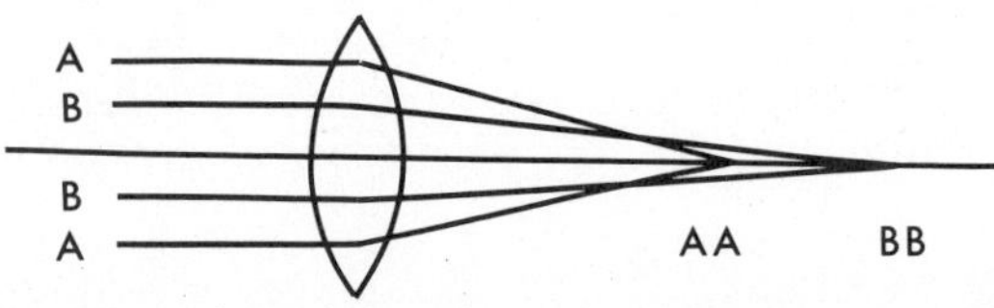

Figure 2–12 Spherical aberration. For a full explanation, see text.

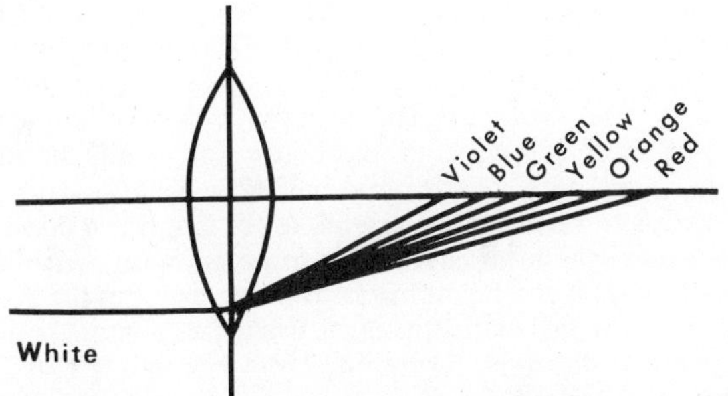

Figure 2–13 Chromatic aberration. For an explanation, see text.

flint glass for the positive and negative lenses, respectively). This will neutralize the magnification of the lens to some degree. Although the correction of a lens is based upon this method, it is actually a very complex problem requiring a complex solution.

Chromatic Aberration. This defect is based upon the fact that white light is composed of the colors of the spectrum, each of which vibrates at a different wavelength. On entering a lens (an optically dense medium) these component colors, because of their differing energy levels, will be affected to differing degrees, with the red end of the spectrum (600 to 700 nm) being affected the least, and the violet and blue end of the spectrum (350 to 450 nm) being affected the most. In the diagram (Fig. 2–13) the violet light rays come to a point of focus closer to the lens than the red, which are farthest away. Using a prism, this is how the spectrum was, and is, demonstrated. A screen placed at "Red" in Figure 2–13 will show a red spot surrounded by a halo of spectral colors; a screen placed at "Blue" will show a blue spot with a halo of spectral colors, the reverse of those seen at "Red." Some correction of chromatic aberration can be achieved by the use of additional lenses, as for spherical aberration. Such a lens is known as an *"achromatic lens"* and is corrected for *two wavelengths of light* in the green-blue region. The incorporation of fluorite, which gives the glass additional color dispersion properties in the secondary lenses, allows correction of three wavelengths of light. Such lenses are known either as *fluorite lenses*, or, if they are as completely corrected for all the aberration as is possible, they are called *apochromatic lenses.* Many more lenses are added to the original lens to achieve such corrections, and their shapes, composition, and design are complex, each company using its own formulae for its lenses.

Optical Components of the Microscope

Oculars (Eyepieces). To understand the function of the ocular, it should be realized that the objective first magnifies the object, producing a virtual image, which is then *remagnified by the ocular* to produce the image seen by the eye. The farther away from the objective the ocular is placed (optical tube length), the greater the magnification of the objective. The eyepiece magnification, however, is constant, since it always receives the image it magnifies in the same plane.

Types of Ocular. There are two principal types of ocular in use: (1) the *Huygenian* and (2) the *Ramsden.*

The Huygenian. The Huygenian type of ocular was designed originally by C. Huygens for use with the telescope, and it is the most popular. It consists of two simple lenses (planoconvex), the lower of which (the field lens) collects the image and focuses it very slightly above the plane of the fixed diaphragm. The field lens is about two-thirds of the way down the eyepiece wall and can be seen by removing the top lens. The image from the field lens is magnified by the top lens to produce the virtual image seen by the eye. Since the objective image is focused just above the fixed diaphragm, it follows that an optically plane glass disc, carrying an engraved scale, e.g., a micrometer eyepiece or grid, will be seen (in focus) superimposed upon the object image.

Ramsden Ocular. These are usually composed of doublet or triplet component lenses, instead of the single lens at top and bottom of the ocular, with the plane side of the bottom lens (lenses) toward the object—which is the reverse of the Huygenian. Most compensated oculars are of this type. They are also used for micrometer eyepieces, since they give less distortion to the scale.

Wide Field, High Eye-Point Oculars. Improvements in optical design have led to the development of lenses with a wider, flatter field. These may be constructed by a formula that gives a higher eyepoint, enabling people who normally wear glasses to use the microscope without removing them.

Compensated Oculars. These originally were designed for use solely with apochromatic objectives, but they may now be used with all modern objectives. They are fully corrected and give a flatter field. They are usually marked "Comp," or "K" if of German origin.

For reasons that are made clear further on, it is inadvisable to use eyepiece magnifications in excess of × 12.5.

The Objective. This screws into the bottom of the body tube by means of a standard thread; although this feature makes all objectives interchangeable, the practice should be avoided because many manufacturers use the objective and ocular interdependently to correct some aberrations.

Objectives usually are marked with their magnifying power (× 4, × 10, × 40, × 100), but it should be remembered that this applies only when they are used at a fixed tube length (i.e., distance from the top of the eyepiece slot to the nosepiece, where the objective screws in), which is normally 160 mm. Divinding the tube length by the focal length will give the magnifying power of the lens. For example, the high dry lens has a focal length of 4 mm, which divided into 160 mm = × 40; if this were used in a system with a tube length of 200 mm; the image would be × 50.

The focal length of a simple lens is the distance from the front of the lens of the object; with compound lenses (composed of several lenses) the focal length is taken from a point between the component lenses. This has led to the use of two descriptive terms, the *focal distance* (focal length) and the *working distance* (the measurement from the object to the front of the lens when it is in focus, which is the same for a simple lens but different from a compound lens).

The Aperture. The quality of an image is dependent upon the amount of light admitted by a lens from each point of an object, and this is directly dependent upon the aperture of the lens. A lens with double the aperture size will admit twice as much light and therefore will give better resolution; with camera lenses this is known as the "f" value. An f 2.0 lens, having a greater aperture (and diameter), is better and costs much more than an f 3.5 lens. Objective lenses are rated by their *numerical aperture* (NA), which is a mathematical method of expressing the aperture of an objective, whether it is used with immersion oil or "dry." The formula is n sine u, where n = RI of the material between the object and lens (e.g., air = 1.0 and immersion oil = 1.51), and sine u is the sine of one-half the angle formed by the front lens and the object. The NA of an objective is important because it limits the resolving power of the lens. The formula for this is: resolution = wave-length of light being employed, over twice the numerical aperture, e.g., $\frac{500\text{ nm}}{2.5} = 200$ nm; this would be smallest definable distance (separation between lines or dots) using an oil-immersion objective (with NA = 1.25) and blue light with a wavelength of 500 nm. A useful general rule is that the maximum useful magnification that can be used is 1000 × NA, that is, × 1250, with an NA of 1.25. If total magnification in excess of these limits is attempted, there is progressive loss of resolution: this phenomenon is known as *empty magnification*. Numerical aperture also affects the *flatness of the field* (when the whole field is in sharp focus, from one side to the other), and the *depth of focus* (when, even when two cells are one above the other, every component seen is in sharp focus); as the NA increases, these decrease in quality.

Objective Types

Achromatic. This is the standard type, which is a reasonably corrected lens and is color corrected for two wavelengths of light.

Fluorite Lens (Semi-Apochromat). This is a well-corrected lens, incorporating fluorite in the component lenses to correct for three wavelengths of light.

Apochromat. The best type of lens, with every possible correction being incorporated; it *must* be used with compensated oculars.

Aplanatic. This well-corrected lens is mostly designed for photomicrography to give a flat field.

Condensers

Condensers must be as well corrected as the objectives with which they are used; they should form a perfect image of the light source and *have the same numerical aperture as the objective with which they are being used.* For years the two-lens Abbé condenser (having no top lens that is easily removable) has been the most common. Best results will be given by a three-lens condenser with a "flip-out" top lens that is as good as the objectives with which it is employed. Immersion oil should be used between the condenser and the slide when an immersion-oil objective is being used. The condenser usually has a built-in iris diaphragm to control the cone of light passing through the object, and a filter carrier. It may also have a "swing-in" negative lens to increase the size of the field illuminated, for use with very low power scanning objectives (e.g., × 2.5).

Binocular Prisms

Until 1950 most microscopists used monocular microscopes, but today these are rarely seen except in high schools or those institutes or universities at which the monoculars have yet to "wear out." The prism system is designed to divert alternate light rays to each of the oculars. The heart of the system is a semisilvering process that allows one light ray (or small bundle) through and reflects the neighboring one; these rays are then directed by further prisms up through the oculars. The prisms should never be tampered with, with the exception of light brushing to remove any dust. Should a microscope fall or be knocked, the prism system should be checked for misalignment; this will cause the two fields to be slightly different and is a common cause of headaches in microscopists, especially those who spend several hours a day at their microscopes.

Adjusting the Binocular Microscope. Since the distance between the pupils of the eyes varies from person to person, the eyepieces on a binocular microscope must be capable of adjustment to accommodate this variable, called the *interocular distance*. Furthermore, the sight of both eyes will not necessarily be the same, and the binocular attachment must be able to accommodate such differences; this is achieved by having one (or both) eyepieces held in adjustable sleeves. The microscope is focused so that the object is in sharp focus using only the eye looking through the fixed eyepiece, and then the image is made sharp for the other eye by using only the focusing sleeve, without touching the main adjustments of the microscope. If both eyepieces are adjustable one is set at the midpoint of focus and it is then used as the fixed eyepiece; if necessary, if there is great disparity between the eyes, this can be readjusted and the exercise repeated.

Illumination

Most microscopes have built-in illumination, with the lamp (or a prism reflecting the lamp image) in the optical path below the condenser. The source of illumination should be uniformly intense, and this is usually achieved by using a diffusing screen (ground glass) and a lens that ensures that the whole of the back lens of the condenser is flooded with light.

Supporting and Adjusting Structure

The early microscopes had a body tube that was focused by means of rack and pinion adjustments. With the development of the modern binocular microscope, the stand and body tube became larger, heavier, and a great deal more stable. It was then realized that focusing could be achieved by movement of the stage (with the object) and the substage (with the condenser, and so forth), giving more precision and longer wear. This movement is actuated by a coarse (fast) and a fine (slow) control; these are usually two immediately adjacent separate controls, but both Leitz and Reichert have models with a single control for both functions.

The Stage. The stage is a metal platform with an aperture of 1 to 1½ inches in diameter. It is usually movable by means of two controls for back and forward and for lateral movement. Mechanical stages usually have scales for recording the position of a slide in either direction, e.g., 0 to 80 for lateral movement and 90 to 120 for the back and forward direction. Each of these scales has a vernier scale that is attached parallel to the main graduated scale. The vernier scale is marked 0 to 10, and it will be found that the 10 graduations of the vernier scale are just equal to 9 on the larger scales: the zero of the vernier gives the reading in whole figures, and the graduation of the vernier scale exactly opposite any of the major scale markings gives the decimal place.

Circular rotating stages, gliding stages (which slide in any direction) and even hot stages (which keep preparations at a predetermined temperature), are available for most microscopes.

Using the Microscope

Provided certain basic rules are followed, using a microscope is fairly simple:

1. The condenser must be focused, and, on those instruments with a centering substage, it must be centered. Failure to do this may result in an untrue image (a circle may appear as an oval with an off-center condenser) or a fuzzy image when the condenser is too high, resulting in some peripheral rays' exceeding the critical angle (see section on Refraction) and being trapped between the slide and coverslip.
2. The light source with a compound lamp (i.e., a lamp with its own lens system) should be focused upon the back lens of the condenser. This is usually done with a built-in light source.
3. The iris diaphragm should be closed to that degree (the cone of light limited) at which only that area of the object being examined is illuminated.
4. Never focus a high-power objective, especially an oil-immersion objective, by racking it down; instead, place it very close to the object and, while looking through the oculars, rack it up and away from the object until it is in focus.
5. Keep the microscope clean and dust free. Never leave immersion oil on a lens; to be certain of remembering, clean it each time you finish examining a slide. Always check that you did not accidently get some immersion oil on the high dry (× 40) objective. Clean lenses with a dust-free, soft tissue, using xylene to remove oil if necessary. Never use *alcohol*; it dissolves some cements.

Critical Illumination

By use of the following steps, critical illumination should be checked every day and not altered.

1. Switch on the lamp, and adjust it to the correct voltage, if necessary; having it too bright will burn out lamps in a shorter time.
2. Place an object on the stage and focus with the × 10 or × 40 lens, with the top lens of the condenser in the optical path.
3. Close the iris diaphragm, which will be near the lamp or at the base of the microscope, at the aperture from which the light emerges. If there is no diaphragm, mark a cross with a grease pencil or felt pen on a slide, and place it over the light source. Rack the condenser up and down until a sharp image of the diaphragm (or cross) appears, without changing the focus of the objective. In practice, it has been found that the best position for the condenser is just below that position giving a sharp image of the light source. This is the *Nelson method* for *critical illumination*, and no lamp condenser is used. If at this point the light source is focused with a lamp condenser on the back lens of the substage condenser (this can be seen by holding a piece of white paper in place; if necessary, adjust the lamp lens so that the lamp filament is seen on the paper), then the microscope is critically illuminated by the *Köhler method.*

Magnification

The magnification of the microscope is the product of two separate systems, the objective and the ocular. With the standard microscope, with a fixed tube length (160 mm), it is simply a question of multiplying the objective magnification by that of the ocular, e.g., × 10, 40 or × 100 objective by × 10 ocular, which equals × 100, × 400, or × 1000. If the tube length can be adjusted, then magnification will be:

$$\frac{\text{Tube length}}{\text{Focal length of objective}} \times \text{ocular magnification}$$

In the example given, this would be:

$$\frac{160\text{ mm}}{16\text{ mm}} \times 10 = 100$$

It should be remembered that microscope magnifications are linear, that is, a structure which is 60 μm long will appear to be 6000 μm long, but since it is magnified in all directions the actual magnification will be 100 × 100, and therefore 10,000 times, viewed through the system described immediately above.

Micrometry

Micrometry is the science of measuring objects under the microscope. To practice micrometry one needs an arbitrary scale in the eyepiece—a *micrometer eyepiece*—and a measured engraved scale on a slide—a *stage micrometer*. The latter can be a proper stage micrometer, which will be a millimeter scale divided into 1/10th and 1/100th graduations, or a hemocytometer.

To measure an object:

1. Place the micrometer eyepiece on the microscope or insert a micrometer eyepiece disc into one on the oculars by unscrewing the lens and putting it on the fixed diaphragm.
2. Using an objective that is appropriate for the object to be measured (e.g., oil-immersion objective for RBC's, or low-power objective for an artery), focus on the stage micrometer scale.
3. Determine the number of divisions of the eyepiece scale that are exactly equal to any given number of stage micrometer divisions, and calculate the value of an eyepiece division. For example, if 10 stage divisions equal 100 eyepiece divisions, then since 10 stage divisions = 1/10 of a mm = 100 μm, 100 eyepiece divisions = 100 μm, and 1 eyepiece division = 1 μm.
4. Remove the stage micrometer and replace it with the object to be measured, *taking care not to change the objective.* Count the number of divisions spanned by the object and calculate the size.

An alternative method is to photograph a stage micrometer and then photograph objects with the same lens system. Duplicate photographs of object and scale can then be measured with a ruler, and the size of objects in the photograph can be calculated.

The Dark-Ground Microscope

As the name implies, this microscope is dependent for contrast upon its black background, against which objects that scatter light are seen; the objects are illuminated by oblique light rays that do not enter the objective. This was the first type of microscope that enabled microscopists to examine living, unstained specimens, and it was the first, and remains the best, method for the demonstration of spirochetes, such as *Treponema pallidum*.

A *special dark-ground condenser* is necessary to provide only oblique light rays; if used with oil-immersion objectives, these must have an NA less than 1.0, because it is almost impossible to produce a condenser that will provide light rays sufficiently oblique (and bright) to give satisfactory results. A special oil-immmersion objective fitted with a diaphragm can be used or, alternatively, a small, thin, metal tube (funnel stop) can be inserted into the back of a routine oil-immersion objective.

Immersion oil must be used between the condenser and the slide to ensure that the maximum light strikes the object without entering the lens.

The light source should be fairly intense, since scattered or reflected light will form the image. It should be realized that such an image will give misleading impression of relative sizes because of a halo effect. Furthermore, great care is necessary in the preparation of specimens, since air bubbles, RBC's, and so forth will scatter a great deal of light and cause the contrast to be lost.

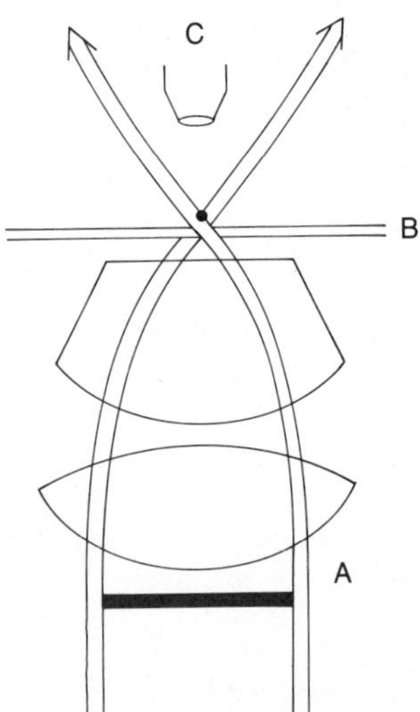

Figure 2–14 The optics of dark-ground illumination. All the central light rays are stopped by an opaque disc *(A)*. A cone of light is made by the condenser above the disc; this light illuminates the object *(B)* but does not enter the microscope objective *(C)*. Thus, the object is seen as a bright image on a black background

The Polarizing Microscope

The basic principle underlying this type of microscope is that light normally vibrates in all planes, at right angles to that of propagation. However, after passing through certain types of crystalline structure, light will be composed of two sets of rays, each vibrating in only a single plane, at right angles to each other: such light is said to be *plane-polarized.* The *Nicol prism,* composed of Iceland spar (calcite), will reflect one of the rays (the extraordinary ray) out of the prism, thus giving rise to a single ray (ordinary) that is plane-polarized. The Nicol prism has now largely been replaced by the Polaroid disc, which is composed of ultramicroscopic crystals of herapathite in nitrocellulose, this suspension being mounted between glass or plastic sheets. These Polaroid discs have the characteristics of a single crystal of herapathite, which has the power to absorb the extraordinary ray, passing only a single ray of plane-polarized light; the plane of vibration of the ray is marked on the disc. If plane-polarized light is directed into such a disc, the light will pass through if it is vibrating in the same plane as the disc (as an ordinary ray) but will be absorbed if it is vibrating in the opposite direction (as an extraordinary ray). Various amounts of light will be passed between these points (total absorption or total passing of light), depending upon the degree of difference.

These microscopes are employed to determine *birefringence,* or the ability to convert light vibrating in all planes, or in only one plane, into two rays vibrating at right angles. A substance (silica) or tissue component (hair, collagen) is detected by examining it between Polaroids (or Nicol prisms) that have their planes of polarization crossed (called *crossed Polaroids*), when the crystal or structure will appear bright against a dark background.

One disc is placed in the optical axis below the object (in the condenser filter carrier or on top of the light source) and is known as the polarizer; the second disc is

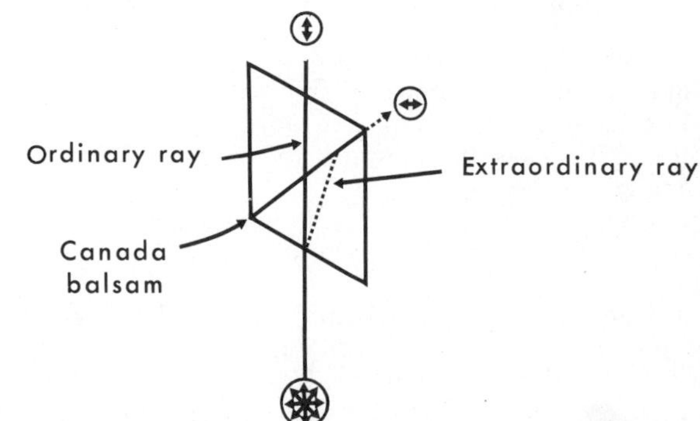

Figure 2–15 The Nicol prism. Only the ordinary ray of light in one plane will pass through the system. The extraordinary ray will be reflected out of the system. Birefringent substances will rotate light that may pass through the prisms as a polarized beam, whereas light not so rotated will be treated as the ordinary ray and be absorbed. Thus birefringent objects will appear as bright light sources on a black background.

placed in the ocular or inserted in the body tube and is known as the analyzer. A special stage is fitted on a proper polarizing microscope so that the crystal or structure can be rotated to determine the degree and angle of rotation.

The Phase-Contrast Microscope

This microscope was devised by Zernike in 1935, for which he was subsequently awarded the Nobel Prize. It is used for the examination of unstained material and is based upon the conversion of slight differences in refractive index within the specimen into differences in amplitude or brightness.

The contrast in the final image in the phase-contrast microscope is due to the fact, as was shown by Abbé, differences in refractive index between adjacent structures (cell wall and cytoplasm) give rise to out-of-focus images that are out of phase by one-quarter of a wavelength, by comparison with the normal image. These images come together in the final image that is seen by the eye, but since the eye is insensitive to phase differences, they are not appreciated. Zernike used a hollow cone of light (produced by an annulus in the condenser) and a phase plate, which exactly matches the image of the annulus, in the back focal plane of the objective. This phase plate further retards the out-of-focus image by a ¼ wavelength (λ), because the direct light (normal imaging rays) goes through a ditch in the plate. Therefore, the diffracted rays (out-of-focus image) go through the inside and outside of the ditch and are further retarded by another ¼ λ by the extra thickness of glass. When light rays arising from the same point are differentially out of phase by ½ λ, destructive interference will take place and little or no light will result.

The Fluorescent Microscope

Fluorescence is the property, possessed by certain materials, of converting short-wavelength light, which is invisible to the human eye, into light of a longer wavelength, which is visible. The light source usually employed is ultraviolet light, although a short-wavelength visible light (blue-violet) may be used.

A fluorescent microscope may be employed to demonstrate naturally occurring fluorescent materials (lipids, elastic fibers, and so forth) or preparations stained with fluorescent dyes, or to localize antibodies carrying a fluorescent lable (*fluorescent antibody technique*).

Fluorescent microscopes normally are equipped with an ultraviolet light source (an Osram HBO 200 lamp unit is ideal), immediately in front of which must be a filter (or filters) to limit the light to set a wavelength (usually a BG 12 filter to give light with a wavelength of approximately 365 nm). Such filters are called *exciter filters*, because the wavelengths of light that they pass excite the molecules and cause them to fluoresce. Since ultraviolet light can cause extensive damage to the eye, fluorescent microscopes must have barrier filters (which will pass only light in the visible range) fitted in the optical path above the object, usually in the body tube, although they may be fitted into the bottoms of oculars. With such equipment a routine microscope can be converted to a fluorescent microscope. While some workers use a normal light condenser, we prefer a dark-ground condenser to give increased contrast.

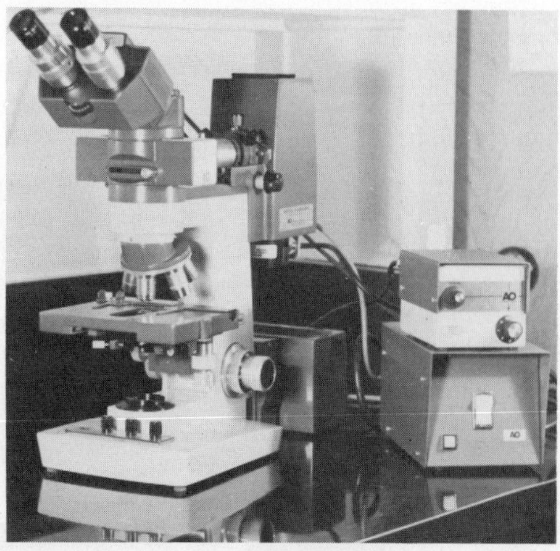

Figure 2–16 Fluorescent microscope. Illustrated is the American Optical Microstar* microscope, which can be used both for regular transmitted light microscopy and for fluorescent microscopy with incident short-wave (ultraviolet) illumination. In the picture, the ultraviolet lamp is housed in an upper lamphouse just behind the binocular part of the microscope. The lamphouse containing a regular incandescent lamp is attached to the lower part of the microscope stand behind the pedestal. To the right, the lower power supply box controls the UV lamp and the upper one controls illumination by ordinary transmitted light. Barrier filters in the ocular part of the microscope prevent unwanted and harmful radiation from reaching the microscopist's eyes when UV light is used.

*American Optical Corp. Buffalo, N.Y. 14215 and Belleville, Ontario K8N 5C6.

Fluorescent microscopy has found its place in the laboratory in direct-staining procedures, such as the fluorescent dye method for the staining of *M. tuberculosis* or for amyloid, and more widely when fluorescing agent is attached to antibody and used as a specific serological agent (see p. 548).

The Electron Microscope

The resolution of the light microscope has been shown (pp. 31 and 34) to be limited by the numerical aperture and the wavelength of light employed. Because the degree of correction in glass lenses is very high, the main limitation is imposed by the light (e.g., half the wavelength of light), giving a normal resolution of approximately 250 nm, and when ultraviolet light is used, a resolution of about 100 nm. By the substitution of an electron beam for light rays, a much greater degree of resolution can be obtained, since at an acceleration of 50,000 volts electrons have a wavelength of only .001 nm; therefore a theoretical resolving power of .0005 nm could be attained, which would enable molecules to be seen. Unfortunately, the degree of correction that is currently possible with transmission electron microscope (TEM) lenses will permit a resolution of only 0.25 nm, but this is still a thousand times greater than that possible with the light microscope.

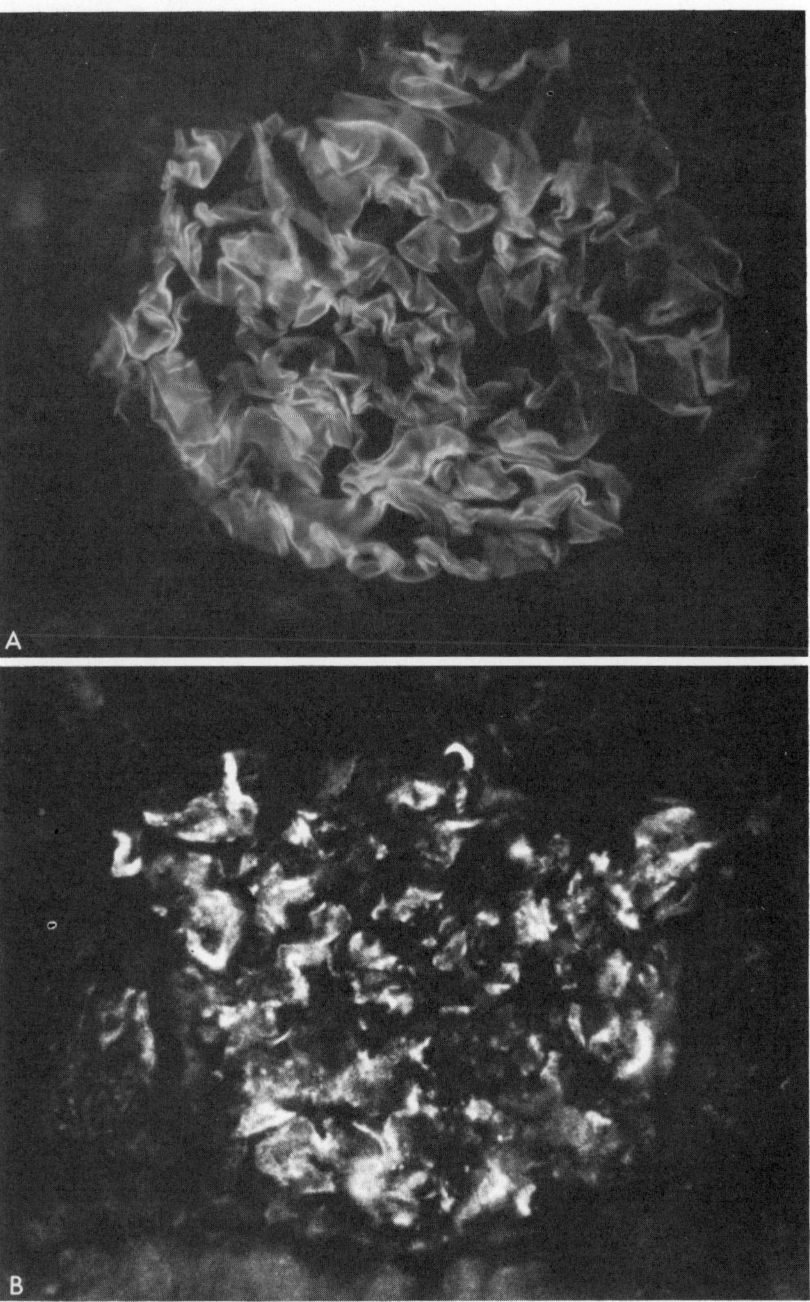

Figure 2–17 Cryostat sections of kidney stained with fluorescent-tagged goat antihuman IgG. *A* shows an even-stained glomerular basement membrane in Goodpasture's syndrome. *B* demonstrates the relative "lumpy" distribution of antibody in membranous glomerulonephritis, although this feature is more marked in acute glomerulonephritis. (Courtesy of Dr. W. H. Chase, Dept. of Pathology, University of British Columbia.)

A further problem with the TEM is that, since electrons have poor penetrating power, the sections to be examined must be very thin—less than 50 nm thick. This necessitates the use of special hard embedding media (plastics) and special ultramicrotomes to cut such thin sections. Steel knives cannot be used to cut these sections; either glass or diamond knives are used.

CHAPTER 2—REVIEW QUESTIONS

1. Give examples of methods for reducing the risk of acquiring hepatitis in the laboratory. In the event that material possibly contaminated with hepatitis virus spilled on the laboratory bench, how would you deal with it?

2. Explain the terms *TC, TD, to deliver with blow out,* and *between two marks* in relation to pipettes. Describe one method to determine the accuracy and precision of pipettes.

3. Define the terms *sterilization, disinfection,* and *antiseptic*. Name four chemical agents that are used in disinfection, and describe their mode of action. Describe the principle of autoclaving. How is the quality of the process controlled?

4. Name four anticoagulants used in hematology. Explain how each prevents blood clotting. List the precautions to be observed in venipuncture to avoid hemolysis of the specimen.

5. Explain the terms *spherical* and *chromatic* aberration. Describe micrometry and the materials necessary to perform it. Give examples of the usefulness of fluorescent and polarizing microscopy.

Section

I

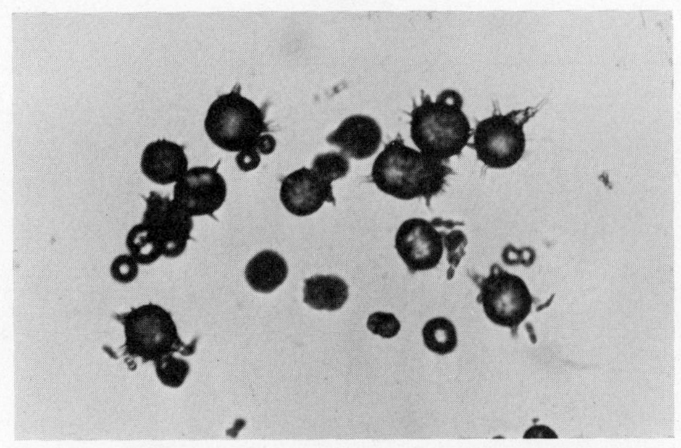

CHEMISTRY

3

QUALITY CONTROL AND STATISTICAL ANALYSIS

INTRODUCTION

Whatever the philosophical attitude of the clinical laboratory worker toward the ever-increasing demand for laboratory tests, his basic responsibility is the same whether the workload is 10 procedures per day or 500. Every effort must be made, by constant checking and assiduous search for error, to produce data of firmly established reliability. The pressure to monitor and maintain laboratory performance has been considerably increased by the imposition of external regulatory systems, which often link the maintenance of adequate standards with licensing powers. The moral and scientific justification for quality control has now been supplemented by statutory and legal liability factors.

OBJECTIVES OF QUALITY CONTROL

1. To provide a continuous record of the *precision* of laboratory results.
2. To give early warning of trends and shifts in control results so that remedial action may be taken *before* serious loss of precision occurs.
3. To permit valid judgments on the *accuracy* of results by monitoring precision and permitting continuous comparisons of assay values on "known" sera with stated levels.
4. To facilitate comparisons between different techniques for the assay of a constituent, and thus to derive a justifiable choice between methods.
5. To monitor the performance of equipment, especially automated analyzers.
6. To provide some indication of technologists' analytical skills.
7. To accumulate a body of information about laboratory performance with which the challenges of external monitoring organizations can be met.

DEFINITIONS IN QUALITY CONTROL

Accuracy. Theoretically, accuracy means exact agreement of a test result with the "true" value. The difficulty lies in the determination of what is true. In a serum sample, the true uric acid value is unknown; we endeavor to report a value which, when carefully checked against the result obtained by a competent analyst using a well-established reference method, lies within specified tolerances. The next problem is to define "specified tolerances." The practical approach has merit; the result reported should be close enough to the true result that any difference would not affect the clinical interpretation and significance. For some analyses the tolerance is very small; in the diagnosis of hyperparathyroidism, for example, the determination of serum calcium ideally should be correct to ±0.1 mg per dL. Fortunately, having regard for the extent of normal biological variation, agreement within ±5% is adequate for many routine biochemical analyses, except for those of electrolytes.

Establishing accuracy by comparison with a reference method has some disadvantages. One of the requirements for a good reference method is a high degree of specificity for the substance being assayed. If the routine method is less specific, there will be a bias in values obtained therewith vis-à-vis those obtained by the reference procedure. In the case of uric acid, if a routine method using the ability of uric acid to reduce phosphotungstate to tungsten blue is compared with a reference method employing the specific conversion of uric acid to allantoin by the enzyme uricase, the latter method will give results about 1 mg per dL lower, because the routine method includes some chromogens other than uric acid.

In practice, if the result of a determination on a commercial control serum prepared with a weighed-in amount of the constituent is within ± two standard deviations of the given value (the standard deviation used having been obtained by a statistically valid process on the method in use), the degree of accuracy is acceptable for clinical purposes.

Precision. Precision is a statistically derived measure of all the random errors affecting the result of an analysis; it is a measure of reproducibility only. The timing of the actions of a high school drill team may be very precise; this precision is quite unaffected by the fact that they all may be marching in the wrong direction. It is quite possible for a method to exhibit excellent precision but poor accuracy; the converse is not true.

Mean. The mean generally used in basic statistical work is the arithmetic mean, which is the sum of the items of data divided by the number of items. It can be used as a measure of the central tendency of the data, that is, of the most typical property. For this purpose, however, its value can be unduly influenced by the presence of "wild" values or "outliers," items of data that diverge so much from the rest that their validity is suspect.

Mode. The mode is the value that occurs most frequently in a list of items of data. It is not affected by extreme values or outliers. In some sets of data there may be two values that occur so much more frequently than any of the rest that a bimodal distribution of the data may be suspected, and this may imply that the data are drawn from two populations rather than one.

Median. If the items of data are arranged in either ascending or descending order of magnitude, the item that occupies the middle position in the list is the median. If the number of items is an even number, the median is the average of the two central items. It is less influenced by wild values than the mean.

In a set of data that are distributed exactly in the "normal," or Gaussian, manner, the mean, median, and mode coincide. If the pattern of distribution of the data is not symmetrical—that is, if it is "skewed"—the three measures of central tendency described will not coincide.

Centile. A centile, or percentile, value is greater than a specified percentage of the list of values. Thus the 75th percentile value in a list of data has 75% of the items below it in value. The 50th percentile will lie in the middle of the list, and hence is equal to the median. One method for determining a normal range is to take only those values from a large list of results of determinations on normal people which lie between the 2½ and 97½ percentiles.

Standard Deviation. This is strictly a mathematical concept, a statement of the extent of random variation in any series of measurements. Because of the simplicity with which it is calculated, its inherent assumptions are often forgotten: that the scatter of the values is symmetrical about the arithmetic mean and that the graphical plot of the values has the special shape, the so-called bell curve, associated with a Gaussian pattern of distribution (Fig. 3–1). The distribution is symmetrical, and the mean, median, and mode coincide. Gauss' formula illustrated an ideal situation, but the data obtained from real results quite frequently do not fit his elegant mold. It will be seen later how this divergence is handled.

Calculation of Standard Deviation. The example illustrates the procedure. (See Table 3–1.)

1. In column 1, list the values, preferably 40 or more. Determine their sum (symbol Σ x) and divide by the number of values to obtain the mean (symbol $\bar{x}$) ("x bar").

2. In column 2, list the absolute values of the differences between each item and the mean value (symbol $\bar{x} - x$).

TABLE 3–1 CALCULATION OF STANDARD DEVIATION—MANUAL GLUCOSE METHOD

Col. 1 Values	Col. 2 Differences	Col. 3 Differences^2
94	6	36
108	8	64
92	8	64
108	8	64
97	3	9
95	5	25
101	1	1
104	4	16
100	0	0
93	7	49
105	5	25
101	1	1
99	1	1
98	2	4
108	8	64
94	6	36
106	6	36
97	3	9
108	8	64
92	8	64
20)2000		632
100 = Mean		

Standard Deviation $= \sqrt{\frac{632}{19}} = \sqrt{33.26} = 5.767$, rounded off to 5.8.

Coefficient of Variation $= \frac{\text{S.D.}}{\text{Mean}} \times 100 = \frac{5.8}{100} \times 100 = 5.8\%$.

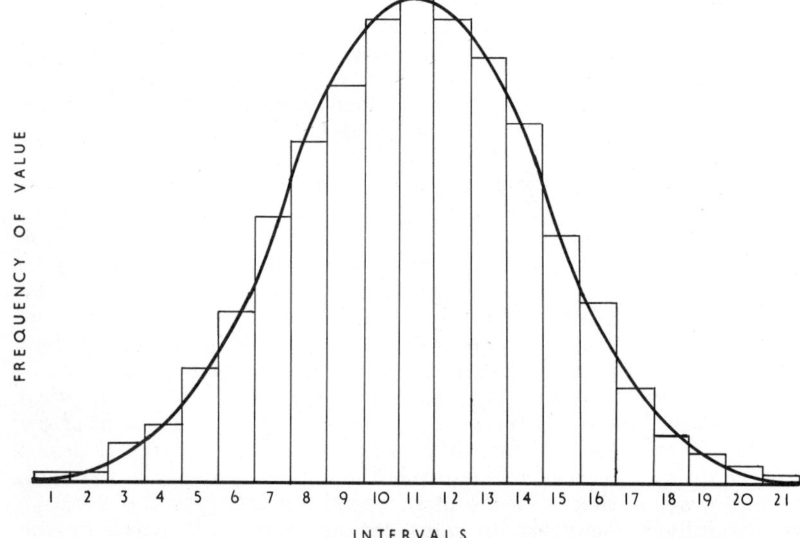

Figure 3–1 Gaussian curve of normal distribution fitted to histogram.

("Absolute value" means ignoring the algebraic sign of the difference.)

3. Square the differences (column 3) and find the sum of the squares (symbol $\Sigma(\bar{x} - x)^2$).

4. Divide the sum of the squared differences by one less than the number of original items of data (symbol $n - 1$).

5. Extract the square root. The result is one standard deviation (symbol s or S.D.). One S.D. either side of the mean includes 68.27% of the items; 2 S.D.s, 95.45%; 3 S.D.s, 99.73%.

A simple method of obtaining the standard deviation from a small group of results is that of Dean and Dixon. The result is only approximate, but it will give some idea of the magnitude of the S.D. For example, if a new method for blood glucose has been in use for six days, and the six values for a control serum are 98, 96, 99, 103, 97, and 98, the range, i.e., the difference between the highest and lowest results, is $103 - 96 = 7$. For a group of six results, the range multiplied by 0.4 ($7 \times 0.4 = 2.8$) is an estimate of the S.D. If the values were 95, 104, 93, 97, 108, and 105, with a range of $108 - 93 = 15$ and an approximate S.D. of $15 \times 0.4 = 6.0$, this could be taken as a warning that the method may not be in good control, since the coefficient of variation is 6%. The multiplying factors for other small groups are:

Group	Factor
4	0.486
5	0.430
6	0.400
7	0.370
8	0.351
9	0.337
10	0.316

This approximation should not be used with groups of more than 10.

If the standard deviation is divided by the mean and the result multiplied by 100, the value obtained is called the coefficient of variation (C.V.). It is used to express the *relative* magnitude of variability when, for example, we wish to compare two different methods of determining the same substance. If one method gave a mean result of 100 mg per dL, with S.D. 2.5, the C.V. would be $\frac{2.5}{100} \times 100 = 2.5\%$. If the second method gave a mean of 90 mg per dL, with S.D. 2.7, the C.V. would be $\frac{2.7}{90} \times 100 = 3.0\%$; the second method shows a greater variability (i.e., a poorer precision) than the first.

Calculation of S.D. Using Paired Values. If the same control serum is analyzed in duplicate on successive days, the S.D. can be calculated as follows (see example below):

1. List the pairs in columns.
2. Determine the difference between each pair of values.
3. Square the differences.
4. Find the sum of the squares.
5. Divide this sum by twice the number of pairs.
6. Extract the square root. This is the standard deviation.

ALKALINE PHOSPHATASE VALUES—ABBOTT VP ANALYZER

Values	Difference	Difference^2
89, 92	3	9
89, 90	1	1
86, 83	3	9
88, 90	2	4
88, 91	3	9
86, 89	3	9
93, 89	4	16
91, 90	1	1
94, 94	0	0
89, 89	0	0
89, 86	3	9
87, 89	2	4
88, 92	4	16
91, 89	2	4
87, 86	1	1
2674		92

$$\text{Mean} = \frac{2674}{30} = 89.13$$

$$\text{S.D.} = \sqrt{\frac{\text{Sum of the squares of the differences}}{\text{Twice the number of pairs}}}$$

$$= \sqrt{\frac{92}{30}} = \sqrt{3.07} = 1.75 = 1.8 \text{ to two significant figures}$$

$$\text{C.V.} = \frac{1.8}{89.13} \times 100 = 1.96\% = 2.0\% \text{ to two significant figures}$$

Note: If the standard deviation were calculated on all 30 values by the method previously described, the result would be larger (2.5, with C.V. 2.8%), since this reflects the "between-day" variation. The "difference-between-pairs" S.D. shows only "within-day" variation. One of the effects of automation, especially of such assays as those of enzymes, is that the difference between the two S.D. values is reduced. Indeed, for some determinations for which automated precision is very good, such as serum sodium by ion-selective electrode, there may be no significant difference between the two S.D.s. It is also not unusual to find that the C.V. within-day at elevated levels may not be significantly greater: by use of the same instrumentation and a control serum with a mean value of 198.4, the C.V. was also 2.0%. For an enzyme such as alkaline phosphatase the chief clinical advantage of C.V.s as low as this value is the much improved ability to detect reliably small changes in the patient's values with time.

In some cases the mathematical manipulations may be made less tedious by using another form of the expression for calculating the S.D.

$$\text{S.D.} = \sqrt{\frac{\text{Sum of the squares of the values} - \frac{(\text{Sum of values})^2}{\text{Number of items}}}{\text{Number of items} - 1}}$$

This is represented symbolically:

$$\sqrt{\frac{\Sigma x^2 - \frac{(\Sigma x)^2}{n}}{n - 1}}$$

Using the values from the above example:

$$\text{S.D.} = \sqrt{\frac{238{,}524 - 238{,}342.5}{29}} = \sqrt{\frac{181.47}{29}} = \sqrt{6.26} = 2.50$$

The distinction between within-day precision and between-day precision illustrated in the preceding example should be carefully noted. Estimates of within-day precision, whether obtained by the analysis of paired samples or by assaying a large batch of the same control serum on one day, do not include any systematic errors in the S.D. and C.V.; the S.D. and C.V. thus obtained are indications of the levels attainable under the best conditions, and therefore they give some information about the method of analysis as a method. If large S.D. and C.V. values are obtained on a within-day basis, the between-day values will inevitably be even larger.

Averaging S.D. Values. If we have two sets of control serum results, from two months, the true average S.D. is found from the formula:

$$\sqrt{\frac{(\text{First S.D.})^2 + (\text{Second S.D.})^2}{2}}$$

If the number of items from which each S.D. was found is different, the calculation has to be changed to give more relative importance to the S.D. based on the larger number of items. The formula then becomes:

$$\sqrt{\frac{(n - 1)\,\text{S.D.}_1^2 + (n - 1)\,\text{S.D.}_2^2}{2}}$$

Variance. Variance is the square of the standard deviation. It is not used statistically merely as a statement of variability but to detect significant differences in the extent of variation between groups of data and to determine the contributions of various factors to the total variation. Variances can be added directly, unlike S.D.s.

Population and Sample. The use of statistics to derive information from collections of very large numbers of items was originally applied to demographic data such as birth and death rates, morbidity from various diseases, and age group differences, and the term *population,* meaning literally "all the inhabitants of a geographically defined area," was extended to refer to "all people in a specified category" and finally to "a complete, well-defined group of items of data." In scientific work the statistical approach was applied to produce general laws governing the behavior of very large numbers of items showing a range of variation of properties, such as the molecules of a gas having different kinetic energies.

In the application of statistics to clinical laboratory results we cannot wait until we have collected a set of data sufficiently large to provide an exact determination of the population standard deviation—the population might be "all the plasma glucose determinations from one year." We must select a smaller group, or *sample,* with characteristics *representative* of the true population, with the intention of deriving a standard deviation (symbol s or S.D.) that is close enough to the true standard deviation of the population (symbol σ) to act as a valid measure of precision. From statistical studies of this problem of valid sample size it appears that the sample should be not less than 40 items and that the probable error is not greatly reduced if the sample size is increased to 60 items. In practice, an *estimate* of the *within-day* S.D. of a method can be made from a single batch of 30 determinations: this estimate can be modified if necessary from the accumulated daily values over a 30-day period. After two months, with 50 to 60 items of data, the S.D. should be established firmly enough for practical purposes and some information about possible trends should be apparent. Recalculation of the S.D. at the end of six or twelve months yields information of largely historical interest: quality control is a day-to-day matter.

TYPES OF ERRORS IN QUALITY CONTROL

It is convenient to classify laboratory errors as either random or systematic. Random errors increase the extent of variability of results; that is, they increase the S.D. value, but the mean of the results is largely unaffected. Systematic errors displace the mean value in one direction, which may be up or down, but do not affect the overall variability as shown by the S.D. value. It is also possible to encounter errors that exercise both types of effect.

Typical random errors are those inherent in pipettes and volumetric glassware with manufacturing variations, in the electronic and optical variations in instruments such as spectrophotometers, in variation in cuvettes, in timing and temperature control, in the effects of light, evaporation, and temperature on serum samples, and in interferences from other substances in the analyzed sample. Typical systematic errors, although their effect may change slowly with time, arise from instability of reagents, inaccuracy of standards, and nonspecificity of a method. Some systematic errors are characteristic of a particular analyst, for example, in the convention adopted for rounding off values or reading a meniscus. Inaccuracy of the wavelength scale of a spectrophotometer may not have an appreciable effect on a method that employs a standard, but it will introduce a systematic error in procedures in which the wavelength setting is critical, such as in the kinetic determination of enzyme activity at 340 nm or the assay of porphyrins, where the molar absorption coefficient is used as a "standard." An undetected misadjustment of a recorder zero will cause a systematic error, and deterioration of a tube in a recorder amplifier can produce a random or systematic variation.

Clerical errors should be regarded as almost completely avoidable, in contrast to the random errors mentioned above. A low incidence of mistakes such as taking blood from the wrong patient, incorrect labeling of samples, delays in specimen transport, and incorrect calculations and transcriptions of results to report forms is evidence of a well-trained, alert, and conscientious technical staff, using a good work organization plan, well-designed worksheets, and thorough checking.

It should be noted that even a systematic error may not be a *constant* one; its magnitude can vary from day to day, from analyst to analyst, and from laboratory to laboratory. Differences between laboratories, often of astonishing magnitude, reflect the accumulated effect of all random and systematic errors, with differences in methodology, instrumentation, and caliber of staff making the greatest contributions.

USE OF QUALITY CONTROL CHART TO LOCATE SOURCE OF ERROR

When a procedure is out of control, or, preferably, when a trend indicates that loss of control is imminent, careful study of the quality control chart often will provide a lead. For example, the occurrence of six or eight successive values on the chart that are not evenly distributed on either side of the mean raises the possibility of a shift in the mean value—a systematic error. The probable causes are incorrectly made standards, an instrumentation change (such as a new filter or light source), or a reagent problem. If the change is an increase in variability, not to the point where control values are outside the usual ± 2 S.D. limits, but with less than two-thirds of the plotted points within ± 1 S.D. of the mean, there is excessive random error. This can be more difficult to locate. If the method has been in good control and the increase in variability is sudden, check for coincidence with a change of technologist doing that test, use of glassware of lower quality, or sudden increase in workload causing "corner cutting." A common cause of increased variability is sheer overwork. If the test is automated, the problem may be a pumping manifold about to expire, a faulty thermostat in a dialyzer or heating bath, or a spectrophotometer lamp about to fail. If the automated system is a discrete analyzer, a faulty piston in a sample pick-up or reagent dispensing syringe or pump is a possible reason. A gradual shift in the mean value is often caused by reagent deterioration or by the use of a bottle of control serum over a period too long for maintenance of content stability. This is particularly true in systems that are "standardized" by a serum "standard."

Sudden, extremely out-of-range values on a control chart, with the values on either side within control, indicate a problem such as the use of an incorrect control serum, a new batch with a different serial number, an error in a procedure run by someone unaccustomed to it, incorrect wavelength setting, or incorrect cuvette size. In practice, the occurrence of the out-of-range value should lead to a repeat analysis of that batch of tests under senior supervision, which normally would locate the source of error.

THE PROBLEM OF OUTLIERS

In a listing of control serum values for S.D. calculation, there may be one or more values that *appear* to be outliers; that is, results are so far from the main set that they are suspected of being caused by a "wild" error, a single occurrence not typical of the procedure. If such outliers are included in the S.D. calculation, they have a disproportionate influence on the size of the S.D. The decision to exclude a value from the calculations may be made by intuition; if the difference between the outlier value and the next nearest value is large compared with the range of the remaining values, it can be excluded. It is preferable to have a better basis for the decision, and for sets of values greater than 25, Chauvenet's criterion can be used (Crymble, 1971). The method, in effect, tests the compactness of the data.

1. Determine the mean and S.D. in the usual way, including the suspected outliers (see example on p. 44).
2. From the F table (Fig. 3–2), determine the F factor corresponding to the number of items used to calculate the S.D.

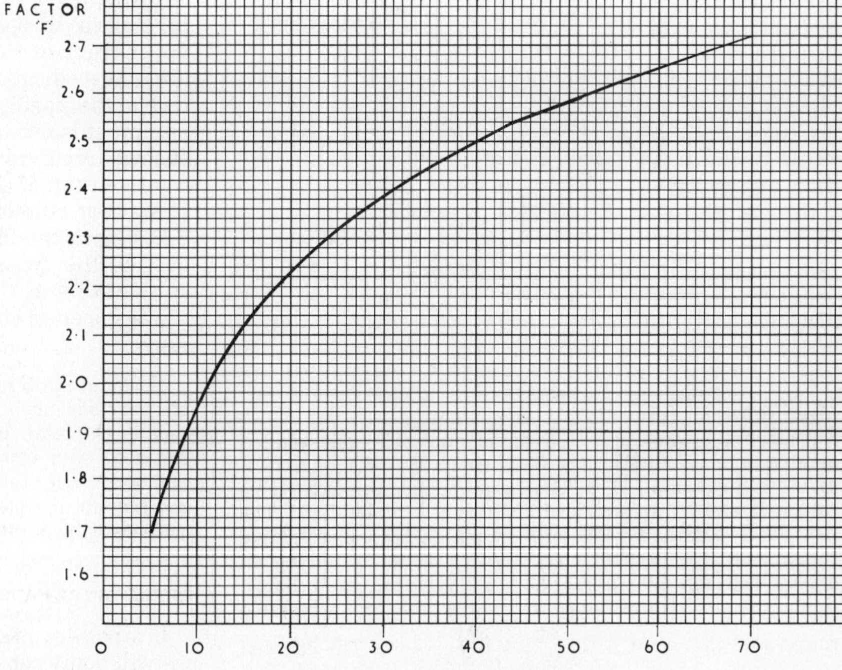

Figure 3–2 Graph of "F" values for use with Chauvenet's method of detecting outlier values.

3. Multiply the S.D. by the F factor to obtain the "acceptable" range.
4. If this acceptable range excludes the outlier, reject it.
5. Redetermine the S.D., omitting the rejected value.
6. Determine the acceptable range as before.
7. If this new range does not exclude any values in the list remaining after the rejection made in 4, the S.D. thus found is correct.
8. If another outlier is found, repeat the process until rejection does not occur.

If the coefficient of variation is calculated before and after rejection of outliers, the effect of the process is readily seen (see example below). It should be noted that the determination of acceptable range using the F value is used only for location of true outliers; the range for quality control purposes will still be the mean ± 2 S.D.s, if this is the convention adopted (see "Deciding on the Range").

Example. Using control serum values for lactate dehydrogenase obtained on 29 successive days, arranged in order of size:

78
78
67
66
65
65
65
63
63
63
62
62
62
62
61
61
61
60
60
60
59
59
59
59
59
58
58
57
57

Mean value, 62; S.D., 5.1; C.V., 8.2%.
The acceptable range derived from the graph of F values plotted against number of items (Fig. 3–2) is ± 2.38 × 5.1 = ± 12.1, giving a range of 50 to 74. The values outside this acceptable range, 78 and 78, are excluded, and the S.D. recalculated. The new S.D. is 2.8; the F value for 27 items is 2.35; the acceptable range is ± 2.35 × 2.8 = 6.6, rounded off to 7.0, giving an acceptable range of 61 ± 7, or 54 to 68. (Note the small change in the mean.) All the values are now within this acceptable range, and the new C.V. is $\frac{2.8}{61} \times 100 = 4.6\%$. The effect of the outlier values on the S.D. and C.V. is clearly evident.

MAGNITUDE OF RESULT VARIABILITY: DECIDING ON THE RANGE

The allowable variability of a product—and most of our products in a clinical chemistry laboratory are analytical values—depends on the purpose or usage of that product. Laboratory results are aids to medical decision making; the ultimate test of their reliability is their power of discrimination between normal and abnormal. The permissible magnitude of variability must therefore be related to the amount of change in the value that is clinically significant.

The common approach to fixing the allowable extent of variation is to calculate the mean and S.D. from a number of determinations on a pool serum, specifying that the limits extend for two S.D.s on either side of the mean. These limits are supposed to include 95% of all results on the pool serum; that is, it is accepted that up to one result in each 20 may be outside these limits without indicating significant loss of control of the procedure. This procedure assumes that the distribution of values is Gaussian and that the same limits are valid for normal, low, and elevated results. This may not be true. We have found that in the automated assay of the aminotransferases, using a discrete system measuring absorbance decrease at 340 nm, the *actual units* of variability about the mean are closely similar at elevated values that are three times the upper limit of normal and in the middle of the normal range. This means that the coefficient of variation is about 15% at low enzyme levels and 3.3% at higher levels. This pattern is inherent in the instrumentation; the absorbance change at low enzyme levels is very small, and the inevitable electronic "noise" in the amplifier of the photometric system is relatively large. At higher levels of enzyme activity, the absorbance change, and hence the signal produced by the photometer, is much greater, but the level of electronic noise is unchanged. Our practice is to use controls with values just above the upper limit of the normal range, which is the critical area for medical decision making. We accept that at low levels the coefficient of variation is high (where we assume it is not important), and that at very high levels such as occur in hepatitis, the information is more of relative than of absolute clinical significance.

Another rule of thumb sets the 95% limits at ± 2.5 S.D.s, with the idea of thus accommodating values just outside the typical Gaussian distribution. Like many rules of thumb, it will function after a fashion, but it is always open to challenge, to which there is no scientific reply.

Most statistical methods used for determining normal ranges are very dependent on the assumption that the data distribution is Gaussian in form. Often this assumption cannot be justified, even using logarithmic and other transformations. Nonparametric statistical methods make no such assumption, and they form a powerful and valid alternative to parametric methods. For an introduction to this topic, see Gindler (1975).

SIGNIFICANT CHANGE

If a patient has a normal blood urea nitrogen (BUN; we will delay consideration of the term "normal" for the time being), there is a certain probability that he does not have renal disease. If his serum creatinine, creatinine clearance, serum uric acid, routine urinalysis, urine culture, serum protein electrophoresis, and total serum protein are all normal, it is most improbable that he has any common type of renal disease. The value of reliable laboratory determinations is in shortening the odds for the diagnostician; that is, in assigning low rates of probability to all but one or two explanations for a patient's illness. The physician is also interested in early detection of disease because of the greatly increased chances of effective treatment. The question that arises is the significance that should be assigned to a result. If the normal range for BUN is 8 to 18 mg per dL, is an elevation to 22 significant? If a patient with chest pains has a creatine phosphokinase (CPK) value of 55 and the normal range is 30 to 50, does this indicate a possible myocardial infarction? If a patient with hepatitis shows a decrease in serum alanine aminotransferase (ALT) from 800 to 750 units, is he improving?

To answer these queries, we could state the reliability of the data in terms of the S.D. If a BUN result of 22 mg per dL is quoted, this value is reproducible to ± 2 mg per dL with a probability of 95%, which means that in one instance in 20, the error could be larger. If we widen the range to ± 3 mg per dL, the true value could lie from 19 to 25 mg per dL, and the value of 22 mg per dL does not seem so abnormal now in relation to a maximum normal range value of 18 mg per dL.

When considering what is a significant change in a result, we could use the C.V. and state that if the percentage change is greater than three times the C.V., the change is probably real. As we have seen, however, the methodology may influence the size of the C.V. It would appear useful, therefore, to have some knowledge of the C.V. at different levels: normal, slightly elevated, moderately elevated, or greatly elevated.

Laboratory data are only an adjunct to clinical decisions. We can indicate the order of reliability of our results as shown, but we cannot draw sharp lines of demarcation between change caused by random variation and that caused by real biological alterations.

Normal Range (Reference Range)

The ideal laboratory test would give neither false positive results (the inclusion of a normal person in the diseased group) nor false negative results (categorizing a sick person as being normal). To attain this end, the range of results with healthy people would not overlap the set of values occurring in disease. The range of results for many biological measurements shows an area of overlap between the apparently healthy and the possibly sick, and the region of analytical doubt often coincides with the zone of clinical uncertainty. In addition, the very concept of a "normal" range is being challenged. With more precise analytical methods and the ability with modern automation to amass very large sets of data, our ability to discriminate between different segments of the population with respect to sex, age, race, dietary habits, life style, geographic location, and occupation has been improved to the point where any statement of "normal range" that ignores these factors is open to serious challenge. It follows that any attempt to derive a valid set of normal ranges (or, to use the current semantic term, *reference values*) requires considerable laboratory resources and access to the large numbers of healthy people in the various classes selected that would be essential to permit reliable statistical analysis of the raw data. In a text at the basic level, extensive discussion of the establishment of normal ranges cannot be encompassed: we will limit our account to the elementary statistical techniques for the display and analysis of collections of patient results from which a check on a normal range in use can be derived.

Histogram

The simplest graphical representation of the pattern of distribution of a set of data is the histogram.

1. Examine the list of values and locate the highest and the lowest. The difference between them is the range (of the data, not the normal range!).
2. Divide this range into a series of equally sized intervals. The number of these will depend on the data; for example, with plasma glucose values from a large sample population in a range from 60 to 120 mg per dL, the interval could suitably be 3 mg per dL. The intervals would be named 59 to 61, 62 to 64, 65 to 67, 68 to 70, and so on. By the usual check mark system, determine the number of values in each interval group. The total number of check marks in each interval group is called the frequency of that group, F (see Table 3–2).
3. Plot the totals from each interval as bar graphs, with each column centered on the middle value of each interval group (see Fig. 3–1).
4. Inspect the histogram to see if a smooth Gaussian curve can be fitted to the bar graphs; if so, the pattern of distribution is probably normal and will have the characteristics previously described (p. 44).

If the curve has to be "skewed," that is, distorted, in order to fit the histogram, the data may have to be transformed. It is known that some biological data follow a log-normal distribution; in this case, the logarithms of the data values are used to replot the histogram and to determine the upper and lower limits of normal by the following method. When the process has been completed, the antilogarithms are determined to convert the data into usable form.

Probability Paper

Referring to the examples of data (see Table 3–2) used to draw the histogram in Figure 3–1, the numbers in the column headed *Frequency "F"* are the total number of check marks (items of data) in each interval. In the column headed *Cum. F,* the values are found by adding to the F value for that interval all the preceding F values. In the next column, each of the cumulative frequency values is expressed as a percentage of the total number of items of original data. The final value in this column should be 100%.

Using a special graph paper called probability paper* (Keuffel and Esser 46–8000), the cumulative frequencies on the horizontal abscissa are plotted against the corresponding highest value of each interval on the vertical ordinate. If the data follow a Gaussian distribution, the

*Probability paper is analogous to semilog graph paper in that it converts a nonlinear function to a linear form.

TABLE 3–2 PLASMA GLUCOSE RESULTS USED TO CONSTRUCT THE HISTOGRAM OF FIGURE 3–1 AND THE CUMULATIVE FREQUENCY PLOT OF FIGURE 3–3

Interval No.	Limits of Interval (mg/dL)	Frequency "F"*	Cum. F	% Cum. F
1	59–61	1	1	0.22
2	62–64	1	2	0.45
3	65–67	4	6	1.35
4	68–70	6	12	2.69
5	71–73	12	24	5.38
6	74–76	18	42	9.42
7	77–79	28	70	15.70
8	80–82	36	106	23.77
9	83–85	42	148	33.18
10	86–88	49	197	44.17
11	89–91	51	248	55.60
12	92–94	49	297	66.59
13	95–97	45	342	76.68
14	98–100	38	380	85.20
15	101–103	26	406	91.03
16	104–106	19	425	95.29
17	107–109	10	435	97.53
18	110–112	5	440	98.65
19	113–115	3	443	99.33
20	116–118	2	445	99.77
21	119–121	1	446	100.00

*The frequency "F" is the number of times a value between a particular set of limits occurs in the set of 446 values; that is, for interval 15, there were 26 results of 101, 102, or 103.

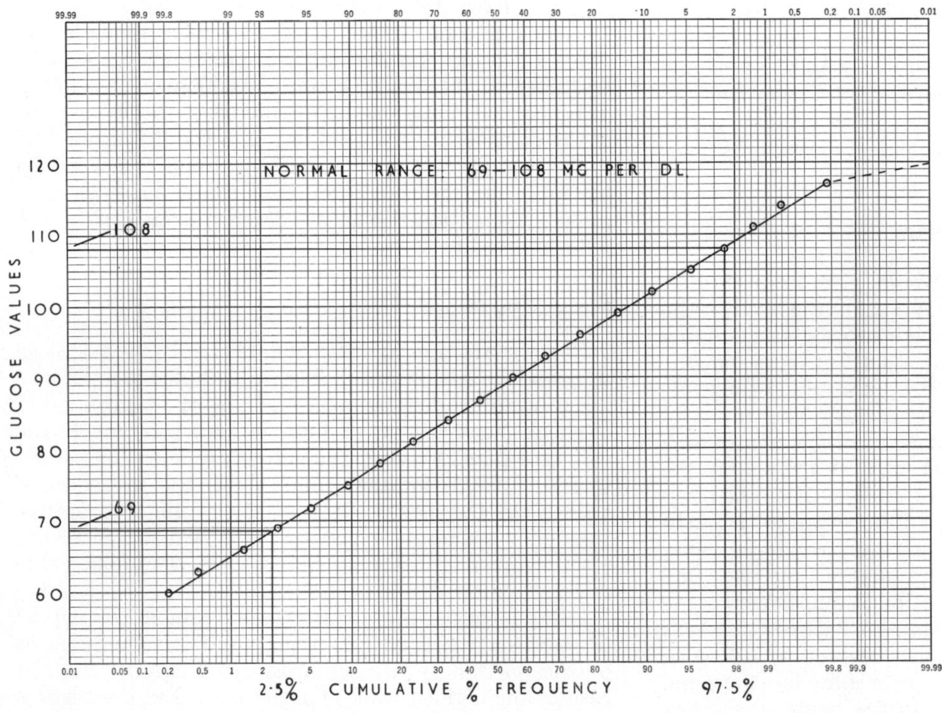

Figure 3–3 Cumulative frequency plot of plasma glucose values for determination of normal range.

TABLE 3–3 DATA USED TO CALCULATE CUMULATIVE FREQUENCY PLOT OF CPK VALUES

Midpoint of Interval	Frequency	Cumulative Frequency	Per Cent Frequency
3	1	1	0.3
8	6	7	2.15
13	17	24	7.38
18	31	55	16.92
23	45	100	30.76
28	47	147	45.23
33	42	189	58.15
38	41	230	70.77
43	40	270	83.08
48	32	302	92.92
53	6	308	94.77
58	7	315	96.92
63	5	320	98.46
68	2	322	99.08
73	2	324	99.69
78	0	324	99.69
83	1	325	99.99
88	1	326	99.99

plot will be a straight line (Fig. 3–3). If the set of data contains values from two different populations, such as normal and abnormal values, the plot on probability paper will show a change in the slope of the line.

Using the fact that the large majority of the results of most routine laboratory tests are normal, it is possible by the use of the cumulative frequency plot to discriminate between the normal and abnormal results. The normal results will tend to be relatively concentrated within a narrow range of values, whereas the abnormal results will be scattered over a wider range and have a different pattern of distribution. The data in Table 3–3 were derived from 326 successive routine creatine phosphokinase (CPK) determinations. The range of normal values quoted for the method was 5 to 50 units. The cumulative frequency plot clearly shows the change in slope. To determine the normal range from the plot, the criteria of Hoffman (1963) were used. The straight line fitted to the lower portion of the plot is extended to meet verticals drawn from the 2.5% and 97.5% points on the abscissa. Horizontals were drawn from the points of intersection to cut the scale of values on the left-hand ordinate, and these values were taken as the limits of the normal range (see Fig. 3–4). The normal range thus derived was 8 to 53 units, which agreed reasonably well with the quoted figures.

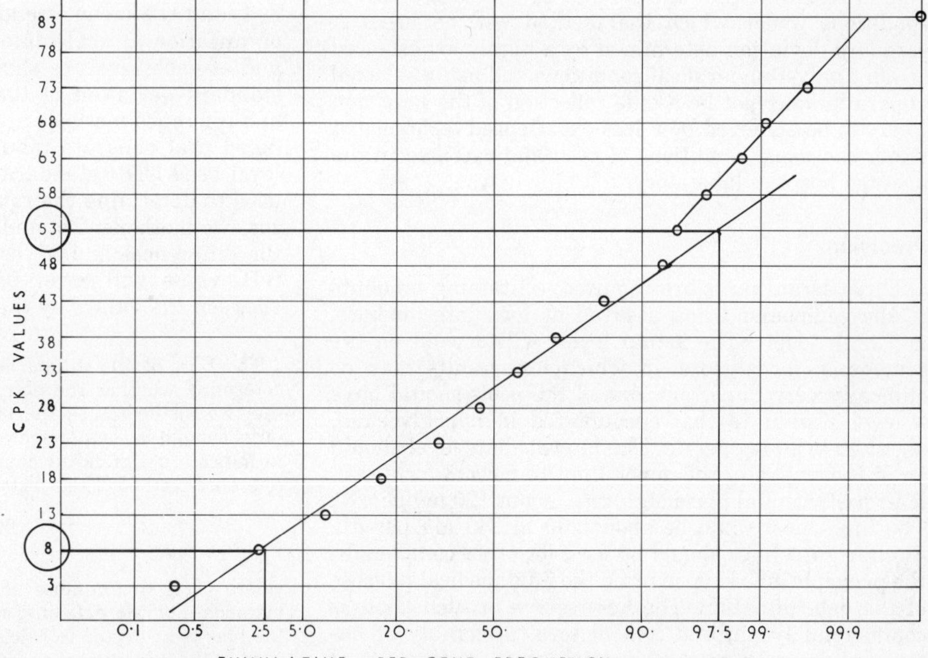

Figure 3–4 Cumulative frequency plot of mixed population, showing both normal and abnormal values of creatine phosphokinase results.

EVALUATION AND COMPARISON OF METHODS OF ANALYSIS

A change in the method for a clinical laboratory analysis may be instituted because of dissatisfaction with a procedure whose clinical reliability is suspect, realization that a method has become outmoded and does not meet diagnostic needs, continuing difficulties in meeting realistic quality control requirements, or replacement of a manual method by an automated instrument. If, after due weight has been given to the qualitative factors (such as cost, availability, and stability of reagents; equipment requirement; staff training; and safety matters), no clear advantages of the new method over the old have become apparent, the choice will rest on the quantitative aspects of accuracy and precision, as in fact it should. The procedure to be described (Barnett and Youden, 1970) is intended for assays of substances available in pure form. The assessment of enzyme methods is a more difficult matter and will be discussed separately.

It should be emphasized that statistical analysis in this and other problems provides *comparative* information. The choice ultimately depends on a summation of factors not readily amenable to statistical analysis. Graphical presentation of data may reveal limitations caused by nonlinearity and errant points.

PROCEDURE (BARNETT AND YOUDEN, 1970)

Three basic questions require answers. These are: (1) What is the precision, under conditions similar to those of routine use, of the proposed new method? (2) What is the accuracy of the proposed new method, as assessed by comparison with an accepted reference procedure and by determinations of recovery of added material? (3) How do results obtained by the existing method and by the proposed new method compare when run in parallel on patients' samples?

It is essential that the results be applicable to the conditions under which the method will be used. A standard deviation determined by a highly experienced senior analyst under ideal conditions and using selected apparatus may not be a true reflection of the precision likely to be achieved by a less experienced technologist under the usual conditions of rush and overload in the average hospital laboratory.

Precision

Three serum pools are required, containing amounts of the compound being assayed at low, intermediate, and high levels. The actual levels will depend on the compound; for glucose, in which low results may be clinically very important, one of the pools should have a level similar to that encountered in hypoglycemia, about 40 to 50 mg per dL. The intermediate level should be in the region of the upper limit of normal for a two-hour postprandial plasma glucose, about 120 mg per dL. The high level could be about 200 to 240 mg per dL. Similar guidelines should be used for other compounds; the principle is to keep in mind the final medical purpose of the determination. The best source of such pools is commercial lyophilized control sera, preferably of human origin, such as the Versatol series. A quantity of each pool sufficient for the complete series of assays should be obtained. In order to obtain the necessary levels, mixtures of two pools may be required. If this is done, the volumes should be measured very accurately. From a pair of pools with glucose values of 40 and 240 mg per dL, a series of mixtures can be prepared. Equal volumes of the pools will give 140 mg per dL; three volumes of the 40 mg per dL pool and one volume of the 240 mg per dL pool will give 90 mg per dL. The general formula for making the mixtures is:

$$\frac{xa + yb}{x + y} = \text{mg per dL in final mixture}$$

Where x = volumes of pool 1
a = mg per dL of pool 1
y = volumes of pool 2
b = mg per dL of pool 2

If a required level cannot be obtained easily by mixtures, existing pool values may be boosted by the addition of small volumes of concentrated solutions of the compound required. Thus, if one volume of a 500 mg per dL solution is mixed with four volumes of a 100 mg per dL pooled serum, the resultant concentration, using the above formula, will be 180 mg per dL. The only objection to this procedure is that the protein level of the mixture will not be the same as for the rest of the pools.

Once the three pools have been prepared, they are analyzed for the chosen component on 20 successive days by both the method under evaluation and a reference method. (The choice of a reference method may be made by reference to standard texts, by consultation with an experienced analyst, or by reference to published papers on evaluations of methods for the same compound.) It is not advisable to try to curtail the work by doing all the paired analyses on one or two days; this does not correspond to the usual pattern of tests on patients, which are rarely done more than twice on the same day. The results are tabulated as shown in Table 3–4, and the mean, standard deviation, and coefficient of variation are calculated separately for each method and at each level; as shown in the table, the bias and standard deviation of the difference between the test and reference methods are also calculated. (It should be noted that separate tabulations are required for each level used.) The standard deviation of the difference is used to determine the range of the differences between the two methods, test and reference. Thus, if the S.D. of the differences is 4.55, as shown, a range of twice this S.D. value will cover 95% of the actual differences between the values by the two methods.

The S.D. of the differences is also used in a "t" test to determine whether the observed average difference between the two methods, i.e., the bias, is a real difference, that is, large enough in comparison with the number of determinations to indicate a significant change in mean values from test to reference method. The t factor is calculated from:

$$t = \frac{\text{bias} \times \sqrt{N}}{s}$$

where N is the number of specimens assayed by the two methods. For the data in Table 3–4, bias = −5 (the sign of the bias is neglected in calculation of the t factor); N = 20; s (S.D. of the differences between the results by the two methods)

TABLE 3–4 COMPARISON OF PRECISION OF TEST AND REFERENCE METHODS

Analysis	Reference Result R	Test Method Result M	Difference R − M	(R − M) − Bias	([R − M] − Bias)²
1	115	117	−2	+3	9
2	117	123	−6	−1	1
3	118	125	−7	−2	4
4	121	129	−8	−3	9
5	115	128	−13	−8	64
6	127	126	+1	+6	36
7	119	118	+1	+6	36
8	120	127	−7	−2	4
9	117	127	−10	−5	25
10	119	129	−10	−5	25
11	122	119	+3	+8	64
12	124	128	−4	+1	1
13	117	122	−5	0	0
14	123	124	−1	+4	16
15	118	126	−8	−3	9
16	119	128	−9	−4	16
17	127	124	+3	+8	64
18	124	128	−4	+1	1
19	121	129	−8	−3	9
20	117	123	−6	−1	1
					394
Means	120	125			
Bias (Reference − Test) = −5			S.D. of Differences $= \sqrt{\frac{394}{19}} = 4.55$		
S.D.s	3.52	3.72	$t = \frac{5 \times \sqrt{20}}{4.55} = 4.91$		
C.V.s	2.93%	2.98%			

$= 4.55$. Then $t = \frac{5 \times \sqrt{20}}{4.55} = 4.91$. From a table of t values (Arkin and Colton, 1963), the value of t that could arise from chance alone with a probability of 95% is 2.09. The larger t value obtained indicates that the bias difference between the methods reflects a real difference. An estimate of the relative precision of the two methods is obtained by calculating the F factor, which is the ratio of the variances. From the data in Table 3–4, the variance (which equals the square of the S.D.) for the test method is 13.84; for the reference method it is 12.39. The ratio $\frac{\text{Test variance}}{\text{Reference variance}} = 1.12$. From the table of F values (Arkin and Colton, 1963), the critical value of F for 20 paired tests (19 degrees of freedom) is 3.0 at the 95% significance level. The calculated F value is smaller than this, indicating that there is no significant difference in the precision of the two methods. It is possible, of course, for the test method to give a lower variance than the reference method (it may simply be a better method!), and in this case, the F ratio is calculated with the reference variance as the numerator.

Accuracy

For assessment of accuracy, the ability of the test method to show acceptable recovery of added substance to a base serum pool is measured. In this procedure, "acceptable" means that the difference between the amount added and the amount recovered is less than twice the standard deviation of the differences between the methods as determined from the data of Table 3–4. The recovery studies are made at three levels, and when the acceptability of recovery at each level is assessed, the S.D. of the differences appropriate to that level must be used. The best way to do this is to arrange the recovery experiments so that the increments of substance used are close to the three levels of the precision determination described earlier. In order to be brief, we will illustrate the procedure at one level only.

Preparation of Recovery Pool. To the original 120 mg per dL pool, add one volume of a 700 mg per dL solution of glucose to four volumes of pool serum. The glucose value obtained is 236 mg per dL, and the added glucose is 116 per dL. The two pools are analyzed by the test method in triplicate, and the results are tabulated as shown:

Base Pool	Recovery Pool	Recovery	Difference (Recovered − Added)
118	242	124	+ 8

The allowable difference, 2 s at this level, is 2 × 4.55 = 9.1 mg per dL. The recovery is within limits. The percentage recovery, 106.9%, may be used, but it does not take into account the level.

Patient Sample Study. For this procedure, at least 40 patients' sera are analyzed by both methods, taking not more than five per day in order to include such between-day variations as the skill of the analyst, instrumental variations, and stability of reagents. The variances by both methods and the s values of the differences can be calculated and assessed as in the precision studies, but often a graphical display of the results will reveal the essential facts. The results on the sera by the reference method are plotted against those by the test method, with the horizontal scale for the reference values and the vertical for the test results. Each point on the graph is the intersection of the reference value with the test value for the same serum (see Fig. 3–5). A line is drawn that represents the average slope of the points as closely

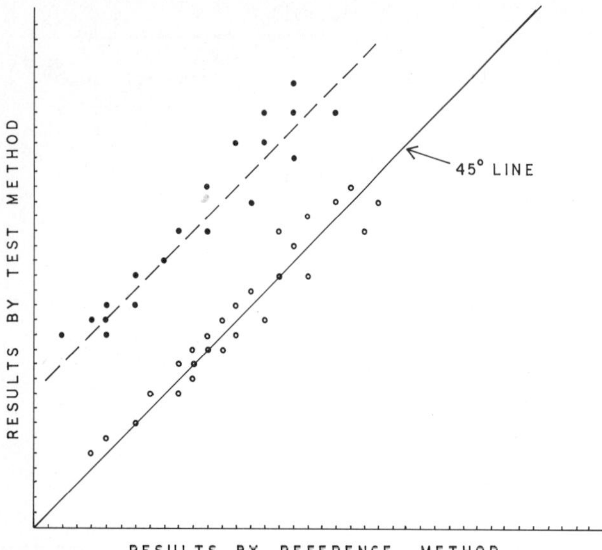

Figure 3–5 Comparison of results by two methods. The open circles show good correlation between the two procedures. The closed circles show that the test method has a positive bias when compared with the reference method.

as possible. A second line is drawn from the origin at 45° to the abscissa. If the average slope of the points is close to this ideal line, this indicates a good agreement between the two methods. If the average line is parallel to the ideal but at some distance above or below it, this indicates a significant bias of one method vis-à-vis the other. If the angle of slope deviates from the ideal, the bias varies with the serum level of the substance. If the points are quite scattered, making drawing an average slope line difficult, there are one or more random sources of variation present.

QUALITY CONTROL AND EVALUATION OF ENZYME DETERMINATIONS

The methods for control of precision in enzyme assays are similar to those used for other substances, with the addition of extra care in protecting the control sera from deterioration after thawing or reconstitution. If a single control serum is used, the level at which control is exercised should be in the region of critical medical decision; frequently this is in the slightly to moderately elevated range. If we are trying to compare two methods by the procedures described above, or if we wish to check the accuracy of an enzyme estimation, the lack of pure preparations of enzymes of human origin constitutes a major problem. Dilution of a serum with a very high activity of the enzyme of interest poses the question of what diluent to use. Water, saline, or buffer will change protein content and alter the levels, usually unknown, of activators and inhibitors. Use of a serum diluent whose enzyme activity has been destroyed introduces another factor in the procedure used to achieve this. Mixtures of a high-level commercial control serum with a normal human serum may not yield the expected values because of the different reaction characteristics of nonhuman enzymes in the commercial serum or even different proportions of isoenzymes. The value of a control serum can be determined by a very carefully controlled kinetic method, but this value cannot easily be converted to serve as a check on a method using quite different conditions of substrate concentration, reaction temperature, presence of activators, and so on.

Some factors mitigate the problem. First, the degree of precision required for an enzyme assay to provide valid clinical information is in many cases of the order of ± 10%. Second, for enzyme assays in which good precision and accuracy are required at levels just above the normal range, e.g., aspartate aminotransferases, creatine phosphokinase, and lactate dehydrogenase, the methods usually employed involve a change in the oxidation-reduction state of a coenzyme such as nicotinamide-adenine dinucleotide (NAD) or nicotinamide-adenine dinucleotide phosphate (NADP). These coenzymes are obtainable in a high state of purity, and provided that a high-resolution, narrow band-pass spectrophotometer using precision cells is available, kinetic methods can be checked with the known molar absorbancies of the coenzymes involved. For example, if a method involving the reduction of one mole of NAD to NADH for each mole of substrate converted is carried out in a 1-cm cell at 340 nm in a total volume of 3.0 mL and a serum sample of 0.2 mL, the theoretical absorbance change for a serum containing 40 milliunits per mL will be found as follows: The absorbance in a 1-cm cell of 1 micromole of NADH per mL at 340 nm is known to be 6.22. In a total volume of 3.0 mL, the absorbance would be $\frac{6.22}{3} = 2.07$. Thus $\frac{\text{Absorbance change}}{2.07} = \text{micromoles}$ of NADH changed. For the stated sample size of 0.2 mL, $\frac{\text{Absorbance change}}{2.07} \times \frac{1.0}{0.2} = \text{micromoles of NADH}$ changed per mL of sample. The International Unit (I.U.) is defined as a change in substrate or associated coenzyme of 1 micromole per minute. It is generally accepted to use the liter as the volume involved, and hence we may define the International Unit as the change of one micromole per minute per liter. Therefore

$$\frac{\text{Absorbance change per minute}}{2.07} \times \frac{1.0}{0.2} \times 1000 = \text{Enzyme activity in I.U./L}$$

Equating this expression to 40 gives as the theoretical absorbance change per minute for a serum enzyme activity of that value:

$$\frac{\text{Absorbance change}}{2.07} \times \frac{1.0}{0.2} \times 1000 = 40$$

The calculated absorbance change is 0.0166. Third, some reactions used for enzyme assays use synthetic substrates of known composition, and the accuracy of the method can be checked by using the product in pure form. The Bessey-Lowry-Brock method for alkaline phosphatase and the Babson phenolphthalein monophosphate procedure for the same enzyme both involve the release of substances of which pure solutions for calibration purposes can be prepared: p-nitrophenol and phenolphthalein, respectively. It has been argued that this approach is invalid, since the substrates are not the physiological forms; but since the normal ranges are derived by the same methodology and patient results are compared with these, the requirements of clinical diagnosis are served.

The practice of some producers of control sera of stating the values for the commonly determined enzymes obtained by a number of the most widely used procedures is helpful, but the basic lack of primary standards remains. We therefore can compare enzyme methods in terms of their precision and in terms of the general considerations of ease, speed, convenience, and cost. The only test for accuracy is the performance in clinical usage.

One aspect in the evaluation of enzyme procedures, new or current, is the delineation of the limits of zero-order kinetics. Since the activity of an enzyme is affected by a wide variety of factors (see "Enzyme Kinetics," p. 151), which can only be established for the initial stages of the reaction, the relationship between enzyme level and the extent of measured change, such as in absorbance at 340 nm, will be constant only over a certain range of values. In the assay of a pure substance, linearity is easily established by adding known amounts to serum samples and by determining and plotting the values obtained against the known quantities. For enzyme assay linearity, only the enzyme level must vary, and hence mere preparation of a set of dilutions of a very high-activity serum will not suffice. A better approach is to use mixtures of two control sera, with very high and low activities, respectively, thus maintaining the concentrations of other factors, such as protein, constant. For example, using control serum A with a lactate dehydrogenase activity of 500 units and serum B with 50 units, the following series can be made:

Volume of A	+	Volumes of B	=	Final Value
1		1		275
1		2		200
1		3		163
1		4		140
1		5		125
1		6		114

The formula used to find the value of the mixtures is:

$$\frac{X \times \text{value of A} + Y \times \text{value of B}}{X + Y}$$

where X and Y are the volumes used.

After the assays are run in duplicate, the actual results are plotted against the calculated values, as shown in Figure 3–6. The point of inflection denotes the point where linearity has been lost; any enzyme assay results above this value must be repeated after suitable dilution with saline. It is true that such dilution introduces some possibility of error, but at such elevated levels of activity clinical interest is more in the direction of changes than of absolute values. The range of linearity obtained in a particular procedure is affected by the composition of the reaction mixture, and most manufacturers of enzyme reagent systems have adopted one of the so-called "optimization" formulae. Some disagreement still persists, however, concerning the relative merits of the various formulations.

In view of the difficulty of comparing results obtained with a particular local method with stated normal ranges derived from other techniques, a pragmatic approach is to determine a local range of normal values. If enough volunteers can be obtained (the average hospital will provide a good range of age groups up to about 55 years), an initial set of 50 duplicate analyses will provide a working estimate of the local method's normal range. If the list of data is kept open and supplemented as opportunity presents itself, the normal range can be refined by a larger sample population and by one more representative of the local mixture of ethnic and socioeconomic groups from which the hospital patient intake is derived. The practice in some institutions of screening new staff members with a routine health examination also could provide a suitable source of samples. This approach is mentioned here as a suggestion, not as a proven solution.

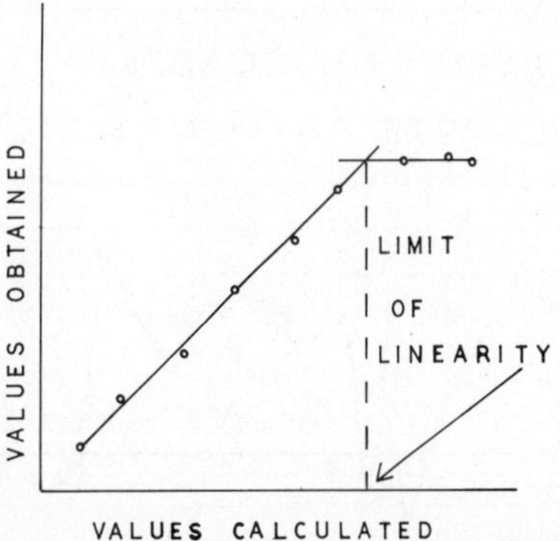

Figure 3–6 Determination of limit of linearity.

THE ORGANIZATION OF A QUALITY CONTROL PROGRAM

An effective quality control program should demonstrate that the results provide reliable information about the patient to the clinician and that the levels of technical expertise and instrument performance are equal to that task and should be able to satisfy the expectations of external monitoring agencies. An effective program cannot be run by remote control: it demands the active, interested cooperation of the technical staff. It is closely related to good instrument maintenance, to equitable allocation of the workload, and to continuing in-service training and knowledgeable supervision.

The basic requirements for a quality control program are:

1. A supply of control sera sufficient for at least six months and preferably for a year. No system that entails redetermination of mean values and standard deviations at frequent intervals will function satisfactorily.
2. Mean values and standard deviations for all the analytes routinely measured by the laboratory, based on a minimum of 30 determinations on separate days. (For methods, see p. 45.)
3. Control sera with values at two levels as the minimum requirement: the levels should relate to the clinical uses of the individual tests as far as is practicable.
4. Clearly defined rules about the manner of use of the control sera—i.e., mode of reconstitution, frequency and location of controls in automated methods, imme-

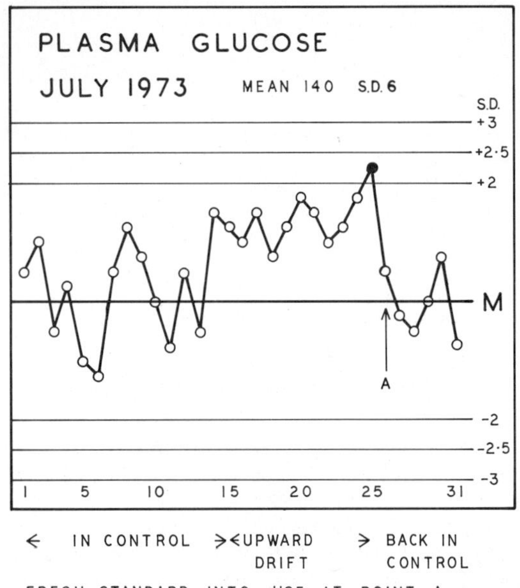

Figure 3–7 Quality control chart showing an upward drift caused by use of an outdated standard, and return to control following introduction of a fresh standard.

diate plotting of control results, and action to be taken as soon as an out-of-control result is noted. A close watch must be kept on the pattern of control results as they accumulate on the display charts. The plotted points should be evenly distributed on either side of the mean, and about two-thirds of the points should fall within ± 1 S.D. Shifts in the general pattern of distribution of the values may indicate a new random error: shifts in the mean value when recalculated at the end of the monitoring period (e.g., one month) may be due to a new systematic error (Fig. 3–7).

5. In addition to the routine controls as described above, a variety of extra checks, especially when the results from those controls are subject to unconscious bias, that is, the *involuntary* tendency to modify the reported or plotted value based on prior knowledge of the correct reading. This point may elicit indignant denials that such a process occurs: however, many studies have demonstrated that it can be detected, mainly in manual analyses. Such extra checks should include processing commercial control sera disguised as patient samples, running mixtures of patient sera and known control sera, analyzing patient sera in duplicate in widely scattered sections of automated determinations and, when feasible, exchanging samples with another laboratory. The fact that such special controls are part of the day's work load cannot be concealed, and indeed it should not be. The controls should be presented as a challenge to responsible professional analysts, not as a threat to subordinate test processors. The results of all such special and occasional checks should be recorded in a quality control journal, together with such data as batch numbers of regular control sera, dates of introduction, notations of problems, and the corrective actions taken.

6. Laboratory participation in at least one external quality control scheme. In some areas an external authority may combine such participation with legislated licensing powers: whether the laboratory enrolls in an additional scheme is a local decision based on workload, economics, and availability.

The maintenance of stable S.D.s and C.V.s, good results with control sera of known values, and acceptable performance in a survey system constitute reasonable grounds for confidence in the reported test results.

In very large, heavily automated clinical chemistry laboratories, some extra controls should be run to determine the interaction between samples (the extent to which the result of a test is affected by a previous high-value specimen). This is particularly important in analytical systems employing the continuous-flow principle and in discrete analyzers using very small sample sizes. Interaction is determined by running in sequence two water "samples," one normal-level control serum, a high-value serum, and the normal-level control again. The high-value serum should be at least three times the normal level control and should be a serum, not an aqueous standard that could have different viscosity characteristics. The per cent interaction is given by the expression:

$$\frac{\text{(Result for the second normal-level control} - \text{Result for the first)} \times 100}{\text{Result for the high-level serum}}$$

For example, if the high-value serum gave a glucose value of 300 mg per dL; the first normal control, 100 mg per dL; and the second normal control, 105 mg per dL, the interaction would be:

$$\frac{105 - 100}{300} \times 100 = 1.67\%$$

When large volume analyzers are being used to process multiple batches of samples or are in action 24 hours a day, it is essential to include additional controls at fixed positions in the sample trays in order to detect the slow changes in results usually referred to as "drift." Comparison of these extra controls, which are analyzed at constant time intervals, will detect gradual shifts in accuracy that, if not investigated and corrected, will lead to out-of-control situations and costly reprocessing of samples.

At this point, a knotty problem has to be discussed: enzyme controls. The lack of primary human enzyme standards and of control sera incorporating such standards—together with the absence of international agreement on a standard assay temperature, substrate composition, and other analytical variables—has led to such anomalies as the reporting of enzyme test results in interlaboratory surveys in such dubious terms as "percentages of your upper limit of normal." A further complication is the assiduous promotion of a new reporting unit, the katal, defined as "the catalytic activity of any catalyst (including an enzyme) that produces the transformation of one mole of substrate per second under defined conditions." The katal is related to the International Unit by the expression

1 I.U. = 16.67 nkat; that is, I.U. × 16.67 = nkat

The conversion formula is derived from the expression

$$\frac{\text{I.U.}}{60} = \mu\text{mol/s}$$

$$\frac{\mu\text{mol/s}}{10^6} = \text{mol/s} = \text{kat}$$

$$\text{Kat} \times 10^9 = \text{nkat}$$

The majority of manufacturers of control sera provide enzyme values determined by a range of commonly used instruments and assay methods, and this mitigates the problems of control of enzyme analyses. At least it is possible to select control sera with levels appropriate to clinical diagnostic needs, typically a normal level and a moderately elevated value. This permits control of precision: monitoring of accuracy is in theory possible only if the laboratory uses one of the instrument and reagent set combinations listed in the control serum package insert. Inspection of the differing values assigned to the same control serum by the manufacturer will illustrate the problem.

The development of high-precision photometric systems and the use of narrow band-pass filters in some discrete analyzers permit standardization by the use of factors based on the molar absorbance of the coenzyme NADH in assay systems where the transformation of one micromole of substrate is accompanied by a corresponding change of oxidation-reduction state of the coenzyme. (See calculation on p. 54.) The apparent simplicity of this approach overlooks a basic requirement of the method: that the absolute accuracy of the photometric system can be determined and fixed. One advantage of this approach is that the laboratory can check the factor given by the instrument manufacturer by making multiple determinations of the enzyme using the same reagent set in a narrow band-pass double-beam spectrophotometer, in cuvettes of certified path length, and employing meticulous technique and temperature control.

Until the differences of opinion regarding analytical variables and reporting units have been resolved, some practical suggestions for control of enzyme assays can be made:

1. If the laboratory's method of assay is identical *in every respect* to that used by the manufacturer of an enzyme control serum, or if the difference is only in the units used for reporting (which are convertible by taking into account only factors such as time, molar concentration, and volume), for control purposes accept the stated values as being correct.

2. The levels at which control is exercised should be related to the medical usage of the test; generally speaking, these will be in the normal range and in the moderately elevated range.

3. If the laboratory's assay method differs from that used by the manufacturer of the control serum, the serum can only be used initially as a check on precision. However, if the technologist takes the greatest possible care with every aspect of the manual method, considering timing, temperature control, precise pipetting, matched cuvettes, and a thorough check of the spectrophotometer, a value in International Units can be assigned to a commercial enzyme control serum; this value can then be used to monitor the accuracy of the automated procedure.

In addition to the control procedures and extra checks already mentioned, the cooperation of the medical staff should be sought in assessing the reliability of the laboratory data in relation to the quality of diagnosis and treatment. An essential part of a quality control program is the careful investigation of any complaints and criticisms; the first indication of a problem may come in just such a manner.

The quality control records in the laboratory should be kept and reviewed after three and six months. Careful comparisons of means and S.D.s over longer periods may detect very slow drifts in instrument performance or changes in technical expertise. We have noted a very slow rise in the C.V. of methods on a discrete analyzer over a period of four years, probably indicating the effects of wear in various mechanical components or change in electronic circuitry. The slow development of worn spots on the mechanism of digital read-out dials on a flame photometer, caused by the clustering of readings within a small range of values, showed up as a small but persistent loss of precision.

The most important feature of any quality control program is the attitude of the technologists involved in both its organization and its implementation. If errors are vigorously sought and honestly recognized, and if corrective action is immediate and effective, almost any reasonable program will fulfill its purpose, even taking into account such problems as unconscious bias.

PRESENTATION OF QUALITY CONTROL DATA

The standard method for presenting quality control data is to use a linear chart, usually covering one month, with three lines, indicating the mean value and the upper and lower allowable limits, usually ± 2 S.D.s (see Fig. 3–7). It is also proposed that the limits should be ± 3 S.D.s (Barnett, 1971), on the grounds that with the ± 2-S.D.s limits the control chart will show one value in each 22 as out of control because the limits encompass only 95.4% of all values. A workable compromise is to show limits of 2, 2.5 and 3 S.D.s on the charts and to regard the occurrence of a value between the 2- and 2.5-S.D. lines as a warning to investigate immediately the procedure concerned.

SAMPLE IDENTIFICATION

A computer-controlled, high-output automatic analyzer is merely an expensive ornament unless it is supplied with the correct samples from the correct patients, taken at the correct time and handled in a correct fashion. The types of error, excluding actual analytical mistakes, include:

1. Clerical errors in identification of patient and tests required.

2. Sample-labeling errors.

3. Sample type errors (e.g., serum or plasma) and use of wrong anticoagulant.

4. Sample condition errors (hemolysis; lipemia from nonfasting samples; changes due to excessive use of tourniquet, contamination with IV fluids or remnants of previously administered substances, such as xylose or bromsulphthalein dye). Overlong pressure from a tourniquet can give false elevations of total protein and calcium values.

5. Failure to maintain unequivocal continuity of identification between blood sample, serum or plasma derived therefrom, analyzer sample cup or spectrophotometer cuvette, analyzer chart or printed result, or reported result and the original patient from whom the test was requested.

A wide variety of patient identification systems and corresponding sample identification methods are in use, and the student must be fully aware of their use. Whatever the system used, it is the direct responsibility of the technologist or IV team member to match the name on the test requisition and specimen label with the identification on the patient. A verbal identification by a member of the nursing staff, another patient, or anyone else should *never* be accepted, except in emergency, when an unidentified casualty or unconscious person may require urgent laboratory work. Any such temporary identification should be replaced by positive information as soon as possible: "John Doe" is merely an expression of ignorance. This requirement for maintenance of continuity of identification extends to such simple points as direct comparison of blood sample tube and serum tube before actual transfer of serum, inclusion of water cups or known controls at regular intervals in sample trays for automated equipment to permit certain identification of results on printer read-outs, and special attention to unusual sources of error such as patients with the same or closely similar names.

SERUM AND PLASMA SEPARATION

Ideally, the sample used for analysis should reflect as accurately as possible the composition of the blood before removal from the vein or artery. The widespread introduction of automatic analyzers and the universal trend to "miniaturization" to permit more tests on smaller sample volumes have imposed more stringent conditions on the quality of the samples. The adverse effects of hemolysis, turbidity, incomplete coagulation, and imperfect preservation must be minimized. The methods employed to achieve this include:

1. Improvements in venipuncture technique and equipment.
2. The use of plastic bead or silicone gel barriers to separate clot from serum and permit easy transfer.
3. The increasing use of plasma obtained with such noninterfering anticoagulants as lithium heparin.
4. The use of serum-clarifying filter devices.
5. The use of glucose-preserving compounds such as lithium iodoacetate, which do not interfere with sensitive enzymatic methods for plasma or serum urea nitrogen.

No matter which system is used, excessive trauma to the blood specimen by such things as overvigorous "ringing" of the clot in clotted samples or overlong exposure of the specimen to high ambient temperatures must be avoided. Serum or plasma should not be allowed to remain in contact with the clot or cells for longer than 30 minutes: potassium levels can be erroneously increased by as much as 2 to 8 millimoles per liter without visible hemolysis, even in the refrigerator. Glucose values in quickly separated plasma or serum will remain stable under refrigeration for at least four hours: losses on the order of 10% per hour can occur in plasma left in contact with cells at room temperature. Samples for serum or plasma hormone analyses may require even more stringent handling, such as immediate freezing. The student should be aware of any special requirements for serum or plasma handling as detailed in test methodologies.

One special problem that has been reported in the operation of automated analyzers is interference with fluid movement in fine-bore peristaltic pump tubing from traces of silicone gel barriers. It would seem that even after apparently adequate centrifugation, very small particles of the barrier gel may remain in the separated serum or plasma and that these remnants adhere to tubing walls. The only effective actions are increase of centrifugation speed and time or use of another serum-plasma separating agent.

The process of serum separation affords an opportunity for the exercise of alert observation. In addition to noting sera with severe hemolysis and lipemia because of the analytical problems and errors they may cause, the technologist should note sera of unusual color. Dark brown serum may indicate intravascular hemolysis with the formation of methemalbumin; this may occur in severe sepsis, hemolytic crisis of sickle cell anemia, and paroxysmal nocturnal hemoglobinuria. Dark green serum often indicates the presence of biliverdin; this may arise from the rupture of bile cysts in the liver in patients with severe obstructive jaundice. The observation is useful because biliverdin does not react with the diazo reagent, and hence the result of a bilirubin assay may appear falsely low. The appearance of turbidity in a serum sample that was clear when first separated may indicate the presence of cryoglobulins, although this phenomenon is more usually noted after the serum has been refrigerated. A serum sample that appears more viscous than normal should be checked for paraprotein; in some cases of multiple myeloma, the serum protein level may rise as high as 13.0 g per dL, and this will produce a discernible change in the serum. A serum sample that shows fibrin threads after separation may have come from a patient treated with heparin or other anticoagulant drugs, which will delay the clotting process. A rare cause of a brown tint in the serum is the presence of myoglobin following major muscle injury or myositis. A serum that appears more brightly yellow than normal may contain drugs such as vitamin preparations. The sera from women taking one of the wide variety of contraceptive pills may have a green tint caused by increased ceruloplasmin levels. Jaundiced sera should be handled with special care to minimize the risk of hepatitis (see p. 17). If the yield of serum after centrifuging is unduly small, the patient may have hemoconcentration, and a determination of osmolality would provide useful clinical information. Another possibility in like circumstances is polycythemia. The technologist who observes such significant changes and alerts other departments of the laboratory, for example, hematology, may accelerate the diagnostic process.

THE INTERNATIONAL SYSTEM OF UNITS (LE SYSTEME INTERNATIONAL D'UNITES)*

At a series of General Conferences of the International Bureau of Weights and Measures from 1954 to 1971, a new system for definition and measurement of fundamental physical units was developed. The so-called CGS system, based on the centimeter, gram, and second, was an earlier attempt in this direction, but it was only coherent for length, mass, and time. (In this connection, the term *coherent* means "internally consistent" or "rational.") In the CGS system, compound terms could be derived by combinations of the basic units; the unit of force, the dyne, was defined as that force which would change the velocity of a mass of one gram by one centimeter per second in one second. The SI system extends the definitions of its basic units to embrace all physical measurements and includes modifying prefixes and rules by which further units may be formed for any scientific and commercial need. The SI system is legally established in a number of countries, and its extension to the rest is only a matter of time and agreement. Apart from the inevitable problems, political as well as technical, in converting to a new system, some areas of particular difficulty are recognized.

Definitions of the Basic SI Units

METER. The meter is the length equal to 1 650 763.73 wavelengths in a vacuum of the radiation corresponding to the transition between the levels $2p_{10}$ and $5d_5$ of the krypton-86 atom (symbol m). (There has been a recent proposal to redefine the meter as the distance traveled by light in a vacuum in 1/299 792 458 of a second.)

KILOGRAM. The kilogram is the unit of mass, equal to the mass of the international prototype of the kilogram (symbol kg).

SECOND. The second is the duration of 9 192 631 770 periods of the radiation corresponding to the transition between the two hyperfine levels of the ground state of the caesium-133 atom (symbol s).

AMPERE. The ampere is that constant current which, if maintained in two straight parallel conductors of infinite length and of negligible circular cross-section, and placed one meter apart in a vacuum, would produce between these conductors a force equal to 2×10^{-7} newton per meter of length (symbol A).

KELVIN. The kelvin, the unit of thermodynamic temperature, is 1/273.16 of the thermodynamic temperature of the triple point of water (symbol K).

CANDELA. The candela is the luminous intensity, in the perpendicular direction, of a surface of 1/600 000 square meter of a blackbody at the temperature of freezing platinum under a pressure of 101 325 newtons per square meter (symbol cd).

MOLE. The mole is the amount of substance of a system that contains as many elementary units as there are carbon atoms in 12 grams of carbon 12 (symbol mol).

Comments on the Units

With the exception of the kilogram, all the above units are independent of any kind of arbitrary standard; they are based on unchanging, observable phenomena that can be checked or redetermined at any time. The kelvin is equal in magnitude to the degree Celsius, which seems likely to remain in use for purposes other than thermodynamics. The definition of the mole reflects the statement that the number of atoms in a mole of an element is equal to Avogadro's number, 6.0228×10^{23}, and that the differences in atomic and molar weights result from different weights of the constituent atoms. A mole of hydrogen and a mole of uranium contain the same *number* of atoms; the uranium atom is 238.03 times as heavy as the hydrogen atom. It should be noted that in the definitions of the meter and the second, spaces are substituted for the commas; thus, 1 650 763.73 is used for 1,650,763.73. This change accommodates the general European practice of using a comma to indicate the decimal point and is intended to prevent confusion. The North American use of a period to indicate the decimal point, either on the line or at half a character height above it, may be replaced by the use of the comma. In the present period of transition to SI units, this is but one of many minor points yet to be settled.

Derived Units

A wide variety of compound units can be derived from the basic units by simple combination and algebraic manipulation. The formal SI unit of concentration is moles per cubic meter (mol/m^3) although, as we shall discuss later, this is impractical for most biological measurements. Chemical reaction rates can be stated in moles per second (mol/s). Events such as emission of particles from a radioactive atom can be stated in the unit s^{-1}, that is, the number per second. This unit is an example of one that is used so frequently that it has been assigned a special name and symbol: hertz, symbol Hz. It is this property of the SI system, the ability to derive units by simple combinations of the basic set without use of factors, that makes it a coherent system. The other derived units with special names are listed in Table 3–5.

TABLE 3–5 DERIVED UNITS WITH SPECIAL NAMES

Name	Symbol	Formation from Basic Units	Quantity Measured
hertz	Hz	s^{-1}	frequency
newton	N	$m.kg.s^{-2}$	force
pascal	Pa	$m^{-1}.kg.s^{-2}$	pressure
joule	J	$m^2.kg.s^{-2}$	energy, heat
watt	W	$m^2.kg.s^{-3}$	power

*Sources for the following description of the SI system are:

Lansley, T. S. Everyone's Guide to SI. The Gazette of the Institute of Medical Laboratory Technology, August, 1971.

The Royal College of Pathologists of Australia and The Australian Association of Clinical Biochemists. Broadsheet No. 14. October, 1973.

The Royal Society of Medicine. Units, Symbols and Abbreviations. A Guide for Biological and Medical Editors and Authors. London, 1971.

Lippert, H. and Lehmann, H. P. SI Units in Medicine. Urban and Schwarzenberg, Baltimore, 1978. Recommended as an excellent description of the system and an exhaustive compilation of conversion tables.

The origin of the complex terms in Table 3–5 can be made somewhat clearer if they are dissected. The unit of force, the newton, combines the unit of length or distance, the meter, with the unit of mass, the kilogram, and the term "s^{-2}," which can be read as "per second per second." Thus the newton is that amount of force which will increase the speed of a one-kilogram mass by one meter per second within the space of one second. If this force of one newton is applied over an area of one square meter, this produces a pressure of one pascal; that is, one pascal is one newton per square meter. If we divide the basic units formula for the newton by m^2, we obtain the basic unit definition of the pascal:

$$\frac{m.kg.s^{-2}}{m^2} = m^{-1}.kg.s^{-2}$$

In actual usage, the pascal is inconveniently small, and the kilopascal (symbol kPa) is used.

The new unit of energy or heat, the joule, is derived from the product of force times distance. This can be visualized as a force of one newton acting with a "leverage" of one meter. The use of the joule as a unit of heat stems from the demonstration by James Prescott Joule that there is a direct relationship between heat and mechanical work. The main significance of the joule in clinical laboratory medicine is its replacement of the calorie in calculations of metabolism and energy changes in reactions.

The set of SI units is completed by the unit of angle, the radian (2π radians = 360°), and the unit of three-dimensional or solid angle, the steradian, which is used in statements of intensity of energy emitted from a source.

Prefixes

By the use of suitable prefixes an extremely wide range of multiples and subdivisions of SI units can be produced. For example, in units of length we need to cover a range from atomic diameters to planetary orbits. Table 3–6 lists the approved prefixes.

Some "old" units, because of wide usage and acceptance, are retained in the SI system. The liter as a unit of volume is more convenient for many biological purposes than the cubic meter; it is redefined as equal to one cubic decimeter. The former definition of the liter as the volume occupied by one kg of water at its point of maximum density is no longer valid. As already noted, the degree Celsius is retained for expressing temperatures; it is simply more convenient for most purposes than the kelvin. New units have been proposed for expressing radioactivity. The curie (symbol Ci), equal to the amount of radioactive material that produces 3.7×10^{10} disintegrations per second, is replaced by the becquerel (symbol Bq), which is a simple statement of the number of such disintegrations per second. Thus, the microcurie of 3.7×10^4, or 37,000, disintegrations per second is replaced by 37 kilobecquerels (37 kBq). The new unit of radiation dose, replacing the rad, is the gray (symbol Gy), defined as the transmission of energy at the rate of one joule per kilogram of tissue. (The rad corresponded to 10^{-2} J/kg.) The measure of ion dose, the roentgen, is replaced by a statement of coulombs per kilogram. This "unit" does not have a special name.

TABLE 3–6 Prefixes for Use With SI Units

Factor	Prefix	Symbol
10^{12}	tera-	T
10^9	giga-	G
10^6	mega-	M
10^3	kilo-	k
10^2	hecto-	h
10^1	deka-	da
10^{-1}	deci-	d
10^{-2}	centi-	c
10^{-3}	milli-	m
10^{-6}	micro-	μ
10^{-9}	nano-	n
10^{-12}	pico-	p
10^{-15}	femto-	f
10^{-18}	atto-	a

As with any language, there are rules of grammar for the SI system:

1. When a prefix is used (see Table 3–6) to indicate a multiple or subdivision of a basic unit, the combination is written as one term. One thousandth of a meter = one millimeter (abbreviation mm); one thousand grams = one kilogram (abbreviation kg).
2. Unit symbols keep the same form whether singular or plural: one centimeter = 1 cm; ten centimeters = 10 cm. The abbreviation is followed by a period only if it concludes a sentence.
3. If a combination of prefix and basic unit is raised to a power, it is regarded as a complete symbol. Thus cm^3 = centimeter cubed, not one hundredth (10^{-2}) of a cubic meter (m^3).
4. When a combination of a number and a basic SI unit is written, it is preferable to include a suitable SI prefix so that the associated numerical value falls within a convenient range. "Convenient" in this context means having a compact form with not more than four figures.

Examples. 17,100 g—preferred form 17.1 kg; 0.0045 m—preferred form 4.5 mm; 0.000074 mg—preferred form 74 ng.

5. When a unit involves the type of expression "units per unit" (for example, milliliters per second for creatinine clearance), two alternatives are recognized. In the example, these could be mL/s or $mL.s^{-1}$. If three units are involved, the solidus (/) is used only once. The International Unit for reporting enzyme activity (micromoles of substrate converted per minute per liter of sample) becomes in SI units μmol/min L or μmol min^{-1} L^{-1}.
6. It will be noted that some basic and special SI units have capitalized symbols, for example, A (ampere) and K (kelvin). This prevents possible confusion with SI prefixes: a for atto- = 10^{-18} and k for kilo- = 10^3.
7. The unit of concentration, mg/dL (milligrams per deciliter), does not conform to SI nomenclature, since this precludes the use of prefixes elsewhere than in the numerator. (The kilogram is an exception to this rule because it is a basic unit of the SI system.) The form mg/dL should be replaced either by mg/L or by the proposed new unit of concentration, mmol/L (millimoles per liter). (See below under "Application of SI Units to Clinical Medicine.")
8. Such dubious compound units as "millimicrons" for

wavelength and "micromicrograms" for erythrocyte hemoglobin content are barred; the correct prefix should be substituted. For wavelengths, nanometers (abbreviation nm = 10^{-9}m) are used; for a millionth of a millionth of a gram, picogram (abbreviation pg = 10^{-12} g) is used.

APPLICATION OF SI UNITS TO CLINICAL MEDICINE

This section is being written during a period of transition. In some countries, the SI system is not only officially recognized but is in varying degrees of practical usage. Outside Europe, a notable example of active progress toward implementation in the medical field is Australia. In many cases scientific journals require strict adherence to the system in submitted papers. It is inevitable that the speed and completeness of conversion to SI units will depend on local initiative, and the process is bound to be uneven. The problems indicated below are largely technical and semantic and the suggested solutions, tentative.

Units of Concentration: General and Special Problems

As noted above, the strict SI system uses the cubic meter as the unit of volume, and hence strict protocol would require kilograms per cubic meter as units of concentration. In biological work, however, this unit is too unwieldy. In addition, if concentrations are expressed in moles, many important interrelationships become more apparent. Similarly, the substitution of the liter makes the unit more easily applicable to physiology and biochemistry. For many substances routinely determined in serum and urine, millimoles per liter (mmol/L) is a convenient mode of expression. For the univalent electrolytes such as sodium, potassium, and chloride, the new unit is numerically equal to milliequivalents per liter, and the conversion would go almost unnoticed. It is mathematically simple to convert mg per dL into mmol per L or μmol per L; the problems arise in the administrative and educational aspects of any conversion scheme. The list of conversion factors in Table 3–7 includes tentative "significant change" values. It covers routine procedures only; the conversion factors are also given with the individual methodologies.

Some special problems arise. When the substance being determined is actually a mixture, it is not possible to use the mole as a basis. For example, serum proteins will be reported in grams, but per liter rather than per dL.

As usual, enzyme units pose a special problem. Until the question of a standard temperature has been settled, any scheme must be tentative. If the International Unit (that amount of enzyme which will catalyze the transformation of one micromole of substrate per minute per liter) is retained, it is readily convertible to the corresponding SI unit of micromoles per second per liter by division by 60, provided that all the conditions of the assay are specified. One proposal creates a new unit, the katal (abbreviation kat), which would be used for all catalytic activities, including enzymatic processes; it is defined as that amount of catalytic activity that produces the transformation of one mole of substrate per second under defined conditions. By this rule, one International Unit would be equal to 16.67 nkat (nanokatals). The katal would appear to be a superfluous creation; Occam's "razor" ("entities should not be multiplied without necessity") remains a useful principle. The same principles apply to substances assayed by indirect methods, such as renin. The error-free transmission of clinical information must be the paramount consideration, and retention of existing units, however arbitrary, is preferable to possibly dangerous confusion and delay.

The Use of SI Units in Hematology

In order to conform to SI units, cell counts should be expressed per liter. The present system for leucocyte counts, thousands (10^3) per microliter (cubic millimeter), translates simply into billions, (10^9), per liter, with the same basic value, that is, $9.5 \times 10^3/\mu L = 9.5 \times 10^9/L$. Red cell counts convert similarly: $4.8 \times 10^6/\mu L = 4.8 \times 10^{12}/L$. Platelet counts are still reported at present as complete numbers without use of exponents, e.g., 340,000/μL (mm^3). If this is converted to exponential notation, it becomes $3.4 \times 10^5/\mu L$. Expressed per liter, this becomes $3.4 \times 10^{11}/L$. Whether this is a better form than $0.34 \times 10^{12}/L$ remains to be decided. It would appear that the implied degree of precision, $0.01 \times 10^{12}/L$, corresponding to 10,000 per mm^3 in current usage, is of the right order. The hematocrit, being a dimensionless number, is not subject to SI rules; it is suggested that its expression as a percentage is not necessary and that

TABLE 3–7 Conversion Factors

Substance	Old Unit	New Unit	Factor	Significant Change Value
Albumin	g/dL	g/L	10	3 g/L
Bilirubin	mg/dL	μmol/L	17.1	5 μmol/L
Cholesterol	mg/dL	mmol/L	0.026	0.5 mmol/L
Creatinine	mg/dL	mmol/L	0.088	0.02 mmol/L
Fibrinogen	g/dL	g/L	10	1 g/L
Glucose	mg/dL	mmol/L	0.056	0.5 mmol/L
Iron	μg/dL	μmol/L	0.179	3.0 μmol/L
Magnesium	mg/dL	mmol/L	0.411	0.1 mmol/L
Phosphate, inorganic	mg/dL	mmol/L	0.323	0.1 mmol/L
PCO_2, PO_2	mm Hg	kPa	0.133	0.5 kPa
Total protein	g/dL	g/L	10	3 g/L
Uric acid	mg/dL	mmol/L	0.06	0.02 mmol/L
Urea nitrogen	mg/dL	mmol/L	0.167	0.5 mmol/L
Calcium	mg/dL	mmol/L	0.25	0.05 mmol/L

the decimal form is adequate. Thus, 44% would be written as 0.44. As an interim measure, it is suggested that hemoglobin be reported as grams per liter; when a definite consensus of opinion emerges among hematologists, the final unit may be millimoles per liter. The conversion involves the fact that each of the four heme units in a molecule of hemoglobin contains an iron atom and carries a molecule of oxygen. Therefore, the functional molecular weight of the molecule from an oxygen-carrying point of view is one-quarter that of the entire molecule. The conversion factor from grams per dL to mmol per L is then 0.621. Thus, 15.6 g/dL = 9.7 mmol/L. One of the debatable issues in determining the consensus mentioned above is this treatment of the molecule. For the red cell parameters, it is convenient to convert the units to SI nomenclature. Mean cell volume in cubic micra becomes femtoliters (fL); mean cell hemoglobin, micromicrograms, becomes picograms (pg); mean cell hemoglobin concentration is converted from grams per dL to grams per liter (g/L). In each case, the numercial value remains the same, apart from that of the last-named item, which increases by a factor of 10.

The Use of SI Units to Express Physical Quantities

Pressure. The change from millimeters of mercury to the SI unit, kilopascals, may have to wait until the practical problems of recalibrating instrument scales have been solved. The conversion factor from mm Hg to kPa is 0.133; thus, a normal P_{CO_2} of 40 mm Hg becomes 40 × 0.133 = 5.32 kPa. The use of mm Hg to report blood pressures seems likely to persist; it is true that the old unit is more manageable than the new, and this factor cannot be legislated out of existence.

Osmolality. Despite its physiological usefulness, this unit is not directly translatable into the SI system, since it combines molar concentration per kg with a factor determined by the number of particles produced by ionization and an activity coefficient that varies with concentration. It appears that a good case could be made for leaving well enough alone and accepting that the osmol and milliosmol express valid information in a useful format.

pH. This is another dimensionless quantity that can be retained. Hydrogen ion concentration could be stated in nanomoles per liter. For example, the calculation for pH 7.4 is:

$$7.4 = \log \frac{1}{[H^+]}$$

Taking antilogs of both sides:

$$\frac{1}{[H^\times]} = 10^{7,4}$$

$$[H^\times] = 10^{-7,4}\ g/L = 10^{-7,4}\ \text{mole per liter}$$

Converting to nanomoles per liter, multiply by 10^9:
$[H^\times] = 10^9 \times 10^{-7.4} = 10^{1.6} = 39.8$ nm/L.

The general formula for calculation of conversion factors is:

$$\text{From mg per dL to mmol per L: } \frac{\text{mg/dL} \times 10 \times 1000}{\text{M.W. in g} \times 1000}$$

$$\text{From } \mu\text{g per dL to } \mu\text{mol per L: } \frac{\mu\text{g/dL} \times 10 \times 10^6}{\text{M.W. in g} \times 10^6}$$

The monovalent electrolytes (sodium, potassium, chloride, and bicarbonate) translate directly into mmol per L without factors, since for these ions 1 mEq per L = 1 mmol per L.

For pressure conversions (Broughton and Sewell, 1970): To convert mm H_2O to Pa (pascals = N/m²): × 9.806; mm Hg to Pa: × 133.322; Atmospheres to kPa: × 101.325; Pounds per sq. in. to kPa: × 6.895; Millibars to Pa: × 100. For energy/heat: kilocalories to kiloJoules (kJ): × 4.187.

CHAPTER 3—REVIEW QUESTIONS

1. Given a list of the quality control results for one test over the period of a month, describe how to calculate the standard deviation and coefficient of variation, how to check the data for outliers, and how to present the data graphically.
2. Sketch a quality control chart and mark thereon sets of points to show a period of acceptable control, a period of excessive random error, a shift, and a trend. Suggest possible reasons for each of the unacceptable sets of values.
3. Describe how to determine the frequency distribution of a large number of items of data, how to present the distribution graphically, and how to determine if that distribution is probably Gaussian.
4. Discuss the special problems of quality control of enzyme determinations.

ANALYTICAL SYSTEMS AND APPLICATIONS

In order to overcome the considerable problems in analyses of biological fluids, the instrumentation and methods of the clinical laboratory make use of all the major analytical principles. The most frequently used procedures involve the interaction of matter and radiation, for example, spectrophotometry, or emission of energy by matter such as flame photometry and radioimmunoassay. The picture is constantly changing; the dramatic growth in the practical application of the last-named technique exemplifies the process. The proliferation of automatic analyzers has proceeded to the point where one is not sure which came first—the considerable increase in laboratory workload or the sophisticated machinery to handle it. In this chapter it is only possible to review the available systems and to indicate briefly their features.

PRIMARY STANDARDS

Three groups of analyses can be recognized: qualitative (Is substance A present?), quantitative (How much substance A is present?), and semiquantitative (Is there enough substance A present to warrant further investigations?). Even with the first category, it is good technique to standardize roughly the quantities of sample and reagents to permit comparisons with previous results.

Some factors are basic to all analyses, regardless of purpose. Chemical cleanliness of apparatus, from the simple test tube to the pumping systems of a complex automatic analyzer, is often considered only when serious loss of precision or accuracy has occurred (see notes on cleaning, p. 73). This concern extends to spectrophotometer cells and cuvettes, since these become part of the optical system of the spectrophotometer (see p. 72). Glassware should be of a grade appropriate to the procedure, especially in ultramicro work. The grade of chemicals should also be suitable for the test in which they are used. This applies particularly to primary standards, for which the following requirements must be met (Young and Mears, 1968):

1. The substance should be readily purified, if possible to the "four nines" level, that is, 99.99% pure, or at least to 99.95% pure.
2. It should not be hygroscopic (tending to absorb atmospheric water) or efflorescent (spontaneously losing water of crystallization).
3. It should be readily soluble.
4. It should have a relatively high equivalent weight.
5. It should not undergo any side reactions or color changes that might interfere with the reaction for which it is the standard.
6. The elements in the substance should be such that disturbances of the natural isotope abundance would not materially affect the molecular weight.
7. It should be preferably nonbasic, completely ionized in solution, and suitable for direct titration. (For examples of primary standards, see Appendix F.)

Purity of Water

Because of the often serious errors that may be introduced in the growing list of critical assays made in the clinical chemistry laboratory (electrolytes, calcium, magnesium, phosphate, iron, enzymes, and trace elements such as zinc) by interfering and unwanted substances in the water used to prepare reagents and make dilutions, the preparation, checking, and storage of water of adequate quality have assumed a much more important role in laboratory practice. In 1976 the College of American Pathologists proposed minimum standards of purity for reagent water, and these are summarized in Table 4–1. To obtain water that satisfies these standards, a variety of systems have been developed.

Distillation. Condensation of the steam produced by vigorous boiling of the water theoretically produces "pure" water, with the impurities remaining in the boiling chamber. In practice, the need to prevent carryover of droplets and volatile impurities and to provide rapid and efficient cooling of the steam has entailed some complexity in the design of the still without leading to a complete solution of the problems. Large amounts of energy are required—several kilowatt-hours per gallon of distillate—as well as large volumes of feed and cooling water. If the feed water is "hard" (that is, contains appreciable amounts of calcium salts), the still requires frequent cleaning. The quality of the product depends on the exact conditions and design of the system.

Ion Exchange. The development of mixed-bed ion-exchange resin columns, which combine both cation- and anion-removing qualities (see p. 99), provides a simple method for production of high-quality water. The columns for producing water of Type I quality (Table 4–1) are costly, and if the feed water is taken directly from

TABLE 4–1 Reagent-Grade Water Standards—College of American Pathologists (CAP)

Property	Type I	Type II	Type III
Conductance:			
micromhos/cm			
maximum (25°C)	0.1	2.0	5.0
Resistivity:			
megohms/cm			
minimum (25°C)	10	0.5	0.2
Silicate:			
mg/L maximum	0.01	0.01	0.01
Heavy metals:			
mg/L maximum	0.01	0.01	0.01

Note: Similar standards have been specified by the American Society for Testing and Materials (ASTM), the American Chemical Society (ACS), the United States Pharmacopia (USP), and the National Committee for Clinical Laboratory Standards (NCCLS). The CAP standards are given here, since they were established with the needs of clinical laboratory analysis in mind. The allowable levels of silicate reflect the difficulty of complete exclusion of this analytically unimportant ion from any system that includes glass tubing or storage vessels.

the domestic supply frequent replacement or regeneration will be required. Ion exchange, as its name implies, will not remove un-ionized organic impurities, and the flow through the column may be impaired by growth of bacteria and fungi. If the ion-exchange system is fed with water that has already been distilled, it will yield high-quality water at a low cost, exceeding in the best case Type I standards.

Carbon Adsorption. One method for removal of organic impurities and also chlorine derived from the chloramine T used to treat domestic water supplies is to pass the water through a column of activated charcoal. This step is usually used as part of a complete system.

Ultra-filtration. Filters made from cellulose acetate or polyamide, with pore sizes as small as 0.1 micrometer, can be used in a water purification system for the initial removal of suspended particulate matter from the feed water and for final "polishing" of the effluent, which may include removal of microorganisms. With use this type of filter tends to become clogged, necessitating either replacement or cleaning, although new designs employing bundles of hollow fibers mitigate this problem.

Reverse Osmosis. With the recent development of semipermeable membranes with sufficient mechanical strength to withstand high pressures in the region of 200 psi (pounds per square inch), equivalent to 1379 kilopascals in the SI system, it is possible to force the feed water through the membrane and remove a large proportion of the impurities, including inorganic ions, most organic compounds, bacteria, and viruses. Some small ions, such as nitrates, are not efficiently removed, and dissolved chlorine derived from chlorination compounds can pass through. The process is most efficiently used as an early stage in a complete water purification system.

Water Purification Systems. It can be seen that a suitable combination of the systems briefly described—using the best features of each—can produce high-quality water at reasonable cost and a good flow rate. A typical system would include a prefilter with a 5 micrometer pore size, a reverse osmosis unit, a combined charcoal and ion-exchange mixed-bed resin column and a final 0.45 micrometer pore size membrane filter to extract bacteria. Such a system (Milli-R/Q Water Purifier*), can produce water of at least CAP Type II quality. A similar system (Milli-Q) using reverse osmosis, a carbon cartridge filter, and two ion-exchange resin units, with a final 0.22 micrometer pore size membrane filter, will deliver water exceeding in purity CAP Type I. Water of this degree of purity will rapidly pick up carbon dioxide and airborne particulate matter in the average laboratory, and its purity, as determined by its specific resistance, will deteriorate. In a modern system the water is continuously recirculated through the chain of membranes and columns to maintain its quality.

Checking the Purity of Water

The standard method for checking the quality of water is to measure its specific resistance, which is defined, in theory, as the electrical resistance measured between opposing faces of a one centimeter water cube. In practice the measurement is made between two platinum electrodes coated with colloidal platinum black, each one square centimeter in area and held a fixed distance apart. (If the distance is not exactly 1 cm, the measuring instrument compensates for this fact.) Alternatively, the conductance of the water under the same conditions can be expressed in micromhos/cm: in the stated units, resistance and conductivity are reciprocals of each other. A specific resistance of 10 megohms/cm equals a conductance of 1/10 or 0.1 micromhos/cm. Absolutely pure water has a specific resistance, calculated from ionization constants and equivalent conductances of the ions, of 23.92 megohms/cm at 20° C and 18.21 megohms/cm at 25° C. The water purification system itself can incorporate a meter calibrated either in resistance or in conductivity or in some cases a simple lamp indicator that is extinguished when the quality of the water falls below a predetermined level. The resistivity meter should be used only for checking the quality of distilled or deionized water: the black colloidal platinum coating on the electrodes will deteriorate if the sensing head is immersed in other solutions, and recoating the electrodes is expensive.

For practical purposes, the absolute minimum grade of water purity for clinical laboratory analyses is CAP Type II, specific resistance 0.5 megohm/cm (Table 4–1), and for all critical analyses, CAP Type I. CAP Type III is suitable for routine rinsing of glassware after washing and for the preparation of noncritical reagents. Glassware used in critical analyses should be rinsed in the appropriate grade of water before use. To illustrate the potential errors from the use of lower grade water, a specific resistance of 0.1 megohm/cm corresponds to a content of dissolved ionized substances of 5.0 ppm. (The unit "ppm," or "parts per million," is an industrial measure: it corresponds to one milligram per million milligrams, or one milligram per liter.) If we assume that one half of the ionized impurities is sodium ion and that the water was used in a flame photometer employing a 1 in 200 dilution of tests and standards, previously

*Millipore Corp., Bedford, Mass. 01730 and Mississauga, Ont. L4V 1M5.

set to zero with CAP Type I water, the error in sodium assays could be as large as 21.7 mEq/L. This level would, in some instruments, exceed the capacity of the zero setting control, and the instrument could not be operated. Similar errors would occur in any assays of inorganic constituents, such as calcium, phosphate, and magnesium, and critical determinations such as those of enzymes could also be affected, especially if the impurities included ions of heavy metals such as lead, copper, and zinc. A source of imprecision in assays using antibodies as reagents, such as radioimmunoassays, is bacterial contamination, providing another reason for the incorporation of membrane filters of very small pore size in water purification systems.

THE ANALYTICAL BALANCE

The modern single-pan analytical balance is capable of the most precise and accurate measurements available to the laboratory analyst. The usual precision of ±0.1 mg in a total load of 100 g corresponds to 1 ppm, permitting the preparation of standard solutions whose accuracy is at least 100 times better than that of the actual method of analysis. To make use of this quality, the balance should be located, ideally, in an air-conditioned room where temperature and humidity variations are at a minimum and where it is protected from drafts, direct sunlight, heat, and corrosive fumes. The support must be solid, and its construction should be massive enough to damp out any external vibration. In some situations it is helpful to locate the balance on a vibration-damping base.

The following general precautions are important for the best performance of the balance:

1. Do not shake or jar the beam, pan support, or case.
2. Weigh with the balance doors closed, except when actually adding or removing material.
3. Hot objects such as evaporating dishes and oven-dried chemicals should be allowed to cool in a desiccator before weighing.
4. Always use weighing bottles or plastic weighing boats; nothing should be placed on the pan that might cause corrosion.
5. Check the leveling before use.
6. Return all internal weights to zero after use.
7. Do not overload the balance; for a stated capacity of 160 g, do not exceed 100 g.
8. Avoid weighing powdered stains or dyes; even the slightest spillage of such materials will contaminate the inside of the case, and effective cleaning is difficult.
9. Keep a large camel's-hair brush close to the balance for removal of spills inside the case. From time to time, wash the brush in warm water and detergent, rinse, and dry with a hot air-stream.
10. If separate weights are used, handle them only with bone- or plastic-tipped forceps, never with the fingers; perspiration is acid and will cause corrosion.

Top-Pan Balance. (Also called top-loading balance.) A convenient balance for weighing out chemicals for bulk reagent preparation is a top-pan balance with taring (preset subtraction of the weight of the weighing boat) and optical scale for subdivisions of grams. A useful size is 1 kg maximum, sensitive to ± 10 mg. The type with a close-fitting plastic cover to protect the mechanism from accidental spills is recommended.

Ultramicro Balance. The standard type of analytical balance using the beam principle is limited in sensitivity by the mechanical elements of its design. In order to make accurate weighings down to the microgram level, balances using a different principle have been devised. The ultramicro balance will weigh up to 1.0 g ± 0.1 microgram or up to 2.5 g ± 1.0 microgram, using electrical detection of the deflection of the balance beam as the load is applied: no weights are used.

Gravimetric analysis, in which a substance is extracted from the original specimen with solvents or precipitated as an insoluble salt and then quantified by direct weighing, is little used in clinical analysis because of its time-consuming nature and requirement for a large sample. It is still used for assay of total fecal lipids.

Volumetric analysis, in which the concentration of an ion in a solution is measured by determining the volume of a solution of known concentration with which it will react in a detectable manner, is used for preparation of standard solutions and in a few analytical methods such as estimation of free hydrochloric acid in gastric fluids. (For preparation of standard solutions, see Appendix F.)

MEASUREMENT OF HYDROGEN ION CONCENTRATION—THE pH METER

Glass may be regarded as a combination of negatively charged silicate ions and a variety of small positively charged ions such as sodium. Small positive ions can enter the glass by displacing sodium ions, but negative ions are repulsed. Because of this and other features of its molecular structure, a very thin (about 0.1 mm) sheet of glass can be penetrated almost exclusively by hydrogen ions. When hydrogen ions are thus adsorbed at one surface of the glass, the impermeability of the glass to negative ions results in a net difference of electrical charge between the two surfaces of the glass, and the size of this difference of electrical charge, the potential, is related to the hydrogen ion concentrations in the solutions on either side of the glass sheet.

If the thin glass is formed into a bulb (usually filled with 1 M hydrochloric acid) containing an electrode and connected by a conducting solution (usually potassium chloride) to a reference cell of which the voltage is exactly known, by suitable electronic means the potential developed across the glass bulb by reason of the hydrogen ion concentration of the solution into which it dips can be compared with the known potential. (The electrical resistance of the glass bulb is very high, and the cell current has to be amplified enough to operate a meter; most of the internal details of a pH meter consists of the necessary stable and precise amplifier circuits.) The reference cell most commonly used is the calomel cell, which contains calomel (mercurous chloride) in contact with metallic mercury. The solution is saturated with potassium chloride, since the potential developed by the calomel cell depends on chloride ion activity, and by keeping this at saturation point, the chloride effect is kept constant.

In order to use the combination of the glass-bulb

electrode and the associated calomel cell as a pH meter, the electrical potential of the calomel cell has to be exactly known. This has been determined experimentally by reference to a cell made from a platinized platinum gauze over which hydrogen gas is flowing. To this cell the electrical potential of zero has been assigned, and other cells such as the calomel cell are assigned electrical potentials as determined by comparison with the platinum-hydrogen cell. Thus the calomel cell with saturated potassium chloride is rated at + 0.2458 volt at 25°C.

So far, we have assembled a system that will measure the *difference* in potential between a glass-bulb electrode dipped in a solution containing hydrogen ions and a calomel cell. In order to convert this potential difference to a hydrogen ion concentration value, i.e., to a pH value, we need a solution of known pH that can be used to relate the measured potential difference to actual hydrogen ion concentration. The determination has been made for several primary standards, particularly potassium hydrogen phthalate, by measurements based on ionization constants plus some assumptions. Thus when we "standardize" a pH meter, we are assigning to a particular potential difference developed between the glass electrode and the calomel cell a pH value shown on a bottle of "standard" whose value has been determined by comparison with one of the primary pH standard buffers, whose value in turn has been determined by a process involving several assumptions. The precision of our pH measurements is determined largely by the quality of the instruments; their accuracy depends on the care with which the calibrating buffer was checked against the primary standard buffer. The National Bureau of Standards assigns a pH value of 4.01 to a 0.05 M potassium-hydrogen-phthalate solution at 25°C, pH 4.03 at 40°C, and pH 4.06 at 50°C. For a solution that is 0.025 M with respect to potassium dihydrogen phosphate (anhydrous) and disodium hydrogen phosphate (anhydrous) (KH_2PO_4 and Na_2HPO_4), the assigned values are pH 6.88 at 20°C, 6.84 at 40°C, and 6.83 at 50°C.

The potential difference between the glass-bulb electrode and the calomel half-cell, often loosely called the "reference electrode," includes small potentials developed at liquid junctions plus what is called the "asymmetry" potential, caused by variation of the structure of the glass bulb resulting from the manufacturing process. At constant temperature these small potentials are constant, and provided the buffer used for calibration of the pH meter has the same temperature as any solutions tested, they introduce no errors. The calomel reference cell will have its stated potential value, provided the contact between its calomel and mercury components is intact and its solution content is kept saturated with potassium chloride. Most reference cells have some means of making effective electrical connection with the solution under test, which at the same time minimizes dilution and contamination of the potassium chloride solution. Early pH meters used agar gels made with potassium chloride solutions; modern instruments employ various forms of porous plugs or fibrous tufts, which serve the same purpose.

One limitation of the glass-electrode pH meter is the so-called sodium error. In alkaline solutions above about pH 10, a high concentration of sodium ions will permit the displacement of hydrogen ions from the glass by sodium ions. The net result is that the indicated pH is less than the true value. When working at these high pH values, one must use either a correction derived from a nomogram (relating scale reading, sodium ion concentration, temperature, and correction necessary) or a special glass electrode whose composition minimizes the sodium error. Theoretical study of the effect of the composition of the glass on the susceptibility of the electrode to cations other than hydrogen ions has led to the development of electrodes that can be used to measure the concentrations of sodium, potassium, calcium and other cations, and anions such as chloride.

These ion-selective electrodes (ISEs) take advantage of several principles. In addition to the formulation of special glasses that favor the entry of a particular ion, and hence its measurement, and that are mainly used for cations, solid state and impregnated membrane electrodes have been developed. These consist basically of a slightly soluble salt made with the anion to be determined (sulfide, bromide, chloride, or iodide), which has been fixed in a synthetic rubber matrix. When immersed in a solution of the particular anion, a process of ionic entry into the membrane and measurement of the resultant potential similar to that of the pH electrode occurs. For potassium ions, knowledge of the influence of valinomycin-type antibiotics on the transport of potassium across mitochondrial membranes has been used to develop electrodes incorporating the antibiotic, which have a selectivity for potassium over other cations of the order of 10,000 to 1. Use of sodium- and potassium-selective electrodes and microprocessor-controlled sample pumping systems has greatly facilitated complete automation of the assay of these two electrolytes.

Comparison of Serum Electrolyte Assays Using Flame Photometry and ISEs

A careful distinction should be made between the flame photometer, which determines the concentration of sodium and potassium in serum or plasma after high dilution (typically 1 in 200), and the two modes of the ISEs. (In one mode the determination is made directly on the undiluted sample; in the other there is considerable predilution.) The three methods differ in the extent to which their results are affected by increased levels of lipids and proteins in the sample.

In the serum/plasma sample the electrolytes are dissolved in the water content and are largely excluded from the lipid content because of their insolubility therein. The standards used to calibrate the flame photometer do not include lipids or proteins. If the autodilutor is set to a dilution ratio of 1 in 200, this ratio will be exactly mirrored in the true concentrations of the electrolytes in the standard solution as delivered to the flame. Thus if the standard sodium content was 140 mEq/L, the actual level reaching the flame would be 140/200 = 0.7 mEq/L. If the serum sample contains 1.0% of lipids *by volume,* the electrolytes will be confined to the remaining 99% of serum water. Thus what appears to be a 1 in 200 dilution of serum is really

$$\frac{0.99 \text{ (True serum water proportion)} + 199 \text{ (diluent)}}{0.99 \text{ (True serum water)}} = \text{(1 in) } 202$$

Therefore the serum sample has been more highly diluted than the standard, and if the sodium concentration in the serum sample was originally 140 mEq/L, it will be underestimated in the ratio of 200/202 and will give a result of 200/202 × 140 = 138.6 mEq/L. (Potassium results will be affected to the same extent.) It will be apparent that the error will be clinically significant only when serum or plasma lipid levels are greatly elevated. In a severely lipemic serum, the volume occupied by the lipids may approach 5%, and the resulting error in the dilution ratio can make a serum sodium of 140 mEq/L read out as 133.3 mEq/L.

If the ion-selective analytical system employs high dilution, errors of similar magnitude from lipemia may be expected. Instruments such as the NOVA series,* which use direct contact between the electrode and the undiluted sample, are not affected by the lipid and protein content of the serum or plasma and measure the electrolytes directly on the serum or plasma water. This reflects the physiological action of the electrolytes in their influence on fluid balance through the osmotic pressure differences across cell membranes. The effect of serum/plasma protein levels on electrolyte assay results is less than that of lipids, because the proteins are partially soluble in serum/plasma water. However, in patients with multiple myeloma, in whom serum/plasma protein levels may be as high as 12 to 13 g/dL, the values for sodium and potassium will be erroneously reduced; it would appear that the correct results would be obtainable only by use of a direct ISE system.

It should be noted that these electrodes measure the *activity* of the ion rather than the *concentration;* for potassium, the difference in serum is very small, but for calcium in serum, about half of which is complexed with protein and citrate, the ISE measures only the ionized fraction. The electrode for calcium is made with an ion exchanger, the calcium salt of didecyl phosphoric acid dissolved in didecylphenyl phosphonate, separated from the test solution by a membrane permeable to small ions. The entry of calcium ions from the sample into the ion exchanger produces the measured potential, which is converted into calcium ion concentrations by reference to suitable standards. The theoretical response of the electrode can be calculated, but actual response is affected by a variety of factors. At present, ISEs are available for bromide, cadmium, calcium, chloride, cupric ion, cyanide, fluoride, fluoroborate, iodide, lead, nitrate, perchlorate, silver, sulfide, potassium, and sodium.†

Use of the pH Meter

In addition to the operating instructions provided by the manufacturer of the particular instrument, some general points should be noted:

1. A new glass electrode should be conditioned by soaking in a pH 7.0 buffer for several hours and thereafter kept in pH 7.0 buffer between measurements. The glass bulb is easily scratched and should be handled gently, as a scratched bulb will often result in severe instability of readings. Avoid using the standard glass electrode at pH values above 10.0. Do not use the standard glass electrode above its stated temperature range. Rinse the electrode thoroughly after use.
2. The calomel reference electrode should be kept capped when not in use. The porous plug should be kept scrupulously clean. Maintain the potassium chloride solution level as recommended by the manufacturer and ensure that a small amount of solid crystalline KCl is always present. If the solid KCl content is allowed to become too great, gaps that may interfere with electrical contact may develop. The excess KCl can usually be gently loosened (with a fine plastic probe inserted through the filling hole) and shaken out, and the level of saturated KCl re-established.
3. The pH meter should be standardized at the temperature at which it is to be used. If it is an expanded scale instrument and the measurements are to be made on this range, standardize with expansion. Many modern pH meters have excellent electronic stability, so a single standardization will suffice for a large batch of measurements. The pH of the standardizing buffer, an aliquot of which must be poured from the bottle and discarded after use, should be within ± 1.0 pH unit of the measurement range expected. Especially when measuring pH of very dilute or weakly buffered solutions, rinse the electrodes thoroughly after standardization.
4. If the pH meter is being used for titrations such as the titration of gastric fluids to pH 7.0, arrange the magnetic stirrer "flea" to prevent damage to the electrodes. Accidental damage to the electrodes can be reduced by making plastic "beakers" by cutting off and discarding the top halves of small plastic bottles.

One symptom of deterioration of one or of both the electrodes is a loss of linearity. If the pH meter is standardized with a buffer of pH 8.0, it should give the value of a buffer of pH 5.0 within ± 0.05 pH unit. Substitution of each electrode in turn with spares whose linearity is known to be good will locate the offender. If moderate to marked instability of the readings is encountered, before embarking on a trouble-shooting search, check if the operator is wearing a synthetic fabric uniform or lab coat. In conditions of low humidity, static charge accumulation on such garments can cause erratic operation. If the instrument has a grounding terminal, connection of this to a suitable ground will often reduce the instability. The majority of pH meters of recent date are grounded via the power plug and electrical outlet, but the grounding system may not be adequate. The hospital electrician will check this on request.

ELECTROCHEMICAL METHODS

In addition to pH measurement and the use of ISEs, there are other procedures that use the electrical activity associated with chemical change to measure the concentration of one of the reactants. The type of electrical activity measured may be voltage or current. In this context, the positive electrode, the anode, is regarded as the site of oxidation, and the negative electrode, the cathode, as the site of reduction. Some examples are given below.

pH End Point. When titrating such fluids as gastric contents, which may contain both strongly and feebly

*NOVA Biomedical, Inc., Newton, Mass. 02164.
†Orion Research, Inc., Cambridge, Mass. 02139.

ionized acids, it is possible to determine the strongly ionized hydrochloric acid by using the pH meter to detect the end point (see p. 65).

Coulometric Titration. Strictly speaking, coulometry involves the measurement of the quantity of electricity by such means as determining the weight of a metal plated to an electrode from a solution by the passage of a known current for a known time. This is based on the relationship that 96,494 coulombs (one coulomb = a current of 1 ampere per second) will deposit one gram equivalent weight of a metal on an electrode. (The quantity 96,494 coulombs is called one faraday.) For laboratory work, coulometric titration involves the production of a titrating ion by the passage of a constant current through suitable electrodes. This is the method used to produce silver ions for the estimation of chloride in the Cotlove titrator. Since the silver ions are produced at a constant rate, the time taken for complete reaction with the chloride ions present will be directly related to the concentration of chloride. The completion of the reaction is shown by the release of free silver ions, which is detected amperometrically, that is, by a sharp increase in current flow in the reaction mixture. The change is used to trigger a relay and to stop a timing device. Comparison with the titration time of a standard permits calculation of the chloride content of the sample. In later versions of the instrument the calculation is made automatically, giving direct read-out of chloride in milliequivalents per liter. The titrating mixture contains nitric acid for good conductivity, acetic acid to enhance precipitation of the silver chloride formed, and gelatin to equalize the reaction rate over the electrode surface.

SPECTROPHOTOMETRY—BASIC PRINCIPLES

Photometry is the measurement of the intensity of light under specified conditions, as in the light meters used in photography. Spectrophotometry investigates the *pattern* of absorption of light energy by a substance, that is, which sections of the available range of wavelengths are most strongly absorbed and which can be used as a means of identification. Thus bilirubin absorbs light strongly at 455 nm; oxyhemoglobin absorbs light strongly at 540 and 578 nm. For analytical purposes, we are interested in the *extent* of absorption of light energy by solutions of the same compound in known and unknown concentrations under identical conditions, which can be used to determine the unknown concentration. In this discussion, the term *light energy* refers to electromagnetic radiation with wavelengths in the range from about 200 nm to about 1000 nm. The term *visible light* indicates the range typically detected by the human eye, from about 400 nm to about 700 nm. The wavelengths below 400 nm are referred to as *ultraviolet,* those above 700 nm as *infrared.* The apparently anomalous use of the prefixes *ultra,* meaning "above" or "beyond," and *infra,* meaning "below," arises from their original application to the frequency of the radiation (the number of cycles per second) rather than to the wavelength (the distance covered by one complete cycle of the radiation). See Figure 4–1.

Light energy of a single wavelength is called "monochromatic light," but the only sources that approach this in quality are the hollow cathode lamp and the laser, both of which are now being employed in spectrophotometers. In most laboratory spectrophotometers the width of the "slice" of the spectrum of energies that can be isolated is determined by the design, and is usually defined by the term *band pass* or *band width.* Strictly speaking, the terms are not synonymous. *Band width* (more correctly, "spectral band width") refers to the range of wavelengths issuing from the exit slit of a monochromator with a monochromatic light source, and it is an indication of the quality of the monochromator. *Band pass* refers to the width of the slice of the spectrum that passes through the sample: it is determined by the shape of the absorbance curve plotted against wavelength and is defined as the width at the absorbance values half way to the peak absorbance (Fig. 4–2). In practice, it is specified that in order to obtain theoretic absorbance values for a pure colored substance in solution, the spectral band width of the *instrument* should be no greater than one-tenth of the *band pass* of the substance (American Society of Clinical Pathologists). Thus, when the course of an enzyme reaction is being followed by the change in the absorbance of NADH at

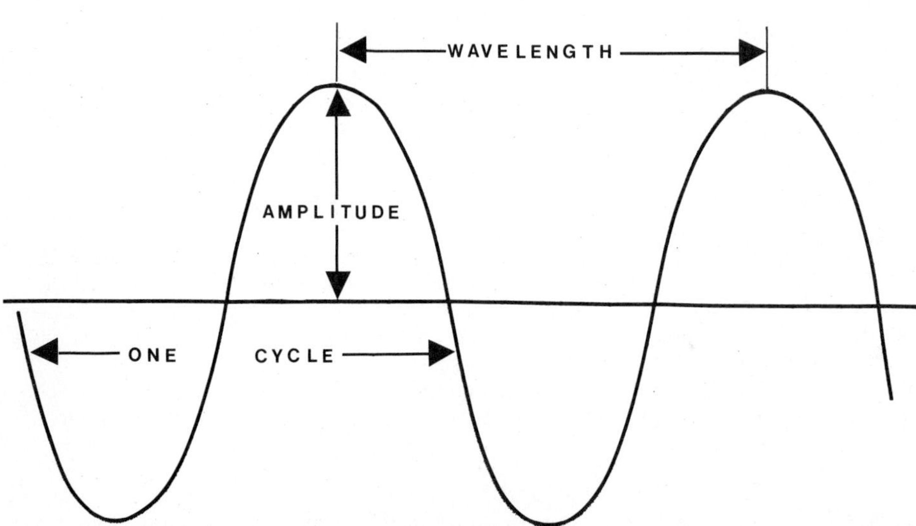

Figure 4–1 Terms used to describe the characteristics of radiant energy.

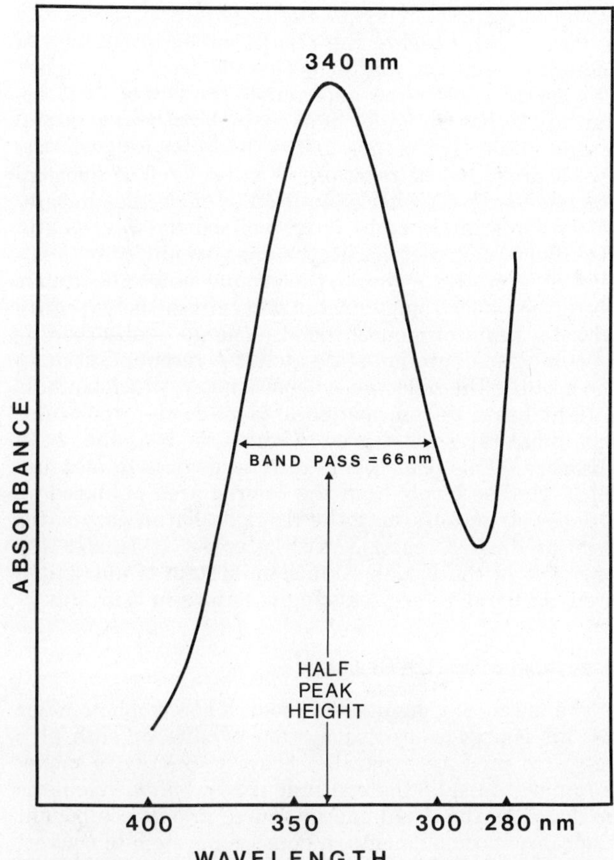

Figure 4–2 Spectrophotometric "scan" of NADH showing determination of spectral band pass.

340 nm and the method is standardized by reference to the theoretical molar absorbance of NADH, it is necessary that the band width of the spectrophotometer be no greater than 6 nm, because the band pass of the reduced coenzyme is about 60 nm (Fig. 4–2).

The Laws of Light Absorption

In a discussion of the theoretical aspects of light absorption, it is assumed that the light source is monochromatic, that the solvent in which the absorbing substance is dissolved is homogeneous and inert with reference to the substance and transparent at the wavelength used, and that the molecules of the absorbing substance do not change state in any way that would affect their light-absorbing properties. Given these conditions, **Lambert's law** states that the fraction of the power of the light entering the solution that is absorbed by the solute is independent of the absolute value of the light intensity. Thus, if a colored solute absorbs 10% of the light in the first 1-cm depth of the solvent, the second-cm depth will absorb 10% of the remaining 90%, or 9%, and the third-cm depth will absorb 10% of the remaining 81%, or 8.1%. **Beer's law** states that the extent to which the light beam is absorbed depends only on the number of absorbing molecules in the light path. Although the two laws are mathematically equivalent, Beer's law is more obviously relevant to the practical application of clinical colorimetric chemistry. The original expression of Beer's law relates the absolute values of the radiant energy of the light beam before and after it passes through the solution, and since it is not practical to make such absolute measurements, the original form,

$$I = I_0 10^{\,abc}$$

where I = light leaving the solution, I_0 = light entering the solution, a = a constant determined by the nature of the colored solute and the wavelength of light used, b = length of light path, and c = concentration of solute in the solvent, is converted mathematically to a more useful form. For this purpose, the absolute light-energy values, I and I_0, are replaced by the ratio of the energy transmitted by the colored solution to that transmitted by the solvent alone set to 100%. The logarithmic form of the original expression, with signs reversed,

$$\log(I_0/I) = abc$$

then becomes, with the substitution of the % transmittance (%T) for the light energy transmitted by the solution and with 100 representing the light energy entering the solution (the spectrophotometer is set to 100% T with the solvent alone),

$$\log(100/\%T) = abc$$

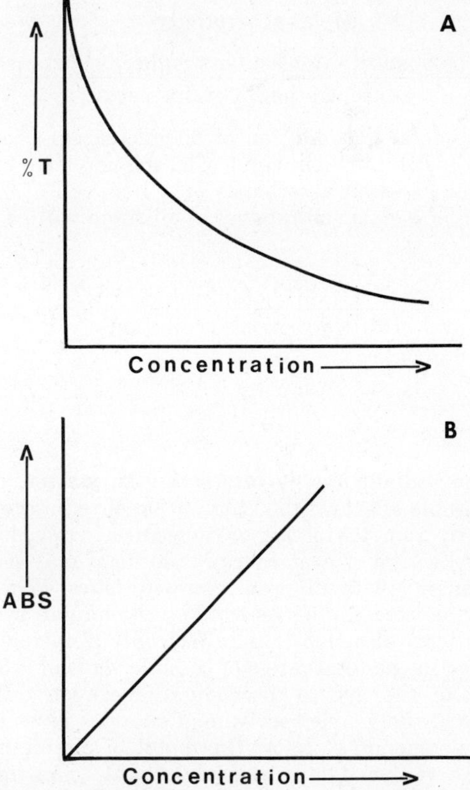

Figure 4–3 *A,* Relationship between %transmittance (%T) and concentration.
B, Relationship between absorbance (ABS) and concentration.

See Figure 4–3*A*. Since log 100 = 2.0, this expression simplifies to

$$2 - \log \%T = abc$$

The product, abc, is defined as the absorbance, A. If the cuvette path length is fixed, and since for a particular substance at a specified wavelength the individual property of that substance, the absorptivity a, is constant, we can substitute a constant k for the product ab, and the final form of the expression, A = kc, states that the absorbance is directly proportional to the concentration of the colored solute, *provided* the conditions listed in the opening sentence of this paragraph are met (see Fig. 4–3*B*). Therefore, the ratio of the absorbances of test and standard solutions will be equal to the ratio of their concentrations. (The absorbance can be converted to %T, and vice versa, using the expression

$$A = 2 - \log \%T$$

Thus an absorbance of 0.5 corresponds to a %T value of 31.6%; 50% T corresponds to an absorbance of 2 − log 50 = 2 − 1.699 = 0.301.) The terms *optical density* and *extinction* have been used with the same meaning as absorbance, but absorbance is preferred. The molar absorptivity (also called the molar extinction coefficient) is defined as the absorbance of a molar solution of a substance in a cuvette with a 1-cm light path at a specified wavelength. In practice, of course, the substance may not be soluble to this extent, and the molar absorptivity is calculated from the formula:

$$\text{Molar absorptivity} = \frac{\text{Absorbance} \times \text{Molecular weight of substance}}{\text{Concentration in grams per liter}}$$

For example, if a dilution of 50 microliters of serum with a known bilirubin value of 21 mg per dL in 3.0 mL of buffer gives an absorbance in a 1-cm cell of 0.32 at 455 nm, the molar absorbance of bilirubin will be given by:

$$\frac{0.32 \times 584 \text{ (MW of bilirubin)}}{0.21 \times 1/61 \text{ (correction for dilution)}} = 54{,}284$$

Color

When radiant energy interacts with matter, one of the possible effects is the stimulation of radiant energy emission from the atoms or molecules involved. Thus the application of heat energy to a metal may produce light energy with different characteristics. When the energy emitted can be detected by the human eye it is called light, although it is in fact only a narrow band included in the total range of possible wavelengths; the ability of the eye to discriminate between different regions of the visible spectrum of energies gives rise to the phenomenon of color. Our habit of distinguishing between visible light, ultraviolet "light," and infrared "light" merely reflects the limitations of our physiological detector, the retina, and its associated optic nerve and brain region. The instrumentation of the laboratory is subject to less stringent limitations, and our ability to detect and measure the results of the interaction of radiant energy and matter is thereby greatly extended. The spectrophotometer determines the pattern and extent of the absorption of light by molecules in solution: if this absorption occurs in the detection range of the eye, it produces the reaction we call *color*. The fluorometer measures the energy emitted by molecules in solution when stimulated by energy of shorter wavelength. The flame photometer uses the energy emitted by heat-excited atoms returning to the ground state. The atomic absorption spectrophotometer determines the extent to which a beam of monochromatic energy is absorbed by a population of ground-state atoms. A recent addition to the group is the reflectance densitometer, which bounces a light beam off an opaque area of colored molecules and quantitates the degree to which the beam has been absorbed. (This principle is used in devices to measure blood glucose levels from the colored area produced on a paper strip containing the reagents for an enzymatic, color-producing reaction with glucose. It is also the principle of the Kodak Ektachem system of automated analysis using color-producing reactions in thin films.)

Spectrophotometer Design

The main components of a modern spectrophotometer are an energy source, a system of slits or slits plus lenses to produce a parallel beam of energy, a monochromator to split the continuous band of wavelengths produced by the usual energy source into its component monochromatic elements, a detection system to convert energy from the form produced by the source into a form that can be displayed, and some means to make this display.

Energy Sources

Tungsten Lamp. The tungsten lamp produces a range of energy wavelengths from about 340 nm to 700 nm, although the output at 340 nm may be low enough to require the greater sensitivity of the double-beam instrument. The amount of heat produced requires the use of cooling fans to protect delicate optical components.

Quartz Halide Lamp. To prevent the deposition of vaporized tungsten from the very hot filament, the bulb contains a small amount of a halogen such as iodine. (The dark film of tungsten seriously reduces the energy output, especially below 400 nm.) As tungsten atoms "boil off" the filament they form tungsten halide, which is volatile and immediately decomposes at the filament surface, redepositing itself on the filament. This extends the working life of the lamp and prevents loss of output. The quartz bulb transmits a higher flux of the shorter wavelengths.

Deuterium Discharge Lamp. To provide an energy source with a high output in the ultraviolet range, deuterium ("heavy hydrogen") is provoked to emit short wavelength energy by an electrical discharge. The high level of short-wavelength ultraviolet energy is dangerous to the unshielded eyes and is demonstrated by the strong smell of ozone produced when the lamp is in use. Two emission lines at 486.1 nm and 656.3 nm can be used to check the accuracy of the wavelength scale of the instrument.

Infrared Energy Sources. Seldom used in clinical chemistry, energy sources for use above 800 nm include the Nernst glower, an electrically heated rod of rare earth element oxides, and the Globar, which uses silicon carbide.

Mercury Vapor Lamp. This emits narrow bands of energy at well-defined places in the spectrum, and some of these are sufficiently close to the absorbance peaks of final reaction colors in routine assays that they serve as high-energy sources that do not require further spectral selection. This type of lamp is found in some European spectrophotometers.

Hollow Cathode Lamp. For some special applications that require monochromatic light, hollow cathode lamps similar to those used for atomic absorption work have been used successfully.

Laser. This method of providing the energy for a photometric system has been used in nephelometers.

Slit System

The ideal energy source would originate from a perfect point, but this is not possible. The spectrophotometer incorporates narrow slits that confine the energy beam to a narrow path and also help to exclude energy from extraneous sources known as stray light. The width of the slit in the light beam emerging from the monochromator, in conjunction with its dispersion (see below), determines the "slice" of the spectrum that passes through the specimen cuvette. It also determines the actual quantity of energy reaching the detector system of the instrument; thus, if the slit is set at too narrow a value, there will be insufficient energy reaching the detector, and the scale cannot be set to zero absorbance (100% T). Since the energy value of the longer wavelengths is less than that of the shorter, wider slit settings are usually required in the yellow to red regions, unless the power of the amplifier section of the detection system can compensate for this. If the blank solution has a very high absorbance, it may not be possible to set the instrument to zero absorbance. The use of very stable, high-power solid state amplifiers in modern spectrophotometers has largely overcome this problem in double-beam instruments; single-beam instruments are still limited to fixed slit widths that correspond to band-pass values of 8 nm and above.

Monochromator

In the simple photoelectric colorimeter of 20 years ago, selection of the wavelength range to be used for a particular measurement depended on the quality of optical filters, which were made of colored glass or dyed gelatin sheets mounted between glass plates. The band pass of such filters was in the range of 35 to 50 nm, and the concomitant inability to meet the monochromatic conditions for the validity of Beer's law often produced nonlinear calibration curves. The need for better spectral selection was first met by the use of prisms, quartz in the best instruments, which produced greater dispersion of the spectrum at the blue end; if a constant band pass was required, variable slits were also needed, adding to the cost of the instrument. In some cases, the back face of the prism was given a reflective coating, so that the incident light was passed through the prism twice, giving a greater dispersion. The prism system is still used in the highest quality spectrophotometers; for more reasonably priced instruments, the method of production of the spectrum is the diffraction grating. The master grating is made by ruling a pattern of fine parallel lines on an optically flat surface with a device called a ruling engine. The lines must be quite close together, about 15,000 per cm. When light passes through the series of very narrow slits produced by such a grating, the emerging wave fronts interfere. (If the edges of two steel rulers are held together and a bright light source viewed through the narrow slit thus formed, the interference bands can be seen.) The result of the interaction between the wavefronts is that certain wavelengths reinforce each other and others cancel each other out. The different wavelengths are diffracted to different extents, and the net result of the two processes of diffraction and interference is the production of a series of spectra. The blue end of one spectrum overlaps the red end of the next; hence, in spectrophotometers using diffraction gratings, internal filters are required to cut off the blue end of the second-order spectrum to prevent its interfering with the red end of the principal spectrum. The spectrum produced by a diffraction grating is of constant dispersion; that is, it has the same width per nm throughout the spectrum. A grating spectrophotometer, therefore, can often function with a fixed slit width over its entire spectral range. Since the master ruled grating can be precisely copied by various methods, diffraction grating spectrophotometers can be produced more cheaply than prism instruments.

For instruments designed to operate at fixed wavelengths, such as some types of automated analyzers, an adequate degree of spectral selection is achieved by the use of interference filters. These consist of a layer of transparent material such as magnesium fluoride coated on each surface with a thin film of silver. Each silver-film layer reflects about half of the incident light and transmits the other half. Part of the light that passes through the first silver layer is repeatedly reflected in the thickness of the magnesium fluoride, but some is reflected outward. This emergent light is "out of step" with the incident light transmitted by the outer surface of the filter. For wavelengths that are exact multiples of the thickness of the magnesium fluoride layer, the emergent rays reinforce each other; all other wavelengths cancel each other out. (The same process occurs when light falls on the very thin film of a soap bubble. The thickness of the bubble is only a few wavelengths of light, and it changes as the bubble evaporates: the interference between light reflected from one side of the bubble and that from the other produces the colors, and the thickness at a particular point determines which color predominates. Another example is the irregular area of colors produced when two flat glass surfaces, such as microscope slides, are squeezed together: the internal reflection takes place in the very thin film of air between the two glass surfaces. The phenomenon, known as "Newton's rings," is used to compare lens surfaces against a master complementary surface during grinding. The more nearly circular the pattern of colored rings, the better the match of the lens against the master surface.) The net effect is that the filter transmits light over only a narrow spectral band, usually about 20 nm wide. In use, the filters are sealed between glass plates to protect them from damage and moisture. An interference filter whose silvered surface appears wrinkled or discolored should be replaced.

Detection Systems

The light detector used in photoelectric colorimeters was the *barrier-layer cell,* consisting of a metal plate onto which is deposited a semiconductor such as selenium, which is covered in turn with a very thin, transparent layer of silver. When light falls on the selenium layer, electrons are emitted from the layer and move toward the metal back plate. This creates a potential difference, or voltage, which is proportional to the intensity of the light and can be measured with a sensitive galvanometer or with a milliammeter in a low-resistance circuit. The barrier-layer cell is simple, requires no external power source, and is relatively rugged. The stability is good, but if exposed to high light intensity for long periods, the output decreases.

Phototubes. These are diodes, two-element tubes, in which the cathode is a semicylindrical sheet of a combination of cesium oxide and silver, or rubidium and rubidium oxide or silver on a cesium-oxide-silver surface. The anode is a single wire placed along the axis of the semicylinder. When light falls on the cathode, it varies the electron flow between this and the anode; this change is detected and amplified by external circuits. Phototubes can be made with different ranges of sensitivity to regions of the spectrum; some spectrophotometers use two phototube detectors with overlapping spectral sensitivity ranges. An external power source is required. The speed of response of a phototube to changes in light intensity is much greater than that of the slow barrier-layer cell, and hence its energy output can be "chopped," that is, converted from a steady signal to an intermittent one and then amplified by the more stable AC circuits.

Photoresistive Diodes. These diodes are devices that change in their resistance to electrical current when light falls on them. In laboratory apparatus their use is largely confined to flame photometers.

Photomultipliers. These are similar in principle to phototubes, but instead of a single unit of semicircular cathode and wire anode, they have a series of such units arranged in a vacuum housing in such a way that the electrons produced in the first unit by the incoming light are aimed at the cathode of the second unit, thus producing an increased electron flow. This process is repeated as many as six to 10 times, producing an amplification of the original signal as great as 10^6. This system can detect and measure very small light intensities and amplify them considerably without loss of stability. It is also highly sensitive to small changes in light intensity, making it possible to measure such changes in the presence of a large background absorbance. If a photomultiplier is exposed to normal room light with its associated high-voltage source still switched on, it can easily be burnt out from overload. The photomultiplier reacts rapidly to changes in light intensity; this property is important in the so-called scanning spectrophotometers. These instruments make a continuous recording of the light-absorbing properties of a substance in solution as the wavelength setting is being moved through a range of values. For this purpose, both the detection system and the recording device must be able to react swiftly to the rapid changes that occur as the wavelength setting approaches a point at which the absorbance spectrum has a sharp peak.

Display

The simplest method of displaying the output of the detection system is a meter, usually a current meter working in the milliamp or microamp range. Both absorbance and %T scales are usually marked, but the former is the more practical, since readings are directly proportional to concentration. A variant on the meter uses some form of digital voltmeter, which converts the output of the detection system into binary coded signals that are then displayed as illuminated numbers. By suitable circuitry the digital read-out can be set to give concentration values by insertion of a standard value or to read out such information as the temperature of a thermostatically controlled cuvette.

Cuvettes and Specimen Holders

Although the cuvette or tube used to hold the solutions whose absorbance is to be determined is a separate item, as soon as it is inserted into the cuvette or tube carrier of the spectrophotometer, it becomes part of the optical system, and frequently it is the component of that system of the poorest optical quality. The most sophisticated double-beam instrument can only utilize its expensive optics and electronics if the cuvette is of equal caliber.

The standard cuvette is made of optical quality glass, borosilicate (hard) glass, or quartz. The most commonly used length of light path is 10 mm, and in a good-quality cuvette this is accurate to ± 0.001 cm. The cuvette walls are parallel and optically flat, without flaws. The best quality cuvettes are sold in matched sets, with a manufacturer's certificate stating the extent of variability in light path lengths and the range of the spectrum transmitted. The type of cuvette used depends on the wavelength range to be used. Optical glass does not transmit enough energy below 340 nm; some special types of glass such as Corex transmit down to about 320 nm. Below this point, quartz cells have to be used. (For care of cuvettes, see p. 73.) Recently, plastic cuvettes have been developed with a wide range of spectral transmission; they have the advantage of cheapness and strength but are easily scratched. They are also used in some types of automatic analyzers. Flow-through cuvettes (see below) are available with the same high optical qualities as the standard 10-mm cuvettes, but they are very expensive and rather difficult to clean. For some purposes, usually involving spectrophotometry of dense solutions, cuvettes with shorter light paths, 0.5 to 0.1 cm, are used.

For many routine analytical purposes, especially when the color reactions are carried out completely in one tube and the readings are made in the visible range of the spectrum, the considerably cheaper tube-type cuvette is used. The quality of these varies greatly; some are supplied in matched sets, with absorbance values when filled with a suitable test solution such as dilute potassium dichromate that agree to within ± 1% of the mean value of the set. Manufacturers' claims of matching to ± 0.25% are, in our experience, optimistic. A more serious source of errors with tube-type cuvettes is the orientation in the light path. If the tube is not accurately round, small errors in its positioning in the spectrophotometer can give large variations in absorbance readings. It is instructive to fill a tube-type cuvette with a dichromate solution that gives an absorbance of about 0.40 against a water blank and then slowly rotate the tube in the instrument holder and watch the changes in absorbance reading. Tube-type cuvettes also vary in wall thickness from batch to batch.

For speed, various designs of flow-through cuvettes are available for routine grade spectrophotometers. They have the advantage that tests, blanks, and standards are measured in identical conditions, and large batches can be read quickly. When linked with a turntable-type sampler and a recorder, flow-through cuvettes can expedite manual procedures. One drawback is that the sample is lost after reading and cannot be rechecked for errors caused by turbidity. In use, the main problem is cleanliness. Even with good flushing after use, stubborn films become deposited on the internal optical surfaces. The unit should be well soaked with a good "stripping" detergent from time to time, and after its soaking and thorough flushing, its absorbance against water with a standard chromate solution such as that used for checking spectrophotometer performance (see p. 75) should be determined. It is best to clean flow-through cuvettes immediately after use so that they are not forgotten. The need for cleanliness extends to the vacuum system used to aspirate solutions into the cuvette; blockage may lead to tubing breakage within the spectrophotometer and possible expensive internal acid damage. Most types of plastic tubing tend to harden with use and time, so it should be inspected and replaced regularly.

Double-Beam Spectrophotometers

Although recent design improvements in single-beam spectrophotometers have reduced some of their limitations, such as the effects of variation in the energy output of the lamp, reduced photometric accuracy at high and low absorbances, and the need to reset blanks with wavelength changes, the most precise and accurate spectrophotometry requires the double-beam system (Fig. 4–4). The great majority of modern instruments of this type use the "double-beam-in-time" layout: after selection of the appropriate wavelength with a monochromator, the light beam is directed alternately through test and reference cuvettes by a rotating disc or mirror. The resulting two streams of light pulses are recombined into a single beam, which is converted into electrical energy pulses by the photomultiplier. (The photomultiplier is essential for the necessary very rapid response to light energy changes.) The energy pulses corresponding to the absorbance of light in test and reference cuvettes are electronically "sorted out," and by various means their ratio is determined. When compared with the ratio determined with the same solvent or blank solution in both cuvettes, the absorbance of the test solution can be derived and displayed on a scale or, in most modern instruments, by LED (light-emitting diode) figures. Since the instrument monitors the energy of the reference cuvette pulse and holds it constant, there is no need for continual resetting of the zero absorbance by the operator, and hence coupling a wavelength drive mechanism with a suitable recorder permits the production of spectral "scans"—graphical displays of the pattern of light energy absorbance by a substance in solution. If the wavelength is held constant, the changes in the absorbance of a solute can be similarly recorded: this principle is used to make kinetic enzyme assays by following the change in absorbance of the coenzyme at 340 nm.

Solvents for Spectrophotometry

When making absorbance measurements or spectral transmission scans in the ultraviolet region, the technologist should be aware that many common solvents show absorption of energy in this part of the spectrum. The list below gives the wavelength below which the solvent has a %T of less than 10 (absorbance greater than 1.0) in a 10-mm cuvette (quartz) against air.

Water	200 nm
Ethanol	210 nm
Methanol	210 nm
Isopropanol	210 nm
Ethyl ether	220 nm
Cyclohexane	210 nm
Chloroform	245 nm
Carbon tetrachloride	265 nm
Acetone	330 nm
Benzene	280 nm
Toluene	285 nm

Wavelength and Wave Number

The expression used to specify a particular region of the electromagnetic spectrum varies with the general nature of the region. For light in the visible and near visible region, the use of the nanometer (10^{-9} meter) yields "convenient" figures. For radio waves, in the broadcast band, frequency (the number of waves per second) is used; for high frequency, where the use of

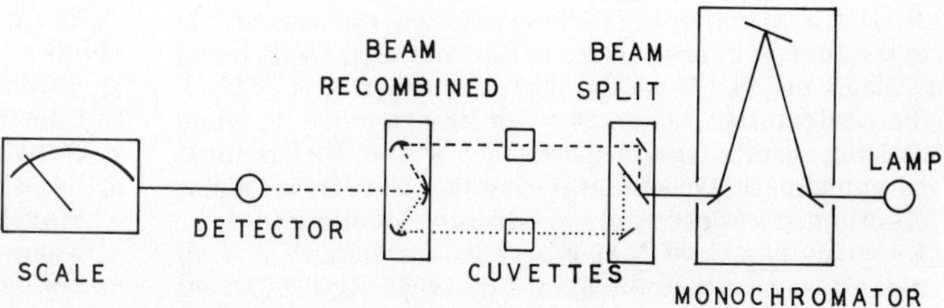

Figure 4–4 Main components of a double-beam-in-time spectrophotometer. The "beam split" and "beam recombined" sections are purely diagrammatic.

kilohertz (thousands of waves per second) would give inconveniently large numbers, the wavelength in meters is used. In laboratory work using infrared radiation, identification of the segment of the energy spectrum in use by the wavelength in nanometers is replaced by the wave number, which is defined as the number of waves per centimeter. Since there are 10^7 nanometers in 1 cm,

$$\text{Wave number} = \frac{10^7}{\text{Wavelength in nm}}$$

For example, energy of wavelength 5 micrometers (microns), or 5000 nm, would have a wave number of 10^7 divided by $5 \times 10^3 = 2000$.

Calibration and Checking of Spectrophotometers

The spectrophotometer can be used in four principal modes:

(i) As an instrument for precise *comparison* of the absorbance of a test solution with that of a standard.

(ii) To produce a scan or graphical plot of the pattern of absorption of light of a solution over a selected region of the spectrum

(iii) To make *absolute* measurements of absorbance when the activity of an enzyme or the concentration of a solute is measured by reference to the known molar absorbance of either a coenzyme or a solute.

(iv) For differential spectrophotometry, in which the difference in the absorbance of a solute measured under different conditions (e.g., pH levels) is a more reliable measure of its presence or concentration than its absorbance at a single condition.

In all four modes, accuracy of the absorbance scale is essential. The requirements for accuracy of the wavelength scale vary with the application. For example, in mode (i) for many analyses an error in the wavelength scale of as much as 10 or even 15 nm would not introduce a serious error in the final answer, since the majority of the colored end products in routine biochemical analyses have relatively broad absorbance maxima; because test and standard are being measured under identical conditions, the relationship between their absorbances will not change appreciably over a range of wavelength settings.

In the other three modes accuracy of the wavelength scale is essential. In mode (ii) the identification of a solute may rest on an exact determination of its absorbance peak wavelength: for example, separation of coproporphyrin from uroporphyrin requires discrimination between two peaks only about 6 nm apart. In mode (iii) the activity of several commonly assayed enzymes involves very exacting measurement of the absorbance change that accompanies the oxidation of NADH to NAD at 340 nm, or the reverse reaction, and conversion of the change in absorbance to International Units using a factor derived from the molar absorbance of NADH. (See calculation on p. 54.) For this method to yield reliable results, the measurement of the NADH must be made at the specific wavelength at which its molar absorbance was determined, typically 340 nm. Since the absorbance peak of NADH at this wavelength is very narrow, so that a small change in wavelength produces a large change in absorbance, absolute accuracy of the wavelength scale, plus a narrow band width (see p. 68) and a cuvette of exactly known path length, are essential.

Errors in the wavelength scale of a spectrophotometer may arise from the following:

(i) Defects in the mechanical system that connects the optical part of the monochromator with the wavelength display. Stretching or slippage of flexible belts, loosening of pulleys and tensioning devices, or excessive "play" in gear trains can result in loss of the precise relationship between the monochromator and the display.

(ii) Failure of the display itself. This may be mechanical in a decimal counter type or electrical in an illuminated display of the "Nixie" tube or LED (light-emitting diode) type. In the latter case, loss of one of the bar elements composing the figures can change "8" into "0."

(iii) Damage to the mounting of the diffraction grating in the monochromator, producing variability in its positioning in relation to the slit.

Errors in the accuracy of the absorbance reading may arise from the following:

(i) Slow changes of the electrical properties of components in the amplifier circuits.

(ii) Excessive levels of stray light, that is, energy reaching the detector system from sources other than the beam traversing the cuvette.

(iii) Dirty or defective optical elements in the light path, including the cuvette, which may be the component in the system that is of the poorest optical quality.

(iv) A light source on the point of burning out, producing major fluctuations in the energy of the beam, most noticeably with single-beam instruments.

(v) Imperfect centering of the light source on the entrance slit of the system, particularly with ultraviolet energy sources.

(vi) Mechanical defects in meter-type absorbance displays or electrical faults in "Nixie" tube or LED-type displays.

(vii) Defective light-sensitive devices (photomultipliers, phototransistors, phototubes) that do not produce an electrical output proportional to the incident light.

(viii) In double-beam spectrophotometers using a vibrating mirror method of direction of the light path alternately through the reference and sample cuvettes, an inconstant period of vibration.

(ix) During the use of micro cuvettes, in which the maintenance of a 10-mm light path using a restricted volume of sample is achieved by reducing the internal width of the cuvette to less than 4 mm, incorrect alignment of the cuvette may produce reflection of the incident light beam on the internal vertical surfaces, with reduction of its intensity not related to the concentration of the absorbing solute. (This is called "vignetting.")

The chief sources of spectrophotometer error are as follows:

Accuracy of absorbance measurement
Linearity of instrument response
Stray energy
Band width
Wavelength setting accuracy
Noise
Drift

For a full discussion of these factors, see the Technical Improvement Service Bulletin, No. 27, from the American Society of Clinical Pathologists. We shall concern ourselves here with those factors amenable to checking without special equipment.

Accuracy of Absorbance Measurement. For regular checking of the accuracy of the absorbance scale of a spectrophotometer, the following solutions are suggested.

Solute	Solvent	Wavelength	Absorbance
Potassium chromate $K_2Cr_2O_4$ 50.5 mg/L	0.05 M KOH	340 nm	0.400
Cobalt ammonium sulfate $CoSO_4 \cdot (NH_4)_2SO_4 \cdot 6H_2O$ 4.0% w/v	1% v/v H_2SO_4	510 nm	0.480
Cupric sulfate $CuSO_4 \cdot 5H_2O$ 4.0% w/v	1% v/v H_2SO_4	650 nm	0.448

The stated absorbances were obtained in 1.0-cm path-length cells against blank settings using the same batch of solvent in a narrow band-pass (1.0 nm) spectrophotometer. The potassium chromate working solution was made by 1 in 10 dilution with 0.05 M KOH of a stock solution containing 505 mg/L. The three solutions were chosen to cover the usual working range of wavelengths and to have absorbances close to the region of maximum sensitivity of the instrument, that is, 0.43 absorbance.

(A variety of commercial solutions and special filters are available for checking not only absorbance scale accuracy but also linearity, stray light, and wavelength scale accuracy. The solutions listed above are an inexpensive alternative.)

Linearity. The linearity of response of a new instrument should initially be checked by making accurate dilutions—1 in 2, 1 in 3, and 1 in 4—of the solutions listed above with the corresponding solvents and plotting the absorbances obtained against concentration. If the plots are all straight lines, future checks can be limited to dilutions of one of the test solutions: the potassium chromate solution at 340 nm is suggested in view of the critical nature of measurements at this wavelength.

Wavelength Setting Accuracy. A very precise check of the wavelength scale of a narrow band-pass spectrophotometer can be made with a pencil-type mercury vapor lamp.* If the lamp is inserted into the cuvette well of the instrument, whose own light source should be blocked off, and the wavelength dial turned to detect points of maximum transmittance of energy, the readings on the wavelength scale can be checked against the following values of strong emission lines of the mercury lamp, which have been rounded off to the nearest nanometer. (CARE! Shield eyes from direct exposure.)

Major Emission Lines of Hg Lamp	
254	405
270	408
302	436
313	547
334	577
365	579

*PenRay Lamp, A. H. Thomas Co., Philadelphia, Pa. 19105, Cat. No. 6323—M.

If the instrument uses a deuterium lamp for ultraviolet spectrophotometry, two prominent lines in the spectrum of the lamp can be similarly used. Their wavelengths are 486.1 nm and 656.3 nm. The spectrophotometer should be set in the single-beam mode, with a narrow slit setting of 0.15 to 0.25 mm, and the spectrum on either side of the two wavelengths slowly scanned. (If a recorder is used, set to a chart speed of 20 or 40 mm per minute.) The reading of the wavelength scale should be noted when maximum deflection of the read-out scale, that is, maximum transmittance, is obtained. The sharp peaks should occur within ± 1.0 nm of the stated values. One source of error is "backlash" of the mechanism of the wavelength setting control. If this is present, the location of the peak will be different when approached from higher values than when approached from lower readings. If the mechanical slack cannot be removed by a service technician, users of the instrument will have to adopt a procedure of always setting the wavelength scale from the same direction.

For checking of the accuracy of the wavelength scale over a wide range of the visible and ultraviolet spectrum, the best device is a filter made with holmium oxide. This provides a number of narrow absorbance peaks at well-spaced wavelengths (Table 4–2). Holmium oxide glass filters are expensive but will last indefinitely with care. They are most conveniently employed in spectrophotometers with double-beam design and an automatic wavelength change drive ("scanning" spectrophotometer). If the spectrophotometer is coupled with a suitable recorder, a permanent record of the absorbance spectrum of the filter is easily and rapidly produced, and the observed absorbance peaks can be compared with the stated locations. In single-beam spectrophotometers the zero absorbance setting will have to be determined in the vicinity of a chosen series of peaks and then, after insertion of the holmium oxide filter, the wavelengths of actual peak absorbance found by very slow movement of the wavelength setting dial on either side of the expected value. The reading of the scale at which the peak is located can then be compared with the stated value.

If a quick check on the wavelength scale is required, a solution of oxyhemoglobin can be used. Prepare it by lysing a small amount of washed red cells in a 0.05% v/v solution of ammonia in distilled water. Shake well and filter. Adjust the solution by addition of either water or more red cells until it gives an absorbance reading of about 0.4 to 0.5 at a nominal wavelength setting of 576 nm. Determine the absorbance of the solution at 2-nm

TABLE 4–2 ABSORBANCE PEAKS OF HOLMIUM GLASS

Peak in nm	Tolerance ± Peak Value
241.5	0.2
279.4	0.3
287.5	0.35
333.7	0.55
360.9	0.75
418.4	1.1
453.2	1.4
536.2	2.3
637.5	3.8

intervals against a water blank over the range from 530 to 580 nm. If the wavelength scale calibrations are accurate, the peak readings should be obtained within 2 nm of 540 nm and 576 nm.

If errors in the accuracy of the wavelength scale are suspected from the above tests, the assistance of the instrument manufacturer in correcting the calibration should be sought. It should be noted that problems of this kind may also be due to other factors that are more difficult to check, such as stray energy. Stray energy is defined as light of other than the desired wavelength, passing through or around the sample at the time of measurement. Its usual effects are loss of linearity and, at ultraviolet wavelengths, displacement of absorption peaks. Detection is by the use of special filters with a very sharp cutoff point, that is, whose passage of light drops to zero at a clearly defined wavelength. If the instrument still shows light transmission below the cutoff point, this can only be stray light that is reaching the photometric detection system.

Noise and drift are defects of the photometric system, usually in electronic amplifiers and light detectors. The usual effect of noise is to produce small random variations in the readings, often seen most easily if a recorder is being used. Variations caused by drift are usually slower and commonly in one direction. The use of double-beam systems and solid state AC amplifiers in modern instruments has reduced these problems to negligible proportions.

Care of Spectrophotometer Cells

If spectrophotometer cells or cuvettes acquire protein films, deposits of salts, or other contaminants, or if their optical surfaces become etched from strong acids or bases, there will be reduced transmission of light through the cell. Residues in the cell may contaminate other sample solutions. These sources of photometric error are often most serious in the region of the spectrum used for critical measurements, for example, at 340 nm in the kinetic methods for enzyme determinations. If the cell walls become scratched, there will be reduced light transmission as a result of scattering. A clean silica cell filled with distilled water should give an absorbance reading of less than 0.15 at 270 nm after the spectrophotometer has been set to read zero absorbance with an air space. A good-quality Pyrex cell should give a similar performance at 320 nm or 340 nm.

A badly scratched or etched cell must be discarded, and the high cost of this item makes it obligatory to follow these simple rules:

1. *Immediately* after use, rinse out the cell *repeatedly* with distilled water. (If the measurements were made in an organic solvent, initial rinsing with the same solvent is advisable.) The rinsing must be thorough to prevent protein film formation. Do not use any mechanical means for cleaning; even the softest brush will scratch the precision optical surfaces. Do not use an ultrasonic cleaning bath; this may damage the cemented edges of the cell.

2. Allow the cell to dry in an inverted position on a clean gauze pad or in one of the special soft plastic cell holders. Remember to keep matched sets together. Do not use an air blast to accelerate drying; most compressed air supplies contain traces of oil and/or dirty water.

3. If the cell is filmed or stained, as detected by visual inspection or by the transmission test above, soak for not more than two hours in a filtered weak solution of a mild detergent, followed by a thorough rinse with distilled water. For a stubborn protein film, soak in a warm solution of pepsin or similar enzyme. (Two suitable sources are the papain solution used in blood bank or the enzymic cleaning solutions for automated blood gas analyzers.) It is good practice to give the cells a short treatment with weak detergent (Contrad 70* in a 2.0% v/v solution) at the end of each working day before the final cleaning.

4. If a solution has been allowed to evaporate in the cell, leaving a hard deposit, try the detergent soak, extended to three or four hours if necessary, followed by thorough rinsing. If the cell is not clean, soak in 70% ethanol to which has been added one drop of concentrated hydrochloric acid per 10 mL. If the deposit contains protein from dried serum dilution, try the enzyme treatment; since the pH of the enzyme solutions is close to neutral, overnight soaking is permissible. The best treatment, however, is prevention.

It is not essential that cells be completely dry before re-use if they are rinsed with a small aliquot of the test solution, which is discarded before refilling the cell for the actual measurement. The cells should be carefully wiped off before being placed in the spectrophotometer; fingerprints or test solution on the outside will cause measurement errors or contamination of the instrument cell carrier. Use a good-quality soft paper tissue or an old, repeatedly laundered cotton handkerchief.

FLUOROMETRY

An atom can be excited to a temporarily higher energy state with subsequent return to the ground state and re-emission of energy by several means. In flame photometry the external energy source is the *heat* energy of a flame, and the atoms excited are mainly simple cations. A wide variety of compounds can absorb energy of the correct characteristics from a *light* source (extending the term *light* to include ultraviolet radiation). The excited compound may re-emit the extra energy either almost instantaneously, after less than 10^{-8} second, or after a longer period. In the process of absorption and re-emission some energy is lost; thus the quantum size of the emitted energy is smaller and the wavelength is correspondingly longer. Typically the exciting radiation is high-energy, large quantum size, ultraviolet radiation, and the emitted energy is smaller quantum size, visible light. If the re-emission of energy occurs in less than 10^{-8} second, the phenomenon is called fluorescence; if the re-emission is delayed, it is called phosphorescence.

Since the characteristics of the exciting radiation have to be "tailor made" for a particular molecular structure, and since the properties of the emitted radiation are similarly determined, fluorometry provides a means of identifying compounds. The presence of coproporphyrin in a urine sample is detected by irradiating the urine

*Harleco, Philadelphia, Pa. 19143.

with "long" wavelength, ultraviolet light of about 354 nm and observing the typical salmon-pink fluorescence produced. The green fluorescence of the zinc-urobilin complex serves to detect urobilin in urine. The process of energy conversion is very efficient; if the source is intense, all the susceptible molecules present can be excited to fluoresce. The phenomenon provides a means of specific quantification of substances that either fluoresce or can be converted to fluorescent derivatives. The intensity of the emitted radiation is high, and fluorometry provides a highly sensitive method of analysis. The main problem, especially with biological fluid samples, is the frequent occurrence of other compounds, especially drugs, that have excitation and emission spectra similar to those of the compound being estimated.

Fluorometers

A simple fluorometer employs narrow band-pass filters to isolate the exciting and emitted wavelengths. A spectrofluorometer, which uses monochromators to achieve much better selectivity, has greater sensitivity because it irradiates the sample with energy exactly "tuned" to the compound being measured, and this same selectivity helps to reduce interference from compounds with excitation and emission spectra similar to those of the desired compound. The use of two monochromators entails much higher cost, and since the energy flux is lower, the detection system is also more complex. The nature of the optical path, that is, measurement of radiation emitted at right angles to the line of the incident radiation (Fig. 4–5), enables the spectrofluorometer to be used as a very sensitive nephelometer (see p. 80). The primary monochromator for the light source is set to 468 nm, which is the point of maximum output of the xenon lamp, and the secondary monochromator, which isolates the emitted radiation in the normal mode of use, is set to 470 nm to exclude nonspecific fluorescence.

FLAME PHOTOMETRY

The work of Albert Einstein on the emission of electrons by certain metals when illuminated with light (the photoelectric effect) explained the observation that the energy of an emitted electron was determined by the wavelength of the incident light through the concept of quantization of energy. A source of radiant energy is not a continuous stream, like water from a garden hose, but a succession of discrete packets called quanta. There is a fixed relationship between the wavelength of the radiation and the size of the quanta of which it is composed: the shorter the wavelength, the larger the size of the quanta.

In flame photometry the heat energy of the flame excites atoms by promoting high-speed collisions. The excited state is unstable, and the atom rapidly returns to the stable "ground" state by ejecting the extra energy. However the ejected energy can be released only in quanta of a specific size determined by the internal structure of the particular element. The net result is that the wavelength of the emitted light—which is determined by the quantum size of the energy—is fixed and typical of that particular element. This phenomenon is the basis for the use of spectroscopy for the detection of elements both in the laboratory and in the stars.

Flame Photometers

The basic components and design features of modern flame photometers vary little from manufacturer to manufacturer. To the basic layout of burner, sample aspirator, detectors, and wavelength selection has been added a variety of specimen dilutors, automatic sample handlers, read-out devices, and printers. To consider the essentials first:

1. The burner and aspiration system. The flame serves two purposes. It is the source of the exciting energy; the maximum value depends on the particular fuel-oxidant mixture used. Air-propane attains 1925°C; air-acetylene, 2200°C; oxygen-acetylene, 3050°C. It is a fortunate coincidence that the energy level needed for the adequate excitation of the two elements of greatest physiological importance, sodium and potassium, is readily attainable by the air-propane flame.

The flame also converts the element from its ionic form in the sample into the uncharged atomic state, which can then be excited to light emission. To achieve this, the water of the sample is evaporated, leaving the solutes as microcrystals; these are then fragmented into ions, which pick up electrons from the flame and become atoms. The temperature of the flame should be high enough to do this rapidly, but it must not be so high that the atoms are excited to the point where the outer electrons are lost. The design of the burner and the aspiration system that introduces the sample must pro-

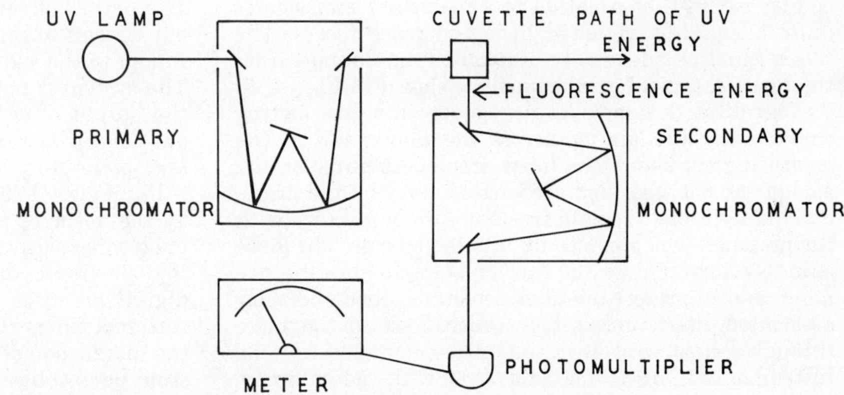

Figure 4–5 Main components of a spectrofluorometer.

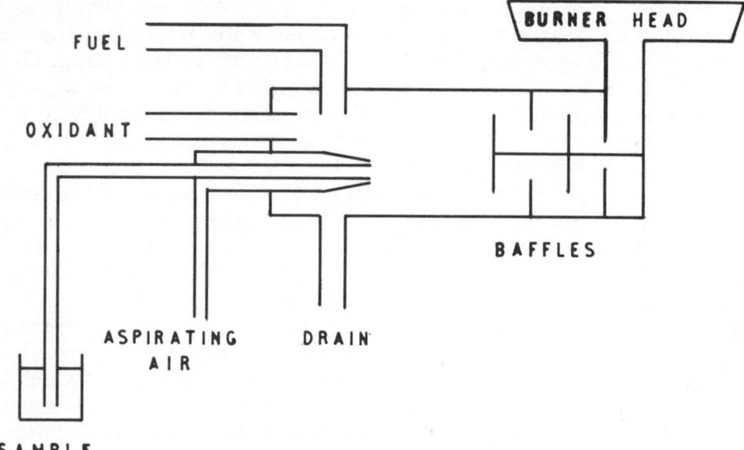

Figure 4–6 Schematic drawing of a premix burner. Note that after mixing of the sample, fuel, and oxidant, the larger droplets of the sample are intercepted by the baffles and drained away.

duce a large enough population of atoms so that the energy output from the extremely small proportion that becomes excited is adequate for accurate measurement, while not producing such a high concentration that the population of atoms in the flame exceeds the available excitation energy. This condition is called "flame saturation," and it precludes the linear relationship between concentration and emitted energy on which the method is based.

In the *premix burner* (Fig. 4–6), which is now in general use, the fuel, oxidant, and atomized sample are mixed together in a special chamber *before* being fed to the burner head. The chamber incorporates some system of baffles or a swirl space, which deflects to waste the large droplets and permits only the small droplets to reach the flame. The small droplet size improves pyrolysis, although a large proportion of the sample is wasted "down the drain." The main advantage is a much quieter flame, both audibly and in the character of the electronic signal produced in the detection system. This permits the use of higher amplification and better sensitivity. The premix burner has to be carefully designed to prevent explosive blowback; safety devices for the same purpose are built into the flame photometer itself.

2. Wavelength selection and detection system. The wavelengths of emitted energy from the three elements usually determined by flame photometry (sodium, 589 nm; potassium, 766 nm; and lithium, 671 nm) are sufficiently well separated in the spectrum, and the emissions of other elements from the serum are sufficiently weak, that isolation of a particular emission is quite adequately obtained by interference filters. The filters must be adequately protected from damage from the heat. A typical arrangement is shown in Figure 4–7. The diluted sample is drawn up into the mixing chamber by the air jet across the upper end of the aspirating capillary. The large droplets impinge on the side of the chamber and are carried away by the drain; the small droplets remain free and form a mixture with the propane, which passes up into the burner. The glass chimney surrounding the burner helps to stabilize the flame and to protect the photosensitive tubes and their associated interference filters, which "look at" the flame through a clear window in the frosted chimney. In some instruments there is a second window in the chimney, which permits monitoring of the flame by a photocell; if the flame becomes extinguished for any reason during operation of the flame photometer, the sudden loss of light falling on the monitoring cell triggers relays that cut off the gas and air flow to prevent explosion.

The three photosensitive tubes detect emitted energy from excited atoms in the flame. The filters determine that one phototube detects the light from sodium atoms, one from potassium atoms, and one from lithium atoms. (This description applies to modern instruments using lithium as the internal luminosity reference; flame photometers employing direct measurement of emitted energy and its comparison with that from a standard solution are now obsolete, except when an atomic-absorption spectrophotometer is used in the flame emission mode.) Since the samples and standards are diluted, either manually or with some type of autodilutor, with the same lithium solution, the energy emitted in the flame by excited lithium atoms is *constant.* The energy emitted in the flame by sodium and potassium atoms is compared with that of the lithium atoms.

The comparison is made by initially setting the digital or other read-out devices to zero, with distilled water aspirating into the flame. Since the distilled water is diluted with lithium solution in the same manner as standards and samples, the only energy emission in the flame is that of the excited lithium atoms. Setting the lithium level meter to the marked point introduces a reference voltage into the electronic circuitry and also corrects for background current in the three phototubes. The action of setting the sodium and potassium read-out devices to zero adjusts the outputs of the amplifiers linked to the sodium and potassium phototubes to zero. The system is now in a state of electronic balance, with the output of the lithium phototube holding the read-out devices at zero. When a solution containing sodium and potassium ions is aspirated into the flame, the lithium signal remains constant, but it is now opposed by the voltages produced in the sodium and potassium phototubes with their associated amplifiers. The resulting electronic imbalance is amplified and drives the digital or other read-out devices until the balance is restored. Since the degree of imbalance will depend on the magnitude of the signal from the sodium and potassium phototubes, the change in reading on the read-out

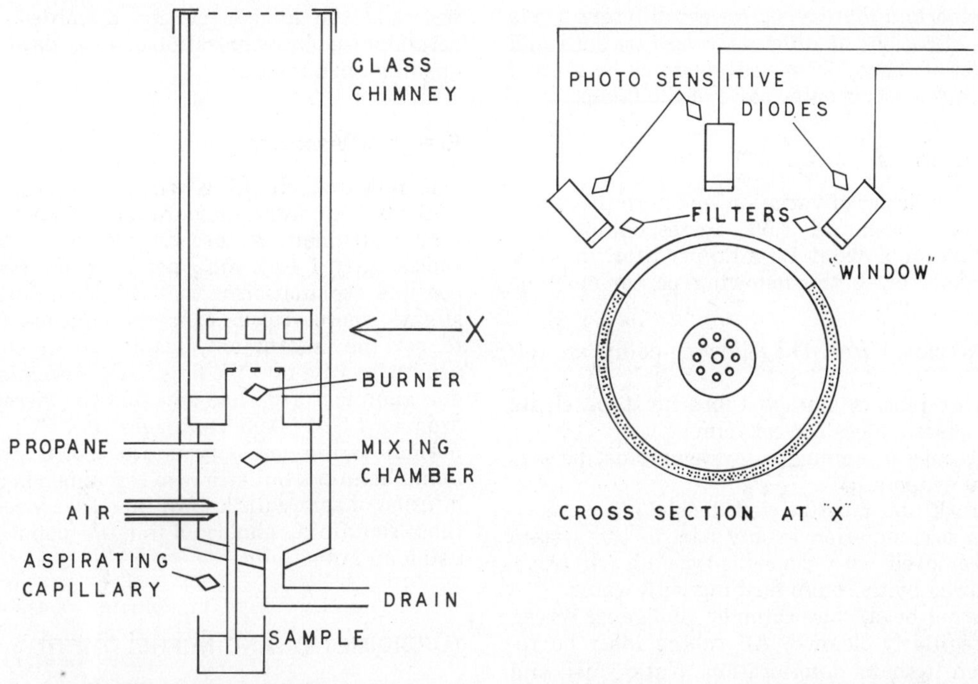

Figure 4–7 Arrangement of mixing chamber, burner, and detectors in a modern flame photometer.

devices will be proportional to the concentration of sodium and potassium in the aspirated solution. When standards are being aspirated, a portion of the output of the amplifiers that increase the size of the signal from the phototubes is fed back by the standard setting controls so that the values on the read-out devices can be made to correspond with the known standard values. When unknowns are being aspirated, the signals they produce in the phototubes will be similarly related to the standard values, and the read-out devices will display the serum concentrations. The range switch used when measuring urine electrolytes introduces a fixed resistance into the potassium amplifier feedback circuit, which automatically makes a tenfold change in the effect of the standard setting control, thus permitting adjustment of the read-out device over a tenfold greater range.

The above brief description is based on the widely used Model 343 Flame Photometer.* The later versions are basically similar, the main improvements being in the electronics and the use of cesium as the internal luminosity reference.

Sources of Error and Problems

Radiation Interference. This is due to the presence in the sample of an element or compound that produces radiation in the flame close in wavelength to that of the desired element. With the use of narrow band-pass interference filters this is not a serious problem, since serum does not contain appreciable amounts of any cation that emits energy when excited at a wavelength close to those of the elements of interest.

Excitation Interference. In addition to the atoms of the element being determined that are excited by flame energy, a further increment of emission can arise because of energy transfer to the element being assayed from excited atoms of another element. For example, the emission signal from excited sodium atoms is enhanced by the transfer of energy from excited potassium atoms. The effect is to make the energy emission of sodium atoms dependent not only on sodium concentration, which is the desired effect, but also on potassium concentration. The usual methods of correction of this problem are to include potassium in the standards at about the same level as in the tests, or to include another cation, called a radiation buffer, in the solutions. The usual cation used is lithium in high concentration, which successfully competes with the sodium atoms for the excitation energy from the potassium atoms. The lithium in the usual internal luminosity reference system therefore serves two purposes.

Background Interference. This originates from compounds that produce a wide-band spectrum of emitted energy in the flame, especially nonionic compounds such as carbohydrates, proteins, and lipids. The effect of this type of interference is minimized by high dilution of the sample and good spectral isolation of the emitted energy of interest.

Chemical Interference. In some cases, the stability of an ionic compound may be high enough to resist pyrolysis in the flame, for example, calcium phosphate. Instead of producing neutral atoms that can be excited to emit energy, the substance forms microcrystals, which are carried away in the burnt gases of the flame. This is one of the reasons for the relatively poor success in determination of calcium by flame photometry. When atomic absorption is used for calcium assay, cations such as strontium or lanthanum are used to combine with the phosphate, thus preventing calcium phosphate formation.

*Instrumentation Laboratory, Inc., Lexington, Mass. 02173.

Two less important sources of error are different levels of ionization of cations at different concentrations and the absorption of energy from excited atoms by ground state atoms in the cooler outer parts of the flame.

General Precautions

The target coefficient of variation in determination of serum sodium is about ± 1.0%, corresponding to a standard deviation of about 1.5 mEq per liter. In order to maintain this level, the following points must be observed:

1. Chemical cleanliness. The following points are relevant:
(a) Serum or plasma storage tubes must be clean: disposable plastic tubes are convenient.
(b) Sample cups in automated systems must be protected from evaporation.
(c) The autodilutor must be well flushed after use.
(d) Protein accumulation in any part of the system must be removed with domestic-type bleach treatment, followed by thorough flushing with water.
(e) The burner head, glass chimney, and gauze screen must be regularly cleaned. All tubing must be replaced when it shows deterioration. Water, fuel, and air line filters should be replaced on a regular basis.
(f) Bottled propane fuel must be a special clean grade for flame photometry.
(g) Compressed air from a bench supply must be filtered to preclude oil and water contamination.
The de-ionized water used for dilution and standard preparation should have a specific resistance of at least 5 to 10 megohms per cm.

2. Standards. Since the majority of routine electrolyte determinations in the clinical laboratory fall within the normal range, the common practice of using a single standard having values of 140 mEq per liter for sodium and 5.0 mEq per liter for potassium may appear acceptable. However, the most important results clinically are those falling outside this range, and it is better technique to have available at least two other standards—120 mEq per liter sodium plus 3.0 mEq per liter potassium, and 150 mEq per liter sodium plus 7.0 mEq per liter potassium—in order to obtain better accuracy with sera with values above and below the normal range. Sodium and potassium chlorides of analytical grade purity or better are available; these should be oven dried overnight at 110°C, then immediately transferred as a thin layer in a clean glass or porcelain dish into the vacuum desiccator to cool. The correct amounts should be weighed as rapidly as possible without sacrificing accuracy (see Standard Values below) and transferred quantitatively to volumetric flasks that have been thoroughly cleaned. It is convenient to use the new plastic volumetric flasks, since these can be cleaned easily. After being made to volume and mixed in the usual manner, standards should be stored in polypropylene bottles. A small amount should be poured out into a plastic bottle of 25- or 50-mL capacity for each day's use, and the unused portion discarded. This reduces errors caused by evaporation of a standard from repeated opening during use.

Effect of Viscosity

If repeated checking with a range of commercial controls from different sources indicates that the particular instrument in use is yielding results that are consistently 1 to 2 mEq per liter low for sodium, one possible explanation is that the serum dilution used is slightly more viscous than the aqueous standard used to set the instrument, leading to a slightly slower aspiration rate into the flame and less emission. At least one manufacturer* has adjusted the viscosity of standards to 1.8 ± 0.05 centipoise at 25°C; the range of normal serum viscosity is 1.5 to 2.0 centipoise. The manufacturer's bulletin also recommends using manual dilution of sera with known increased viscosity, such as those containing abnormal immunoglobulins, instead of using an autodilutor.

TURBIDIMETRY AND NEPHELOMETRY

Turbidimetry measures the extent to which a beam of light in a photometer or spectrophotometer is attenuated by the presence of suspended solid particles in the sample cuvette. Nephelometry measures the amount of light scattered at right angles to the light path by particles in the beam. Turbidimetry can thus be used in a spectrophotometer without special equipment; the nephelometer requires a detector placed in the right angle position, analogous to a fluorimeter; indeed, in some applications using Technicon continuous flow systems a fluorimeter is used as a nephelometer. Turbidimetric methods are still widely used as simple ways of measuring low levels of protein in urine and cerebrospinal fluid, although procedures employing dye binding could displace the older methods. (See p. 216.) The chief disadvantages of turbidimetric methods are the difficulty of reproducing the exact conditions of protein precipitation, the small range of concentrations over which the procedure is linear, and the relatively large sample required. The adoption of a rigidly unvarying technique is essential, and if possible, standards with a distribution of fractions that is similar to that of the test sample should be used.

With the introduction of more sophisticated nephelometers, using high-intensity light sources such as lasers plus improved optical systems, it is now practicable to measure protein levels in such high dilution that the difficulties attendant on precipitation are minimized, and the concomitant availability of specific antisera has led to the development of automated systems for immunoglobulin assays.

*Instrumentation Laboratory, Inc., Lexington, Mass. 02173, Bulletin 25571, 1973.

Standard Value	120	140	150	3.0	5.0	7.0
Weight of sodium chloride per liter	7.0128g	8.1816g	8.766g	—	—	—
Weight of potassium chloride per liter	—	—	—	0.2237g	0.3728g	0.5219g

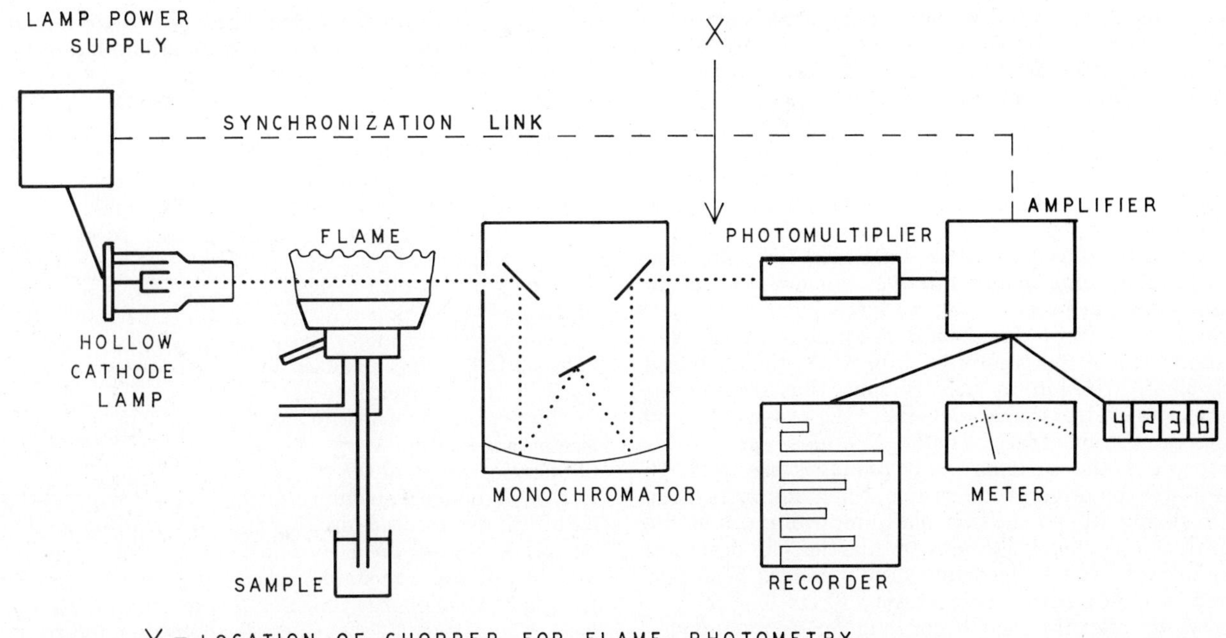

Figure 4–8 Main components of a single-beam atomic absorption spectrophotometer.

ATOMIC ABSORPTION SPECTROPHOTOMETRY

Kirchhoff's law states that if an element can be excited by external energy to emit radiation of a specific wavelength, that element in the ground state will absorb radiation of exactly the same wavelength. (The "ground state" of an atom is its condition of lowest energy and greatest stability.) The specificity of the radiation emitted by an excited atom as it returns to the ground state is the basis for the flame photometer. In 1952 Walsh pointed out that flame photometry makes use of only the very small proportion of atoms that can become excited—often less than 1 in 100,000. Atomic absorption spectrophotometry depends on energy from an external source being absorbed at a specific wavelength by the greatly preponderant ground state atoms. In addition to the inherent advantages of sensitivity and specificity, atomic absorption spectrophotometry is independent of temperature and less susceptible to spectral interference and to matrix effects. (These are problems caused by the presence of other substances in the analyzed material.)

For a practical instrument to utilize these principles, four basic components are required (Fig. 4–8):

1. An intense, stable source of the radiation that is specifically absorbed by the atoms of the element to be determined. The only true source is excited atoms of the same element, since it is only to energy thus produced that the ground state atoms will be "tuned." The standard source is the hollow cathode lamp, incorporating a tubular cathode made of or with the element to be determined and filled with an inert gas such as neon. When electrically excited, the cathode sputters off atoms of the metal of which it is composed, and the energy excites them to emit their specific radiation. The band width of energy emitted is very narrow indeed, on the order of 0.001 nm. The emergent beam is focused as a narrow cylinder by the shape of the cathode plus optical means. For reasons to be discussed later, the power supply to the lamp is not continuous but is pulsed at a frequency in the region of 285 cycles per second (285 Hz).

2. A method for producing an atomic vapor of the element to be determined. To obtain the best degree of absorbance of the energy from the hollow cathode lamp, as large a proportion of the atoms as possible must be in the ground state. Since in biological fluids inorganic substances are present in the form of ions or protein complexes, the process of production of the atomic vapor must include conversion of ions to uncharged atoms and the disruption of complexes. The most convenient method is to nebulize the sample into a flame, most commonly an air-acetylene flame; for some analyses nitrous oxide–acetylene, air-hydrogen, air–coal gas, or air-butane have been used. The sequence of events after introduction of the sample solution into the flame is complex, involving desolvation (removal of water), liquefaction, and vaporization of the solid thus produced and atomization to produce uncharged ground state atoms.

The use of a flame is convenient, but it introduces some problems. Some of the atoms produced in the flame will become excited and emit their specific energy wavelength, just as in the flame photometer; and some of the energy spectrum of the flame itself will fall into the same region. These two unwanted energy emissions are constant in character, and the signal they produce in the detection system is a steady signal. As we have seen, the energy from the hollow cathode lamp is pulsed at a fixed frequency, and the amplifier in the detection system is triggered by the same pulses. The amplifier responds, therefore, only to signals that originate in absorbance of the pulsed hollow cathode lamp energy; it does not detect the steady signal from flame background or any excited atoms in the flame.

If the process of atomization in the flame is incomplete,

the extent to which the hollow cathode light is absorbed will be reduced. This can occur in three main ways. The flame conditions may not be adequate for complete release of protein-complexed ions; this is usually overcome by prior precipitation of protein or by incorporation of perchloric acid in the diluent. Some ions such as calcium may form thermostable microcrystals with anions such as phosphate; this is offset by including in the diluent a large excess of an ion that forms stable complexes with phosphate, thus rendering the latter ion unavailable for combination with calcium. The usual cations used are lanthanum and strontium.

Most atomizers for atomic absorption spectrophotometry are of the premix type, in which the aspirated sample is carried into a spray chamber that incorporates devices to control the droplet size to the range of 3 to 30 microns. Various types of baffles and glass spray beads onto which the entering spray impinges are used. To minimize corrosion in the system, the atomizer is made of resistant alloys such as platinum-iridium, and the spray chamber of glass or inert plastic. The design of the burner head is important. The standard head produces a very narrow, stable flame, 10 cm long for air-acetylene mixtures and 5 cm long for nitrous oxide–acetylene mixtures. To resist corrosion, the burner head is made of titanium or similar metal and is of heavy construction to prevent distortion of the narrow slot with high temperatures. It is desirable that the burner head can be adjusted in three directions: vertically, laterally, and in rotation. The flame is very narrow, about 2 mm, and the sensitivity of the instrument depends on the precision with which the lamp beam is aimed along the flame length. The vertical control of burner position is necessary to locate the particular region of the flame that gives the best analytical results. The events in the flame that govern the location of the highest concentration of the atomic vapor are complex, and trial and error remains the best approach.

If atomization is incomplete, with the persistence in the flame of molecular compounds of the element being analyzed, there will be absorbance of the energy from the hollow cathode lamp of a nonspecific nature. In the more sophisticated instruments with double-beam systems, one of the beams may be used to monitor nonspecific absorbance from this cause.

The most suitable mixtures of fuel and oxidant for analysis of a particular element have been well established, although they vary with the particular instrument and type of burner head. The technologist will find that in some analyses the acetylene flow setting is critical in obtaining the best precision and linearity, and he must expect to determine the optimum values for his own instrument.

The sensitivity of an atomic absorption method depends, among other things, on the concentration of the atomic vapor attainable. In some methods the rate of atomization of the sample is increased by using a diluent other than water, such as butanol, thereby improving the quantity of element released in the flame per unit of time. The use of an organic solvent may be coupled with the conversion of the ion to be measured into an organometallic complex that is soluble in, and extractable by, the solvent. Some degree of concentration of the element to be measured can thereby be obtained.

3. A system to select and isolate the specific energy emission of the hollow cathode lamp, excluding all other spectral lines. In order to utilize the unique relationship between the emitted energy of the lamp and its absorption by the element being determined, all other spectral lines emitted by the lamp must be excluded from the detection system. The standard instrument for achieving this is a grating monochromator. A grating is used in preference to a prism because its dispersion of the spectrum is linear and it is less expensive to manufacture. In addition, a grating monochromator has a higher efficiency in the ultraviolet region, and since the mass of the glass grating is relatively small, it is not distorted by temperature changes to the same extent as a prism. (The shift in setting caused by temperature change is usually called monochromator drift.)

The operation of the monochromator can be briefly summarized as an energy "sieve." From the broad band of energies entering the monochromator, only that very narrow band corresponding to the monochromator setting will be focused on the exit slit leading to the detection system. In a good instrument the slit width and height are adjustable, permitting some control of the quantity of energy reaching the detection system.

4. A sensitive, stable system for detection and measurement of the changes in the energy of the lamp beam. If the element being determined does not absorb to a great degree, or is present only in a very small amount, the *difference* in energy of the lamp beam will be small. (The situation is roughly analogous to measuring small increments of color in the presence of a large blank value in colorimetry.) It is the object of good methodology to overcome this problem; we have already mentioned such devices as the use of organic solvents to enhance absorption. The operator should endeavor to adjust the conditions so that the final readings on meter or recorder fall within the range of 20 to 70% of full scale.

The energy detector is usually a photomultiplier (PM) tube or, in some cases, a pair of tubes with overlapping ranges. The inherent amplification of the PM tube is further boosted by a very stable AC-type electronic amplifier, which, as we have seen, is "in step" with the pulsing frequency of the lamp. Most instruments incorporate a scale expansion feature; this varies the power of the amplifier, either in steps or continuously over a range of × 1 to × 10. The use of the full × 10 expansion is usually accompanied by some increase in "noise," but this is partly offset by various types of damping controls, which minimize the amount of meter needle or recorder flutter. In the more elaborate instruments, signal averaging or integrating circuits are used and, most recently, peak detection circuits.

The final display can be a meter or recorder. With a meter, it is convenient if the original signal, a *decrease* in the energy of the light beam, is electronically inverted so that the meter reading becomes directly proportional to concentration. The recorder mode of read-out is best suited to instruments with automatic feed of samples to the atomizer, although it can be helpful in determining the true peak reading when working at a high scale expansion.

In addition to the main design features listed above, the atomic-absorption spectrophotometer requires fuel and oxidant controls that can be reproducibly set to stable flow rates, provision for mounting of hollow cathode lamps (this may be in the form of a turret, with provision for maintaining lamps not in use in a "warm-up" mode to save time when changing from one element to another), and safety devices to prevent ignition of the fuel-oxidant mixture in the premix chamber (blowback, which can cause an explosion in some instruments). With good design the last-named problem does not arise; we have operated our present instrument for more than 10 years without a single incident of this nature. Operation using nitrous oxide as the oxidant is rather more critical, but in recent designs, conversion from air to nitrous oxide is achieved automatically.

METHODOLOGY

The details of methods will vary with the instrument in use, and the manufacturers provide manuals with suggested methods.

General Points

All pipettes must be scrupulously clean. Immediately after use they should be rinsed free of serum, soaked at least one hour in 20% v/v hydrochloric acid, repeatedly rinsed in distilled water, and dried. If available, an autodilutor that can be set to a suitable ratio will expedite the making of dilutions, but the precision of the dilutor must be extremely good, that is, ± 0.2% or better. We have found that disposable stoppered or capped plastic tubes are chemically clean and obviate the problems of removing tightly adherent contamination, which occurs with glass tubes. Measurements of serum can also be made using the hand-operated pipettors with disposable plastic tips, but a wash-out technique has to be used because of the differing viscosities of serum samples and aqueous standards. Strict attention must be paid to recommended cleaning and maintenance schedules for the particular instrument. The burner head should be treated carefully during cleaning to prevent distortion of the narrow slit. Hollow cathode lamps should be operated at the lowest current that gives acceptable stability and sensitivity. Ample warm-up time must be allowed. The intake tube of the aspirating capillary should be kept in distilled water at all times during instrument operation, except when aspirating a sample or standard. This helps to maintain the burner head at a constant temperature. The acetylene used must be of the highest purity, so-called white spot grade. It is advisable to replace the tank when the pressure has fallen to about 90 lb per sq in. If the tank is used at lower pressures, there may be problems with stability or entry of the acetone, in which the acetylene is dissolved, into the flame. (Acetylene gas cannot be compressed: it explodes spontaneously.) Each time a new tank is put into use, the junction with the reducing valve should be checked for leaks with a soap solution.

OSMOMETRY

If a substance, any substance, is dissolved in a pure solvent, several of the *physical* properties of that solvent are changed. The amount of change in such properties as specific gravity and refractive index depends on both the concentration of solute and its chemical nature. Four other changes—freezing point, boiling point, osmotic pressure, and vapor pressure—depend only on the *number* of particles in solution and are independent of the chemical nature of the particles. In addition, they can be shown to be related mathematically. For this reason, they are named the colligative properties (Latin *colligare* = to bind together). When one mole of any nonionic solute is added to one kilogram of water, the freezing point is lowered by 1.86°, the osmotic pressure increased by 22.4 atmospheres, the boiling point raised by 0.52°, and the vapor pressure decreased by 0.3 mm Hg. (It should be noted that in this connection "osmotic pressure" does not have the same meaning as "colloid osmotic pressure," or oncotic pressure, which is a measure of a pressure difference owing to differing numbers of large particles, typically proteins, on either side of a membrane through which they cannot pass. (Instruments for measuring colloid osmotic pressure are available, but they are in limited use only.) A solution made by dissolving one mole of a nonionic solute in one kilogram of water, called a molal solution, will freeze at −1.86°C. Thus, for a single solvent solution, determination of its freezing point permits calculation of the molality.

$$\text{Molality} = \frac{\text{Depression of the freezing point below } 0^\circ\text{C}}{1.86}$$

(The use of the freezing point merely reflects that this is the most common measurement made for this purpose; recently, instruments for determining osmolality by the decrease in vapor pressure have been introduced.)

The theoretical osmolality of a solution, based on the equation above, is modified in practice by the production of more than one particle per molecule owing to ionization and the occurrence of electrostatic attraction between the ions. The formula then becomes:

$$\text{Osmolality} = \text{Concentration of solute in moles/kg of water} \times N \times C$$

where N = the number of particles produced per molecule of solute and

C = the activity coefficient

Thus, for sodium chloride, 8.5 g/kg of water, yielding two particles per molecule on ionization and an activity coefficient of 0.93, the osmolality is:

$$8.5/58.5 \times 2 \times 0.93 = 0.270 \text{ osmols or } 270 \text{ mOsm/kg}$$

DETERMINATION OF OSMOLALITY

In order to determine the freezing point of the test solution to the required accuracy—about 0.001°C—it must be cooled slowly in a programmed manner to allow for the brief phase of supercooling and the slight rise in temperature associated with the release of heat of fusion as crystallization takes place. The necessary accuracy and sensitivity of temperature measurement at this critical point are achieved by the use of a thermistor, a solid state device that changes its electrical conductivity with change in temperature. The conductivity at the critical point can be compared with a standard value previously set in the instrument, and the difference converted to milliosmols per kilogram. In practice, a precision of ± 2 mOsm/kg can be achieved at levels of about 300 mOsm/kg.

CLINICAL OSMOMETRY

It must be emphasized that measurements of osmolality on biological fluids such as serum and urine are only of comparative value. These fluids are complex mixtures of both ionized and unionized solutes, and it is not possible to relate concentration, specific gravity, and osmolality.

Specimens for Osmometry

Blood samples should be obtained with minimum stasis, using clean, dry equipment. The serum should be separated as soon as possible and recentrifuged at high speed to remove all solid particles. If the determination cannot be made immediately, the serum will be stable for up to 10 hours in the refrigerator, preferably in a small tube filled to the top and tightly sealed or capped. Urine samples are collected without preservatives and centrifuged until crystal clear. The determination should be made immediately. If a period of refrigeration causes precipitation of solutes, warm the sample to redissolve these before centrifugation.

The procedure for osmolality determinations will depend on the particular instrument, but some points are of general application. The samples must be completely clear and free of any solid particles. The sample vessel used in the osmometer must be scrupulously clean and dry. The instrument must be carefully standardized with suitable known solutions; enough for each standardization should be poured from the bottle and any excess discarded. Use standards close to the expected results. If the ethylene glycol–water mixture in the cooling bath is old, the rate of cooling will be slow and the results unreliable. The fluid should be completely changed at least every three months.

Normal Values

Serum: 281 to 297 mOsm/kg. Females average 5 mOsm/kg lower than males.

Urine: Since urine osmolality varies greatly with diet and fluid intake, four groups of normals have been suggested:

- Healthy males: 392 to 1090 mOsm/kg (767 to 1628 mOsm/24 hr).
- Healthy females: 301 to 1093 mOsm/kg (433 to 1146 mOsm/24 hr).
- Convalescent patients: 273 to 896 mOsm/kg (340 to 900 mOsm/24 hr).
- Ward patients on standard diet: 288 to 884 mOsm/kg (261 to 900 mOsm/24 hr).

Osmometry provides a rapid check on the composition of intravenous fluids; for example, physiological saline of 0.9% w/v composition should have an osmolality of 285 mOsm/kg. Since the proteins on a molar basis contribute little to the osmolality of a solution, spinal, pleural, and peritoneal fluids have osmolalities close to that of serum taken at the same time.

CHROMATOGRAPHY

Starting with the work of the Russian botanist Tswett in 1903 with the plant pigments chlorophylls and xanthophylls, the problem of separating and identifying the individual members of a closely related group of compounds, often easily denatured, has been solved by the use of chromatography. The original mixture of substances, either in solution or converted to volatile derivatives, is moved through or past a stationary porous or fibrous medium. The resultant interaction between the substances and the support medium, plus other forces such as adsorption, differences in partition coefficient, and sieving at the molecular level, sorts out the substance molecules by their differing speeds of movement, so that they are finally located at different places on a fibrous support medium or issue from the chromatographic system in sequence at different time intervals. Of the systems briefly described below, paper and thin-layer chromatography, gas-liquid chromatography, and to some extent high-performance liquid chromatography are in general, routine use: the remaining methods are mainly used in research.

PAPER CHROMATOGRAPHY

In paper chromatography, a mixture of substances, which are often related chemically, is initially confined to a small starting region, or spot, at one end of the porous filter paper strip. When this spot is percolated by a moving solvent in which members of the mixture are soluble, the substances will be picked up from the starting spot and carried along in the interstices of the porous paper support. Adsorbed to the paper support is a small amount of water, in which the members of the test mixture are also soluble. A process of exchange occurs, whereby the substances from the original spot are distributed between the mobile solvent and the water in the paper according to their differing solubilities.

After completion of the separation process, the application of suitable color reactions will locate the position on the strip of each pure substance spot. These can be identified by comparison with similarly treated known pure compounds or by comparison with the R_f values of pure standards as shown in the formula at the top of p. 85.

The use of paper as the support medium is exemplified by the method for detection of sugars in urine on p. 000. The fibrous structure of the support has the disadvantage that it tends to cause diffusion of the separated substances, giving less well-defined and separated spots.

THIN-LAYER CHROMATOGRAPHY

Stahl in 1958 introduced practical methods for thin-layer chromatography (TLC), which substitutes for the paper a thin layer, typically 0.25 mm, of very finely powdered silica gel, microcrystalline cellulose, alumina, polyacrylamide gel, dextran, or kieselguhr, bound to a glass plate or other flat support. The chromatographic

$$\text{The } R_f \text{ value} = \frac{\text{Distance traveled from the starting spot by the unknown}}{\text{Distance traveled from the starting spot by the moving solvent}}$$

process in TLC is more closely akin to that on columns, in which adsorption phenomena are predominant, than to that on paper. One advantage of the glass backing is the ability to use more drastic methods of locating the separated substances, such as treating the TLC plate with sulphuric acid and heating to char the organic substances to black carbon spots. In routine laboratory work, the use of TLC is shown by the method for separation of amino acids on p. 151.

Nomenclature—A Note

Tswett's original term ("chromatography") arose from his work with substances naturally colored. By "developing solvent" he meant the liquid passed through his column to carry the mixed substances along the column for the separation processes to operate. In the great majority of paper chromatography and TLC today, the substances are colorless and not directly visible on the chromatogram. In order to locate them, a variety of reagents are used to produce colors with the spots, plus, in some cases, illumination with ultraviolet light. In some ways, the reagents used to detect the spots could be regarded as "developers," but to prevent confusion they are usually called "detection" or "location" reagents. Thus, "development" of a chromatogram is the initial physical separation of the components of the applied sample. Some attempts have been made to introduce a more generally applicable terminology such as "sorptogram" for "chromatogram," but Tswett's terminology seems likely to survive, which is some recognition of his work.

Gas-Liquid Chromatography (GLC)—Principles

If a substance in the form of a vapor is in contact with a liquid of low vapor pressure, a proportion of the vapor molecules will dissolve in the liquid phase. For any given combination of vapor and liquid, the proportion of the former that transfers into the latter is fixed under specified circumstances. The ratio

$$\frac{\text{Weight of substance per unit volume of liquid phase}}{\text{Weight of substance per unit volume of vapor phase}}$$

is called the partition coefficient.

If the liquid phase is held stationary as a very thin layer on some kind of inert support, and if the vapor is carried over the liquid surface by a stream of inert gas (carrier gas), some of the vapor molecules at the leading edge of the vapor mass will transfer into the liquid phase. Since they cannot move in the liquid phase to any appreciable extent, they are retarded in their movement; the rest of the vapor molecules travel further on and are in turn taken up in the liquid phase. At the rear edge of the moving vapor mass, the space above the liquid phase is now occupied by carrier gas only, and the molecules of vapor that originally dissolved in the liquid will now be released and returned into the carrier gas (see Fig. 4–9). The net effect is that the original mass of vapor molecules will travel along as a compact body.

If the single vaporized substance is replaced by a mixture of two substances with different partition coefficients, the same processes of solution and release will take place, but the extent to which each substance is retarded in its movement by those processes will differ, and the original homogeneous mixture of two vaporized substances will be separated into two distinct, moving masses of pure vapor. To use an analogy, in a race over snow, a man in snowshoes, who is less hindered by its softness than a man in boots, will soon pull ahead.

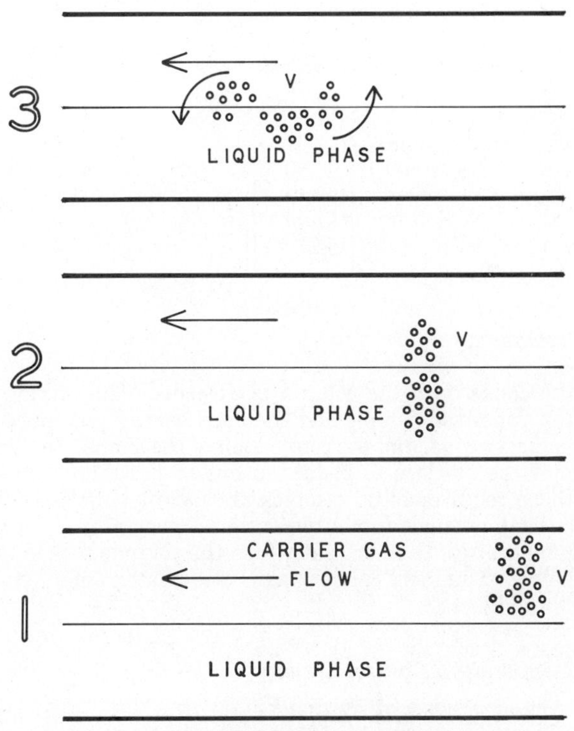

Figure 4–9 Diagrammatic sequence of events in gas-liquid chromatography. In 1, the vaporized sample is carried into the space above the stationary liquid phase. In 2, the sample partly dissolves in the liquid phase. In 3, as the initially undissolved portion of the sample moves along the column and enters the liquid phase, the previously dissolved portion of the sample re-enters the space above the liquid phase.

The Gas Chromatograph *(Fig. 4–10)*

The basic components of a gas chromatograph are (1) sample injection system; (2) temperature control system; (3) carrier gas flow control system, including flow meter; (4) column; and (5) detection system and recorder.

Sample Injection System

The sample must be in vapor form when it enters the column, all the components of a mixture must be completely vaporized, and the quantity of sample must be adequate for reliable measurement but not so large that

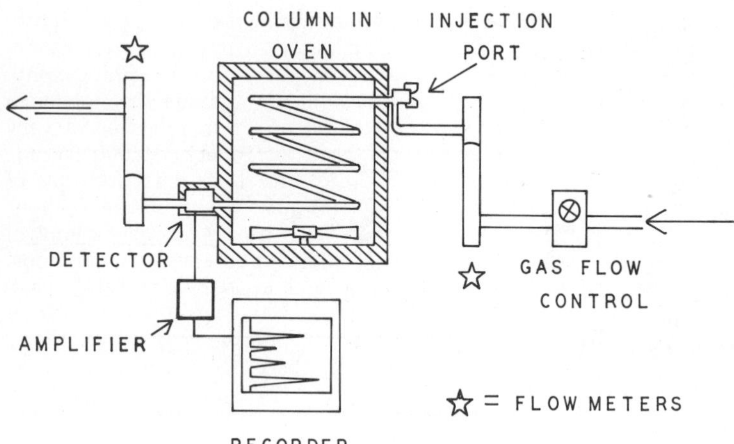

Figure 4–10 Main components of a simple gas chromatograph.

the capacity of the column is exceeded. The mixing of the vaporized sample and the inert carrier gas must be homogeneous, and the conversion of the sample to vapor must be as close to instantaneous as possible. To meet these requirements, samples are usually injected with special syringes into a block that is heated to a higher temperature than that at which the column is held (see below). The inert carrier gas is also heated before entry to the block.

Temperature Control System

The requirements are stringent. Not only must high temperatures of up to 350°C be possible, but they must be controlled within narrow limits of ± 1°. In addition, for some methods the temperature must be raised at a rapid rate and in a predetermined sequence and lowered under similar control. The usual method of meeting these requirements is an insulated hot air oven in which rapid equilibration of temperature is achieved by high-volume fan circulation.

Carrier Gas System

The inert carrier gas, which sweeps the vaporized sample through the column, may be nitrogen, argon, or helium; for some applications, hydrogen and carbon dioxide have been used. The gas must be pure, free of water vapor and hydrocarbons. In some instances, the carrier gas used depends on the detection system to be employed (see below).

Column

The column is the site of interaction between the sample and the absorbing liquid. Since the sample in vapor form is transported by the carrier gas, it is referred to as the mobile phase; the absorbing liquid is held in some form of support and is therefore called the stationary phase. The efficiency of the interchange processes between mobile and stationary phases, which determine the effectiveness of the GLC system, requires that the absorbing liquid is distributed in a thin layer. There are two main methods: (a) the packed column and (b) the capillary column.

(a) Typical dimensions of a packed column are about 2 meters long, internal bore 2 to 9 mm, usually coiled to permit more compact design of the temperature control oven. The stationary phase is coated on a porous solid such as diatomaceous earth, crushed firebrick, glass beads, ground teflon, special fluorocarbon polymers, and even a porous matrix produced by heating commercial detergent powder. The column itself may be glass, copper, stainless steel, or aluminum. The stationary phase liquid is coated on the packing support solid, usually prior to packing, by dissolving it in a volatile solvent, covering a thin layer of the packing solid, and removing the solvent by heat or forced evaporation. Typical stationary phase liquids are long-chain hydrocarbons such as squalane, silicone oils, and greases, esters such as dinonylphthalate, and polyalcohols such as polyethyleneglycol.

(b) In a capillary column, the support for the stationary phase is the inner surface of the tube itself. Capillary columns are narrow bore, 0.1 to 0.25 mm, and can be very long, up to 30 meters, and for special purposes, even as long as several hundred meters. They are made of glass or stainless steel, and the coating of stationary phase liquid is very thin, measuring from 0.5 to 5.0 micrometers.

Before the detection systems used in GLC are described, some definitions are required. *Retention time* is the time elapsed from the insertion of the sample into the column to the appearance of a particular component at the detector.

Another identifying property of a substance in GLC is its *retention volume.* If a substance takes 15 minutes to reach the detector with a carrier gas flow rate of 20 mL per minute, the volume of gas required to move that substance through the column is 15 × 20 = 300 mL. This is the retention volume. In practice, the retention volume is affected by so many variables that it is easier to express it as a fraction of the retention volume of a known substance. The fraction

$$\frac{\text{Retention volume of unknown}}{\text{Retention volume of reference}}$$

is called the *relative retention.*

Detection System

The successful application of GLC to the separation and identification of the components of mixtures relies on the availability of systems able to detect very small amounts of pure substances in the effluent stream of the carrier gas. A modern detector is sensitive to 10^{-10} to 10^{-13} g. This sensitivity is achieved by using detectors that produce an electrical signal in response to the appearance of substances in the effluent carrier gas; this signal can be electronically amplified to drive a recorder pen. The thermal conductivity detector, also called a katharometer, employs a heated wire or an electronic device called a thermistor, whose electrical resistance varies with temperature. If the wire temperature is set at a steady level by the application of a constant electrical current, and if the flow rate of carrier gas past the wire is constant, the rate of heat loss from the wire by the cooling effect of the gas flow is also constant. When a vaporized substance is eluted from the column in the carrier gas, its presence changes the rate at which the hot wire is cooled in the gas flow. The associated change in the temperature of the sensor wire produces a change in its electrical resistance, which can be detected and amplified electronically.

The flame ionization detector depends on the very large increase in electrical conductivity of a flame when the hydrogen-oxygen mixture used to produce it is contaminated with very small amounts of organic compounds.

In another type of detector, the ionization of the carrier gas, argon, is produced by beta particles emitted from a radioactive nickel foil. The free electrons released from the argon produce an excited energy state in ground state argon atoms, which in turn produce ionization of organic molecules derived from the GLC column. The net result is an increased number of ions and hence an increased current, which can be amplified.

The final component of the system is the recorder, which must be sensitive to voltages in the millivolt range and have a rapid response time. The duration of the signal from the detector for a component in the column effluent may be only a second or so, and unless the recorder pen can respond quickly, the full height of the peak may not be recorded.

Quantification

The read-out from a GLC system is a series of peaks on a recorder tracing. The separated compounds are identified by their different retention times, often by comparison with that of an internal standard. The quantity of a component producing a peak is proportional to the area under the peak, and various means of determining the areas under the peaks are used. A common approximation is to multiply the peak height by the peak width at a point halfway up the peak; this assumes that the shape of the peak is that of the Gaussian distribution.

High-Performance Liquid Chromatography (HPLC)

In order to take full advantage of the ability of columns incorporating such principles as adsorption, ion exchange, gel permeation, and liquid-liquid partition to separate labile compounds that would be seriously denatured by such methods as gas-liquid chromatography, the inherently slow movement of fluids through such columns can be accelerated by the application of very high pressures on the order of 4000 to 10,000 pounds per square inch (27.5 to 69 MPa.) Through the use of changes in the ultraviolet absorption in the effluent from the column, excellent and rapid separations of many labile biological compounds—such as peptides, lipids, antibiotics, drugs, catecholamines, and steroids—can be made. For assay of the last three groups of substances this technique is coming into use in many routine clinical chemistry laboratories.

Gel Permeation Chromatography (GPC)

In gel permeation chromatography, the column is packed with very small beads of special polymers. When swollen with water, the pores and channels in the beads have a range of sizes determined by the characteristics of the polymers. Since the pores are of molecular size, if a mixture of compounds of high molecular weights is passed through the column, the smaller molecules will become temporarily trapped in the pores of the beads and hence delayed in their movement; larger molecules will tend to bypass the pores. The net result is that the larger molecules will leave the column first, followed by the other compounds in ascending order of molecular size, although the sequence is also affected by molecular shape. The GPC method is still largely a research technique used to separate mixtures of peptides, proteins, haptoglobins, nucleic acids, and other important biological compounds. It has also been used to determine the approximate molecular weight of proteins. Components of a mixture separated on a GPC column are usually detected by ultraviolet absorbance or by differences in refractive index or electrical conductivity.

Ion-Exchange Chromatography

The principle of ion exchange between anions or cations in a solution and charged side-groups on synthetic resin molecules has a much wider range of uses than the production of deionized water or isolation of compounds prior to analysis. If a suitable ion-exchange resin is used as a column packing, its particular affinities for members of a group of ionized compounds can be used for their separation. The principle has been most extensively applied to inorganic ion separations, but it has one important use in biochemistry. If a solution containing a mixture of amino acids is applied to a column of a suitable ion-exchange resin, the amino acids become linked to the resin by exchange with its active side-groups. The firmness of the attachment, however, varies, and if the column is subsequently washed through (eluted) with a series of buffers of different pH values, the individual amino acids can be eluted from the column in sequence and quantified by their reaction with ninhydrin. The entire process can be automated, permitting the detection and quantification of the amino acids in complex mixtures such as hydrolysates of proteins, and urine.

ELECTROPHORESIS

If an electrical force is created in a tube of fluid containing charged particles by means of electrodes at the ends of the tube, the particles will migrate in the fluid toward the electrode whose polarity (negative or positive property) is opposite in sign to the charge on the particles. The attractive force is proportional to the product of the charge on the particle and the potential (power) of the electrical force in volts per centimeter of tube length. The speed of movement of the charged particles depends on their distance from the attracting electrode; they tend to accelerate as they get closer to the electrode. This tendency is opposed by the increase in the retarding effect of the viscosity of the fluid as the speed of the charged particles increases. (Viscosity can be thought of as the "internal friction" that resists changes in the flow of a fluid.) The two forces will be in balance, and therefore the velocity of the charged particles will remain constant during the entire trip down the tube, at one particular value for the rate of migration of the particles. The actual rate of migration is determined directly by the electrical charge on the particle and inversely by its ionic radius. Thus, the greater the charge and the smaller the ionic radius, the faster the rate of migration of a particle for a particular voltage. Particles that differ either in electrical charge or in ionic radius can therefore be separated. It should be noted that the ionic radius of a particle may be much larger than its molecular size, owing to the particle's tendency to pick up water molecules and solute molecules from the fluid. This effect is particularly important with proteins.

Electrophoresis in a tube of fluid can be done (this is the classical Tiselius method), but it is technically difficult. Routine methods of electrophoresis minimize diffusion of the separated fractions or groups of charged particles by holding the fluid medium in some kind of solid support such as paper, cellulose acetate, starch gel, agar, agarose gel, or polyacrylamide gel. After separation of the groups of charged particles, they can be easily detected by fixing them onto the support medium and using specific stains.

Electrophoresis on a support medium (zone electrophoresis) is affected by several factors that determine the effectiveness of the separation. These are:

Electro-Osmosis. This is the movement of the buffer fluid itself under the influence of the applied voltage. The cellulose acetate tends to acquire a negative charge, and the water molecules in close association with the cellulose acetate become positively charged and are attracted toward the negative electrode or cathode. The negatively charged protein molecules move toward the anode, but the electro-osmotic flow of the buffer fluid moves the entire pattern back toward the cathode. The visible effect on the stained pattern is that the slowest moving component, the gamma globulins, is carried toward the cathode side of the point of application.

Heating Effect. The applied current produces some heating of the support medium, with evaporation of the fluid medium from its upper surface. (This is the source of the condensed moisture seen on the under surface of the electrophoretic tank lid.) As the fluid evaporates, capillary action draws fluid from the buffer compartments, producing a fluid flow in the cellulose acetate strip toward the center. The net result of this and other flow variations is to make the distance of travel of a particular component vary with varying points of application; thus the quality of separation of hemoglobins on cellulose acetate depends on the point of application. The heating effect, if allowed to become excessive, can cause severe distortion of the final pattern, and if a procedure requires a high voltage or current, the cell may have to be directly cooled.

Adsorption. In some cases, there is an attraction between the charged particles being separated and the molecules of the support medium. The effect is "tailing," that is, undue spreading of the separated fractions. One of the reasons for the clearer separations on cellulose acetate is that its adsorptive capacity is lower than that of paper.

Gel Pore Size. With starch gel, polyacrylamide gel, and Sephadex (a synthetic polymer; see under "Gel permeation chromatography" on p. 87), the spaces between the gel particles are quite small and can act as a sieve of molecular dimensions. A second separation process is operative, and this can be seen in the much larger number of fractions obtained: about 30 on polyacrylamide as compared with five on cellulose acetate for serum proteins.

Practical Factors Affecting the Quality of Electrophoretic Separations

Buffer pH, Ionic Strength, and Composition. The pH of the buffer will determine the states of ionization of the charged groups of the constituent amino acids of proteins, and hence their electrical charges. Because of the cathode-directed movement of the fractions caused by electro-osmosis, and in order to obtain good separation of the proteins for detection and quantification, it is usual to use a buffer of high pH, usually about 8.6, since at this value all the proteins are negatively charged and move toward the anode. The ionic strength of the buffer is a compromise. High ionic strengths yield distinct separations, but the mobilities of the fractions are low, giving crowded patterns; low ionic strengths give faster rates of migration but more diffuse patterns. A typical value using a barbital buffer is 0.075. (For calculation of ionic strength, see Appendix F.)

The composition of the buffer affects the quality of separation to only a small extent. Barbital-based buffers are almost universal for proteins; TRIS buffers are used for hemoglobins.

Evaporation and Heating. If the enclosed volume of the electrophoretic tank (Fig. 4–11) is kept small and the tank is carefully sealed, the atmosphere inside will rapidly become saturated and further evaporation from the strip will be minimized. Since heating is proportional to the square of the current flowing, the voltage used should be just adequate to give good separations in a reasonable working time. If higher voltages are necessary, e.g., for hemoglobins, the process should be carried out in the cold room or refrigerator.

Sample Application. In order to minimize diffusion of the separated protein fractions the majority of sample applicators carry the material held by capillary attraction between two parallel wires or thin bars: when these

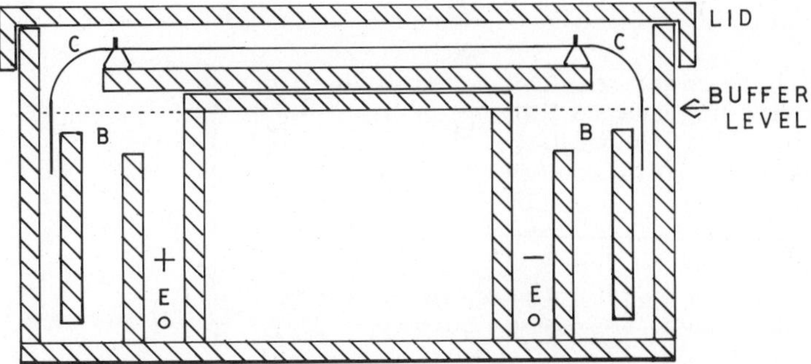

Figure 4–11 Cross-section of a simple electrophoresis apparatus. *E*, electrodes; *B*, baffle system to minimize diffusion of breakdown products of buffer; *C*, cellulose acetate membrane on carrier.

are brought into controlled contact with the surface of the support medium, the sample is transferred as a sharp, narrow band. The applicator must be scrupulously clean and undistorted. The controlled force of contact between the applicator and support medium surface prevents retention of some of the sample at the application point, with the consequent production of an artefactual band in the final stained pattern. In agarose gels and starch gels, a narrow slot is cut or formed in the gel, and the sample is transferred with a fine pipette or serrated plastic edge, or inserted soaked into a small strip of filter paper.

STAINING AND CLEARING. One of the chief advantages of cellulose acetate as a support medium is the ease with which the separated fractions can be stained and the background dye washed out, plus the ability to make the membrane crystal clear for subsequent scanning of the pattern of separated fractions. For the best results, the combined stain-fixative should not be used more than about eight to 10 times, and the dehydration and clearing baths should be changed after every third use. The procedure used for dehydration and clearing will depend on the particular apparatus and system in use; methanol-acetic acid, cyclohexanone, and dioxane have all been used, although the last-named is somewhat toxic. The time and temperature of the heating step are critical, and close control of oven temperature must be maintained.

SCANNING AND QUANTIFICATION. Most laboratories use some type of scanner, a device that moves the stained, cleared strip past a light source–filter–slit-photometer system, which produces an electrical signal proportional to the intensity of staining of each fraction and feeds this signal to the pen of a strip chart recorder. A typical recording is shown in Figure 6–10. More sophisticated versions incorporate an integrator, which is a mechanical or electronic system that measures the area under each peak of the tracing, plus a calculator and a printer that produces a typed report showing the actual serum concentration of each fraction. No matter how elaborate the system, however, it depends on the quality of the stained and cleared strip of cellulose acetate. Even very small artefacts will give errors, as will incomplete removal of solvents or overloading of the strip with protein. An old, dirty batch of dye will deposit small, darkly staining specks on the strip; incomplete clotting of the same prior to application will give rise to an extra peak of fibrinogen on the strip between the beta and gamma fractions.

ELECTROPHORESIS OF SAMPLES WITH LOW PROTEIN CONCENTRATIONS

Although it is possible to process samples such as urine and cerebrospinal fluid directly using a highly sensitive protein stain such as nigrosin, it is technically simpler to concentrate the sample until the protein level approaches that of a serum sample. Thus, if a CSF with a protein level of 50 mg per dL can be reduced to 1/100 of its volume, the protein concentration is now $\frac{50 \times 100}{1000} = 5.0$ g per dL, which is quite adequate for separation and quantification of the fractions. The most convenient method for concentration, which should not denature the proteins, is membrane filtration.

Membrane Filtration. The requisite conditions for rapid ultrafiltration, i.e., large working area of the semipermeable membrane and efficient removal of water and permeating solutes, are obtained in the Minicon–B concentrator* by making the membrane the rear wall of a plastic cell and backing it with an absorbent pad. The working area of the membrane is 22 cm^2, and the pad can absorb at least three times the filling volume of the cell, which is 5 mL. The cutoff point of the membrane (which is stated as the molecular weight above which solutes will not pass through the membrane) is 15,000, so that all proteins of interest, including Bence Jones protein, are retained in the cell. The cell is tapered so that the sample is finally concentrated in its tip, where the membrane is made impermeable to prevent complete desiccation of the sample. The cell is filled with 5 mL of CSF or filtered urine and refrigerated overnight (Figs. 4–12 and 4–13). If the initial protein level is greater than about 70 mg per dL, it may be necessary to terminate the process when the sample has been concentrated down to the 25 or 50 × mark. After concentration, the sample is removed with a fine capillary pipette and used for electrophoresis or immunoelectrophoresis.

This method is simple and economical, and the gain in sensitivity is such that Bence Jones protein can be detected at levels far too low for detection by the usual tests. When introducing samples into the cell, care must be taken not to scratch the very thin membrane forming the rear face.

*Amicon Corporation, Danvers, Mass. 01923 and Oakville, Ont. L6H 2B9.

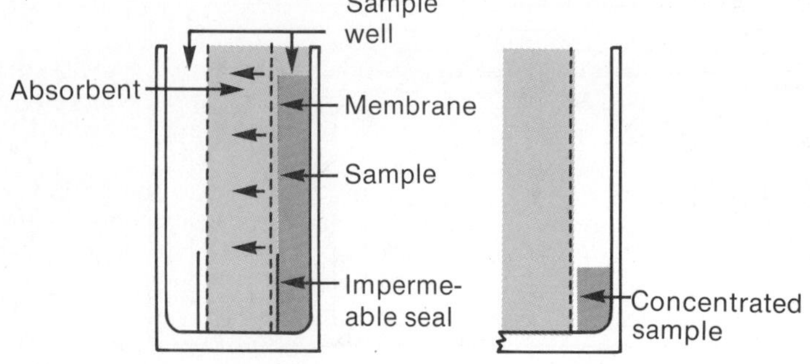

Figure 4–12 Cross-section of "Minicon"-type concentration cell. (Courtesy of Amicon Corp., Danvers, Mass. 01923.)

The process does not give quantitative recovery of solutes with molecular weights above the cutoff point; this must be noted if the concentrate is to be used for immunoelectrophoresis.

PROBLEMS WITH ZONE ELECTROPHORESIS

The cellulose acetate system has been in use for more than 10 years, and the majority of clinical laboratories are familiar with the procedure, assisted by the excellent instruction manuals of the manufacturers. The experience and judgment of the technologist are still required for detection and correction of the causes of poor results and for scrutiny of the patterns for abnormalities.

The chief causes of poor results are:

CROWDED PATTERNS. Voltage too low; incorrect ionic strength of buffer; poor electrical contact between cellulose acetate strip and buffer compartments; loose electrical contacts to the platinum wire electrodes; or insufficient running time.

DIFFUSE, INDISTINCT PATTERNS. Voltage too high; running time too long; incomplete blotting of strip prior to sample application; faulty batch of cellulose acetate; incorrect ionic strength of buffer; denaturation of sample from bacterial contamination or overlong storage; use of a staining bath from which the fixative has been omitted.

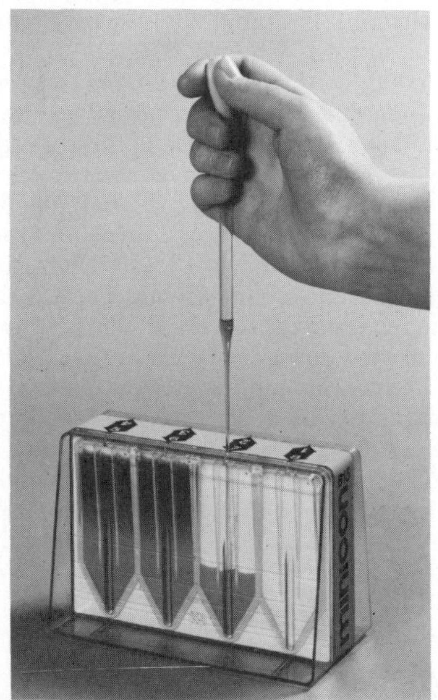

Figure 4–13 Placing sample into "Minicon" cell for concentration (Courtesy of Amicon Corp., Danvers, Mass. 01923.)

DISTORTED PATTERNS. Overheating owing to a too high current setting; uneven wetting of cellulose acetate strip prior to sample application; dirty sample applicator; excessive load of sample (sera with very high protein levels owing to large monoclonal components should be diluted with buffer); uneven tension of the strip on the carrier; buffer spots on the strip caused by excessive condensation in the tank; fingerprints on the strip during removal from storage box, immersion in buffer or sample application; or presence of mucoprotein strands in such samples as pleural fluid and joint fluids.

NO SEPARATION OF FRACTIONS. Failure of power supply; faulty electrical connections; strip not making contact with buffer compartment containing electrodes. It should be noted that a reading on the *voltmeter* on the power supply does not prove that the electrical connections are in order; there must be *current* flow. Substitution of saline or other fluid for the correct buffer should be detected by excessive current flow and overheating.

WEAK OR UNEVEN STAINING. Old or overused staining solution; or poor technique in floating strip on dye surface causing uneven penetration.

PATCHY OR CLOUDY CLEARING OF STRIP. Excessive use of clearing solution or evaporation; poor technique in applying strip to glass plate; leaving strip too long in clearing bath; oven too cold; or trapped air bubbles under strip.

GROSS DISTORTION OR WRINKLING OF CLEARED STRIP. Incorrect composition of clearing solution; or excessive oven temperature.

EXTRA BAND ON STAINED STRIP. Incomplete clotting of sample with residual fibrinogen; excessive application force owing to defective sample applicator's marring of surface of cellulose acetate; or lipemic serum with large content of chylomicrons.

The interpretation of plasma protein separations is discussed in Chapter 6, p. 147.

IMMUNOELECTROPHORESIS (IEP)

This technique, which involves the detection and quantification of individual proteins by combining the separative power of electrophoresis with the specificity of the antigen-antibody reaction, is described on p. 550.

LIGAND ASSAYS (COMPETITIVE PROTEIN-BINDING ASSAYS)

Definitions

Ligand—Any substance that will become bound to a specified binding agent, forming a ligand-binding agent complex.

Binding agent—A substance possessing one or more sites on its molecule that can hold a ligand.

Label (marker, tracer)—A substance that can be used to indicate the presence of a ligand and to differentiate ligand molecules thus labeled from those not so labeled.

Antigen—Any substance that will provoke the production of a specific immune response in an animal.

Antibody—An immunoglobulin produced in response to an antigen and having a specific binding affinity for it.

Hapten—A small organic nonprotein molecule, incapable of provoking any immune response itself, but which in combination with a protein can stimulate the production of an antibody specific for the combination.

Affinity—The strength of the attraction of the ligand and the binding agent.

Avidity—The strength of the attachment of the ligand to the binding agent after binding has occurred.

Capacity—The number of binding sites on the molecule of a binding agent.

Specificity—The ability of a ligand assay to determine a single analyte without interference from other substances.

Sensitivity—The smallest amount of an analyte that can be discriminated from a blank value with a specified degree of reliability.

Types of Ligand Assays

Ligand assays are subdivided into the following:

1. *Competitive protein-binding assays,* which are in practice taken to indicate those procedures in which the binding agent is a naturally occurring plasma protein.
2. *Radioimmunoassays (RIA),* a subgroup of competitive protein-binding assays in which the binding protein is an artificially provoked antibody to the analyte and the label used to detect the ligand is a radioisotope.
3. *Fluoroimmunoassays (FIA),* which employ a fluorescent substance as the ligand label.
4. *Enzyme immunoassays (EIA, ELISA),* which use an enzyme-substrate system as the ligand label.
5. *Viroimmunoassays (VIA),* which label the ligand with a bacteriophage that is rendered inactive (unable to produce plaques on suitable bacterial colonies) when linked to an antigen ligand. The bacteriophage-labeled antigen ligand competes with the unlabeled ligand (the analyte) for the limited number of binding sites on the binding agent, which is an antibody. This method has had only very limited application.

The use of ligand assays will be illustrated by reference to the two most widely employed—radioimmunoassay and the EMIT (Syva) version of enzyme immunoassay. (The ELISA version of enzyme immunoassay, using enzyme-labeled antigens or antibodies attached to a solid support, such as glass beads, is mainly applied to the detection of microbiological ligands.)

PRINCIPLE OF RADIOIMMUNOASSAY (RIA)

Radioimmunoassay combines the high specificity of an antigen-antibody reaction with the great sensitivity of detection and quantification of compounds tagged with a radioactive "label" atom.

If there is in a solution a mixture of three components, i.e., a "natural," or unlabeled, antigen, the same antigen with one of its atoms carrying a radioactivity label, and a quantity of antibody specific for the antigen that is insufficient to bind all the unlabeled and labeled antigen molecules present, the two forms of the antigen will compete for the available binding sites. Thus, if the number of labeled and unlabeled molecules is the same, each type has an equal chance of finding a free binding site; half the available antibody binding sites will carry labeled antigen and half will carry unlabeled antigen (Fig. 4–14*A*). If the number of unlabeled antigen molecules is greater than the number of labeled ones, a larger number of the antibody binding sites will become occupied by unlabeled antigen molecules (Fig. 4–14*C*). Thus, the larger the number of unlabeled antigen molecules in the mixture, the smaller the fraction of the original quantity of labeled antigen that will become bound by antibody. Since the firmly bound combination of antigen and antibody can be separated from the remaining components of the original mixture and its radioactivity determined and compared with that of the original labeled antigen addition, and since the relative amounts of bound and free labeled antigen will depend on the number of unlabeled antigen molecules originally present, a calibration curve can be made by adding known amounts of unlabeled antigen to the system of labeled antigen and antibody, separating, determining the ratio of radioactivity of bound to original labeled antigen, and plotting this ratio against the known amounts of added unlabeled antigen. If a sample containing an unknown amount of natural (unlabeled) antigen is then mixed with the same amounts of labeled antigen and antibody as in the calibration curve mixture, the antigen-antibody complex separated and the ratio of its radioactivity determined when compared with that of the original amount of labeled antigen, this ratio, usually expressed as a percentage, when referred to the calibration curve, will give the amount of unlabeled (natural) antigen in the sample.

The unique combination of specificity and sensitivity of the RIA principle makes it particularly suitable for the assay of substances such as insulin, growth hormone, thyroxine, testosterone, progesterone, angiotensin, aldosterone, and drugs such as digoxin in serum or plasma at the level of nanograms per mL.

The procedures involved in radioimmunoassay differ in the radioactive element used as the label, in the method used to separate the antigen-antibody combination from the unbound antigen, and in the standardization. The majority of current methods use ^{125}I (radioactive iodine) or ^{3}H (tritium, the radioactive isotope of hydrogen) as the labels. For separation of the antigen-antibody combination, charcoal coated with dextran is used. The dextran acts as a molecular sieve that passes only unbound antigen molecules for retention by the charcoal; the antigen-antibody combinations are too large to cross the dextran coating. After centrifuging, the relatively dense charcoal grains with their adsorbed

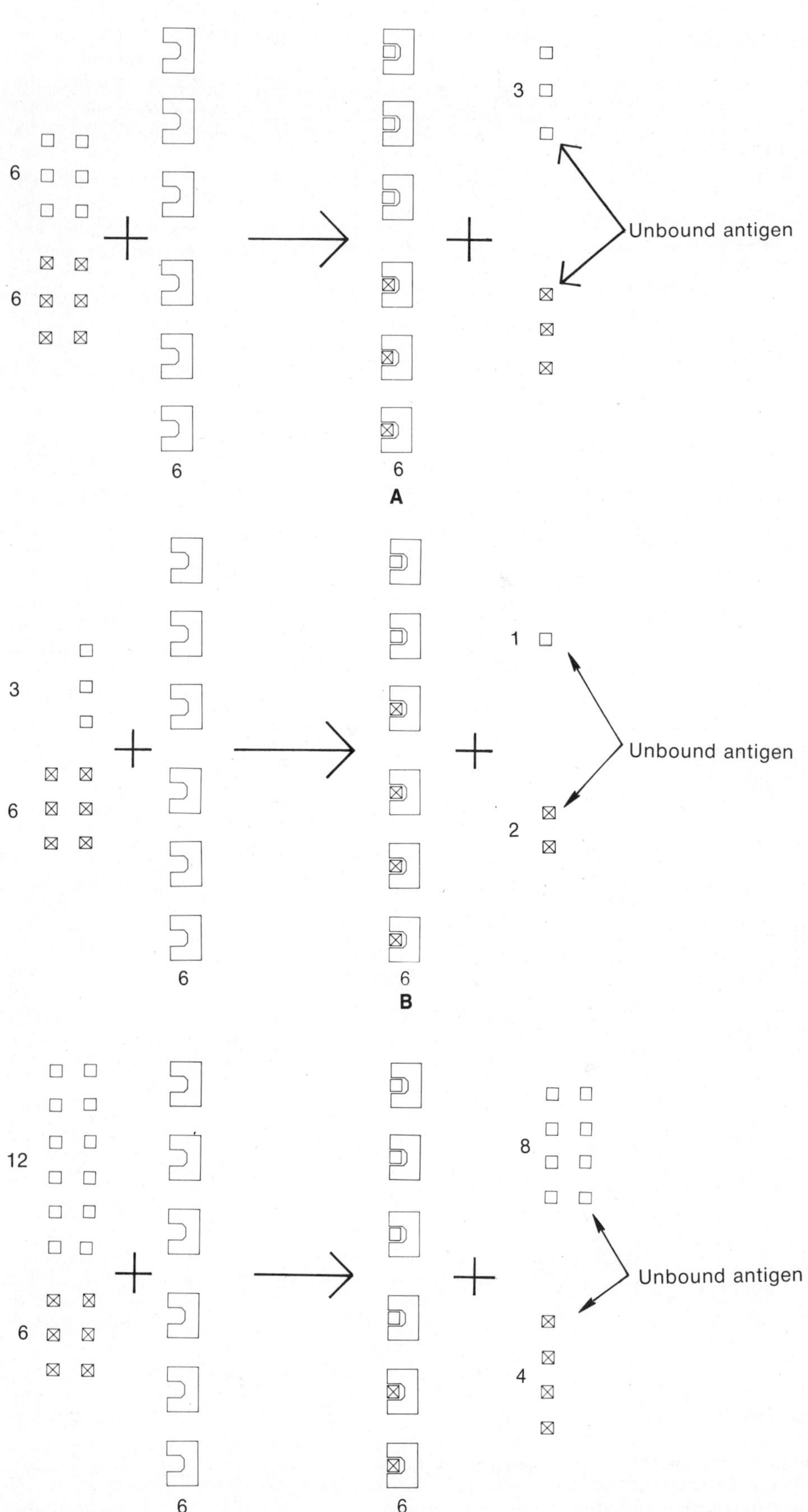

Figure 4–14 *A,* Principle of RIA. The initial concentrations of unlabeled and labeled antigen are equal, and the radioactivity of the bound and free antigen is in the ratio 1 to 1. Percentage bound, 50%.

B, The initial concentrations of unlabeled and labeled antigen are in the ratio 1 to 2, and the radioactivity of the bound to free antigen is in the ratio 2 to 1. Percentage bound, 67%.

C, The initial concentrations of unlabeled and labeled antigen are in the ratio 2 to 1, and the radioactivity of the bound to free antigen is in the ratio 1 to 2. Percentage bound, 33%.

Note that the proportion of bound antigen *decreases* as the number of molecules of unlabeled antigen *increases.*

antigen molecules will be packed at the bottom of the tube, and the supernatant containing the antigen-antibody combinations can be separated. Measurement of the ratio of radioactivities of the two components completes the assay. A more sophisticated method of precipitating the antigen-antibody combination is to add a second antibody prepared to react with the protein of the first antibody, usually a gamma globulin. The resultant complex can then be separated either by centrifugation or cellulose acetate filters. Standardization can be done as described in the description of general principles above.

The RIA technique promises to provide reliable data by relatively simple methods about biological substances that present considerable analytical problems when more orthodox procedures are used. In practice, of course, RIA has its own sources of error. These include

1. Lability of the compound analyzed.
2. Antibody cross-reaction with related antigens.
3. Interfering substances in the sample, e.g., urea and bilirubin.
4. Poor pipetting technique (good pipetting technique is critical, because of the very small volumes).
5. Inefficiency of the centrifuging steps.
6. Contamination of the equipment from extraneous radioactive materials.
7. Change in the antigen's chemical or immunological identity owing to the process of adding radioactive label to the antigen.

RIA methods measure the amounts of particular molecular structures, not their biological activity.

Measurement of Radioactivity

The radioactive atoms used as labels produce different types of emitted radiation. ^{125}I emits short-wavelength, high-energy gamma rays; ^{3}H (tritium) produces beta-type radiation, which is actually high-speed particles, positively or negatively charged electrons. Gamma rays are detected by a so-called scintillation counter, which consists of a large sodium iodide crystal that contains thallium as an activator. The crystal is in close contact with a photomultiplier tube (see p. 72), and when an emitted quantum of gamma radiation strikes a sodium iodide molecule in the crystal lattice, it produces a photon of light energy. This light is picked up and amplified by the associated photomultiplier tube and converted to a pulse of electrical energy. The *number* of pulses is proportional to the quantity of radioactive material in the sample; the power or *energy* of the pulse is determined by the energy of the original gamma ray. The scintillation counter incorporates "discriminators," which pass through only those pulses whose energy levels correspond to those of the gamma radiation emitted from the particular radioactive atom whose detection is required. Finally, the scintillation counter uses a scaler to count the number of pulses arriving in a preset time or to determine the time required for a preset number of pulses to occur.

To detect beta particles, which have less energy than gamma radiation, a liquid scintillation system is used. The sample is mixed in a so-called scintillation cocktail, which contains substances that are excited to emit light when struck by a beta particle. These compounds, sometimes called "fluors," are dissolved in special grade solvents such as toluene and hexafluorobenzene; the latter is used when a liquid scintillation system is used to count gamma radiation. The fluors are referred to by abbreviations: thus, POPOP is 1,4-di-2-(5-phenyloxazoyl)-benzene; BBOT is 2,5-bis-(5′-tertiary-butylbenzoxazolyl-(2′)-thiophen. The light emissions are detected by a pair of photomultiplier tubes, which are arranged so that only those light flashes that are picked up simultaneously by both photomultipliers are recorded; any energy pulses that occur in the photomultiplier tubes from external radiation sources are ignored. One advantage of the liquid scintillation system is that it can be used for detecting gamma radiation as well as beta particles. The gamma radiation stimulates the molecules of the solvent to emit so-called Compton electrons, which in turn cause light emission from the fluor. The chief problem with liquid scintillation systems is called "quench." This is a general term for effects of temperature, color, ionic strength, and the amount of water present, which reduce the counting efficiency of the system. Counting efficiency is that percentage of the actual radioactivity of the sample that is detected; even under the best conditions it is only about 60%, and any standardization methods must take this into account.

Substances Assayed by RIA

Any list is inevitably provisional because of the dramatic growth in the use of the RIA principle. The following procedures are representative of those available as commercial kits:

Renin Activity	Human Placental Lactogen
Cortisol	Follicle Stimulating Hormone
Insulin	Luteinizing Hormone
Vitamin B_{12}	Folate
Cyclic AMP	Morphine
Digoxin	IgE
Digitoxin	Human Chorionic Gonadotropin
Human Growth Hormone	Testosterone

Principle of the Enzyme Multiplied Immunoassay Technique (EMIT)*

In order to make use of the principle of competition for the active sites on an antibody by molecules of the corresponding antigen from two sources, it is necessary to label in some way the antigen molecules from one of the sources. In radioimmunoassay (see p. 91) the label is a radioactive atom, and the location in the analytical system and the quantity of labeled fraction of the antigen can be determined by measurement of the characteristic radiation emissions from the label. There are two disadvantages to this approach: the radioactive label is detectable only for a limited time, determined by the decline in the very radioactivity by which it is measured, and special detection equipment (gamma counter, scintillation counter) is required. The EMIT method over-

*Syva Company, Palo Alto, Calif. 94304.

comes both disadvantages by using an enzyme as the label and the change in absorbance associated with its action on a substrate (as measured in a spectrophotometer at 340 nm) for quantitation.

For each compound assayed by this method a specific antibody is produced. The reaction mixture is prepared to contain the serum sample with its content of the "free" (that is, unlabeled) form of the drug, a restricted amount of the antibody to the drug, an enzyme substrate and the requisite coenzyme, and a fixed amount of a combination of the drug and an enzyme with activity against the substrate. There are thus two forms of the drug in the mixture: the free drug from the patient's serum and the added drug-enzyme combination. Since the amount of antibody is limited, the two forms of the drug (the antigen) compete for the available reaction sites on the antibody molecules. If the drug-enzyme combination gains access to the active site on the antibody, a change is induced in the three-dimensional form of the enzyme that destroys its ability to attack the substrate. As the number of molecules of the free drug increases, more of the active sites on the antibody are occupied and correspondingly fewer of the enzyme-drug combination molecules are able to bind to the antibody. The enzyme-drug combination molecules that are thus left free in the mixture will react with the substrate and produce a change in the coenzyme and hence a change in the absorbance at 340 nm. Thus, the higher the concentration of the free drug, the greater the number of drug-enzyme molecules left free and the larger the change in absorbance at 340 nm associated with activity against the substrate. The absorbance produced in the mixture containing the unknown serum sample can be compared with a calibration curve produced by running the procedure with known amounts of the free drug. The method has been successfully applied to the assay of such drugs as theophylline, phenytoin, phenobarbital, digoxin, and morphine and to the determination of thyroxine.

RADIOACTIVE ISOTOPES

Although modern knowledge of the structure of the atomic nucleus has shown it to be most complex, it is convenient here to regard it as containing two main kinds of elementary particles: positively charged protons and uncharged neutrons. The proton has unit mass and a single positive charge; the neutron has the same mass but is uncharged. The total positive charge of the nucleus, which equals the number of protons therein, is balanced by an equal number of negative electrons in orbit around it. (Again, the situation is much more complex than this, but the picture is adequate for our purposes.) The sum of the mass units of protons and neutrons equals the atomic weight of the element, the weight of the electrons being negligible. The chemical properties of an element are determined by the number of orbital electrons. It is possible, therefore, to have a group of elements with the same number of electrons (and therefore identical chemical natures) but differing in the number of neutrons in the nucleus, and therefore in their atomic weights. Such a group of elements constitutes a family of isotopes. The element tin occurs in 10 different isotopic forms, all with 50 orbital electrons, but with atomic weights ranging from 111 to 125. The existence of isotopes for many elements explains why naturally occurring elements do not have atomic weights that are exact whole numbers; their atomic weights are the weighted averages of the isotopes composing them.

As a result, probably, of the increasing complexity of nuclear structure with increasing atomic weight, all elements with atomic weights above 209 or atomic numbers (the number of positive charges on the nucleus) above 83 show the phenomenon of spontaneous nuclear decay, or radioactivity. In this process, the unstable nucleus achieves temporary stability by the emission of radiation or high-speed elementary particles. If the emission of the particle changes the nuclear mass or charge, either another isotope of the element or a new element is formed. The existence of radioactive atoms in nature, as opposed to those artificially produced in the intense neutron flux of the nuclear reactor, is not limited to the heavier atoms; the well-known technique of dating organic materials by measurement of their content of radioactive carbon is based on its natural occurrence.

The use of radioisotopes for diagnosis depends on the ability to detect and measure the element, no matter in what chemical combination it may occur, by means of its emitted particles or radiation. These emissions can be of three types: alpha particles, which are identical to the nuclei of helium atoms, with a mass of four units and a positive charge of two units; beta particles, which are high-speed electrons with velocities that may approach the speed of light, negligible mass, and a single negative or positive charge (the latter is sometimes called a positron); and gamma radiation, which is very short-wavelength electromagnetic radiation similar to x-rays. (The origin of beta particles from a nucleus stated to contain protons and neutrons may appear to be a contradiction. It is believed that the negative beta particle arises by fission of a neutron, producing a proton and the beta particle; the positron is produced by a similar breakup of a proton, releasing a neutron as well.)

All three types of emission can be detected by suitable equipment, and the intensity measured in terms of the number of emitted particles ("counts per minute") or bursts of energy per unit time. In addition, the characteristic energies of the emitted particles or rays can be measured as a means of identifying the particular isotope that emitted them.

Symbols

An isotope, radioactive or stable, is identified by the usual chemical symbol for the element with a subscript showing the atomic number (number of protons in the nucleus = number of orbital electrons) and a superscript showing the atomic weight (more correctly, the mass number). Thus, one of the radioactive isotopes of iodine used in nuclear medicine is commonly referred to as ^{131}I. The complete symbol is $^{131}I_{53}$.

Each individual isotope having its own unique atomic number and mass number is called a nuclide. There are over 800 nuclides, including the manmade elements beyond uranium in the periodic table.

Units of Radioactivity

The original unit, the curie, symbol Ci, equaled 3.7×10^{10} radioactive disintegrations per second, which is the radioactivity of 1 g of radium. This unit was divided into the millicurie, symbol mCi, 3.7×10^7 disintegrations per second, and the microcurie, symbol μCi, 3.7×10^4, or 37,000, disintegrations per second. The unit under the SI system is the becquerel, defined as "reciprocal seconds," that is, the number of events per second, with the symbol Bq. Thus, 1 microcurie equals 37 kBq (kilobecquerels). Generally speaking, the quantities of radioactivity encountered in analytical procedures involving radioisotopes are in the kilobecquerel range, and more sensitive detection equipment permits measurements at such a low level of activity that any associated radiation danger is negligible.

Modes of Use of Radioisotopes

As Tracers. If one or more atoms in the molecule of a substance are radioactive, that substance or its metabolites can be followed through any chemical or other processes by detecting its characteristic radioactivity. For example, carbon dioxide in which the carbon atom is radioactive can be taken up by a bacterium, and after allowing sufficient time for the organism to incorporate the CO_2 in its metabolism, the various metabolites can be extracted from a culture of the organism, separated, and identified by such techniques as thin-layer chromatography (see p. 84), and those into which the CO_2 was incorporated can be detected by their radioactivity. By techniques of this type, the metabolic pathways of the organism can be investigated.

As Locators. Some types of tumor tissue selectively take up certain elements from the circulation, and if a patient is surveyed by suitable detection equipment after administration of a nontoxic compound of such an element, the tumor can be located. By scanning techniques, in which the detection system is moved in a systematic pattern over the area of interest, such as the head, thyroid, or liver, a pattern of radioactivity that will map the particular organ and show regions of increased or decreased uptake of radioactivity can be obtained.

As Labels. If a quantity of a substance that has been labeled by making one of the atoms in its constituent molecule radioactive is subject to two possible directions or reactions in a procedure, the proportions of the original quantity that take each route can, with a high degree of accuracy, be determined by radioactivity measurements. The largest application of this principle is in radioimmunoassay, where the distribution of a labeled reactant is a measure of the quantity of its natural unlabeled analogue (see p. 91).

Radiation Hazards

The charged particles and rays given off by radioactive isotopes produce their effects on living tissue by causing the creation of pairs of ions along their path in the tissue. If the intensity of the radiation is such that the ionization produces abnormal molecular or atomic fragments in the cells, tissue damage will result. If the exposure to the radiation is minimal, there will be no visible effects. Larger doses will produce the syndrome of radiation sickness: nausea, vomiting, decrease in white cell count, and reddening of the skin in the area immediately affected by the radiation. These effects, however, will last only a fairly short time. Still larger doses will cause permanent cell damage: interference with cell division, eye damage, severe, possibly fatal, anemia, and, at a later date, malignant changes.

Because of increased sensitivity of detection instruments, the amounts of radioactivity required in diagnostic procedures are far too small to be dangerous in themselves. As far as possible, modern methods use radioactive elements with short half-lives. The half-life of a nuclide is the period of time it takes for its initial activity to fall to half its value. It is typical of a particular nuclide; indeed, some of the manmade nuclides are recognized only by their pattern of radioactive emissions and their extremely short half-lives. The only reason that some natural radioactive elements such as radium, uranium, and thorium are still found is that their half-lives are very long, and they have not yet decayed completely. One uranium nuclide has a half-life of 4.5×10^9 years, but diagnostic isotopes' activity after introduction into the body or in laboratory use falls off rapidly.

Despite this, strict precautions must be taken to avoid accidental ingestion or skin contamination with radioactive materials. Scrupulous technique, regular monitoring of work areas, thorough cleaning and decontamination after spills, and strict adherence to the "no smoking–no eating" rule in the laboratory are essential.

INDICATORS

Indicators are substances used to detect the end point (attainment of chemical reaction completion) when the concentration of one solute is determined by the measured addition (titration) of a reacting solute of known concentration. Examples are acid-base titrations, chloride ion determination, and oxidation-reduction reactions. In the last-named case, a typical reaction is the titration of oxalic acid with potassium permanganate in the Clark-Collip method for assay of serum calcium. The titrant, permanganate, also serves as the indicator, since it becomes colorless when reduced by the oxalic acid, and the end point is signaled by the first small excess of purple permanganate ion.

For acid-base titrations, in which the reactants are usually both colorless, an indicator is required that shows a sharp color change at the equivalence point: the majority of commonly used indicators for this purpose are weak acids whose degree of dissociation depends on pH. Thus over a range of about two pH units, centered on a pH value equal to the ionization constant of the acid indicator, the indicator changes from its undissociated form to its conjugate base form with a concomitant shift in color. In many cases, one of the forms of the indicator has a resonance or quinonoid structure that confers intense color on the molecule, and only a very small amount of indicator is required.

Selection of Indicators for Acid-Base Titrations

When a strong (highly ionized) acid is titrated with a strong base, the rate of change of pH as the equivalence

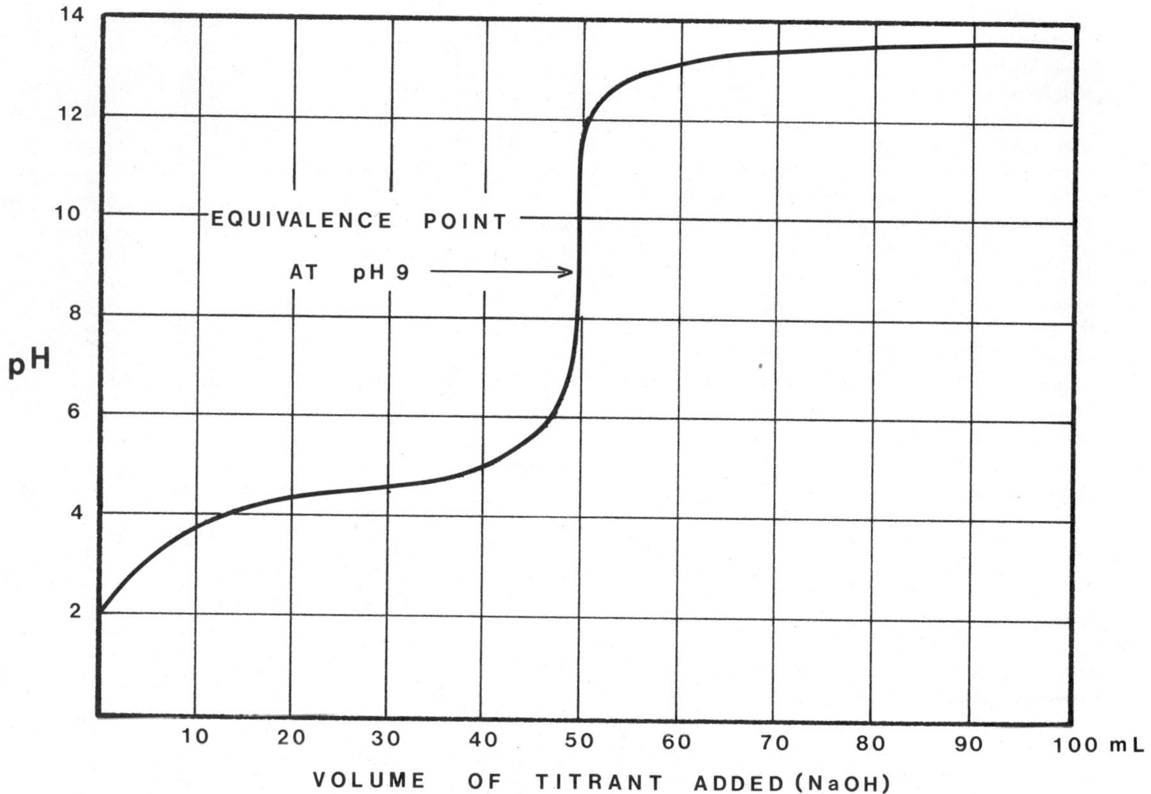

Figure 4–15 Titration curve showing the pattern of pH change when a weak acid, for example, acetic acid, is titrated with a strong base, such as sodium hydroxide, of equal molarity. Volume of acid used, 50 mL.

point is approached is so great that a number of indicators will signal the end point: the indicator is changed completely from one colored form to the other by one drop of titrant. When weak acids and bases are being titrated, an indicator must be used whose range of color change brackets the pH value at which equivalence of the reactants occurs. This critical pH value is initially determined by addition of the titrant in small, equal-volume aliquots and simultaneous recording of the pH with a pH meter (electrometric detection of end point). When the added volume of titrant is plotted graphically against pH, a curve similar to that in Figure 4–15 is obtained, and the pH corresponding to the middle of the inflexion point (see figure) designates the required characteristics of a suitable indicator.

For example, if a weak acid is titrated with a strong base, such as acetic acid with sodium hydroxide, the pH at the equivalence point is greater than pH 7.0 because the reaction in solution of the product of the process (sodium acetate) is about 9.0, and an indicator such as phenolphthalein, with an effective range pH 8.0 to 9.6, is appropriate. Conversely, when a weak base is titrated with a strong acid, such as ammonia in solution with hydrochloric acid, the reaction product is ammonium chloride, and its solution is acidic (pH 5.0) because of the presence of the ammonium ion NH_4^+. The correct indicator would be methyl red, with an operating range of 4.2 to 6.3. With very weak acids and bases the rate of change of the pH in the area of equivalence is so slow that titration using an indicator is not practical. (For chloride ion titration, see p. 197.)

In the presence of colloidal charged particles or molecules such as proteins, the color of an indicator may be shifted from that shown in a buffer free from colloids. This "protein error" of indicators can be used to detect protein in urine. The paper strip contains an indicator plus a buffer and, when wetted with urine, will show a typical hue. If protein is present, the charged molecules preferentially combine with one of the alternative forms of the indicator, causing a color shift. The extent of this shift is roughly proportional to the protein concentration. A typical system for this purpose is tetrabromthymol blue buffered to pH 3.0 with citrate; the protein molecules combine with the anionic (blue) state of the indicator, promoting an increased ionization of the yellow form. The resultant increase of the blue component of the system changes the original yellow to shades of green.

Other sources of interference with the action of some indicators are temperature and salt effects. The methyl red and methyl orange indicators change their dissociation constants (analogous to the ionization constants of the weak acids) with increase of temperature, thereby altering their effective ranges; salt concentrations above about 1 M have a similar effect. Some indicators show a slight shift in range when in alcohol solution, but in the usual titrations in aqueous solution, the small amount of alcohol derived from an indicator in that solvent is negligible.

PREVENTIVE MAINTENANCE

As the volume and scope of clinical laboratory work increase, the disruption of output produced by instrument failure becomes more unacceptable, particularly with the high-volume automated analyzers. An organized program of preventive maintenance, with responsibility clearly assigned and full records kept, is essential. Log books should be maintained for each major instrument with details of problems and actions taken and a copy of the serviceman's report. Even if an operating problem is successfully cleared by the technical staff, clear notes of the incident will accelerate the handling of similar difficulties in the future. In-service training on new equipment must include the specified maintenance, and compliance will be facilitated if the essential points are displayed in brief on a card attached to the instrument.

The list of equipment that follows is not exhaustive, and each laboratory must determine its own needs. It is intended only as an outline.

Automated Analyzers and Cell Counters

Carry out the manufacturer's schedule as the minimum, supplemented by further points based on the laboratory's own log book. Scrupulous cleanliness should be automatic: any sample or reagent spills must be cleaned up immediately. Avoid placing any container of any fluid (including coffee!) where a spill could gain access to electronics, particularly the control keyboard. When a reagent container requires refilling, flush it out thoroughly before filling. Check plastic reagent lines for kinks. Check that cooling fans are working, and clean any air filters regularly. Do not leave loose sample cups where they may jam moving parts. Investigate even the smallest fluid leak immediately. Keep records of calibration settings and ADC (analogue to digital conversion) numbers when available—sudden changes often precede instrument failures. If the records indicate that a source lamp in the photometric section of the instrument has a typical life of about seven or eight months, change it every six months. Change printer paper rolls as soon as the usual warning stripe of color appears. Clean paper residue and dust from printers with an air blast. Check waste lines and waste channels frequently for signs of solids accumulation.

Balance

The balance is used as a source of absolute accuracy for the preparation of standards. In addition to its careful placement in the laboratory, it must be kept scrupulously clean at all times. Merely brushing out spilt reagent chemicals is not enough: the last traces must be carefully and thoroughly removed with slightly dampened tissues and then the case interior dried. The analytical balance should not be used for stains and dyes. All weighings must be in either plastic weigh boats or weighing bottles: nothing should ever be placed directly on the pan. The balance should be protected from physical insult and rough handling. It should be checked and overhauled at least once yearly.

Blood Gas Analyzer

The critical nature of the clinical information provided by the blood gas analyzer, especially for neonates, entails a rigid maintenance routine on a daily, weekly, and monthly basis. The frequency of some service attentions—membrane changes, calibration gas changes, tubing changes—may be related to the level of use of the instrument. Arrange a service contract that includes a complete overhaul every six months. Pay particular attention to cleaning of blood residues from waste lines, waste containers, and entrance ports and valves. Change electrode membranes on a regular basis rather than waiting for signs of poor response. Check all gas line tubing at regular intervals for any signs of deterioration or splitting—this can produce obscure intermittent faults. If the manufacturer's manual details any electronic performance checks as part of the trouble-shooting routines, make these checks on a regular monthly basis. If the plumbing systems of the instrument use pinch valves compressing plastic tubing, inspect these on a monthly basis for crimps or splits. A hand lens may be necessary.

Centrifuge

Balance all loads. Clean out all spills or tube breakages immediately, and include disinfection with 2% glutaraldehyde. Check the condition of brushes monthly, and lubricate as specified by the manufacturer. Do not leave electrical braking systems turned on for long periods. If a tachometer is available, check the accuracy of the revolutions per minute indicator, if present, at least every six months.

Deionizers

If the quality of the effluent from a deionizer column is checked regularly with the conductivity meter and recorded, a reliable estimate of the average working life of the column can be derived, and thereafter the column can be changed or recharged on a time-determined basis. In many cases, the column becomes less efficient from channeling or bacterial growth rather than from actual exhaustion, and regular replacement is preferred to recharging.

Desiccator

Do not wait until the desiccant shows visible signs of exhaustion, such as caking or change of the indicator in a silica gel packing. Change the desiccant every six months or more frequently if the desiccator is opened often.

Dilutors and Dispensers

The simple piston-operated dilutors and dispensers, employing ball valves, should be checked for precision every three or six months, depending on the usage. Weighing of repeated deliveries of water permits calculation of the mean volume and the precision. The dilutor may similarly be checked by repetitious dilution of the same electrolyte standard solution and estimation of the sodium content in the flame photometer. The ball valves eventually wear, and this will show as a loss of precision and of a clean "cutoff" at the end of each delivery. Problems with dilutors of this type can be reduced by filtering all solutions before filling the reservoir. Unless the dispenser is rated for the purpose do not use it for strong bases. If the piston is not specially coated to prevent sticking, it may need regular treatment with a very thin coat of a silicone grease.

Interval Timers

The accuracy of the commonly used plastic-cased clockwork timer should be checked against a good stop-watch every six months.

Osmometer

The fluid in the refrigeration bath of the freezing point osmometer should be changed every three months after allowing the instrument to warm up to thaw any ice crystals. If the instrument is heavily used, an indication that the bath fluid needs changing is a slowing down of the freezing cycle. The thermistor detector should be inspected for damage regularly. The accuracy of the calibrations should be checked every three months.

pH Meter

Since careful cleaning after each use should be normal practice the only regular maintenance a pH meter needs is the checking of the level of potassium chloride solution in the reference electrode and occasional inspection of the glass electrode with the hand lens for surface scratches. Most modern pH meters incorporate circuits for checking the electronics.

Pipettors

The air displacement type of hand pipettor (Oxford, Eppendorf) should have the internal O ring that provides the piston seal lubricated every two weeks and replaced every two months, assuming normal usage. Each pipettor should bear a local serial number or letter, and its precision should be checked by weighing 20 deliveries of water every six months. The aperture in the tip should be cleaned when the O ring is lubricated.

The micro pipettes that use a plastic-tipped plunger that completely empties a glass or plastic capillary tip (SMI, Labindustries) usually signal the need for a tip change by leakage of fluid past the tip into the capillary. Each time the tip is replaced, the calibration of the pipette should be checked with the gauge supplied and adjusted if necessary.

Refrigerator

Apart from regular cleaning and clearing out of outdated kits and reagents, the temperature of the refrigerator should be checked with a maximum-minimum thermometer every three months. A rise in the overnight value may indicate the need for service attention to the refrigeration unit. Failure to defrost automatically has the same implication.

Spectrophotometers

The requirement for regular checking of absorbance scale, wavelength scale, and linearity has already been noted. (See p. 74.) In addition, the tungsten source lamp should be inspected for accumulation of a dark film of vaporized tungsten: this is a signal to change the lamp. The quartz halide lamp largely obviates this problem. The cell compartment should be cleaned out weekly or as required. If a flow cell is fitted, it should be flushed after every use and soaked in weak stripping detergent followed by thorough flushing daily. If the spectrophotometer is fitted with a thermostatically controlled flow cell or cell compartment, the actual temperature attained should be checked every three months. In some instruments this facility is built in: if this is not the case, allow a cuvette of distilled water to come to temperature equilibrium and check the value with a small clinical thermometer. Precise checking of temperature settings other than 37°C will require a remote sensing electronic thermometer and the services of the manufacturer's field engineer.

Do not attempt to clean any mirrors in the optical system of the instrument: the surfaces are extremely susceptible to damage, and expert service assistance is essential. If a tungsten or deuterium lamp is changed, it must be carefully realigned so that the beam enters the optical system without "vignetting," that is, without striking the side wall of the cuvette. The manufacturer's manual will provide instructions. This procedure is particularly critical if micro cuvettes are being used, since they usually retain the standard 1.0 cm path length by reducing the cuvette width. After changing the lamp in a spectrophotometer, carefully clean off all fingerprints before turning on the power.

As a simple alternative to the procedures detailed on p. 75 for checking the linearity of the spectrophotometer, the method of Frings (1976) can be used. The method also permits a check on the accuracy of the wavelength scale. A stock solution is made containing 0.10 mL of French's green food coloring* diluted up to 200 mL with distilled water. This solution is stable for up to six months in a brown glass bottle at room temperature. On each day of use the following dilutions are made:

Tube No.	5.0 mL of	5.0 mL of	% of stock concentration
1	Stock		100
2	Stock	Water	50
3	Tube 2	Water	25
4	Tube 3	Water	12.5

The absorbances of all tubes are measured against a water blank at the three peak wavelengths of 257 nm, 410 nm, and 630 nm. Absorbance versus concentration should be plotted on graph paper for each wavelength. The plots should be linear over the whole range. Since the absorbance peaks are narrow, manual scanning to either side of the nominal peak wavelength settings will indicate any serious error in wavelength scale accuracy.

*R. T. French Co., Rochester, N.Y. 14609.

Water Baths

To prevent the accumulation of deposits on the heater elements and thermostat sensor of a 37°C water bath it should be emptied out every month and refilled with distilled water to which a suitable rust inhibitor and fungicide have been added. Water lost by evaporation should be replaced with distilled water only. In the closed-circuit circulator baths found in some automated analyzers a mixture of water and ethylene glycol may be preferable, subject to the manufacturer's instructions.

Boiling water baths require cleaning out at least weekly if in constant use, and the seal that insulates the heater element from the body of the bath should be inspected for any signs of leakage.

It should be reiterated that the above recommendations are intended only as a guide and are open to modification based on local experience, actual usage, and the requirements of legislation or government regulation. The main requirement is for some organized, recorded program with allotted responsibilities and conscientious performance. The technologist should also recognize that preventive maintenance extends beyond instrumentation to include the checking of reagents and kits for expiration dates.

ION-EXCHANGE RESINS

The process of ion exchange is the reversible interchange of ions in solution with ions of the same electrical sign in the molecular structure of an insoluble solid. The process occurs to some extent in glass; heavy metal ions in a solution stored in a glass bottle can interchange with sodium ions in the glass. For an effective ion-exchange process, however, the availability of the ions in the solid must be increased by a sort of "molecular engineering," which creates a molecule with the required exchange ability, for example, anions or cations, and produces it in a physical form providing easy access for the solute ions.

The naturally occurring ion exchangers such as zeolite (a hydrated aluminum silicate used to remove calcium ions from water) have been replaced by synthetic resins, polymers of styrene and divinylbenzene in the form of small beads, varying from 1 to 2 mm in diameter down to colloidal levels. Ion-exchange resins are usually used in the form of columns, since a solution as it passes down has the maximum opportunity to undergo the exchange process. For production of ion-free water, a mixed-bed resin incorporating both anion and cation exchangers is used. Special formulations have been produced for processes such as the adsorption of amino acids followed by their sequential elution (washing out) by buffers graded to remove them according to their affinity for the resin. Substances in urine that interfere with sensitive reactions can be selectively removed by ion-exchange resins.

A complete treatment of the processes involved in ion exchange is beyond the scope of this text. A simple approach is to regard the active cationic or anionic groups of the synthetic resin as being relatively "loose" because of the large size of the polymer molecule, so that if an ion in the surrounding solution has a greater affinity for the active group on the resin than the original structural ion, it will displace it. Once attached to the resin molecule, the solute ion can only be removed either by displacing it with another solute ion with even stronger affinity for the resin functional group or by eluting it with a great excess of a solute that is less strongly bound. (See Figure 4–16.)

A special type of ion exchanger, not a resin, is the high molecular weight, water insoluble, liquid variety, which is used in some of the ion-selective electrodes (see p. 66). The insoluble nature of such ion exchangers is derived from the hydrocarbon basis of their molecules, and their ion-exchanging ability from acidic or quaternary ammonium groups.

ULTRAMICRO ANALYSIS

The availability of a range of discrete-type automated analyzers capable of providing precise determinations of the majority of the routinely determined analytes using sample volumes of 20 microliters or less has greatly reduced the need for manual ultra-micro analyses in the general hospital laboratory. For example, the Beckman ASTRA 8 analyzer* will deliver a complete test panel (sodium, potassium, chloride, total CO_2, glucose, urea nitrogen, creatinine, and calcium) from a micro sample cup containing only 200 microliters of serum or plasma, and this level of performance can be matched by other instruments of recent design. However, since in certain circumstances the technologist may have to cope with severely restricted specimen volumes due to an inability to obtain venous blood, as with severe burn cases or very small premature infants, some general guidelines are given here.

General Principles

The method used to obtain the blood sample becomes of great importance, since a contaminated or hemolyzed specimen may produce more serious errors than with macro methods. The puncture site may be the finger tip or ear lobe in small children or adults, or the heel in infants. When the heel is used for blood sampling it is essential, especially with premature infants, that the puncture be confined to the areas shown in Figure 4–17 and that it be not more than 2.4 mm deep. The puncture should not be made on the posterior curvature of the heel or through a previous puncture that could be infected. The risk is of osteomyelitis of the calcaneus, the future weight-bearing heel bone (Blumenfeld et al., 1979). The skin surface must be thoroughly cleaned with an alcohol swab and dried with a brisk motion with a dry sterile cotton ball. The use of an iodine-containing skin antiseptic is not recommended because of possible contamination. The friction with the cotton ball should be sufficient to promote free capillary circulation, but without excessive pressure. The puncture is made with a sterile disposable lancet (Becton-Dickinson Long Point type) and should be made firmly and deliberately at right angles to the skin surface. To prevent contact of the blood with the skin—one cause of hemolysis—a *very*

*Beckman Instruments, Inc., Fullerton, Calif. 92634 and Toronto, Ont. M8Z 2G6.

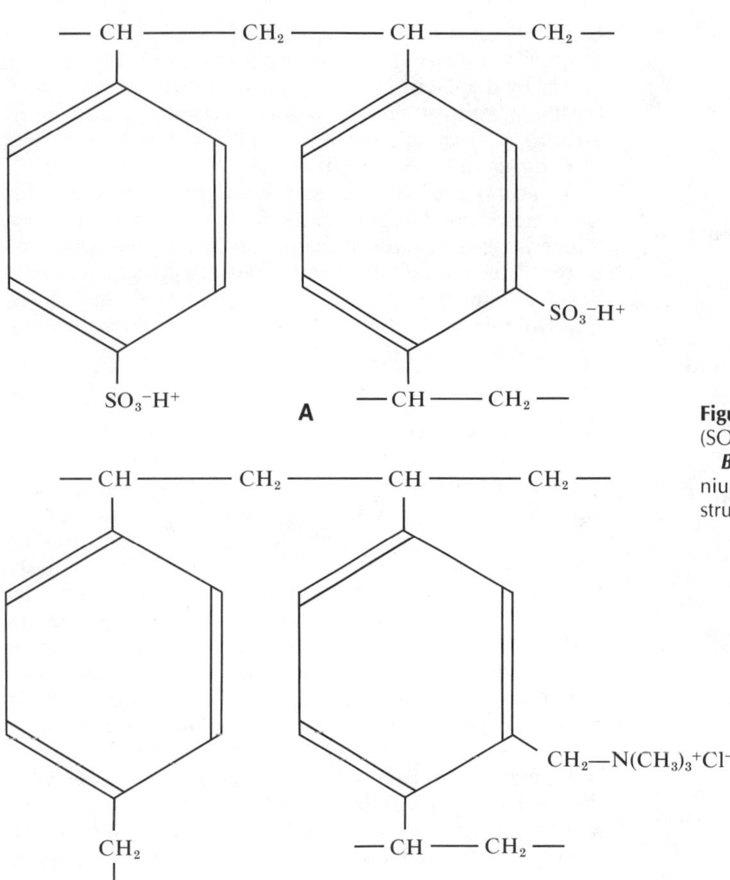

Figure 4–16 ***A,*** Cation-exchanger resin structure. The sulfonic ($SO_3^-H^+$) groups are the active exchanging structures.

B, Anion-exchanger resin structure. The quaternary ammonium (—$N(CH_3)_3^+$ $C1^-$) groups are the active exchanging structures.

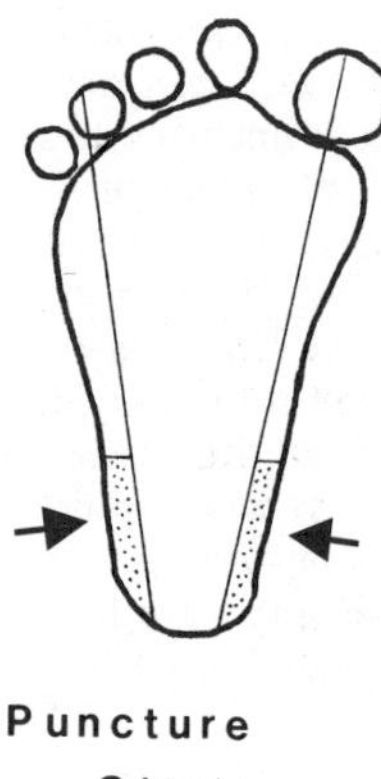

Figure 4–17 Lower surface of foot of neonate showing the recommended sites for taking blood samples *(dotted areas).*

thin film of sterile Vaseline can be applied to the skin before the puncture is made. To obtain good samples without hemolysis or contamination with tissue fluid, the blood flow must be quite free; any "milking" of the puncture site must be avoided. With infants, using heel puncture, if the blood flow slows after some drops have been obtained, it may be restored by *gentle* pressure by the thumbs on the heel surface, stretching the skin *away* from the puncture site. The use of various commercial pastes intended to promote free capillary circulation is not advised, owing to the risk of contamination. If difficulty is experienced in obtaining a free blood flow, try to improve the circulation by application of gentle warmth, or, in the case of infants, by massage of the leg toward the foot.

Blood Collection Tubes

Whenever possible, the collection tube should be heparinized, since a better yield of plasma will be obtained than serum from the same blood quantity. We have tried a variety of methods of blood collection for ultramicro work, and none is perfectly satisfactory.

To combine easy heparinization of the sample with easy filling of the tube and simple centrifugation, we suggest the following system (Fig. 4–18). A heparinized Caraway collection tube is placed, tapered end uppermost, in a small plastic centrifuge tube. (Ammonium heparin is used, which does not interfere with electrolyte determinations.) After skin puncture, the blood is allowed to run down the Caraway tube into the bottom of the plastic centrifuge tube, preventing air locks. One full Caraway tube yields about 0.35 mL of blood. On return to the laboratory, the Caraway tube is removed

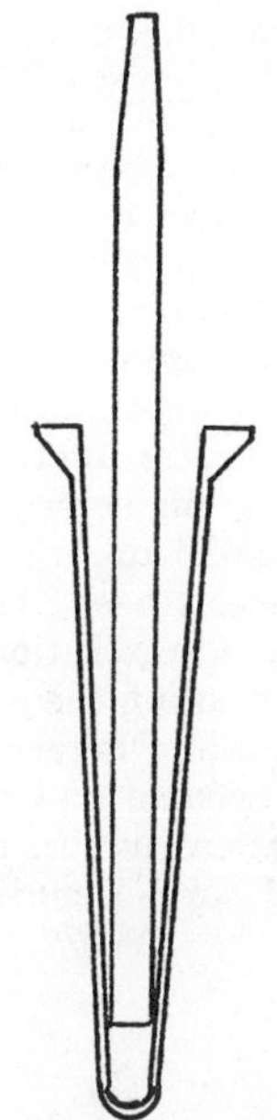

Figure 4–18 Heparinized Caraway blood collection tube in position in small plastic centrifuge tube for pediatric sampling. See text for details of use.

and discarded (the small drop remaining in the tube may be gently blown out with a mouthpiece and rubber tube, if desired) and the plastic centrifuge tube spun in the Fisher Model 59 centrifuge. The centrifuge tubes are very strong and will withstand 4000 g; two minutes at this setting will give good separation of plasma.* About 110 to 130 microliters of plasma are obtainable. If a nonheparinized Caraway tube is used, the yield of serum is about 80 to 100 microliters. The plasma or serum should be transferred immediately to a small glass or plastic test tube with a fine-tipped Pasteur pipette. The plastic test tube should be the type with a stopper.

Instrumentation

Spectrophotometer. A good quality instrument is essential. It should have a range of at least 340 to 700 nm, a band pass of 8 nm or less, and a cuvette holder that will accept precision microcuvettes having a light path of 10 mm with a contained volume of 0.5 mL or less and excellent stability. If a double-beam instrument is to be used, the cuvette holder should be adjustable so that the light beams pass accurately through the center of the microcuvettes, or masks should be available to serve the same purpose. If the light beams do not traverse the cuvettes precisely they may be reflected from the internal glass surfaces, and the attendant deflection of the emergent light beams will cause serious errors in photometry. (This source of error is termed "vignetting.")

Reaction Vessels. One of the most serious sources of error in ultramicro analysis is contamination. Ions and protein tend to become firmly adsorbed to glass test tubes and are difficult to remove. Disposable plastic test tubes offer a good solution; in our experience their chemical cleanliness is excellent.

Pipettes. The most convenient positive displacement–type micro pipettors employ a glass capillary tip with complete expulsion of the serum or plasma sample by a plastic plunger that extrudes slightly from the glass capillary.* If the tip is wiped with a tissue between measurements, it can be used repeatedly over the course of a working day. When rigid blood precautions are necessary, a similar pipettor with a plastic capillary tip that can be fitted and discarded without being touched can be used.† These types of micropipetting devices are slim enough to permit serum or plasma sampling directly from small plastic centrifuge tubes.

For measurement of diluents and reagents, standard Class A volumetric pipettes are used. If a large number of tests are to be processed, the new Model M (1.0 to 3.0 mL) and Model S (0.2 to 0.8 mL) Oxford reagent dispensers are useful.

Centrifuge. A small, high-speed bench model centrifuge with a special head for microtubes is necessary.

Work Area. Ultramicro analysis is exacting and requires a well-lit, comfortable work area, set apart from the busier parts of the laboratory. Some workers prefer to sit, others to stand; suitable benching should be available. All the equipment should be reserved for this type of work and kept in dust-free storage. The extent of the special provision for this kind of work will depend on the demand; in a pediatric hospital the provision of a separate laboratory would be justifiable.

Personnel. Reliable results from ultramicro methods can only be produced by meticulous, patient, and practiced technologists. The limitations of available sample often mean that doubtful results cannot be repeated.

Analytical Principles (Natelson, 1961; Meites and Faulkner, 1962)

(i) *Simplicity.* Ideally, the method should involve only one measurement of sample, one reagent, and one reaction tube, which also serves as the photometer cuvette. As far as possible, precipitation of proteins should be avoided, and the removal of aliquots from one reaction tube to another should be minimized. Direct chemical reactions should be used rather than complex conversions; for example, measurement of plasma bilirubin in neonates by direct spectrophotometry is better than the use of a diazo reaction method. If removal of a precipitate is required, use centrifugation rather than filtration.

(ii) *Specificity.* The reaction used should be specific for the substance measured. An enzymatic method for glucose is better than one based on chemical reduction of cupric ions.

(iii) *Standards and Controls.* Since most ultramicro methods avoid protein precipitation, standards (in some procedures) and controls should both be in a serum base. The values of standards should ideally bracket the expected test values, that is, the standard levels should

*Hurden Laboratory Products, Ann Arbor, Mich. 48106; 250, 400, and 550 microliter sizes. Beckman Instruments, Inc., Spinco Division, Palo Alto, Calif. 94304.

*"Micro/Pettor," Scientific Manufacturing Industries, Emeryville, Calif. 94608.

†Labindustries, Berkeley, Calif. 94710.

be chosen so that they cover the probable range of test values. Standards and controls should be run with every batch of tests.

(iv) *Spectrophotometry.* The absorbance readings obtained should be of the same order as those found with a macro procedure using the same chemical principles. This may be done in two ways. If the ultramicro method is a scaling down of a macro procedure, the ratio of sample to final volume should be maintained constant. In some cases the production of a reaction may be measured at a wavelength giving better sensitivity; for example, in the determination of inorganic phosphate a great increase in spectrophotometric sensitivity is obtained by reading the absorbance of the phospho-molybdate ion in the ultraviolet instead of using its reduction product in the red region of the visible spectrum. As previously mentioned, a spectrophotometer with a narrow band pass is essential.

The final colors used for spectrophotometry should be stable, and the relationship between absorbance and concentration must be linear over the ranges of interest. The use of flow-through cuvettes in the spectrophotometer avoids errors owing to size variations in cuvettes, but most systems involve loss of the sample after the reading; this may be a disadvantage. Flow-through cuvettes for ultraviolet work are expensive.

(v) *Mixing.* Mixing is preferably done by vibration unless the mixture is very viscous; in the latter case glass-stoppered microtest tubes or stoppered plastic tubes may have to be used. Whichever method is used, violent agitation, which traps air bubbles in the mixture, should be avoided.

Methods. The procedures described below are only suggestions, using methods that we have found practical and reliable. Suitable adaptations of other macrotechniques will suggest themselves to the technologist to meet particular problems.

Alkaline Phosphatase

Principle. The alkaline phosphatase of the sample hydrolyzes a phenolphthalein monophosphate substrate, and the released phenolphthalein is measured spectrophotometrically after addition of a stabilizing buffer.

Procedure. The method described on p. 172 is modified as follows:

(i) Reduce the sample size to 20 microliters.
(ii) Increase the incubation time to 20 minutes.
(iii) Reduce the volume of stabilizer to 2.0 mL.

Standardization is made by running suitable quality control sera at normal and elevated levels in the same way as the tests, and using the expression

$$\frac{\text{Absorbance of Test}}{\text{Absorbance of control serum closer in value}} \times \text{Value}$$

of control serum = alkaline phosphatase in I.U. Suitable sera are Versatol-E and Versatol-E-N.*

Total Bilirubin

The regular direct spectrophotometry method detailed on p. 249 can be scaled down to use 25 microliters of plasma instead of 50 and 2.0 mL of phosphate buffer instead of 3.0 mL. The final result will have to be multiplied by the factor $\frac{0.050}{0.025} \times \frac{2.025}{3.050} = 1.33$. (The first term corrects for the smaller sample size; the second term corrects for the difference in final volume, that is, if a quantity of bilirubin is diluted in a *smaller* volume than that used for the standardization procedure, it will give a correspondingly *higher* absorbance; if the standardization factor is to remain valid, this difference has to be compensated by the ratio of the new and original volumes.) If regular 1 cm square cuvettes are used, check that the final 2.025 mL volume is sufficient for the particular instrument used. This may be done by adding a dilute dichromate solution to the test cuvette in aliquots of 0.2 mL, reading the absorbance at 400 nm against a water blank, and determining at what total volume the readings become and remain constant. Alternatively, a semi microcuvette can be used with a total volume of 1.0 mL for a 1 cm light path.

Urea Nitrogen

The manual procedure detailed on p. 217 can be used with the following modifications to permit a sample size of 10 microliters.

1. In addition to using only 10 microliters of sample, reduce the volume of working standard and control to 10 microliters.
2. Reduce the volume of distilled water added in step 5 to 5 mL.
3. Measure the final absorbances in 1 cm square precision cuvettes rather than round tubes; the small sample size makes very precise photometry essential.

Calcium

The calcein-EDTA titration method on p. 261 can be used as described. In most pediatric work the clinical information sought is not so critical as that required for detection of hyperparathyroidism, and coefficients of variation on the order of ± 3% are acceptable. Advantage can be taken of the precise pipetting abilities of discrete-type automatic analyzers to process even very small batches of ultra-micro calcium assays. With some adroitness on the part of the operator, the system may be induced to sample two or three times from the same small sample cup, thus improving the precision of the determination. For reasons of limited demand, the number of models of automatic calcium titrators on the market has sharply declined, presumably as a result of the increased use of discrete-type analyzers.

The use of atomic absorption spectrophotometry has the advantages of fewer reagents and less demanding technique. Whether it can be used for ultramicro calcium assays will depend on the sophistication of the available instrument. The average single-beam type requires about 2.0 mL in order to obtain a reliable reading, with a serum sample of 50 microliters and maximum scale expansion and damping, and appropriate standards made in the same manner.

---

*General Diagnostics Division, Warner-Lambert Co., Morris Plains, N.J. 07950.

Cholesterol

The enzymatic cholesterol method described on p. 137 is readily scaled down to use a sample size of 10 μL if required.

Creatinine

The situation with determination of serum or plasma creatinine, that is, the analytical unsuitability of the Jaffe reaction, with its high blank and low sensitivity, is aggravated by the limitations of sample size involved in ultramicro analysis. In our experience, with rigid attention to technique it is possible to obtain reliable results with a scaled-down version of the manual procedure (see p. 219) using 0.2 mL of plasma or serum, and microcuvettes. Methods based on measurement of the rate of formation of the creatine-alkaline picrate complex encounter problems resulting from nonspecific reactions that have rates both faster and slower than that of creatinine itself. The best solution is found in the semi-automated instruments that determine the instantaneous reaction rate at a time when the nonspecific reactions have either gone to completion or not started. Accurate creatinine determinations on 25 μL samples are practical.*

Glucose

Principle. The glucose of the sample is converted to glucose-6-phosphate by the enzyme hexokinase. The glucose-6-phosphate is in turn converted to 6-phosphogluconate by the enzyme glucose-6-phosphate dehydrogenase. The hydrogen ions removed from the glucose-6-phosphate are taken up by the coenzyme NADP, which is thereby converted to its reduced form, NADPH, which has a strong absorbance at 340 nm. Since the NADP is converted mole for mole with the glucose-6-phosphate, the increase in absorbance at 340 nm is related directly to the initial glucose concentration, provided that the reaction is allowed to proceed to completion.

Reagents. These are most conveniently obtained as Glucose Stat-Pack.† Each pair of vials, one containing NADP, the other glucose-6-phosphate dehydrogenase, hexokinase, ATP, and buffer, produces 15.5 mL when reconstituted and mixed. Unopened, the vials are stable for up to two years if refrigerated. Unused reconstituted reagent is stable for up to 48 hours at 4°C.

Standard. Dilute a stock 1.0 g per 100 mL glucose solution 1 in 10 with saturated aqueous benzoic acid. This working standard containing 100 mg per 100 mL is stable for months if refrigerated.

Control. Use a commercial control serum with a given value for true glucose in the region of 80 to 100 mg per dL. After reconstitution in the usual manner, dilute with an equal volume of distilled water to obtain a control with a value of about 40 to 50 mg per dL. The preparation used should not contain an increased level of bilirubin. Lab-trol‡ is convenient, since it is already in solution.

Procedure

1. Set up four 1 cm square cuvettes, preferably a matched set. Using a soft pencil on the frosted face, label them test, test blank, standard, and control: T, TB, S, C.

2. Into TB, pipette 3.0 mL saline. Add 20 microliters of specimen (i.e., serum, plasma, urine, CSF), using a micropipette and wash-out technique. Mix by gentle inversion using Parafilm. Measure the absorbance at 340 nm against a water reference. Record the absorbance as Abs_a.

3. Into T, S, and C, pipette 3.0 mL of Glucose Stat-Pack reagent. Measure the absorbances at 340 nm against a water reference. Record the values as T_a, S_a, and C_a.

4. To T, add 20 microliters of specimen; to S, 20 microliters of standard; to C, 20 microliters of control, using the same careful wash-out technique. Mix by gentle inversion; allow to stand at room temperature in the cuvettes for ten minutes.

5. Read the absorbances of T, S, and C at 340 nm against a water reference.

6. To make sure that the reaction has gone to completion, allow the cuvettes to stand a further five minutes and recheck the absorbances. T_b, S_b, and C_b.

Calculation

Factor: $\frac{100}{S_b - S_a}$. This should be close to the manufacturer's stated factor of 435, corresponding to $S_b - S_a = 0.230$. Glucose in specimen in mg per dL $= (T_b - (T_a + Abs_a)) \times$ factor. The correction for the initial absorbance of the specimen Abs_a is equivalent to an error in the glucose value, if it were not considered, of 5 to 15 mg per dL, especially in the presence of bilirubin. Glucose in control $= (C_b - C_a) \times$ factor. At a control level of 50 mg per dL, the allowable error is $\pm$ 4 mg per dL, provided that the spectrophotometer scale can be read to $\pm$ 0.005 absorbance.

Notes

1. If the specimen is not jaundiced, lipemic, or hemolyzed, for most clinical purposes the Abs_a reading can be omitted, thereby using less of the specimen. The probable error is not more than 5 mg per dL.

2. If the absorbance $T_b - T_a$ is greater than 0.8, corresponding to a glucose level greater than about 350 mg per dL, pour the cuvette contents into a small test tube, pipette a further 3.0 mL of reagent into the cuvette, mix by gentle inversion, add to the test tube, and mix this by inversion. Allow to stand for ten minutes. Read the absorbance of the mixture at 340 nm as before against a water reference. The calculation now becomes: $(T_{b2} - T_a) \times$ factor $\times 2 =$ mg glucose per dL. The effect of the initial absorbance of the sample can be ignored at this level.

Glucose—Alternative Method

The procedure described above requires a narrow band-pass spectrophotometer; an alternative method, suitable for routine instruments with band passes from 8 to 20 nm, couples the generation of the NADPH with a colorimetric reaction in which the NADPH reduces phenazine methosulfate; this in turn converts iodonitrotetrazolium (INT) to its reduced form, which can be measured at 520 nm.

---

*Creatinine Rate Analyzer 2, Beckman Instruments, Inc., Fullerton, Calif. 92634 and Toronto, Ont. M8Z 2G6.

†Calbiochem, La Jolla, Calif. 92037.

‡Dade Division, American Hospital Supply Corp., Miami, Fla. 33152.

Reagents. These are available as Glucostrate.* One vial contains buffered enzyme reagent: ATP, hexokinase, magnesium ions, glucose-6-phosphate dehydrogenase, and NADP. The phenazine methosulfate (PMS) and INT are bottled separately. The diluent is 0.1 M hydrochloric acid. The buffered enzyme reagent vial is reconstituted with 10 mL of distilled water according to the manufacturer's instructions.

Standard and Controls. The same as for the previous method. The method is linear up to at least 500 mg per dL.

Procedure

1. Set up five spectrophotometer cuvettes—10 or 12 mm light path—and label them for test, controls (include one in the region of 100 mg per dL and one about 50 mg per dL), standard, and reagent blank: T, C_1, C_2, S, and RB.

2. Reconstitute the buffered enzyme reagent vial with 8.0 mL of distilled water, mix gently to dissolve, and add 2.0 mL of color developer (PMS and INT). Mix.

3. Pipette 1.0 mL of this combined reagent into each tube. Incubate all tubes for 3 minutes at 37°C.

4. Using a micropipette and wash-out technique, add 20 microliters of test serum, controls, and standard to the appropriate cuvettes. Mix well and incubate for exactly ten minutes.

5. At the end of the ten minutes, add rapidly 5.0 mL of 0.1 M HCl to each tube, remove from water bath, and mix by inversion.

6. Read the absorbances of test, controls, and standard at 520 nm setting zero absorbance with the reagent blank.

Calculation

$$\frac{\text{Test Absorbance}}{\text{Standard Absorbance}} \times \text{standard value} = \text{glucose in}$$

mg per dL. Mg/dL × 0.056 = mmol/L.

Use for the calculation whichever standard absorbance is closer to that of the test, using a corresponding standard value in the above formula.

Notes

1. The reconstituted enzyme reagent is stated to be stable for up to three days if refrigerated; stability up to five days has been reported, but this would depend on the number and duration of removals from refrigeration for use during that period.

2. Interference from bilirubin, hemoglobin, and fluoride is minimal.

Magnesium

The sensitivity of the atomic absorption method for magnesium is very good (see pp. 81 and 264), and it can be scaled down for ultramicro purposes by using 50 microliters of serum or plasma and 2.5 mL of trichloroacetic acid solution. The same standards will be valid. If the amount of sample is very small, use 25 microliters plus 2.0 mL of trichloroacetic acid solution, preparing the standards by a similar dilution ratio. If the aspiration rate of the atomic absorption spectrophotometer in use is such that a 2.0 mL volume is insufficient for a reliable reading, increase the trichloroacetic acid volume to 3.0 mL and increase the sensitivity by adjustment of the scaler or similar control. The setting of the damping control may have to be increased to obtain stable readings. The technologist will have to determine the best conditions for his or her own instrument. Standards should be prepared with the same dilution *ratio* as the test, but using greater actual *volumes* to ensure accuracy.

*General Diagnostics Division, Warner-Lambert Co., Morris Plains, N.J. 07950 and Scarborough, Ont. M1K5C9.

Inorganic Phosphate

Principle. The inorganic phosphate of the sample is converted to the phosphomolybdate polyacid by reaction with ammonium molybdate in sulfuric acid. Precipitation of proteins is prevented by the inclusion of a wetting agent, Tween 80. The absorbance of the phosphomolybdate polyacid is measured at 340 nm, obviating the need for the reduction step.

Reagents (Daly and Ertingshausen, 1972)

Sulfuric Acid, 0.60 Molar. Into about 500 mL of cold distilled water in a 1 liter volumetric flask, pipette 33 mL of reagent-grade concentrated sulfuric acid. Mix by swirling, allow to cool, make to volume. Store in a polypropylene bottle.

Molybdate Solution. Dissolve 2.0 g of analytical-grade ammonium molybdate $(NH_4)_6Mo_7O_{24}\cdot 4\ H_2O$ in 1 liter of 0.6 M sulfuric acid.

Stock Tween 80. Mix one volume of Tween 80 with two volumes of distilled water.

Working Reagent. Mix 100 mL of molybdate solution with 0.9 mL of stock Tween 80 solution. Prepare at least 30 minutes before use.

Blank Reagent. Mix 100 mL of 0.6 M sulfuric acid with 0.9 mL Tween 80 stock solution.

Stock Standard. Dissolve 439 mg of analytical-grade potassium dihydrogen phosphate KH_2PO_4 in about 50 mL distilled water in a 100-mL volumetric flask; make to volume, mix. Store in a polypropylene bottle. Preserve with 50 mg sodium azide.

Working Standard. Dilute 5.0 mL of stock up to 100 mL with distilled water. This solution can be used for up to a week if kept refrigerated to retard mold growth.

Control. Use two commercial control sera, preferably without elevated bilirubin levels, with values in the normal and elevated range.

Procedure

1. Set up two rows of specially cleaned cuvettes (see Notes). Label the front row test(s), standard, low control, high control. Label the rear row test blank(s), standard blank, low control blank, high control blank.

2. Into the front row pipette volumetrically 3.0 mL of working reagent. Into the rear row pipette 3.0 mL of blank reagent.

3. Using a micropipette and scrupulous wash-out technique, add 20 microliters of test samples, standard, and controls to the front row, and mix by inversion using Parafilm. Add 20 microliters of the appropriate samples, standard, and controls to the rear row, and mix.

4. Let stand for fifteen minutes.

5. Read the absorbance of each cuvette in the front row against the corresponding blank cuvette in the rear row at 340 nm.

Calculation

$\frac{\text{Test Absorbance}}{\text{Standard Absorbance}} \times 5 =$ mg inorganic phosphate per dL. The controls should give results within ± 0.2 mg per dL of stated values. Mg/dL × 0.323 = mmol/L.

Notes

1. As with any phosphate assay method, contamination is the main source of errors. It is recommended that a special set of acid-washed cuvettes and pipettes be reserved for this procedure.

2. If the method is used for other than pediatric cases, the occurrence of a turbidity that is not cleared by the Tween 80 almost invariably indicates the presence of a paraprotein. This problem is common to all the phosphate methods that do not incorporate a protein precipitation step.

3. The absorbance of the phosphomolybdate complex at 340 nm is considerable; if the available sample is very small, the amount used can be reduced to 10 microliters and the final result multiplied by $\frac{3.01}{3.02} \times 2 = 1.993$. The precision will still be adequate for clinical purposes.

4. Mixing should be by gentle inversion; rapid agitation will cause frothing.

5. If the serum sample contains large amounts of bilirubin, it may not be possible to set the photometer to zero absorbance with the blank. In this case the readings should be made on a more sophisticated instrument, preferably of the double-beam type.

6. The final absorbance readings are stable for at least 1 hour.

7. Severe hyperbilirubinemia, i.e., greater than 25 mg per dL, causes a turbidity that is not cleared by increasing the Tween content.

8. Most commercial heparin preparations contain enough phosphate to give errors; use serum.

9. This method can be adapted to discrete-type automatic analyzers using even smaller sample sizes, but rigid precautions against contamination of the fluid-handling sections of the instrument offset to some extent the working convenience of the procedure.

10. An elegant and very sensitive method for the assay of inorganic phosphate employs an acid solution of molybdate and the dye malachite green. The presence of phosphate changes the brown color of the dye to an olive green (Itaya and Ui, 1966).

Total Protein

The reaction used is that of the manual biuret method on p. 141, with the quantities scaled down as detailed here.

Procedure

1. Use either 100 × 13 mm test tubes or plastic disposable cuvettes.

2. In test, standard, and reagent blank, pipette 1.0 mL of Doumas biuret reagent; in test blank and standard blank, pipette 1.0 mL of alkaline tartrate reagent.

3. Proceed as in the method on p. 141, except that 20 microliter volumes of serum, standard, or deionized water are used instead of 100 microliters.

4. If the spectrophotometer used cannot make absorbance measurements on 1.0 mL volumes, the final colored solutions will have to be transferred to suitable semi-micro cuvettes providing a 1.0 cm light path with a total volume of 0.6 mL or more. A more convenient method is to use a flow cell–type instrument* with a flow-cell volume small enough to permit adequate wash-out from an available sample volume of 1.0 mL.

Sodium and Potassium

Using a standard-type photometer, such as the IL 343,† which aspirates 1.0 mL of diluted sample in 40 seconds, 2.0 mL is sufficient for a steady reading. With the usual 1:200 dilution ratio, the addition of 20 microliters of test serum, standard, and control serum to 4.0 mL of 15 mEq per liter lithium diluent, using scrupulous technique with wash-out, will provide enough fluid for duplicate readings. (Some of the newer instruments routinely aspirate only microquantities of serum and can be used directly.) The 4.0 mL of lithium diluent must be measured with a Class A volumetric pipette.

---

*Stasar III spectrophotometer. Gilford Instrument Laboratories, Inc., Oberlin, Ohio 44074.

†Instrumentation Laboratory, Inc., Lexington, Mass. 02173.

CHAPTER 4—REVIEW QUESTIONS

1. Describe three processes used in the production of pure water. Suggest a system capable of producing CAP Type 1 water.

2. Give a list of precautions that are important in the care of an analytical balance.

3. Explain the "sodium error" of a pH meter and show how this phenomenon has been used for the measurement of ions.

4. Explain the difference between the terms *band pass* and *band width*. How may these factors affect the choice of a spectrophotometer?

5. Discuss the factors that may give rise to errors in wavelength and absorbance readings on a spectrophotometer. How may the occurrence of these errors be detected?

6. Describe the basic components of a gas chromatograph.

7. What are the practical factors affecting the quality of electrophoretic separations?

8. Explain the process of radioactivity and give examples of its use. What are the possible hazards of excessive exposure to radiation?

9. What precautions should be taken when obtaining blood samples by heel puncture in neonates?

10. Discuss the changes that could be made in a manual method to permit reliable results using a very small plasma or serum sample.

5

AUTOMATION IN CLINICAL CHEMISTRY

LABORATORY AUTOMATION

Strictly speaking, replacement of manual operations by mechanical devices in the laboratory is merely "mechanization." Industry reserves the term "automation" for machine systems that incorporate continuous monitoring of the product, with the results of the checking process used to control the entire process. This principle of using the characteristics of the product to regulate the machinery producing it is called "feedback." The term originated in electronics; in a radio transmitter, a small aliquot of the output after amplification is fed back into the primary oscillator circuit to sustain and control its vibrations. The thermostat control of a house heating system works on a similar principle. It senses a drop in room temperature and activates a relay, which switches on the heating system; when the room temperature rises to a predetermined value, the thermostat sensor-relay system turns off the heat.

In an automatic analyzer, the product is information. We control the quality of the information by running samples of known value with every batch, comparing the results with the known levels, and if the difference is outside stated tolerances, taking corrective action. We are aware of a fault in the output only *after* it has occurred; we hope that the change has not been affecting our results for too long. The new generation of automatic analyzers includes microprocessors or small computers. (A microprocessor can be regarded as a small computer with a fixed program of functions and abilities that the instrument operator cannot change except in regard to a few minor features, such as selecting the units of reporting; a computer's RAM [random access memory], as opposed to the microprocessor's ROM [read only memory], can be modified and reprogrammed by the operator.) In addition to controlling the operations of the analyzer (sampling, reagent addition, photometric or other measurements, calibration, and result calculation), the computer facilitates the inclusion of a range of self-checking abilities and diagnostic processes, error detection, and, in the most sophisticated versions, curve-fitting programs for true kinetic enzyme assays, accumulated quality control data for subsequent presentation at weekly or longer intervals, and visual display of calibration curves and quality control values.

It should be realized that computer control of laboratory instrumentation does not automatically ensure greater reliability of results. The most sophisticated multichannel, computer-monitored analyzer is at the mercy of a technologist who cannot reconstitute lyophilized standardization and control sera accurately, and a programming error may produce masses of results that cannot be assigned with certainty to the correct patients.

TYPES OF AUTOMATIC ANALYZERS

There are four main types of automatic analyzers for processing large numbers of routine clinical chemistry tests. (Automated radioimmunoassay instruments will be considered later.)

1. Technicon continuous flow systems
2. Discrete analyzers
3. Centrifugal analyzers
4. Thin-film analyzers

In addition to its classification as above, an analyzer may be either discretionary or nondiscretionary; that is, the test or tests to be run on each sample can be predetermined, or every sample can be processed for a test or set of tests. For example, on the multichannel Technicon analyzers prior to the SMAC, each specimen received identical treatment and the complete panel was run. On the Beckman ASTRA 8, however, the tests to be performed on each sample are programmed through the microprocessor keyboard; any combination can be requested, and the complete program for a set of samples can be reviewed on the CRT (cathode ray terminal). The trend is to provide direct interaction between the operator and the instrument for set-up, calibration, result read-out, and trouble-shooting.

Continuous Flow (Figs. 5–1 and 5–2)

The Technicon Autoanalyzer systems have delivered reliable data in quantity and variety in a wide range of fields, such as clinical chemistry, industrial analysis, pharmaceutical analysis and control, and drug screening, and their development encompasses micro sample capability and full computer control. Almost any manual analytical procedure can be adapted to the continuous flow principle, and recent innovations involving electronic timing of sample pick-up, smaller dialyzers, better pumping systems, electronic sensing of rise times on recorder peaks, and flow-cell design improvements have

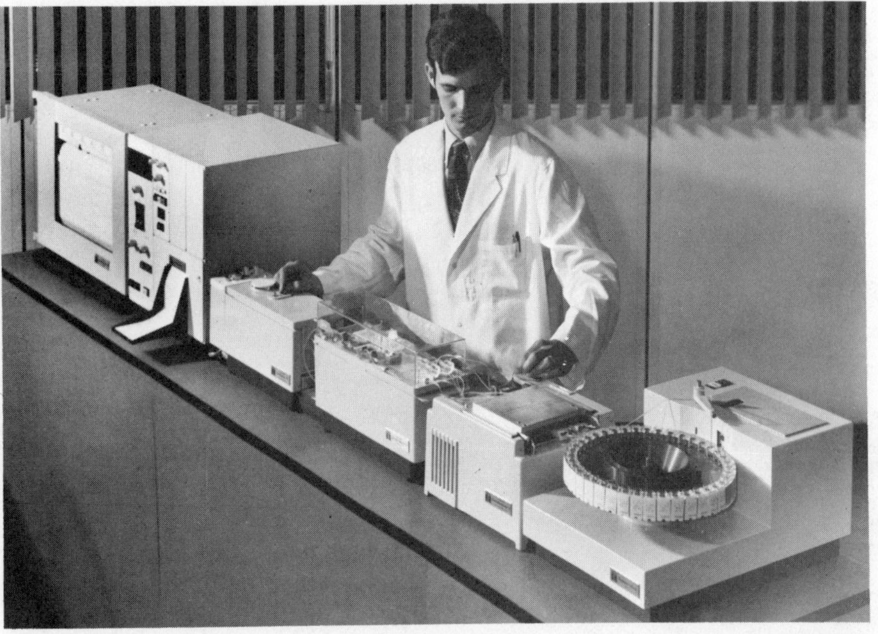

Figure 5–1 The AutoAnalyzer II system, incorporating higher production rates up to 120 samples per hour, interchangeable analytical cartridges, prepackaged reagents, and automatic sample identification. The punch-coded identification labels can be seen attached to the samples on the turntable. Results are printed out automatically, in addition to recorder display of peaks. (Courtesy of Technicon Instruments Corp., Tarrytown, N.Y. 10591.)

increased the number of tests per hour per channel to as high as 150.

Typical Features

1. Continuous pumping of samples and reagents, using peristaltic pumps.
2. Protein removal by dialysis.
3. Segmentation of sample and reagent streams, separation of one sample from the next, and continuous "scrubbing" of tubing by air bubbles.
4. Flow-through cuvettes in an interference filter photometer, using a fixed reference light path.
5. Recorder read-out (in basic systems): collated patient reports in the later systems (SMAC).
6. Modular design, permitting interchanging of major parts.

Discrete Analyzers

The majority of recent designs in automatic analyzers employ the discrete principle, whereby each specimen is handled as a separate process in its own dedicated reaction vessel. This type of system can be regarded as a logical replacement of manual pipetting, hand movement of tubes, mixing, incubation, and photometry of the final colored solution by mechanical measuring devices, transport systems, and transfer mechanisms. In theory, this type of automation should have preceded the continuous flow approach; the delay in its introduction was largely due to design and manufacturing problems. The various solutions to those problems have given rise to a corresponding variety of instruments. Our selection of those described below is intended to illus-

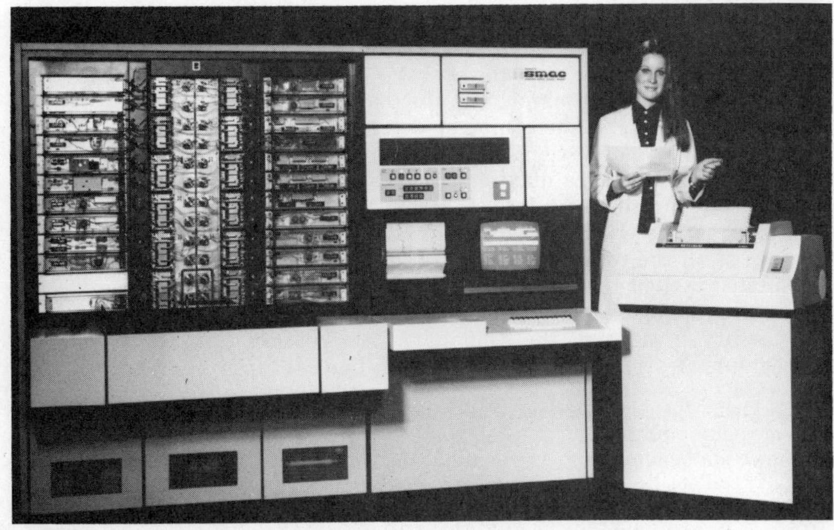

Figure 5–2 The Technicon SMAC computer-controlled high-speed biochemical analyzer, with small sample size and high rate of output—150 samples per hour—of as many as 40 tests per sample. All functions, including start-up, wash, and shut-down, are computer controlled. (Courtesy of Technicon Instruments Corp., Tarrytown, N.Y. 10591.)

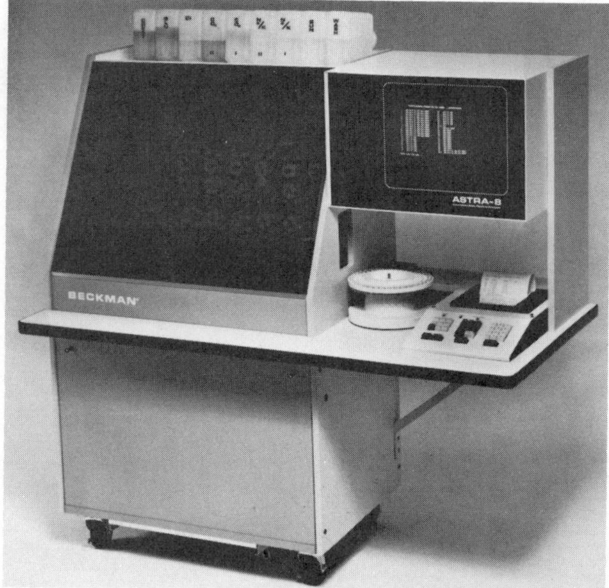

Figure 5–3 The Beckman ASTRA 8 (*A*utomated *S*tat and *R*outine *A*nalyzer). The analytical modules with their associated peristaltic pumps are behind the sloping plastic cover on the left-hand side, and the sample turntable and printer are on the right. The selected test schedule is displayed on the screen above the printer. (Courtesy of Beckman Instruments, Inc., Fullerton, Calif. 92634.)

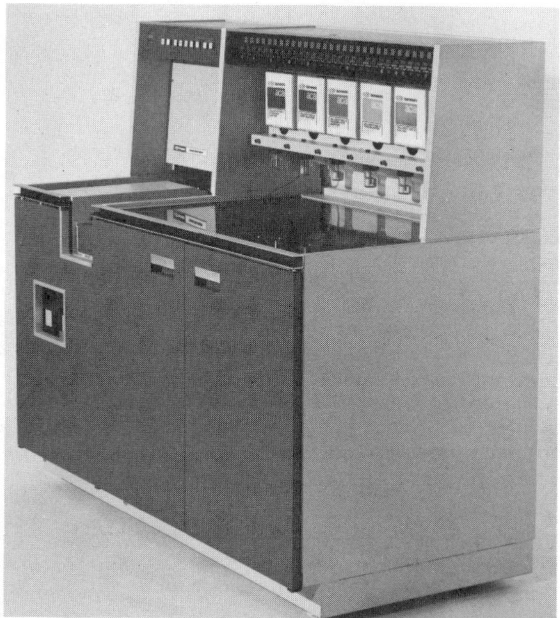

Figure 5–4 The Dupoint ACA Automatic Clinical Analyzer. (Courtesy E. I. Du Pont de Nemours and Co., Inc., Wilmington, Del. 19898.)

trate the differing methods used, not to assess their performance.

Discrete Analyzers with Complete Discretionary Ability

The Beckman ASTRA 8 and ASTRA 4 analyzers* are microprocessor-controlled, ultra-micro sample instruments that have been developed by the concatenation of miniaturized versions of the company's single-test semi-automatic bench model analyzers for glucose, urea nitrogen, chloride, bicarbonate, and creatinine, with the addition of a combined sodium/potassium unit employing ion-selective electrodes. For each sample, any single test or any combination of tests can be preselected using a keyboard. Results are displayed on a screen (CRT) and by printer. The ASTRA is in effect a multichannel analyzer (Fig. 5–3).

The American Monitor KDA† is a computer-controlled, single-channel analyzer. After loading the 90-position, cooled sample tray, the operator programs the required tests for each sample into the computer. When operation commences, the computer determines the sequence in which the various tests will be run, one test at a time, to obtain the maximum speed. Thus it may run all the glucose assays first, then all the urea nitrogen tests, and so on. The use of a full computer permits storage of all the results with the subsequent print-out of collated patient reports.

Another approach to provision of complete discretionary ability is used in the DuPont ACA (*A*utomatic *C*linical *A*nalyzer),‡ shown in Figure 5–4. For each test there is a special plastic pack that incorporates the reagents for the test and a double-walled reaction chamber that is used to form the cuvette for photometry (Fig. 5–5). For each serum sample there is a special pack that acts as a sample reservoir. The top of each test pack is a plastic block that may contain a chromatographic column to remove interfering substances, a gel filtration matrix to retard small molecules, or a protein precipitation column containing porous glass beads coated with a protein precipitant. On the top of each pack is a test name in bold letters plus a binary coded identification that instructs the instrument computer. The sample reservoir pack carries a written label with patient identification, which is reproduced photographically on the final report. The action of feeding a sample reservoir pack into the instrument followed by the reagent packs for the desired tests programs the entire test process.

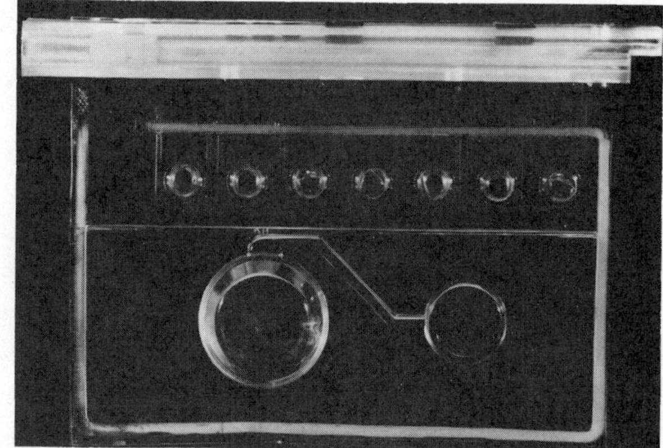

Figure 5–5 Plastic reagent pack with formed cell for photometry. The row of small circular "bubbles" originally contained the reagents. (Courtesy of E. I. Du Pont de Nemours and Co., Inc., Wilmington, Del. 19898.)

*Beckman Instruments, Inc., Fullerton, Calif. 92634 and Toronto, Ont. M8Z 5T2.

†American Monitor Corp., Indianapolis, Ind. 46268.

‡E. I. DuPont de Nemours and Co., Inc., Wilmington, Del. 19898.

Sample volumes vary from 60 to 500 microliters; the instrument can be programmed to use smaller serum volumes if a larger coefficient of variation is tolerable. Enzyme determinations are made by kinetic methods. The final report is a 4½ × 6″ slip upon which the patient's name and other identification data are reproduced photographically and the test results are printed as numerical values with a test identification abbreviation.

Discrete Analyzers without Specific Discretionary Ability

The Abbott ABA–100 Bichromatic Analyzer, ABA–200, and VP Analyzer* incorporate several special features that illustrate particular solutions to some problems of automatic analyzer design (Figs. 5–6 to 5–8). Transfer of final solutions for photometry is avoided by combining the reaction vessels and spectrophotometer cuvettes into a single disposable plastic 32-compartment molding (Fig. 5–9). Incubation with rapid rise to a stable temperature is achieved by complete immersion of the reaction vessel in a water bath. The system uses ultramicro samples, often as small as 5 microliters, and the absorbance changes encountered in the pseudokinetic enzyme assays are consequently correspondingly minuscule. The problem of interference from serum and reagent color is overcome by taking absorbance readings at two wavelengths, the so-called bichromatic system. One reading is taken at or close to the wavelength of maximum absorbance, the other at a point at which the absorbance of the desired chromogen is at a minimum but the absorbances of the reagent and sample are closely similar. Subtraction of the second reading from the first isolates the absorbance produced by the reaction. The problem of measurement of this absorbance remains. Since it originates as an electrical signal from a photomultiplier, it can be precisely compared with the electrical signal produced in a special die-away circuit; the value of this reference signal as it decreases with time is known very exactly. The electrical signals from the photomultiplier—corresponding to the absorbance values at the two wavelengths—mirror in their difference the absorbance produced by the reaction. By direct comparison of the electrical signal difference with the reference signal in the die-away circuit, with its known relationship between magnitude and time, the electrical signal from the photomultiplier can be converted to a time difference, and since the microprocessor, in common with many computer devices, can measure time very precisely by converting it to a count of very short intervals (this is called "digitization"), a similar precise value can be assigned to the measured absorbance and compared with either a predetermined calibration factor or the similar absorbance derived from running a standard solution. This elegant method is claimed to provide a detection sensitivity of 0.00015 absorbance (see Fig. 5–10). In the figure, curve RC represents the change in the reference circuit voltage with time. Point A indicates the higher voltage in the photomultiplier, Point B the lower. When the voltage in the reference circuit has a value equal to that of Point A, the microprocessor starts to count time at very short intervals (on the order of microseconds) until the reference circuit voltage matches that at Point B, stopping the time count. Thus the photomultiplier voltage difference A minus B is converted to the precise time count from T_1 to T_2. The system incorporates an automatic correction for any change in the absorbance of the reagents during the course of a test and can be set to detect nonlinearity of a reaction caused by very high enzyme activities. The ABA–100 incorporates one form of discretionary ability: the operator can select which samples in the loading tray will be processed for a particular test merely by

*Abbott Laboratories, Irving, Tex. 75061.

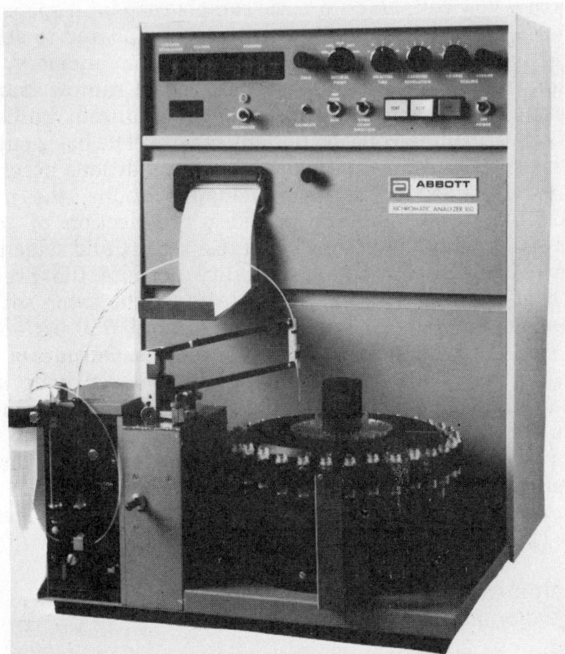

Figure 5–6 The Abbott ABA–100 Biochromatic Analyzer. (Courtesy of Abbott Scientific Products Division, South Pasadena, Calif. 91030.)

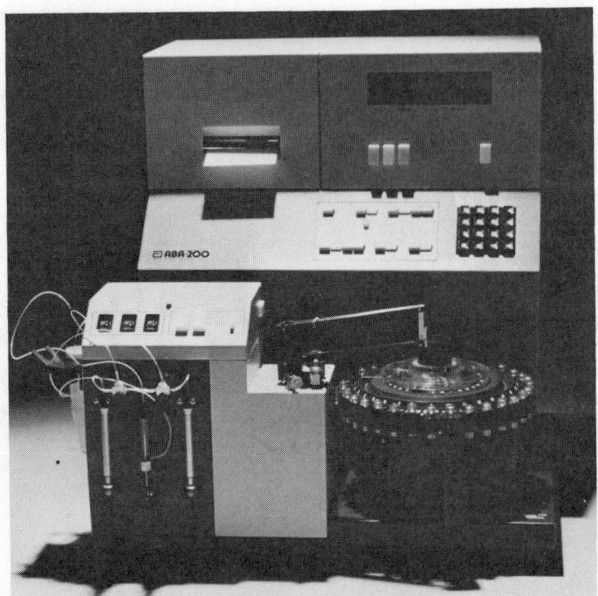

Figure 5–7 The Abbott ABA–200 automatic analyzer. (Courtesy of Abbott Laboratories, Irving, Texas 75061.)

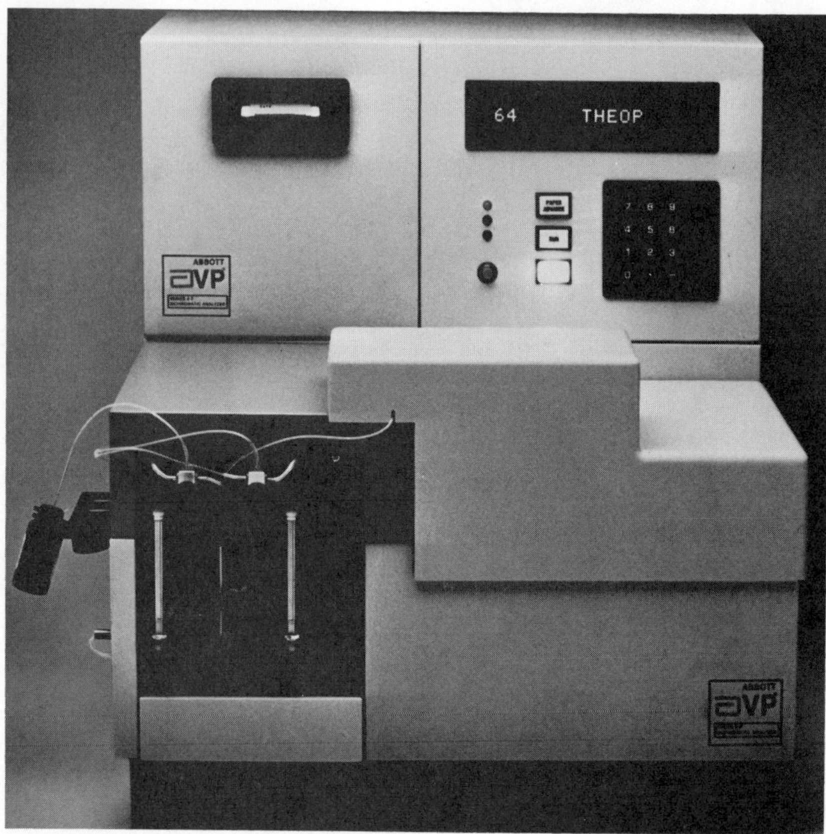

Figure 5–8 The Abbott VP automatic analyzer. The sample turntable and sample pick-up/reagent-dispensing probe are beneath the stepped cover at the right-hand side, minimizing sample evaporation. (Courtesy of Abbott Laboratories, Irving, Texas 75061.)

either raising the serum cups into position or leaving them down.

As a result of increased quantitative and qualitative demands on the smaller laboratory, with the concomitant need for the substitution of automated methods for manual procedures, plus the probability of even further

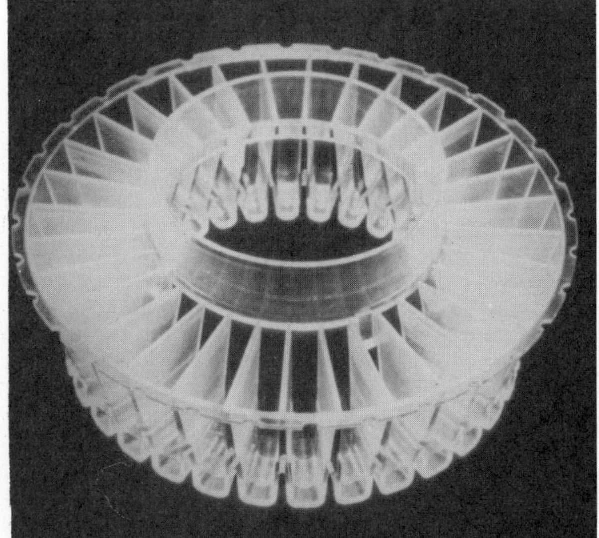

Figure 5–9 Combined 32-compartment reaction vessel and spectrophotometer cuvette unit for the Abbott ABA–100 Bichromatic Analyzer. (Courtesy of Abbott Scientific Products Division, South Pasadena, Calif. 91030.)

expansion, there is a need for analytical systems that can be expanded and updated. The Gilford clinical chemistry analyzers* provide a graded series of systems from a simple combination of a high-grade spectrophotometer with a flow cell, an automatic sample/reagent dispenser, and a controller/printer, which can be updated to store the parameters for a number of tests in memory, to more sophisticated outfits with carousel sample transport and pick-up, multiple reagent addition, built-in diagnostics, and collated patient reports. The basic outfit within any group can be updated as conditions necessitate. Finally, for high-volume applications, the new "IMPACT 400" system provides preselection of test panels, complete automation of test set-up, and selective batching. This last-named ability permits the preselected running of a variety of tests on the same set of loaded sample cups, with storage of up to 250 patients' results and production of collated reports. Outputs of up to 200 enzymes or 450 end-point tests per hour are claimed. One extra advantage of this type of system is its continued usefulness as a "back-up" even after its replacement by high-output analyzers or as the main instrument in a special laboratory for assays such as those for drugs by the EMIT methods (Figs. 5–11 and 5–12).

Automated Electrolyte Analyzers—New Developments

Successful combinations of Technicon continuous flow systems and flame photometers and carousel-type spec-

*Gilford Instrument Laboratories, Inc., Oberlin, Ohio 44074 and Mississauga, Ont. L4W1X9.

Figure 5–10 Principle of the absorbance measurement system of the Abbott ABA–100 and VP analyzers. See text for explanation of diagram.

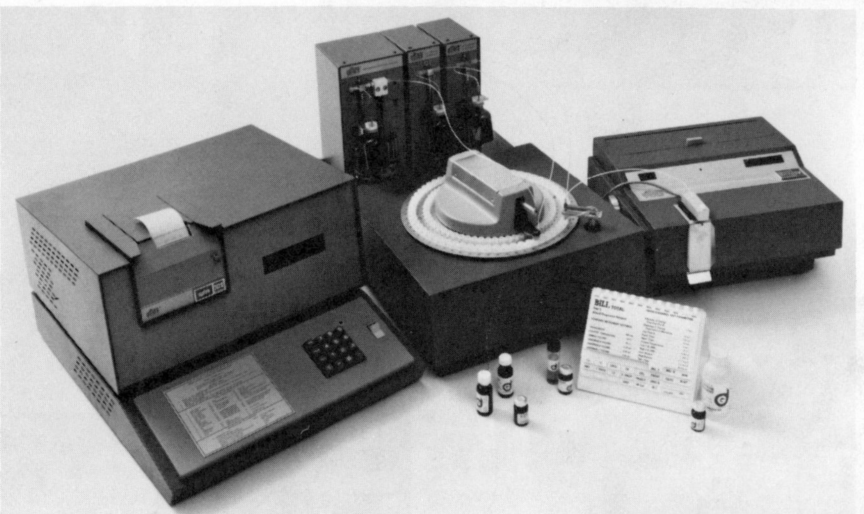

Figure 5–11 The Gilford System 203-S. The modules are, from left to right, the microprocessor control and data collection unit, the 60-place sample turntable with reagent dispensers to the rear, and the flow-cell spectrophotometer. (Courtesy of Gilford Instrument Laboratories, Inc., Oberlin, Ohio 44074.)

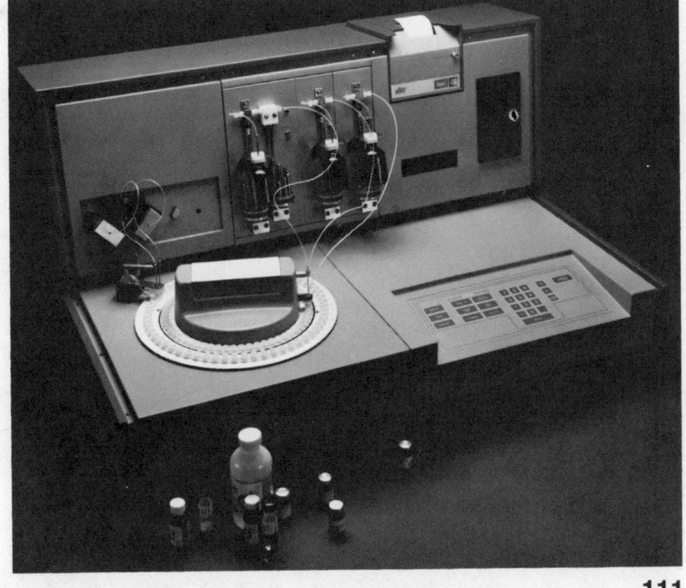

Figure 5–12 The Gilford IMPACT 400 incorporates fully automatic set-up and selective batching of more than 60 tests, collation of patient reports, and compatibility with a formatted printer or a computer system. A dual cuvette system permits outputs of 200 enzymes and 400 end-point chemistries per hour. Note the touch-sensitive keyboard, impervious to accidental spillage of reagents. (Courtesy of Gilford Instrument Laboratories, Inc., Oberlin, Ohio 44074.)

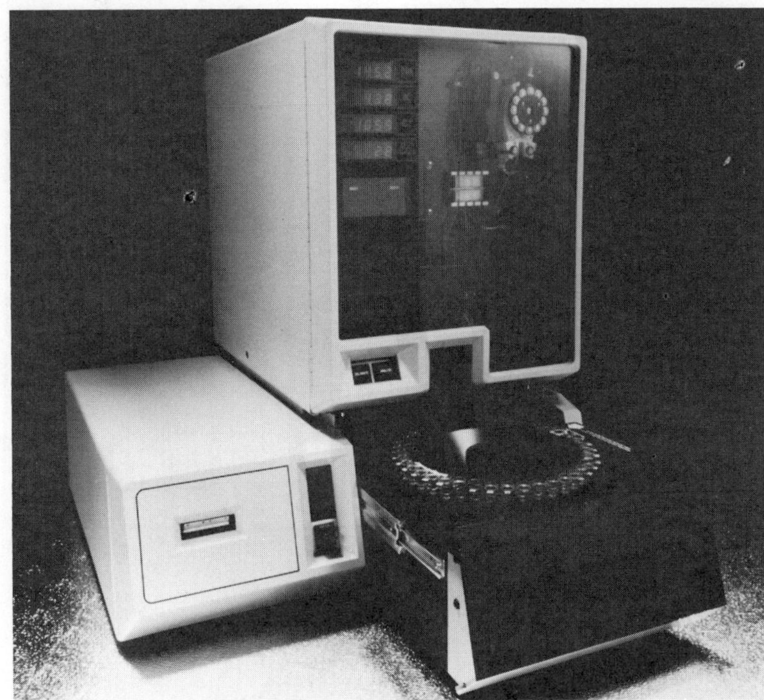

Figure 5–13 The NOVA 4 + 4 automated electrolyte analyzer using ion-selective electrodes. (Courtesy of NOVA Biomedical, Newton, Mass. 02164.)

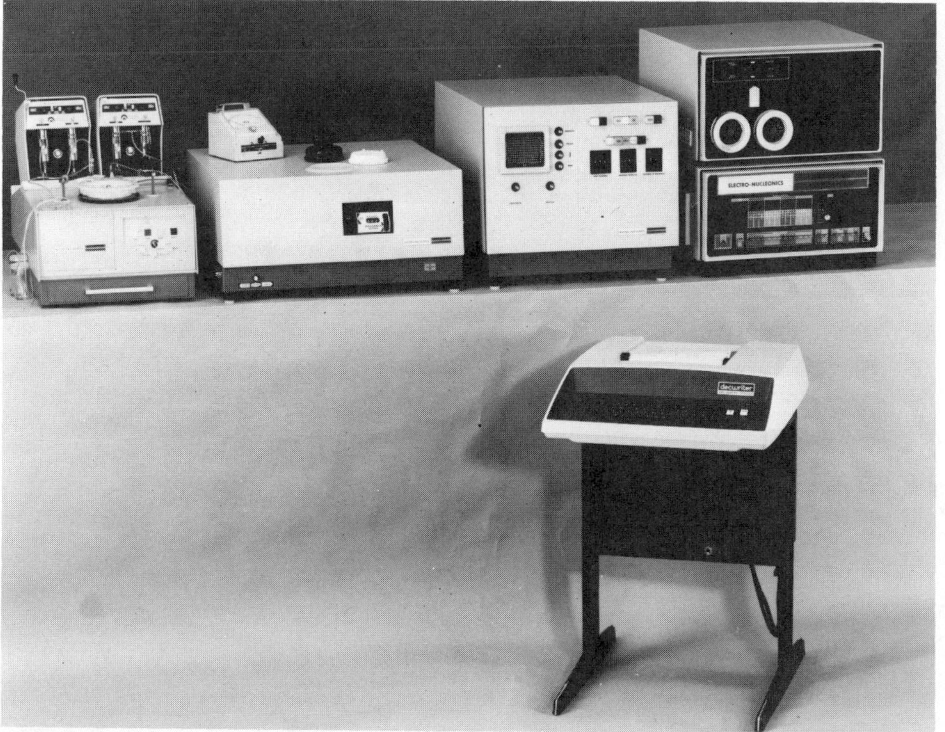

Figure 5–14 The ENI GeMSAEC Automatic Fast Analyzer. (Courtesy of Electro-Nucleonics, Inc., Fairfield, N.J. 07006.)

imen carriers with flame photometers and printers have been in use for at least 15 years. The development of reliable ion-selective electrodes for the four chief electrolytes—sodium, potassium, chloride, and total CO_2—coupled with the precise process control attainable with the new microprocessors has produced such instruments as the NOVA 4.* This instrument, together with its completely automated version, the NOVA 4 + 4, can deliver up to 80 sets of electrolytes per hour by the use of flow-through electrodes. Calibration is automatic, and the instrument is ready for immediate use at all times. Audible and visual alarms of operational problems are built into the program. The lack of discretionary ability is not relevant, since modern clinical practice requires all four measurements (Fig. 5–13).

Automatic Analyzers Using the GeMSAEC Principle

The ENI GeMSAEC Automatic Fast Analyzer,† shown in Figure 5–14, the Rotochem II,‡ shown in Figure 5–15, and the Centrifichem§ are centrifugal analyzers based on the work of Dr. N. G. Anderson. The acronym "GeMSAEC" is derived from the initials of the organizations that provided the main support for the development of the system, the National Institute of *Ge*neral *M*edical *S*ciences and the United States *A*tomic *E*nergy *C*ommission (Anderson, 1969). The three commercial versions operate in a similar manner, differing in the methods of loading and the extent of computer control available to the user.

The heart of the system is a thick Teflon rotor disc about 4″ in diameter, which can be spun at high speed by a vertically mounted electric motor. Into the upper surface of the disc are formed concentric rings of shaped cavities, 16 or 32 in each ring. Each cavity in the inner rings is connected to the corresponding cavities in the outer rings by capillary passages. Of the four rings of cavities, the two innermost contain reagents and/or diluents; the third contains serum samples; the outermost cavities are actually cuvettes, usually of quartz or with quartz windows (Fig. 5–16).

*NOVA Biomedical, Inc., Newton, Mass. 02164

†Electro-Nucleonics, Inc., Fairfield, N.J. 07006.

‡American Instrument Co., Silver Spring, Md. 20910.

§Union Carbide Corp., Tarrytown, N.Y. 10591 and Toronto, Ont. M4P 1J3.

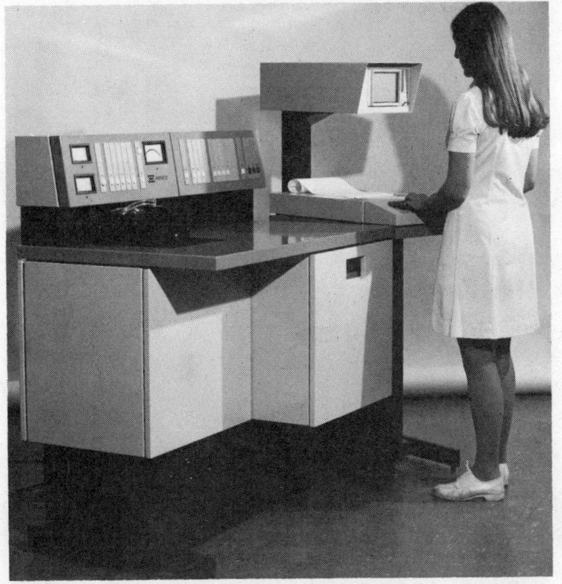

Figure 5–15 The Rotochem II. (Courtesy of American Instrument Company, Silver Spring, Md. 20910.)

After loading of the disc with reagents and samples (see Fig. 5–17), with one set reserved for a blank, the rotor is spun. Centrifugal force transfers the reagents outward through the capillary channels, mixes them with the serum samples, and then transfers them into the photometer cuvettes. Extra mixing may be achieved either by drawing air through the cuvette or by decelerating and accelerating the rotor. As the reaction proceeds in the cuvette rotating at the periphery of the disc, it is monitored by a vertically mounted photomultiplier above the rotor; the light source is below the edge of the rotor disc. The electrical signals from the photomultiplier corresponding to the changes in absorbance of the contents of the cuvette are converted to a binary digit code, which is transferred to a small computer memory. Since the rotor is spinning at high speed, each cuvette is read by the photometric system every 130 milliseconds. The reference or blank cuvette is also read at the same interval, and thus the combined photometric/computer system follows the reaction in the cuvette with great precision. The multiplicity of readings permits averaging of the values so that enough data for an accurate result are amassed in as little as two minutes. With a suitable computer slope search program, the progress of a kinetic enzyme reaction can be continuously monitored, the linear portion located, and the true reaction rate determined.

To make available to the smaller laboratory the better precision of automated analyses and to extend the range of procedures that such a laboratory can provide, one company has produced a miniature centrifugal analyzer, the "Gemeni."* The thick Teflon rotor disc of the GeMSAEC system is replaced by a disposable light plastic 20-cuvette disc that can be loaded, either manually or by an accessory loading device, with samples and reagents. The analyzer is programmed by a coded test card that calls up from the microprocessor memory the relevant chemistry parameters, such as wavelength selection, incubation time, sample blanking, number of data points taken, and data processing. Insertion of the loaded cuvette disc and the appropriate test card initiates the test run, and the results are printed out on the test card. The Gemeni incorporates some internal system checking. The analytical methods are quite sophisticated, with the use of bichromatic readings for blank correction and least squares curve fitting for kinetic assays. The manufacturer claims that with the built-in system checking the operator can locate and rectify the majority of faults, and the instrument signals standard and reagent problems that occur during an analytical run. The design of the disposable cuvette permits unused cuvettes from a small test batch to be used for subsequent batches.

*Electro-Nucleonics, Inc., Fairfield, N.J. 07006.

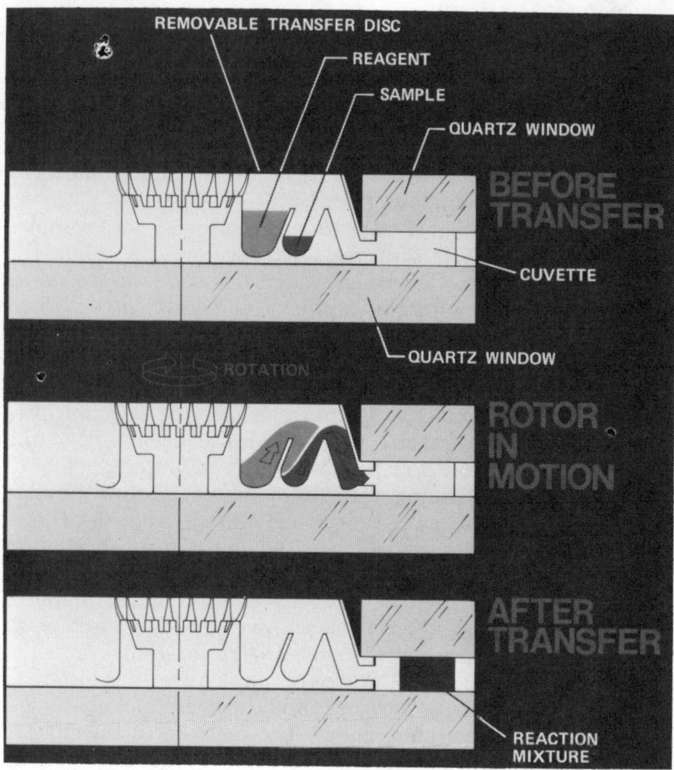

Figure 5–16 Cross-sections of the rotor in a centrifugal-type analyzer, showing the sequence of mixing and transfer of sample and reagents. (Courtesy of Electro-Nucleonics, Inc., Fairfield, N.J. 07006.)

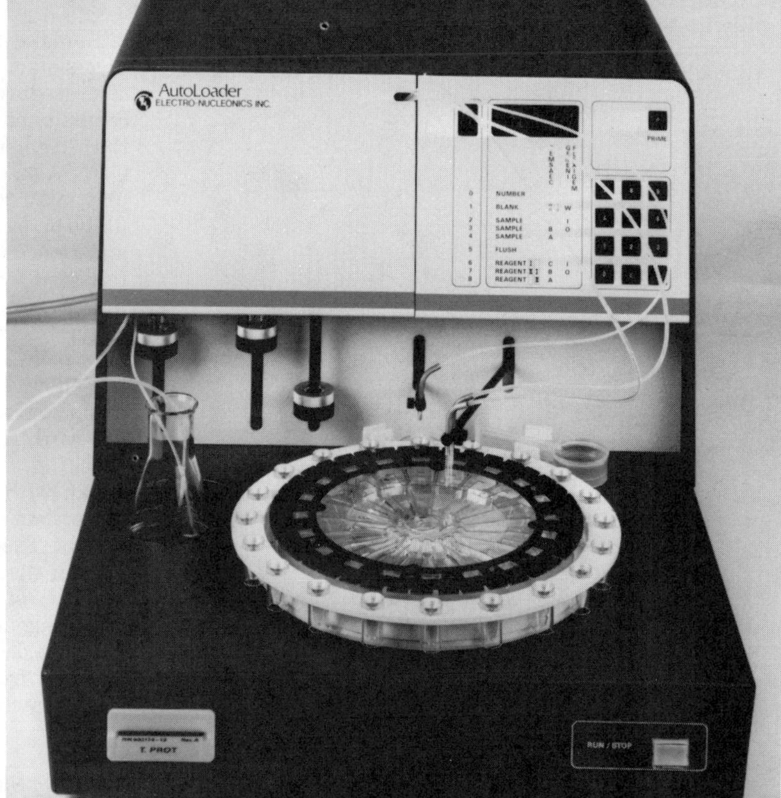

Figure 5–17 The "AutoLoader" for automated loading of samples and reagents into the cuvette-discs of GeMSAEC and Gemeni centrifugal analyzers. (Courtesy of Electro-Nucleonics, Inc., Fairfield, N.J. 07006.)

Thin-film Technology Analyzers

This category of automated clinical chemistry analyzers is represented by the Kodak "Ektachem."* It is unique in several respects: the only fluid used in the system is the serum or plasma sample; exacting measurement of the sample volume has been replaced by drop-wise dispensing; transmission spectrophotometry has been replaced by reflectance spectrophotometry, in which the intensity of color is measured by determining the proportion of a beam of light that is reflected off the colored area; and sodium and potassium measurements are made in disposable ion-selective electrodes.

For each test a 16-mm square chip has been produced, carried in a somewhat larger plastic slide with an obvious resemblance to a mounted photographic transparency. The chip contains several very thin layers, designed to accept a metered drop of serum, spread it evenly into a reagent layer, confine the colored product to a fixed area for reflectance spectrophotometry, and in some cases control the access of analytes to the reactive layers. For sodium and potassium the chip incorporates ion-selective membranes and flat silver/silver chloride electrodes. When the sample is dispensed onto one section of this system it creates a half cell, which is put into connection with an exactly similar half cell onto which a reference solution has been similarly dispensed. The potential difference produced between the two half cells is proportional to the concentration (or, more correctly, the activity) of the sodium or potassium in the sample.

The Ektachem system is completely discretionary: once the sample cups have been loaded the computer can be programmed with the test or tests required on each sample, including preset panels, and as each serum cup arrives at the loading station the appropriate types and numbers of chips, each in its own carrier slide, are delivered from cartridges previously loaded into magazines. The chips are moved to incubation and read-out stations, and after suitable incubation and measurement steps the results are stored in the computer memory. At the completion of the run of samples all results for each patient are automatically collated and printed out on one report. The stated rate of output is 120 tests per hour, and the sample cups can be loaded with as little as 20 μL of serum.

The Ektachem system is an outstanding example of the application of a technology (multiple thin films) developed for one purpose (photography) to a completely different problem, ultra-micro clinical chemistry analyses. Three different analysis modes—discretionary, single-test batching, and "stat"—and a 10 μL sample size would seem to make this system particularly suitable for pediatric analyses.

*Eastman Kodak Co., Rochester, N.Y. 14650.

Other Systems

In addition to the instruments briefly described above, there are also highly specialized systems such as those that combine a computer, a gas chromatograph, and a mass spectrometer to identify drugs.* We have excluded some instruments that might be regarded as partly automated, for example, flame photometers with the addition of AutoAnalyzer components and a recorder or printer to provide sampling introduction and result recording. Some flame photometers can be fitted with a turntable or rack-type specimen handling systems† (Fig. 5–18). The same principle has been applied to atomic absorption spectrophotometers.‡ The full potential of the available range of samplers, data processors, printers, and minicomputers has not yet been utilized, and

*Finnigan Corp., Sunnyvale, Calif. 94086.

†KLiNa Flame, Beckman Instruments, Inc., Fullerton, Calif. 92634; Instrumentation Laboratory, Inc., Lexington, Mass. 02173; and FLM–2, The London Co., Cleveland, Ohio 44145.

‡Varian Instruments, Palo Alto, Calif. 94303.

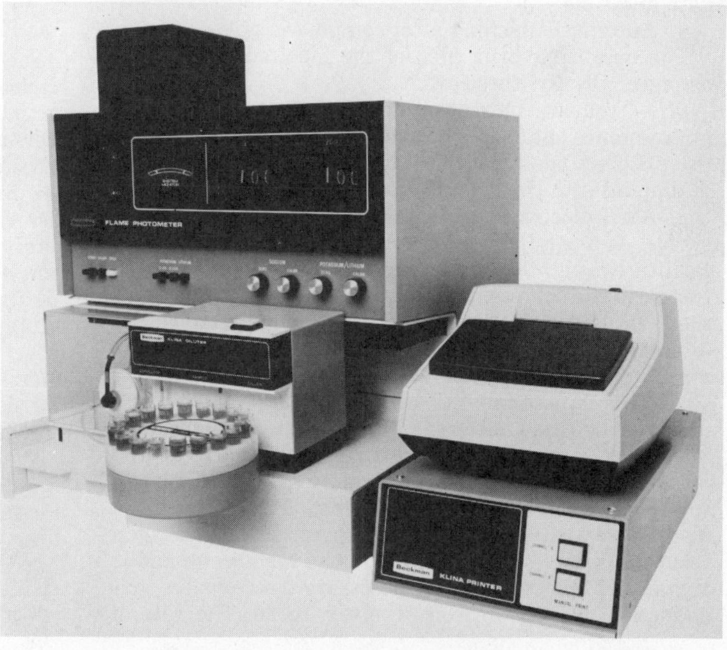

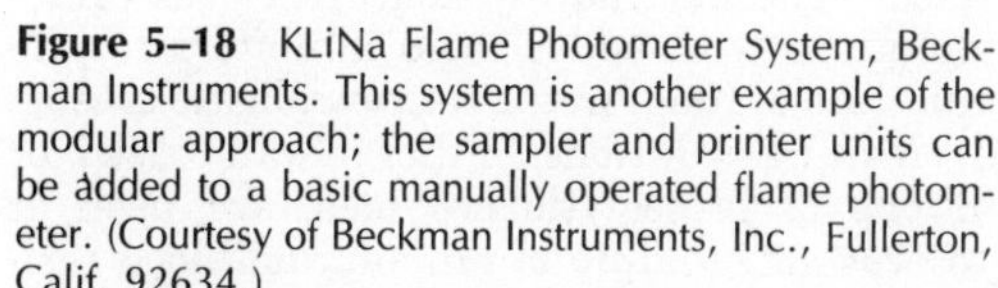
Figure 5–18 KLiNa Flame Photometer System, Beckman Instruments. This system is another example of the modular approach; the sampler and printer units can be added to a basic manually operated flame photometer. (Courtesy of Beckman Instruments, Inc., Fullerton, Calif. 92634.)

there is no reason why a laboratory should not develop an automated system geared to particular local needs.

We wish to emphasize that this is only a very brief survey of a rapidly widening field of automatic analyzers. Some trends in design are becoming evident, but the evolutionary process cannot be regarded as complete until the reliability and service systems of these instruments are good enough that reasonable operator skill and maintenance will hold downtime to a negligible level. "Negligible level" in this context can be defined as the loss of less than half a day of operations in any one month or less than a total of two days in a year.

Blood Gas and Acid-base Analytical Systems

The very rapid growth in demand for accurate measurement of blood pH, Po_2, and Pco_2 (that is, hydrogen ion concentration and partial pressures of oxygen and carbon dioxide) and simultaneous calculation of the derived parameters bicarbonate, oxygen saturation, base excess and total CO_2 has been met by a series of automated instruments that have largely displaced the earlier manual models, except in small laboratories. A typical "state of the art" (that is, incorporating the latest advances in microprocessor and electrode design) blood gas analyzer will provide all the listed information using about 200 microliters of heparinized blood in the "normal" mode or as little as 40 microliters in the "micro" mode of operation. The design of electrodes permits stability of pH electrodes on the order of 0.001 pH unit and measurement of the gases with coefficients of variation of 4% or better. The main features of these instruments are:

1. Microprocessor control of all functions
2. Temperature control of the electrodes to plus/minus 0.05°C
3. Automatic self-calibration and self-checking systems
4. Display of results on CRT or LED (light-emitting diode) panels
5. Automatic print-out of results, sometimes with date and time
6. Automatic flushing after completion of each test

The operating principles of the electrodes have not changed. Briefly, these are:

pH—To meet the requirements of small sample size, maintenance of anaerobic conditions, and rapid response the pH electrode is, in effect, turned inside out. Instead of dipping into the sample, as in the routine pH meter, the glass electrode contacts the blood on the inner surface of a capillary glass tube. This arrangement also facilitates the other needs—small volume, lack of contact with the surrounding atmosphere, and rapid attainment of thermostatic equilibrium. Completion of the circuit with the calomel reference electrode may be made via liquid or fibrous potassium chloride junctions or through a membrane.

Po_2—The Clark electrode for Po_2 measurement has a very fine platinum wire cathode maintained at the specific potential (−650 millivolts) at which oxygen molecules are reduced, and separated from the blood sample by a thin polypropylene membrane. As oxygen from the sample diffuses through the membrane and is reduced at the cathode, the necessary electrons for that reduction are drawn from a silver anode. The rate of oxygen diffusion depends on the oxygen tension (partial pressure) in the blood, and this in turn determines the rate of reduction and hence the rate of electron transfer from the anode. This process of electron transfer is an electric current, and its value in microamperes is proportional to the Po_2 of the sample.

Pco_2—The Severinghaus electrode is essentially a pH electrode whose active glass surface is separated from the blood sample by a membrane that is permeable to uncharged molecules but that will not allow passage of charged particles such as hydrogen ions. Typical membrane materials are silicone rubber and Teflon. Behind the membrane is a porous spacer—usually paper or synthetic fabric—that holds a layer of bicarbonate buffer. As the CO_2 molecules diffuse through the membrane they react with the bicarbonate buffer, producing a small change in pH. The rate of this change depends on the rate of CO_2 diffusion, which in turn reflects the partial pressure of the dissolved CO_2 in the blood sample.

The measured values for pH and Pco_2 are used in the Henderson-Hasselbalch equation to calculate the bicarbonate:

$$\text{pH} = \text{pK}_a + \log \frac{[\text{Salt (bicarbonate)}]}{[\text{Acid (carbonic acid)}]}$$

The value for carbonic acid is from the relationship $H_2CO_3 = 0.03 \times Pco_2$. The dissociation constant of carbonic acid is taken as 6.1, although it has been shown that this is not invariably true, especially in severe disturbances of acid-base balance (see p. 183). Thus the only unknown in the equation is the bicarbonate, which can be calculated by the microprocessor in the instrument. The equation can be rearranged to:

$$\text{Bicarbonate} = \text{antilog}\,(\text{pH} - \text{pK}_a + \log [\text{Carbonic acid}])$$

Thus with pH 7.4, carbonic acid 1.2 mmol/L, and pK_a 6.1:

$$\begin{aligned}\text{Bicarbonate} &= \text{antilog}\,(7.4 - 6.1 + 0.0792)\\ &= \text{antilog } 1.3792\\ &= 23.9 \text{ mmol/L}\end{aligned}$$

The very small electrical signals produced by the electrode are amplified by solid state electronics and compared with stored reference values derived from previous calibrations using buffers of known pH and gases of exactly known composition. Some instruments use fully humidified gases for calibration, some use dissolved gases. The automatic wash cycle uses dilute detergent solutions with added mold inhibitors to prevent accumulation of fungi in the narrow plastic tubing. Additional cleaning solutions, either alkali based or dilute solutions of proteolytic enzymes, are used at intervals to prevent build-up of protein and blood residues. Meticulous cleanliness is essential regardless of the design of the instrument, and a detailed record should be kept of all maintenance and service work.

The sophistication of modern blood gas instruments is well shown by the Corning Model 178,* which uses a microcomputer (Hewlett-Packard HP 85) for data handling, quality control records, automatic print-out of

*Corning Medical and Scientific, Medfield, Mass. 02052.

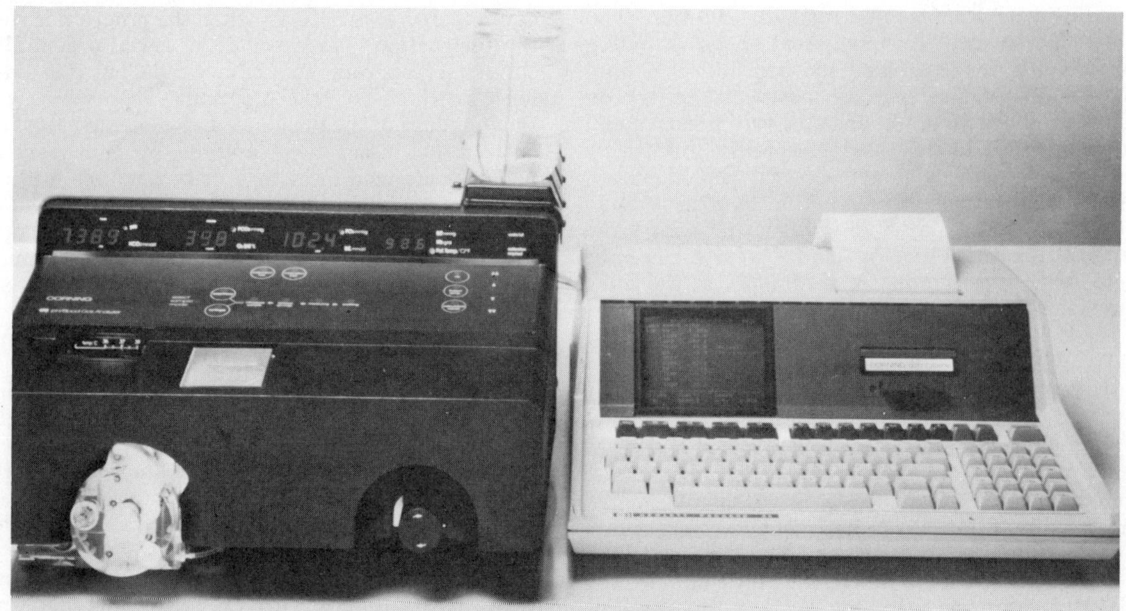

Figure 5–19 The Corning Model M-178 pH/Blood Analyzer with Hewlett-Packard HP-85 microcomputer. (Courtesy of Corning Medical and Scientific, Medfield, Mass. 02052.)

quality control charts, and a variety of operator-initiated activities (Fig. 5–19). The use of a true microcomputer facilitates modification of programs and the potential to add disc storage of patient results. The separation of data handling from instrument operation ensures that problems with the computer system do not prevent the processing of patient samples.

An example of the microprocessor-controlled automatic blood gas analyzer that extends the preprogrammed abilities beyond routine operation is the Radiometer ABL–3.* This instrument incorporates several user-interaction programs, for example, for selection of calibration schedules, checking of liquid sensors, valves, and pumps, and selection of reporting units. The calibration system uses buffers equilibrated with the standard gases that are produced by precise mixtures of room air and pure carbon dioxide. The hemoglobin value used for calculation of base excess is determined by a built-in photometer rather than being assumed (Fig. 5–20).

This review has been limited to the developments in automation in clinical chemistry. The principles have been applied to the special requirements of other departments of the laboratory, particularly hematology. The tedious process of presenting radioactive samples to a scintillation counter has been replaced by combinations of a rotary sample carrier or rack system, a detector, and an automatic printer. Recently the complete process of analyzing samples by radioimmunoassay has been completely automated in systems that require

*Radiometer America, Westlake, Ohio 44145; Bach-Simpson Ltd., London, Ontario N6A 4G7.

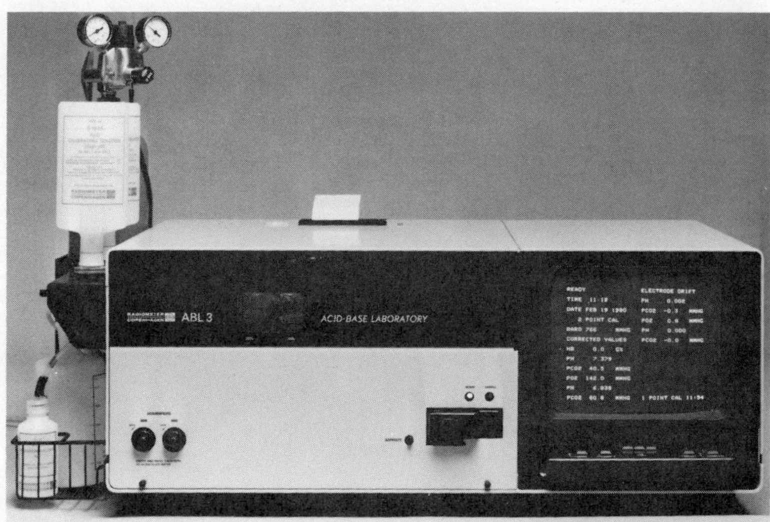

Figure 5–20 The Radiometer ABL-3 Automated Blood Gas Laboratory. (Courtesy of Radiometer America, Westlake, Ohio 44145 and Bach-Simpson Ltd., London, Ontario, Canada N6A 4G7.)

only loading with samples and reagents and that then proceed to perform all the analytical steps, including separations and counting, and the printing of a final report.* Continuous flow analytical systems† have been developed for blood grouping and antibody titration and have been applied to the assay of specific proteins by immunological methods combined with nephelometry. The list of applications of automation is already long, and it grows almost daily. It is also true that some instruments for which glowing claims were made have failed to meet the rigorous requirements of the busy routine laboratory.

LABORATORY COMPUTING AIDS

Programmable calculators are now relatively inexpensive, and no medical laboratory should be without one. They enable even simple, but repetitive, calculations to be performed with far less risk of computational errors than exists when an ordinary calculator is used. For this reason, a type should be chosen that can store the operating programs on magnetic cards or tape, so that they can be rapidly entered into the machine memory. A printer is also a most useful attachment, avoiding transcription and its inevitable inaccuracies.

Many such calculators are capable of most of the statistical procedures required in the average laboratory, for example, correlation coefficient, t test, mean, and standard deviation. Some have sufficient memory to allow the fitting of immunoassay standard curves, to perform nonparametric statistics, and to provide considerable help with quality control calculations.

The *program* of a calculator or minicomputer is a set of numbered instructions: when the program is running, the instructions are executed in serial order. The machine itself operates in a binary code, but it is a difficult form in which to write programs. This coding is called the *language* of the machine, and, to make programming easier, the instructions entered by the operator are usually arranged to be in a more readable form, which is then translated by part of the calculator called the compiler into the binary (or machine) language. The instruction set or language differs from one model of calculator to another and will be found in the manufacturer's instructions.

Minicomputers, sometimes called desk-top computers, are becoming more inexpensive and ubiquitous. They differ from the programmable calculator in having more memory and by operating in what is called a high-level language, such as Fortran, Algol, or Basic. Basic is the language employed by most home and commercial minicomputers: it is based on English words and allows easier writing of programs than does a programmable calculator.

When choosing a desk-top computer for a laboratory, it is wise to purchase a model from a major manufacturer such as Wang, Texas Instruments, or Hewlett-Packard even though they may be a little more expensive than some similar devices, because the reliability of their products is well established and reliability is all-important in the laboratory environment.

It is wise to purchase some of the maker's programs (or software) with the machine, especially for the commonly used statistical procedures. The new machine can then be brought into use quickly, while programming skills can be gradually acquired. For most purposes, this is all the computational power the average laboratory will need. There is a quantum jump between the desk computer and its applications and the question of data processing for the entire laboratory, with major analyzers "on-line." Although most laboratories will eventually acquire such a system, they are at present large, complex, and expensive and cannot be further discussed here. However, the advent of powerful desk-top mini-

*CONCEPT 4 Radioassay Analyzer, Micromedic Systems Division, Rohm and Haas Co., Horsham, Pa. 19044; Technicon STAR, Technicon Instruments Corp., Tarrytown, N.Y. 10591; ARIA II, Becton Dickinson Immunodiagnostics, Salt Lake City, Utah 84115.

†Technicon Instruments Corp., Tarrytown, N.Y. 10591.

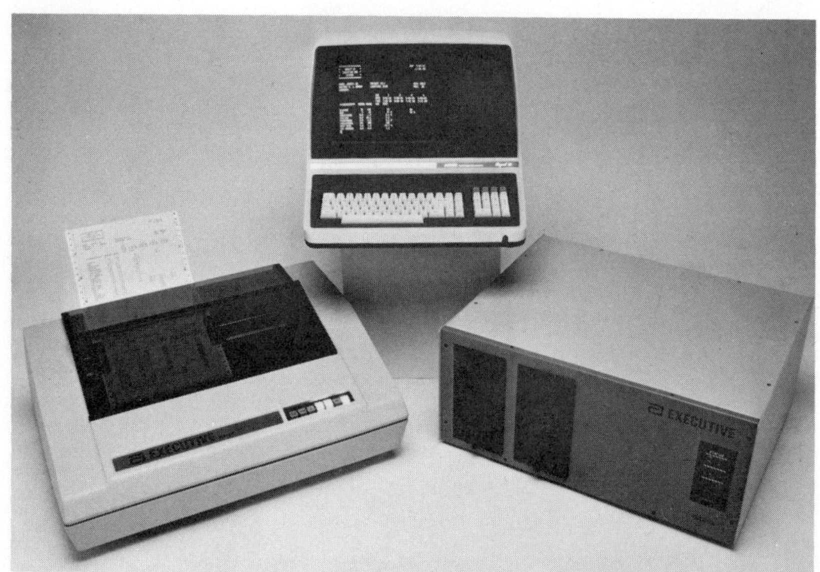

Figure 5–21 The Abbott "Executive" data handling system.

computers means that data handling systems with on-line capability will become available at relatively low cost. The system shown in Figure 5–21 is an example.

CHAPTER 5—REVIEW QUESTIONS

1. Describe the typical features of a continuous flow automatic analyzer.
2. Describe the photometric system of the Abbott series of discrete analyzers that permits precise absorbance measurements.
3. Describe the essential features of a centrifugal analyzer.
4. Describe the special features of the Kodak Ektachem analyzer.
5. What are the main features of the automated blood gas analyzers?
6. Describe the principles of the pH, PO_2, and PCO_2 electrodes used in automated blood gas analyzers.

6

CARBOHYDRATES, LIPIDS, PROTEINS, AND AMINO ACIDS

CARBOHYDRATES

Carbohydrates are compounds of fundamental importance in the body. With a few exceptions they have the general formula $(CH_2O)_n$. The simplest carbohydrates are polyalcohols, which are also aldehydes or ketones; they are usually known as monosaccharides and, for them, in the general formula n usually equals 5 or 6. Monosaccharides can exist as straight chains (Fig. 6–1).

By convention, the carbon atoms are numbered from the aldehyde or ketone end. Note carefully that atoms 2, 3, 4, and 5 of the glucose molecule as depicted are asymmetrical: exchange of the hydrogen and hydroxyl groups on one of these carbon atoms will produce a structurally different molecule. For glucose in the straight chain form there are 2^4, or 16, possible alternate forms, or *isomers*. Although chemically very similar, the isomers may show physical differences so that only one form will react with a specific enzyme (for example, glucose oxidase).

```
    H—C═O                  ┌──────────┐
      |                    ↓          |
    H—C—OH              H—C—OH        |
      |                   |           |
   HO—C—H               H—C—OH        |
      |                   |           O
    H—C—OH             HO—C—H         |
      |                   |           |
    H—C—OH              H—C—OH        |
      |                   |           |
     CH2OH              H—C───────────┘
                          |
                         CH2OH

  D-glucose          α-D-glucopyranose
```

Figure 6–1 Straight chain and ring forms of D-glucose.

The straight chain formula is a simplification of the usual structure, because in solution and in most biological reactions, the molecule exists as a ring structure (Fig. 6–2).

Two major ring forms exist: a *pyranose* form, with six carbon atoms in the ring (the most usual configuration), and a *furanose* form, with five carbon atoms (as in fructose). The presence of asymmetrical carbon atoms causes the isomers to show optical activity: they may rotate the plane of a beam of polarized light to the right or the left (dextrorotatory [D] or levorotatory [L] forms, respectively). In the ring form, the carbon atom 1 is also asymmetrical, producing alpha and beta variants (Fig. 6–2).

When two monosaccharides are joined together by a glycosidic link, a disaccharide results; the monosaccharides may be similar or dissimilar:

Maltose	Two glucose residues	Reducing sugar
Lactose	Galactose + glucose	Reducing sugar
Sucrose	Glucose + fructose	Non-reducing sugar

Monosaccharides can join together to form long chains, which may be straight or may show complex branching, to produce macromolecules called *polysaccharides*. These are important compounds in the body: a good example is glycogen, which is a storage form of glucose composed

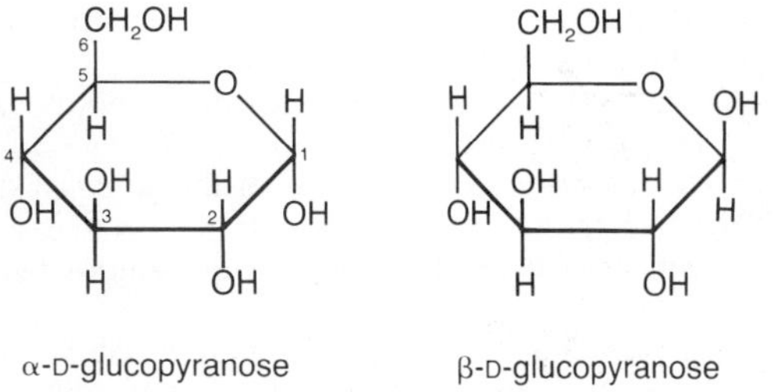

Figure 6–2 Stereoisomers of D-glucopyranose.

of numerous glucose residues combined in a strongly branched form.

Starch is the polysaccharide storage form of glucose in plants. In mammalian organisms, other, often very complex, polysaccharides are found as blood group substances and in mucin, cartilage, the matrix of bone, and many other tissues. Furthermore, most extracellular proteins have varied proportions of carbohydrate molecules attached to them, possibly to provide greater molecular stability outside the cell.

Reducing Properties

It has been known for almost 200 years that certain sugars have reducing properties (e.g., alkaline copper sulphate is reduced to brown copper oxide). This property is conferred on monosaccharides and disaccharides by the presence of the aldehyde group. However, only a small amount of the free aldehyde form is present in the equilibrium mixture. The aldehyde group is also in equilibrium with an enol form (Fig. 6–3). The shift to the enol form is favored by a high pH, and the presence of the double bond and negatively charged group confers reducing properties on the molecule. Until quite recently this reaction formed the basis of all chemical methods for the estimation of "reducing sugars." When applied to blood, glucose alone is usually measured, as it is the major monosaccharide in the plasma and red cell. However, there is usually some interference from nonsaccharide reducing substances such as glutathione in the red cells.

The modern preferred method for the measurement of glucose is a specific enzyme assay using glucose oxidase or hexokinase and applied to plasma, not whole blood.

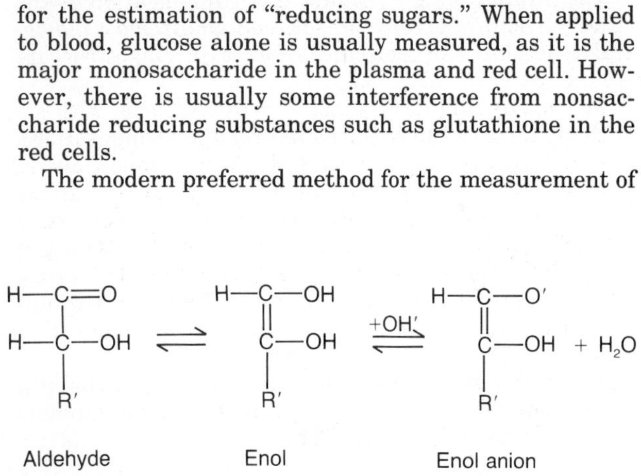

Figure 6–3 Formation of enol group, with reducing properties.

Carbohydrate Metabolism

Carbohydrates are ingested partly as monosaccharides and disaccharides but chiefly in the form of the glucose polymers starch and glycogen. The polymers are digested in the lumen of the gut to oligosaccharides, by the action of amylase from the pancreatic secretions. The intestinal epithelial cells possess a brush border that is in direct contact with the gut contents: this contains enzymes whose action is to reduce the oligosaccharides further to monosaccharides. Thus only monosaccharides, chiefly glucose, fructose, and galactose, are absorbed and pass in the blood of the portal vein to the liver, where fructose and galactose are metabolized to glucose. The major portion of the glucose is stored, either in the form of glycogen in liver and muscle or as neutral fat in the adipose tissue cells.

The oxidative degradation of glucose is the major source of energy for the metabolic activity of all the body cells, chiefly by means of the production of adenosine triphosphate (ATP). This process occurs in two main stages, anaerobic and aerobic. Figure 6–4 shows in outline the major pathways of energy metabolism, including the extremely important links between fats and carbohydrates.

The principal degradative pathway is from glucose, via glucose-6-phosphate, to pyruvate: this is known as the anaerobic (or Embden-Meyerhof) pathway, because the reactions can proceed without any need for oxygen. This series of enzymatic reactions results in the formation of two moles of ATP per mole of glucose; during this process, the coenzyme nicotinamide adenine dinucleotide (NAD+) is reduced to NADH. Pyruvate is next converted to acetylcoenzyme A, which enters the aerobic Krebs cycle by condensing with oxalacetate to form citrate. The Krebs cycle produces 24 moles of ATP per mole of glucose; the ATP is produced by the mitochondrial electron transfer system, which, it should be remembered, requires oxygen as the final electron acceptor. In addition, 12 moles of ATP are derived from other reactions. Altogether one mole of glucose when completely oxidized will produce at least 36 moles of ATP. NADH is also oxidized back to NAD+ by the reactions of the Krebs cycle: this is the ultimate fate of the NADH produced by the anaerobic pathway.

If there should be some limitation of the oxygen supply to the Krebs cycle, a situation that occurs in actively contracting muscle in the normal person or in hypoxic disease states, then the oxidation of NADH to NAD+ (which is essential to maintain the activity of the anaerobic reactions) cannot be achieved in sufficient quantity by the Krebs cycle.

Instead, pyruvate is metabolized to lactate by the following reaction:

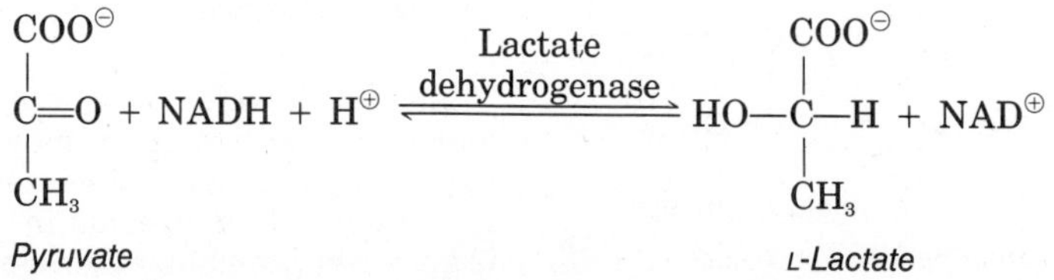

$$\underset{\textit{Pyruvate}}{\begin{array}{c}COO^{\ominus}\\|\\C{=}O\\|\\CH_3\end{array}} + NADH + H^{\oplus} \xrightleftharpoons[]{\text{Lactate dehydrogenase}} \underset{\textit{L-Lactate}}{\begin{array}{c}COO^{\ominus}\\|\\HO{-}C{-}H\\|\\CH_3\end{array}} + NAD^{\oplus}$$

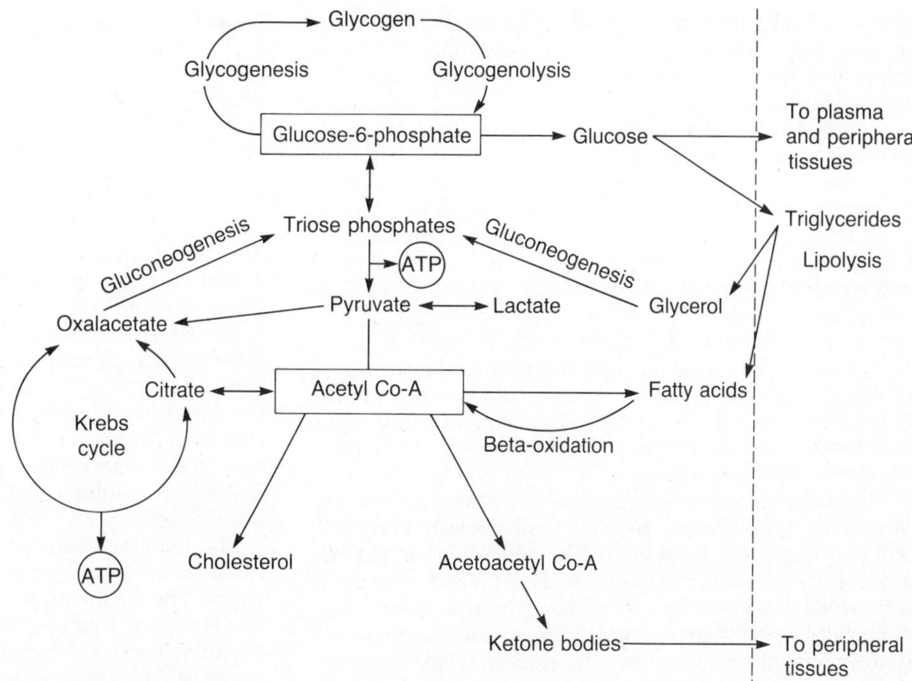

Figure 6–4 Schematic interrelationships of carbohydrate and lipid metabolism in the liver.

The conversion of glucose to lactate is called *glycolysis,* and it is the means by which the so-called oxygen debt is accumulated. Under these particular circumstances, lactate is a virtual metabolic dead end, and it can be converted back to pyruvate only when adequate oxygen supplies become available again to metabolize the NADH produced by the reverse reaction. This conversion usually occurs in the liver, following transport of lactate to that organ from tissues such as muscle (the Cori cycle). This accounts for the high lactate levels in the venous blood flowing from actively exercising muscle and also for the accumulation of lactic acid in hypoxic states.

It will be seen from Figure 6–4 that the 2-carbon compound acetyl coenzyme A is a central point in the metabolism not only of glucose, but also of fats and proteins. The process of lipolysis (conversion of triglycerides [neutral fats] to free fatty acids and glycerol) is inhibited by insulin. Under conditions of relative or absolute lack of insulin, lipolysis increases. The fatty acids and glycerol are transported to the liver, where glycerol can be resynthesized to glucose (forming one of the routes for gluconeogenesis) and the fatty acids enter the spiral sequence of reactions called beta oxidation, which produces ATP.

The end product of beta oxidation is acetyl coenzyme A: large amounts of this are produced if lipolysis is increased, and eventually production can outstrip the ability of the Krebs cycle to metabolize it. Under such conditions, the excess is metabolized, first to acetoacetyl coenzyme A and then to the so-called ketone bodies: acetoacetic acid, acetone, and beta-hydroxybutyric acid.

Glucose Homeostasis

Under normal conditions of nutritional intake and balance, the brain and some other tissues are very dependent on an adequate supply of glucose to maintain their energy supplies. A sudden fall of plasma glucose levels below about 50 mg/dL (2.78 mmol/L) will produce symptoms of hypoglycemia (see below), and a further decline will induce coma. Prolonged elevations, on the other hand, will lead to the vascular and other long-term complications described under diabetes.

Thus it is essential for the body to maintain plasma glucose levels within a rather narrow range despite wide variations in the rate of glucose influx and utilization. Apart from metabolic factors, plasma glucose levels are affected by a number of hormones.

Insulin

Insulin is a polypeptide hormone (approximate MW 6000) that is essential for life and that is secreted continuously by the beta cells of the islets of Langerhans. The islets are clusters of cells scattered through the exocrine tissue of the pancreas. They comprise several different types of cells; the majority (60 to 80%) are designated beta cells, whereas most of the remainder are alpha cells and secrete glucagon.

Insulin is synthesized in the cell as a continuous twisted structure, termed *proinsulin.* A loop of this (the C-peptide, or connecting chain) is removed by a hydrolytic enzyme, producing the insulin molecule, which is composed of two chains (A and B) linked by disulfide bonds. Some proinsulin is present in serum, but it has very little insulin-like activity. However, it is antigenically similar and will be measured in the radioimmunoassay for insulin.

Insulin is stored in granules in the beta cells and is released under the stimulus of various compounds. Glucose is the most potent releasing agent. A glucagon-like hormone is secreted into the blood from the intestine, and this also stimulates insulin secretion; the presence of the hormone is probably responsible for the difference in response between an oral and intravenous glucose tolerance test. Caffeine and leucine also can cause insulin release.

Insulin is the only hormone that will produce a fall in blood sugar levels. It stimulates the uptake of glucose by muscle and fat cells, probably by some direct effect on membrane permeability. It also increases the uptake of glucose into liver cells by stimulating glucokinase activity, since the membrane of the hepatic parenchymal cell is freely permeable to glucose; insulin also inhibits the hepatic output of glucose. It has no effect on the uptake or utilization of glucose by the brain.

In muscle, liver, and fat cells it activates the transport of amino acids and stimulates the synthesis of proteins. It inhibits lipolysis in fat cells and reduces the plasma free fatty acid concentration. In summary, insulin stimulates anabolic processes.

The following hormones have anti-insulin actions: glucagon, epinephrine, cortisol, and growth hormone. All are capable of producing an elevation of plasma glucose by various mechanisms. Even short periods of hypoglycemia are more damaging to the brain than moderately prolonged hyperglycemia, and the fact that more hormones elevate plasma glucose levels than depress them obviously has survival value.

The glycogen in the liver cells is a storage form of glucose: by the enzymatic process called glycogenolysis, free glucose can be rapidly mobilized and secreted into the circulation by the liver. The glycogen reserves are quite limited, however, and under conditions of moderate exercise (e.g., running) they can be consumed entirely within some 20 minutes. Once depletion of the glycogen reserve has occurred, the majority of the tissues can switch over to oxidation of long-chain fatty acids or of ketone bodies to provide their energy requirements, thus decreasing the rate of glucose utilization.

Some tissues (for example the brain) continue to require glucose, especially those with an obligatory anaerobic metabolism, notably the red and white cells, kidney medulla, and the retina. After the glycogen stores are depleted, these tissues are provided with glucose by the process of gluconeogenesis, by which glucose is generated from the metabolism of lactate, glycerol, or amino acid residues. Gluconeogenesis occurs to a major extent in the liver and the kidney cortex, with the kidney becoming quantitatively more important as fasting proceeds.

However, most cells (apart from the obligatory anaerobes) can utilize fatty acids or ketone bodies for almost all of their energy requirements. During prolonged fasting even the brain can ultimately derive up to 40% of its energy from ketone bodies. As this process occurs, glucose utilization and also plasma glucose levels reach minimal levels.

During prolonged fasting insulin levels are considerably reduced, so that the very powerful antilipolytic action of insulin is reduced and mobilization of free fatty acids and glycerol is increased, resulting in increased ketone body formation in the liver. However, enough circulating insulin is present to prevent the severe ketosis seen with diabetes.

Diabetes Mellitus

Diabetes mellitus is a disease characterized primarily by abnormally high levels of glucose in the blood, because of either a relative or absolute deficiency of insulin. The word *diabetes* means literally a "running through," referring to the characteristic diuresis, and *mellitus* means "sweet" or "honey-like": the name refers to the presence of large amounts of glucose in the urine, an important finding in bygone days when gustatory sampling of urine was a necessary part of a physician's diagnostic methods.

Diabetes mellitus may occur as a primary disorder or secondary to certain diseases in which, for reasons other than the lack of insulin, there is some abnormality in the handling of glucose. Whatever the causes, the biochemical finding is that of blood glucose levels that are elevated beyond the physiologically normal, whether fasting or under a glucose load: a state of *glucose intolerance.*

The nomenclature and diagnostic criteria of diabetes mellitus have undergone considerable revision in recent years. The following discussion is based on the report of the National Diabetes Data Group (1979), which should be consulted for detailed information, especially on the diagnosis of diabetes mellitus in pregnancy.

1. The most severe and potentially lethal form of diabetes mellitus is due to an absolute lack of insulin following the destruction of the islet cells in the pancreas. Both islet cell antibodies and viruses have been implicated, but inherited factors are also involved. This type was formerly referred to as juvenile diabetes: however, it can occur at any age and is now classed as *insulin-dependent diabetes mellitus* (IDDM). (Some authors now call it Type 1 diabetes mellitus.) Ketosis is common, and these patients are absolutely dependent on exogenous insulin for their survival.

2. The non–insulin dependent, non–ketosis-prone group is now named non–insulin-dependent diabetes mellitus (NIDDM) or Type 2. Patients in this category may be subgrouped as obese and nonobese. Insulin is not essential in the treatment of this group. Inherited factors are of greater etiological significance than in IDDM.

3. Impaired glucose tolerance can occur secondarily to some systemic diseases: pancreatic disease, if there is destruction of islet tissue; cirrhosis; and endocrine diseases, such as Cushing's disease and pheochromocytoma, because of the anti-insulin action of cortisol and epinephrine, respectively. Many drugs are also capable of impairing glucose tolerance, particularly certain diuretics and psychoactive drugs.

Diabetic Coma

The most severe manifestations of the diabetic state are seen in IDDM. This is the classic form of the syndrome: there is usually a sudden onset, apparently following the rapid destruction of islet cells in the pancreas. The abrupt withdrawal of insulin (the *only* physiological agent that *lowers* blood glucose levels) engenders a series of biochemical changes that explain most of the clinical features of the disease.

The major clinical features are as follows. Affected individuals suffer rapid loss of weight, pass large volumes of urine (polyuria), and drink large amounts of fluid to replace the lost water (polydipsia). They become drowsy and lethargic. The skin is warm but dry, and signs of dehydration may be present. Vomiting also causes further fluid loss. In precoma and coma, deep sighing respirations ("air-hunger") occur; the breath has a sweet, fruity odor. There is a marked predisposition to infections and pruritus.

The major biochemical changes are as follows:

1. The liver continues to secrete free glucose, despite the hyperglycemia, probably because of the action of cortisol with reversal of the glycolytic pathway.
2. The entry of free glucose into muscle and adipose tissue is inhibited, thus preventing its storage as glycogen and neutral fat, respectively. Indeed, because of the unopposed action of growth hormone and cortisol, lipolytic activity is increased and free fatty acids enter the blood in uncontrolled amounts.

The excess of free fatty acid is largely converted to ketone bodies, and the presence of much acetone is responsible for the sweet odor of the breath. The excess ketone bodies cannot be metabolized fast enough, and thus their presence is a major cause of the severe metabolic acidosis that is a marked feature of diabetic coma. A blood pH of 6.9 to 7.0 is not unusual in coma; a pH of 6.8 or less is occasionally seen, but it is usually lethal despite intensive treatment.

Some free fatty acids are converted to triglycerides, and a severe hypertriglyceridemia is usually present. The plasma from a patient in coma may look like thick cream.

3. The inability to store glucose means that, once the plasma level rises above the renal threshold of approximately 180 mg/dL, glucose begins to spill into the urine in large amounts, owing to saturation of the reabsorptive mechanism for glucose.

There is a limit to the reabsorptive capacity of the kidney and to its concentrating powers: it cannot secrete glucose as a dry powder or even as a thick syrup: the maximum osmolality of the secreted urine is about 1200 mOsm/kg. Therefore, because so much glucose is being lost into the urine, large volumes of urine of high osmolality are excreted—a state of osmotic diuresis.

Because the usual amount of water cannot be reabsorbed, an increased amount of glomerular transudate flows through the renal tubules and there is insufficient time for the normal reabsorption of other substances, such as sodium and bicarbonate. These are thus swept out of the body, resulting in significant sodium and bicarbonate depletion. The loss of bicarbonate also contributes to the metabolic acidosis.

The severe dehydration seen in this state is due to (1) osmotic diuresis, (2) vomiting, and (3) hyperventilation. The first two causes also produce a severe sodium deficiency. The hyperventilation lowers the blood P_{CO_2} to provide some compensation for the metabolic acidosis (see Chapter 8), and a P_{CO_2} of 15 mm Hg may be seen. The plasma is also hyperosmolar, a feature that disturbs brain function and is, in part, responsible for drowsiness and coma.

The severe dehydration causes a fall in plasma volume, with the onset of hypotension and cardiovascular shock. The resulting poor perfusion and subsequent hypoxia of the tissues are major factors in the elevation of lactate levels; a pH of less than 7.2 is usually associated with a significant hyperlactacidemia.

Occasionally, ketosis is absent: this is a proven finding in some cases of hyperosmolar coma, but it should be remembered that in this state severe hypoxia results in a disproportionate production of beta-hydroxybutyric acid, which is *not* detected by the usual chemical tests based on the Rothera nitroprusside reaction. This may account for some cases of apparent nonketotic diabetic coma.

The non–insulin dependent type shows similar changes biochemically, although in a much milder form, without ketosis or coma. Recurrent infections, peripheral neuritis, and pruritus may be presenting features.

Both forms share the same long-term complications, notably, severe atherosclerosis, cataract, retinal damage, pyelonephritis, and glomerulonephritis. The precise reasons for these chronic changes are still obscure; however, the present view is that all are almost certainly related to prolonged elevation of glucose levels alone. It seems now beyond debate that better control of plasma glucose levels is associated with fewer long-term vascular complications.

Diagnostic Criteria

The present consensus is that significant glucose intolerance has been overdiagnosed in the past: the following criteria have been established to avoid this, and they agree closely with European experience and recommendations. The figures given below are based on venous plasma or venous whole blood, using a "true glucose" method (glucose oxidase or a hexokinase), preferably in automated instruments, such as a centrifugal analyzer, which give greater precision.

Any *one* of the following is considered to establish a diagnosis of a diabetic state severe enough to warrant treatment.

1. Presence of the classic signs and symptoms already described, with grossly elevated plasma glucose levels.
2. An elevated *fasting* glucose concentration, on more than one occasion, that fulfills the following criteria:

$$\text{Venous plasma} \geq 140 \text{ mg/dL } (7.8 \text{ mmol/L})$$
$$\text{Venous whole blood} \geq 120 \text{ mg/dL } (6.7 \text{ mmol/L})$$

If the fasting values meet these criteria, then a glucose tolerance test is *not* needed.

3. A fasting glucose concentration less than in (2) but showing a *sustained* elevation during the oral glucose tolerance test on more than one occasion. *Both* the 2-hour sample *and* some other sample drawn between the

ingestion of glucose and the 2-hour sample must meet the following criteria:

Venous plasma ⩾ 200 mg/dL (11.1 mmol/L)
Venous whole blood ⩾ 180 mg/dL (10.0 mmol/L)

For criteria defining impaired glucose tolerance insufficient to require treatment, and for the diagnosis of diabetes in pregnancy, see the study referred to above (p. 122). See also the cautionary notes in the following section.

The Oral Glucose Tolerance Test

It should now be understood from the above discussion of diagnostic criteria that an oral glucose tolerance test (OGTT) may not be needed in order to establish a diagnosis of diabetes mellitus. The OGTT is, at best, an unsatisfactory test with poor reproducibility, posing severe difficulties in interpretation.

The test is designed to evaluate the endogenous insulin response to a physiological glucose challenge. As the glucose is absorbed from the gut, the plasma level rises and triggers the release of preformed insulin from the beta cells, keeping the peak level at 150 mg/dL or less in the normal person. Despite the fact that poor absorption from the gut may affect the test, the challenge of glucose entering the body *via* the gut and portal vein is a more physiological stimulus than the intravenous tolerance test, which is not recommended for ordinary diagnostic purposes.

Preparations

1. The patient must be ambulatory and free from pyrexia, acute illness, or trauma for at least two weeks; drugs such as birth control pills, salicylates, steroids, and diuretics should be discontinued during the three-day dietary preparation period at least. If the patient is already under treatment with hypoglycemic drugs, i.e., insulin, or the sulfonylurea group, these should be discontinued, at least on the day of the test.

2. Dietary preparation. The patient must have a diet containing at least 150 g carbohydrate per day for three days prior to the test. Normal persons who have been on a low carbohydrate diet may give a diabetic-type response to the OGTT because the beta cells of the pancreas have not been accustomed to coping with a high carbohydrate load.

3. If not already done, it is advisable to determine the patient's fasting plasma glucose level prior to the OGTT in case a definite state of hyperglycemia exists; administration of a large dose of glucose may be contraindicated, and the physician ordering the OGTT should be advised.

Procedure

A fasting venous sample should be obtained first; it is advisable to measure the glucose level of this immediately if no other glucose values are known for that particular patient. If the result is more than 150 mg/dL, then an OGTT need not be performed, with resulting economies in time and materials.

For adults, a dose of 75 g of glucose is given by mouth. This should be dissolved in at least 300 mL of water; a flavoring may also be used. Some commercial preparations are satisfactory, but their constituents should be known precisely. For children, give 1.75 g/kg up to a maximum dose of 75 g. Zero time is the beginning of the drink, which should be imbibed over a period of about 5 minutes. Blood samples should then be collected at 30-minute intervals for a period of 2 hours.

It is customary to collect urine samples at the same time as the plasma samples; the main advantage of this is to provide a correlation between any glycosuria and the corresponding plasma glucose levels. If glucose appears in the urine when the plasma level is below 180 mg/dL, then the patient probably has a lowered renal threshold for glucose, a harmless condition known as renal glycosuria, but one that may be interpreted as diabetes if only the urine is tested for glucose (as, for example, during an examination for life insurance).

Interpretation

If *both* the 2-hour sample *and* some other sample taken after the 75-g glucose load meet or exceed the following levels, the diagnosis of diabetes is substantiated.

Venous plasma ⩾ 200 mg/dL (11.1 mmol/L)
Venous whole blood ⩾ 180 mg/dL (10.0 mmol/L)

Occasionally, in about 5% of normal people, a flat curve is obtained with glucose levels remaining at, or close to, the fasting level. Sometimes a very early peak has been missed, but, provided that the drink has been taken and that there is no gastrointestinal disease or injury such as a pyloric stenosis or previous gastrectomy, a flat curve appears to be of no special significance.

It must be remembered that many variables can affect the observed plasma levels. Factors that can modify the result and cause poor reproducibility with consequent difficulties in interpretation are the state of nutrition, the diet before the test, preceding exercise or inactivity, fear, blood flow through the muscle mass (affected by posture and exercise during the test), and the presence of fever and infection. Gastric emptying and intestinal absorption may be profoundly affected in a pregnant woman, which, together with the hormonal changes, makes the diagnosis of diabetes during pregnancy a matter for extreme caution even for the expert physician.

It should be noted that the revised criteria for interpretation of the OGTT are much more conservative than those previously employed. The less stringent criteria of the past have been the cause of many normal persons' being classified as diabetic.

Glycosylated Hemoglobin

The monitoring of patients with diabetes mellitus over long periods of time is usually achieved by regular urine testing and occasional plasma glucose estimations. In many patients this is unsatisfactory because significant fluctuations in glucose levels may not be detected; yet, after much debate, it now seems reasonably certain that the late vascular complications of diabetes mellitus can be avoided or ameliorated by achieving better control of plasma glucose levels. The significant value seems to be the mean plasma glucose level over a 24-hour period; however, it is just this value that cannot easily be estimated with any certainty.

Recently, claims have been made that this mean glucose level can be assessed indirectly by determining the proportion present in blood of a component known as glycosylated hemoglobin (G-Hb). This form of hemoglobin was discovered in diabetic patients in 1958. It is sometimes called fast hemoglobin—more accurately, hemoglobin A_{1c}. It represents a hemoglobin A molecule to which a glucose residue has become attached. If blood glucose levels are on average consistently higher than normal, then a greater proportion of red cell hemoglobin will become glycosylated. Therefore, since this reaction is apparently irreversible and the red cell has a life span of approximately 120 days, the percentage of G-Hb present in the blood should be an index of the average plasma glucose level over the previous two or three months.

Two other glycoslylated fractions, Hb A_{1a} and Hb A_{1b}, have also been described. All these glycosylated hemoglobins migrate as a "fast" fraction by hemoglobin electrophoresis and can be individually separated by electrophoresis or column chromatography. However, it is technically more convenient and clinically acceptable to measure the three together.

Hb A_{1c} normally comprises less than 8% of the total red cell hemoglobin content. A level of 10% or more is definitely indicative of a poorly controlled diabetic state: well-controlled diabetics show values within the normal range. The test appears to be most useful in assessing the control of the diabetic state over long periods of time. Elevated values indicate a need to revise the treatment regimen; occasionally, especially in young insulin-dependent diabetics, they may indicate a willful failure to take insulin.

Glycosylated hemoglobin has also been proposed as a screening test for diabetes. One recent study showed that the correlation of elevated levels with a diabetic OGTT depended on the criteria for interpretation of the OGTT. The more conservative the criteria, the greater the number of patients with glucose intolerance who also had elevated G-Hb, up to 85% using the most conservative system.

Some caution should be observed in the interpretation of the test results. The column chromatography methods are extremely sensitive to small variations in the ambient temperature: a careful temperature correction is mandatory. Furthermore, lipemia (a not uncommon finding in poorly controlled diabetics) will produce a spurious elevation: if a nonlipemic sample is unobtainable, washing of the cells will reduce the interference. Because Hb F runs in the same position as Hb A_{1c}, the test cannot be used in children under the age of two years or in patients with thalassemia.

Hypoglycemia

Pathologically low blood sugar levels may result from lack of glucose or from relative or absolute hyperinsulinism. In normal people homeostatic mechanisms maintain the blood glucose level during fasting. At first this is accomplished by glycogenolysis, but once the glycogen stores have been exhausted gluconeogenesis from fatty acids and from amino acids occurs. Blood glucose homeostasis is one of the very last of the controlling mechanisms to succumb in starvation.

Causes of Hypoglycemia

Insulinomas. These are rare functional tumors of the beta cells of the islets of Langerhans. They are also called nesidioblastomas and probably comprise a little over half of all islet cell tumors, being only slightly more frequent than the alpha-cell tumors that give rise to the Zollinger-Ellison syndrome (p. 230). Although they may occur at any age, they are most common between 25 and 60 years. About 70% are benign, 10% are obviously malignant, and 20% fall into the doubtful category. Continuous or irregular secretion of large amounts of insulin causes hypoglycemic attacks characterized by Whipple's triad in that: (1) they can always be induced by prolonged fasting (24 to 72 hours); (2) during attacks the blood sugar is below 50 mg per dL; and (3) administration of sugar brings prompt relief. Patients usually learn to abort or prevent their attacks by eating and, as a result, many victims are overweight.

Although many different tests have been proposed for the diagnosis of insulinoma, the best diagnostic maneuver is still that of admitting the patient to hospital and observing the effect of prolonged fasting on the plasma glucose and insulin levels. Two-thirds of insulinoma patients will show a fall of plasma glucose to less than 60 mg/dL (3.3 mmol/L) after such a fast, and they will also exhibit physical symptoms of hypoglycemia.

It is important to look for an elevation of insulin levels inappropriate for the prevailing plasma glucose level. This is best done by calculating the plasma immunoreactive insulin (IRI)/glucose ratio by the following formula:

$$\text{IRI/Glucose ratio} = \frac{100 \times \text{IRI } (\mu\text{U/mL})}{\text{Glucose (mg/dL)} - 30}$$

A value of more than 100 μU/mg is strong evidence for a hyperinsulinemic state. The rare but real possibility of covert self-administration of insulin must also be remembered.

Insulin is now measured by a radioisotope ligand assay: there is usually some cross-reaction with proinsulin, hence the use of the term *immunoreactive insulin.* Normal fasting levels are 5 to 25 μU/mL; the actual reference range depends on the assay system: higher values are found in obese subjects. If a series of samples is to be taken from a patient, it is important to ensure that all the samples are either plasma *or* serum, as most methods show a slight bias depending on the protein matrix.

Hypoglycemia Caused by Nonislet Cell Tumors. A number of such cases have been reported to date. In almost all cases the tumors have been large (800 to 10,000 g), and about 60% of them have been of mesenchymal origin. Some 80% have been located in the retroperitoneal areas, and the remainder in the thorax. About 20% have been hepatic carcinomas. A few have been adrenocortical carcinomas.

Characteristically, the hypoglycemic attacks, which

may be very severe, are relieved when the neoplasm is removed but return with recurrence of the tumor.

Miscellaneous Causes of Hypoglycemia. *Reactive* hypoglycemia can occur 1 to 2 hours following a meal in certain people, especially those who have had gastric surgery. To establish the diagnosis, it is essential to show that the plasma glucose level is low at the time of the appearance of symptoms. A 5-hour oral glucose tolerance test is of value in defining this state.

Hypoglycemia, as defined by a plasma glucose level of less than 60 mg/dL (3.3 mmol/L) concomitant with symptoms, can also occur in cirrhosis, alcoholism, and adrenal failure: a considerable number of rarer causes are also known.

Glucose in Body Fluids

With the widespread use of methods that are specific for glucose and the abandonment of manual methods using whole blood, the distinction between blood glucose, blood sugar, and blood reducing substances is now academic. "Blood" glucose is measured in plasma or serum, with the inclusion of preservatives such as iodoacetate or fluoride. Among the many advantages of the new methods is their direct applicability to such samples as urine, CSF, pleural and paracentesis fluids, joint fluids, and so on. We are aware that such obsolescent procedures as the *o*-toluidine method may still be in use as small-batch manual assays in laboratories with limited resources, and a brief note is included. For the same reason a short description of the continuous flow method using alkaline ferricyanide is given.

For the preservation of the glucose content of samples two additives have been used: a mixture of sodium fluoride and thymol, and iodoacetate, usually as its lithium salt. Both are effective, but the latter is preferred in many systems because, unlike fluoride, it does not interfere with urea nitrogen methods employing urease, and the absence of sodium ion permits use of the serum for electrolyte determinations. It should be noted that immediate separation of plasma or serum from red cells or clot, respectively, and its refrigeration will preserve glucose levels for at least two hours, since in that time under those conditions bacterial action is negligible. Fluoride also interferes with the peroxidase enzyme employed in some glucose oxidase methods.

Review of Glucose Assay Methods

1. Reduction of Alkaline Ferricyanide. In the reduction of alkaline ferricyanide (yellow) to ferrocyanide (colorless) by the glucose dialyzed from a diluted plasma or serum sample in a continuous flow system, the reaction is promoted by heating in a glass coil immersed in an oil bath at 95°C. The loss of yellow color is proportional to the glucose level in the sample, thus limiting the range of values that can be measured by the ferricyanide concentration.

2. *o*-Toluidine Method. The glucose of a trichloracetic acid protein-free filtrate of whole blood, plasma, or serum is reacted with *o*-toluidine in strongly acid solution to produce a green condensation product, probably a glucosamine, with a peak absorbance at 630 nm. For automation, protein precipitation is replaced by dialysis, and less corrosive versions of the reagent, in which beta-hydroxycarballyllic acid is substituted for glacial acetic acid, are employed. The reagent also reacts with xylose, producing a brown chromogen, and this can be used to assay urine xylose.

3. Hexokinase Methods

a. The glucose of the sample is reacted with ATP (adenosine triphosphate) in the presence of hexokinase to produce glucose-6-phosphate and ADP (adenosine diphosphate). The glucose-6-phosphate is reacted with either NADP (nicotinamide adenine dinucleotide phosphate) or NAD (nicotinamide adenine dinucleotide) in the presence of glucose-6-phosphate dehydrogenase to produce NADPH (reduced NADP) or NADH (reduced NAD) and 6-phosphogluconate. The reduced NADP or NAD has a high absorbance at 340 nm that is proportional to the original amount of glucose. The reaction proceeds rapidly to completion and therefore is usually employed as an end-point method (see bottom of page). This reaction is readily adapted to discrete-type automated analyzers and is sensitive enough to assay low glucose levels in urine. It is insensitive to fluoride.

b. The glucose of the sample is reacted with hexokinase as in reaction (a) and then the NADPH is used to reduce an iodonitrotetrazolium (INT) dye through the intermediary compound phenazine methosulfate (PMS) to produce a reddish-purple chromogen with maximum absorbance at 520 nm. The intermediary reactant phenazine methosulfate is used to bridge the oxidation-reduction potential gap between the NADPH and INT dye. The reaction has to proceed by steps that are energetically feasible: direct reduction of the INT by NADPH alone cannot occur.

4. Glucose Oxidase Methods

a. The glucose of the sample is oxidized to gluconic acid and hydrogen peroxide by the enzyme glucose oxidase. The oxygen required is taken up from that dissolved in the reaction mixture, and the rate of oxygen uptake is determined by an oxygen-sensitive polarographic electrode as used for blood Po_2 determinations. Interference from oxygen released by the breakdown of the hydrogen peroxide is prevented by incorporating molybdate and iodate ions in the reagent, thus making the rate of oxygen uptake directly proportional to the glucose in the sample. The method uses a very small sample size—typically 10 μL—and is not sensitive to fluoride in the blood sample. Plasma or serum (or urine) has to be used, because the red cells of whole blood would also take up oxygen from the reagent. The method is used in bench model glucose analyzers* and in at least one discrete automated analyzer.†

*Beckman Glucose Analyzer 2, Beckman Instruments, Inc., Fullerton, Calif. 92634; Yellow Springs Instrument Co., Inc., Yellow Springs, Ohio 45387.

†ASTRA 4 and 8, Beckman Instruments, Inc., Fullerton, Calif. 92634 and Toronto, Ont. M8Z 5T2.

$$\text{Glucose} + \text{ATP} \xrightarrow{\text{Hexokinase}} \text{Glucose-6-phosphate} + \text{ADP}$$

$$\text{Glucose-6-phosphate} + \text{NADP} \xrightarrow{\text{Glucose-6-phosphate dehydrogenase}} \text{NADPH} + \text{H}^+ + \text{6-phosphogluconate}$$

b. A number of methods use glucose oxidase initially and then determine the hydrogen peroxide released in the reaction by coupling it with a variety of chromogens. The chromogens are oxidized by oxygen released from the peroxide by added peroxidase enzyme. (This second stage of the reaction is sensitive to fluoride.) The original chromogen employed was *o*-dianisidine, but this has been replaced by others that are deemed less carcinogenic. The Gochman and Schmitz reaction uses an oxidatively coupled reaction with 3-methyl-2-benzothiazolinone hydrazone and *N,N*-dimethyl aniline to produce an indamine dye with a broad absorbance maximum at 590 nm: this particular second-stage reaction is not affected by fluoride. It has been successfully automated on a continuous flow analyzer by immobilizing the glucose oxidase onto the inner surface of a plastic coil: a 10-cm polyamide tube with an internal diameter of 1 mm provided sufficient enzyme action to permit a test rate of 150 per hour.*

The Trinder reaction couples the hydrogen peroxide with phenol and 4-amino-phenazone to produce a purple color with an absorbance maximum at 515 nm: since peroxidase has to be incorporated, some interference from fluoride would be expected.

The method of Miskiewicz et al. (1973) uses peroxidase to catalyze the oxidation of the chromogen 2,2′-azine-di-(3-ethyl-benzothiazoline-(6)-sulfonic acid [ABTS]). This is the basis of a commercially available set of reagents.†

The above list of glucose methods is not exhaustive but represents the kinds of procedures in common use. Because of its simplicity the manual method detailed below uses hexokinase: one advantage of the procedure when retained as "back-up" for a routine automated system using the same reagent is that the lyophilized reagent has a storage life that often greatly exceeds that claimed by the manufacturer.

Plasma Glucose Estimation Using Hexokinase (Calbiochem S.V.R.‡)

Principle. As in paragraph 3a, p. 126.

Procedure

1. In a water bath set at 30°C set up a rack with a series of 100 × 16 mm test tubes. For each test and control serum set up a Test and a Blank tube. For each batch of tests set up one Reagent Blank tube.

2. Into all Test tubes and the Reagent Blank tube pipette 3.0 mL of prepared reagent: into the Blank tubes pipette 3.0 mL of 0.9% w/v sodium chloride solution. Allow all tubes to equilibrate for five minutes.

3. To each pair of Test and Blank tubes add 20 μL of the corresponding test or control serum, using a positive displacement micropipettor with a disposable tip. Mix by gentle lateral shaking, and leave in the water bath for at least five minutes but not more than 15.

4. At the expiration of the incubation period, measure the absorbances of the contents of all tubes in a 10-mm light path cell in a narrow band-pass spectrophotometer at 340 nm, setting zero absorbance with distilled water. Record the absorbance readings.

5. If the absorbance of the Reagent Blank tube is greater than 0.5, the reagent is unsuitable for the assay, and the test run must be repeated using fresh reagent.

Calculation. For each test and control determine the corrected absorbance:

Test absorbance − (Reagent Blank absorbance + Sample Blank absorbance)

The corrected absorbance corresponds to the increase in absorbance due to the production of reduced NADP in the reaction, less the initial absorbance of the reagent and the absorbance of the sample itself. If the corrected absorbance is greater than 1.150, repeat the test using a 10-μL sample size in both Test and Blank tubes. The final result will have to be multiplied by two.

Corrected Absorbance × 437 = Glucose in mg per dL
Corrected Absorbance × 24.26 = Glucose in mmol per dL

The factor of 437 is derived from the following calculation.

The conversion of one micromole of glucose to 6-phosphogluconate as shown in paragraph 3a, p. 126, is accompanied by the production of one micromole of reduced NADP. The absorbance increase after incubation, after correction for the reagent and sample blanks, can therefore be converted to micromoles of reduced NADP by dividing by its known molar absorptivity. The micromoles of reduced NADP are related to glucose using the molecular weight thereof, 180.16. The other terms in the formula correct for the actual reaction volume, 3.02 mL; the path length through which the absorbance was determined, 1.0 cm; and the sample size, 0.020 mL. The complete expression is:

$$\frac{\text{Abs. increase} \times 3.02 \times 180.16 \times 100}{6.22 \times 0.02 \times 1 \times 1000} = \text{Abs. increase} \times 437$$

Example

Reagent Blank: 0.05
Sample Blank: 0.05
Final test absorbance: 1.045
Corrected absorbance: 1.045 − (0.05 + 0.05) = 0.945 × 437 = 413 mg/dl

Note that if the absorbance of the sample blank were not subtracted, the final result would have been too high by 22 mg/dL.

Normal Values (Fasting)

Plasma or serum: 55 to 90 mg/dL (3.05 to 5.00 mmol/L)
Cerebrospinal fluid: 45 to 75 mg/dL (2.50 to 4.16 mmol/L)
(If the plasma glucose is elevated the CSF glucose is about 80% of the plasma level.)

Reagent. The reagent for this procedure is available commercially as "Glucose–S.V.R."* Vials are available in 6.5 mL and 15.0 mL sizes.

*"Autozyme" and "SMAC," Technicon Instruments Corp., Tarrytown, N.Y. 10591 and Montreal, Que. H4T 1P5.

†GOD-POD, Boehringer Mannheim Diagnostics, Indianapolis, Ind. 46250 and Dorval, Que. H9P 1A9.

‡Calbiochem, La Jolla, Calif. 92037.

*Calbiochem, La Jolla, Calif. 92037.

Notes

1. Suitable controls should be run with every batch of tests, preferably at low normal, normal, and moderately elevated levels.
2. The procedure can be used with serum, provided that it was separated from the clot as quickly as possible and kept refrigerated until the assay is made.
3. Plasma obtained with any of the routine anticoagulants may be used: if fluoride is used there may be a small delay in the test absorbance value's attaining its final level. With the majority of assays the final test absorbance is reached quickly, typically after three minutes at 30°C.
4. Determination of the test blank value should not be omitted, particularly with hemolyzed, lipemic, or icteric samples.
5. The only hexose that may interfere and might be found in plasma is fructose.
6. The range of linearity without using a reduced sample size is up to 500 mg/dL.
7. When reconstituting the reagent vial, use only the highest quality deionized water and dissolve by gentle inversion: do not shake vigorously.
8. Slight hemolysis will not cause errors: severely hemolyzed samples should not be used. In our experience the hemolysis has to be serious enough to give the plasma or serum a light cherry red color before interference is encountered.
9. The lyophilized reagent stored at refrigerator temperature is remarkably stable, often well beyond the stated expiry date. Though it is not acceptable laboratory practice to use an outdated reagent, in an emergency a batch of vials of reagent that is not more than three months beyond its stated expiry date may be used, provided its activity is checked with a standard solution of glucose of 400 mg/dL. Because the hexokinase enzyme is specific for β-D-glucose, any aqueous standards must be allowed to stand at room temperature for at least 90 minutes for the process of mutarotation to go to completion. (Glucose in solution exists in an equilibrium between two forms that differ in their optical rotation of polarized light: α-D-glucose and β-D-glucose. The process whereby this equilibrium is attained is called mutarotation.) Similarly, lyophilized control sera must be allowed to stand after reconstitution before being assayed for glucose by either a hexokinase or glucose oxidase method. The mutarotation may be accelerated by the presence of a mutarotase enzyme as a contaminant in glucose oxidase preparations.
10. The spectrophotometer must be a narrow bandpass instrument (8 nm or less); otherwise the factor used in the calculation, based on the molar absorptivity of reduced NADP, will not be valid.
11. The method can be applied to urine after clarification by centrifugation. For 24-hour collections the urine should be preserved by adding either 5.0 mL of glacial acetic acid or 5.0 g of sodium benzoate. By use of a spectrophotometer with a digital absorbance readout stable to 0.002, urine glucose values as low as 10 mg/dL can be determined.
12. The coefficient of variation of the method at normal and elevated plasma glucose levels is about 3%.

This method is detailed here to illustrate the use of enzymes to achieve specificity in an analysis, the simplicity of such methods when contrasted with chemical assays, the ability to use ultra-micro sample sizes, the often unsuspected sources of error as typified by the mutarotation problem, and a reaction that can be applied unchanged to either manual or automated analyses.

Blood Lactate and Pyruvate

Blood lactate assays are made in the investigation of lactate acidosis in diabetic and cardiac disease or after widespread tissue hypoxia (lack of adequate oxygen supply) and, in combination with pyruvate determinations, in the diagnosis of severe deficiencies of the B group of vitamins. Elevated lactate values have been reported in some neuromuscular disorders and in leukemia. Raised pyruvate levels have been reported in congestive heart failure, but the chief use of this assay is in the investigation of thiamine deficiency.

Lactate is measured on a perchloric acid protein-free filtrate of whole blood, prepared immediately after the blood has been obtained and kept chilled until assayed. After the addition of a lactate dehydrogenase suspension the amount of reduced NAD produced as the lactate is converted to pyruvate is a measure of the lactate level. The reaction is driven to completion by the inclusion in the reagent mixture of glutamate and alanine aminotransferase, which convert the pyruvate to alpha-ketoglutarate and alanine.

Pyruvate is determined by the reverse reaction. Added lactate dehydrogenase converts the pyruvate to lactate in the presence of reduced NAD, which supplies the necessary hydrogen ions for the process: the decrease in absorbance at 340 nm reflects the extent of this reduction and hence is proportional to the pyruvate level. This pair of methods illustrates the bidirectional property of enzymes and the ability to direct the reaction in a required orientation by the incorporation of either the oxidized or reduced form of the associated coenzyme.

Normal Values

Blood lactate: 5 to 20 mg/dL (0.56 to 2.24 mmol/L)
Blood pyruvate: 0.3 to 0.9 mg/dL (0.034 to 0.102 mmol/L)

Inborn Errors of Carbohydrate Metabolism

A number of inherited disorders affecting the metabolism of carbohydrate compounds other than glucose are known. All of them are of considerable rarity and, with two exceptions, will not be further considered here.

Galactosemia

This inherited disorder is characterized by an inability to convert galactose to glucose. This normally occurs by way of the reactions shown in Figure 6–5. In this disease, there is a deficiency of the enzyme galactose-1-phosphate uridyl transferase. Symptoms appear within a few days or weeks of beginning milk feeding, since galactose is a component of the disaccharide lactose. The disorder is characterized by vomiting, diarrhea,

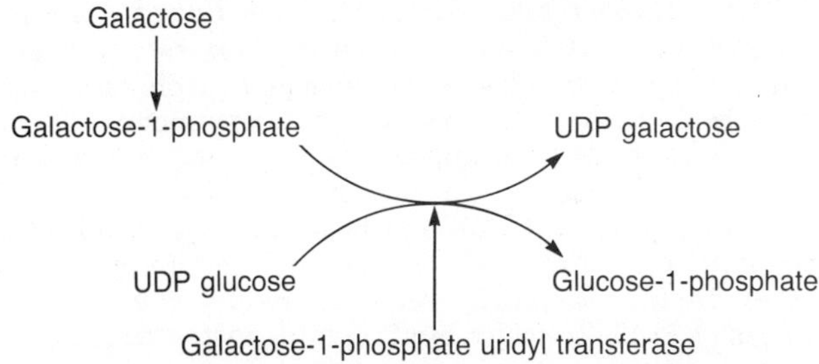

Figure 6–5 Galactose metabolism. UDP, uridine diphospho-.

jaundice, hepatosplenomegaly, cataracts, and mental retardation. If the disease is untreated, fatal cirrhosis of the liver develops rapidly. Damage to the renal tubules also produces the Fanconi syndrome of phosphoglucoaminoaciduria.

Early withdrawal of galactose and lactose from the diet will effectively prevent further development of the disease, although tissue damage already present may not be reversible.

Glycogenoses

More than six inherited disorders of glycogen synthesis or degradation are known: all are rare and have been shown to be due to specific enzyme deficiencies. Although these conditions may be suspected on the basis of the clinical findings and some of the more common laboratory tests, a definitive diagnosis requires measurement of the enzyme activities in liver and muscle by a laboratory experienced in such techniques.

LIPIDS

Definition

Lipids are organic substances that are compounds of, related to, or associated with fatty acids, and that are insoluble in water.

Classification

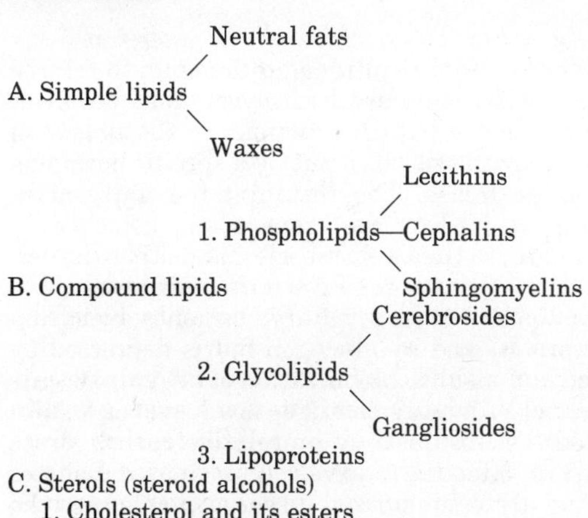

2. Steroids
3. Bile acids

D. Substances associated with lipids
1. K vitamins
2. Carotenoids
3. Tocopherols (vitamin E)

Classification

Neutral Fats. These consist of the trihydric alcohol ($OHCH_2CHOHCH_2OH$) glycerol, all three hydroxyl groups of which are esterified with fatty acids. The latter are straight-chain carbon compounds having a terminal COOH group and an even number of carbon atoms, for example, palmitic (16C), stearic (18C), oleic (18C). Fatty acids may be saturated, as in most animal fats (butyric, palmitic, stearic), or unsaturated, as in vegetable oils (oleic, linolenic, arachidonic). Soaps are metallic (sodium, potassium, magnesium, calcium) salts of fatty acids.

Waxes. Waxes are fatty acid esters of alcohols other than glycerol.

Lecithins. A typical lecithin consists of glycerol esterified with two fatty acids, one of which is generally unsaturated (usually arachidonic). The third OH of the glycerol is esterified to phosphoric acid, which, in turn, is bound to the organic base choline, $(CH_3)_3{\equiv}\overset{+}{N}CH_2CH_2OH$. The phosphocholine groups make lecithins less insoluble in aqueous solutions and facilitate combinations with proteins. Lecithins are important in the transport of fats in the plasma and in brain and general cell structure.

Cephalins. These resemble lecithins except in the base attached to the phosphoric acid; instead of choline they have either ethanolamine ($HOCH_2CH_2NH_2$) or the amino acid serine ($HOCH_2\overset{NH_2}{\overset{|}{C}}HCOOH$). Cephalins are important in brain structure. Those with the phosphatidyl ethanolamine group form the lipid component of the various thromboplastins.

Sphingomyelins. These resemble cephalins, except that the base, sphingosin, is attached, on the one hand, by its amino group to the fatty acid and, on the other, by its OH group to choline phosphoric acid. Sphingomyelins are important components of brain tissue. In Niemann-Pick disease great excess of sphingomyelin and lesser amounts of lecithin and cephalin are deposited in many tissues (brain, spleen, liver, bone marrow, and lymph nodes). Neither lecithins, cephalins, nor sphingomyelins are soluble in acetone.

Glycolipids. The best-known subgroup, the cerebrosides, resemble sphingomyelins except that the sphingosin is attached by its OH group, not to choline phosphoric acid, but to galactose. Cerebrosides are very abundant in myelin. Abnormal storage (thesaurosis) of cerebrosides (mainly kerasin) occurs in the spleen, liver, lymph nodes, and bones in Gaucher's disease.

Gangliosides are more complex than cerebrosides and are composed of fatty acids, sphingosine, glucose, galactose, and neuraminic acid. They are deposited in excess in the brain and spleen in Tay-Sachs disease.

Steroids and Sterols. These all share as their basic structure the cyclopentano-perhydrophenanthrene nucleus. Many important biological compounds belong to this group, for example, cholesterol, bile acids, vitamin D, the large numbers of steroid hormones produced by the ovaries, testes, and adrenal cortex, digitalis cardiac glycosides, and many carcinogens.

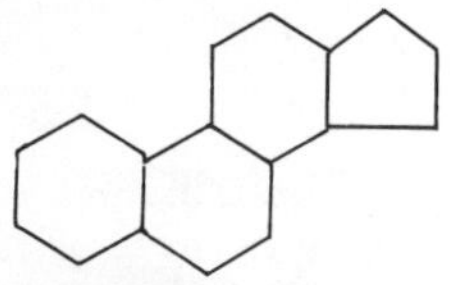

Cyclopentano-perhydrophenanthrene nucleus

Metabolism of Lipids

Apart from digestion and absorption (p. 236), this may be considered under three headings—transport of lipids in the plasma, catabolism and anabolism in the liver, and depot fat—all three of which are normally in dynamic equilibrium.

Transport of Lipids in Plasma. (Essential additional information on plasma lipoproteins will be found on p. 131.) Most lipids are nonpolar and therefore require carrier systems to permit their transport in the aqueous phase plasma. Specific plasma proteins act as carriers, and certain lipids (lecithins, sphingomyelins, and cholesterol and its esters) aid in stabilizing the lipoprotein systems. Thus all lipids and lipid-soluble substances are transported as lipoproteins.

TRANSPORT OF DIETARY (EXOGENOUS) LIPIDS. Absorbed and resynthesized dietary lipids are transported by two different methods and routes. Short-chain (less than 10 or 12C) glycerides disperse reasonably well in aqueous media and pass from the intestinal mucosal cells directly into the capillaries of the portal system in which, bound loosely to albumin, they are carried to the liver. Longer-chain glycerides, that is, the bulk of dietary fat, and more complex lipids, plus fat-soluble vitamins A, D, E, and K are "packaged" in chylomicrons by the intestinal mucosal cells. These fatty particles then are excreted into the lamina propria of the mucosa and gain access to the lacteals, which carry them to the cisterna chyli. From there they ascend in the thoracic duct to enter the blood in the left subclavian vein. The great majority of chylomicrons ultimately reach the liver.

Chylomicrons. These are spherical particles from 0.1 to 0.5 μm in diameter. They consist of an outer beta-lipoprotein envelope containing beta-polypeptide, phospholipid, cholesterol, and some (probably absorbed) albumin and alpha-polypeptide. Their lipid content is 95% triglyceride, 3% phospholipid, and 2% cholesterol. The ratio of free to ester cholesterol is higher in chylomicrons than in any other lipoprotein. Because of their very high triglyceride content, chylomicrons are the lightest of all lipoproteins (density < 1.006), and they belong to the S_f 400+ class (most are $S_f\ 10^5$ or more). Characteristically, when electrophoresed on paper in Veronal buffer containing 1% albumin, they show little or no mobility, that is, they remain at or near the point of application of the serum aliquot. They may be visualized by dark-field microscopy. Of all lipoproteins, the chylomicrons contribute most to turbidity or lactescence of serum or plasma.

Plasma Lipoprotein Lipase (Clearing Factor). From 3 to 6 hours after a meal containing moderate to large amounts of fat, the plasma becomes first turbid and then lactescent (milky) because of chylomicronemia. This lactescence quickly disappears following heparin injection. This postheparin clearing is caused by the enzyme lipoprotein lipase (LPL), which is produced in adipose tissue, liver, heart, vascular endothelium, and possibly other tissues. Heparin seems to act by causing the release of LPL from its binding sites in the tissues, so that it becomes active at the surface of cell membranes and leaks into the blood. LPL hydrolyzes glycerides and is almost certainly concerned in the uptake of glycerides by cells. Normally it exerts no significant lipolytic activity in plasma. It is inactivated by high concentrations of sodium chloride, by protamine, and by diisopropylfluorophosphate.

Normal postabsorptive plasma does not contain any LPL, and the only fat-splitting enzyme activity present is that of serum "lipase," that is, esterases that are capable only of hydrolyzing short-chain glycerides. Persons on almost fat-free diets, chronic alcoholics, those with malabsorptive states, and possibly also those with chronic pancreatitis exhibit reduced PHLA (postheparin lipolytic activity).

Fate of Absorbed Dietary Lipids. Our knowledge is far from complete, but evidence suggests that most dietary fat is handled by the liver, an unknown but lesser amount by adipose tissue, and small quantities by other tissues such as voluntary and heart muscles, which may be able to take up chylomicrons directly. The liver also may take up a small amount of fat in chylomicron form, but it assimilates most, and adipose tissue all, triglycerides only after hydrolysis, which presumably takes place on the surface of or within the cell membrane.

ENDOGENOUS LIPID METABOLISM AND TRANSPORT (Fig. 5–4). Within the liver cells the components of dietary fats, most of which have been split before adsorption by the hepatocytes, are resynthesized into glycerides, phospholipids, and so forth and then are transported from the liver to adipose and other tissues mainly by the prebeta-lipoproteins. Those lipids in excess of energy requirements are taken up (after hydrolysis) by the fat cells, within which they are resynthesized to triglycerides. Since fat cells are unable to phosphorylate glycerol, they must provide glycerophosphate by simultaneous glycolysis.

Free Fatty Acids (Unesterified or Nonesterified Fatty Acids). When energy requirements demand, the stored triglycerides of fat cells are hydrolyzed, not, however, by lipoprotein lipase (which functions in the *uptake* of free fatty acid by the tissues), but by a specific hormone-sensitive tissue lipase. The resultant free fatty acids (FFA) (UFA or NEFA) are transported, attached to plasma albumin, to the liver, muscles, and other tissues. This lipolytic mobilization of FFA is promoted by growth (somatotrophic) and other pituitary hormones, by adrenocortical steroids, and by glucagon but is depressed by epinephrine and insulin. Mobilization of FFA also occurs in the presence of hypoglycemia or low levels of insulin in the blood, i.e., in absolute or relative carbohydrate lack, as occurs in fasting, starvation, untreated diabetes mellitus, and glycogen storage disease. In this case the "mobilization" is actually caused by cessation of fat synthesis as a result of unavailability of alpha-glycerophosphate. Although the concentration of FFA in the plasma after an overnight fast in adults is only 0.3 to 0.7 mEq per liter, they represent the major endogenous lipid transport system.

Plasma Phospholipids. These constitute the largest single fraction of plasma lipids, amounting to 150 to 300 mg per dL until the age of 30. Their composition is: phosphatidyl choline, 70%; sphingomyelin, 20%; the remaining 10% is made up of phosphatidyl ethanolamine, phosphatidyl serine, lysolecithin, and inositol phosphatide. The phospholipids are one of the main stabilizers of the lipid cargoes on the lipoprotein transport vehicle, because lecithins and sphingomyelins both act as mild detergents.

Plasma Glycerides. These are mainly triglycerides and are highest during absorption after meals, when dietary fats are transported in chylomicrons. Endogenous glycerides of the plasma represent almost exclusively those in transit from the liver to other tissues; these form the great bulk of plasma glycerides in the postabsorptive state. Normal triglyceride levels after overnight fast are 25 to 150 mg per dL.

CHOLESTEROL

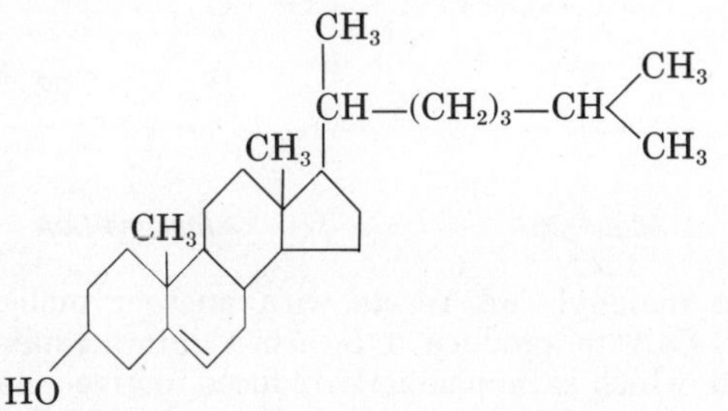

As its formula shows, cholesterol is a steroid alcohol, the OH group making it, systematically, an alcohol, and the hydrocarbon side chain attached to carbon atom 17 conferring lipid-like solubility in ether, choloroform, and so forth. Practically every cell in the body can manufacture cholesterol from simple two-carbon compounds (acetates). The liver, adrenal cortex, ovaries, and testes, and also the intestinal epithelium, are particularly active in the synthesis of cholesterol. The adrenal cortex, ovaries, and testes use cholesterol and its esters for the manufacture of steroid hormones. In addition to manufacturing cholesterol, the liver also esterifies it, converts part of it to cholic acid, and excretes it in the bile (just under 1 g per day). Although the body synthesizes cholesterol with great ease, it appears to have great difficulty in degrading it. Transport and excretion of cholesterol are promoted by estrogens; testosterone seems to have the opposite or no effect in this regard.

The rate of hepatic cholesterol synthesis appears to be related inversely to the amount of chylomicron cholesterol reaching the liver. In bile duct obstruction, bile acids do not reach the gut, and both cholesterol absorption and chylomicron formation are reduced, and the hepatic synthesis of cholesterol increases 2 to 3 times.

TABLE 6–1 Usual Mean (and 90% Limits) Cholesterol and Phospholipid Plasma (Serum) Levels for Both Sexes

Age	Total Cholesterol	Phospholipids
Newborn	70 (45–100)	90 (70–165)
1 mo–1 yr	130 (65–165)	165 (95–230)
1–30 yr	180 (110–250)	220 (150–300)
*30–39 yr	210 (150–280)	270 (205–340)
*40–49 yr	245 (160–325)	275 (185–355)
*50–59 yr	250 (140–340)	305 (225–380)

*Total plasma lipids: 400–1000 mg per dL

*Values from Fredrickson and Lees, 1966.

About 70% of the plasma cholesterol is esterified, chiefly with linoleic acid; this apparently occurs mainly in the plasma under the influence of an enyzyme *lecithin-cholesterol acyl transferase,* which is released from the liver. In severe hepatic disease the enzyme activity in the plasma falls, and the proportion of esterified cholesterol also diminishes. Formerly, the ratio of free to esterified cholesterol was used as an index of severe liver failure, but it is quite unreliable for this purpose.

Table 6–1 gives reference ranges for serum cholesterol levels at different ages; these are based on apparently healthy North American adults. Similar ranges have been obtained in European studies, but not all industrialized societies show such high means and upper limits. It is still not clear whether these levels, although normal, are desirable. Some of the epidemiological evidence suggests that levels above 220 mg per dL may be a factor in the development of vascular disease. However, until more evidence is available, it is convenient to apply the values in Table 6–1 according to age and sex.

PLASMA LIPOPROTEINS

Plasma Albumin

Albumin constitutes the main transport vehicle for free fatty acids, the direction being mainly from adipose tissue to liver, muscle, and other tissues.

True Lipoproteins

These are the alpha-, beta-, and prebeta-lipoproteins and the chylomicrons. To all of them the general rule applies that as their density diminishes, their triglyceride content increases and their protein content declines.

Alpha$_1$-Lipoproteins. These are the high-density lipoproteins (HDL; density, 1.063 to 1.21). They are manufactured by the liver and contain less sphingomyelin and more lysolecithin than the low-density lipoproteins (LDL). Genetically determined absence of HDL results in Tangier disease, a rare disorder in which cholesteryl esters accumulate in the reticuloendothelial tissue and which is characterized by complete absence of the alpha-lipoprotein band on electrophoresis.

Low-Density Lipoproteins

BETA-LIPOPROTEINS. These are the S_f* 0 to 20 (density, 1.006 to 1.063) lipoproteins, often subdivided into S_f 0 to 12 (density, 1.019 to 1.063), normally amounting to about 350 mg per dL, and the S_f 12 to 20 (density, 1.006 to 1.019), normally amounting to about 75 mg per dL. These most important lipoproteins are manufactured by the liver and probably also by the intestinal mucosal cells in which they are used to form chylomicrons. The lipid of the S_f 0 to 12 group consists of cholesterol, 55%, phospholipid, 30%, and triglyceride, 15%. They also carry the plasma carotenoids, and the increments in cholesterol and phospholipids observed with increasing age apply also to the beta-lipoproteins. They are noted, too, for their antigenicity.

PREBETA-LIPOPOPROTEINS (VERY LOW-DENSITY LIPOPROTEINS). These are the S_f 20 to 400+ lipoproteins. They contain both alpha- and beta-polypeptides, and this accounts for their prebeta mobility on electrophoresis. They are subdivided into: (1) the larger, S_f 20 to 400 subclass of lipoproteins, which amount to about 150 mg per dL and contain 20% cholesterol, 30% phospholipid, and 50% triglyceride; and (2) the S_f 400 to 10^5 subclass, which contain 60% triglyceride and 20% each of cholesterol and phospholipid. Normally, the S_f 400 to 10^5 lipoproteins are absent from postabsorptive serum. Both subclasses of the prebeta-lipoproteins contribute to plasma turbidity, the S_f 400 to 10^5 more so because of their greater content of triglyceride. For the same reason, quantity for quantity, neither contributes as much to turbidity or lactescence as do chylomicrons.

CATABOLISM (DEGRADATION) OF FATTY ACIDS IN THE LIVER AND KETOGENESIS

By a series of enzymic reactions, initiated or "sparked" by adenosine triphosphate (ATP) and coenzyme A (CoA), fatty acids are degraded stepwise to acetyl-CoA. Normally, the great majority of this acetyl-CoA is taken up by the carbohydrate tricarboxylic acid (Krebs) cycle and is combusted, with the production of energy, carbon dioxide, and water. However, a small amount of the acetyl-CoA is condensed thus (ketogenesis):

$$2\ \text{acetyl-CoA} \rightarrow \text{acetoacetyl-CoA} + 1\ \text{CoA}$$

This acetoacetyl/CoA is then hydrolyzed to acetoacetic acid and CoA, most of the acetoacetic acid so formed being reduced by the liver to beta-hydroxybutyric acid.

$$CH_3COCH_2COOH \xrightarrow{NAD.H_2} CH_3CHOHCH_2COOH$$

Acetoacetic acid *β-Hydroxybutyric acid*

The three substances, acetoacetic acid, beta-hydroxybutyric acid, and acetone are collectively called ketone bodies or acetone bodies. The acetone is formed by spontaneous decarboxylation of small amounts of acetoacetic acid:

$$CH_3COCH_2COOH \rightarrow CH_3COCH_3 + CO_2$$

Acetone

*The S_f notation refers to the ultracentrifugal flotation rates of lipoproteins in salt solutions of density 1.063, expressed in Svedberg units (10^{-13} cm/sec/dyne/g).

ANABOLISM (SYNTHESIS) OF FATS

The process of synthesis of fats is not a simple reversal of the catabolic processes. It is true that the end product of lipid catabolism, acetyl-CoA, is also the starting point for synthesis; but since both processes may be going on in the same cells under the same conditions, the two pathways must be kept separate. The sequence for lipid synthesis involves a special intermediate compound, malonyl-CoA, which does not occur in the catabolic chain of events. The basic requirements for the anabolic sequence are different from those for the catabolism of fats; they include two enzyme complexes and four cofactors—adenosine triphosphate as an energy source, carbon dioxide, reduced nicotinamide-adenine dinucleotide phosphate, and manganese ions. The catabolic process requires oxidative enzymes and magnesium ions but not carbon dioxide.

The initial step in the synthetic process involves the coupling of acetyl-CoA with carbon dioxide to form the very reactive substance malonyl-CoA.

$$CH_3\text{—}CO\text{—CoA} + CO_2 \rightarrow HOOC\text{—}CH_2\text{—}CO\text{—CoA}$$

Acetyl-CoA *Malonyl-CoA*

The malonyl-CoA reacts with another molecule of acetyl-CoA to produce a 5-carbon intermediate compound, which is immediately reduced to give a 4-carbon fatty acid combined with CoA, butyryl-CoA. This compound, since it is still activated by its CoA group, can react again with acetyl-CoA to give a 6-carbon fatty acid. The process repeats itself, and the fatty acid chain grows by 2 carbon atoms at each step, until the 16-carbon fatty acid, palmitic acid, is produced. This appears to be the longest-chain fatty acid produced by this route of synthesis. It is interesting to note that the molecule of carbon dioxide that is required for the initial reaction is released again when butyryl-CoA is formed, and thus functions as a catalyst. The condensation between acetyl-CoA and carbon dioxide requires biotin, one of the B vitamins, as a catalyst. The whole process of fatty acid synthesis takes place in the microsomes, and is thus segregated in the cell from fatty acid catabolism, which takes place in the mitochondria. The further steps, in which the fatty acids are combined with glycerol, phosphate, and choline to form such lipids as lecithin, probably take place in the mitochondria.

DEPOT FAT

At body temperature fat is liquid and is stored (chiefly as neutral fat) in the adipose tissue cells in such places as beneath the skin, in the breasts, and in the mesentery and retroperitoneal tissues. It serves as a great energy reserve (9.3 Cal/g), and for insulation and padding.

ALTERATIONS OF PLASMA LIPIDS IN DISEASE

Note. Alterations in blood lipids affect the plasma components almost exclusively, and for this reason estimations are carried out on plasma or serum, usually the latter.

Low Blood Cholesterol

Low levels of plasma cholesterol (also total lipids) are found in the newborn and infants, in severe anemias, and in prolonged or severe wasting diseases. The ester fraction of cholesterol falls precipitously (to 10 to 50% of total) in hepatocellular damage. In hyperthyroidism, plasma cholesterol tends to be in the low normal range. Most blood lipid fractions tend to be low in malabsorptive states. Plasma cholesterol falls in old age. It is also very low in alpha-lipoprotein deficiency (Tangier disease).

High-Density Lipoprotein Cholesterol (HDL Cholesterol)

It has gradually become clear in recent years that measurement of the cholesterol contained in the alpha-lipoprotein fraction (high-density lipoprotein) is of greater value in predicting an increased risk of coronary heart disease (CHD) than is the assay of total cholesterol or of triglycerides.

Factors such as increasing age, male sex, obesity, smoking, and lack of exercise all increase significantly the risk of CHD, probably by a variety of different mechanisms. One such mechanism appears to be alterations in HDL levels. It seems reasonably certain that HDL functions to transport cholesterol *from* the tissues *to* the liver, where it is excreted in the bile. Extensive epidemiological studies have shown that *low* HDL levels are associated with an *increased* risk of CHD (Gordon et al., 1977); furthermore, it does appear that measurement of HDL cholesterol is of some value in identifying the high-risk individual.

Simple examination of the alpha band of a lipoprotein separation can demonstrate very low levels of the HDL fraction; however, a quantitative method of measurement is preferable. Apart from ultracentrifugation (which is expensive) and scanning of an electrophoretic strip stained for lipids (which gives erratic results), a number of methods are available whose principle is to precipitate the lipoproteins other than HDL and then to measure the cholesterol content of the supernatant.

Manganese-heparin precipitation can work well, but it is very dependent on the quality of the heparin. Magnesium-dextran sulfate, or magnesium-phosphotungstate methods work well but appear to give a slightly lower reference range. Since the cholesterol content in the alpha fraction is low, even in normal people, a sensitive and precise method for the determination of cholesterol is required: a cholesterol oxidase technique using a centrifugal analyzer is recommended.

A level of 45 mg/dL in a male (55 mg/dL in a female) indicates an average risk of developing CHD. Probably of more significance is the ratio:

$$\frac{\text{Total cholesterol}}{\text{HDL cholesterol}}$$

TABLE 6–2 THE RELATIONSHIP BETWEEN THE RISK OF CORONARY HEART DISEASE AND THE RATIO OF TOTAL CHOLESTEROL/HDL CHOLESTEROL

Risk	Ratio of Total Cholesterol/HDL Cholesterol	
	Men	*Women*
Below average (1/2)	3.4	3.3
Average	5.0	4.4
Above average (2×)	9.6	7.0
Above average (3×)	23.4	11.0

From Castelli et al. (1977).

(See Table 6–2.) Note that a *high* ratio is associated with a *high* risk. In our experience, the HDL cholesterol level and ratio in any one individual remain remarkably constant. Levels of HDL cholesterol of 70 mg/dL or more are associated with the longevity syndrome.

However, although still a question of some debate, it does appear that the level and ratio can be altered (and the risk of CHD correspondingly reduced) by the familiar measures of weight loss, low saturated fat intake, cessation of smoking, and increased physical exercise.

Both estrogens and alcohol will elevate plasma levels of HDL cholesterol, probably by stimulation of synthesis of the apoprotein in the liver. Many epidemiological studies have shown some protective effect on the development of CHD by a moderate alcohol intake, especially in the form of wine. Indeed, it is an old pathological observation that persons dying from alcoholic cirrhosis very seldom have significant atheromatous degeneration of the coronary arteries. The critical level below which there is still protection against CHD but above which there is a definite and increasing risk of cirrhosis is approximately 80 g ethanol per day, equivalent to 9 oz. of 40 proof spirit or 30 oz. of wine.

Elevated Plasma Lipids

Since lipids are always transported in association with carrier proteins, the terms *hyperlipemia* and *hyperlipoproteinemia* are virtually synonymous; hyperlipoproteinemia seldom occurs without hyperlipemia. Elevation of plasma lipids may occur as a primary inherited disorder or secondary to some disease state. It is possible to separate the hyperlipoproteinemic states into a number of different types, and this is usually essential in planning therapy.

In the following pages a general description will be given of various disease states in which an elevation of plasma lipids is found, followed by a description of the WHO system of lipoprotein phenotyping and a discussion of the primary inherited hyperlipoproteinemias.

Secondary Hyperlipemia

Peak plasma lipemia occurs 3 to 6 hours after a normal mixed meal and mainly involves neutral fats. There appears to be a slight gradual rise in plasma cholesterol levels with aging. In the latter half of pregnancy plasma cholesterol is about 30% above the woman's normal value. Generally, men have total blood cholesterol levels higher than women (estrogens tend to lower plasma cholesterol).

In hypothyroidism, both the free and ester cholesterol are raised above the normal range for the particular person, but other lipids are unaffected. In the nephrotic syndrome, alpha$_1$-lipoproteins are diminished, but beta-lipoproteins are greatly elevated and total plasma lipids may exceed 2 g per dL (the plasma may be frankly lipemic or even "milky"); cholesterol, neutral fats, and also phospholipids are raised. Alpha-lipoproteins are reduced, but the beta-lipoproteins, and sometimes also the prebeta- and rarely even the chylomicron lipoproteins, are elevated. In lipoid nephrosis, total plasma cholesterol ranges from 300 to 1000 mg per dL (average 500 to 600).

Blood lipids are increased in ketosis generally, including untreated diabetes, in which all major lipid fractions are usually elevated. Total plasma lipids in untreated diabetics commonly range from 0.7 to 2.0 g per dL (values as high as 22 g per dL were recorded in the preinsulin era; in such cases the plasma is milky or even creamy). The simplest explanation for lipemia in ketosis and diabetes is that it represents excessive mobilization of lipids.

Lipoprotein Phenotyping and the Familial Hyperlipoproteinemias

This discussion is based largely on the WHO memorandum (1972). For further reference, the chapter by Bierman and Glomset (1981) is recommended. Lipoprotein phenotyping is a procedure that is becoming less and less useful; however, a description is retained for completeness. Lipid electrophoresis can also be of use in checking a very low or high HDL cholesterol level and in screening for Tangier disease and abetalipoproteinemia.

As already described, it is possible to divide the plasma lipoproteins into four major classes: (1) chylomicrons; (2) beta-lipoproteins, or low-density lipoproteins (LDL); (3) prebeta-lipoproteins, or very low-density lipoproteins (VLDL); and (4) alpha-lipoproteins, or high-density lipoproteins (HDL). The classification of hyperlipoproteinemia according to the system of Fredrickson requires quantitation of these four classes. This can be done reliably only by ultracentrifugation in salt solutions of varying density, measuring the flotation rate of the different fractions. This requires expensive apparatus which is not available in most hospital laboratories; however, some commercial laboratories offer this service.

Failing this, lipoprotein phenotyping generally can be accomplished by combining a number of simpler observations. The appearance of the plasma sample after standing overnight at 4°C should be noted. The plasma may be quite clear, or it may be turbid throughout; if chylomicrons are present these will form a cream layer at the top of the sample, and the infranatant then may be clear or turbid. Turbidity is related to triglyceride levels. A minor degree of turbidity is easily missed, and some experience in observation is required to detect it. A major discrepancy between triglyceride levels and turbidity suggests some analytical error. The cholesterol and triglyceride content should be determined, and the cholesterol/triglyceride ratio calculated. Lipoprotein electrophoresis provides valuable additional information, as described further on.

Plasma samples for lipid determinations should be taken from a patient on his usual diet after *at least* a 12-hour fast; a shorter fast period chiefly interferes with triglyceride determinations, since cholesterol levels rise only some 3% after a meal. The anticoagulant used should be EDTA, and the plasma can be stored for several days at 4°C without the lipoprotein pattern changing. Longer storage periods, or repeated freezing and thawing, should be avoided. Estimations of phospholipids or free fatty acids do not provide any clinically useful information.

Many different media have been suggested for lipoprotein electrophoresis; at present paper and agarose gel are still the best media, the latter having the advantage of speed in separation and improved definition. Many excellent commercial methods are available, and therefore no method description will be given here. Quantitation of the four classes by scanning of the electrophoretic strip has been advocated by some, but it generally has not proved satisfactory in practice.

Quantitation of beta-lipoproteins is possible by precipitation with dextran sulfate but is difficult to calibrate and standardize without an ultracentrifuge. Techniques have been described for quantitative estimation of classes of particles of different size and triglyceride content by nephelometry after filtration through cellulose acetate membranes of known pore size. These also are difficult to calibrate and standardize.

Once the above data have been obtained, it is generally possible to classify hyperlipidemia into one of six phenotypes. These patterns may be caused by a primary familial disorder, or they may be acquired in the course of some disease process, as described earlier. However, final interpretation should always be made by the clinician in the light of the clinical data.

Normal Pattern

The normal cholesterol range has been discussed above; for the purposes of classification in North America and Europe, it is convenient at present to take the upper limit of the normal range for age and sex, as given in Table 6–1. The normal range for plasma triglycerides is 10 to 140 mg per dL, the upper limit rising to 170 to 180 mg per dL in the fifth and sixth decades. After a 12-hour fast, the plasma is normally water clear, and the electrophoretic pattern shows only alpha and beta bands (Fig. 6–6). However, in 10% of normal people a faint prebeta band will be seen. This is designated as a "sinking" prebeta; its significance is not clear.

The Hyperlipoproteinemias

Type I. In this type there is an inability to clear chylomicrons from the plasma. The standing plasma exhibits a cream layer over a clear infranatant. There is usually some rise in cholesterol levels, but the triglyceride levels show striking increases, up to 15 g per dL or so. On electrophoresis a broad heavy chylomicron band is present at the origin (Fig. 6–6), the alpha and beta bands may not be visible, whereas the prebeta band may be absent or present in normal intensity. These changes usually establish this pattern; it is quite rare but is occasionally seen secondary to diabetes mellitus, dysgammaglobulinemia, pancreatitis, or alcoholism.

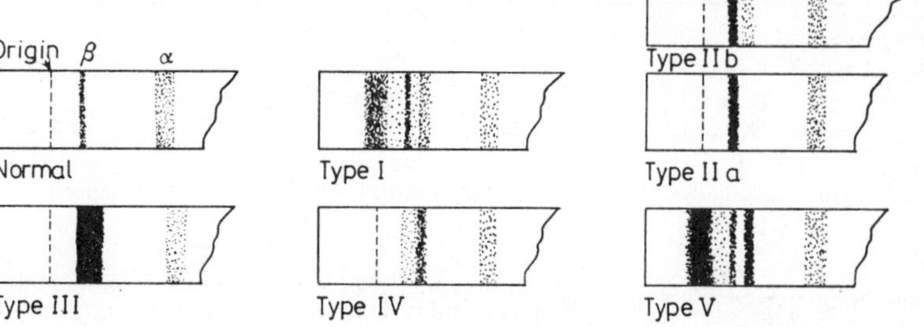

Figure 6–6 Plasma lipoprotein patterns obtained by paper electrophoresis according to the WHO classification. (From Hyde, T. A., and Draisey, T. F.: Principles of Chemical Pathology. London, Butterworth, 1974.)

PRIMARY TYPE I HYPERLIPOPROTEINEMIA (BÜRGER-GRÜTZ DISEASE). This is caused by a deficiency of the enzyme lipoprotein lipase, which is activated by heparin, and it clears chylomicrons from the plasma. The defect is inherited as a recessive character. Extremely high chylomicron and triglyceride levels are present in the plasma of the homozygous individual from the early weeks of life and usually are associated with lipemia retinalis, hepatosplenomegaly, and bouts of abdominal pain and pancreatitis. Xanthomata are generally present.

Type II. This is characterized by an increase in beta-lipoprotein (LDL), which generally is apparent as an elevation in the serum cholesterol level. Occasionally, hyperbeta-lipoproteinemia can occur with normal serum cholesterol concentrations if the level of HDL is low. Two subgroups are now distinguished.

TYPE IIA. There is an increase in LDL, but not VLDL. The plasma is clear, and serum cholesterol levels are elevated (see the discussion of normal ranges on p. 131). Serum triglyceride levels are within normal limits. The cholesterol/triglyceride ratio is always more than 1.5. On electrophoresis an intense beta band is present. Chylomicron and prebeta bands are absent, and the alpha band is of normal intensity.

TYPE IIB. Both LDL and VLDL are elevated. The plasma is faintly turbid, there is a modest increase in triglycerides, and the cholesterol/triglyceride ratio is variable. On electrophoresis the beta band is intensely stained, and a prebeta band is also present, usually more intense than the faint prebeta seen in some normal individuals. This is usually sufficient to establish the diagnosis, but if there is doubt, ultracentrifuge studies should be performed to confirm whether there is an elevation of LDL.

The type II pattern is encountered with some frequency. Most often it is secondary to a number of disorders, including hypothyroidism, nephrotic syndrome, obstructive liver disease, dysgammaglobulinemia, and occasionally in women taking oral contraceptives.

Primary type II hyperlipoproteinemia formerly was designated familial hypercholesterolemia. It is recessively inherited. In homozygous individuals the plasma cholesterol reaches 500 to 900 mg per dL, and they develop numerous tendinous and tuberous xanthomata and die prematurely of atherosclerotic disease, usually in the first two decades of life. Heterozygous individuals show similar features, but the total serum cholesterol is lower, in the range of 250 to 500 mg per dL, and the vascular complications develop more slowly. A sharp distinction between normal and heterozygous type II individuals sometimes is possible only by LDL measurements.

Type III. This is a rare pattern, and usually is found as a primary disorder. It is characterized by the presence of VLDL of abnormally high cholesterol content, and abnormal electrophoretic mobility ("floating" prebeta).

The standing plasma is turbid and often has an overlying chylomicron layer. Both cholesterol and triglyceride levels show a moderate elevation, the cholesterol/triglyceride ratio being close to one. On electrophoresis a broad beta band that extends into the prebeta position is present. Occasionally a prebeta band is present. Definitive diagnosis requires ultracentrifugation.

Type IV. This type is characterized by an increase in VLDL (prebeta) without any concomitant rise in LDL (beta). The standing plasma is usually turbid, occasionally clear, with no chylomicron layer. The plasma cholesterol is generally normal, but the triglycerides are elevated, and the chylomicron/triglyceride ratio may show considerable variation on repeated samples from an individual, a point of diagnostic importance. In some patients, modest elevation of cholesterol is found; if this is in the LDL region, the patient has type IIb; if, on the other hand, the LDL cholesterol is in the normal range, the patient has type IV. On electrophoresis the beta and alpha bands may be normal or decreased, whereas the prebeta band shows greater intensity.

The type IV pattern is not uncommon and is seen most frequently secondary to a considerable number of disorders. The most commonly encountered of these are listed in Table 6–3. A transient type IV pattern may be seen after acute myocardial infarction, pancreatitis, and burns.

As a primary disorder, the type IV pattern is less frequent. Both sporadic and familial types are seen, and in the latter, type III and type V individuals may be related. Affected individuals have premature atherosclerosis, and there appears to be a fairly close relationship in this group between ischemic heart disease and fasting triglyceride levels. Although cerebrovascular disease is also more common, its relationship to triglyceridemia is less clear. Eruptive xanthomas, hyperuricemia, and acute pancreatitis also occur.

Type V. This is a relatively uncommon pattern, characterized by an increase both in VLDL (prebeta) and chylomicrons. The standing plasma is turbid, with an overlying chylomicron layer; this is diagnostic if type III is excluded. A marked increase in the endogenous prebeta particles is present, and this shows trailing to the origin, where it may fuse with the chylomicron band. The LDL is also reduced. Both cholesterol and triglyceride levels are elevated, the cholesterol/triglyc-

TABLE 6–3 LIPOPROTEIN PHENOTYPING

Type	Confirmatory Observations	Diseases in Which the Lipoprotein Pattern May Be Present as a Secondary Feature
I	Triglyceride levels are usually very high, and there is no change in the electrophoretic pattern after heparin (see text).	Diabetes mellitus, dysglobulinemia, alcoholism
IIa	The plasma should be free of turbidity. The beta band is sharp and stains intensely.	Myxedema, nephrotic syndrome, dysglobulinemia, cholestasis
IIb	The beta band is sharp and intense, a distinct but not elevated prebeta is present.	As for IIa
III	A broad, deeply staining beta band is present, extending well into the prebeta zone. Confirmation by acrylamide gel electrophoresis, or by ultracentrifugation is essential.	Thyroid and liver disease, myeloma
IV	Beta band usually diminished, prebeta is distinct and more intense than normal. Triglycerides always elevated.	Myxedema, diabetes mellitus, nephrotic syndrome, pancreatitis, alcoholism, dysglobulinemia, pregnancy, obesity, some oral contraceptives
V	Prebeta lipoproteins increased, with trailing of lipid toward origin. Beta band may be indistinct. The presence of chylomicrons over a turbid infranatant is diagnostic if Type III can be excluded.	Diabetes, pancreatitis, alcoholism, nephrotic syndrome, dysglobulinemia, myxedema
—	Probably unclassifiable, but considered biliary tract disease.	—
—	Normal or unclassifiable. Check whether patient was adequately fasted. Check for intercurrent disease, especially of malignant nature. Check alcohol intake. *Note:* A faint prebeta band is present in about 10% of normal samples.	—

eride ratio lying between 0.15 and 0.6. The triglyceride levels tend to be in the 1000 to 3000 mg per dL range. This pattern is sometimes seen secondary to diabetes mellitus, pancreatitis, alcoholism, nephrosis, myxedma, and dysgamma-globulinemia.

Liver Disease

The lipoprotein pattern in obstructive disease of the hepatic bile ducts is unusual. Cholesterol and phospholipid levels are high, and triglyceride and free fatty acid levels are normal. The pattern simulates the type IIa. An abnormal low-density lipoprotein, "LP-X," is present in the plasma.

Plasma Lipid Methodology

Color Reactions Used in Cholesterol Determinations

Before 1975, the majority of methods in routine use were variants of two basic reactions: the Liebermann-Burchard (L-B) and Zak reactions. These processes are essentially oxidative, the oxidizing agent in the L-B reaction being SO_3, and in the Zak reaction, Fe^{3+}. The two methods produce different final colors, i.e., green and reddish violet, respectively, because each is a step-by-step process, with successive introduction of double bonds into the cholesterol molecule. In the L-B reaction, the green product is a pentaene, with five double bonds; in the Zak reaction, the process stops after the addition of four double bonds to form a tetraene. The later change from green to yellow in the L-B reaction accompanies the final change to a hexaene, cholestahexaene sulfonic acid. The chromogens are believed to be formed from the pentaene or tetraene by conversion to carbonium ions by the action of the strong acids present. The greater amount of color per unit quantity of cholesterol produced by the Zak reaction is a result of its greater efficiency. The Zak reaction proceeds almost to completion, whereas the L-B reaction is only about one-seventh complete at the pentaene stage.

The disadvantages of these methods, such as the corrosive nature of the reagents, the difficulties in their automation, the instability of the final colors, and problems with standardization, have been largely overcome by the development of enzymatic procedures. The enzyme cholesterol esterase, EC 3.1.1.13, splits cholesterol esters to release free cholesterol plus fatty acid anions. The free cholesterol is then oxidized by the enzyme cholesterol oxidase, EC 1.1.3.6, originally isolated from higher bacteria of the *Nocardia* group, to produce 4-

$$\text{Cholesterol ester} \xrightarrow{\text{Cholesterol esterase}} \text{Free cholesterol} + \text{Fatty acid anion}$$

$$\text{Cholesterol} + O_2 \xrightarrow{\text{Cholesterol oxidase}} \text{4-Cholesten-3-one} + H_2O_2$$

$$2\,H_2O_2 + \text{4-Aminoantipyrine} + \text{Phenol} \xrightarrow{\text{Peroxidase}} \text{Quinoneimine dye} + H_2O$$

cholesten-3-one and hydrogen peroxide. The hydrogen peroxide is then measured by a reaction with 4-aminoantipyrine and phenol catalyzed by peroxidase, EC 1.11.1.7. The final colored product is a quinoneimine dye with an absorbance maximum at 505 nm. The reaction takes place in mild conditions—pH 6.7 at 37°C—and the final color is stable for at least 30 minutes. The method is readily automated on discrete-type analyzers or continuous flow instruments, and excellent coefficients of variation are obtainable. For standardization either solutions of pure cholesterol in isopropanol or the molar extinction coefficient of the quinoneimine dye can be used. The method can be summarized as shown above.

A detailed method will not be given here, since commercial kits of reagents for both manual and automated use are available. It should be noted that standardization using the molar absorbance coefficient of the quinoneimine product can be used in a manual method only if the spectrophotometer has a band width of 10 nm or less, negligible stray light, and a regularly checked wavelength accuracy.

The procedure that follows is included as an example of a reference method, illustrating the meticulous technique required for such a determination. Saponification to convert cholesterol esters to free cholesterol and solvent extraction to exclude compounds in the serum that might interfere with the color reaction are replaced in the method outlined above by specific enzymes. See Table 6–1 for reference ranges.

It should be noted that some authorities report a sex difference in cholesterol normal ranges, whereas others have not found this to occur.

Determination of Serum Cholesterol—Reference Method (Abell et al., 1952)

Principle. After conversion of the esterified cholesterol to free cholesterol by treatment with alcoholic potassium hydroxide (saponification), the free cholesterol produced, together with that already present in the serum, is extracted into petroleum spirit (petroleum ether). After removal of the solvent the cholesterol is determined by the green color produced with the Liebermann-Burchard reaction.

Procedure

1. Set up a 25-mL glass-stoppered centrifuge tube for each test, for each standard, and for control serum. Into tests and control pipette 0.5 mL of serum; into high and low standards pipette 5.0-mL and 2.5-mL aliquots of the working standard, respectively. To tests and control add 5.0 mL of alcoholic potassium hydroxide; stopper and mix. To high standard add 0.3 mL of 33% potassium hydroxide. To low standard add 2.5 mL ethanol and 0.3 mL of 33% potassium hydroxide; stopper and mix.

2. Heat all tubes for 55 minutes in the 37°C water bath.

3. Cool to room temperature. Add to all tubes 10 mL of petroleum spirit, and mix. Add to all tubes 5.0 mL of distilled water, stopper, and shake well for 1 minute. Centrifuge at low speed—1000 to 1500 rpm—for five minutes.

4. For tests and control, transfer 4.0 mL of petroleum spirit layer (upper) into correspondingly marked 150 × 19 mm tubes or similar. From standards transfer 3.0-mL aliquots into similar tubes.

5. Place unstoppered tubes in a water bath in the fume hood at 60°C. Evaporate off the petroleum spirit with a gentle stream of either nitrogen or dried filtered air. Allow to cool.

6. Place all tubes plus an empty tube for reagent blank into a 25°C water bath. At one-minute intervals add 6.0 mL of fresh Liebermann-Burchard reagent, mix on vortex-type mixer, seal with Parafilm, and place back in water bath.

7. Using a high-resolution spectrophotometer set at 620 nm and *absolutely dry* 10 mm cuvettes, determine the absorbancies of tests, control, and standards against the reagent blank with the same timing and sequence as in step 6, commencing exactly 30 minutes after the first addition of reagent in step 6. Protect the tubes from strong direct light.

Calculation

$$\frac{\text{Test Absorbance}}{\text{Standard Absorbance closer in value}} \times \text{Standard value}$$

$$= \text{Cholesterol in mg/dL} \times 0.026 = \text{mmol/L}.$$

High Standard value = 300 mg/dL = 7.8 mmol/L.

Low Standard value = 150 mg/dL = 3.9 mmol/L.

Normal Values. See Table 6–1.

Reagents

Petroleum Spirit (also called petroleum ether). Reagent grade, boiling point range 60 to 80°C.

Ethanol. Reagent grade absolute ethanol. For preparation of standards, keep a 1-liter glass bottle of ethanol with a layer of anhydrous sodium sulfate in the bottom to keep it anhydrous.

Concentrated Sulfuric Acid and Acetic Anhydride. Reagent grade.

33% Potassium Hydroxide. Dissolve 20.0 g of reagent-grade potassium hydroxide in 20 mL of distilled water, mix well, cool.

Alcoholic Potassium Hydroxide. Just before required, mix 3.0 mL of 33% w/w potassium hydroxide and 47 mL of absolute ethanol. Discard the unused portion.

Cholesterol Standard. Dissolve 100 mg of highest purity cholesterol in, and make up to 250 mL with, reagent-grade absolute ethanol. Keeps up to 2 months at 4°C. Store in a glass bottle with a well-fitting stopper.

Liebermann-Burchard Color Reagent. This is made freshly within one hour of use. In a round-bottomed flask supported in a bath of ice chips and water, chill 20 volumes of acetic anhydride. When the temperature is down to about 5°C, add *slowly* 1 volume of concentrated sulfuric acid with gentle swirling to mix. Allow to remain chilled for 9 minutes, then add 10 volumes of glacial acetic acid, swirl well to mix, and allow to come to room temperature. Rubber gloves should be worn during this operation.

Notes

1. The above technique follows that described in Henry, 1974.
2. The average hospital piped air supply often contains water, which is known to interfere seriously with the color reaction. The evaporation of the petroleum spirit can be hastened if a simple manifold is made to lead air or nitrogen into the tubes.
3. It has been noted that concentrated sulfuric acid is very hygroscopic, and a frequently opened large bottle will absorb enough water to interfere with the color reaction. The use of small polypropylene screw-capped bottles, completely filled, to hold a suitable volume for preparation of the color reagent will overcome this problem.

Serum Triglycerides Determination

Because the triglycerides of the plasma or serum constitute a group of substances rather than a single compound, all current methods require conversion of the members of the group to one common form for assay. This is achieved by hydrolysis, either chemical or enzymatic, of the triglycerides to free glycerol, followed by determination of the glycerol, again by either chemical or enzymatic reactions. (A variation substitutes transesterification using sodium ethoxide for the hydrolysis. The triglycerides are split to yield glycerol and ethyl esters of the fatty acid portions of the molecule.) Prior to chemical hydrolysis or transesterification, the triglycerides may be extracted from the plasma or serum with isopropanol or chloroform-methanol in the presence of an adsorbent such as silicic acid or zeolite (sodium aluminum silicate), which removes interfering substances such as bilirubin, glucose, monoglycerides, diglycerides, and phospholipids. The practical difficulties of automating such a process have stimulated the development of fully enzymatic hydrolysis, using either lipase plus an esterase or lipase plus alpha-chymotrypsin, in the presence of a surfactant.

Following release of the glycerol, it can be determined by one of the following reactions:

(i) Oxidation to formaldehyde can be done using periodate; the formaldehyde is reacted with chromotropic acid (4,5-dihydroxy-2,7-naphthalenedisulfonic acid) to give a pink derivative with maximum absorbance at 565 nm.

(ii) Oxidation to formaldehyde with periodate can be done, followed by combination with ammonium ion and acetylacetone (Hantsch reaction), producing a yellow lutidine derivative with maximum absorbance at 410 nm. The lutidine derivative can also be determined fluorimetrically.

(iii) The glycerol can take part in the sequence of enzymatic reactions shown below.

The final reaction is associated with a change in the coenzyme from the reduced to the oxidized form with a concomitant decrease in absorbance at 340 nm. The rate of this reaction reflects the amount of glycerol, since all the other reactants are present in excess. (The glycerol is referred to as the "rate-limiting" constituent.) This reaction (Bucolo and David, 1973) is readily adaptable to automation, and kits of reagents are available commercially.*

(iv) In order to replace the measurement of a rate reaction at 340 nm with an end-point determination in

*Calbiochem, La Jolla, Calif. 92037.

$$\text{Glycerol} + \text{ATP} \xrightarrow{\text{Glycerol kinase}} \text{Glycerol-3-phosphate} + \text{ADP}$$

$$\text{ADP} + \text{Phosphoenolpyruvate} \xrightarrow{\text{Pyruvate kinase}} \text{ATP} + \text{Pyruvate}$$

$$\text{Pyruvate} + \text{NADH} + \text{H}^+ \xrightarrow{\text{Lactate dehydrogenase}} \text{Lactate} + \text{NAD}$$

ATP: adenosine triphosphate
ADP: adenosine diphosphate
NADH: reduced form of the coenzyme nicotinamide adenine dinucleotide
NAD: oxidized form of NADH

$$\text{Glycerol} + \text{ATP} \xrightarrow{\text{Glycerol kinase}} \text{Glycerol-3-phosphate} + \text{ADP}$$

$$\text{Glycerol-3-phosphate} + \text{NAD} \xrightarrow{\text{Glycerol phosphate dehydrogenase}} \text{Dihydroxyacetone phosphate} + \text{NADH}^+ + \text{H}^+$$

$$\text{H}^+ + \text{NADH}^+ + \text{INT} \xrightarrow{\text{Diaphorase (lipoamide dehydrogenase)}} \text{Formazan} + \text{NAD}$$

INT: iodonitrotetrazolium dye
Formazan: red reduction product formed from INT with peak absorbance at 500 nm

---

the visible range, which is more convenient for manual assays, the glycerol released from the triglycerides by the action of bacterial lipases (derived from *Pseudomonas* and *Chromobacterium* spp.) can be determined by the series of reactions as shown above.

The absorbance produced in this series of reactions by serum samples is then compared with that produced by a suitable standard, such as triolein or glycerol. The complexity of current reagent kits is well illustrated by the sources of the enzymes: lipase from microbial sources, glycerol kinase from *E. coli*, glycerolphosphate dehydrogenase from rabbit muscle, and diaphorase from *Clostridium kluyveri*.* A manual method using this series of reactions is described below. A procedure using a colorimetric end-point is described, since it is more convenient for those spectrophotometers capable of making accurate absorbance measurements in the range from 0.0 to 1.0 absorbance: methods involving the reaction described in paragraph (iii) above, in which the reagent initially contains a high level of reduced NAD, require either a spectrophotometer able to make readings at absorbances above 1.5 or the use of special blanks to shift the test absorbance range below 1.0.

Principle. See paragraph (iv) above.

Procedure

1. Set up one 100 × 16 mm test tube for each serum sample, one for reagent blank, one for standard, and one for a control.

2. Using a plastic-tipped positive displacement pipettor, add 2.0 mL of reconstituted reagent (see under *Reagents*) to each test tube.

3. Using a positive displacement pipettor with a glass capillary tip† and wiping off the tip between measurements, add 10 μL of deionized water to the reagent blank and 10 μL of each test serum, glycerol standard, and control serum to the appropriately labeled tubes. Mix by gentle lateral shaking, cap or cover with Parafilm, and incubate for 15 minutes in a 37°C water bath.

4. Set the spectrophotometer to zero with deionized water at 500 nm. Determine the absorbances of tests, reagent blank, standard, and control, using 10-mm light path cells (see *Notes*).

5. Subtract the absorbance of the reagent blank from the absorbances of tests, standard, and control to give the corrected absorbances.

*Diagnostic Chemicals Ltd., Charlottetown, P.E.I., Canada ClA 4H5; Diagnostics Division, Fisher Scientific Co., Orangeburg, N.Y. 10962.

†SMI (Scientific Manufacturing Industries), Emeryville, Calif. 94608.

Calculation

$$\frac{\text{Corrected test absorbance}}{\text{Corrected standard absorbance}} \times \text{Standard value} = \text{Serum triglycerides in mg/dL}$$

For SI units, mg/dL × 0.0113 = mmol/L (based on the molecular weight of triolein 885.4).

Reagents. These are available commercially.* For use, one vial of the triglyceride color reagent is dissolved in 20.0 mL of Tris buffer by gentle inversion. Keep the dissolved reagent in the brown bottle until used. It is stable for at least 48 hours at 2 to 5°C: temporary storage at room temperature is not recommended.

Standard. Because the triglycerides in the serum are a group of related compounds rather than a single substance, it is not possible to make a true standard. For practical purposes it is assumed that the triglycerides can be represented as triolein (glyceryl trioleate). Because one mole of triolein releases one mole of glycerol on hydrolysis, and in order to provide a more stable standard solution, glycerol is used as the standard, based on the relationship that 92 mg of glycerol corresponds to 885.4 mg of triolein; that is, 1.0 mg glycerol corresponds to 885.4/92, or 9.62, mg of triolein. The commercial set of reagents includes a glycerol standard containing 20.79 mg/dL, corresponding to 20.79 × 9.62 = 200 mg/dL triolein. The method is linear to at least 400 mg/dL, and a single standard is adequate. The normal range is 30 to 160 mg/dL for young adults (0.34 to 1.81 mmol/L). Values up to 210 mg/dL (2.37 mmol/L) may be obtained in older people. It is preferred practice for each laboratory to establish its own normal range based on the local population.

Notes

1. If the absorbance of the reagent blank is found to be reproducible at about 0.1 (with freshly made reagent), the spectrophotometer can be set to zero with the reagent blank, thus simplifying the calculation.

2. The method includes any pre-existing glycerol, monoglycerides, and diglycerides in the serum: these are estimated to constitute from 5 to 10% of the measured "triglycerides" in adults and as much as 10 to 25% in children. Elevations of triglyceride levels of as much as 45% have been associated with the use of oral contraceptives.

3. The best sample is fresh serum from blood taken after a 14-hour fast. Storage for up to four days at 2 to 5°C is adequate. Fresh plasma from blood taken using

*Diagnostic Chemicals Ltd., Charlottetown, P.E.I., Canada ClA 4H5; Diagnostics Division, Fisher Scientific Co., Orangeburg, N.Y. 10962.

heparin or EDTA can be used: fluoride or oxalate plasma is unsuitable. Moderate hemolysis does not interfere.

4. The selection of a suitable control serum presents some difficulties. If control of precision alone is intended, a commercial control serum that has a value in the region of the upper end of the normal range and that is not visibly lipemic on reconstitution will be adequate. If some indication of accuracy is required a control serum for which the manufacturer provides a value obtained by *exactly the same method employed in the assay* may be used. The problem is well illustrated by the wide range of values quoted for the same serum, typically from 206 to 337 mg/dL. Another complication is the presence in some commercial control sera of unspecified amounts of free glycerol.

5. The test serum should be reassayed after suitable dilution with saline if the original result exceeded 400 mg/dL or if the sample showed visible lipemia. In sera showing separation of chylomicrons on standing, high dilution of the sample after thorough mixing will be required before assay; otherwise the amounts of lipases may not be adequate for complete hydrolysis of the triglycerides.

6. This method is readily automated on a discrete-type analyzer.

7. The spectrophotometer should be a modern instrument with a narrow band pass (10 nm or less), low stray light value, good stability, and a digital-type read-out sensitive to 0.001 absorbance. If a flow cell is used, great care must be taken with cleaning, since the reddish formazan dye produced by the reaction tends to become deposited on glass or plastic surfaces and may be difficult to remove. It may be removed by allowing a warm 25% dilution of commercial hypochlorite bleach to sit in the cell for 15 to 30 minutes and then thoroughly flushing the cell with a detergent solution and finally with deionized water. Alternatively, the set of solutions from the determination may be measured in a disposable plastic cuvette, which is then discarded.

This method illustrates the considerable simplification of a previously complex assay by the use of enzymes, the importance of good micropipetting technique, the subtle problems associated with quality control and standardization, and the necessity of adopting a method appropriate to the available instrumentation.

Thin-Layer Chromatography of Serum Lipids

A detailed technique for the separation of the neutral fats and phospholipids of serum, including the cholesterol and cholesterol ester fractions, is given in the previous edition of this text. It has no practical application in routine clinical biochemistry. Separation of lecithin and sphingomyelin in amniotic fluid in the estimation of fetal lung maturity is discussed on p. 274.

PROTEINS

Proteins are essentially polymers, composed of amino acids, linked together by peptide bonds to form polypeptide chains. The general structure of an amino acid is shown in Figure 6–7. The genetic code recognizes 20 amino acids for incorporation into proteins. Ten of these

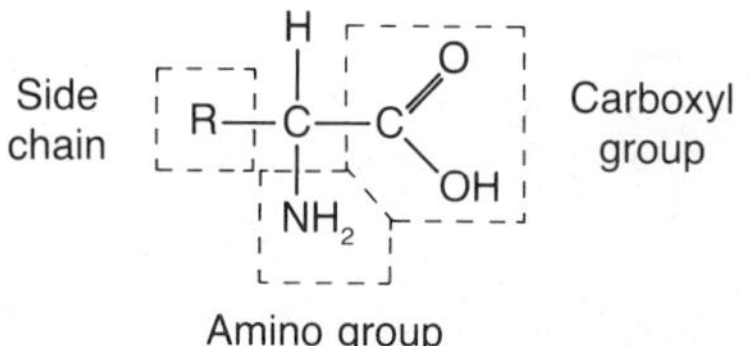

Figure 6–7 General structure of an amino acid.

can be synthesized by the body; of the remainder, eight are called essential amino acids; they cannot be synthesized but must be obtained from ingested food. These are isoleucine, leucine, valine (the three branched chain amino acids), lysine, methionine, phenylalanine, threonine, and tryptophan. Arginine and histidine are essential amino acids in infancy.

Most proteins are either structural elements (e.g., collagen) or enzymes. Others function as hormones, antibodies, and so forth. Proteins are synthesized in the ribosomes of the rough endoplasmic reticulum, with messenger RNA produced in the cell nucleus acting as the coding template.

The peptide bond that links the amino acids together is formed by the condensation of the amino ($-NH_2$) group of one molecule with the carboxyl ($-COOH$) group of the other (Fig. 6–8). Once the polypeptide chain is formed, other bonds may occur between adjacent elements:

1. Hydrogen bonds between $-NH$ or $-OH$ groups
2. Ionic interactions between charged groups ($-NH_3^+$)
3. Hydrophobic interactions
4. Disulfide ($-S-S-$) bonds between cystinyl residues

Protein chains are described as having primary, secondary, tertiary, and quaternary structures. *Primary* structure refers to the ordered arrangement of amino acids in the polypeptide chain; conventionally these are numbered in sequence, beginning with the terminal amino group and ending at the end of the chain that bears the free carboxyl group. *Secondary* structure refers to the twisting of the chain into shapes such as that of the alpha helix of the keratins found in wool and hair. *Tertiary* structures are complex nonlinear foldings of the protein chain to form globular shapes such as that of the hemoglobin molecule. *Quaternary* structure refers to cross-linkages (usually disulfide bonds) between two or more separate polypeptide chains (e.g., insulin).

Proteins are charged molecules: the isoelectric point of any particular form depends mainly on the primary structure of the protein, and an alteration in even one amino acid can change it. Advantage is taken of this property in the separation of protein mixtures (e.g., plasma) by techniques such as salt fractionation and electrophoresis.

Proteins are catabolized in the body to the component amino acids. These may then be reutilized in the synthesis of new protein, or else the amino group may be removed (deamination) and processed in the liver to form the waste product *urea*, which is excreted in the urine. The skeleton remaining after deamination is then used in the synthesis of glucose (gluconeogenesis) and other carbohydrates.

$$R_1\text{—}\underset{\displaystyle H}{\overset{\displaystyle COOH}{C}}\text{—}NH_2 + COOH\text{—}\underset{\displaystyle H}{\overset{\displaystyle NH_2}{C}}\text{—}R_2 \quad R_1\text{—}\underset{\displaystyle H}{\overset{\displaystyle COOH}{C}}\text{—}NH.OC\text{—}\underset{\displaystyle H}{\overset{\displaystyle NH_2}{C}}\text{—}R_2$$

Figure 6–8 Formation of the peptide bond.

Plasma Proteins

The functions of the plasma proteins are:

1. To maintain osmotic pressure in the blood (albumin accounts for 75% of the colloid osmotic pressure of plasma).
2. To act as a reserve of protein for tissue repair and growth.
3. To act as pH buffers (plasma proteins, but especially hemoglobin).
4. To act as transport mechanisms, e.g., transport of lipids and lipid-soluble substances (bilirubin, vitamins A, D, and E, steroid hormones), carriage of metals, e.g., iron by transferrin; also, about half the blood calcium is bound to protein.
5. To act as immunological agents. Gamma globulins contain the antibodies against disease-causing organisms. The blood group agglutinins are associated with the beta-2 globulins.
6. To provide factors necessary for normal blood coagulation, e.g., fibrinogen, prothrombin, antihemophilic factor, factors V and VII, plasma thromboplastin component (PTC), plasma thromboplastic antecedent (PTA), and so forth.
7. To provide necessary enzymes in the blood. Many of the clotting factors behave as enzymes. Other enzymes in the blood are proteinases (e.g., plasmin), peptidases, amylase, acid and alkaline phosphatases, deoxyribonuclease, histaminase, choline esterase, beta-glucuronidase, transaminases, dehydrogenases, and so forth.

Increased plasma protein levels may be found in hemoconcentration or may be the result of the presence of abnormal proteins, usually globulins, as in plasma cell myeloma. Reduced levels of plasma proteins may be caused by (1) excessive loss, as in severe albuminuria (e.g., nephrosis), extensive burns (the hypoproteinemia here may be masked by hemoconcentration), prolonged undernutrition (starvation, kwashiorkor, sprue), and in protein-losing lesions of the gastrointestinal tract; or (2) liver damage leading to reduced protein synthesis, e.g., cirrhosis.

Estimation of Plasma and Serum Proteins

It is more usual to estimate serum proteins, since it is usually easier to obtain good clear serum than plasma. The difference between the two is that serum lacks fibrinogen.

Methods of Estimation

The available methods of serum protein determination include assay of nitrogen content by Kjeldahl digestion, determination of specific gravity, measurement of the tyrosine content by the reaction of the phenolic group of this amino acid with Folin and Ciocalteu's phosphotungstomolybdic acid reagent, and measurement of the ultraviolet absorbance of the peptide bond at 215 nm or the aromatic ring structures of tyrosine and tryptophan at 280 nm. In the main, however, this determination is made either by correlating the refractive index measurement of total solids with the protein content or by the biuret reaction.

Refractometry

When a beam of light crosses the boundary between two transparent media, such as air and a fluid, as a result of the change of its velocity it undergoes a change in direction. The extent of this change depends on the nature of the fluid and its solute content. The higher the solute content, the greater the increase in refractive index. The magnitude of the change is also affected by temperature. In a refractometer used for serum protein determinations, the necessary correction for temperature is achieved by using a liquid crystal system, and the assumption is made that the solutes in serum other than protein remain relatively constant, so that the refractometer reading of total solutes can be related empirically to protein level. This assumption does not hold true if the serum is abnormally pigmented, contains a very high urea level, is hemolyzed, or is lipemic. In other cases the correlation is good enough for clinical purposes.

The Biuret Reaction

This reaction — which owes its name to the somewhat irrelevant fact that the nonphysiological substance biuret produces the same color—is the formation of a complex between cupric ions and the peptide bonds of protein in an alkaline solution. All substances with three or more peptide bonds give the reaction, and the intensity of the purple color produced is proportional to the number of such bonds present and hence to the amount of protein.

Serum Protein Determination (Doumas, 1975)

Principle. When a solution containing proteins is reacted with tartrate-complexed cupric ions and alkali, the copper binds to the peptide bond structure of the proteins, forming a purple chromogen with an absorbance maximum at 540 nm. The absorbance of this color can be compared with that produced by solutions with a known protein content.

Procedure

1. Set up five large test tubes labeled Test, Test Blank, Standard, Standard Blank, and Reagent Blank.

2. Into Test, Standard, and Reagent Blank pipette 5.0 mL of biuret reagent. Into Test Blank and Standard Blank pipette 5.0 mL of alkaline tartrate.

3. To Test and Test Blank add 100 microliters of test serum. To Standard and Standard Blank add 100 microliters of Standard. To Reagent Blank add 100 microliters of deionized water. Mix all tubes on a vortex mixer and let stand 30 minutes at room temperature.

4. Determine the absorbances of all tubes at 540 nm in a spectrophotometer with a band pass of 8 nm or less, using a 1.0 cm cell or flow cell and setting zero absorbance with alkaline tartrate solution.

5. Determine the corrected absorbance for the test: Test abs − Test Blank abs. − Reagent Blank abs.

6. Determine the corrected absorbance for the standard: Standard abs. − Standard Blank abs. − Reagent Blank abs.

Calculation

$$\frac{\text{Corrected Test absorbance}}{\text{Corrected Standard absorbance}} \times \text{Standard value} = \text{g protein per dL of Test}$$

For SI units (g per liter) multiply this result by 10.

Normal Values

Adults: 6.3–8.2 g/dL (63–82 g/L).
Full-term infants: 4.6–7.0 g/dL (46–70 g/L). Adult levels are attained at about the third year.

Reagents

Sodium Hydroxide, 6 Molar. Dissolve 240 g of analytic-grade sodium hydroxide pellets in about 700 mL of deionized water, with constant swirling and cooling. When all is dissolved, make up to 1 liter with deionized water; mix and store in a polypropylene bottle, tightly stoppered.

Biuret Reagent. Put about 500 mL of deionized water in a 1-liter volumetric flask and dissolve completely therein 3.0 g of cupric sulfate, $CuSO_4 \cdot 5H_2O$. Add 9.0 g of potassium sodium tartrate, $KNaC_4H_4O_6 \cdot 4H_2O$, and swirl to dissolve completely. Add 5.0 g of potassium iodide, KI, and swirl to dissolve. When solution is complete, add slowly with swirling 100 mL of 6-molar sodium hydroxide solution; make to volume, and mix well by repeated inversion. Store in a polypropylene bottle. This solution is stable at room temperature for at least six months.

Protein Standard Solution. The source of the bovine serum albumin used to prepare the standard is important. The preparation from the National Bureau of Standards, SRM 927, ranks as a primary standard, but it is expensive. For routine analyses BSA Cohn Fraction V* is suitable. Dissolve 80.0 g in sodium chloride/sodium azide diluent (see below) and make up to 1 liter with the same. Mix well by repeated gentle inversion; dispense into small tightly stoppered plastic vials, completely filled; and store in the refrigerator. Take out one vial per day and discard the unused portion. For the best economy, since only about 220 microliters are required for a batch of tests, dispense the standard in 250-microliter stoppered plastic micro centrifuge tubes and limit the volume made to 100 mL.

Sodium Chloride/Sodium Azide Diluent. Dissolve 9.0 g of sodium chloride, NaCl, and 0.5 g of sodium azide, NaN_3, in, and make up to 1 liter with, deionized water. **Caution:** Sodium azide is toxic. Exercise care in weighing and handling. If any solution containing an azide is to be discarded, it must be diluted with large amounts of water and flushed away thoroughly. Azides can react with metal plumbing — copper or lead — to produce explosive metallic azides.

*Sigma Chemical Co., St. Louis, Mo. 63178

Notes

1. The method is linear to serum protein values of 14.0 g/dL.
2. Plasma may be used, but the result will include the fibrinogen.
3. If large batches of determinations are to be run, the addition of serum and standard to the tubes should be made at timed intervals, and the absorbance readings made similarly.
4. Interference from hemoglobin and bilirubin is negligible unless the levels are unusually high.
5. The presence of dextran from plasma volume expanders produces a turbidity with the reagent: centrifuge the final colored solution and determine the absorbance of the clear supernatant.
6. The use of a tourniquet during phlebotomy tends to increase protein levels in the serum sample by about 0.5 g/dL.
7. The correction by the test blank for lipemia in the sample is not adequate at high levels of chylomicrons in the blood. In such cases the acetone precipitation method can be used (Chromy and Fischer, 1977). Briefly, 100 microliters of serum is mixed with 500 microliters of water and 10 mL of acetone. The precipitated proteins are separated by centrifugation, the supernatant is decanted off, and the protein is redissolved in 5.0 mL of biuret reagent as in the routine procedure.

Plasma Protein Fractionation

At the present time, opinion is divided over the value of serum protein electrophoresis. Many laboratories perform and report a separation on cellulose acetate quantitated by a scanning densitometer. Others maintain that such a procedure has no real value and that the specific proteins of interest should be determined quantitatively, usually by some form of immunoassay.

We believe that serum protein electrophoresis still has a place in clinical chemistry. It has the advantages of speed and relative economy; furthermore, it may not uncommonly reveal some unsuspected problem. However, it is most important that the separations be inspected *visually* by the clinical chemist or an experienced technologist before they are quantitated and reported. The reason for this is that the trained eye is far more perceptive of the position and intensity of the protein fractions than is a densitometer. We feel that a simple mechanical quantitation *without* such inspection is almost valueless. Any anomalies should be brought to the attention of the clinical chemist or pathologist and a descriptive note added to the outgoing report.

Adequate distinction between beta-gamma fusion ("bridging") and polyclonal and monoclonal gammopathies can usually be made only in this way. Furthermore, the careless use of plasma instead of serum will be seen immediately. Fibrinogen migrates immediately behind the beta band and may be interpreted by the inexperienced (especially on a scan) as an abnormal band or M-band, thus possibly leading the clinician seriously astray.

If unusual features are reported, then further investigation by immunoassay may be warranted. It should be remembered that such methods are still expensive and should not be used indiscriminately.

Interpretation

In general, abnormalities of the electrophoretic separation involve only one of the classic fractions. However, two patterns are seen that affect more than one band.

Acute Phase Reaction

This is a common pattern, and every technologist should be able to recognize it. The changes consist essentially of a marked reduction in the intensity of the albumin band and of an equally marked increase in the $alpha_1$ and $alpha_2$ bands, occasionally with some increase in beta.

This pattern is generally indicative of acute severe illness, e.g., burns or septicemia. Occasionally it may be supporting evidence for a subacute condition such as endocarditis or nephrotic syndrome.

Liver Failure

Because the liver is the source of albumin and almost all of the globulins, with the exception of the immunoglobulins, severe liver failure can produce a decline in all these fractions. It should be emphasized, however, that the reserve capacity of the liver is considerable and that such reductions are usually seen only in terminal states.

Albumin

The following disease states frequently produce a reduction in serum albumin levels:

Malnutrition, starvation, and malabsorption
Stress (surgical, burns, and infection)
Cirrhosis
Hypergammaglobulinemia
Hypothyroidism
Hepatic toxins such as carbon tetrachloride

Analbuminemia is a rare inherited disorder in which the albumin band is faint or absent. It is usually harmless: affected persons do not suffer from edema, because the globulin fractions rise to give a normal total protein level and thus a normal oncotic pressure.

Bisalbuminemia is an uncommon condition characterized by two intense, rather narrow bands in the albumin position. Unless the sample is run together with a control serum, it may cause some confusion as to which end is which. Visual inspection should easily resolve this problem.

Abnormal elevations of albumin apparently do not occur. It is important to remember that the level of serum albumin is of no value as an index of overall liver function or of its ability to synthesize albumin.

$Alpha_1$ Globulins

Most of this band is composed of a protein called $alpha_1$-antitrypsin, which appears to have the function of removing trypsin and other potentially damaging enzymes from the plasma. A much diminished or absent band should be reported, because it suggests the possibility of $alpha_1$-antitrypsin deficiency. Elevations occur as part of the acute phase reaction.

$Alpha_2$ Globulins

Elevations usually occur as part of the acute phase reaction; however, very prominent bands suggest the possibility of a severe chronic inflammatory disorder or an occult malignancy, especially if there is some elevation of the gamma fraction. Because a major component of the band is haptoglobin, a decrease suggests the possibility of hemolytic anemia.

Beta Globulins

Increased beta globulin is usually due to elevated beta-lipoprotein levels, which can be confirmed by lipid assays and lipid electrophoresis. Transferrin, the iron-transporting protein, runs in this region, but changes in its plasma level rarely show on protein electrophoresis. It should be noted that occasionally, especially with fresh buffer, the beta band may appear on inspection to be split; this is of no pathological significance.

Gamma Globulins

It is important not to forget that (1) the gamma globulin band is broad and diffuse because it is composed of proteins that, although antibodies, nonetheless show sufficient variation in their structure to migrate at many different rates, and (2) immunoglobulins (gamma globulins) are almost the only plasma proteins *not* manufactured by the liver.

Careful inspection should be made for diminished or apparently absent gamma bands. This may be the first indication of a hypogammaglobulinemia (p. 534).

Abnormal *elevations* of immunoglobulins are of three main types, which are easily recognized by inspection of the separation strip.

1. Monoclonal gammopathy. A single very intense band is seen on the strip, most commonly in the slow gamma region, but it can appear anywhere up to the zone between the beta and $alpha_2$ bands. When very intense, it may have a curly edge, particularly toward the cathode.

This is sometimes called an M-band, because in approximately 50% of cases it is indicative of myeloma, a malignant proliferation of plasma cells. It now seems certain that all of the malignant cells originate from one malignant parent cell, thus forming a clone. Because all of the cells produce immunoglobulin, the net result is the presence in the plasma of large amounts of immunoglobulin of one, and only one, specific molecular structure, thus producing a sharp band on electrophoresis.

Inspection will usually show a deficiency or absence of other immunoglobulin species; thus the IgG band around the M-band is pale or even apparently absent.

M-bands can also appear in a wide variety of chronic diseases, and they may be the first indication of an occult neoplasm. Occasionally, especially in elderly people, they appear to have no pathological significance and may stay the same over many years or just disappear.

2. Polyclonal gammopathy. Here there is an elevation of all or most of the immunoglobulin species, forming a broad, intense band that is yet distinguishable visually (though not reliably by densitometry) from the beta band. Such elevations are indicative of chronic inflammatory disorders, especially rheumatoid arthritis and related conditions.

3. Beta-gamma fusion. In this pattern, the gamma band shows a polyclonal elevation that is so broad that it runs into the beta band, making it impossible to separate the two, even by visual inspection.

This pattern is almost pathognomonic of portal cirrhosis; it should always be looked for and reported. True fusion is not usually seen with other types of cirrhosis (e.g., posthepatic scarring). It apparently takes some time to develop. The elevation of many IgG species is thought to occur because the blood from the gut, which normally carries small amounts of ingested foreign (and thus antigenic) protein, by-passes the damaged liver. The normal filtering action of the Kupffer cells on such proteins is thus lost, and stimulation of a multiple antibody response occurs.

Methods

It is usual and convenient to separate the plasma proteins by a zone electrophoresis method, as described on p. 88. Table 6–4 gives reference values, and Figures 6–9 to 6–11 show typical patterns obtained by scanning.

TABLE 6–4 NORMAL VALUES IN ELECTROPHORESIS OF SERUM PROTEINS*

Adults (Cellulose acetate electrophoretic system, Smith, 1960)

Total	6.3–8.2
Albumin	3.5–5.2
Alpha-1 globulin	0.1–0.4
Alpha-2 globulin	0.4–0.8
Beta globulin	0.5–1.0
Gamma globulin	0.6–1.3

Infants and Children (O'Brien and Ibbott, 1962)

Premature Infants

	first week	*4 months*	*12 months*
Total	4.32–7.63	4.74–6.17	5.80–7.12
Albumin	2.81–3.91	2.78–4.92	3.22–4.48
Alpha-1 globulin	0.13–0.47	0.05–0.45	0.19–0.46
Alpha-2 globulin	0.25–0.65	0.37–0.83	0.50–1.11
Beta globulin	0.31–1.16	0.41–1.13	0.64–1.08
Gamma globulin	0.48–1.56	0.12–0.67	0.33–1.20

Full-Term Infants

	first week	*12 months*	*4 years and above*
Total	4.65–7.41	6.08–6.72	6.15–8.10
Albumin	3.32–5.13	4.07–5.03	3.72–5.50
Alpha-1 globulin	0.12–0.32	0.15–0.35	0.12–0.30
Alpha-2 globulin	0.25–0.47	0.41–0.66	0.35–0.95
Beta globulin	0.17–0.61	0.52–0.83	0.47–0.92
Gamma globulin	0.40–1.41	0.45–0.66	0.53–1.20

*In grams/dL.

LIVER FUNCTION TESTS BASED ON FLOCCULATION OF SERUM PROTEINS

A number of empirical tests of liver function have been used for many years, based on turbidity or flocculation reactions of various substances with serum. These reactions appear to depend largely on the elevation of serum immunoglobulin levels in liver disease. Those most commonly employed have been the thymol turbidity test, the cephalin-cholesterol flocculation test, and the zinc sulfate turbidity test.

With modern rapid and inexpensive methods of protein electrophoresis, the continued use of these tests no longer can be justified. Consequently they will not be described here.

AMINO ACIDS

Amino acids are nitrogen-containing compounds of the general formula:

$$\begin{array}{c} NH_2 \\ | \\ R\text{—}CH \\ | \\ COOH \end{array}$$

When united in long chains by peptide bonds, they form proteins. The great majority of mammalian proteins are constructed from various combinations and permutations of some 23 amino acids. Proteins in food are mostly broken down by digestive enzymes to their constituent amino acids, which, attached to a carrier protein, are then absorbed across the gut wall by a process of active transport. Four major types of carrier protein exist, each of which is specific for one of the four major groups of amino acids. These groups are:

1. Neutral amino acids. These are monoamino-monocarboxylic acids and include alanine, valine, leucine, isoleucine, serine, threonine, tyrosine, phenylalanine, tryptophan, histidine, asparagine, methionine, cysteine, and citrulline. The carrier protein for this group is thought to be defective in Hartnup disease.

2. Dibasic amino acids. These are diamino-monocarboxylic acids and include arginine, lysine, and ornithine. The transport of these (and of cystine) is defective in cystinuria.

3. Acidic amino acids. These are the dicarboxylic acids, aspartic and glutamic acid, for which no syndrome of defective transport is known to exist in man.

4. Imino-glycine group. This comprises the two imino acids, proline and hydroxyproline, and glycine.

Similar, if not identical, carrier proteins exist in the proximal tubule of the kidney, their function being to reabsorb the amino acids filtered through the glomerulus.

A number of disorders of amino acid metabolism and transport are recognized; these are almost all rare, and therefore only a quite general discussion of pathogenesis and diagnostic procedures will be given.

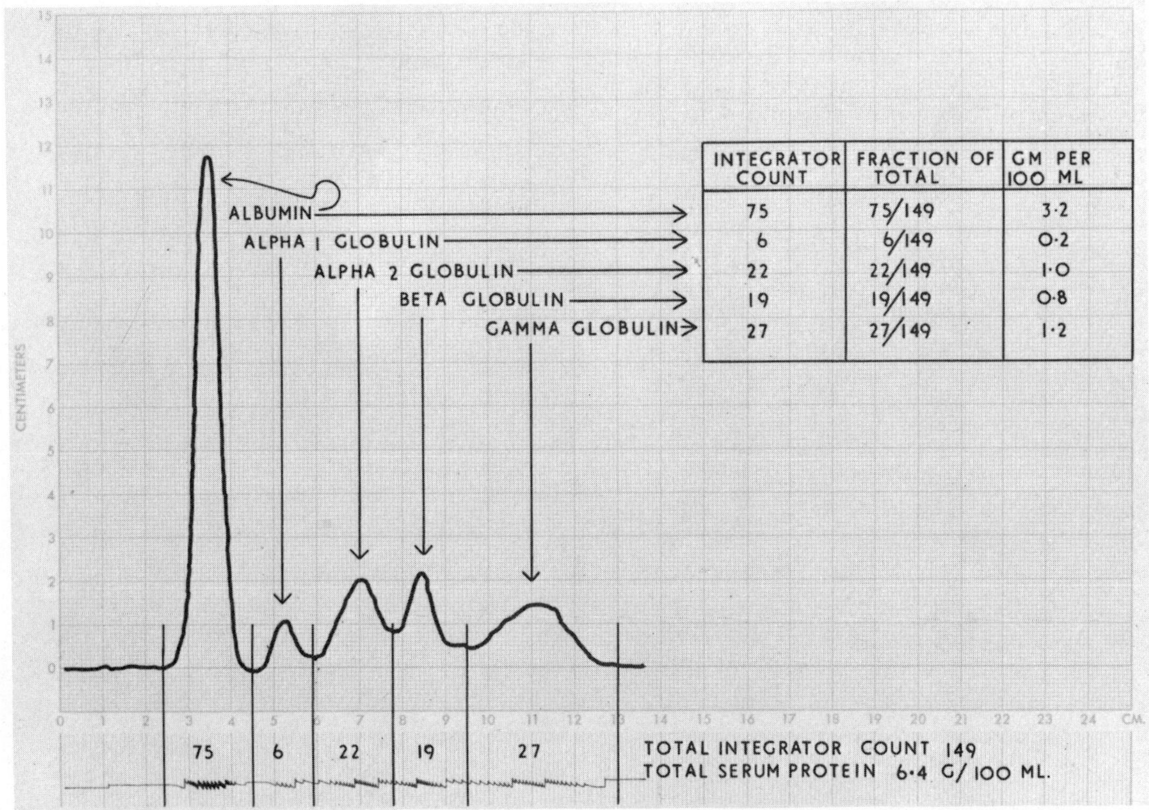

Figure 6–9 Quantitation of serum protein fractions by integration of the areas under the peaks of a densitometric tracing. Each unit of integration corresponds to 0.1 cm². The total serum protein value was obtained by the biuret method.

Normal Amino Acid Values and Patterns

Fasting plasma contains 4 to 6 mg per dL of α-amino acid nitrogen. Within 3 hours of ingestion of a protein-rich meal this rises by about 2 mg per dL. In the urine, a normal adult excretes a total of 300 to 650 mg of amino acids per 24 hours, and glycine accounts for about 25 to 30% of this. Actually, glycine, histidine, taurine, 1-methylhistidine, glutamine, serine, alanine, 3-methylhistidine and alpha-aminoisobutyric acid make up 80 to 90% of the total urinary amino acid excretion in normal adults. Only small amounts of lysine, tyrosine, leucine, isoleucine, and phenylalanine are excreted, with traces of proline, cystine, valine, and tryptophan.

TABLE 6–5 Classification of Defects of Amino Acid Metabolism

A. *Secondary (Generalized) Aminoaciduria*
  - Acquired defect
  - Inherited defect

B. *Primary (Specific) Aminoaciduria*
  - Overflow aminoaciduria (defect of catabolism)
  - Renal aminoaciduria (defect of transport)
  - Defects of urea synthesis

Disorders of Amino Acid Metabolism (Table 6–5)

Secondary Aminoaciduria

Aminoaciduria may occur in association with any disease state that interferes with the normal function of the proximal tubule. Whether secondary to either inherited or acquired disease, there is a generalized rise in excretion of amino acids, with no increase in any particular group being observable on chromatography. The determination of total alpha-amino nitrogen excretion is therefore of some value in diagnosis.

Acquired Form. A considerable number of factors may cause renal tubular damage and aminoaciduria. The more important of these are: heavy metals, such as lead; poisons, such as Lysol; renal disease, such as nephrosis and acute tubular necrosis; and deficiency states, such as scurvy and rickets. In some instances the amino acid excretion may revert to normal with appropriate treatment (e.g., in scurvy), but more often permanent renal damage occurs and the aminoaciduria will persist.

Inherited Form. A number of inherited disorders of metabolism occur in which renal tubular damage may be a facet of the disease process; examples are von Gierke's disease, galactosemia, Wilson's disease, and cystinosis. The aminoaciduria is not present at first, but appears and gradually intensifies as the disease state progresses.

Secondary aminoaciduria does not always occur as an isolated phenomenon, but may be associated with other

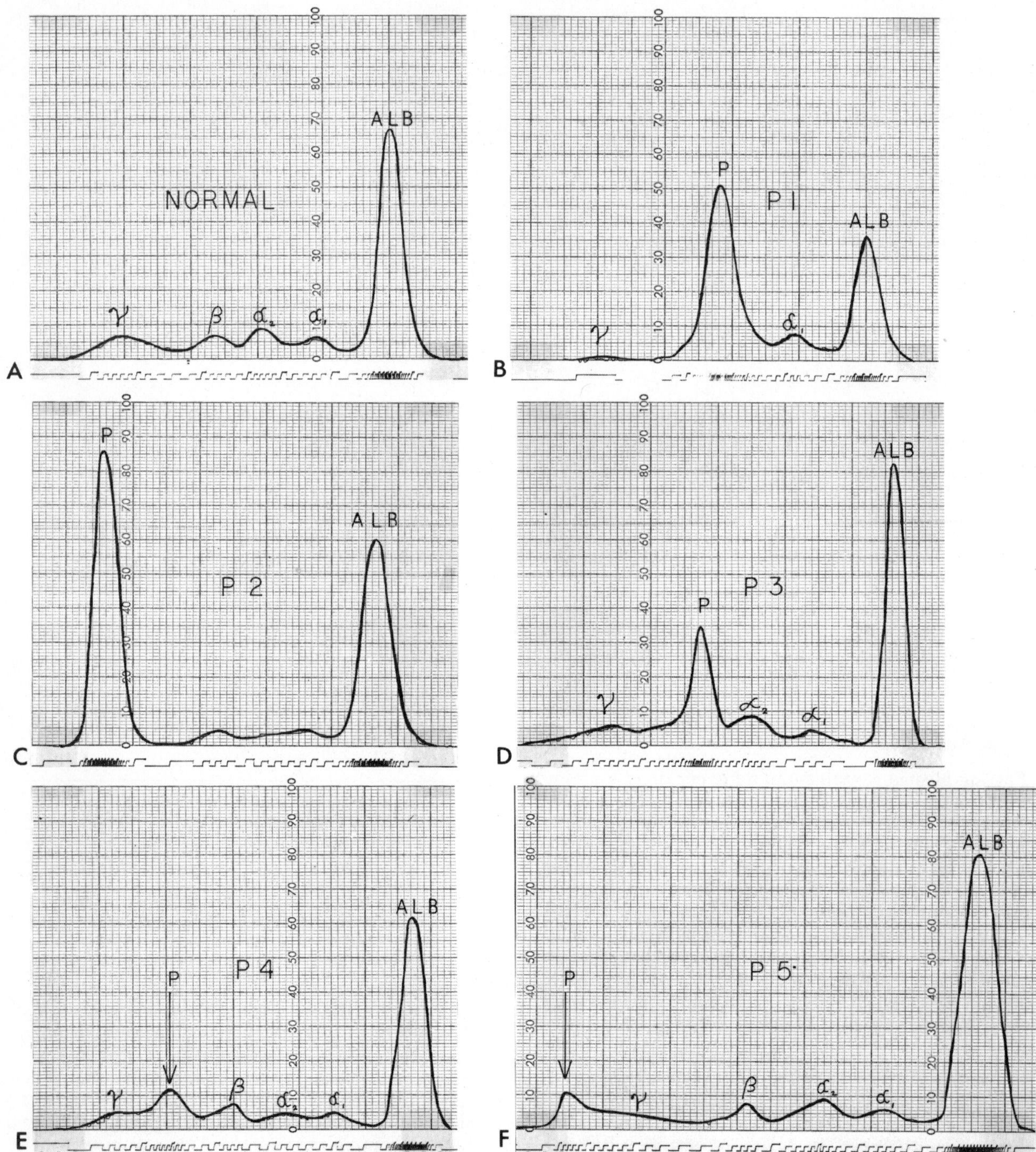

Figure 6–10 Densitometric scans of serum protein electrophoretic strips. **A**, Normal serum. **B**, Large monoclonal protein peak, *P*, in the beta globulin region. **C**, Large monoclonal protein peak, *P*, in the gamma region. Note apparent absence of alpha$_2$ globulin. **D**, Medium-sized monoclonal protein peak, *P*, in the beta globulin region. The gamma globulin fraction is not as severely reduced as in **B. E,** Small monoclonal protein peak, *P*, in the fast gamma globulin region. **F**, Very low monoclonal protein peak in the slow gamma globulin region. This was barely visible after the cellulose acetate strip had been cleared for densitometry, but after staining and washing, was detected against the white background of the uncleared strip.

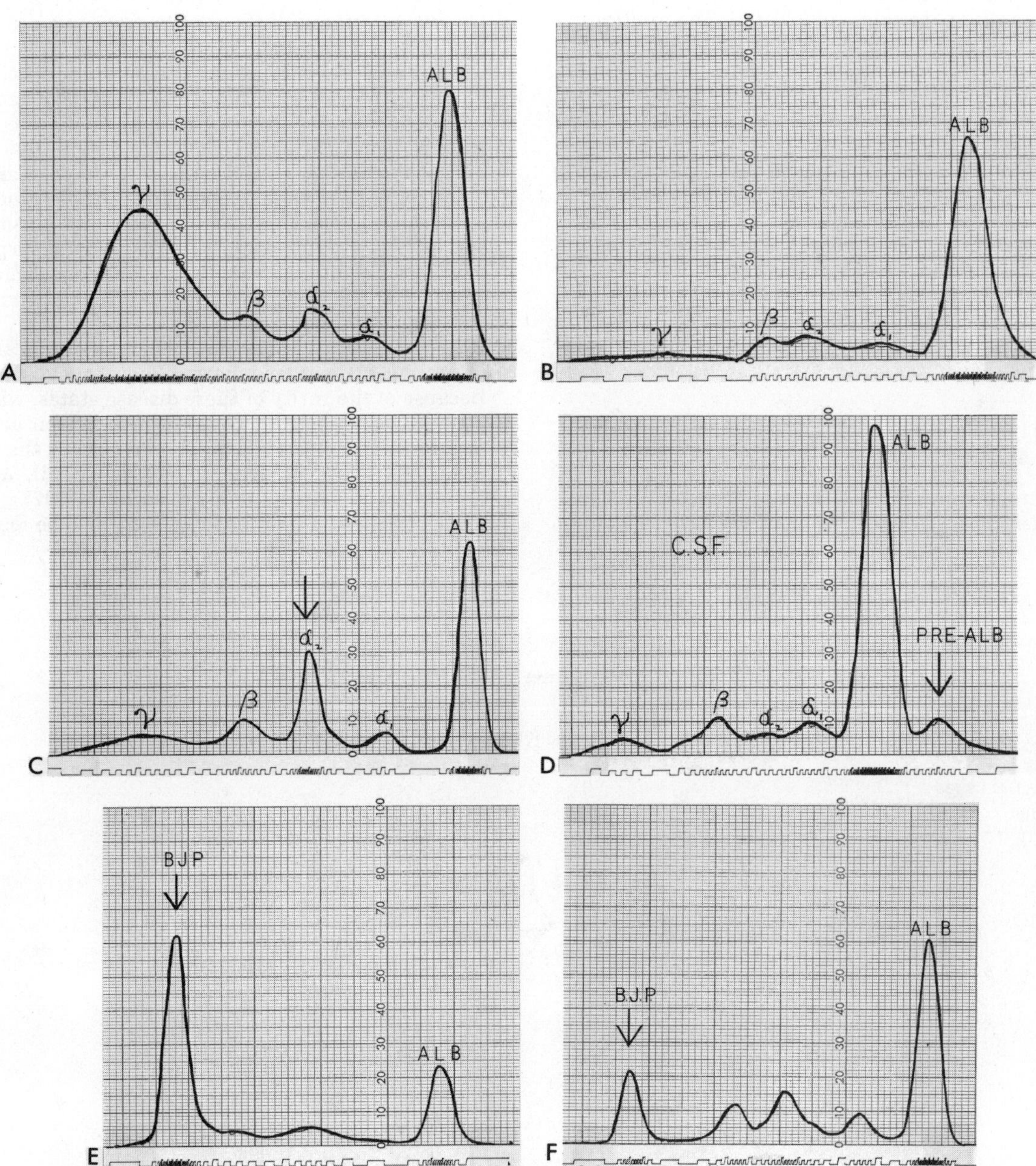

Figure 6–11 Densitometric scans of protein electrophoretic strips. **A**, Cirrhosis with greatly elevated gamma globulins fraction. **B**, Hypogammaglobulinemia. **C**, Elevated $alpha_2$ globulin fraction. This type of narrow peak may resemble that of a monoclonal protein. **D**, Normal cerebrospinal fluid, concentrated 100-fold. Note the pre-albumin or rho protein fraction, which is typical of CSF. **E**, Urine concentrated 50-fold, showing presence of Bence Jones protein. The screening test of heating at 56°C with a pH 4.9 buffer was negative/doubtful trace. **F**, Urine concentrated 50-fold, showing small Bence Jones protein peak. The remainder of the pattern closely resembles that of serum.

defects of tubular reabsorption. This association is known as Fanconi's syndrome.

Fanconi's Syndrome (Synonym: Phosphoglucoaminoaciduria). Fanconi's syndrome is characterized by a generalized aminoaciduria and a variable but elevated renal excretion of glucose, phosphate, bicarbonate, calcium, potassium, protein, and water. The continuing loss of these substances is associated clinically with hypophosphatemic rickets (unresponsive to vitamin D), hyperchloremic acidosis, and hypokalemia, the latter often with severe muscle weakness. Infants and children fail to show normal physical or mental development. Indeed, the presence of Fanconi's syndrome always should be considered in any infant who fails to thrive.

In adults, the disease develops rather more insidiously, and severe osteomalacia (which is the adult equivalent of rickets) may be the presenting feature.

Fanconi's syndrome is a biochemical diagnosis established by demonstrating the metabolic abnormalities described. In order to define its etiology in any particular patient, further investigations would be required.

Primary Aminoacidurias

This group of disorders comprises genetically determined defects of metabolism or of transport of amino acids. Although all of these diseases are rare or uncommon, they have assumed a position of importance in recent years, partly because they demonstrate the far-reaching effects of a single gene mutation and partly because many of them will respond to treatment, especially if the diagnosis can be established early enough.

Overflow aminoaciduria results from some primary block in the catabolism of a particular amino acid, whereas *renal aminoaciduria* results from specific defects of the transport mechanisms in the renal proximal tubule. The overflow group often may be detected more readily by examination of the plasma, especially in mild forms, whereas the renal group exhibits only an aminoaciduria with normal plasma amino acid values. For this reason it is important to examine both plasma and urine in any patient when this diagnosis is suspected. A number of additional simple screening tests should be performed at the same time, such as the ferric chloride test for certain organic acids.

These methods are described below; they will also aid in detecting some other inherited metabolic disorders.

Because of the rarity of these disease states, with one exception no further description will be given here; for reference purposes the reader should consult the standard texts by Scriver and Rosenberg (1973), and by Stanbury, Wyngaarden, and Fredrickson (1977), where further references to methodology will also be found.

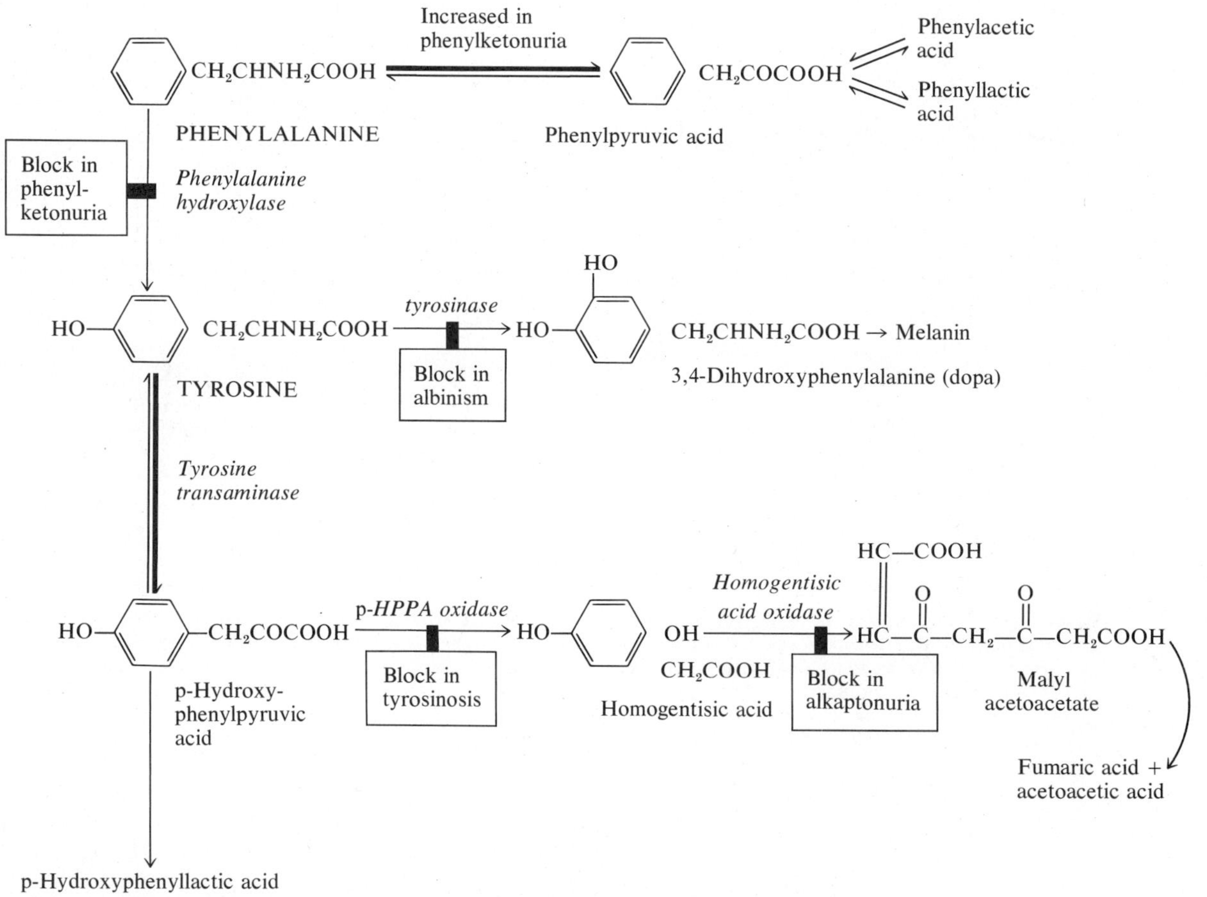

Figure 6–12 Metabolism of phenylalanine and tyrosine.

Phenylketonuria (PKU)

This aminoacidopathy is not rare: the severe classic form occurs in 1:10,000 live births, and a number of milder variants have been reported. Its present importance lies in the fact that early diagnosis and treatment are essential. A brief description will be given here.

Affected children are fair-haired and fair-skinned; they show severe and progressive mental retardation and reduced growth. The disease is inherited as an autosomal recessive trait with no significant sex difference.

The primary cause is a severe or complete deficiency of phenylalanine hydroxylase. This enzyme converts phenylalanine to tyrosine, which is the precursor of important compounds such as thyroid hormones, catecholamines, and melanin. It will be seen from Figure 6–12 that because phenylalanine cannot be metabolized to tyrosine, plasma levels of phenylalanine rise and increased synthesis of the organic acid metabolites phenylpyruvic acid and phenyllactic acid occurs.

All three compounds also appear in the urine, where the presence of phenylpyruvic acid is responsible for the mousy odor. (Other amino acid disorders characterized by an unusual odor are listed in Table 6–6.) Ferric chloride added to the urine will react with the phenylpyruvic acid to give a green color, and this can be used as a screening test in neonates. The principle is employed in commercial stick tests.

A more reliable, sensitive, and specific screening procedure is the Guthrie test. This uses a dried blood spot as the specimen and is widely employed in mass screening programs.

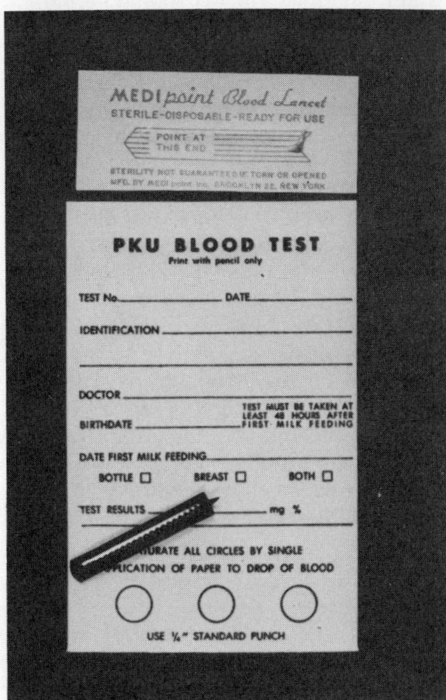

Figure 6–13 Card for PKU testing with small sterile lancet removed from the package. Blood drawn with the lancet is allowed to fill the small circles at the foot of the card. Information about the patient is written in the spaces designated on the card, including the date of birth and the date that the blood sample was drawn.

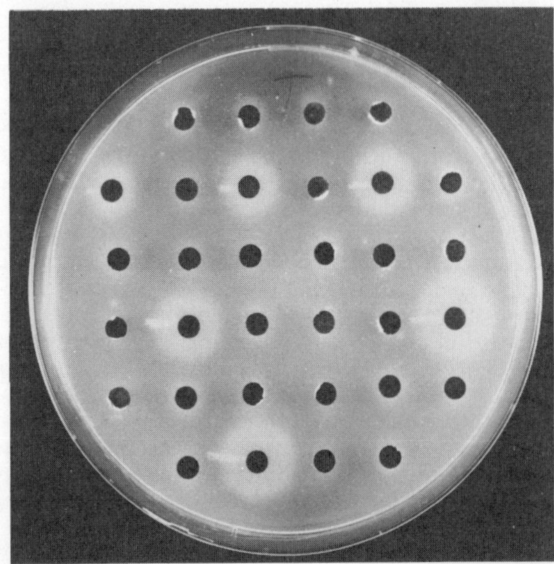

Figure 6–14 The PKU plate after incubation. The white areas around some of the discs are growths of *Bacillus subtilis*.. These are the control discs with concentrations of phenylalanine of 2 mg (least growth) to 20 mg per dL (most growth). All the test discs are negative.

Principle of the Test. Beta-2-thienylalanine prevents the growth of *Bacillus subtilis* (American Type Culture Collection No. 6051); but this inhibition does not occur in the presence of phenylalanine. A medium (Demain's medium) containing the inhibitor is seeded with spore suspension. Discs of blotting paper (Fig. 6–13) impregnated with the infant's blood, taken at least 48 hours after the first feeding and preferably as late as possible before discharge from the hospital, are placed on the medium with control discs and incubated at 37°C overnight (Fig. 6–14).

Growth will be seen around the control discs containing different concentrations of phenylalanine. The amount of growth around the disc containing 4 mg per dL phenylalanine is used for comparison. Test discs supporting a similar amount of growth or more are from patients who must be investigated further for PKU.

Positive Guthrie test results are also found in patients in whom, for some reason, development of liver phenylalanine hydroxylase is delayed, possibly in some heterozygotes, and in infants who, although free of PKU, initially have high blood levels of phenylalanine acquired through the placenta from afflicted mothers. These instances emphasize the importance of follow-up and confirmatory investigation.

Normal blood levels of phenylalanine are less than 1 mg/dL; in affected untreated individuals values up to 60 mg/dL may be seen. Quantitative determinations must be made to confirm a positive screening test result.

Although the cause of the mental retardation is still not certain, treatment with a phenylalanine-free diet will prevent (but not reverse) the mental deterioration. Thus it is essential that the diagnosis be established and treatment instituted within the first few days of life. For this reason comprehensive screening programs have been established in many countries, the cost of these being much lower than the lifetime institutional care of untreated children.

Methods for the Detection of Aminoaciduria and Some Other Inborn Errors of Metabolism

Chemical Tests—Urine

Note. Samples of urine preferably should be absolutely fresh and in the case of infants free from fecal contamination. (Feces contain free amino acids.) Use of acid as a preservative may cause anomalous patterns and is best avoided. If the urine has to be stored before processing, refrigeration is the method of choice for short periods and deep-freezing for long storage. Some sources of errors must be borne in mind. Methionine may appear in the urine of an infant ingesting a feeding formula that has been supplemented with DL-methionine or taking an oral preparation containing the same amino acid for treatment of diaper rash. Some antibiotics, for example, ampicillin, will produce one or two spots that stain with ninhydrin on chromatograms. The occurrence of increased urinary amino acids does not necessarily indicate an inborn error of metabolism; it can occur in liver disease and renal tubular abnormalities. Finally, the timing of the test procedures may be important. It is of little use to try to detect galactose in the urine if the infant has been taken off milk-containing foods; if treatment of the inborn error already has commenced, or if the condition is not fully manifest, equivocal results may be encountered.

In some cases the urine from a patient with an inborn error of metabolism will have a characteristic odor, distinct from the slightly aromatic smell of a normal fresh urine (see Table 6–6).

A negative result from the battery of chemical tests described below will eliminate the possibility of the following compounds' being present, in abnormal amounts, in the urine: Reducing substances including glucose (see p. 128), phenylpyruvic acid, phenylalanine, phenolic acids, valine, leucine, isoleucine, tyrosine, homogentisic acid, cystine, homocystine, and acid mucopolysaccharides. The ninhydrin test will also detect a significant generalized amino aciduria.

Reagents and Procedures

Ferric chloride reagent. Dissolve 1.0 g of ferric chloride, $FeCl_3 \cdot 6H_2O$, and 1.0 g of ferrous ammonium sulfate, $Fe(NH_4)_2(SO_4)_2 \cdot 6H_2O$, in 100 mL of 0.02 M hydrochloric acid.

Place 1.0 mL of reagent in a small tube, add 10 drops of urine, shake to mix. Observe within two to three minutes. Phenylpyruvic acid (in phenylketonuria) and imidazolepyruvic acid (in histidinemia) produce a green color; p-hydroxyphenylpyruvic acid (in tyrosinosis) is not detected. Ingestion of salicylates will give a purple or brownish purple color.

Benedict's qualitative reagent. This is most conveniently purchased commercially. To 5.0 mL of the reagent in a test tube add 0.5 mL urine; heat in the boiling water bath for five minutes. An abnormal amount of a reducing sugar is indicated by a yellow or orange precipitate; further identification may be made by chromatographic procedures. The most important sugars detected are glucose and galactose, in diabetes mellitus and galactosemia, respectively.

Cyanide-nitroprusside test. Mix 5.0 mL of urine and 2.0 mL of a freshly made 5.0% aqueous solution of sodium cyanide. Let stand five minutes. Add 5 drops of a freshly made 5.0% w/v aqueous solution of sodium nitroprusside, and mix. The immediate appearance of a magenta color, which may vary from a medium to a very dark tint, indicates the presence of cystine (in cystinuria) or homocystine (in homocystinuria).

Dinitrophenylhydrazine test. Dissolve 0.15 g of 2,4-dinitrophenylhydrazine in 40 mL of methanol, and then add a mixture of 5 mL of concentrated hydrochloric acid and 5 mL of water. Shake well to dissolve, filter if not clear, and keep in a brown bottle in the refrigerator. Check the urine for the presence of ketones, using one of the commercial stick or tablet tests; acetone and acetoacetic acid will give false positive reactions. To 1.0 mL of clear urine (centrifuge if necessary) add three drops of the reagent, mix by lateral shaking, let stand at room temperature; inspect for a pale yellow cloud or precipitate after 30 and 60 minutes. Positive reactions are obtained in any condition in which keto acids are excreted in the urine.

Cetyltrimethylammonium bromide test. Dissolve 1.995 g of citric acid and 12.205 g of sodium citrate dihydrate in about 80 mL of distilled water. Dissolve therein 5.0 g of cetyltrimethylammonium bromide, make up to 100 mL with distilled water, and mix. The pH should be 6.0.

Clear the urine by centrifuging, and to 5.0 mL of urine at room temperature add 1.0 mL of the reagent. Mix and let stand for ten minutes. A heavy flocculent precipitate indicates an increase in urinary mucopolysaccharides (gargoylism: excretion of chondroitin sulfate B and heparitin sulfate).

Nitrosonaphthol test. (i) Mix one volume of concentrated nitric acid with 5 volumes of distilled water. (ii) Dissolve 2.5 g of sodium nitrite in 100 mL of distilled water. (iii) Dissolve 100 mg of 1-nitroso-2-naphthol in 100 mL of 95% ethanol. The last two reagents should be kept refrigerated. To 1.0 mL of reagent (i) in a small test tube, add one drop of reagent (ii), followed by 0.1 mL of reagent (iii), and mix. Add immediately 3 drops of fresh urine; mix again. If the original yellow tint is replaced by an orange-red color within 2 to 5 minutes, the urine contains excessive amounts of one or more of the following: tyrosine, p-hydroxyphenylpyruvic acid, or p-hydroxyphenylacetic acid, indicating possible tyrosinosis.

TABLE 6–6 Inborn Metabolic Errors Associated with Characteristic Odor

Disorder	Odor
Phenylketonuria	Musty; mousey
Maple syrup urine disease	Maple syrup; burned sugar
Methionine malabsorption	Oast house; dried celery
Tyrosinemia; tyrosyluria	"Methionine"
Isovaleric acidemia	Sweaty feet; locker room
Short-chain fatty acid oxidation defect (Sidbury et al., 1967)	Sweaty feet

NINHYDRIN TEST. **Add 3 drops of urine (the specific gravity should be about 1.020—very concentrated urines should be diluted, and the test is unreliable with very dilute samples) to 1.0 mL of a 0.2% w/v solution of ninhydrin (triketohydrindene hydrate, indanetrione hydrate) in ethanol; mix and let stand for two minutes. A definite blue or purple color suggests an increased amount of amino acids.**

Chromatography

1. A semiquantitative fractionation of amino acids in urine and plasma may be made using paper or, preferably, thin-layer chromatography. One- or two-dimensional separation may be employed. Details will be found in the previous edition of this text and in Scriver and Rosenberg (1973).
2. A quantitative fractionation of all the amino and imino acids present in a plasma or urine sample can be made using a specialized form of column chromatography. The sample is passed through a column of synthetic ion-exchange resin beads, and the amino and imino acids become attached to the beads. The amino and imino acids are then sequentially eluted from the column with buffers of graded pH and reacted with ninhydrin. The colored products of this reaction are measured spectrophotometrically and the absorbances displayed on a recorder. Each peak on the recorder trace corresponds to a single amino or imino acid, permitting not only identification but quantitation. For complete details see Scriver and Rosenberg (1973).

CHAPTER 6—REVIEW QUESTIONS

1. Describe the principles of two methods for assay of plasma glucose.
2. What were the analytical disadvantages of the Liebermann-Burchard and Zak reactions used for the assay of cholesterol and how have they been overcome?
3. What is the clinical value of analysis of plasma lipids?
4. Describe the protein fractions obtained by zone electrophoresis and the changes that may occur in them in disease states.
5. Describe the metabolic changes that occur in the body at the onset of acute diabetes mellitus.
6. How is the diagnosis of diabetes mellitus established by laboratory tests?

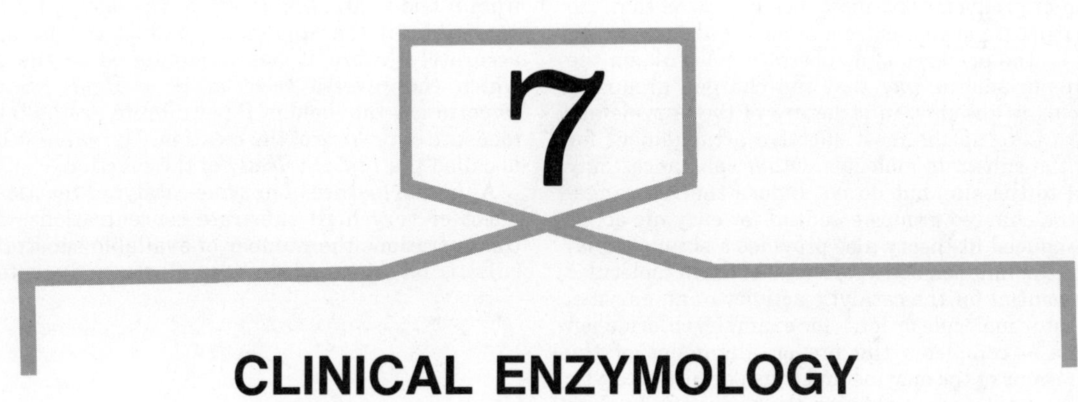

CLINICAL ENZYMOLOGY

INTRODUCTION

The purposes of this chapter are to describe both the process of enzymatic catalysis of biochemical reactions—how the features of that process affect the methods and problems of enzyme assays—and the associated difficulties with primary standardization and true quality control. The enzyme determinations in current use for clinical diagnosis will be outlined, including the practical application of isoenzyme separations.

ENZYME KINETICS

The study of enzyme kinetics is fundamental to an understanding of the biological machinery of the living cell. The study is concerned with *active* processes, largely continuous during the life of the cell. An analogy may be made to an automobile. The cell and the automobile engine are both energy conversion machines; the automobile converts the stored chemical energy of a fossil fuel into mechanical motion by a violent process, explosive oxidation in a confined system of piston and cylinder. The cell releases stored chemical energy, typically of carbohydrates, by a controlled stepwise oxidation system at low pressure and temperature. The oxidative process in the automobile is triggered by a high-voltage electrical spark; the essential agents in the energy release system of the cell are the organic catalysts called enzymes.

A working definition of an enzyme might be "A protein whose molecular structure incorporates regions or sites capable of catalyzing particular chemical reactions through specific activation of the reactants."

In order for any chemical reaction to take place, some of the molecules of the reactants must be in an energy state higher than that of the average molecule present. The necessary increment of energy is called the activation energy. A common method of achieving this is the introduction of energy from an external source in the form of heat; in the case of an automobile engine, the high-voltage spark serves this purpose. The enzyme promotes a reaction by forming a temporary union of reactant and enzyme that has a lower activation energy than the reactant alone, thus permitting a reaction to take place under lower free energy conditions than otherwise would be required. It should be noted that an enzyme cannot initiate a reaction that is energetically impractical; it merely facilitates and accelerates an existing reaction. It is true that in some cases a reaction may proceed, in the absence of the enzyme, at an almost negligible rate under biological conditions.

The phenomenon of specific activation can be studied from several aspects. In the last decade the three-dimensional architecture of some enzyme proteins has become better known, and it appears that the rigid relationship between enzyme and substrate implied by Emil Fischer's "lock-and-key" analogy needs to be modified to explain such facts as the binding to the active site of the enzyme of substances either larger or smaller in molecular size than the true substrate, without the formation of products. The most recent view is that the protein structure of the enzyme is not rigid, but can be modified by the presence of a substrate molecule on the active site in such a way that the charged groups of amino acids in the protein structure of the enzyme are induced to take up the most effective arrangement for splitting the substrate molecule. Other substances may be bound to the site, but do not induce the rearrangement of the charged groups essential for enzymic activity. The induced fit theory also provides a simple explanation for the function of activators, i.e., small molecules or ions essential for the catalytic activity of an enzyme. The activator molecule or ion—for example, chloride ion for amylase—completes the proper alignment of the charged groups of the enzyme and thus permits catalytic action. The activator may bind to the active site in close association with the substrate molecule, or it may bind at another location, inducing the necessary change in the three-dimensional shape of the enzyme. (This change in the properties of an enzyme induced by the binding of some compound to sites on the molecule is called the allosteric effect.) A somewhat similar process occurs when oxygen is being taken up by the hemoglobin molecule; the uptake of the first oxygen molecule subtly alters the three-dimensional structure of the heme portion and facilitates the union with three more oxygen molecules.

Another method of study of the enzyme-substrate relationship is based on the phenomenon of inhibition. Complete, irreversible blocking of enzyme activity usually involves distortion of the three-dimensional form of the enzyme either by attachment of the inhibitor to its surface or by inactivation of side chains, essential for attack on the substrate, by substances that form strong covalent derivatives thereof. The forms of inhibition that are reversible involve competition for the active site by a compound of similar structure to that of the typical substrate, or combination with a region of the enzyme molecule other than the active catalytic site. Careful study of the reversible types of inhibition has yielded much useful information about enzyme activity.

To examine the operation of a catalytic system, such as an enzyme reaction, it is convenient to do this at a time when the various stages of the process can be regarded as going on at a steady speed. In order to do this, Briggs and Haldane in 1925 proposed a simple scheme of enzyme action to which this "steady state" idea could be applied. In this scheme the enzyme, E, forms a complex with the substrate, S; this ES complex then breaks down to yield the product, P, and releases the enzyme unchanged. This relationship is shown by the equation:

$$E + S \underset{K_2}{\overset{K_1}{\rightleftharpoons}} ES \underset{K_4}{\overset{K_3}{\rightleftharpoons}} E + P$$

The arrows indicate that *each step* of the process is reversible. The simplifying assumption is that the formation of the ES complex takes only a fraction of a second, and that it breaks down to give E and P at a similar rate. In these circumstances the concentration of the ES complex will remain constant. It is also assumed that the reverse reactions, whereby E and S are derived from breakdown of ES, and ES is formed from E and P, are, *in the very early stages of the reaction*, negligible. If the amount of product can be measured accurately before it has accumulated to the point at which the reverse reaction $E + P \rightarrow ES$ assumes importance, the yield of P per minute can be taken as a measure of the *rate* of the reaction. The value so obtained is called the *initial velocity* of the reaction.

A unique feature of enzyme-catalyzed reactions is the effect of very high substrate concentrations. At these concentrations the number of available substrate molecules is large enough to keep all the active sites of the

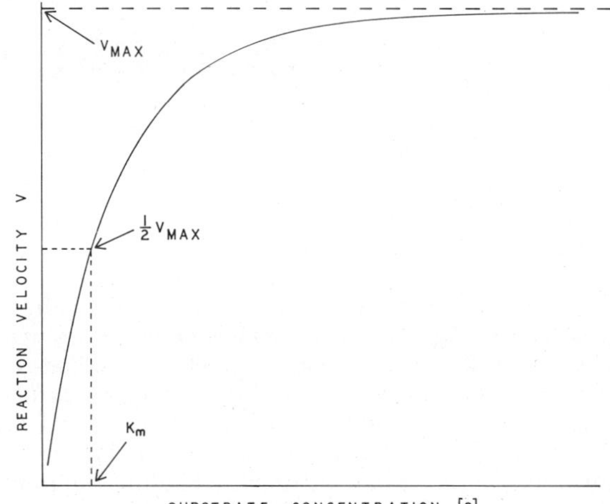

Figure 7–1 The relationship between the initial velocity of an enzyme reaction and the substrate concentration. The horizontal dotted line is drawn at the reaction velocity equal to half the maximum attainable; it intersects the curve at the point that corresponds to a substrate concentration equal to the value of the Michaelis-Menten constant, K_M.

enzyme busy. The evidence that this is the case is the leveling-off of the reaction; further increase of substrate concentration produces no increase in reaction rate. If the initial velocity of an enzyme-catalyzed reaction is measured at a wide range of substrate concentrations, and the relationship plotted, a curve is obtained of the form shown in Figure 7–1.

From consideration of the reversible reactions in the equation $E + S \underset{K_2}{\overset{K_1}{\rightleftharpoons}} ES \underset{K_4}{\overset{K_3}{\rightleftharpoons}} E + P$, calculation of the various rates of formation and breakdown, and application of the assumption that in the steady state condition the rate of the reverse reaction $E + P \underset{K_4}{\rightharpoonup} ES$ is negligible, an expression can be formulated that combines the three other rate constants, k_1, k_2, and k_3, into one lumped constant, K_M, called, after its originators, the Michaelis-Menten constant. Using this lumped constant, a relationship can be derived between v, the initial reaction velocity, at substrate concentration S, V_{max}, the theoretical maximum reaction velocity, and K_M.

$$v = \frac{V_{max}[S]}{K_M + [S]}.$$

This is the Michaelis-Menten equation. By some simple mathematical transformations, expressions of practical value can be obtained. For example, if we substitute the Michaelis constant for [S], the equation simplifies to:

$$v = \frac{V_{max} \times K_M}{K_M + K_M}$$

$$= \frac{V_{max} \times K_M}{2\ K_M}$$

$$= \frac{V_{max} \times 1}{2} \text{ or}$$

$$= \tfrac{1}{2}\ V_{max}$$

This means that if we wish to carry out an enzyme reaction in conditions approximating maximum velocity, the lowest possible value for the substrate concentration is equal to K_M. If we make S equal to five times K_M, then

$$v = \frac{V_{max} \times 5\ K_M}{6\ K_M}$$

Dividing both sides by V_{max}, the ratio of the actual velocity v to the maximum V_{max} equals $\frac{5K_M}{6K_M} = 0.83$, i.e., the actual velocity is 83% of the maximum. If we make [S] equal to 50 K_M, the actual velocity equals 98% of maximum. Thus we can determine the best substrate concentration for an enzyme assay to yield reaction rates close to the theoretical maximum.

Another feature of the Michaelis-Menten constant, K_M, is the information it gives on the reactivity of a substrate vis-à-vis an enzyme. If, for example, there are two enzymes that will attack the same substrate, the enzyme with the smaller K_M value will have the greater activity for that substrate, since at any given substrate concentration the ratio between this concentration and that required for maximum reaction rate V_{max} will be higher for the enzyme with the lower K_M; therefore its reaction rate, as a fraction of V_{max}, will be greater.

Note. Since the Michaelis-Menten constant, K_M, is derived from expressions involving concentrations of reactants and intermediates, it has the dimension of moles per liter. Thus it is valid to express the concentration of a substrate, [S], in terms of a factor times the K_M value for a particular enzyme.

In order to determine the K_M and V_{max} values for an enzyme, in theory we should make a large number of measurements of the reaction velocity at various substrate concentrations and draw or derive the hyperbolic curve shown in Figure 7–1. In practice, the values of v and [S] from a small number of measurements covering a wide range can be plotted as a straight line by a mathematical transformation known as the Eadie-Hofstee plot, from which the values of K_M and V_{max} can be directly determined (Fig. 7–2). Another, similar mathematical variation and plot is the Lineweaver-Burk method, in which the reciprocals of v and [S] are displayed (Fig. 7–3). This method is useful in the investigation of the effects of inhibitors. (See later.)

Inhibition

Substances that interfere with activity of an enzyme may do so by an irreversible molecular injury to the enzyme. For example, iodoacetamide disrupts the essential three-dimensional structure of the enzyme molecule by forming stable combinations with the —SH groups that are frequently found as points of linkage in adjoining peptide chains. If the inhibitor is present in sufficient quantity, all the enzyme molecules will become inactive after enough time has elapsed. If the inhibitory effect can be overcome by increasing the concentration of substrate molecules, however, the phenomenon can be regarded as an equilibrium situation, which can be expressed mathematically in equations similar to the Michaelis-Menten equation. This type of effect is called *competitive* inhibition; the inhibitor is usually a compound structurally similar to the substrate and therefore

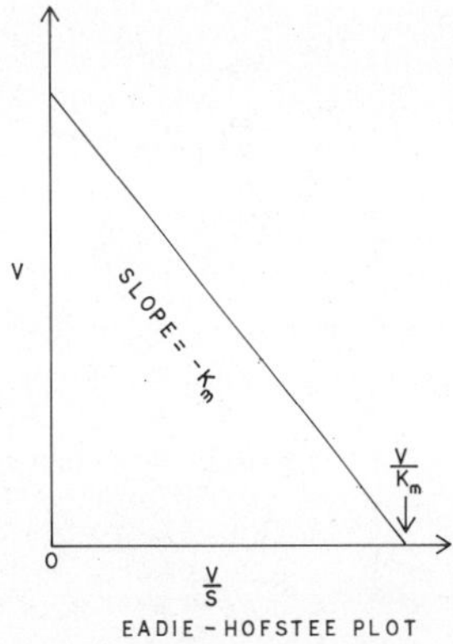

Figure 7–2 Eadie-Hofstee plot of velocity against velocity/substrate concentration ratio. The important measurements, K_M and V_{max}, are given by changing the sign of the plotted slope and the value of the intercept on the vertical axis.

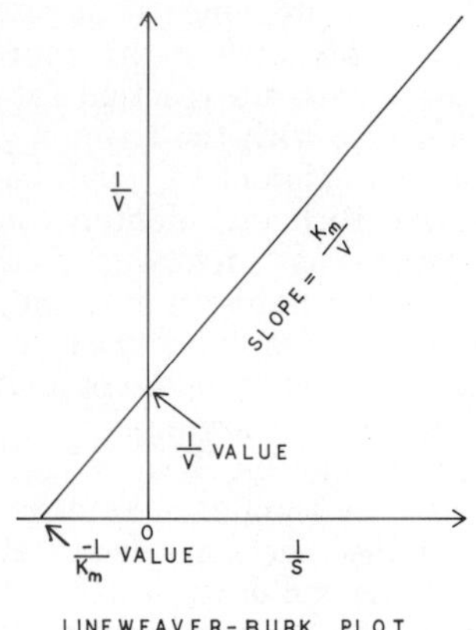

Figure 7–3 Lineweaver-Burk plot. The reciprocal of the velocity of the reaction at a particular substrate concentration is plotted against the reciprocal of that concentration.

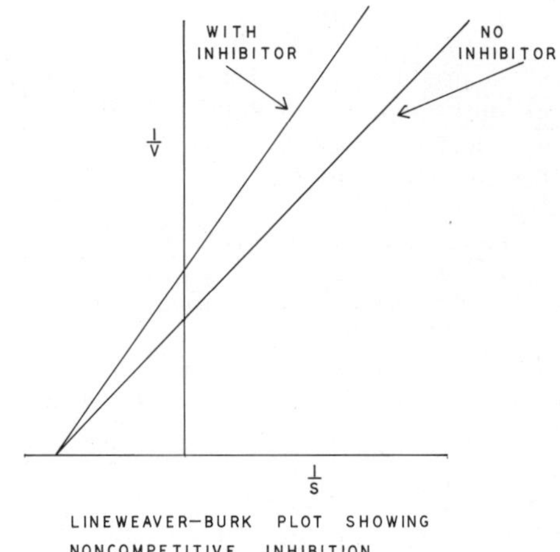

Figure 7–5 Lineweaver-Burk plot showing noncompetitive inhibition.

capable of binding to the active site of the enzyme. Once formed, however, the enzyme-inhibitor complex cannot proceed with the formation of a product and release of the enzyme. This type of inhibition is often important in the intracellular control of reactions, in which the rising concentration of the end-result of a series of linked reactions slows down the earlier stages in order to limit the final concentration of the product. Competitive inhibition is studied by constructing a series of Lineweaver-Burk plots in the presence of rising concentrations of the inhibitor. The typical features of such a plot are shown in Figure 7–4. The slopes of the lines increase (indicating reducing activity, since this is a reciprocal plot), but the intercept on the vertical axis, which is a measure of the V_{max}, does not change. This means that no matter how much inhibitor is added, in theory V_{max} for the enzyme always can be obtained by increasing the ratio of substrate molecules to inhibitor molecules. The effect of the competitive inhibitor is to change the apparent K_M value.

If a similar series of Lineweaver-Burk plots is produced by the addition of a substance to an enzyme-substrate mixture, but the form of the graph is as shown

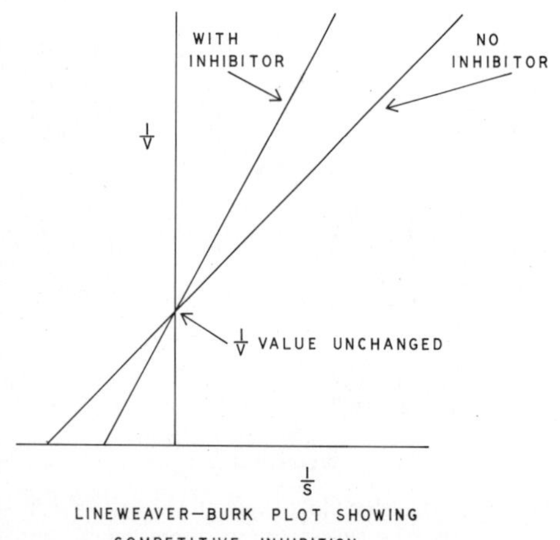

Figure 7–4 Lineweaver-Burk plot showing competitive inhibition.

in Figure 7–5, and if the effect *cannot* be reversed by increasing substrate concentration, the inhibition is said to be *noncompetitive*. Competitive inhibition is fairly easy to visualize; two structurally similar molecules compete for an active site that is unable to distinguish between them, and the effect on the enzyme activity will depend on which of the two compounds has the larger number of molecules available for combination. In noncompetitive inhibition, the interference with enzyme action is not caused by permanent disruption of essential three-dimensional structure, as with iodoacetamide, but probably involves binding of the inhibitor to a region of the enzyme molecule distinct from the true active site or chelation by a compound such as ethylenediaminotetraacetate (EDTA) of a metal ion necessary for enzyme activity. The rapidly lethal effect of the cyanide ion to a large extent is owing to its combination with ferric or ferrous ions essential to the cytochrome system of nearly all cells.

Isoenzymes

The general importance of the enzyme lactate dehydrogenase in cell metabolism is shown by its occurrence in all tissues of the body, including red cells. The basic reaction catalyzed is the same—the removal of two hydrogens from lactate to yield pyruvate:

$$\begin{array}{l} CH_3 \\ | \\ CHOH \\ | \\ COO^- \end{array} + NAD^+ \rightleftharpoons \begin{array}{l} CH_3 \\ | \\ CO \\ | \\ COO^- \end{array} + NADH + H^+$$

The released hydrogen ions are taken up by the coenzyme nicotinamide-adenine dinucleotide (NAD), which is thereby reduced to NADH. The course of the reaction can be followed by monitoring the rate of NADH production at 340 nm. If the kinetic characteristics of lactate dehydrogenase extracted from different tissues are determined, different K_M values are obtained. The effect of varying substrate concentration is different, and the effect of inhibitors such as urea varies. In addition, the various members of the lactate dehydrogenase group differ physically, as demonstrated by their different electrophoretic mobility based on variations in molecular charge.

Consideration of the above leads to a working definition. If a particular reaction is catalyzed by an enzyme that exists in different tissues of a single species in a group of genetically determined separable forms, the members of that group are called isoenzymes. It should be noted that this definition excludes enzymes with catalytic activity against a group of chemically related substances, such as the esterases. The lactate dehydrogenase enzyme molecule can be split by such agents as 12 M urea or 5 M guanidine hydrochloride into four subunits, each with a molecular weight of about 35,000. Coupled with the demonstration that the five types of lactate dehydrogenase isolated from various human tissues showed a pattern of amino acid composition that paralleled their electrophoretic mobility (the types with the higher proportion of acidic amino acids such as valine and aspartic acid migrated toward the positive electrode with the higher velocity), this led to the theory, since amply confirmed, that the five varieties of lactate dehydrogenase were derived by combining in different ratios two basic kinds of subunits, usually called M and H. From these two subunits, five different arrangements can be made: 4 M's, 3 M's plus 1 H, 2 M's plus 2 H's, 1 M plus 3 H's, and 4 H's. The type with 4 M's has the slowest electrophoretic mobility, is typical of muscle and liver, and is often called LDH_5; the variety with 4 H's has the fastest electrophoretic mobility, is typical of heart tissue, and is often called LDH_1.

Although the existence of isoenzymes has been demonstrated in most of the enzymes of medical importance, their separation as an aid to diagnosis is used for lactate dehydrogenase, creatine kinase, and, to some extent, alkaline phosphatase. This aspect will be discussed in more detail as part of the description of the individual enzymes.

One practical problem in assay of enzymes, that of suitable standards and controls, is caused, at least in part, by the addition of enzymes of animal origin, with kinetic and isoenzyme properties differing from those of human enzymes, to commercial control sera. If the stated assay values were determined by the manufacturer using the optimum conditions for the *animal* enzyme, it is obviously questionable to use the value to control an assay system designed for *human* enzymes. This point will be discussed later on.

Enzyme Determinations—Practical Considerations

The overall purposes of determinations of enzymes in body fluids are to provide evidence of a disease process, of the anatomical location of the abnormality, assistance in delineation of the cause of the illness, assessment of the extent and severity of the problem, control of treatment, and, as often as possible, proof of recovery. The same or similar purposes could be assigned to most laboratory procedures; enzyme assays have the special advantage of reflecting intracellular processes more closely. Determinations of serum sodium give some information on sodium levels in the interstitial fluid, and indirectly in the intracellular fluid, but this information is secondhand at best. A sharp rise in the LDH_1 moiety of serum lactate dehydrogenase indicates a lesion in the heart muscle with high specificity. A rise in serum gamma-glutamyltranspeptidase is nearly specific for liver disease. The main limitation of the clinical usefulness of enzyme assays is the mass of practical difficulties inherent in the methodology.

Problems with a piece of laboratory equipment, especially an automated one, may arise from the design characteristics. Autodilutors employing peristaltic pumps are much more prone to blockage than types using syringes, for example. Similarly, difficulties with enzyme determinations are usually associated with the inherent properties of a catalytic protein.

Properties of Enzymes

1. The statement that "all enzymes are proteins" is still unchallenged. The success in preparing enzymes as pure crystalline proteins, initiated by Sumner in 1926, has reinforced the dogma. The main reason for not regarding the nonprotein coenzymes as enzymes is that the activity they exhibit is based on their function as carriers; they do not possess the elaborate three-dimensional molecular structure necessary for specific activation. Enzymes have the general chemical and physical properties of proteins, including instability to heat, radiation, violent agitation, extremes of pH, organic solvents such as alcohol, and strong oxidizing and reducing agents. The specific effects of strong urea and guanidine hydrochloride solutions in splitting proteins into separate subunits, usually long polypeptide chains, have already been mentioned in connection with isoenzymes. (The fact that enzymes can be separated by electrophoresis does not prove their protein nature; the same property is shown by amino acids, for example.)

2. Many enzymes will operate only with the assistance of a nonprotein cofactor. This cofactor may be a simple inorganic or metallic ion, in which case it is called an "activator"; a good example is the association of amylase and the chloride ion. If the chloride ion is removed from a preparation by dialysis, the amylase becomes inactive; the activity is restored if the chloride ion is replaced.

When the cofactor is a complex organic compound, often a nucleotide (a combination of a nitrogen-containing heterocyclic compound such as the purine adenine, a sugar, usually ribose, and one or more phosphate groups), the relationship with the enzyme is rather more complex. Since such a substance (called a coenzyme) does undergo some chemical change during the reaction, typically from its oxidized to its reduced form, it might be regarded as a substrate; but since at the end of the series of linked reactions it reappears unchanged, it is also a cofactor. In some cases the coenzyme is so closely attached to the enzyme, for whose activity the close attachment is essential, that it is called a "prosthetic group." The implication of the term is that the coenzyme functions as a "tool" for the action of the enzyme. In these cases the enzyme, inactive alone, is called the "apoenzyme"; in active combination with its prosthetic group it is called the "holoenzyme." For example, the heme group is essential for the activity of such enzymes as the cytochrome oxidases and peroxidases. (The reaction usually employed for the detection of occult blood in feces utilizes the ability of the heme portion of hemoglobin to catalyze the release of oxygen from a peroxide, mimicking the action of a peroxidase.) It has been suggested that the criterion for differentiation between true prosthetic groups and coenzyme carriers is their behavior during the complete catalytic cycle. A prosthetic group remains firmly attached to its apoenzyme; a coenzyme carrier shuttles from one enzyme to another.

3. A conspicuous feature of enzyme-catalyzed reactions is their speed. The term "turnover number" has been used as a measure of the quantity of substrate changed; owing to the development of two different methods of stating this parameter, based respectively on the number of molecules of substrate per molecule of enzyme or per number of active catalytic sites, the Commission on Enzymes of the International Union of Biochemistry proposed two new definitions:

MOLECULAR ACTIVITY. The number of molecules of substrate transformed per minute by one molecule of enzyme.

CATALYTIC CENTER ACTIVITY. The number of molecules of substrate transformed per minute per catalytic center. The value of the molecular activity can vary from as low as 50 per minute to as high as 5×10^6. The highest known molecular activity is that of carbonic anhydrase: 3.6×10^7. This is not surprising in view of the role of this enzyme in catalyzing carbon dioxide release from the red cell during its very brief time in the lung circulation, a matter of a few seconds at most.

4. Enzyme reactions are customarily referred to as reversible. A distinction should be made between an enzyme reaction carried out as an isolated system in a test tube and the same reaction taking place in the highly complex circumstances of the living cell. In the first case, by altering the conditions, i.e., nature of substrate, type of coenzyme present, and reaction, lactate dehydrogenase can be used either to remove two hydrogens from lactate to form pyruvate or to add two hydrogens to pyruvate to form lactate. Both directions have been used as the basis of assay methods. In the cell, an enzyme reaction does not take place as an isolated phenomenon but as an integral part of a scheme for energy production, synthesis, mechanical motion (muscle), or electrical activity (nerve). In the red cell, the reaction goes mainly in the pyruvate to lactate direction. The concentration of lactate is some 50 to 60 times that of pyruvate. In the liver cell, the conversion of lactate to pyruvate is the first step in the synthesis of glucose needed to restore glycogen reserves used up in heavy muscular activity. In addition, the direction of an enzyme reaction may be governed by the availability of coenzymes and their restriction from some regions of a cell by poor diffusibility in and out of the mitochondrion. From a practical point of view, the direction of a reaction used for assay purposes is ensured by providing correct substrate level, adequate coenzyme concentration, and in some cases a means of removing the reaction product to prevent this from inhibiting the reaction.

5. Although it is true that enzymes exhibit greater specificity than inorganic catalysts, complete specificity of an enzyme for a single substrate is unusual. The best common example is urease, which is quite specific for urea and will not attack even closely related compounds. The majority of enzymes show specificity of function; i.e., a dehydrogenase catalyzes an oxidation-reduction reaction involving hydrogen transfer, but the substrate is often a member of a group whose members are chemically related. Lactate dehydrogenase will attack betahydroxybutyrate, which is similar in structure to lactate.

$$\begin{array}{c} CH_3 \\ | \\ CHOH \\ | \\ COOH \end{array} \qquad \begin{array}{c} CH_3 \\ | \\ CHOH \\ | \\ CH_2 \\ | \\ COOH \end{array}$$

Lactic acid *Beta-hydroxybutyric acid*

One of the isoenzymes of lactate dehydrogenase, the "fast" LDH_1, shows this ability to a greater extent than the other four variants, and an increase in total serum LDH that arises mainly from this fraction is regarded as indicative of heart tissue as the source.

The ability of such enzymes as alkaline phosphatase to split inorganic phosphate from a wide range of organic phosphate esters has permitted the development of an equally wide range of methods for assay. In some instances the lack of true specificity leads to problems. It is difficult to be sure that the determination of cholinesterase is not affected by the presence of less specific esterases in the sample. In one respect enzymes show remarkable specificity. If a substrate exists as two stereo-isomers, differing only in the spatial arrangement of their constituent atoms, only one form is subject to enzyme attack. Thus lactate dehydrogenase will not attack the D stereo-isomer of lactic acid, only the L form. This type of specificity reflects the high degree of discrimination shown by the substrate recognition site on the enzyme molecule.

6. Some enzymes, typically those produced for digestion, are synthesized in inactive forms called "zymogens." The gastric proteolytic enzyme pepsin is manufactured in the chief cells of the gastric mucosa, with its activity masked by an extra 42-member amino acid chain attached to its NH_2 terminal end. This "pepsinogen" is rapidly converted to the active form, initially by the high acidity of the gastric fluids, followed by an "autocatalytic" activity of the pepsin thus formed on the remaining pepsinogen. In this process the masking chain is split off. The conversion of the acid-catalyzed initial pepsinogen to pepsin does not take place inside the chief cells, because the hydrogen ion concentration there is too low.

7. The following factors affect the rate of enzyme reactions.

Temperature

The majority of chemical reactions are accelerated by increase of temperature, since the increased molecular activity increases the frequency of molecular contact, and the number of molecules with sufficient energy to react increases. With enzyme reactions, two main processes are operating; one is the increase in the number of molecules with a high energy value as the temperature is raised; the other, the increasing effect of heat denaturation of the enzyme protein. Thus the velocity of the reaction will increase almost linearly with temperature for a time; thereafter the activity will decrease and finally cease. Over the temperature range in which protein denaturation is not serious, enzymes typically double their rate of activity for a temperature rise of 10°C. It is obvious that close control of temperature in enzyme assays is essential. The actual temperature chosen for an assay will depend on several factors. It must be well below denaturation temperature; it must be high enough to produce a rate of change susceptible to accurate measurement (one of the problems with serum aldolase measurement is the low activity at temperatures below 37°C); and the rate of reaction should not be so rapid that the practical range of values measurable is limited. Owing to the effect of changing substrate concentration on enzyme activity, too rapid a reaction rate will deplete the substrate to the point where the reaction is no longer linear (see *Substrate Concentration* below). The chosen operating temperature must be maintained closely; the variation should not be more than ±0.1°C.

Substrate Concentration

For accurate measurement of the rate of an enzyme reaction, it is necessary that that rate does not change during the course of the assay. We have already seen how the Michaelis-Menten equation can be used to calculate the ratio of reaction velocity at a given substrate concentration to the velocity that would be obtained at a substrate concentration sufficient to saturate the enzyme with substrate molecules. If we make the substrate concentration 20 times the K_M value for a particular enzyme, the reaction velocity will be 95% of maximum. If the reaction is allowed to proceed for a length of time that will permit accurate measurement of the product, and if this causes the concentration of substrate to fall by 10%, we can calculate the effect this fall will have on the reaction rate. At the starting concentration $= 20 \times K_M$, $v = 0.95$, or 95% of the maximum. At the end of the reaction time, substrate concentration has fallen to $18 \times K_M$, and the reaction velocity $v = 94.7\%$ of the maximum. The change is small and could be ignored. The practical problem arises with a substrate of limited solubility and an enzyme with a high K_M.

Hydrogen Ion Concentration—pH

Although some enzymes maintain high activity over a range of pH values, for example, the hydrolysis of sucrose by invertase, the majority of enzymes of clinical significance show a peak activity at a well-defined pH value. Changes in pH affect the state of ionization of those portions of the three-dimensional shape of the enzyme molecule that are concerned with the catalytic activity and may also influence the features of the substrate molecule that are similarly involved. There may also be a direct effect of pH on the K_M value of the enzyme.

The so-called optimum pH for an enzyme will vary according to the substrate and buffer used in a particular assay method. This is one of the factors that make interconversion of units between methods a matter of some difficulty.

The buffer system used in an assay must be able to maintain the pH within ±0.05 unit during the course of the procedure. It should not interfere with the reaction, and it should be chemically stable.

Activators and Inhibitors

In practical terms, activators are simple substances, often inorganic ions, that accelerate a reaction. If the presence of the substance is essential for the reaction, it is more properly regarded as a cofactor. Amylase requires chloride ion in order to function. Alkaline phosphatase does not have such an absolute requirement for magnesium ions, but their presence produces greater catalytic activity. It is obvious that a known activator should be incorporated in an enzyme assay system.

Inhibitors present a different problem. We have seen previously that an inhibitor may be a permanent enzyme "poison," and if a substance of this type is present in a reaction mixture, the result of the assay is liable to be nil. The effect of a competitive inhibitor is to change the apparent K_M value; thus a substrate concentration calculated to be sufficiently large to give a reaction rate close to maximum will, in the presence of a competitive inhibitor, be less than adequate, leading to results both too low and nonlinear. The noncompetitive type of inhibitor affects the actual velocity of the reaction, but the end result—low values—will be the same. In some cases excessive levels of an activator may cause inhibition. From a practical point of view, an attempt should be made to exclude such known inhibitors as heavy metal ions (silver, mercury, copper, lead), and arsenic and cyanide. Only reagents of high purity should be used to make enzyme assay substrates and buffers.

Time

The general rule that a longer reaction time gives a greater product yield is offset in enzyme determinations by the fall in reaction velocity as the substrate concentration drops; incubation times have to be kept as short as possible to avoid this source of error. The widespread use of automatic analyzers with sensitive photometric systems permits reaction times as short as 30 seconds, and the incorporation in the control programs of these instruments of detection of substrate depletion alerts the operator to the need to dilute the original sample for a repeat analysis. The automation of enzyme determinations also provides precise timing of incubation and termination of the reaction when end-point rather than kinetic measurements are being made. If a manual method is used, the technologist must establish accurate timing of the method by such techniques as the mixing of sample and substrate at timed intervals, with termination of the reaction in an identical manner. The possibility of inaccuracy of the timer used should not be overlooked, and periodic checking against a good stopwatch is advisable.

Enzyme Concentration

Logically, if a test serum contains twice as much of an enzyme as another sample, it should produce twice the amount of measurable chemical or other change in the substrate, and in the majority of cases this is true. When there are apparent deviations from this condition, the reasons often lie in the method of assay. In the kinetic method of determination of the aminotransferases, when the reaction catalyzed by the enzyme being measured is coupled to another reaction, also enzymatic, which involves a change in a coenzyme (NADH to NAD), this can be followed by the absorbance decrease at 340 nm. If the activity of the aminotransferase is very high, the overall velocity of the system may be limited by the capacity of the second reaction. This problem can be overcome quite simply by reducing the size of the sample.

Factors Affecting Choice of Method

The "ideal" method for assay of an enzyme would have the following features:

1. Simplicity, involving the minimum number of pipetting and other operations.
2. Accuracy adequate for the purposes of the determination (e.g., clinical diagnosis), and precision adequate to justify confidence in the results.
3. Ready adaptability to automated or semi-automated techniques. Suitability for batch working.
4. Ready availability of stable reagents.
5. Linear relationship between measured chemical or other change and enzyme concentration over a wide range of values.
6. Availability of suitable standards and controls.
7. Specificity for the enzyme to be assayed.

It is doubtful if any method meets all these criteria, but the situation has been considerably improved by the development of so-called optimized methods that combine the best available substrates and buffers to meet the features listed above, by improvements in the commercial products in respect to lyophilization and stability, and, most important, by the strides in automation, making true or pseudokinetic assays practical. (By "pseudokinetic" is meant a procedure in which the enzyme reaction is monitored between two fixed times and the linearity during that time is assumed.) Even where manual methods are still in use, the availability of sensitive, high-purity synthetic substrates such as phenolphthalein and thymolphthalein monophosphates and *p*-nitrophenyl phosphate plus the provision of narrow band-pass, stable spectrophotometers fitted with flow cells provide clinically useful determinations.

Enzyme Unit Values

The problem of reporting enzyme estimation results remains. Each method has its own arbitrary unit, valid for that procedure alone. It is not practical—or in most cases even possible—to determine the actual concentration of an enzyme, and measurements can be made only in terms of the amount of measurable chemical or other change that the enzyme produces under fixed conditions. Some attempt has been made to bring order into the confusion of enzyme activity units, and the recommendations of the International Union of Biochemistry are described here.

For most clinical chemistry determinations, suitable standards in pure form are available. In contrast, pure preparations of enzymes are either nonexistent, very expensive, or not identical to the enzyme being estimated. At the present time the only clarification possible of the rather chaotic situation in enzyme reporting is more precise definition of the arbitrary units. To this end the Joint Subcommission on Clinical Enzyme Units of the International Union of Biochemistry and the International Union of Pure and Applied Chemistry recommend that the activity of an enzyme be expressed as the micromols of substrate transformed per minute by one liter of serum or other fluid under specified conditions of time, temperature, pH, substrate concentration, presence of activators, and ionic concentration. In cases in which the exact molecular weight of the substrate is not known, the micromols of measured product released may be used. For enzymes determined by reference to the measurement of absorbance change caused by change in the associated coenzymes from the oxidized to the reduced form or vice versa, the activity is defined in terms of the micromols of reduced nicotinamide-adenine dinucleotide (NADH) or of reduced nicotinamide-adenine phosphate dinucleotide (NADPH) formed or destroyed per minute per liter of serum or other fluid.

The following examples illustrate the calculations. In the Bodansky method for determination of alkaline phosphatase, one Bodansky unit is equivalent to 1 mg of phosphorus released from beta-glycerol phosphate in one hour by 100 mL of serum. One milligram of phosphorus contains 1000/31 micromols; dividing by 60 gives the micromols per minute, and multiplying by 10 gives the amount per liter. Thus one Bodansky unit corresponds to $\frac{1000}{31} \times \frac{1}{60} \times 10 = 5.38$ micromols inorganic phosphorus released per minute per liter of serum. Therefore Bodansky units multiplied by 5.38 equals International Units (I.U.) of enzyme activity.

Isocitric dehydrogenase (ICD) activity is measured by following the increase in absorbance at 340 nm owing to the formation of reduced NADP resulting from the action of the enzyme on isocitrate in the presence of manganous ions at 25°C. One micromol (i.e., one millionth of a mol) of reduced NADP has an absorbance in a 1-cm cuvette of 6.22 at 340 nm. If the absorbance change per minute is divided by 6.22, this will give the micromols of reduced NADP formed, when the total volume of the reaction mixture and the amount of serum are taken into account. The final expression is:

$$\frac{\text{Absorbance increase per minute}}{6.22} \times \frac{\text{Volume of mixture}}{\text{Volume of serum used}} \times 1000 = \text{Micromols of reduced NADP formed per minute per liter}$$

If the reaction mixture volume is 3.0 mL, and this contains 0.5 mL serum, each increase in absorbance of 0.001 corresponds to 0.96 micromol of reduced NADP formed per minute per liter, and this equals 0.96 I.U.

In the *Recommendations (1972) of the Commission on Biochemical Nomenclature on the Nomenclature and Classification of Enzymes together with their Units and the Symbols of Enzyme Kinetics,* new proposals were made in the field of expression of enzymatic-catalytic activity. The new unit advocated is the "katal," defined as the amount of activity that converts one mole of substrate per second. One International Unit (that amount of enzyme which will catalyze the transformation of one micromole of the substrate per minute under standard conditions) is equivalent to 16.67 "nanokatals" (symbol nkat). It is not possible to decide at this time whether the International Unit or the katal will become the accepted usage. The katal has the advantage of better consonance with the Système International (SI) set of basic units, but the introduction of International Units into laboratory medicine has created enough problems to make the practical laboratory scientist hesitate before making still another change.

Nomenclature of Enzymes and Coenzymes

The initial proposals for standardization of unit values have been discussed, and these brief notes are designed to introduce the technologist to the recommendations of the International Union of Biochemistry for the systematic naming of enzymes and coenzymes. The necessity of this procedure arises from the existence of at least 1770 well-characterized and distinct enzymes. Only time will determine if the new names will displace the old trivial ones in common clinical and laboratory usage. The replacement of the coenzyme names diphosphopyridine nucleotide (DPN) and triphosphopyridine nucleotide (TPN) by the new names nicotinamide-adenine dinucleotide (NAD) and nicotinamide-adenine dinucleotide phosphate (NADP) is already generally accepted, mainly because the old names were chemically inaccurate. The nomenclature of the cytochromes is still under review, with only pro tempore recommendations, but this does not greatly affect clinical biochemistry at present.

The guiding principles of the new system may be briefly stated as follows:

The overall reaction catalyzed by the enzyme is the basis of the name.

Each enzyme will be specifically designated by a code number with four elements. The first figure in the code places the enzyme in one of six main groups:

1. Oxidoreductases
2. Transferases
3. Hydrolases
4. Lyases
5. Isomerases
6. Ligases (synthetases)

Oxidoreductases are enzymes catalyzing oxidation-reduction reactions; the commonest examples are the dehydrogenases. Transferases catalyze the transfer of a chemical group from one substance to another. The common example is aspartate aminotransferase. Hydrolases are hydrolyzing enzymes that split a substrate, such as an ester, by the introduction of the elements of water into the structure. An example is acetylcholinesterase. Lyases remove groups from substrates without hydrolysis, leaving double bonds in the molecular structure of the product. Decarboxylases, such as pyruvate decarboxylase, are typical members of this class.

Isomerases catalyze intramolecular rearrangement of the substrate compound. A typical member of this group interconverts glyceraldehyde-3-phosphate and dihydroxyacetone phosphate.

Ligases catalyze the joining together of two substrate molecules, with the simultaneous breakdown of a pyrophosphate bond in adenosine triphosphate or a similar substance. At present no enzyme of clinical importance belongs to this group.

The second figure element of the code gives more specific information about the enzyme. For example, in the transferase group the second figure element indicates the nature of the group transferred.

The third figure element of the code gives more specific detail about such things as the type of acceptor molecule for an oxidoreductase or the precise chemical type of the group transferred by a transferase.

The fourth figure element is the serial number of the enzyme in the class as indicated by the third figure element.

For example, the enzyme with the code number 2.6.1.2 is a member of group 2, the transferases. The second figure element, 6, indicates that the type of group transferred is a nitrogen-containing group. The third figure element indicates that the nitrogen-containing group is an amino group. The fourth figure element indicates that this enzyme is the second member of the amino-group transferases. Its complete systematic name is L-alanine:2-oxoglutarate aminotransferase. Its recommended trivial name is alanine aminotransferase, or ALT. Its old name was glutamic-pyruvic transaminase, or GPT.

For complete details of the nomenclature rules, the published recommendations of the International Union of Biochemistry should be consulted. (Enzyme Nomenclature, Recommendations 1972 of the International Union of Biochemistry. American Elsevier Publishing Co., New York, 1973.)

Abbreviations for Names of Enzymes

For ease of communication, both verbal and written, a variety of abbreviations of enzyme names are commonly used. It is probable that many clinicians will still be using "OT" for aspartate aminotransferase and "PT" for alanine aminotransferase for some time to come, and rigid insistence on the part of the laboratory staff on the use of either the new names or the proposed new abbreviations, AST and ALT, will not hasten their general acceptance. Only the test of usage will determine the viability of a technical term. We include here some items from the proposed list but do not actively advocate their unilateral replacement of the older terms (Table 7–1).

Nomenclature of Coenzymes

As noted previously, the nicotinamide nucleotide coenzymes are now known by names that are chemically correct. Thus diphosphopyridine nucleotide (DPN, coenzyme I, cozymase) is now called nicotinamide-adenine dinucleotide (NAD), and triphosphopyridine nucleotide (TPN, coenzyme II, phosphocozymase) is now designated nicotinamide-adenine dinucleotide phosphate (NADP). The reduced forms of the coenzymes are expressed as reduced NAD and reduced NADP, unless the actual change in ionization is to be indicated. In the latter case the forms NADH + H^+ and NADPH + H^+ are used.

TABLE 7–1 ABBREVIATIONS FOR NAMES OF SOME ENZYMES OF DIAGNOSTIC IMPORTANCE

E. C. Number	Trivial Name	Abbreviation
1.1.1.1	Alcohol dehydrogenase	AD
1.1.1.27	Lactate dehydrogenase	LD
———	Hydroxybutyrate dehydrogenase	HBD
1.1.1.42	Isocitrate dehydrogenase	ICD
1.1.1.49	Glucose-6-phosphate dehydrogenase	GPD
1.11.1.6	Catalase	CTS
2.1.3.3	Ornithine carbamyl transferase	OCT
2.6.1.1	Aspartate aminotransferase	AST
2.6.1.2	Alanine aminotransferase	ALT
2.7.1.40	Pyruvate kinase	PK
2.7.3.2	Creatine kinase	CK
3.1.1.3	Lipase	LPS
3.1.1.8	Cholinesterase	CHS
3.1.3.1	Alkaline phosphatase	ALP
3.1.3.2	Acid phosphatase	ACP
3.1.3.5	5′-Nucleotidase	NTP
3.2.1.1	Amylase	AMS
3.4.11.1	Leucine aminopeptidase	LAS
3.4.23.1	Pepsin	PPS
3.5.3.1	Arginase	ARS
3.4.21.4	Trypsin	TPS
3.5.4.3	Guanine deaminase	GDS
4.1.2.13	Aldolase	ALS
4.2.1.1	Carbonic anhydrase	CAS

STANDARDIZATION OF ENZYME DETERMINATIONS

Even though there is at least partial agreement on a definition of a unit of enzyme activity, as long as the only *practical* way of measuring the enzyme content of a sample is in terms of the amount of chemical change produced, there will be a problem of standardization. The trend in standardization of automated methods on some of the new multichannel instruments is to use sera whose content of such chemically well-defined substances as glucose and urea has been accurately established by reducing the original level to very low values by various means and then "weighing in" the desired amounts. The use of a similar system for enzyme standards has brought forth the objections that the weighed-in enzymes are of animal rather than human origin, with different reaction characteristics and isoenzyme patterns. If an enzyme assay system involves a coenzyme such as NAD or NADH, since the transformation of one mole of substrate is usually accompanied by that of one mole of coenzyme, the majority of automated methods use a factor derived from the known molar absorbance of the coenzyme, converting the measurement of absorbance change during the course of the timed reaction into its equivalent in micromoles of substrate transformed per minute. (See under *Enzyme Unit Values* above.) The objection can be raised that there is no absolute check on the purity of the coenzyme used to determine its molar absorbance. In some instances, e.g., *p*-nitrophenyl phosphate as a substrate for alkaline phosphatase determination, the product of the reaction, *p*-nitrophenol, is obtainable in pure form, and the method can be calibrated by reference to its known micromolar concentrations. It must be pointed out that this is not a true primary standardization; this could only be done with pure human alkaline phosphatase enzyme, if it were available. The same problems arise in obtaining suitable controls for enzyme determinations. If the control serum is a lyophilized human serum, the enzymes are of human origin but the assayed values are not known with absolute certainty; if it is an animal serum, with weighed-in enzymes from animal sources, its characteristics may differ from those in the test samples. However, such controls are adequate for their primary purpose, which is to check on precision, and careful inspection of the control charts for shifts in the mean will at least raise the possibility of a loss of accuracy (see p. 47). The use of control sera as standards has been advocated, since this would correct errors due to temperature or timing faults; but the use of nonhuman sources of the added enzymes involves the problems mentioned above. The reliability of commercial enzyme controls has improved to the point where recovery of the stated levels with the specified equipment and methodology affords acceptable confidence in patient results.

Temperature Correction Factors

The instruction leaflets included in many commercial kits and reagent sets for assay of enzymes usually have a table purporting to provide a convenient set of multiplying factors to convert results obtained at one temperature to the values that would be obtained at the chosen temperature of the procedure. However, the situation is not as simple as it is made to appear. As the temperature of assay changes, the conditions for optimal conditions also change, such as substrate concentration and pH. The reason is partly the occurrence of most enzymes as families of isoenzymes, whose individual optimal conditions differ. To quote King, "an assay performed under optimal conditions at 25° and then corrected to 30° will not yield the same value as an assay conducted at 30° under the optimal conditions pertaining to 30°." In practical terms the point is perhaps a minor one, but it is one more argument for international agreement on a firm standardized assay temperature. One proposal is to use the melting point of the rare metal gallium (approximately 29.77°C) as the standard temperature, since this would provide a fixed reference at a temperature suitable for the majority of clinical enzyme assays. Implementation of this suggestion would require both international acceptance of the principle and technological solution of the practical difficulties.

Interference with Enzyme Assays

When this is known it will be noted in the discussion of the individual enzymes. Charts summarizing the effects of common anticoagulants are published by at least two commercial sources.* For at least four enzyme assays it has been shown that there is no significant difference in the accuracy and precision when either water or saline is used to dilute high-activity sera prior to reassay.

Enzymes as Reagents

The use of enzymes as analytical reagents has greatly increased since the days, over 30 years ago, when the urease contained in finely ground soya or jack beans was used in the Van Slyke–Cullen method for urea nitrogen determination. Some enzyme properties—such as specificity for substrate, activity at low temperatures, and sensitivity when the reaction can be measured or followed by the large absorbance changes at 340 nm associated with oxidation-reduction state changes in coenzymes—appear well suited to biochemical analyses. In some cases, an enzymatic method requires fewer steps. A good example is the development of enzymatic systems for serum triglyceride and cholesterol determinations which can be completed in one tube and automated. Such enzyme properties as lack of stability, inactivation by metallic ions, and at times uncertain degrees of purity can produce a new spectrum of problems and sources of error. These errors can be subtle. We have been led astray by a commercial urease preparation that had enough activity for normal and moderately elevated urea nitrogen levels (including *both* our controls), but that seriously underestimated higher values. If a procedure uses coupled enzyme reactions, for example, in the assay of creatine kinase (p. 165), the primary reaction with a serum of very high activity may "take off" at a rate that exceeds the ability of the subsequent reactions in the sequence to "catch up," and the process never achieves a true linear rate. Unlike problems with purely chemical reactions, these and other problems are not self-advertising. In the methods described in this text, the effects of deterioration of enzyme reagents will be noted when known.

A recent application of the "enzyme reagent" principle is the so-called EMIT method (see p. 93).

The use of enzymes as reagents is not, of course, confined to clinical chemistry. The proteolytic enzymes bromelin, papain, and trypsin are used extensively in blood bank procedures. Histological staining procedures for polysaccharides are controlled by processing duplicate sections in which the substance concerned is converted to nonstaining products by such enzymes as diastase, hyaluronidase, or sialidase. The use of the enzymatic equipment of the yeast cell in the manufacture of bread and the conversion of fermentable sugars to ethyl alcohol give the principle a respectable tradition.

*Boehringer Mannheim Diagnostics, Inc., Indianapolis, Ind. 46250 and Dorval, Que. H9P 1A9; Gilford Instrument Laboratories, Inc., Oberlin, Ohio 44074 and Mississauga, Ont. L4W 1X9.

Urinary Enzyme Determinations

Apart from amylase, uropepsin, and arylsulfatase A (in detection of metachromatic leukodystrophy), urine enzyme assays have not been used widely in diagnosis. The reasons are partly technical (i.e., urine contains unknown enzyme inhibitors that have to be removed by dialysis, and the levels of enzymes are often low) and partly clinical (i.e., evidence of renal disease usually is sought by other means). The development of reliable methods for the assay of enzymes specifically related to renal tissue, such as arginine-ornithinetransaminase and *N*-acetyl-beta-glucosaminase, could change this picture. For a discussion of this topic, the technologist is referred to the review article by Raab (1972).

CHARACTERISTICS AND MEASUREMENT OF SERUM ENZYMES OF CLINICAL IMPORTANCE

In the following discussion, unavoidably brief, attention is concentrated on the enzymes whose presence in the serum generally reflects their release in above normal amounts from damaged cells. It is pertinent to consider the processes by which cellular enzymes gain access to the serum or plasma, especially with the recent growth in the use of panels of tests designed to pinpoint a particular organ as the site of a disease process. (The following is based on the review article by Posen, 1970, which should be consulted for greater detail.)

Under normal conditions, the level of an enzyme in the circulating plasma remains reasonably constant. This implies that there is an equilibrium between the processes of release into the blood and the mechanisms of removal. If the level rises, this could imply either increased release—the usual assumption—or decreased removal; it may also involve change in the isoenzyme pattern in which a component of high activity in the assay system used replaces one of lower activity.

Three processes may be involved in removal of enzymes from the circulation: binding or trapping by tissues close to the circulation system, mixing of plasma enzymes into the fluids of other compartments, and denaturation by peptidases or other unknown processes. The existence of factors other than simple excessive release and removal can be suspected from the poor correlation in many instances between the enzyme pattern of a tissue and that of the plasma following a lesion of that tissue. In some cases there is a purely quantitative effect, e.g., the amount of aspartate aminotransferase released from a few grams of infarcted heart muscle obviously will be much smaller than that released from several hundred grams of diseased liver.

In the case of amylase, this enzyme has a relatively low molecular weight (about 45,000) and is rapidly excreted by the kidney, although this does not account completely for the rate of removal. The exception to this is the occurrence of an abnormal form of amylase with a much greater molecular weight (about 200,000); its inability to pass the glomerular membrane produces the condition of macroamylasemia, with elevated serum amylase and reduced urine amylase. It has been postulated that the increased molecular size of the macroamylase is caused by the formation of a complex of normal amylase bound to an 11S IgA globulin, possibly as the result of a unique autoimmune reaction.

Another factor that may influence the pattern of plasma enzymes after damage to a particular tissue is the intracellular location. Normally the enzymes of the mitochondria, microsomes, cell wall, and nucleus remain in those structures. It is possible that one or more of these cell organelles is more fragile or more susceptible to damage by a disease process, and this would be reflected by the entry into the plasma of a disproportionate amount of the enzymes associated with that organelle.

In some cases the elevation of a serum enzyme level is iatrogenic, i.e., caused by some medical or surgical procedure. Intramuscular injections of volumes greater than one mL can increase serum CK values to as much as three to five times normal levels. Administration of morphine, codeine, and meperidine causes constriction of the sphincter of Oddi at the junction of the common bile duct and duodenum, and the associated increase in intraductal pressure may elevate levels of serum amylase and lipase. Opiates may raise intrabiliary tract pressure sufficiently so that serum AST and LDH levels may rise, and only the concurrent normal CK value may preclude a diagnosis of myocardial infarction. Extensive surgery of almost any type can elevate the CK from associated muscle trauma. The technologist should bear in mind that increased levels of an enzyme in the serum are not necessarily caused by the "usual" reasons. Very high CK values are found in cerebrovascular accidents as well as in myocardial infarction; high LDH results can be associated with an intravascular hemolytic process, such as sickle cell anemia, or with red cell damage in an artificial heart valve; and very high alkaline phosphatase results, equaling or even exceeding those encountered in obstructive jaundice, may be found in a nonicteric serum in Paget's disease of bone. Details of the stability of various enzymes under different storage conditions are given in Table 7–2.

Enzyme Levels in Cerebrospinal Fluid

The upper limits of normal in I.U. per liter are 13.5 for aspartate aminotransferase (AST), 40 for lactate dehydrogenase, and 58 for malate dehydrogenase. The AST and LDH values are high in bacterial meningitis,

TABLE 7–2 STABILITY OF ENZYMES

Enzyme	Room Temperature	Refrigerator	Deep-Frozen
Acid phosphatase (with added buffer)	5 days	5–7 days	8 days
Alkaline phosphatase (see notes)	5 days	7 days	
Aldolase	5 hours	5 days	15 days
Amylase	5 days	3 months	
Argininosuccinate lyase	6 hours	6 hours	6 days
Cholinesterase	7 days	14 days	3 months
Creatine kinase	12 hours	5 days	1 month
Gamma-glutamyltranspeptidase	5 days	7 days	1 month
Guanase	3 days	14 days	6 months
Isocitrate dehydrogenase	5 days	2 weeks	
Lactate dehydrogenase (see notes)	4 days	Unstable	Unstable
Leucine aminopeptidase	5 days	7 days	1 month
Lipase	7 days	6 weeks	3 months
5′-Nucleotidase	4 days	4 days	3 months
Ornithine carbamoyltransferase	1 day	7 days	6 months
Oxytocinase	4 hours	Unstable	Unstable
Phosphohexose isomerase	4 hours	14 days	
Aminotransferases	3 days	7 days	2 weeks

Stability of Enzymes on Storage

Notes

1. The above table is based on various sources plus our own experience. The figures given are only a guide: there is still much argument in this area.
2. The rate of loss of activity in some cases is related to the height of the initial level.
3. The integrity of isoenzyme patterns is often much less than the stated values: if at all possible sera for such procedures should be processed immediately.
4. The storage of alkaline phosphatase at low temperatures is complicated by the tendency for values to increase (see p. 173).
5. The true stability time will be affected by the handling of the sera—if a rack of sera is removed from refrigeration each day, left out on the bench for even an hour and then returned, the stability of the samples will understandably deteriorate.
6. It has been reported that lactate dehydrogenase has its poorest stability at 0°C (Henry, 1974).
7. The erratic nature of enzyme behavior in storage—as well as other serum constituents—has been shown by various studies.
8. The most extensive and complete source of data on enzyme stability is found in Henry, 1974.

in contrast with the normal or slightly elevated levels that occur in viral infections. Simple concussion does not elevate AST; brain contusion produces elevations of AST and LDH in proportion to the damage. Malignant metastases in the brain elevate AST and LDH values; benign tumors do not. In noncerebral carcinomatous lesions, the associated neuromyopathy typically elevates cerebrospinal fluid AST but not LDH.

In the section that follows, no attempt has been made to give a complete methodology for all enzymes previously discussed. For this, more specialized texts should be consulted (Tietz, 1976; Henry, 1974). The methods given in full illustrate such basic principles as effective buffering, inclusion of activators, preparation of a standard curve, and calculation of units. In actual practice the great majority of enzymes are assayed in the laboratory using the wide range of commercial sets of reagents, usually referred to as "kits." The trend is to the production of such kits designated as "optimized," that is, with that combination of substrate, buffer, coenzyme, activators, and so on that will yield the highest activity and hence the best sensitivity. It should be noted that there is not, as yet, unanimity about what constitutes optimization. Analytical and other sources of incorrect results are less obvious in enzyme assays, and the inclusion of controls, preferably at two levels, is essential, whether the method is an infrequently performed manual procedure or an automated high-volume determination. Whereas in nonenzyme measurements it may be sufficient to run controls at the beginning of the batch, with enzyme assays the controls should also be processed at the end to check for the slow change in accuracy and/or precision usually called "drift."

In the following survey of enzymes of clinical diagnostic importance, the number used in the *Recommendations (1972) of the Commission on Biochemical Nomenclature on the Nomenclature and Classification of Enyzmes together with their Units and the Symbols of Enzyme Kinetics,* published under the title *Enzyme Nomenclature* by Elsevier Publishing Company, New York, 1973, is identified as the E.C. number. The term "trivial name" indicates the shortened form of the full enzyme name suggested for convenience of communication. The name or initials that follow the trivial name are those in common laboratory and medical usage and may be subject to some local variation. The full format is as follows:

Trivial Name (Initials)
E.C. Number Full systematic name
Isoenzyme pattern
Optimum activity pH
Substances that interfere with assays

Data on isoenzyme constitution are taken from the text, *Isoenzymes* (Wilkinson, 1970).

FRUCTOSEBIPHOSPHATE ALDOLASE (ALDOLASE)

E.C. 4.1.2.13 Fructose-1,6-biphosphate D-*glyceraldehyde-3-phosphate lyase*

At least five isoenzymes, formed from three basic subunits. Two isoenzymes in normal serum are demonstrable.

Optimum pH range 6.8 to 7.2.

Citrate and oxalate may give slight interference.

Tissue Sources. Aldolase is found in all cells, since it is an essential enzyme of the glycolytic system, but it is most abundant in skeletal and heart muscle. Within the cell, aldolase is found mainly in the nonparticulate fraction. The liver contains comparatively much less activity, but it has a related enzyme, fructose-1-phosphate aldolase, which, unlike muscle aldolase, is active against both fructose-1-phosphate and fructose-1,6-biphosphate.

Reaction Catalyzed

$$\begin{array}{l} CH_2O\cdot PO(OH)_2 \\ | \\ CO \\ | \\ HOCH \\ | \\ HCOH \\ | \\ HCOH \\ | \\ CH_2O\cdot PO(OH)_2 \end{array} \rightleftharpoons \begin{array}{l} CH_2O\cdot PO(OH)_2 \\ | \\ CO \\ | \\ CH_2OH \end{array} + \begin{array}{l} CHO \\ | \\ HCOH \\ | \\ CH_2O\cdot PO(OH)_2 \end{array}$$

Fructose-1,6-biphosphate *Dihydroxyacetone phosphate* *Glyceraldehyde phosphate*

Range of Normal Values. With the kinetic procedure (see further on) the normal range is 1 to 6 I.U. per liter, using 0.2 mL serum and 3.0 mL substrate at 37°C. (The aldolase activity of normal serum is low, and absorbance change per minute at temperatures below 37°C is too small for accurate measurement. Even at this temperature a kinetic test run time of ten minutes is required.)

Clinical Significance. Serum aldolase levels are greatly elevated in Duchenne-type pseudohypertrophic muscular dystrophy, in contrast to other diseases of muscle. The pattern of the increase is similar to that for creatine kinase; it is highest in the early stages, falling progressively as the disease process advances. It has been postulated that the elevated aldolase values may be caused more by increased permeability of the muscle cells than by increased destruction of muscle tissue.

Serum aldolase is elevated in the early stages of acute hepatitis of either viral or toxic origin. The changes parallel those in the aspartate aminotransferase and alanine aminotransferase. Aldolase levels are usually normal in cirrhosis and obstructive jaundice. There is some evidence that serum aldolase levels may be increased in the presence of an actively growing tumor.

Methods of Estimation. The preferred method for assay of aldolase uses fructose-1,6-biphosphate as the substrate. The enzyme splits the substrate to yield two triose phosphates, dihydroxyacetone phosphate and glyceraldehyde-3-phosphate. The glyceraldehyde-3-phosphate is converted to dihydroxyacetone phosphate by the enzyme triosephosphate isomerase, included in the reaction mixture. A second enzyme in the reaction mixture, glycerolphosphate dehydrogenase, converts the dihydroxyacetone phosphate to glycerol phosphate, a reaction that requires the coenzyme reduced NAD as a source of hydrogen ions. The change in the coenzyme from the reduced to the oxidized form is accompanied by a decrease in absorbance at 340 nm, and the rate of this change is a measure of the activity of aldolase in the serum sample. A commercial kit is available for this method.* Infants have aldolase levels about four times that of adults, and children about twice.

*Calbiochem, La Jolla, Calif. 92037.

CHOLINESTERASE (CHOLINESTERASE)

E.C. 3.1.1.8 *Acylcholine acyl-hydrolase*

Five to seven isoenzymes reported, depending on the technique of separation.

Optimum pH 8.6.

Oxalate, fluoride, and high levels of heparin inhibit the enzyme.

Reactions Catalyzed. The body contains two groups of esterases that are capable of hydrolyzing esters of choline (a nitrogenous alcohol) with various organic acids, such as acetic. The group that hydrolyzes acetylcholine preferentially, with the E.C. number 3.1.1.7. and the systematic name acetylcholine hydrolase, is typically associated with nervous tissue and red blood cells and is of physiological interest because of its possible role in the removal of acetylcholine released at nerve endings during the transfer of nerve impulses to muscle cells in order that further nerve impulses may, in turn, stimulate muscle contraction. Its determination has no clinical applications at present. The reaction shown can be taken as illustrating the general ability of both acetylcholine hydrolase (also called true or Type I cholinesterase) and the enzyme with which we are clinically concerned, cholinesterase (also called pseudocholinesterase or Type II).

$$\underset{\text{Acetylcholine}}{CH_3{\cdot}COOH_2{\cdot}CH_2{\cdot}N(CH_3)_3} + H_2O \rightarrow \underset{\text{Acetic acid}}{CH_3{\cdot}COOH} + \underset{\text{Choline}}{HOCH_2{\cdot}CH_2{\cdot}N(CH_3)_3}$$

Range of Normal Values. The range of normal values depends on the method. With a procedure available commercially* (see under *Method of Estimation*) using butyrylthiocholine iodide as the substrate, the range of normal values at 30°C is 3714 to 11,513 I.U./L, and at 37°C, 4659 to 14,443 I.U./L.

In the investigation of the genetic variants of the enzyme by the use of various inhibitors (see below) the results are reported as percentages of the activity without inhibition.

Clinical Significance. Determinations of serum or plasma cholinesterase activity are usually made in the investigation of poisoning due to organic phosphate insecticides, such as the parathion group, and in cases of sensitivity to the suxamethonium group of muscle relaxant drugs. Decreased levels of plasma or serum cholinesterase are found in liver cell damage, both acute and chronic, but this is not of material diagnostic importance.

In poisoning from organic phosphate compounds the physiological sequence involving acetylcholine release and removal at the neuromuscular junction is blocked by inactivation of the acetylcholinesterase enzyme by the phosphate group. This causes accumulation of acetylcholine at nerve endings and excessive stimulation of the muscle. Both forms of cholinesterase—plasma and red cell—are reduced in blood.

In a small percentage of patients to whom the muscle relaxant suxamethonium (succinylcholine) is administered, the usual rapid hydrolysis of the drug by the serum cholinesterase, which effectively limits its period of action, is impaired, producing a prolonged apneic state necessitating artificial resuscitation. It is now known that the problem is caused by existence of a number of genetic variants of the enzyme. The four possible genes—E_1^u, E_1^a, E_1^s, E_1^f— give rise to 11 different phenotypes (the so-called silent genotype $E_1^s\ E_1^s$ exists in two variants), seven of which are believed to be associated with sensitivity to suxamethonium. Determination of the genotype is done by measuring the extent to which the enzyme activity is affected by inhibitors such as dibucaine and fluoride, plus different buffers such as TRIS and phosphate. In general, the normal type enzyme is inhibited by both dibucaine and fluoride to about 85% and 81%, respectively; the genetic variants causing sensitivity to suxamethonium are inhibited to the extent of about 5 to 77% by dibucaine, while showing varying reactions to fluoride that permit their genotyping.

Method of Estimation. A typical commercially available method* uses butyrylthiocholine iodide as the substrate in a phosphate buffer at pH 7.7. The cholinesterase of the sample splits the substrate to yield thiocholine and butyrate. The reactive sulfhydryl group of the thiocholine reacts with dithiobis (nitrobenzoate) to produce a yellow compound, 2-nitro-5-mercaptobenzoate, with a high absorbance at 410 nm. The level of absorbance after a fixed time or, preferably, the rate of development of the yellow product, is proportional to the activity of the enzyme in the sample. The method is calibrated by reference to the known molar absorbance of the 2-nitro-5-mercaptobenzoate.

ALPHA-AMYLASE (AMYLASE)

E.C. 3.2.1.1 1, 4-αD-*Glucan glucanohydrolase*

Two isoenzymes, associated with pancreatic and salivary origin.

Optimum pH range 6.9 to 7.0.

Citrate, oxalate, fluoride, and EDTA all inhibit amylase.

Tissue Sources. The main sources are pancreas, salivary glands, and perhaps liver; the last-named source is still disputed.

Reaction Catalyzed. Amylase hydrolyzes a wide range of starches, polysaccharides, and the liver storage polymer, glycogen. Starch contains a high proportion of amylose, in which the glucose units are linked between the C-1 of one molecule and the C-4 of another: it is amylose that gives the typical blue color with iodine. Starch also contains amylopectin, which has a branched structure. Whereas amylase can break down amylose almost entirely to the disaccharide maltose, the branched structure of amylopectin limits the attack of the enzyme so that in addition to maltose, some small polymers called "limit dextrins" remain.

Range of Normal Values. See under methods of estimation, p. 234. The use of arbitrary units persists because the calculation of an International Unit would require an accurate molecular weight for the substrate—starch or amylose—plus correction for the incomplete hydrolysis noted earlier.

*"Cholinesterase C-system," Boehringer Mannheim Diagnostics, Inc. Indianapolis, Ind. 46250 and Dorval, Que. H9P 1A9.

*"Cholinesterase C-system," Boehringer Mannheim Diagnostics, Inc. Indianapolis, Ind. 46250 and Dorval, Que. H9P 1A9.

Clinical Significance. See under *Gastrointestinal Tract*, p. 232.

Methods of Estimation. See p. 234. Serum amylase determinations have been successfully automated, using the starch-iodine reaction and the newer methods described on p. 234.

Creatine Kinase (CK)

E.C. 2.7.3.2 ATP, Creatine N-Phosphotransferase

Three isoenzymes have been detected in serum—one originating in muscle, one in brain, and a hybrid formed from one dimeric subunit from each. They are designated, respectively, MM, BB, and MB types. Rather surprisingly, the elevated CK levels found in a variety of acute central nervous system disorders, such as encephalitis and meningitis, have been shown to be caused by the MM isoenzyme.

Optimum pH 9.0 for the creatine to phosphocreatine reaction; optimum pH 6.8 for the phosphocreatine to creatine direction. Oxalate and fluoride inhibit the enzyme; it is also light-sensitive.

Tissue Sources. CK is found mainly in brain, skeletal, and cardiac muscle.

Reaction Catalyzed

Creatine + ATP (adenosine triphosphate) ⇌ Phosphocreatine + ADP (adenosine diphosphate).

Range of Normal Values. The range of normal values depends on the assay system used, and initially the manufacturer's values should be used. With the accumulation of a sufficiently large number of patient results, the locally valid normal ranges, male and female, can be determined by the cumulative frequency plot method. (See under *Quality Control and Statistical Analysis,* p. 49.) Using the method described below, the expected normal range at 37°C is stated as 32 to 250 I.U./L. At 30°C the range is 18 to 164 I.U./L.

Clinical Significance. In addition to the three sources named above, only very small levels of CK are found in other tissues, such as liver, spleen, and red cells. Elevated serum values are thus almost entirely caused by lesions of either cardiac or skeletal muscle. The most striking increases in CK occur in the early stages of Duchenne-type progressive muscular dystrophy, in which levels may be 400 times normal; the elevated serum values often precede definite clinical signs and usually show a slow decrease as the disease limits the physical activity of the patient.

The defective gene responsible for Duchenne-type dystrophy is carried on the X chromosome; thus, as in hemophilia, the condition is exhibited in the affected males and transmitted by the females.

Serum CK assays are widely employed in detection of myocardial infarction. Typically the serum level increases sharply within two to six hours following the infarction to from three to six times the upper limit of normal; the peak elevation occurs about 24 to 36 hours after the event, and thereafter the values rapidly fall until after 48 hours they may be within the normal range. The maximum level attained may be as high as 10 times the upper limit of normal range, and it is roughly correlated with the extent of the infarction. The test is therefore valuable in early diagnosis, but after 36 hours the more sustained elevations of AST and LDH are of more diagnostic significance.

The increased CK values in cerebrovascular accidents (strokes) are often very high (we have seen values of 700 I.U./L) but are not of critical diagnostic importance. A large proportion of hypothyroid patients have elevated CK values, and transient elevations occur after vigorous muscular activity and during labor (obstetrical variety). The effect of intramuscular injections has already been mentioned.

The estimation of serum CK activity is of some value in screening for patients at risk of developing *malignant hyperpyrexia* (also called malignant hyperthermia). During, or shortly after, a general anesthetic, affected individuals develop muscle spasms and an elevation of central body temperature, sometimes as high as 44°C. The mortality is high, even after correction of the associated acidosis and hypovolemia. Many affected individuals have elevated serum CK levels, usually 1.5 to 2 times the upper limit of normal, and many have overt signs of myopathy. Unfortunately, at least 20% of affected individuals have normal serum CK values and no discernible myopathy.

Methods of Estimation. The most practical routine method utilizes the reverse reaction. Initially the CK reacts on creatine phosphate in the presence of ADP to produce creatine and ATP:

$$\text{Creatine phosphate} + \text{ADP} \rightarrow \text{Creatine} + \text{ATP}$$

The ATP then provides the high-energy phosphate to promote the conversion of glucose to glucose-6-phosphate by the enzyme hexokinase:

$$\text{ATP} + \text{glucose} \rightarrow \text{Glucose-6-phosphate} + \text{ADP}$$

To this point there has been no *measurable* change: by reacting the glucose-6-phosphate to 6-phosphogluconate with the enzyme glucose-6-phosphate dehydrogenase, the associated coenzyme NAD is reduced to NADH, and the associated increase in absorbance at 340 nm can be monitored as an index of the overall reaction and hence the activity of the CK.

$$\text{Glucose-6-phosphate} + \text{NAD} \rightarrow \text{6-phosphogluconate} + \text{NADH}$$

It is the practice in methods for CK assay to incorporate added sulfhydryl (—SH) groups in the reaction mixture, usually in the form of cysteine, mercaptoethanol, or dithiothreitol (also called Cleland's reagent). These substances are designed to stabilize the enzyme by maintaining its —SH type cross-linkages, but it has been pointed out that in addition to this effect there is an apparent increase in enzyme activity plus a changed pattern of results in myocardial infarction, producing greater elevations that persist for a longer time. The latter effect should not be overlooked when interpreting results. Another problem is the loss of linearity after dilution of very high-activity sera with water or saline, leading to erroneously high values. The phenomenon is caused by an inactivator normally present in the serum that becomes less effective after dilution.

CK assays have been adapted to automation by suitable modification of manual methods.

GAMMA-GLUTAMYLTRANSPEPTIDASE (GGTP)

E.C. 2.3.2.2 (*γ-Glutamyl*)*-peptide: amino-acid γ glutamyltransferase*

Three isoenzymes isolated, one major and two minor components. By some techniques, up to seven fractions have been isolated, but it is not certain whether these are true isoenzymes.

Optimum pH range 8.0 to 8.5.

Oxalate, citrate, and fluoride cause slight inhibition.

Tissue Sources. The kidney, liver, and pancreas have the highest amounts of GGTP, but because of its function in amino acid transport across cell membranes, it is found in all cells.

Reaction Catalyzed

GGTP catalyzes the cleavage of the terminal glutamyl residue from a peptide having such a structure and its transfer to another peptide or in some cases an amino acid. A typical peptide that supplies the gamma-glutamyl group is glutathione—gamma-glutamylcysteinylglycine. Glycylglycine is a typical recipient peptide.

Range of Normal Values. By the method of Szasz detailed below, normal values for males are quoted as 12 to 38 I.U./L and for females 9 to 31 I.U./L, at 30°C.

Clinical Significance. Although the highest levels of GGTP are found in renal tissue and pancreas, interest in GGTP levels has been largely confined to hepatic disease. The occurrence of elevated GGTP levels in myocardial disease, when these are found, is believed to reflect primarily associated liver involvement rather than a direct release from heart tissue. It has also been noted that elevated GGTP values in the absence of recent renal surgery or known liver disease are suggestive of a rejection of transplants.

The elevation of GGTP levels is found in all types of liver disease, i.e., viral hepatitis, toxic hepatitis, alcoholic liver damage, malignancies, cirrhosis, and obstructive liver conditions (which yield the greatest elevations), and in conditions that often involve the liver, such as acute pancreatitis and pancreatic carcinoma, and infectious mononucleosis. Involvement of the liver by sarcoidosis and miliary tuberculosis produces elevated GGTP values. Except in some types of renal malignancy, GGTP values rarely are elevated in renal disease.

Methods of Estimation. The majority of published methods use a variety of synthetic substrates, usually combinations of a gamma-glutamyl group with a substance that can be determined after its release from the combination by the action of the enzyme. The procedure of Szasz described later, in which the GGTP splits gamma-glutamyl-*p*-nitroanilide to release the measured yellow *p*-nitroanilide, has the disadvantage of limited solubility of the substrate, and recent commercial procedures* employ more soluble substrates such as gamma-glutamyl-3-carboxy-4-nitroanilide, based on later work of Szasz and Persijn. (The reaction product *p*-nitroanilide is more correctly called 5-amino-2-nitrobenzoate.) Earlier methods, which determined the alphanaphthylamine released from gamma-glutamylnaphthylamide by its reaction with a stable diazonium compound, Fast Blue B, are not used today. The method detailed below is given as an example of a kinetic assay rather than as representing current laboratory practice.

Determination of Serum Gamma-Glutamyltranspeptidase (GGTP) (Szasz, 1969)

Principle

The serum activity of GGTP transfers the gamma-glutamyl portion of a gamma-glutamyl-*p*-nitroanilide to a glycylglycine receptor, and the reaction is followed by the increasing absorbance at 405 nm owing to the released yellow 5-amino-2-nitrobenzoate.

*"C-system" Gamma-GT. Boehringer Mannheim Diagnostics, Inc. Indianapolis, Ind. 46250 and Dorval, Que. H9P 1A9.

COOH						COOH
HC—NH_2						HC—NH_2
CH_2						CH_2
CH_2						CH_2
C=O		COOH		COOH		C=O
NH		CH_2		NH		CH_2
HS—CH_2—CH	+	NH	→	HS—CH_2—CH	+	NH
C=O		C=O		C=O		C=O
NH		CH_2		NH		CH_2
CH_2		NH_2		CH_2		NH_2
COOH				COOH		
Glutathione		*Glycylglycine*		*Cysteinylglycine*		*Glutamyl-glycylglycine*

Procedure

1. Prepare the working substrate as described under *Reagents*.

2. Pipette 3.0 mL of substrate into a 10-mm light path cuvette, and equilibrate to 30°C in the thermostatted sample compartment of a narrow band-pass spectrophotometer (see Note 1).

3. With a positive-displacement pipettor, add 0.1 mL serum; mix by gentle inversion using Parafilm, and replace the cuvette in the spectrophotometer.

4. After two minutes, record the absorbance at one-minute intervals over a period of five minutes, or make a continuous tracing with a recorder set to a chart speed of about 6 cm per minute.

5. Determine the average absorbance increase per minute over the period.

Calculation

$$\frac{\text{Absorbance change/min} \times 1000 \times 3.1 \times 1000}{9900 \times 1 \times 0.1}$$

In the conditions used, with a serum sample of 0.1 mL, total reaction volume of 3.1 mL, molar absorptivity of 5-amino-2-nitrobenzoate 9900, the formula simplifies to:

Absorbance change/minute × 3131 = I.U./L

Range of Normal Values

Males: 12 to 38 I.U./L at 30°C
Females: 9 to 31 I.U./L at 30°C

Reagents

Ammediol Buffer, 0.05 M, pH 8.6. Dissolve 526 mg of 2-amino-2-methylpropane-1,3-diol in about 80 mL distilled water. Using the pH meter, adjust the reaction to exactly pH 8.6 by means of dropwise addition of 1-molar HCl, and make up to a final volume of 100 mL with distilled water; mix.

Substrate. Warm 50 mL of ammediol buffer to 60°C and place on a magnetic mixer. With constant stirring add 63.2 mg L-gamma-glutamyl-*p*-nitroanilide, 145.4 mg glycylglycine, and 111.9 mg magnesium chloride $MgCl_2.6H_2O$. This solution is cooled to 30°C for use.

Any unused substrate from the day's tests can be kept at room temperature and will be usable for up to two days. There is a slow rise in the initial absorbance over this time. Owing to precipitation, the substrate becomes unusable after this time.

Notes

1. The spectral absorbance curve of 5-amino-2-nitrobenzoate is very steep in the region of the chosen wavelength, 405 nm, and a high-resolution instrument is essential for reproducible results.

2. Do not overheat the substrate during preparation; this will accelerate deterioration.

3. A suitable control serum is Validate-E.

4. The reaction product, 5-amino-2-nitrobenzoate, is highly toxic, and contact with the skin or mucous membranes should be avoided, even with the low concentrations encountered.

5. If the assay is made at a different temperature, the results can be related to the normal range at 30°C by using the factors:

Assay Temperature	Factor to Convert Results to Values at 30°C
25°C	1.31
37°C	0.69

6. The method is linear up to about 8 times the upper limit of normal.

Comment

The probable physiological role for GGTP is indicated by the need for an acceptor peptide, glycylglycine, in the reaction mixture: in its absence the activity of the enzyme appears to be limited to hydrolytic breakdown of the substrate only, with a much reduced rate of apparent activity. The requirement for a narrow band-pass spectrophotometer arises from the use of the molar absorbance of the released product for standardization: the value stated—9900—is valid only with an instrument of that caliber. The procedure using the more soluble substrate is readily automated, but if the analyzer employs the bichromatic principle (see p. 109) the molar absorbance used to calculate the results has to be determined under those circumstances. The original paper of Szasz (1969) provides an excellent example of the methods for determination of the Michaelis-Menten constant and of optimum pH and type of receptor peptide.

Glucosephosphate Isomerase (PHI, Phosphohexose Isomerase)

E.C. 5.3.1.9 D-*Glucose-6-phosphate ketol-isomerase*

Isoenzymes have been separated in mice; none has been reported in human serum.

Optimum activity at pH 9.0.

No data on effect of anticoagulants: serum used for assay.

Tissue Sources. Widely distributed in many body tissues; high in liver and muscle, erythrocytes.

Reaction Catalyzed

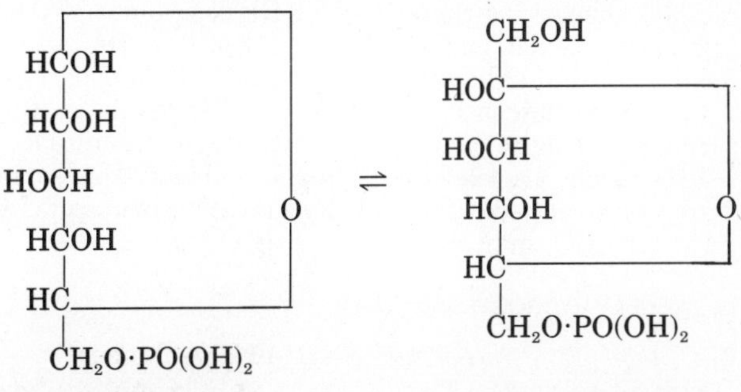

Glucose-6-phosphate *Fructose-6-phosphate*

The important role played by this enzyme in glycolysis explains its presence in all cells.

Clinical Significance. The chief clinical use of PHI assays is in following the course of treatment of cancer, particularly when there are metastases. Increases in PHI levels correlate well with progressive deterioration, and a satisfactory response to treatment is shown by declining levels of the enzyme.

ISOCITRATE DEHYDROGENASE (ICD)

E. C. 1.1.1.42 *Threo-D_s-Isocitrate: $NADP^+$ oxidoreductase (decarboxylating)*

Four isoenzymes reported.
Optimum pH range 7.0 to 7.8.
Oxalate, fluoride, and heparin inhibit the enzyme.

Reaction Catalyzed

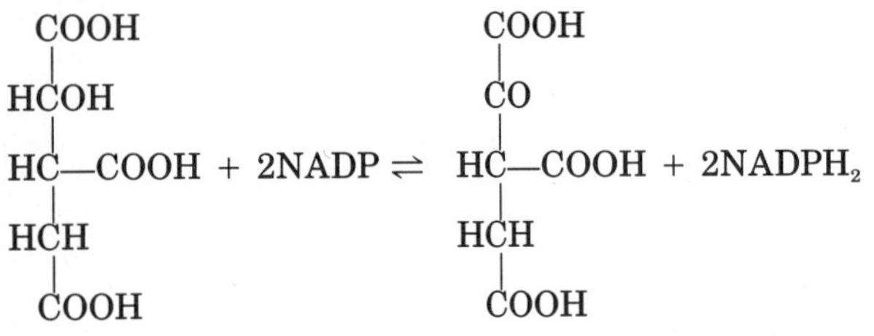

$$\begin{array}{l} COOH \\ | \\ HCOH \\ | \\ HC\text{—}COOH \\ | \\ HCH \\ | \\ COOH \end{array} + 2NADP \rightleftharpoons \begin{array}{l} COOH \\ | \\ CO \\ | \\ HC\text{—}COOH \\ | \\ HCH \\ | \\ COOH \end{array} + 2NADPH_2$$

Isocitric acid *Oxalosuccinic acid*

The oxalosuccinic acid spontaneously converts to alpha-ketoglutaric acid.

$$\begin{array}{l} COOH \\ | \\ CO \\ | \\ HC\text{—}COOH \\ | \\ HCH \\ | \\ COOH \end{array} \rightarrow \begin{array}{l} COOH \\ | \\ CO \\ | \\ HCH \\ | \\ HCH \\ | \\ COOH \end{array} + CO_2$$

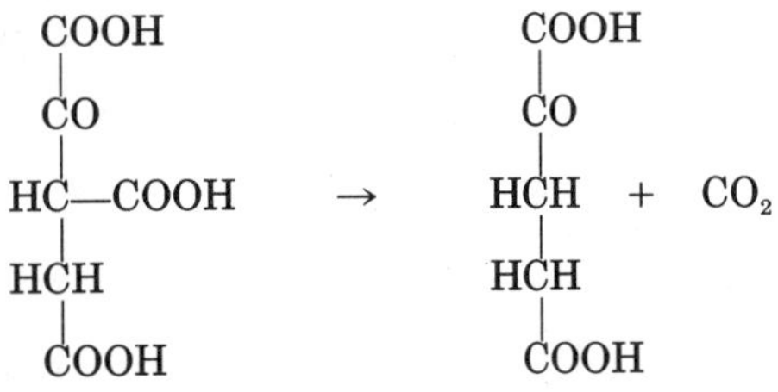

Oxalosuccinic acid *Alpha-ketoglutaric acid*

Tissue Sources. There are two main types of ICD; one, found in the mitochondria, requires NAD as coenzyme; the other, found in the soluble nonparticulate fraction of the cell contents, requires NADP. Both forms require manganous (Mn^{++}) ions as activators. The NADP-dependent type is found in many tissues, especially liver, heart, and skeletal muscle. Red blood cells and platelets contain large amounts.

Range of Normal Values. With the spectrophotometric method, measuring the rate of NADP to reduced NADP conversion at 340 nm at 25°C in a reaction volume of 3.0 mL, normal values range from 1 to 7 I.U./L of serum.

Clinical Significance. Changes in ICD levels in the serum are of significance almost entirely in liver disease.

ICD levels are elevated, often tenfold, in the early stages of viral hepatitis, and this elevation is one of the most sensitive indicators of this stage of the disease.

LACTATE DEHYDROGENASE (LDH)

E. C. 1.1.1.27 *L-Lactate: NAD^+ oxidoreductase*

Five isoenzymes. (A sixth occurs only in mature testicular tissue.)

Optimum pH lactate to pyruvate 8.8 to 9.8; pyruvate to lactate 7.4 to 7.8.

Oxalate and heparin interfere to some extent, the latter only at high levels. EDTA inhibits the enzyme by chelating a metallic activator, possibly Zn^{++}. The inhibitory effect of urea varies with the nature of the isoenzyme, the slowest-moving LDH_5 component being the most affected.

Reaction Catalyzed

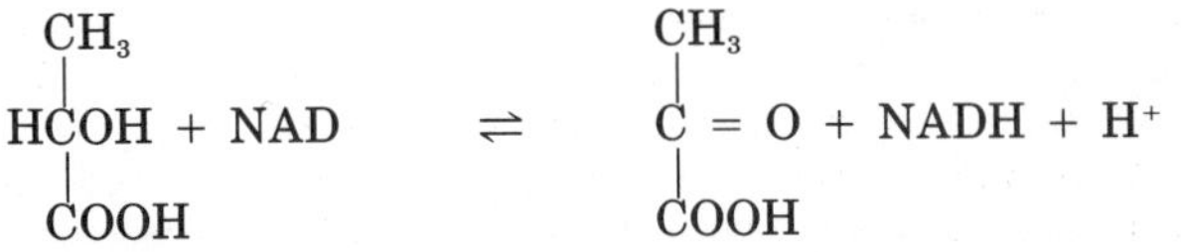

$$\begin{array}{l} CH_3 \\ | \\ HCOH \\ | \\ COOH \end{array} + NAD \rightleftharpoons \begin{array}{l} CH_3 \\ | \\ C = O \\ | \\ COOH \end{array} + NADH + H^+$$

Lactic acid *Pyruvic acid*

The lactic and pyruvic acids are present in solution as their anions, and are more accurately represented by the structures:

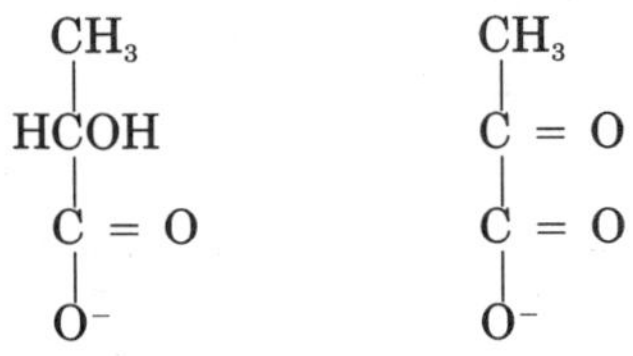

$$\begin{array}{l} CH_3 \\ | \\ HCOH \\ | \\ C = O \\ | \\ O^- \end{array} \qquad \begin{array}{l} CH_3 \\ | \\ C = O \\ | \\ C = O \\ | \\ O^- \end{array}$$

Lactate *Pyruvate*

Tissue Sources. LDH is a cytoplasmic enzyme found in all tissues; the main difference lies in the particular isoenzyme of LDH that predominates in a tissue. The red and white blood cells contain large amounts, as do skin, heart muscle, kidney, and liver.

Range of Normal Values. Using the lactate to pyruvate direction, with the formation of reduced NAD, at 30°C with the procedure of Wacker et al., as packaged by Calbiochem, the normal range is 30 to 110 I.U./L. With the system of Wroblewski and LaDue, using the pyruvate to lactate direction, at 30°C as packaged by Calbiochem, the normal range is 85 to 185 I.U./L. It will be noted that any range of normal values cited will, because of the plethora of methods and kits, have to be related specifically to the exact method and conditions used. Some procedures employing the pyruvate to lactate direction yield numerically higher values than the method cited above.

Clinical Significance. Because of the almost universal distribution of LDH in the tissues and blood cells, measurements of total LDH activity are of doubtful clinical value. Indeed it has been suggested that such determinations (if elevated) merely serve to indicate that the patient has an active disease process, in much the same way as does an elevated sedimentation rate. Moderate elevations occur in myocardial damage, and since the elevation persists for a somewhat longer period than that of the serum AST—up to 7 to 12 days—it is sometimes of use when investigations were not carried out within the first 48 hours of the onset. Moderate elevations occur in acute liver disease but are not specific unless isoenzyme separation is done (see the next section). Moderate to large increases are found in untreated pernicious anemia. Small elevations may be found in hemolytic anemias.

The elevations in malignant disease are often very great, especially in the presence of extensive metastases, in which levels of over 10,000 I.U./L. have been observed. LDH levels in the spinal fluid are about one-fifth of the serum levels; increases have been reported in meningitis and head injuries and in some cases of malignant processes of the central nervous system. Simultaneous determinations of LDH, AST, and serum bilirubin have proved of value in the differentiation of pulmonary from myocardial infarction. In the former case, AST is normal, but LDH and bilirubin are elevated; in the latter, both AST and LDH are elevated, but the bilirubin is normal.

Methods of Estimation. Methods using the forward, or lactate-to-pyruvate, reaction can be purely spectrophotometric, following the rate by the associated increase in absorbance at 340 nm as the coenzyme NAD changes to reduced NAD. Similarly, the reverse reaction, pyruvate to lactate, can be followed by the loss of absorbance at 340 nm. These procedures can be applied to large batches in discrete-type analyzers. A useful end-point assay couples the reduced NAD to a tetrazolium dye, INT (2-*p*-iodophenyl-3-*p*-nitrophenyl-5-phenyl tetrazolium chloride). This is done by using phenazine methosulfate (PMS) as an electron carrier, which reduces the INT to a stable formazan as it simultaneously oxidizes the NADH to NAD. The final color of the formazan—a reddish-violet—is measured in the spectrophotometer and compared with that produced by a suitable enzyme-in-serum standard.

LDH Isoenzymes

By electrophoresis on cellulose acetate, in agar gel or agarose gel, it can be shown that the LDH of serum is a mixture of five distinct isoenzyme fractions. The fastest-moving component—the one that is detected closest to the anode—is called LDH_1; the slowest, LDH_5; with LDH_2, LDH_3, and LDH_4 evenly spaced between them (see Fig. 7–6). LDH_1, sometimes called the "fast" fraction to avoid confusion with the alternative European nomenclature in which the sequence of numbering is reversed, is associated with the myocardium, and LDH_5, the "slow" fraction, is associated with the liver.

It has been shown that the five fractions are built up from two different kinds of monomeric units. Each isoenzyme contains four of these units, each of which has a molecular weight of about 35,000. LDH_1 contains four identical monomers, all type H; LDH_5 contains four type M monomers. The other isoenzymes are composed of different combinations: LDH_2 is H_3M, LDH_3 is H_2M_2, and LDH_4 is HM_3. A sixth LDH isoenzyme, found in postpubertal human testes, is composed of a different type of monomeric subunit; its close affinity with the serum LDH group is shown by the ability of their monomeric units to combine with those of the testicular variety of LDH to form a new series of tetramers with different electrophoretic and other properties. Various techniques have been published for the separation and quantitation of LDH isoenzymes. They differ in the nature of the support medium used—agar, agarose, cellulose acetate—and in the method of detection—colorimetric or fluorimetric. The method summarized below produces clear-cut patterns that provide good "scans" for quantitation of the fractions (see Fig. 7–6), and has the further advantage of employing the same buffer and apparatus as that used for routine serum protein electrophoresis.

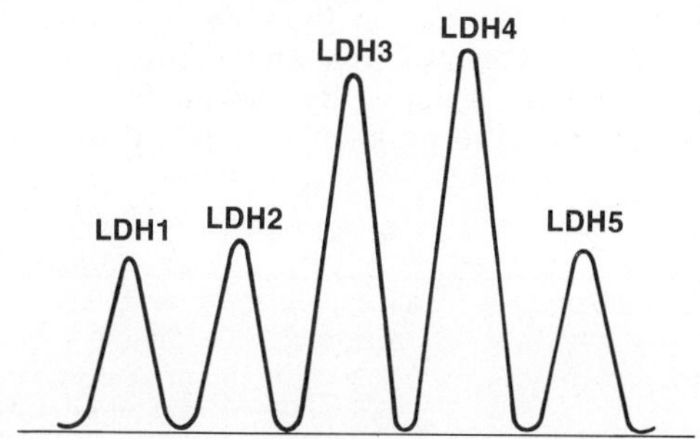

Figure 7–6 Tracing of densitometric scan of LDH isoenzymes separated on cellulose acetate by the method described. The sample was heparinized plasma from a newborn.

The LDH isoenzymes are demonstrated, after electrophoretic separation for 20 minutes at 250 volts, by the following reaction. The cellulose acetate strip with the separated fractions is incubated with a mixture of lactate, the coenzyme NAD, nitro blue tetrazolium, and phenazine methosulfate. The isoenzyme converts the lactate to pyruvate (the reverse, pyruvate-to-lactate reaction may be inhibited with cyanide), and the NAD is simultaneously converted to its reduced form, NADH + H^+. The phenazine methosulfate transfers the hydrogen atoms from the NADH + H^+ to the nitro blue tetrazolium, which is thereby reduced to an insoluble violet dye called violet formazan. The various isoenzyme fractions appear as violet bands in the support medium and can be quantitated by scanning.

The normal ranges for the LDH isoenzyme fractions, expressed as percentages of total LDH activity, are as follows:

Isoenzyme	Percentge of Total LDH
LDH_1	18–33
LDH_2	28–40
LDH_3	18–30
LDH_4	6–16
LDH_5	2–13

Normally, LDH_1 is less prominent than LDH_2; reversal of this pattern occurs in myocardial infarction and also in megaloblastic and hemolytic anemias. LDH_5 is usually hardly visible; it becomes increased and prominent in hepatitis and other acute hepatocellular disease. A midzone increase (LDH_3 and LDH_4) occurs in malignancy and also in severe disease associated with general tissue necrosis.

A fairly widely used variant of the isoenzyme approach to better clinical usefulness of LDH assays is the determination of the so-called hydroxybutyrate dehydrogenase activity. This is in reality an assay of the fast-moving LDH isoenzymes associated with myocardial damage by taking advantage of the greater activity against a chemical relative of lactate, alpha-ketobutyrate. The HBDH activity is measured by its catalytic effect on the conversion of alpha-ketobutyrate to alpha-hydroxybutyrate with the concomitant absorbance decrease owing to associated reduced NAD to NAD change.

$$CH_3{\cdot}CH_2{\cdot}C = O{\cdot}COO^- + NADH + H^+ =$$

Ketobutyrate

$$CH_3{\cdot}CH_2{\cdot}CHOH{\cdot}COO^- + NAD$$

Hydroxybutyrate

Suitable sets of reagents are available commercially*; the normal range for the Calbiochem procedure is 96 to 210 I.U./L at 30°C.

Leucine Aminopeptidase (LAP)

E.C. 3.4.11.1 α-Aminoacyl-peptide hydrolase (cytosol)

Three isoenzymes demonstrable in normal serum, six or seven in various pathological states.

Optimum pH 7.2 to 7.5.

EDTA inhibits the enzyme.

Reaction Catalyzed. The true aminopeptidases attack the end of a peptide chain that has a free amino group, releasing the amino acid that carries the group. Leucine aminopeptidase hydrolyzes peptides with a leucine residue as the terminal group. A wide variety of compounds are attacked, including natural peptides and various synthetic compounds such as leucylglycine, L-leucylglycylglycine, and L-glutamyl-L-leucinamide.

Tissue Sources. The main source of LAP is the cells of the pancreas, in which it is produced for the further breakdown of peptides released during digestion by the proteolytic enzymes. This enzyme is not assayed in most laboratories because of its minimal diagnostic usefulness.

Lipase (Lipase)

E.C. 3.1.1.3 Triacylglycerol acyl-hydrolase

Isoenzyme pattern uncertain owing to problems of substrate specificity.

Optimum pH 7.8 to 8.0, but to some extent substrate dependent.

Anticoagulants do not inhibit.

Tissue Sources. The main source is the pancreas, with small amounts in the intestinal wall and gastric mucosa. Adipose tissue contains a special lipoprotein lipase that hydrolyzes the triglycerides of circulating lipoproteins prior to their storage. Lipases are also present in blood cells.

Reaction Catalyzed. Lipase hydrolyzes triglycerides, which are combinations—esters—of the trihydric alcohol glycerol and three long-chain fatty acids. The enzyme preferentially attacks the alpha positions—those at either end of the three-carbon backbone of glycerol—to produce two molecules of free fatty acids and one molecule of an ester of glycerol with one molecule of fatty acid attached in the center or beta position (see diagram below).

Clinical Significance. See in *Gastrointestinal Tract*, p. 233.

Methods of Estimation. See p. 233.

*Calbiochem, La Jolla, Calif. 92037.

5′-Nucleotidase (5′N)

E.C. 3.1.3.5 5′-Ribonucleotide phosphohydrolase

Isoenzymes have been detected.

Optimum pH 7.5 to 7.9, depending on buffer used.

EDTA inhibits by chelating magnesium ions, which activate the enzyme.

Reaction Catalyzed

Adenosine-5′-phosphate

5′-Nucleotidase specifically splits off the phosphate group from adenosine-5′-phosphate and similar nucleotides with a phosphate group on the number 5′ carbon of the pentose portion of the molecule. 5′-Nucleotidase can be regarded as a member of the alkaline phosphatase group with a more limited substrate specificity. The ability of other serum alkaline phosphatases to attack adenosine-5′-phosphate entails the inclusion of inhibitory or competitive substances in analytical mixtures. (See under *Methods of Estimation.*)

Tissue Sources. Since this enzyme is concerned with nucleic acid catabolism, it is found in all cells: the catabolic processes will be more active in the metabolically busy liver cells than in the relatively stable bone tissues, and the association between increased serum 5′-N levels and liver disease is understandable.

Range of Normal Values. By the method of Persijn and van der Slik, the range of normal values is 3.5 to 11.0 I.U./L.

$$\begin{array}{l} CH_2{-}O{-}CO{-}(CH_2)_{14}{-}CH_3 \\ | \\ CH{-}O{-}CO{-}(CH_2)_{14}{-}CH_3 \\ | \\ CH_2{-}O{-}CO{-}(CH_2)_{14}{-}CH_3 \end{array} \rightarrow \begin{array}{l} CH_2OH \\ | \\ CH{-}O{-}CO{-}(CH_2)_{14}{-}CH_3 \\ | \\ CH_2OH \end{array} + 2\ CH_3{-}(CH_2)_{14}{-}COOH$$

Glyceryl tripalmitate — *Glyceryl monopalmitate* — *Palmitic acid*

Clinical Significance. 5′-Nucleotidase levels in serum are typically greatly elevated in obstructive jaundice and in liver malignancies; in viral and toxic hepatitis, and also in bone disease, the values are normal or only slightly raised. Determinations of 5′-N would appear to be definitely superior to alkaline phosphatase estimations in the differentiation of the causes of jaundice and in the distinction between liver and bone as the source of an elevated alkaline phosphatase level caused by malignancy. 5′-N values are not affected by drug-induced liver damage.

Methods of Estimation. In order for any assay method to be specific for 5′-N, the action of other phosphatases on the substrate has to be either diverted or compensated for. In one approach, two determinations are made—using adenosine 5′-monophosphate as the substrate—one with added nickel ions in the form of nickel chloride, the other without. The nickel ions selectively inhibit the 5′-N; hence, one determination includes alkaline phosphatase plus 5′-N, the other measures alkaline phosphatase only, and the difference between the two is a measure of the 5′-N activity. The actual measurement made is of released inorganic phosphate.

In the other procedure, only one determination is made, but the substrate includes, in addition to the adenosine 5′-monophosphate, a large excess of either beta-glycerophosphate or disodium phenylphosphate. The K_M value of alkaline phosphatase for these additional substrates is more favorable than for the adenosine 5′-monophosphate; therefore the alkaline phosphatase activity of the sample is diverted to that reaction, while the 5′-N reacts with the adenosine 5′-monophosphate. At the end of the incubation, instead of the released inorganic phosphate's being determined, the adenosine is converted to inosine by adenosine deaminase included in the reaction mixture, and the ammonium ion released by that reaction is determined by the sensitive Berthelot reaction.

The two methods illustrate the practical use of selective inhibition (nickel ions on 5′-N) and of differing K_M values.

Phosphatases (Alkaline Phosphatase, Acid Phosphatase)

E.C. 3.1.3.1 (Alkaline) *Orthophosphoric monoester phosphohydrolase* (alkaline optimum)
E.C. 3.1.3.2 (Acid) *Orthophosphoric monoester phosphohydrolase* (acid optimum)

Alkaline phosphatase isoenzymes. Two patterns have been reported. Some adults show two isoenzymes; others, having blood groups B and O, show three, probably of bone, liver and intestinal origin.

Acid phosphatase isoenzymes. Two isoenzymes can be detected using starch gel electrophoresis, but as many as five using polyacrylamide gel electrophoretic separation.

Alkaline phosphatase: inhibited by EDTA owing to chelation of magnesium ions.

Acid phosphatase: inhibited by oxalate and fluoride. Prostatic acid phosphatase is inhibited by tartrate in some assay systems. (See further below.)

Optimum pH, alkaline phosphatase: varies with the assay system used, but usually in the range of pH 9.6 to 10.0.

Optimum pH, acid phosphatase: varies with the assay system used, but usually in the range of pH 4.8 to 6.0.

Reaction Catalyzed. The phosphatases discussed here are the nonspecific phosphomonoesterases; the substrate-specific 5′-nucleotidase and glucose-6-phosphatase are not included. The nonspecific phosphatases catalyze the general reaction:

$$\text{HO—}\overset{\text{OH}}{\underset{\text{O}}{\overset{|}{\underset{\|}{\text{P}}}}}\text{—O—R} + H_2O \rightarrow \text{HO—}\overset{\text{OH}}{\underset{\text{OH}}{\overset{|}{\underset{|}{\text{P}}}}}\text{=O} + \text{R—OH}$$

Organic phosphate ester → *Inorganic phosphate*

A wide variety of organic phosphate esters are attacked, and some have been used as substrates in estimation of the enzymes: beta-glycerophosphate, disodium phenyl phosphate, disodium *p*-nitrophenyl phosphate, phenolphthalein phosphate, alpha- and beta-naphthyl phosphates, and so forth. The terms *acid* and *alkaline* refer simply to the pH values at which the enzymes have maximal activity. These vary with the nature of the substrate and other analytical factors but are in the region of pH 4.9 for acid phosphatase and 10.0 for alkaline phosphatase.

The phosphatases can also function as transferases, linking the released inorganic phosphate with a suitable acceptor substance. This explains the greater alkaline phosphatase activities found in the presence of buffers, such as the amino alcohols, to which the released inorganic phosphate can be transferred by the transphosphorylating action of the enzyme. The apparent effect is to accelerate the clearance of the phosphate from the active site of the enzyme.

Tissue Sources

Acid Phosphatase. Apart from small amounts in bone, liver, spleen, and kidney, the two main normal sources are the prostate gland (in men) and the red cells. A third variety of acid phosphatase has been found occasionally in the sera of women with cancer of the breast.

Alkaline Phosphatase. This form of the enzyme is found in the osteoblast cells of bone, in liver cells, and in the intestine, kidney, and placenta.

Range of Normal Values. Since the time of the third edition of this text the use of International Units for reporting enzyme activity has become universal. However, normal value ranges are still dependent on the method and its particular combination of substrate, buffer, activators, reaction temperature, and incubation time and on its use of an end-point or kinetic measurement. Table 7–3 shows the conversion factors for some of the most widely used substrates: the widespread use of automated analyzers has promoted the use of methods with *p*-nitrophenyl phosphate as the substrate and the amino alcohol buffers. (See *Comment* later on.) The student should note that universality of reporting units—International Units/liter—does not entail similar coincidence of normal ranges, and that the use of empirical factors to convert results by one procedure into those of another is at best questionable.

TABLE 7–3 Enzyme Unit Definitions for Acid and Alkaline Phosphatase

Bodansky (1954) and Shinowara-Jones-Reinhart (1942)
One unit = release of 1.0 mg inorganic phosphate expressed as P in one hour by 100 mL serum. Expressed as I.U. (micromol/minute/L) Bodansky units × 5.4 = I.U. Normal range 1.5-4.0 Bodansky units = 8-22 I.U./L. Shinowara-Jones-Reinhart units × 5.4 = I.U. Normal range 2.2-6.5 SJR units = 15-35 I.U./L.
King-Armstrong (1934)
One unit = release of 1.0 mg phenol in 15 minutes at pH 10.0 by 100 mL serum. K-A units × 6.94 = I.U. Normal range 3.5-13.0 K-A units = 25-92 I.U./L.
Bessey-Lowry-Brock (1946)
One unit = release of 1 micromol of p-nitrophenol in one hour by 1.0 mL serum. BLB units × 16.7 = I.U. Normal range 0.7 to 2.7 BLB units = 11.7-45.0 I.U./L.
Babson (1965)
One unit = release of 1 micromol phenolphthalein per minute by 1.0 mL serum. Babson unit = I.U. Normal range 9-35 I.U./L.
Roy et al. (Acid Phosphatase) (1971)
One unit = release of one micromol of thymolphthalein per minute/liter. This unit is equal to one I.U./L, or one milliU/mL. Normal range 0.11-0.60 I.U./L.

Clinical Significance

Acid Phosphatase. The serum level of the form of acid phosphatase that is derived from prostatic tissue is usually elevated if a cancer of the prostate has spread to bone. The elevation may be of considerable degree, but it is not invariably present, since if the tumor is very anaplastic with primitive-type cells, these may not be able to manufacture the enzyme. In the presence of known cancer of the prostate, a rise in the serum prostatic acid phosphatase of even 0.5 unit may indicate spread to bone; a fall in the level of the enzyme is a useful indication that hormonal therapy is taking effect. A subsequent rise usually indicates renewed activity of the metastases.

Alkaline Phosphatase. Determinations of alkaline phosphatase activity are most commonly made as an aid to the differential diagnosis of liver disease; this procedure has been an important member of the usual set of liver function tests for more than 30 years. The other area of clinical use is in the investigation of bone disease and hyperparathyroidism.

The association of elevated alkaline phosphatase values with liver and gallbladder disease is well recognized. Very high levels occur in jaundice because of obstruction of the biliary tract, and, at one time, the elevation of plasma levels of alkaline phosphatase was thought to be due to retention of the enzyme, invoking a mechanism similar to that producing elevation of plasma bilirubin levels. However, it has been shown that synthesis of the enzyme by the cells lining the biliary canaliculi is increased when duct obstruction occurs. It would appear that, in all probability, the major cause of the plasma elevation is this induction of enzyme synthesis. It has been demonstrated too that it is the liver, not the bone, isoenzyme that appears in the plasma in obstructive jaundice. Bile alkaline phosphatase is composed partly of the liver isoenzyme, together with a complex of that enzyme with phosphatidylcholine. It appears that the kidney is normally unable to excrete alkaline phosphatase derived from the plasma; the alkaline phosphatase found in urine is derived from renal sources, and elevated values are associated with specifically renal lesions such as carcinoma, nephritis, nephrosis, systemic lupus erythematosus, and infarction.

The general picture may be summarized thus: elevated alkaline phosphatase values in serum occur in both obstructive and intrahepatic jaundice, with the higher activities being found in the former condition, but with some overlap in the ranges found in the two types of disease. The differential diagnosis of jaundice is best made by reference to more specific tests, both enzymatic and others. In the absence of jaundice, raised alkaline phosphatase values can be a useful indication of hepatic lesions such as liver malignancy and drug-induced liver damage and of such uncommon conditions as sarcoidosis, histoplasmosis, and cysts.

The appearance in the serum in the third trimester of a normal pregnancy of an alkaline phosphatase with characteristics different from those usually present, and its origin in the placenta, raised the possibility that its level might reflect the status of the placenta, since it is readily separable from other types of the enzyme by its heat stability and resistance to EDTA inactivation and urea. At present this expectation does not appear to have been well founded.

The serum alkaline phosphatase level in bone diseases is determined by the nature of the process in the bone. If the lesion arises from or affects the osteoblast cells, which are active in bone growth and repair and contain high concentrations of the enzyme, the serum values will be elevated. If the process is primarily osteoclastic—bone destruction—the alkaline phosphatase values will be normal. The contrast is well shown by osteomalacia and osteoporosis. In the former condition the osteoblasts are active, endeavoring to mitigate the processes that are interfering with calcium and phosphorus utilization; in the latter case, the osteoid tissue, containing the osteoblasts, is not producing increased amounts of alkaline phosphatase. In osteomalacia, therefore, serum alkaline phosphatase levels are increased; in osteoporosis, they are normal.

It follows from this that serum alkaline phosphatase levels will be increased in such conditions as Paget's disease (osteitis deformans), rickets, osteogenic sarcoma, healing fractures (slightly raised), and hyperparathyroidism. If the invasion of bone by metastases from a cancer elsewhere in the body stimulates osteoblastic activity, such as occurs with spread of carcinoma of the prostate, the serum enzyme level will rise. In other cases, such as cancer of the breast, the serum enzyme levels are usually normal or at most slightly elevated.

Methods of Estimation. A wide variety of organic phosphate esters have been used for estimation of serum phosphatases. The optimum pH of the enzyme varies with the substrate used, and in the case of the acid phosphatases there are differences in substrate specificity with enzymes of prostatic and red cell origins.

Substrate	Product Measured
Beta glycerophosphate	Inorganic phosphate
Disodium phenyl phosphate	Phenol
Thymolphthalein monophosphate	Thymolphthalein
Phenolphthalein monophosphate	Phenolphthalein
p-Nitrophenyl phosphate	*p*-Nitrophenol

The replacement of the first two substrates listed by the last three, and particularly by the last-named, is due, in part, to the common property of the last three—they are indicators that have a distinct color in the alkaline conditions of the assay—whereas the first two methods entail chemical determinations of the reaction product. In addition, the use of the amino alcohol buffers, which accelerate the reaction (see *Comment* later on), renders the last three methods more suitable for simple automation.

Methods of assay for acid phosphatase have been complicated by the need to determine selectively the enzyme of prostatic cell origin. Other phosphatases active at about pH 4.9, especially those of red cell origin, have no clinical significance as far as is known. Two main approaches have been used: attempts to locate a substrate specific for the prostatic type enzyme and various inhibition techniques, in which formaldehyde was used to inhibit the acid phosphatases other than the prostatic type and tartrate was used to selectively inhibit that type. In practice the results were least informative in just those circumstances in which the best performance was needed, i.e., in early detection of carcinoma of the prostate, its possible spread to bone, and the effects of treatment. The introduction of thymolphthalein monophosphate as a specific substrate for prostatic acid phosphatase has materially improved the situation, and a technique is described further on.

It has been noted that the improved precision of alkaline phosphatase assays attendant on recent improvements in methodology has made more obvious the increase in alkaline phosphatase levels in human serum when stored. Increases of 1.0% per hour in pooled serum when frozen and thawed, and as much as 10% after 96 hours in fresh serum at room temperature, were found; refrigeration decreased but did not abolish the rate of increase.

Serum Alkaline Phosphatase Estimation (Bessey, Lowry, and Brock, 1946)

Principle

The enzyme alkaline phosphatase hydrolyzes the *p*-nitrophenyl phosphate substrate, producing inorganic phosphate and *p*-nitrophenol. The quantity of *p*-nitrophenol released under standardized conditions of time, temperature, and pH is measured by the absorbance of the yellow color it assumes in alkaline solution. The Bessey-Lowry unit of alkaline phosphatase activity is defined as the amount of enzyme that will release one micromol (0.1391 mg) of *p*-nitrophenol per milliliter of serum per hour at pH 10.5. One Bessey-Lowry unit corresponds to 16.7 International Units if the latter are defined as the number of micromols of substrate hydrolyzed per minute by 1 liter of serum.

Procedure

1. Set up two test tubes, marked test and blank. Pipette into each 1.0 mL of a mixture of equal parts by volume of alkaline buffer and substrate (see Note 1).

2. Warm both tubes in the 37°C water bath for five minutes.

3. Using 0.1-mL positive-displacement micropipettes and careful wash-out technique, add 0.1 mL serum to the tube marked test and 0.1 mL distilled water to the blank tube.

4. Incubate for exactly 30 minutes (see Note 2).

5. Remove from the water bath; add immediately and rapidly to both tubes 10.0 mL of 0.02 molar sodium hydroxide. Mix by inversion using Parafilm.

6. Read the absorbance of the test tube at 410 nm, using the blank to set zero absorbance on the spectrophotometer. Add two drops—0.1 mL—of concentrated HCl to both tubes and repeat the absorbance reading. Subtract the second absorbance value from the first, and refer the corrected reading to the calibration curve to obtain the units of alkaline phosphatase activity.

Calibration

1. Set up six test tubes containing the volumes of working standard solution (see *Reagents*) and 0.02 M NaOH as listed:

Tube No.	Working Standard	0.02 M NaOH	Unit Value
1	1.0 mL	10.0 mL	16.7
2	2.0 mL	9.0 mL	33.4
3	4.0 mL	7.0 mL	66.8
4	6.0 mL	5.0 mL	100.2
5	8.0 mL	3.0 mL	133.6
6	10.0 mL	1.0 mL	167.0

2. Mix well by inversion; read the absorbance of all tubes at 410 nm on the spectrophotometer, setting zero absorbance with 0.02 M NaOH.

3. Plot absorbance values along the vertical ordinate of the graph paper against the corresponding units of alkaline phosphatase activity on the abscissa. The shape of the calibration curve will depend on the instrument used; with a narrow band-pass spectrophotometer a straight line will be obtained; with instruments having a wider band pass a curve will result.

Normal Values

Adults. 11.7 to 45.1 I.U./L
Infants 1 to 3 months. 73.5 to 227.1 I.U./L.
Children 3 to 10 years. 56.8 to 152.0 I.U./L
At puberty. 56.8 to 258.9 I.U./L

After puberty there is a steady fall; the adult values are applicable from the age of about 16 years.

Reagents

Alkaline Buffer pH 10.5. Dissolve 7.50 g pure glycine (aminoacetic acid, NH_2CH_2COOH) and 0.203 g pure magnesium chloride, $MgCl_2{\cdot}6H_2O$, in about 750 mL fresh distilled water. Add 85.0 mL M NaOH, mix, dilute to 1 liter with distilled water, and mix again. Check the pH with a pH meter; it should be 10.5 ± 0.1. The buffer is stable at least 6 months in the refrigerator.

Substrate—p-Nitrophenyl Phosphate. The purity of the *p*-nitrophenyl phosphate is critical. By far the best is that supplied by Sigma Chemical Co., St. Louis, Mo. 63178. Dissolve the contents of one capsule—100 mg—in 25 mL distilled water. It is best preserved combined with buffer (see Note 1).

Stock p-Nitrophenol Standard 10 Millimols Per Liter. Dissolve 1.3911 g analytical-grade *p*-nitrophenol, $NO_2C_6H_4OH$, in, and make up to 1 liter with, fresh distilled water. Keeps up to one year in the refrigerator.

Working Standard Solution. Pipette accurately

into a 200 mL volumetric flask 1.0 mL stock standard; make up to 200 mL with 0.02 M NaOH. Mix well. Prepare freshly for making the calibration curve; discard the unused portion.

0.02 M Sodium Hydroxide. Dilute 20.0 mL accurately standardized 1 M NaOH up to 1 liter with fresh distilled water. Mix well; store in a plastic bottle.

Notes

1. The most convenient system is to mix equal volumes of alkaline buffer and substrate solution, pipette 1.0 mL aliquots into suitable test tubes, stopper, and store in the freezer.
2. For determinations on infants and children, with their higher normal values, the incubation time may be reduced to 15 minutes; the result will have to be multiplied by 2. The same procedure may be used to reassay sera with values above 167 I.U./L; there is no appreciable loss of accuracy. If the values are greatly elevated, repeat the estimation using serum diluted 1 in 5 with saline and multiply the result by 5.
3. The addition of concentrated HCl in step 6 abolishes the yellow color of the released *p*-nitrophenol, so that the second reading is a measure of extraneous color due to bilirubin or interference from turbidity.
4. If a narrow band-pass spectrophotometer is used, 1.0-cm light path cuvettes are suitable; with instruments of less precision, 19-mm or ¾-inch tubes or cuvettes must be used. The absorbance of the 167 unit standard in a 1.0-cm cuvette should be about 0.76 to 0.80.
5. Plasma may be used, provided that neither fluoride nor oxalate was used. Heparin is the best anticoagulant.

Comment

This procedure incorporates two important points: the inclusion of magnesium ions as activators of the enzyme and the use of a pure solution of the reaction product, *p*-nitrophenol, for standardization. One disadvantage of the original method is the restricted range of linearity: inspection of the normal ranges will show that determinations on sera from children would often involve dilution of the sample. A typical modern variant* overcomes this problem by the use of 2-amino-2-methyl-1,3-propanediol as the buffer and the bis(2-amino-2-ethyl-1,3-propanediol) salt of *p*-nitrophenol phosphoric acid as the substrate. The extended range of linearity—as high as 1200 I.U./L. on automated equipment—is derived in part from the ability of the buffer to combine with the inorganic phosphate released during the reaction: removal of one of the products of an enzyme-catalyzed reaction drives it in the direction of completion and provides greater sensitivity (more measurable product in the same incubation time.) The adult normal range by the improved method is 36 to 92 I.U./L. The other factor that extends the range of linearity is the use of a kinetic measurement: monitoring the rate of production of the yellow product will provide sufficient data for calculation of the enzyme activity in far less elapsed time than the 30 minutes of the manual method. A shorter reaction time entails less breakdown of the substrate, and thus even at very high activities there is not enough substrate depletion to affect the linearity. This is one of the advantages of automated enzyme assays.

*"a-gent," Abbott Laboratories, Diagnostics Division, South Pasadena, Calif. 91030 and Mississauga, Ont. L4W 2S7.

Serum Prostatic Acid Phosphatase Determination (Roy et al., 1971)

Principle

The prostatic acid phosphatase of serum splits sodium thymolphthalein monophosphate at pH 6.0 to release free thymolphthalein, the blue color of which is determined spectrophotometrically after addition of an alkaline color developer. The absorbance obtained is compared against a calibration curve prepared with pure thymolphthalein.

Procedure

1. For each sample set up two test tubes, labeled test and control. Into each pipette 1.0 mL of buffered substrate and preincubate for 5 minutes in a water bath at 37 ± 0.1°C.

2. Add 5.0 mL of color developer to control tube. Using a 0.2-mL positive displacement pipettor and careful "washout" technique, add 0.2 serum to test tube; mix by gentle lateral shaking, keeping the tube in the water bath. Add 0.2 mL serum to control, and mix by lateral shaking.

3. Exactly 30 minutes after addition of serum to test tube, rapidly add to this 5.0 mL color developer, and immediately mix by inversion using Parafilm.

4. Setting zero absorbance with the control tube, read the absorbance of the test at 590 nm, using 1-cm curvettes.

5. Refer the test absorbance to the calibration curve to obtain the serum prostatic acid phosphatase in I.U. per liter.

Normal Values

Males 0.11 to 0.60 I.U./L

Sera from females show some acid phosphatase activity with this substrate, up to about 0.5 I.U./L, but only males show significant elevations.

Reagents

Citrate Buffer 0.1 M, pH 5.95. Prepare two stock solutions:

SOLUTION A. Dissolve 29.41 g of trisodium citrate dihydrate in about 950 mL distilled water, add 25.0 mL of Brij-35 solution (see further on), and dilute to 1 liter; mix well.

SOLUTION B. Dissolve 2.1 g of citric acid monohydrate in about 95 mL distilled water, add 2.5 mL of Brij-35 solution, dilute to 100 mL and mix well. In a large beaker, put 450 mL of solution A and place on a magnetic mixer. Mixing constantly, add solution B slowly, constantly monitoring with a pH meter until the reaction is exactly pH 5.95. The final solution is stable for up to six months in the refrigerator.

Buffered Substrate. Dissolve 0.185 g of sodium thymolphthalein monophosphate in 100 mL mixed buffer. Final reaction should be pH 6.0. The solution is stable under refrigeration for up to two months.

Color Developer. Dissolve 2.0 g sodium hydroxide and 5.3 g anhydrous sodium carbonate in, and dilute to 1 liter with, distilled water. Will remain stable on the bench for six months.

Thymolphthalein Stock Standard. Dissolve 968.7 mg of thymolphthalein in, and make up to 100 mL with, absolute ethanol. Keep tightly stoppered under refrigeration. Will remain stable for one year.

Serum Preservative: Acetate Buffer, 5 M, pH 5.0. On a magnetic mixer, to a mixture of 50 mL distilled water and 13.0 mL of glacial acetic acid in a small beaker, add 43.5 g sodium acetate trihydrate with constant stirring until dissolved, adding more water if necessary, but not to exceed a total volume of about 95 mL. Adjust the reaction by dropwise addition of glacial acetic acid to pH 5.0 at 37°C. Make up to a final volume of 100 mL. Add 0.02 mL to each mL of fresh serum.

Brij-35 Solution. Dissolve 20.0 g Brij-35 in about 60 mL distilled water with gentle heat; do not overheat. When all dissolved, make up to 100 mL with distilled water. Will remain stable at room temperature for six months. (For occasional assays by this method, a convenient set of prepared reagents is available from Worthington Biochemical Corp., Freehold, N.J. 07728, Catalogue No. 7915.)

Notes

1. With normal sera the absorbance difference between test and control is small, and the technologist may prefer to measure the solutions in a 19-mm or ¾-inch round cuvette. (See Note 3.)
2. The final color is stable for up to two hours.
3. If the absorbance measurement is made with a filter-type of wide band-pass instrument, the calibration curve (see further on) will not be linear; hence the calibration curve must be made using the same photometer as for the assays.

Calibration Curve

This should be remade whenever new reagents are prepared or if the spectrophotometer is changed. In some cases it may suffice to run a check standard of 3 I.U./L.

1. Dilute 1.0 mL of stock thymolphthalein standard up to 50 mL with absolute ethanol.
2. Mix up six test tubes, and into them pipette 1.0, 2.0, 4.0, 6.0, 8.0, and 10.0 mL of diluted standard. Make each tube up to 10.0 mL with absolute ethanol, then mix using Parafilm.
3. Into six further test tubes, marked 1.5, 3.0, 6.0, 9.0, 12.0, and 15.0 I.U./L, pipette 1.0 mL of buffered substrate. Add 0.2 mL of the respective standard tubes, using 0.20 mL wash-out pipettes, and mix by gentle agitation. To all tubes add 5.0 mL of color developer; mix by inversion using Parafilm.
4. Determine the absorbances of all tubes at 590 nm, setting zero absorbance with a mixture of 1.0 mL buffered substrate, 0.2 mL ethanol, and 5.0 mL color developer.
5. Plot the absorbances obtained against the corresponding standard values.

Comment

There are several problems peculiar to the determination of the fraction of serum acid phosphatase of prostatic origin.

1. The enzyme is very unstable; as much as a 50% loss of activity can occur at room temperature in one hour. Acidification to pH 5.0 with acetate buffer helps.
2. The normal range is very low, and clinically significant changes may be so small as to require an analytical precision difficult to attain in an enzyme assay.
3. The presence of acid phosphatases of different, and to some extent unknown, origins entails the use of some form of selective detection of the prostatic fraction. In the method given above, the substrate is believed to have that property; in other procedures selective inhibitors have been included in the reaction mixture, such as formaldehyde to inhibit red cell acid phosphatases or tartrate to inhibit the prostatic fraction. The latter group of methods requires two determinations, with and without the inhibitor, so that the prostatic fraction is the difference between two values, each with its associated errors.

Recently the problem of specificity for the prostatic fraction has been tackled by the use of radioimmunoassay: this improves one aspect of the assay but involves the special instrumentation and techniques of that type of methodology.

Isoenzymes of Alkaline Phosphatase

The proven usefulness of study of the isoenzyme patterns of serum LDH has encouraged the development of sensitive methods for detection of the isoenzymes of alkaline phosphatase and the production of commercial kits. The detection of an abnormal isoenzyme—the "Regan" type—in some cancer patients has also stimulated inquiries in this field. Separation by electrophoresis on cellulose acetate with subsequent detection of the fractions by color reactions similar to those used to determine the enzyme in serum often shows overlap between the bonc- and liver-origin fractions, making interpretation difficult. Better discrimination may be obtained by combining an electrophoretic method with selective inhibition of one of the fractions in the sample. For example, after ten minutes at 56°C more than 80% of the activity of bone alkaline phosphatase is destroyed; if about 50% activity remains after this treatment, the enzyme is more probably of liver origin. It is important to note that this and similar procedures can only help to elucidate the electrophoretic appearances. Another approach that has proven successful is to separate the isoenzymes by electrophoresis in columns of acrylamide gel, in which the molecular sieving effect improves the clarity of the separations.

AMINOTRANSFERASES

These enzymes catalyze the transfer of an amino (NH_2) group from an alpha-amino acid to an alpha-keto acid, forming a new amino acid and a new keto acid. In clinical enzymology, two members of this group are important: aspartate aminotransferase (AST, formerly known as GOT) and alanine aminotransferase (ALT, formerly known as GPT).

Aspartate Aminotransferase (AST)

E.C. 2.6.1.1 L-*Aspartate:2-oxoglutarate aminotransferase*

Five isoenzymes have been demonstrated in human serum concentrate.

Optimum pH 7.4.

Slight interference from oxalate.

Reaction Catalyzed

$$\begin{array}{lclclcl}
\text{COOH} & & \text{COOH} & & \text{COOH} & & \text{COOH} \\
| & & | & & | & & | \\
\text{CH}_2 & & \text{CH}_2 & & \text{CH}_2 & & \text{CH}_2 \\
| & & | & & | & & | \\
\text{CH}_2 & + & \text{CO} & \rightleftharpoons & \text{CH}_2 & + & \text{CH}\cdot\text{NH}_2 \\
| & & | & & | & & | \\
\text{CH}\cdot\text{NH}_2 & & \text{COOH} & & \text{CO} & & \text{COOH} \\
| & & & & | & & \\
\text{COOH} & & & & \text{COOH} & &
\end{array}$$

Glutamic acid — *Oxalacetic acid* — *Alpha-keto-glutaric acid* — *Aspartic acid*

Tissue Sources. The tissue sources are (in descending order of concentration): heart, liver, skeletal muscle, kidney, and pancreas.

Range of Normal Values. The wide variety of methods employed, differing in substrate type and concentration, length of lag phase owing to the coupled reaction system in the spectrophotometric methods, temperatures employed, and side reactions (see further on) and other variables make it difficult to quote normal ranges. Generally speaking, using the coupled reaction system (see further below) at 37°C with optimum substrate concentration, the normal range is about 10 to 30 I.U./L.

Clinical Significance. Serum values are elevated by the release of the enzyme from damaged cells of the myocardium (heart muscle) within 6 to 12 hours after occlusion of a coronary artery. The degree of elevation is roughly proportional to the extent of the damage; an extensive lesion would give AST values over 200 units. The maximal value is reached about 48 hours after the onset, and the level returns to normal in three to five days.

Serum AST values are greatly increased in acute liver cell damage; in viral hepatitis levels up to 1200 units are not uncommon, and in toxic liver damage caused by carbon tetrachloride poisoning even higher values occur. Moderate increases occur in other liver diseases, such as in the later stages of cirrhosis and neoplasms of the liver, but these rarely exceed 300 units. Levels in obstructive jaundice are similar. In infectious mononucleosis the serum AST levels reflect the extent of liver involvement; in severe cases the values may be as high as for acute viral hepatitis.

Serum AST levels are slightly to moderately elevated in certain forms of muscular dystrophy; higher elevations occur in crush injury to muscle and in dermatomyositis.

Methods of Estimation. With the wider availability of narrow band-pass spectrophotometers and of small automated analyzers, kinetic and pseudokinetic procedures can be expected to replace colorimetric methods for assay of the aminotransferases. The colorimetric method summarized below is included to illustrate that approach: in circumstances of infrequent usage and limited facilities it can still provide useful clinical information.

Colorimetric Method. Using a substrate containing aspartate and alpha-ketoglutarate, in which the reaction shown in *Reaction Catalyzed* above is driven from right to left, the amount of oxaloacetate produced in a fixed time is determined by its combination with a reactive diazonium compound, 6-benzamido-4-methoxy-*m*-toluidine chloride or Azoene Fast Violet B. The method can be standardized against a reference serum of preassigned value. Since the measured product, oxaloacetate, will inhibit the AST activity at elevated levels, the reaction tends to depart from linearity. A reagent set for the method ("TransAc") is available commercially.*

Spectrophotometric Method. The same reaction direction as for the colorimetric method is used: as fast as the oxaloacetate is produced it takes part in a second "indicator" reaction with added malic dehydrogenase and is converted to malate. During this conversion the added coenzyme reduced NAD is converted to NAD, a change that is associated with a loss of absorbance at 340 nm and that is monitored spectrophotometrically. Since the malic dehydrogenase and reduced NAD are present in excess, the limiting factor on the reaction velocity and the associated change in absorbance at 340 nm is the AST activity. The method can be standardized by reference to the molar absorbance of reduced NAD, since the coenzyme is converted to the NAD form mole for mole with the amount of oxaloacetate produced. The potential interference with the linearity of the reaction from side reactions with lactate dehydrogenase and keto acids in the serum sample is minimized by the inclusion of LDH in the reaction mixture to drive the side reactions rapidly to completion. In some methods the side reactions are allowed to go to completion before the main reaction is initiated by the addition of alpha-ketoglutarate. The majority of commercial reagent sets for assay of AST contain "optimum" levels of the reactants, although there is some difference of opinion as to what constitutes "optimum."

ALANINE AMINOTRANSFERASE (ALT)

E.C. 2.6.1.2 L-*Alanine:2-oxoglutarate aminotransferase*

Only a single enzyme in serum, but some evidence for two isoenzymes in tissues.

Optimum pH 7.4.

Slight interference from oxalate.

Tissue Sources. The tissue sources are (in descending order of concentration): liver, kidney, heart, skeletal muscle, and pancreas.

Reaction Catalyzed

$$\begin{array}{lclclcl}
\text{COOH} & & & & \text{COOH} & & \\
| & & & & | & & \\
\text{CH}_2 & & \text{CH}_3 & & \text{CH}_2 & & \text{CH}_3 \\
| & & | & & | & & | \\
\text{CH}_2 & + & \text{CO} & \rightleftharpoons & \text{CH}_2 & + & \text{CH}\cdot\text{NH}_2 \\
| & & | & & | & & | \\
\text{CH}\cdot\text{NH}_2 & & \text{COOH} & & \text{CO} & & \text{COOH} \\
| & & & & | & & \\
\text{COOH} & & & & \text{COOH} & &
\end{array}$$

Glutamic acid — *Pyruvic acid* — *Alpha-keto-glutaric acid* — *Alanine*

Range of Normal Values. The same comments as those made on the range of normal values for AST are also

*General Diagnostics Division, Warner-Lambert Co., Morris Plains, N.J. 07950 and Scarborough, Ont. M1K 5C5.

valid for ALT. Using the coupled reaction system, the normal range is about 10 to 35 I.U./L at 37°C.

Clinical Significance. Serum ALT values may be slightly elevated in myocardial damage, but this is probably owing to liver cell damage secondary to impaired blood supply.

Serum ALT levels are greatly increased in acute liver cell damage; in some cases the extent of the rise is greater than that of the AST, and this has led to the view that ALT estimations are more specific for acute liver cell damage than AST measurements. This has not been borne out by experience; the same lack of definite correlation also applies to the idea that the ratio of ALT/AST is greater than unity in viral hepatitis and less than unity in such conditions as cirrhosis, hepatic neoplasms, and hemolytic jaundice. It is true that the elevation of GPT that may occur in myocardial damage is much less than that found in viral hepatitis.

Methods of Estimation. The spectrophotometric and colorimetric methods for ALT estimation are similar to those employed for AST. In the spectrophotometric method the pyruvate produced by the enzyme from alanine and alpha-ketoglutarate is converted to lactate by lactate dehydrogenase. The associated conversion of reduced NAD to NAD is followed by the decrease in absorbance at 340 nm.

DIAGNOSTIC ENZYMOLOGY

Although the interpretation of changes in the levels of individual serum enzymes has already been discussed, it is convenient here to describe briefly the changes that occur in myocardial infarction and in various forms of liver disease.

Myocardial Infarction

Changes in serum CK, AST, and LDH activity are of value in the diagnosis of myocardial infarction. These changes are shown graphically in Figure 7–7. CK activity rises rapidly, commencing four to six hours after infarction and reaching a peak at 24 to 36 hours. By this time AST levels are increasing, and these usually peak at two to three days. LDH levels tend to rise a little later and peak at two to three days, but they usually remain elevated longer, for up to 14 days. Daily estimations of these enzymes for three days following a possible episode of infarction will provide diagnostic and prognostic information and may help to confirm other data, such as that provided by the electrocardiogram, concerning the severity of the infarction and whether fresh necrosis is occurring. However, it seems quite clear that by the use of a combination of LDH and CK isoenzyme separations, a diagnosis of myocardial infarction can be made with great accuracy, sometimes long before any electrocardiographic changes occur.

In myocardial infarction, a reversal of the normal concentrations of LDH_1 and LDH_2 occurs, with LDH_1 being the more prominent ("flipped" LDH). This can also occur in megaloblastic and hemolytic anemias, so it is not pathognomonic of heart muscle necrosis.

Most methods of separating CK isoenzymes show either no MB band in the normal individual or, at most, a faint band amounting to 2–5% of the total. The appearance of a distinct MB band, even without quantitation, is strong evidence for myocardial infarction.

The presence of both an MB band and a "flipped" LDH has a 100% predictive value for myocardial infarction and thus is a very powerful diagnostic combination. Isoenzyme methods are, at present, expensive and tech-

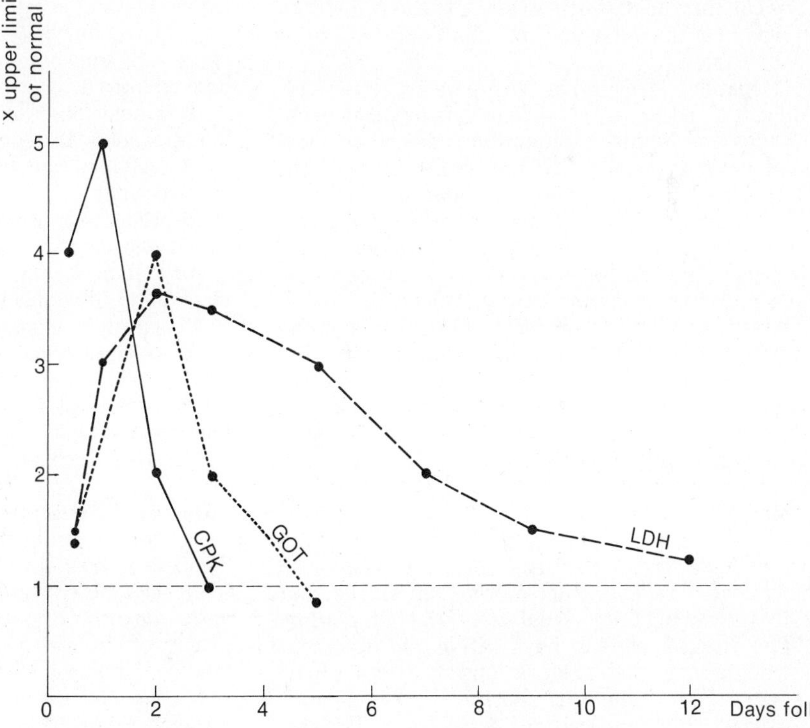

Figure 7–7 Change in serum enzyme activity following myocardial infarction.

TABLE 7–4 Serum Enzyme Patterns in Liver Disease

Condition	AST	ALT	LDH	AP	5N	GGPT
Acute viral hepatitis	15-20	15-20	6-8	1-2	1-2	1-4
Obstructive jaundice (intrahepatic or posthepatic)	3-4	3-4	1-2	3-6	4-6	4-10
Cirrhosis (established portal cirrhosis)	2-3	2-3	1-2	1-2	1-2	1-20
Tumor deposits in liver (without jaundice)	1-2	1-2	1-3	1-3	2-3	4-20

Note: The values given are approximate only and are expressed as a multiple of the upper limit of the normal range (ULN). For example, if the ULN for Serum AST in your laboratory is 40 "units," then the level found in acute viral hepatitis will be on the order of $15 \times 40 = 600$ units.

AST = aspartate aminotransferase
AP = alkaline phosphatase
GGPT = gamma-glutamyltranspeptidase
ALT = alanine aminotransferase
5N = 5′ nucleotidase
LDH = lactate dehydrogenase

nically demanding in terms of time and expertise. However, they provide such conclusive evidence for a diagnosis of myocardial infarction that any laboratory, other than the most basic, should have them available. In the authors' experience, separation by electrophoresis is far superior to column chromatography, partly because interfering factors (such as fluorescent molecules and immunoglobulin complexes) can be recognized and identified more readily.

In other cases of chest pain, such as pneumonia, pleurisy, pulmonary infarction, and dissecting aneurysm, CK and AST levels show little or no alteration, but LDH levels may rise and the LDH isoenzyme pattern may be of diagnostic value.

Liver Disease

The typical enzyme patterns in some of the commonly encountered liver disorders are presented here and summarized in Table 7–4.

Acute Hepatitis. This term covers acute liver cell damage such as occurs in viral hepatitis or after exposure to drugs and toxins. Both aminotransferases show striking elevations; usually ALT tends to be higher than AST. Occasionally, the aminotransferases may remain elevated for months after all other abnormal changes have disappeared. Such "transaminitis" does not necessarily indicate that the hepatitis has entered a chronic phase and may have no prognostic significance.

LDH levels show only a moderate elevation, but the isoenzyme pattern may be diagnostic; characteristically, LDH_5 is increased. The alkaline phosphatase (AP) level does not show any large alteration, unless edema and inflammatory changes induce intrahepatic cholestasis. The gamma-glutamyltranspeptidase (GGTP) activity tends to show only a mild elevation, but this may be quite prolonged.

Cirrhosis. Cirrhosis is a condition in which there is slow loss of liver tissue over long periods of time, and there is variable regeneration of the lost tissue, but eventually increasing fibrosis and shrinking of the organ occurs. The disease tends to have active and quiescent phases; when active, modest elevations of AST and LDH levels appear. For alcoholic cirrhosis GGTP is a much more sensitive index, and initially a raised GGTP level may be the only abnormal biochemical finding.

Hepatobiliary Obstruction. Obstruction of the biliary tract, both within the liver and of the extrahepatic ducts, results in often considerable elevations of AP, GGTP, and 5′-nucleotidase activity. The aminotransferases and LDH show little change unless there is some complicating factor such as infection.

Intrahepatic Tumors. GGTP may be a sensitive indicator of early neoplastic involvement of the liver, followed by rises in AP and 5′-nucleotidase. With large metastatic deposits, LDH levels may be elevated, and the isoenzyme pattern may be helpful.

CHAPTER 7—REVIEW QUESTIONS

1. Explain the terms *specific activation, induced fit, and allosteric effect* in relation to enzymes.
2. Give the basic Briggs and Haldane "steady state" expression and show how the Michaelis-Menten constant is derived from it.
3. Briefly describe the procedure for determination of the Michaelis-Menten constant of an enzyme.
4. What is "inhibition" in enzyme kinetics? Describe the two types.
5. What is an isoenzyme? Give one example of a set of isoenzymes and show how they are constructed.
6. List the main characteristics of enzymes. Describe the chief factors that affect the rate of enzyme reactions.
7. List the features of an ideal enzyme assay method.
8. In an enzyme assay the enzyme releases 120 μg of a product with a molecular weight of 500 in one hour with a serum sample of 50 μL. Calculate the enzyme activity in International Units.
9. Give three examples of the use of enzymes as reagents.
10. Briefly describe a method for the demonstration of the isoenzymes of lactate dehydrogenase, with a diagram of the expected pattern in a patient with severe liver disease.
11. List the enzyme determinations that might be useful in the diagnosis of a myocardial infarction and describe the pattern of changes in their levels over the first seven days following the onset of the infarction.
12. List the changes in enzyme levels that could be associated with (a) hepatobiliary obstruction and (b) cirrhosis.

WATER, ELECTROLYTES, AND ACID-BASE BALANCE

The precise control of the body content of water, electrolytes, acids, and bases is of vital importance in maintaining the integrity of living organisms. The mechanisms involved are intricately interrelated, and the student may find it helpful to read more than one text in order to gain perspective and insight into the problems involved. The texts by Tietz (1976), Davenport (1974), Adams and Hahn (1979), and Collins (1976) are suggested.

It is convenient initially to discuss these constituents more or less separately, although the interrelationships should become clearer toward the end of the chapter.

WATER

The normal human body contains 50 to 70% water. The lean (that is, fat-free) body mass contains 65 to 70%; the proportion is higher in infants and falls with age. The gradual increase of depot fat with age also causes a decline in the percentage of total body water.

Both total body water and osmolality (see p. 207) are maintained within relatively narrow limits. Body water varies by ± 0.2% per day, and osmolality ranges between 285 and 290 mOsm/kg. The osmolality of the intracellular and extracellular fluids must be the same, although the electrolyte concentration is quite different.

Average values for water intake and output are shown in Table 8–1, which is largely self-explanatory. Metabolic water is derived from the oxidation of foodstuffs.

Water, once absorbed, diffuses rapidly and equally through the body. However, because of the osmotic activity of the solutes and the effect of the semipermeable membranes of the cells in producing varying concentrations of such solutes, it is convenient to regard body water as divided into separate compartments. The major divisions are given in Table 8–2. Other small pools are present (e.g., cerebrospinal fluid), and some water is held in a tightly bound form on the surface of the mineral crystals of bone and structural molecules such as collagen.

Methods are available for measuring the volume of the major compartments. With the exception of blood volume, these are largely research methods little used in routine practice and will not be described here.

TABLE 8–1 AVERAGE VALUES FOR WATER INTAKE AND OUTPUT

Water Intake		Water Output	
Water of beverages	1200 mL	Lungs	700 mL
Water content of food	1100 mL	Insensible perspiration	300 mL
Water of oxidation	300 mL	Sweat	100 mL
Total intake	2600 mL	Feces	100 mL
		Urine	1400 mL
		Total output	2600 mL

ANTIDIURETIC HORMONE

The amount of water in the body is largely determined by the total content of sodium and potassium; however, plasma osmolality is maintained by the action of antidiuretic hormone (ADH, vasopressin) on the kidney.

ADH is a polypeptide hormone secreted by the posterior lobe of the pituitary gland. It acts on the epithelial cells lining the collecting ducts of the renal tubules. These cells possess membranes that are normally impermeable to water (and are the only such cells in the body). ADH causes these membranes to become permeable to water, but not to solutes. This allows water to be drawn from the lumen of the collecting tubules into the zone of high osmotic pressure formed by the countercurrent mechanism (p. 202), thus concentrating the urine. Plasma osmolality is monitored by cells in the supra-optic nucleus of the hypothalamus that have direct neural connections with the posterior lobe of the pituitary. These cells synthesize ADH, which is then stored as granules in the axons. The granules migrate

TABLE 8–2 APPROXIMATE FLUID COMPARTMENT VOLUMES IN THE ADULT MALE

Compartment	Volume in Liters	Percentage of Total Body Fluid	Percentage of Body Weight
Total body fluid	42	100	50–70
Intracellular fluid	28	67	30–40
Extracellular fluid (including plasma)	14	33	15–20
Plasma	3	0.7	4.5
Blood	5	1.1	—

in the axon from the hypothalamus to the pituitary gland.

Thus, if plasma osmolality *rises,* ADH is released, making the tubule cells more permeable to water and so causing water retention and increasing the concentration of the urine solutes. The water entering the collecting ducts represents about 10% of the filtered load, or approximately 15 L/day.

WATER DEFICIENCY AND EXCESS

Alterations in body water content alone, with no associated change in the body electrolyte content, are uncommon but can occur.

Water deficiency may be due to reduced intake or to increased loss (this may occur from the skin as perspiration or from the lungs during hyperventilation). Excessive amounts of urine may be passed during an osmotic diuresis, such as may occur in uncontrolled diabetes mellitus or with hypercalcemia.

A partial or complete lack of ADH may occur; rarely as a congenital defect or more commonly following pituitary damage (for example, in car accidents, when the pituitary stalk is sheared by the sudden movement of the brain). This produces a state called *diabetes insipidus,* characterized by the passing of very large volumes of urine of very low specific gravity. Such patients are constantly at risk of dying from dehydration.

Water excess may occur as a result of increased intake (psychogenic polydipsia) or of excessive intravenous infusions of dextrose. It may also occur from water retention produced by increased ADH secretion. This syndrome of *inappropriate secretion of ADH* is not uncommon, especially in hospital patients. Whether the elevated ADH levels are truly inappropriate is debatable; however, it has been definitely established that an increase in ADH secretion occurs in many severe disease states. The more important conditions are bronchogenic carcinoma, head injuries, other cerebral lesions, metastatic carcinoma, and lung disease (especially pneumonia).

Water excess can usually be recognized by inspection of the plasma electrolyte levels; all are low, especially sodium, which is often below 120 mmol/L. The hemodilution is confirmed by the blood urea nitrogen (BUN) level, which will be below 10 mg/dL, and by a comparison of the serum and urine osmolalities (low and high, respectively). Apart from analytical error, this is by far the most common cause of a BUN level of less than 10 mg/dL.

ELECTROLYTES

The term *electrolyte* refers to a solution of charged particles or ions that will conduct an electrical current. The particles may be positively charged (cations) or negatively charged (anions). The common cations in the body are sodium, potassium, calcium, and magnesium; the common anions are chloride, bicarbonate, phosphate, sulfate, and organic acids. The proportion of cations and anions is so balanced that electrical neutrality is preserved. This, it should be understood, is not the same as neutral pH (7) or even normal body pH (7.4).

The SI system requires electrolyte units to be molar. For univalent ions (e.g., sodium) milliequivalents and millimoles are the same. For divalent ions (such as calcium, which generally is reported in mass concentration units in North America) $\text{mmol/L} = \frac{\text{mEq/L}}{2}$. Note, however, that there is no assumption about valency when molar units are used.

The concept of *ionic activity* should be introduced here, although a text of physical chemistry should be consulted for details. The activity of an ion = activity coefficient × concentration (i.e., $a = f \cdot c$), and the ionic activity can loosely be regarded as "effective concentration." In very dilute solutions f approaches unity, but in concentrated solutions it becomes a significant factor, owing to interaction between ions. In fact ionic activities, rather than concentration, are the fundamental quantities for many physiological phenomena, but they have seldom been investigated in clinical work. Pure sodium chloride solutions in the 100 to 150 mmol/L range have an ionic activity coefficient on the order of 0.75 to 0.8, indicating significant interaction. Obviously the presence of protein will affect the ion/water ratio and thus the ionic activity. Indeed, some authors have suggested that electrolyte concentrations should be reported in mmol/L plasma water.

Gibbs-Donnan Equilibrium. When two solutions are separated by a semipermeable membrane through which all the solutes can pass freely, then an equilibrium is established such that the ions are equally distributed in both compartments. Both the total ion concentration and the total concentration of osmotically active particles are the same on both sides of the membrane.

However, if the solution on one side contains charged, but nondiffusible particles such as proteins, then the distribution of the diffusible ions will be unequal. This unequal distribution of the diffusible ions gives rise to a membrane potential. However, the Gibbs-Donnan law states that the *product* of the concentrations of the diffusible ions in one compartment is equal to the *product* of the concentrations of the diffusible ions in the other compartment.

The numerical example below should make this clearer.

In the example Pr^- indicates nondiffusible protein carrying a negative charge.

Note that within each compartment electrical neutrality is preserved but that there is a difference in the sum of the charges on each side of the membrane, creating the membrane potential.

Before Steady State		→	**After Steady State**	
Compartment 1	*Compartment 2*		*Compartment 1*	*Compartment 2*
Na^+ = 3 mmol/L	Na^+ = 3 mmol/L		Na^+ = 2 mmol/L	Na^+ = 4 mmol/L
Cl^- = 3 mmol/L			Cl^- = 2 mmol/L	Cl^- = 1 mmol/L
	Pr^- = 3 mmol/L			Pr^- = 3 mmol/L

Distribution of Ions. The distribution of ions in intracellular and extracellular fluid is shown diagrammatically in Figure 8–1. Sodium is the predominant cation of the extracellular fluid. Small amounts of potassium, calcium, and magnesium are present in the extracellular fluid, whereas carbonate and chloride constitute the greater part of its anion content. Small amounts of organic acids and phosphate are also present. In plasma the anion balance is made up by protein; there is very little protein in interstitial fluid, and there the electrical balance is made up chiefly by an increase in chloride.

The major cation of the intracellular compartment is potassium, although small amounts of magnesium and sodium are also present. These are balanced largely by phosphate. The precise concentrations vary with the different tissues.

Sodium

The total body content of sodium is on the order of 75 mmol/kg. Some 50% of this is sequestrated in bone and is only very slowly mobilized and exchanged with the remainder. The normal plasma sodium concentration is 135 to 145 mmol/L, the content per liter of plasma water being some 8 to 9 mmol/L higher. The average daily intake of sodium is between 50 and 3000 mmol. Sodium is lost from the body in sweat, feces, and urine; under normal circumstances only the latter route is quantitatively significant. The amount of sodium excreted in the urine is under close regulatory control. Of the 15 to 20 mmol/min filtered by the glomerulus, only some 2% appears in the urine. Most of the sodium is passively reabsorbed in the ascending limb of the loop of Henle by an active transport mechanism requiring energy.

The kidney can reduce sodium loss in the urine to just a few millimoles per day, largely under the control of aldosterone. This mechanism is described further on p. 201. Whether there is a salt-losing hormone is still a matter of debate.

Potassium

The total body content of potassium is 50 to 60 mmol/kg; the intracellular concentration is difficult to estimate precisely but is about 160 mmol/L in muscle. The concentration is lower in red cells, about 45 mmol/L, and the plasma concentration is 3.5 to 5.6 mmol/L.

It is vitally important that potassium determinations not be done on hemolyzed blood, because the potassium released from the lyzed cells will artificially elevate the plasma value. For this reason, too, it is preferable to measure potassium in plasma, not serum: the process of clotting causes some release from the red cells. Even plasma may be unreliable, because hemolysis can occur if the specimen is spun for too long (for example, during a coffee break) in a centrifuge that becomes overheated. Obviously, even on a hemolyzed sample, a *low* potassium level is significant.

The average dietary intake of potassium is 50 to 150 mmol/day. The mechanism of renal absorption and excretion is described on p. 300. It is important to remember that hydrogen ions and potassium ions compete for excretion (and are exchanged for sodium). In alkalosis, for example, an excessive loss of potassium occurs from the body, with an eventual fall in plasma levels.

The major plasma anions are chloride and bicarbonate. The bicarbonate concentration is regulated by mechanisms described later in this chapter. Chloride levels tend to vary inversely with the bicarbonate concentra-

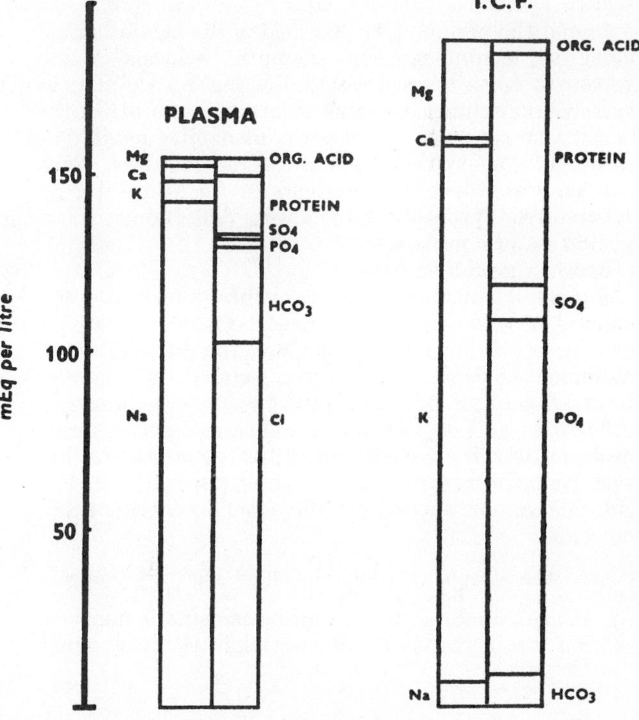

Figure 8–1 The balance of the main cations and anions in plasma and intracellular fluid. Adapted from Black, D. A. K.: Essentials of Fluid Balance, 3rd ed. Oxford, Blackwell Scientific Publications, 1964.

tion and in general depend on the concentration of other ions in order to preserve electrochemical neutrality.

Anion Gap

If the concentrations of the two major plasma anions are summed and subtracted from the sum of the two major cations, a difference of 12 to 18 mmol/L will be obtained in the normal person. This is called the "anion gap."

$$\text{Anion gap} = ([Na^+] + [K^+]) - ([Cl^-] + [HCO_3^-])$$

Some advocate omitting potassium from the equation as an insignificant factor; if this is done, the gap is some 5 mmol lower.

This relationship forms a useful and rapid check on the analytical accuracy of electrolyte determinations, and the technologist should become accustomed to checking results by this calculation, especially outside the routine batches or when the estimations are done on different machines. The clinical significance of abnormalities of the anion gap is described later.

It should be clearly understood that serum or plasma concentrations of electrolytes may not give much guidance as to the total body content. This is especially true of plasma potassium levels, because most of the ion is intracellular. Using plasma levels of potassium as an index of the intracellular levels is rather like trying to pick up a dime at the bottom of a jar of molasses using a stalk of celery; it can be attempted, but the exercise is of dubious value. Only major shifts in potassium balance are reflected in the plasma values. Nonetheless, plasma levels much higher or lower than the reference range are significant in that they can induce cardiac arrhythmias.

ACID-BASE BALANCE

One of the problems in this field is the lack of agreement on terminology. For example, "acidosis" would appear to mean an acid reaction of the intracellular or extracellular fluids, whereas in practice the pH of the blood very rarely falls below the neutrality point. The report of the Ad Hoc Committee of the New York Academy of Sciences Conference on Acid-Base Terminology (1964) proposed the following definitions:

Acid—a proton donor.

Base—a proton acceptor.

Buffer—a substance that in solution increases the amount of acid or base that must be added to cause a change in pH. The buffer value, β, is the ratio of a small increment of strong base to the associated small change in pH. A solution with unit buffer value will change its pH by one unit on addition of one equivalent of strong base per liter. It should be noted that anions and cations such as sodium, potassium, magnesium, calcium, and chloride cannot function as buffers and are neither acidic nor basic.

pH—the simple relationship $ph = \log \frac{1}{[H^+]}$ is purely theoretical; in practice the measurement is made by reference to a standard cell electromotive force, which is affected by temperature. The main practical point is the necessity to maintain close control of temperature when making pH measurements.

Total carbon dioxide concentration—the total carbon dioxide extractable from a biological fluid by treatment with strong acid. It is made up of dissolved carbon dioxide, carbonic acid, bicarbonate and carbonate ions, and carbamino compounds.

P_{CO_2}—the partial pressure of carbon dioxide in a gas phase in equilibrium with a biological fluid.

Carbonic acid—the concentration of carbonic acid, H_2CO_3.

Dissolved carbon dioxide concentration—the concentration of the CO_2 gas in physical solution. In practice, the very small amount of carbonic acid found in biological fluids is included, and the sum of the two is found by multiplying the P_{CO_2} by a factor that is usually taken as 0.03 but that varies with temperature.

Bicarbonate concentration—in the strict chemical sense, the concentration of HCO_3 ion in the biological fluid. In practice, it is usually calculated by subtracting the parameter $0.03 \times P_{CO_2}$ from the total carbon dioxide concentration; thus it includes carbamino compounds and carbonate. The error is not important physiologically, except in intracellular fluid, which is not directly amenable to analysis.

Standard bicarbonate concentration—the HCO_3 ion concentration in blood that has been equilibrated with CO_2 at 40 mm Hg at 37°C. Depending on the method used, the blood sample may be oxygenated in vitro or remain as drawn.

Carbon dioxide combining power—the total carbon dioxide concentration of anaerobically separated plasma equilibrated to a P_{CO_2} of 40 mm Hg at room temperature. This measurement is subject to many experimental variables and is obsolete.

Buffer base—the sum of the buffer anions of whole blood: HCO_3, plasma proteins, and hemoglobins. Minor buffers are not included.

Base excess—originally (Siggaard-Andersen, 1965) the titratable base of whole blood when titrated with strong acid to a pH of 7.40 at 38°C. The Ad Hoc Committee modified this definition by changing the temperature from 38°C to 37°C.

The Committee's report also makes the point that calculations using the Henderson-Hasselbalch equation are valid only for single-phase liquids such as serum or plasma; the relationship cannot be simply applied to whole blood.

Acidosis and Alkalosis. It is proposed that these terms be restricted to the direction of the effect on blood pH that a disturbance would have if it were not compensated for by the physiological control mechanisms. Thus if the accumulation of an acid metabolite would tend to change the pH in a downward direction, even though this tendency is opposed by the buffer systems of the blood, which make the actual pH decrease minimal, the original disturbance is regarded as an acidosis. The source of the disturbance is indicated by either a general adjective—*respiratory* or *metabolic*—or a more specific term—*diabetic*. The general rule is to indicate the nature of the problem from a physiological rather than a purely chemical viewpoint.

ACID-BASE REGULATION

In order to preserve cell life, the factors, both internal and external, that may disturb the conditions essential for continuing cellular function must be controlled. When such control exists, the situation is said to be one of homeostasis. Single-celled organisms can exchange gases and excrete waste products directly into their surroundings; multicellular organisms have had to develop more complex arrangements. The main feature is a transport system carrying oxygen and nutrients to the cells, and removing carbon dioxide and waste products. Since that system must be in intimate contact with the cells, its own composition must be regulated, particularly for those components that have a large effect on cell function, such as hydrogen ion concentration. It would be senseless for a cell to discharge excess hydrogen ions into the transport fluid if they were left free to interfere with another cell's metabolism. There also must be systems for regenerating the components of the control system and for sensitive detection of disturbances in the system of homeostasis that will initiate corrective action.

Although we tend to discuss acid-base regulation as though it were an isolated topic, in fact it is closely bound up with oxygen and carbon dioxide transport, respiratory dynamics, and renal function. From a technical point of view, we need to know what the systems are, the basis of their operation, and how their status can be assessed by laboratory procedures. The prime limitation on such assessment is the inability to sample cell contents or even the interstitial fluid surrounding the cells. We investigate the acid-base state of the blood mainly because it is the only area accessible to sampling. We have to assume that the ready interchange of the active components of the systems between cell, interstitial fluid, and blood makes the blood a reasonable indicator of the other two.

BUFFER SYSTEMS

If a weak acid (weak = only slightly dissociated and therefore yielding only small amounts of hydrogen ion) and a salt of that acid are present in a solution, the salt dissociates to a much greater extent than the acid, producing ions of the conjugate base of the acid. Addition of hydrogen or hydroxyl ions to the buffer system produces changes in the ionic pattern that minimize the acidifying or alkalizing effect of the added ions. The reactions may be summarized as follows (using the carbonic acid-bicarbonate system of the plasma as an example):

$$H^+ + {}^-HCO_3 \rightarrow H_2CO_3$$

The added H^+ ions react with bicarbonate to produce weakly ionized carbonic acid; the small number of H^+ ions from the carbonic acid will have only a small effect on the total H^+ ion concentration, and the drop in pH will be minimized.

$$^-OH + H_2CO_3 \rightarrow {}^-HCO_3 + H_2O$$

The added ^-OH ions reduce the carbonic acid content of the solution; but the quantitative decrease in H^+ ion concentration is small because of the weak ionization of carbonic acid, and therefore the rise in pH will be minimal.

In considering the characteristics of a buffer system, the extent of ionization of the acid component is expressed by the dissociation constant, K′. This depends on the relationship:

$$\frac{H^+ \times {}^-HCO_3}{H_2CO_3}$$

(Strictly speaking the terms in the expression should be stated as ionic activities, not concentrations, but the distinction does not add materially to the basic concepts.)

If the K′ value for the carbonic acid system is required, there is a practical problem: measurement of carbonic acid concentration is very difficult. In practice, since there is a known relationship between carbonic acid content and its dissociation product, carbon dioxide, which *can* be measured, the dissociation constant K can be determined. For the carbonic acid system, it is expressed as its negative logarithm to avoid inconveniently small numbers (such as for the pH notation), and the usual value stated is 6.1. (The true value varies according to the pH and to whether activities or concentrations are used. Siggaard-Andersen distinguishes four pK values but indicates that the differences are trivial for most purposes.)

The importance of knowing the pK value for a buffer acid is related to the buffering ability of the system. A buffer system has its maximum capacity to minimize change of pH at pH values close to the pK. This leads to the question: If the carbonic acid-bicarbonate system is most effective at pH 6.1, what is its suitability at the normal blood pH of 7.4? Although the system is not working at its peak range, nevertheless this apparent disadvantage is offset by the ease with which its components, bicarbonate and carbonic acid (in terms of the dissolved carbon dioxide), can be controlled and adjusted by the kidneys and lungs, respectively. The unique feature of the bicarbonate–carbonic acid buffer system is the fact that one component (bicarbonate) is "fixed" and is regulated by metabolic processes, ultimately in the kidney, whereas the other component is volatile (when converted to carbon dioxide and water by carbonic anhydrase) and can be regulated by the lungs and respiratory mechanisms. The overriding importance of this feature will be realized when we consider the lack of rapid and adjustable methods of controlling the levels of the other buffer systems. In addition to the relationship between the pK values of the acid component of a buffer system and its zone of most effective activity, the other factor governing the power of the system is the actual concentration of its components. If the bicarbonate level of the plasma is depleted by acids in diabetic acidosis, the system becomes progressively less effective until the renal mechanisms replenish the bicarbonate.

The Henderson-Hasselbalch Equation

For any buffer system composed of a weak acid and one of its salts, there is a relationship between the attributes of the system expressed in the equation:

$$pH = pK + \log \frac{[Salt]}{[Acid]}$$

The values for the salt and the acid are expressed as concentrations, although strictly activities should be used. It will be noted that if the concentrations of salt and acid are equal, with a ratio of 1.0, the value for the pH is equal to the pK value (log 1 = 0). Again referring to the bicarbonate–carbonic acid system, the pK used is 6.1; typical values for the bicarbonate and acid concentrations would be 24 mmol per liter and 1.2 mmol per liter. (The carbonic acid concentration is found by multiplying the partial pressure of carbon dioxide, P_{CO_2}, by the factor 0.03.) The ratio of bicarbonate–carbonic acid is thus 24/1.2, or 20/1. The pH determined at this ratio is then:

$$\begin{aligned} pH &= 6.1 + \log 20 \\ &= 6.1 + 1.301 \\ &= 7.401 \end{aligned}$$

Since pK is taken as a constant, the Henderson-Hasselbalch equation contains three unknowns; determination of any two will permit calculation of the third. In practice, as we shall see, it is usual to measure pH and P_{CO_2}, calculate the carbonic acid from the expression

$$H_2CO_3 = 0.03 \times P_{CO_2}$$

and then calculate the bicarbonate. (The term P_{CO_2} for partial pressure of carbon dioxide is written correctly as P_{CO_2}, since the letter p or P stands for "partial pressure"; it does not have the meaning of the p in pH; this designates the term as having a logarithmic derivation.)

The constants of the Henderson-Hasselbalch equation may, in certain circumstances, change or at least appear to change. The factor 0.0301 is the solubility coefficient of carbon dioxide in plasma at 37°C. This numerical value can vary with temperature and also if there is much lipid in the plasma.

It is also now established beyond doubt that in seriously ill patients (particularly when rapid shifts are occurring in electrolyte concentrations), the apparent value for pK'_1 may not be constant at 6.1. Why this is so is still not at all clear, but it does mean that a calculated value for bicarbonate is quite unreliable in such patients. The difference between the analyzed and calculated values may be as much as 8 to 10 mmol/L; furthermore, the calculated (but not the analyzed) value may show wide fluctuations over a quite short period of time, a phenomenon not normally seen.

Most modern blood gas analyzers are programmed to produce a bicarbonate value from P_{CO_2} and pH readings; it is vital to realize that this may be unreliable and that in seriously ill patients a *measured* bicarbonate value should be obtained at least once a day. It is also important to realize that the factor which determines the blood pH is the ratio of bicarbonate–carbonic acid. Before the advent of rapid and accurate methods for measurement of blood pH and P_{CO_2}, for information about the acid-base status of the patient the clinician had to rely on such measurements as the CO_2 combining power and CO_2 content. These two measurements give the *sum* of the bicarbonate and carbonic acid components under different analytical conditions; at best the information is only qualitative and at worst grossly misleading. The CO_2 content determination still has some use in emergency situations, since it will at least indicate a gross deficiency of bicarbonate in such conditions as diabetic coma; in disturbances of the acid-base regulation with a respiratory element, however, it is of little use. We will return to this aspect later.

As mentioned previously, the buffer systems controlling acid-base balance are not solely blood systems. Intracellular buffering is at least as important, both in the red cell and the tissue cells. The intracellular and extracellular systems are similar in components; they differ in the relative preponderance of these components in different locations. The relative importance is governed by the actual concentrations (for example, the amounts of protein are larger than those of other buffers) and by the characteristics of the buffer system. Thus the proteins are important, quite apart from quantity, because their average pK values are close to the normal blood pH of 7.4. The plasma phosphate system has a similar pK value but is less important because the concentrations are much lower. Another factor influencing the biological utility of a buffer system is the ability of its components to pass from plasma to cell and from cell to interstitial fluid. This applies most forcefully to the hydrogen ion, which can travel easily across cell walls. The hydrogen ion is not of course strictly a component of a buffer system, but it is the common factor between the systems, so that the operations of one system affect those of another through the intermediary hydrogen ion. This interconnection of the buffer systems is called the isohydric principle; to quote Guyton, "The buffer systems actually buffer each other."

The Phosphate Buffer System

The "basic," or "salt," component is the monohydrogen phosphate ion; the "weak acid" component is the dihydrogen phosphate ion. Addition of hydrogen ions to the system produces the change:

$$HPO_4^{=} + H^+ \rightarrow H_2PO_4^-$$

The weakly acidic dihydrogen phosphate produced has only a small effect on pH. Addition of basic ions converts some of the dihydrogen phosphate of the system into weakly basic monohydrogen phosphate. The overall effectiveness of the system, despite the fact that its pK is closer to the blood pH of 7.4 than the bicarbonate–carbonic acid system, is limited by the low concentration in extracellular fluids. The concentration of phosphates inside the cells is much greater, and this system assumes correspondingly greater importance.

The Protein Buffer Systems

This can be regarded as a dual system: the proteins of the plasma and cells on the one hand, and the special protein pair hemoglobin/oxyhemoglobin on the other. We will treat them separately, since the latter system has special features.

Proteins derive their buffering ability from the free carboxylic acid and amino groups in their structure. The free groups arise from those amino acids that have acidic and basic groups over and above those required for peptide bond formation. Thus aspartic acid has an extra carboxylic acid group; lysine, an extra amino group. Another source of amino groups is the guanidino structure (—NH—CNH—NH_2) in arginine. We shall see in the case of hemoglobin the importance of the imidazole group of histidine. In solution at a particular pH, the groups will be dissociated to varying extents; the general pattern of their action is the buffering of added basic ions by the hydrogen ions released from the —COOH groups, and of added hydrogen ions by the hydroxyl ions released from the amino groups, whose actual form in the protein is —NH_3OH. The large concentrations of protein both in the plasma and intracellularly make this system probably the most important one quantitatively. Even the intracellular component is involved in the plasma processes, since the bicarbonate ion and carbon dioxide are readily diffusible across cell membranes.

The buffering capacity of hemoglobin is greater than that of other proteins for two main reasons. First, it contains an unusually large proportion (8%) of histidine, the imidazole group of which is particularly effective at physiological pH. Second, the spatial association of the histidine of the hemoglobin molecule with the heme prosthetic group engenders changes in the state of the imidazole group during oxygen uptake and release from the heme, which in turn enhance the buffering ability of the whole molecule.

Uptake of oxygen in the lungs by the heme group of hemoglobin changes the dissociation constant of the imidazole group of a histidine group, and in effect makes it a stronger acid; that is, the dissociation increases, releasing hydrogen ion into the surrounding fluid, in this case the contents of the red cell. It reacts with the bicarbonate, which is the transport form of carbon dioxide released from tissue cells by their metabolism, to produce carbonic acid; under the influence of the enzyme carbonic anhydrase this is "dehydrated" to produce water and carbon dioxide, which passes into the plasma and is excreted in the lungs. In this process the hydrogen ion released during oxygenation of the hemoglobin is effectively buffered.

In the tissues the process operates in the reverse direction. As the oxyhemoglobin releases oxygen, a reaction promoted by the low Po_2 in the tissues, the dissociation of the imidazole group decreases, becoming a weaker acid, and therefore taking up hydrogen ion from the red cell fluid. As carbon dioxide enters the red cell from the tissues, it reacts with water to form carbonic acid. This reaction proceeds very slowly in the plasma, but the enzyme carbonic anhydrase in the red cell accelerates the process more than 200-fold. The carbonic acid then dissociates to give hydrogen and bicarbonate ions; the hydrogen ions are taken up by the change in the imidazole group of hemoglobin noted earlier. The bicarbonate diffuses into the plasma and is replaced by chloride ion in order to maintain the electrical neutrality of the red cell contents. This is usually referred to as the chloride shift.

It might appear that this transfer of bicarbonate ion from the red cell to the plasma would make it unavailable for subsequent excretion in the lungs. When the red cell enters the lungs, the carbonic anhydrase converts the small amount of carbonic acid therein into water and carbon dioxide, as described previously. This promotes the reaction in which bicarbonate is converted to carbonic acid. Bicarbonate migrates from the plasma under the influence of the gradient established and in turn is converted to carbonic acid by the hydrogen released from hemoglobin as it becomes oxygenated. The movement of bicarbonate from plasma to red cell is counterbalanced by a movement of chloride in the opposite direction—this is the other phase of the chloride shift.

It will be noted that the uptake of oxygen and excretion of carbon dioxide are both dependent on the buffering properties of hemoglobin. In addition, about 30% of the carbon dioxide is transported in very loose combination with hemoglobin (and to some extent with plasma proteins) in the form of carbaminohemoglobin. The combination is so loose that in the lungs it is broken rapidly to release the carbon dioxide into the plasma and then to the alveoli. A small amount, about 7%, of the carbon dioxide is carried in true solution in the plasma.

The Carriage of Oxygen in the Blood

The term P_AO_2 is used to indicate the partial pressure (or tension) of oxygen gas in arterial blood (not plasma or serum). The volume of oxygen carried in blood is determined by two factors: the amount dissolved and the amount bound to hemoglobin.

The dissolved fraction, even at high oxygen tensions, is very small: at a P_AO_2 of 100 mm of mercury (13.3 kPa), 100 mL of arterial blood will contain only 0.3 mL of O_2. The cardiac output of blood is approximately 5 L/min; if blood contained only *dissolved* oxygen, the metabolic requirements of an adult male would necessitate a cardiac output of 100 L/min. Clearly, the fraction bound to hemoglobin is of great importance. One molecule of hemoglobin will bind four molecules of oxygen; the degree to which the hemoglobin molecules in the blood have combined with molecular oxygen to become oxyhemoglobin is called the percentage saturation.

The relationship between P_AO_2 and percentage saturation is shown in Figure 8–2; this is known as the oxyhemoglobin association/dissociation curve. Note the sigmoid shape. This means that at high P_AO_2, variations in oxygen tension make very little difference to the oxygen saturation. However, the mixed venous point ($P\bar{v}O_2$) is at about 40 mm of mercury, where the saturation is 75% and the curve becomes very steep. This is the critical point at which oxygen is unloaded into the tissues. It can be seen that, if the shape of the curve is altered (that is, if the relationship between P_AO_2 and per cent saturation varies), the volume of oxygen unloaded to the tissues can change appreciably.

The shape of the curve can change for a number of different reasons. Major shifts will occur if the red cells contain an abnormal hemoglobin or if there is a deficiency of hexokinase or pyruvate kinase. In clinical situations, a shift can occur with changes in pH, Pco_2 (influencing pH), temperature, or the red cell content of diphosphoglycerate (2,3-DPG).

A shift to the right indicates a *decreased* affinity of hemoglobin for oxygen and can be caused by an *increase* in Pco_2, red cell 2,3-DPG, temperature, or hydrogen ion concentration (low pH). Conversely, a shift to the left is produced by a decrease in these factors.

These facts are of clinical importance: in the lungs, carbon dioxide is released, the hydrogen ion concentration decreases, and the affinity of hemoglobin for oxygen

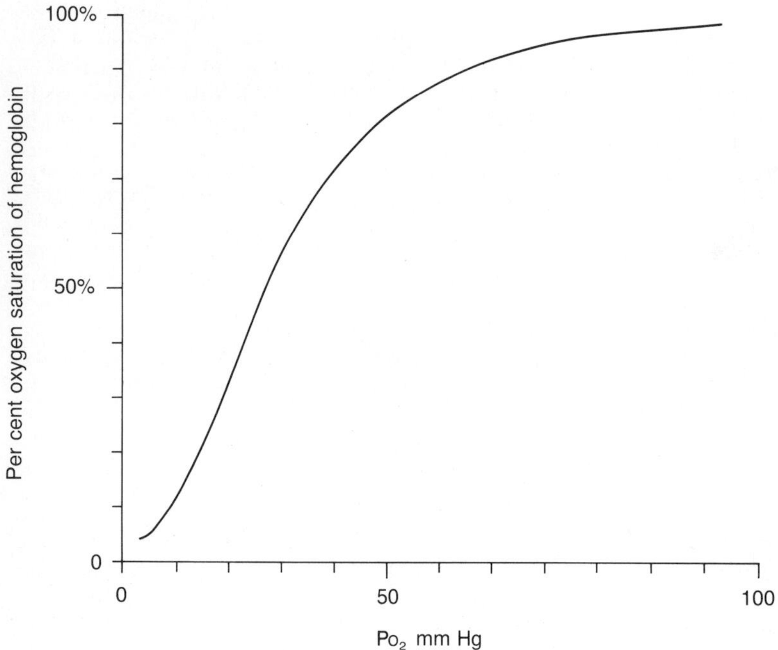

Figure 8–2 The oxyhemoglobin association/dissociation curve.

is increased. The 2,3-DPG content of banked blood is very low, and thus transfused blood that is more than 2 to 3 days old will not release as much oxygen to the tissues as fresh blood. The transfused cells will regain their normal DPG content after a few days, however.

To the respiratory internist and technician, the shape of the dissociation curve is obviously of some clinical importance. This can be defined by measuring the Po_2 at 50% saturation (P 50). To do this requires titration with varying oxygen tensions and simultaneous measurement of the oxyhemoglobin saturation using an oximeter.

It should be clearly recognized that a *calculated* percentage hemoglobin saturation, although usually valid in the normal person, may be quite inaccurate in a sick person. If a true reading of saturation is required, nothing can replace a measured value (see the comments on calculated bicarbonate).

Detection Systems

Control of pH by buffer action is an immediate, on-the-spot action, and in normal circumstances suffices to prevent the additional hydrogen ions produced in digestion and absorption of food from upsetting homeostasis. Changes in lung ventilation that cause retention of carbon dioxide will lower blood pH because of increased carbonic acid formation and reduced oxygen tension in the blood. These changes are detected by several mechanisms.

1. Increase of Pco_2 and hydrogen ion concentration in the blood stimulate the respiratory control center in the medulla of the brain. The increased rate and depth of breathing that results increases carbon dioxide excretion in the lungs, lowering carbonic acid level in the blood and hence raising the pH. This system is very sensitive and can produce effective change in a few minutes, provided that other factors do not impair its operation. This action is assisted by the ability of increased Pco_2 levels to gain access to the spinal fluid (the same is not true of hydrogen ions, however). Once in the CSF the carbon dioxide forms carbonic acid, and there is a special area of nerve fibers that detects the associated rise in hydrogen ion concentration and stimulates the respiratory activity.

2. In the carotid and aortic arteries there are small bodies that are sensitive to chemical changes in blood composition; they are called chemoreceptors. They are sensitive to Po_2 levels—unlike the respiratory center in the brain—as well as to Pco_2 and hydrogen ion levels. A fall in Po_2 level produces a nervous impulse in the chemoreceptors that in turn stimulates the respiratory control center in the brain. The chemoreceptors, although sensitive to Pco_2 and hydrogen ion level changes, are not as important in respiration control as the direct effect of these substances on the control center in the brain.

There are other nervous mechanisms that affect respiration, but these are described in texts on medical physiology.

An important feature of the nervous mechanisms just described is their incorporation of automatic control. When the initial stimulus to increased rate of respiration—raised Pco_2 level—has been reduced by the effect of the response, the stimulus itself decreases and the system returns to normal. This type of control, in which the effect of a reaction to a change is to damp down the initial stimulus, is called "feedback." The term is borrowed from electronics and modern industrial techniques. It implies the use of the output of a device to control the quality of that output by modifying the input. To give an example: an automated lathe can be programmed by a tape to cut a piece of metal to a certain size. As the work proceeds, a measuring system determines the size attained. This measurement is compared with the programmed final size, and this information in turn controls the rate of cutting, so that the work stops as soon as the final size is reached. This process is considered further in connection with laboratory automation (see p. 106).

As we have seen, the reaction of the buffer systems to acid-base disturbances is immediate, and the reaction time of the respiratory systems is a few minutes. The third system, the renal, is the long-term member of the team. Its functions are to replenish buffer ions, especially bicarbonate, used up in buffering excess hydrogen ions, to assist with special systems of its own in dealing with large incursions of acidic or basic ions, and to adjust its capacity for these functions in order to handle a continuing problem.

The renal mechanisms of acid-base regulation are found in the tubules, distal and proximal, and in the collecting tubules (see Fig. 8–3). The main activity is control of bicarbonate level in the plasma. The cells contain carbonic anhydrase and can combine carbon dioxide and water to form carbonic acid. Although this dissociates only to a small extent to give hydrogen and bicarbonate ions, as fast as these are released they are transported out of the cell—the hydrogen ions into the tubular fluid and the bicarbonate into the blood. The cellular mechanisms that move hydrogen ions into the tubular fluid are very efficient, e.g., the pH of that fluid can be reduced as low as pH 4.0. Since the reaction starts off with carbon dioxide, its level in the plasma will control the rate of bicarbonate formation in the tubule cells.

The hydrogen ions thus discharged into the tubular fluid will react with any bicarbonate filtered by the glomerulus, forming carbonic acid, which dissociates into carbon dioxide and water. The carbon dioxide diffuses from the tubular lumen into the cells and can serve as a source of bicarbonate to maintain plasma levels by the mechanism just described. It should be pointed out that for this mechanism to produce a net gain of bicarbonate into the plasma, there must be a plentiful supply of hydrogen ion. In alkalosis, in which a plasma bicarbonate excess is present, a proportion of this ion filtered by the glomerulus will pass out into the urine because of lack of hydrogen ions in the tubular fluid. Thus the mechanism is self-regulating, controlled ultimately by the hydrogen ion content of the blood, that is, its pH.

In order to excrete an excess of hydrogen ions, the tubules have a special mechanism in which these ions are combined with ammonia. The ammonia is manufactured in the tubular cells, mainly from the amino acid glutamine, by a deaminating enzyme. The ammonia reacts with hydrogen ions in the tubular fluid to produce the ammonium ion, NH_4^+. The predominant anion in the fluid is chloride, and the ammonium can be regarded as forming ammonium chloride. This is a neutral salt, and therefore will not affect the pH. The ammonia-synthesizing system can increase in capacity to cope with a continuing load of hydrogen ions, a process that can take about 48 hours. It should be noted that once in high gear, so to speak, the system cannot shut off at short notice; it will take about the same time interval to return to normal operation. In a patient whose metabolic acidosis has been corrected rapidly by vigorous treatment, this can result in excessive loss of hydrogen ion, leading to an alkalosis. These renal mechanisms for regulating H^+ excretion are summarized in Figure 8–3.

THE INTERPRETATION AND CLINICAL SIGNIFICANCE OF ELECTROLYTE AND ACID-BASE DATA

Although not strictly the province of the medical technologist, some knowledge of the significance of the laboratory data should be not only of interest to the technologist but also of potential value in assessing whether a data set is coherent or whether there are

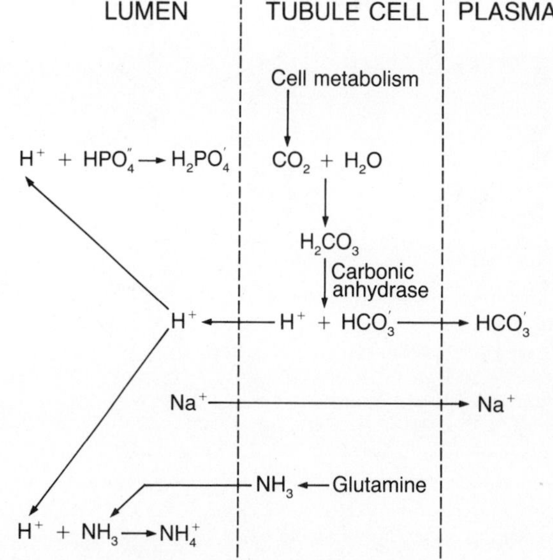

Figure 8–3 Generation of H^+ and HCO'_3, and buffering by phosphate and ammonia, in the renal tubule. From Spencer, F.: Aspects of Human Pathology Theory Relevant to Medical Laboratory Sciences.Reading, Mass., Butterworth, Inc., 1972.

discordant features that might draw attention to analytical problems.

The interpretation of electrolyte and acid-base data is largely a matter of experience, coupled with a comprehensive knowledge of the clinical information available on a particular patient. Nonetheless, an often surprising amount of information may be extracted from the simple numerical values.

In its most basic form the Henderson-Hasselbalch equation can be expressed as

$$\text{pH} \alpha \frac{[\text{Bicarbonate}]}{[\text{Carbonic acid}]}$$

which is equivalent to

$$\text{pH} \alpha \frac{[HCO_3]}{P_{CO_2}}$$

or, in a more general form,

$$\text{pH} \alpha \frac{\text{Metabolic component}}{\text{Respiratory component}}$$

These relationships emphasize that a *fall* in the bicarbonate level or a *rise* in CO_2 tension will cause a *fall* in pH, and *vice versa*. pH is really an inconvenient unit for clinical work: not only is it inverted (a fall in pH means a rise in $[H^+]$), but a difference of 0.3 pH units means a doubling or halving of the H^+ concentration. Some advocate reporting $[H^+]$ in nanomoles (or $[H^+] \times 10^9$). The pH reference range of 7.35 to 7.45 would then be 45 to 35 nanomoles. It is to be hoped that this will become the practice before long.

The extremes of blood pH in life are pH 6.8 (158 nmol/L) to 7.7 (20 nmol/L). The patient's prognosis at such values is very poor, of course; acidosis tends to be tolerated much better than alkalosis, however.

The terms *acidosis* and *alkalosis* have already been defined; it will be apparent from the above simplification of the Henderson-Hasselbalch equation that they can have a metabolic or a respiratory etiology. Four basic states of acid-base imbalance can therefore be defined: metabolic acidosis, metabolic alkalosis, respiratory acidosis, and respiratory alkalosis. In the simplest terms, the loss from or addition to the body of acid or base produces a change in the $[H^+]$ that is reflected in a shift of the blood pH outside the normal range. At this point the state is called *uncompensated.* However, regulatory mechanisms come into operation that attempt to bring the pH back within the normal range. If this happens then the state is *fully compensated:* more usually only partial compensation occurs; that is, the pH is still outside the normal range.

The etiology of the four states will be described briefly, followed by some discussion of their diagnosis from the laboratory data. Reference to Figure 8–4 will perhaps help to visualize the changes. This is based on the Davenport diagram (Davenport, 1974). The X and Y axes represent pH and $[HCO_3^-]$, respectively. The curved lines are the P_{CO_2} isobars, which are related to the X and Y axes by the Henderson-Hasselbalch equation. The sloping line is the buffer titration line: when plasma is exposed to varying CO_2 tensions (under controlled conditions) the bicarbonate and pH values move together along the buffer line. If any two of the three parameters are known, a point indicating the acid-base status can be placed on the graph.

Metabolic Acidosis

This may occur in two ways.

1. Addition of a fixed acid. The main causes are uremia, ketoacidosis, lactic acidosis, and poisoning with salicylate, methanol, or ethylene glycol. (Methanol is

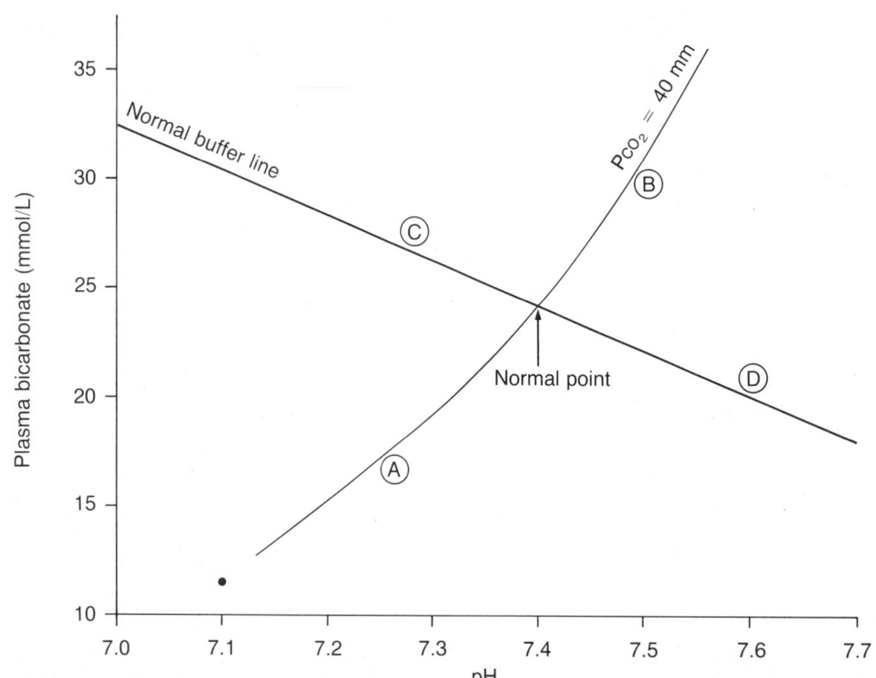

Figure 8–4 Davenport graph. See text for description.

metabolized to formic acid, ethylene glycol to oxalic and hippuric acids.)

2. Loss of bicarbonate. The main causes are diarrhea, renal failure, pancreatic fistula, hyperalimentation, renal tubular acidosis, and ureteroenterostomy (transplantation of ureters into the colon or into an ileal-loop bladder).

The initial change is a fall in pH and bicarbonate, with no change in Pco_2; this is represented by point A in Figure 8–4. However, rapid compensation occurs because of the onset of hyperventilation (a neural response), and CO_2 is "blown off" by the lungs. This tends to increase the HCO_3/Pco_2 ratio and thus elevates the pH. The classic example is diabetic coma: the deep respirations ("air-hunger," Kussmaul respirations) are a very striking feature. A useful rule of thumb in assessing the degree of compensation is that for every 1 mmol fall in the bicarbonate concentration, the Pco_2 should fall 1 mm to achieve maximum compensation. However, complete compensation (in the sense that a normal pH is reached) is the exception in metabolic acidosis, even though compensation may be maximal.

Metabolic Alkalosis

The major causes are as follows:

1. Loss of fixed acid, resulting from loss of gastric secretions through vomiting or aspiration or from chronic potassium deficiency.

2. Increased intake of base, which usually occurs following the ingestion of large amounts of sodium salts of bicarbonate, lactate, or citrate.

The plasma bicarbonate level is elevated, and the pH rises (Point B in Fig. 8–4). Following this, adjustment of the respiratory rate elevates the Pco_2 and produces compensation. The reduction in respiratory rate or volume is not clinically noticeable, unlike the situation in severe metabolic acidosis.

Respiratory Acidosis

The following are the usual causes:

1. Reduced diffusion of carbon dioxide due to intrinsic lung disease.

2. Depression of neural respiratory mechanisms, for example in poliomyelitis or drug overdose.

The reduction in ventilation rate causes retention of carbon dioxide, with elevation of blood Pco_2 levels: this reduces the HCO_3/Pco_2 ratio, and the pH falls (Point C in Fig. 8–4). In order to compensate, the kidney increases its excretion of H^+ and *retains* bicarbonate. This mechanism is slow to operate (unlike the very rapid adjustment of respiration in metabolic imbalance), and it may take 6 to 7 days for the process to achieve maximal efficiency. Again, a useful rule of thumb is that for every 3 mm elevation of Pco_2 above normal, the bicarbonate level should rise 1 mmol for maximal compensation.

Respiratory Alkalosis

This state follows prolonged hyperventilation, which may be caused by emotion, drugs (e.g., salicylates), brain stem lesions, and other neural factors. Initially Pco_2 falls and pH rises (Point D in Fig. 8–4); if the state is prolonged, compensation is achieved by renal loss of bicarbonate.

Mixed Disturbances

In seriously ill patients it is by no means uncommon to have two types of acid-base disturbance present simultaneously. A relatively common combination is respiratory acidosis combined with metabolic alkalosis. This frequently follows the administration of steroids or thiazide diuretics to a patient with respiratory acidosis.

Calculated Anion Gap. The calculated anion gap can provide some additional information. In fact, the calculation should always be made before attempting to interpret acid-base or electrolyte data.

In metabolic acidosis, a high gap distinguishes the group of disorders caused by the addition or retention of fixed acid (e.g., ketoacidosis) from the second group, in which loss of bicarbonate occurs. The "missing" anions are usually ketone bodies, lactic acid, sulfate, phosphate, formic acid, oxalic acid, etc. Sometimes, if bicarbonate has been administered or compensation has occurred, the elevated gap may be the only indication of an underlying metabolic acidosis.

In uremia, the gap is usually elevated, in the range 24 to 29 mmol/L, mostly because of phosphate and sulfate ions. A higher value is suggestive of some additional factor, for example, lactic acidosis.

Metabolic acidosis with a normal anion gap is characterized by a fall in plasma bicarbonate together with a rise in the plasma chloride level. A chloride level of more than 110 mmol/L is very suggestive of this type of acidosis.

Occasionally other anions may cause an elevated gap without any acid-base disturbance; this is seen, for instance, during treatment with carbenicillin and other negatively charged drugs.

A low anion gap is also of some diagnostic value once the possibility of analytical error has been eliminated. Small declines occur in dilutional states (e.g., inappropriate secretion of ADH) and in hypoalbuminemia (e.g., nephrotic syndrome). Perhaps the most important cause of a low anion gap is multiple myeloma, in which large amounts of abnormal proteins are circulating. If these carry a positive charge (being then cations, not anions) the calculated gap may then be very small or even negative. This usually occurs only in the IgG type of myeloma. However, problems may arise with other paraproteinemias if a flame photometer is the analytical instrument, because of viscosity effects altering the rate of aspiration.

For a more extended discussion of the anion gap, see the paper by Emmett and Narins (1977).

Sodium and Potassium Abnormalities

Abnormalities of sodium and potassium levels can indicate a number of possible disorders.

Sodium. A relatively common finding in hospitalized patients is a low plasma sodium level (hyponatremia). This does not necessarily indicate sodium depletion: in many patients it may indicate a dilutional state. The major causes of hyponatremia are listed in Table 8–3. The diagnostic search algorithm (Fig. 8–5) is helpful in distinguishing hyponatremia due to sodium loss from

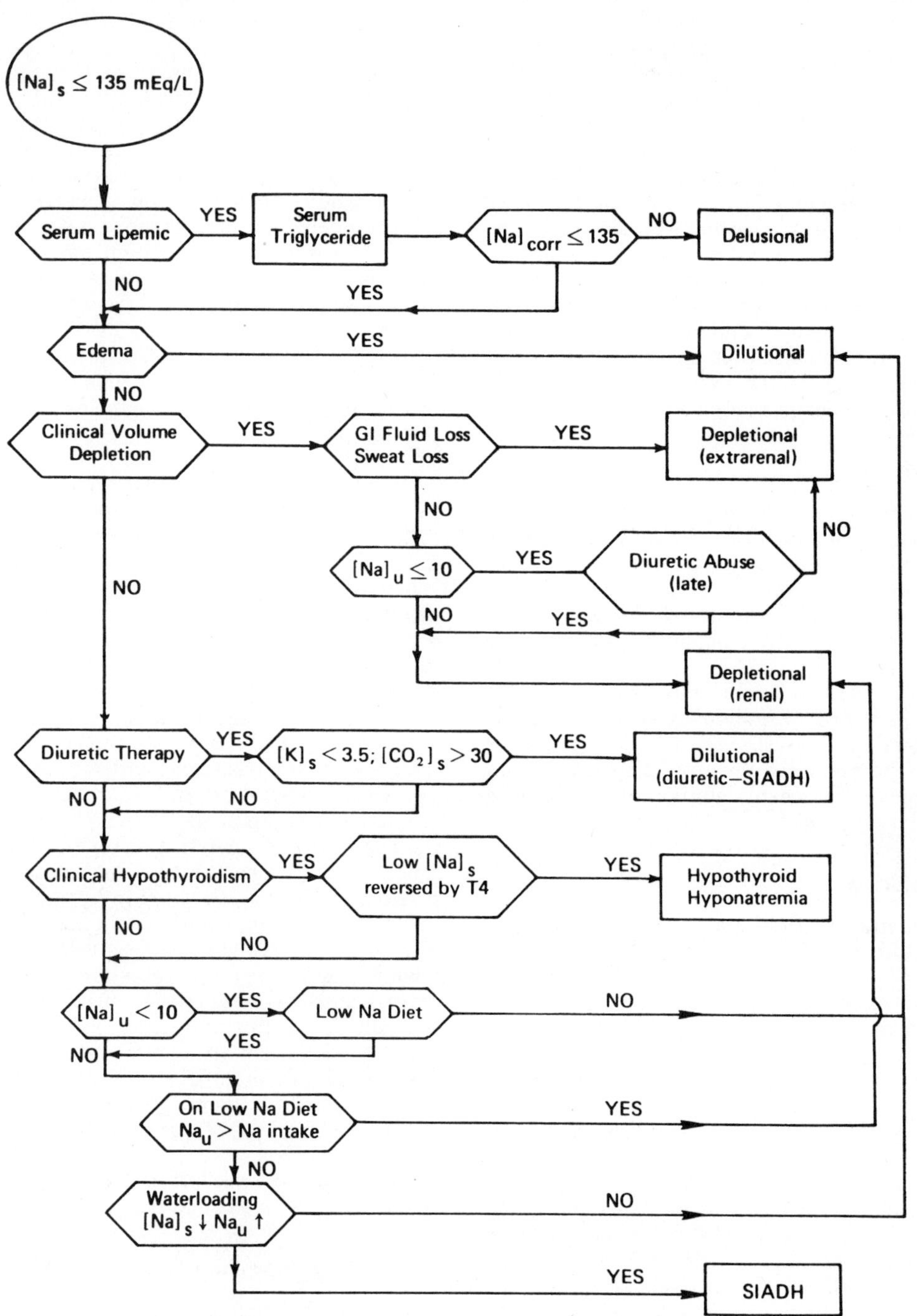

Figure 8–5 Hyponatremia: diagnostic search algorithm. Reproduced with permission from Burke, M. D.: Hyponatremia. American Society of Clinical Pathologists Check Sample (No. CC-103) **17**:10, 1977.

dilutional and other states. Generally, dilutional states are characterized by low serum osmolality, whereas in hyponatremia from other causes the osmolality may be normal or even elevated. Salt-losing nephritis, cirrhosis, and inappropriate secretion of ADH are the most common causes of hyponatremia.

Hypernatremia may follow excessive sodium intake by mouth or by intravenous infusion. However, it most often follows retention of sodium caused by intrinsic renal disease or inadequate renal perfusion (as in congestive cardiac failure).

Potassium. A low potassium level (hypokalemia) is the more common abnormality, and it usually indicates fairly severe potassium depletion. The major causes are listed in Table 8–4, and a diagnostic search algorithm is given in Figure 8–6. The most common causes are diarrhea (due to reduced potassium absorption by the large bowel), diuretics (due to loss in the urine: some non–potassium-losing diuretics are available, however), and the treatment of diabetic ketoacidosis with insulin (the movement of glucose into the cells requires an associated influx of potassium). Also, for reasons already given, hypokalemia is a common finding in metabolic alkalosis, whatever the cause.

Although interpretation should be based on logical considerations, the use of acid-base diagrams can be helpful. Numerous forms of such diagrams have been published: one of the most useful is that shown in Figure 8–7. The shaded bands represent the 95% probability zone for the particular disorder, whether compensated or not.

TABLE 8–3 THE CAUSES OF HYPONATREMIA

I. Depletional
- A. Extrarenal
  1. Gastrointestinal fluid loss
  2. Excessive sweat loss
- B. Renal
  1. Diuretic abuse
  2. Salt-losing nephritis
     - a. Severe chronic renal failure
     - b. Medullary cystic disease
     - c. Polycystic disease
     - d. Chronic pyelonephritis
  3. Renal tubular acidosis
  3. Adrenal insufficiency

II. Dilutional
- A. Edematous
  1. Congestive cardiac failure
  2. Hepatic failure
  3. Nephrotic syndrome
  4. Advanced chronic renal failure
  5. Protein calorie malnutrition
- B. Nonedematous
  1. Potassium depletion
  2. Hypothyroidism
  3. Hypopituitarism
  4. IADH (inappropriate secretion of ADH)
     - a. Small-cell carcinoma of lung
     - b. Pancreatic malignancies
     - c. CNS disorders
     - d. Pulmonary infection
     - e. Drugs: diuretics, chlorpropamide, tolbutamide, vincristine, cyclophosphamide

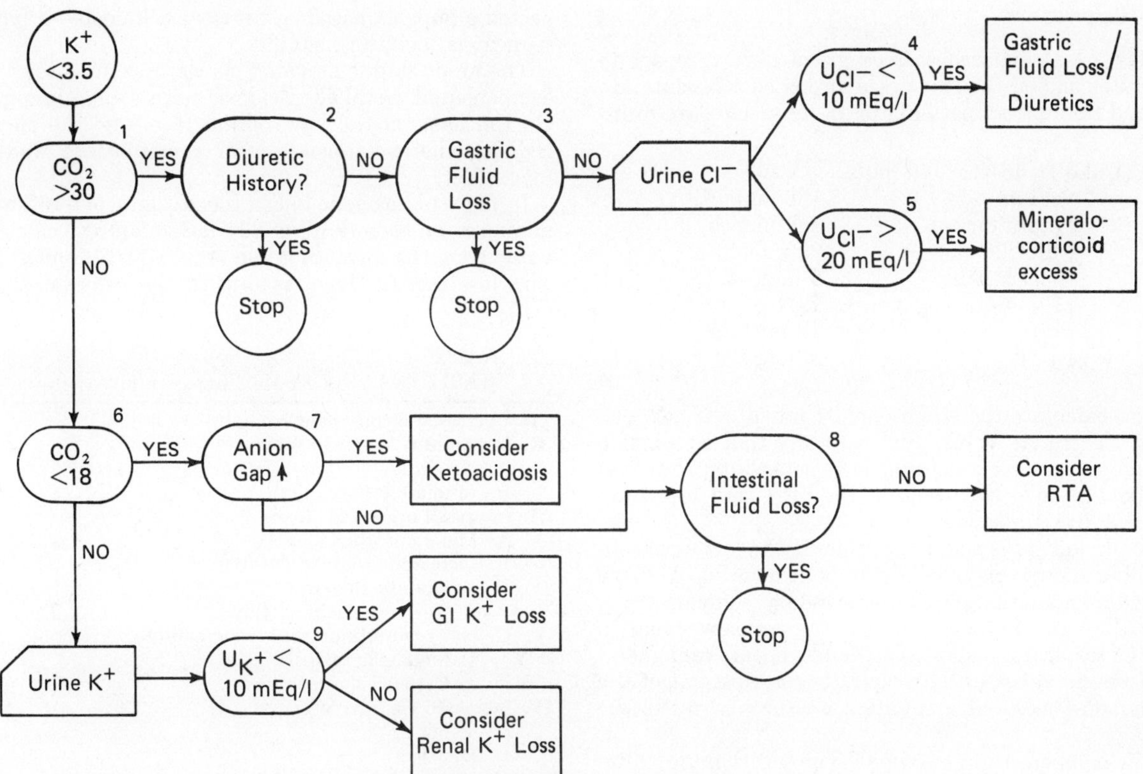

Figure 8–6 Hypokalemia: diagnostic search algorithm. Reproduced with permission from Burke, M. D.: Hypokalemia. American Society of Clinical Pathologists Check Sample (No. CC-111) **18**:6, 1978.

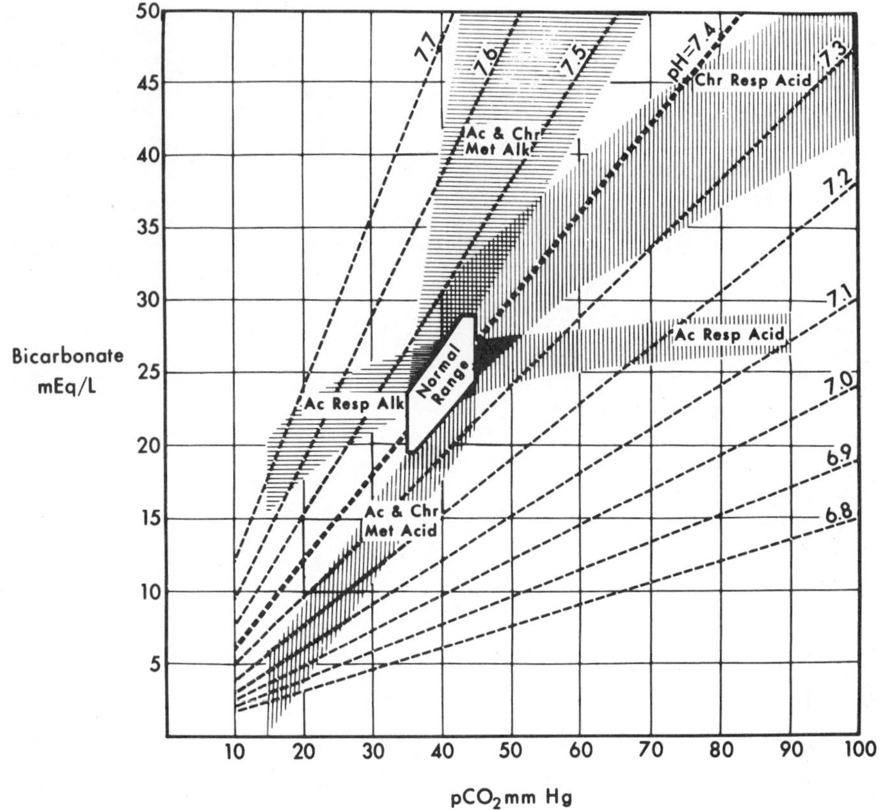

Figure 8–7 In vivo nomogram showing bands for defining a single respiratory or metabolic acid-base disturbance. Reproduced with permission from Arbus G. S.: An in vivo acid-base nomogram for clinical use. Can. Med. Assoc. J. **109**:291, 1973.

Case Histories

A few case histories will be given here in order to illustrate some of the principles discussed. The data are real and taken from patients in an intensive care unit.

Case 1: 46-year-old male

Sodium	128 mmol/L
Potassium	3.0 mmol/L
Chloride	95 mmol/L
Bicarbonate	5 mmol/L
pH	7.04
Pco_2	18 mm Hg
BUN	30 mg/dL

First, calculate the anion gap: 31 mmol/L. Next, look at the electrolyte values and note any that lie outside the reference range: sodium, low; potassium, low; and bicarbonate, low. Next look at the pH—very low—and then the Pco_2—also low.

The pH indicates a state of acidosis, the low bicarbonate value shows this to be a metabolic acidosis. The low Pco_2 value must therefore be a secondary, compensating, event (had the Pco_2 value been the primary event, a state of respiratory alkalosis would appear: remember, a *fall* in the value of the respiratory component of the Henderson-Hasselbalch equation produces a *rise* in the pH).

Is the compensation maximal? The bicarbonate value has fallen 19 mmol and the Pco_2 value by 17 mm Hg, so that compensation is virtually complete. If the Pco_2 value had been lower than this, one would have suspected a superimposed respiratory alkalosis—a pattern seen in salicylate poisoning.

The anion gap is elevated, so we have a state of well-compensated metabolic acidosis with a high anion gap. On the basis of the low sodium level and the elevated BUN, diabetic ketoacidosis or renal failure would be most likely.

In fact this patient had a blood sugar of 1160 mg/dL and a serum osmolality of 330 mOsm/kg (the calculated value from the formula given on p. 83 is 323 mOsm/kg). The low sodium level is due to the osmotic diuresis

TABLE 8–4 The Major Causes of Hypokalemia

I. Decreased dietary intake
II. Increased K^+ entry to cells
- A. Alkalosis
- B. Insulin hypersecretion

III. Increased urinary K^+ loss
- A. Mineralocorticoid excess
- B. Increased distal tubular flow
  1. Diuretic therapy
  2. Salt-losing nephropathy
- C. Na^+ reabsorption with a nonreabsorbable anion
  1. Metabolic acidosis
  2. Carbenicillin therapy

IV. Increased GI tract loss
- A. Vomiting
- B. Diarrhea
- C. Intestinal fistula or tube drainage
- D. Large villous adenomas
- E. Laxative abuse

(sweeping sodium out of the body in the urine before the kidney has time to reabsorb it), and the elevated BUN may represent prerenal uremia (which follows the hypovolemia and fall in blood pressure caused by the severe fluid losses) or, in long-established diabetes, intrinsic renal disease. A further feature of interest is the slightly reduced potassium level following the initiation of treatment with insulin.

Case 2: 82-year-old female

Sodium	143 mmol/L
Potassium	4.8 mmol/L
Chloride	124 mmol/L
Bicarbonate	8 mmol/L
pH	7.22
P_{CO_2}	20 mm Hg
BUN	76 mg/dL

By use of the same observations and reasoning as given for the first example, the data indicate a compensated metabolic acidosis with a normal anion gap. Note, for comparison with the previous case, the high chloride value.

The commonest causes would be chronic diarrhea or bicarbonate-losing nephritis with renal failure. The potassium value would be expected to be lower with chronic diarrhea (the colon normally reabsorbs significant amounts of potassium), and the data would fit the second category.

In fact this patient had had a nephrectomy with implantation of the ureters into an ileal-loop bladder.

Case 3: 70-year-old male

Sodium	137 mmol/L
Potassium	5.6 mmol/L
Chloride	86 mmol/L
Bicarbonate	40 mmol/L
pH	7.28
P_{CO_2}	84 mm Hg

The data indicate that an acidosis is present, and that the anion gap is normal (16 mmol). However, the P_{CO_2} value is markedly elevated, indicating a respiratory source of the disorder. The bicarbonate value is also elevated, indicating that compensation has occurred. Is this maximal? The P_{CO_2} value is 39 mm above the upper limit of normal, and the bicarbonate value is 12 mmol above the upper limit of normal. Using the formula given, 39/3 = 13, so that compensation is maximal and the pH will not return to normal values.

This patient had chronic obstructive lung disease and emphysema.

Laboratory Investigation of Acid-Base Balance

With the availability of reliable instruments for measurement of blood pH, P_{CO_2}, and P_{O_2}, there is no excuse for continued dependence on such methods as CO_2 combining power or CO_2 content, except in emergencies. Determination of pH and P_{CO_2} and knowledge of the hemoglobin level permit the rapid reporting, using nomograms, of actual bicarbonate, standard bicarbonate, and base excess. This last parameter is defined as the titratable base determined by titration of the blood to normal pH of 7.40 at normal P_{CO_2} of 40 mm Hg and at normal temperature of 38°C. It is an expression of the metabolic component of the acid-base system independent of the respiratory component. If there is a deficiency of the metabolic component of the buffer systems, the base excess value will be a negative number; perhaps a better term in these circumstances is *base deficit.* Its value is in assigning a numerical value to the corrective action required.

Although we tend to regard the pH and P_{CO_2} values as the chief source of status information on acid-base balance, the P_{O_2} value is more than an indication of the efficiency of oxygen uptake by the lungs. If the P_{O_2} value is low, from whatever cause, the consequent oxygen lack in the tissues (tissue hypoxia or anoxia) leads to an excess of hydrogen ions. In normal metabolism the hydrogen ions produced during the metabolism of carbohydrates are combined with oxygen to form water as the last step in the electron carrier (cytochromes) system. Lack of adequate oxygen supplies causes an excess of hydrogen ions and hence acidosis. Since the P_{CO_2} value may not be affected seriously, it is not strictly a respiratory type of disturbance. It may occur in severe shock and cardiac arrest.

Source of Blood for pH, Electrolyte, and Gas Analyses: Sources of Analytical Error

The best sample for determinations of blood pH, P_{O_2}, and P_{CO_2} is arterial blood taken with the minimum amount of heparin. Formerly the preferred method for obtaining blood samples for pH and gas analyses used a glass syringe pretreated with a solution of heparin. The mobility of the glass piston in the syringe assisted in confirming that an arterial puncture had been achieved, since the plunger would rise under arterial pressure, whereas that of the standard plastic syringe would not. The introduction of sterile, heparinized plastic syringes* with special pistons designed to move under arterial pressure has facilitated the process. If the blood sample is kept chilled with crushed ice to retard oxygen consumption by the red cells and release of such acidic ions as lactate, the pH and gas values will remain stable for at least 20 minutes. Although loss of oxygen from blood in plastic syringes has been reported, the effect is small (except at very high P_{O_2} values) and can usually be ignored.

Venous blood samples taken with a vacuum-type sampling tube are occasionally used, although the errors in P_{O_2} values consequent on contamination with residual oxygen in the tube and the unstoppering before introduction of the blood into the analyzer make such samples of limited value.

In neonates, especially premature ones, the most convenient source of blood is a catheter in the umbilical artery. This procedure is the responsibility of the pediatric unit or neonatal intensive care unit staff.

The use of capillary blood samples should be confined to cases in which arterial samples are unobtainable. In normal adults and infants, the values obtained for P_{O_2} correlate well using arterial and capillary samples; but in just those kinds of cases in which the condition of the patient may make the use of capillary samples tempting,

*Arterial blood gas syringe No. 5696, Becton, Dickinson and Co., Rutherford, N.J. 07070 and Mississauga, Ont. L5J 2M8.

i.e., severe respiratory distress or shock, the values obtained will be affected seriously by the degree of peripheral vascular shutdown present. This is often obvious at the time of sampling; even with vigorous rubbing of the finger, heel, or earlobe, plus a deep skin puncture, the blood does not flow freely and easily and cannot be regarded as even approximating arterial blood in composition.

The blood must be mixed thoroughly by rapid rotation of the syringe between the palms, interspersed by rotation about the shorter axis. Before introduction of the blood into the sample chamber, the first few drops are expelled as waste. In those instruments in which the sample chamber is not visible, there is a danger of air bubbles becoming trapped against one or both of the electrode membranes. The only preventive is scrupulous cleanliness in the chamber and lead-in tubes. In addition to thorough flushing after use, an enzymic cleaning agent (an acid solution of pepsin) will remove protein film without damage to the delicate electrodes and membranes. To clean the sections of the tubing system other than those leading to the electrode chamber, 1-molar potassium hydroxide is commonly used. Another effective flushing agent is isopropanol.

Standardization and Controls

The following points must be considered.

1. Although modern blood gas analyzers with microprocessor control are automatically standardized at preset intervals using buffers drawn from large bottles in a closed system, the technologist should be aware that the stock of calibrating buffers must be stored away from light and undue heat and should not be used after the expiry date marked thereon. The pH calibration process is reliable only if the temperature of the pH electrode is correct and stable. One reason for the pH values found for three blood gas controls all being too low or too high is failure of temperature control. It should be pointed out that the pH system of a modern blood gas analyzer, reading often to the third decimal place, is more sensitive than that of the usual laboratory pH meter; therefore the latter instrument cannot be used to check the calibrating buffers.

Typical formulae for pH calibration buffers are (National Bureau of Standards):

1.179 g of pure dried potassium dihydrogen phosphate, KH_2PO_4, and 4.302 g of pure dried disodium hydrogen phosphate, Na_2HPO_4, dissolved in carbon dioxide– and ammonia-free deionized water to a final volume of one liter at 25°C. This buffer will have a pH of 7.413 at 25°C, 7.386 at 37°C, and 7.384 at 38°C.

3.388 g of pure dried potassium dihydrogen phosphate, KH_2PO_4 and 3.549 g of pure dried disodium hydrogen phosphate, Na_2HPO_4, dissolved in carbon dioxide– and ammonia-free deionized water to a final volume of one liter at 25°C. This buffer will have a pH of 6.865 at 25°C, 6.841 at 37°C, and 6.840 at 38°C.

2. The gas mixtures used to set Po_2 and Pco_2 ranges must be prepared accurately. Only gases supplied with a certificate of analysis can be regarded as reliable.

3. The rate of gas flow through the humidifiers should not be too rapid; there must be time for complete saturation of the gas by water vapor. The design of the humidifier chambers should produce streams of small bubbles, and the water level must be maintained at the correct level to ensure saturation.

4. Since the response of the Po_2 and Pco_2 electrodes is not instantaneous (see *Principles of Blood pH and Gas Electrodes* below), the microprocessor program in the modern blood gas analyzer may involve one of the following procedures:

a. The electrode output is measured after a fixed time, and the chosen interval is assumed to be long enough for stability to have been reached.

b. The electrode output is continuously monitored until it achieves a plateau, that is, a reading that does not change with time.

c. The electrode output is measured after a fixed time, but the value is compared with the theoretical value based on the characteristics of the electrode and is accepted only if it tallies within specified limits.

Improvements in electrode and membrane design and the microprocessor monitoring programs provide stable readings after shorter time intervals, on the order of 30 to 45 seconds. The usual indicators of a faulty or leaking electrode, a damaged or coated membrane, or faulty temperature control are delayed achievement of stability or severe instability, drifting of readings up or down, sudden jumps in the displayed response, or incorrect results with controls. The modern instruments incorporate electronic systems for detecting and signaling such problems, in addition to electrical contact fluid level sensors for adequate buffer bottle levels and full waste containers. The trend in design is to reduction of the length and complexity of hydraulic tubing systems, which can be the source of subtle operating problems.

Quality Control of Blood pH and Gas Analyses

An error in the determination of plasma glucose of 3% would not lead to any clinical or diagnostic problems; a similar inaccuracy in a blood pH measurement would be completely unacceptable, converting a normal value of 7.40 to that of a severe uncompensated acidosis, 7.18, or of an equally serious alkalosis, 7.62. The accuracy requirements for Po_2 and Pco_2 measurements are not quite so stringent, although errors in the Pco_2 determination will produce inaccuracies in the calculated bicarbonate value. For example, with a measured pH of 7.40 and Pco_2 of 36 mm Hg, the bicarbonate value calculated from the Henderson-Hasselbalch equation is 21.5 mmol/L. With the same pH and a Pco_2 determined as 40 mm Hg, the bicarbonate value becomes 23.9 mmol/L. The clinical effects of errors in Po_2 measurements are most serious in the region of 40 mm Hg, since the sigmoidal shape of the oxygen saturation curve is reflected in larger changes in oxygen saturation for a given change in Po_2.

The various types of blood gas quality control materials now available—aqueous buffers equilibrated with

NORMAL Po_2 (mm Hg)

Age	Mean Po_2	Range
20–29 yrs	95	80–110
30–39 yrs	90	78–108
40–49 yrs	86	76–104
50–59 yrs	82	71–100
60–69 yrs	78	67– 95

gas mixtures in ampoules,* fluorocarbon emulsions,† and aqueous buffers pre-equilibrated with known gas mixtures and stored in double-walled, pressurized, valve-tipped cans‡—are all adequate for checking the precision of blood gas analyzers. The differences of opinion and the thrust of commercial promotion rest on the suitability of the products for determination of accuracy and sensitivity to factors such as temperature errors. For example, the use of TRIS buffers instead of phosphate buffers increases by a factor of about three the sensitivity of the control to temperature errors in the instrumentation. The inclusion of hemoglobin§ or preserved red cells is claimed to detect the effects of protein deposition on electrode membranes.

From the laboratory point of view some other factors are relevant. The cost of blood gas controls entails some limitation on their use: this is a local decision. The technique of opening the ampoule-type controls and transferring their contents to the analyzer is exacting, and in some cases the pressure can–type may be preferred. On balance, the most realistic philosophy emphasizes the regular use of controls, rather than being overly concerned with the particular brand, and, most important, rigorous application of control results to ensure the provision of clinically valid data.

Sources of Error in Blood Gas Determinations

Sampling Errors

1. Blood taken from wrong patient.
2. Blood taken from patient during changes in ventilation therapy or during period of hyperventilation induced by patient stress.
3. Failure to keep sample cool during transit. **Note**: Do not use gel-type freezer packs—after solidifying in the freezer they are cold enough to produce hemolysis of the blood.
4. Undue delay in analysis.
5. Large air bubbles left in syringe sample: an air bubble equal to 10% of the sample volume will increase the Po_2 reading by about 11 mm Hg.
6. Excessive amount of heparin; this can reduce the Pco_2 reading by as much as 40% and can change the pH.
7. Insufficient mixing before introduction into analyzer.

Operational Errors

1. Use of contaminated or date-expired calibrating buffers.
2. Bacterial contamination of electrode chambers and tubing.
3. Air bubbles trapped on electrode membranes.
4. Protein-coated membranes.
5. Impending failure of battery supplying −600 mV polarizing voltage for Po_2 electrode in some instruments.
6. Incorrect calibration due to:
   a. Low tank pressure.
   b. Leaks in tubing conveying calibration gases to instrument.
   c. Room air leak into system—if a Po_2 value greater than 100 mm Hg is obtained on a patient not hyperventilating and not receiving an increased oxygen intake, suspect this type of error.
   d. Incorrect connection of calibration gas tank.
   e. Incorrect calibration buffer bottle. (Some instruments automatically check for these errors.)
   f. Loss of saturation of potassium chloride bridge solution in pH electrode. When the saturation is achieved by the insertion of a solid "doughnut" of KCl, its complete dissolution will introduce a small bias and slightly low pH results.

Temperature Errors

1. Loss of thermostatic control of the electrodes.
2. Failure to correct displayed results for patient body temperature. If patient temperature is 30°C and the instrument readings are made at 37°C, the pH value will be 0.1 low, a Pco_2 value of 29 mm Hg in the patient will read out as 40 mm Hg, and a patient oxygen value of 51 mm Hg will read out as 77 mm Hg. As a guide, if the patient's body temperature differs from normal by more than 2°C the displayed results should be corrected. Modern analyzers incorporate the ability to do this automatically, since the correction equations are complex. For a patient temperature of T°:

$$\text{pH at T°C} = \text{pH at 37°C} + (-0.0147 \times [T - 37])$$

$$Pco_2 \text{ at T°} = Pco_2 \text{ at 37°C} \times 10^{(0.019 \times [T - 37])}$$

$$Po_2 \text{ at T°} = Po_2 \text{ at 37°C} \times 10^{f(T - 37)}$$

$$\text{where } f = 0.0052 + (0.0268 \times [1 - e^{-0.3(100 - \%O_2 \text{ Satn})}])$$

Instrumental Errors

The majority of the sources of error listed above are avoidable with adequate maintenance or detectable by regular quality control checks. The existence of problems in the complex electronics of blood gas analyzers may be realized by recording the amplifier read-out values that can be obtained with some instruments: a large change in one or more of these check values indicates a serious electronic problem. Impending failure of an electrode system may be signaled by an unusually short working life after the electrode has been serviced and remembraned or by erratic performance. The microprocessors that control the automatic functions of blood gas analyzers are sensitive to very short duration "spikes" of high voltage in the main power supply. If problems are traced to this source, some type of spike suppressor should be fitted. It is not possible to cover all the possible sources of error and operating problems in this brief discussion. The main considerations are correct maintenance, regular quality control checks, correct sampling procedures, and an alert scrutiny of results for anomalies.

*G.A.S. Controls, General Diagnostics Division, Warner-Lambert Co., Morris Plains, N.J. 07950; "contrIL," Instrumentation Laboratory Inc., Lexington, Mass. 02173.

†"abc," Instrumentation Laboratory, Inc., Cidra, Puerto Rico 00639.

‡"Confirm," Corning Medical and Scientific, Medfield, Mass. 02052.

§"PRIME," Fisher Diagnostics, Orangeburg, N.Y. 10962.

Principles of Blood pH and Gas Electrodes

Strictly speaking, the term *electrode* should be reserved for the conductor through which the electrical activity associated with an electrochemical process enters or leaves the system: by that definition the term *pH electrode* is a misnomer, since pH measurements are associated with potentials (voltages) and not with currents (movements of electrons). However, in the absence of a simple alternative the word *electrode* will serve.

The blood pH electrode uses the same basic principles as the routine pH meter electrode (see p. 65), but it has been modified to meet the special requirements of its use: very small sample size, maintenance of anaerobic conditions, rapid response, and close control of temperature. In the modern blood gas analyzer these requirements have been met in one of two ways.

1. The special "pH-sensitive" glass of the usual pH meter electrode is formed into a fine capillary that can be completely filled by less than 100 μL of blood: in effect, the electrode has been turned inside out. Close temperature control is ensured by a circulating water jacket (in the older designs), a fan-driven air bath, or, most commonly, metal heating blocks. The electrical contact between the blood sample and the reference electrode is made via a liquid potassium chloride junction, in some instruments separated from the blood by a membrane.

2. The pH electrode is essentially a miniaturized version of the standard type, but the sample volume is kept very small by leading the blood sample across the face of the electrode, using very small capillary channels. The Po_2 and Pco_2 electrodes are similarly arranged, so that the three form a chain of small chambers connected by the channels. This arrangement has the advantage of allowing visual inspection of the blood sample while it is being measured so that air bubbles and clots can be seen. The electrical connection with the reference electrode is made via a membrane.

The Po_2 electrode (Clark electrode) operates on the polarographic principle; i.e., when a substance is reduced at a metal electrode, once a critical voltage that is typical of the substance has been reached, the current flow is related to the concentration of the substance. A very thin—25 μm—platinum wire cathode is mounted in a glass carrier so that only its very small cross-section is exposed. This exposed tip dips into a buffered solution of potassium chloride held as a very thin layer between the electrode tip and a polypropylene membrane. The circuit is completed by a silver–silver chloride anode. As the oxygen atoms diffuse from the blood through the membrane, they are reduced by a −600 millivolt potential applied to the electrode.

$$O_2 + 2H_2O + 4\,e^- \rightarrow 4OH^-$$

Each oxygen molecule requires four electrons for its reduction, and these come from the silver–silver chloride anode. The rate of reduction and hence the rate of electron flow depend on the rate of oxygen diffusion via the membrane into the zone of active reduction close to the platinum wire cathode, which in turn is governed by the partial pressure of the oxygen in the blood sample. If the temperature is controlled, the system attains a steady state in less than a minute, and the constant electron flow, i.e., current, is a measure of the blood Po_2. The buffered potassium chloride solution has the typical composition of 5.1 g disodium hydrogen phosphate, 2.5 g potassium dihydrogen phosphate, and 1.0 g potassium chloride per dL of water.

The Pco_2 electrode (Severinghaus electrode) makes use of the special properties of a Teflon or silicone rubber ("Silastic") membrane to permit the passage of small uncharged molecules, such as carbon dioxide, while barring the entry of charged particles such as hydrogen ions. The main body of the electrode is simply a pH electrode with a thin layer of a bicarbonate plus sodium chloride solution held in a porous layer between the Teflon or silicone membrane and the pH electrode. The carbon dioxide molecules diffuse through the Teflon or silicone and react with the bicarbonate to form carbonic acid, which dissociates to release hydrogen ions with a consequent pH change. Once the system has reached equilibrium, the pH shift is proportional to the rate of entry of carbon dioxide molecules and hence to the partial pressure of the CO_2 in the blood sample outside the membrane. The solution used to receive the carbon dioxide as it diffuses through the membrane has the composition 0.042 g sodium bicarbonate and 0.116 g sodium chloride in 100 mL of water.

ESTIMATION OF PLASMA CARBON DIOXIDE CONTENT

Titration Method

Principle

A known amount of acid is added to plasma or serum. The amount of acid required to liberate the carbon dioxide from the bicarbonate of the plasma is determined by titrating the mixture back to the original pH of the plasma.

Procedure

Blood is obtained as directed at the beginning of this section. Heparinized plasma should be used in an emergency.

1. In a 125 mL Erlenmeyer flask place:
M/100 hydrochloric acid—5.0 mL.
Serum or heparinized plasma—1.0 mL.
Caprylic (secondary octyl) alcohol or antifoam—1 drop.

2. Swirl gently for 2 minutes to facilitate release of CO_2.

3. Incubate for 30 minutes at 37°C.

4. Add 20 mL of CO_2 free distilled water and 3 drops of PSP indicator.

5. Titrate with M/100 sodium hydroxide until the color changes from the original yellow to a pink tint; excess of NaOH is shown by a further change to magenta or reddish purple. Detection of this end point requires a little practice.

Calculation

$$(5.0 \text{ mL} - \text{titer of M/100 NaOH in mL}) \times 10 = \text{mmol/L}$$

BASIC CALCULATIONS.

1. 1 liter of M/100 HCl ≡ 1 liter of M/100 $BHCO_3$ ≡ 1/100 equiv. $BHCO_3$

2. 1 mL of M/100 HCl ≡ 1/1000 × 1/100 equiv. $BHCO_3$ ≡ 1/100 mEq $BHCO_3$

3. If A = mL of M/100 acid neutralized by the $BHCO_3$ of 1.0 mL of plasma, then A × 1/100 = mEq of $BHCO_3$ per mL of serum and A × 1/100 × 1000 = A × 10 = mEq (mmol) $BHCO_3$ per liter of plasma.

Reagents

M/100 Hydrochloric Acid. This is most conveniently prepared by accurate volumetric dilution of a commercial M/10 stock solution.

M/100 Sodium Hydroxide. This should be prepared each week, by diluting a M/10 solution of sodium hydroxide 1 in 10 with CO_2-free distilled water, and checked against the M/100 hydrochloric acid.

Phenolsulfonphthalein (PSP) Indicator. Dilute one ampoule of the Hynson, Westcott, and Dunning* phenolsulfonphthalein solution (1.0 mL contains 0.6 mg of the dye), to 10 mL with distilled water.

Caprylic (Secondary Octyl) Alcohol. This is used to prevent foaming and should be analytic reagent grade.

Normal Values

Normal values are 24 to 34 mmol/L.

Automated methods for serum or plasma carbon dioxide content have been developed. On the Technicon AutoAnalyzer† the carbon dioxide released by acidification of the dialyzed sample is bubbled through a solution of phenolphthalein, and the resultant change in color of the indicator is measured colorimetrically. On a discrete-type automatic analyzer‡ the carbon dioxide released by mixing the plasma with an acid reagent diffuses through a membrane into a bicarbonate solution. The rate of change of the pH associated with this process, as determined by a micro pH electrode, is compared with a standard pH produced by a reference pH electrode.

ESTIMATION OF PLASMA OR SERUM CHLORIDES

The chloride ion is the most important anion, quantitatively, of the extracellular fluids of the body; it is the main anion counterbalancing the major cation, sodium, to maintain electrical neutrality of the body fluids. As already explained, the movement of the chloride ion into and out of the red cell is essential for the movement of the bicarbonate ion to and from the plasma in response to the changing amounts of carbon dioxide therein (see *Chloride Shift,* p. 185).

Semi-automated Methods for Estimation of Chlorides

The methods used to estimate chlorides can be divided into three groups: manual, semi-automated, and fully automated. A manual titration method is given in detail later on, with discussion of its chemical principle.

The semi-automated methods in widespread use involve two principles.

1. In the *Cotlove-type titrator,* the sample or standard solution is diluted with a nitric acid–acetic acid solution containing gelatin and is placed in a small titration vessel, into which two pairs of electrodes dip. One pair, of which one member is a silver wire, generates silver ions at a constant rate; the other pair, sensing electrodes, detects changes in the electrical conductivity of the solution. A stirring paddle maintains good mixing. When the instrument is switched on and set, silver ions, released at a constant rate, combine with the chloride ions of the sample to form insoluble silver chloride. As soon as all the chloride ions have been thus removed from solution, the next increment of silver ions will rapidly increase the conductivity of the solution. This rapid change is detected and activates a relay that stops a timer or counting device. Since the release of silver ions proceeds at a constant rate, the time they take to combine with the chloride ions of the sample or standard solution is related directly to the quantity of chloride present. The later models of the instrument automatically convert the measured time into millimoles of chloride ion per liter. If the initial calibration and daily checks are carefully made, and the practical points listed here are followed, the Cotlove Chloridometer will estimate chloride ion content of serum, CSF, and other samples with a standard deviation of ± 2 mmol per liter under routine working conditions. This degree of precision can be bettered if duplicate samples are run.

OPERATING POINTS

a. All glassware and pipettes must be scrupulously clean; a preliminary soaking in 20% nitric acid is advised.

b. The same positive-displacement micropipette should be used to measure both tests and standards, with a careful washout technique plus prerinsing with each solution before measurement. The pipette must be checked for accuracy and must be absolutely grease-free.

c. The silver wire electrode must be kept clean, and a fresh length drawn down into service whenever it appears thinned or corroded. Avoid the use of domestic-type silver cleaners that incorporate antitarnishing agents such as silicones: these may coat the electrode and interfere with its function.

d. The gelatin reagent must be kept refrigerated in small aliquots and not refrozen.

e. At least two "warmup" runs must be made before the actual determinations are made.

Normal Values

Normal values are 99 to 108 mmol/L or 580 to 630 mg per/dL (as NaCl).

2. The *Zall color reaction* has been used in semi-automated chloride analyzers (IL 279 chloride analyzer*) and in continuous flow fully automated procedures. The reagent contains mercuric thiocyanate and ferric nitrate. The chloride ions of the sample or standard displace the thiocyanate ions to form soluble but undissociated mercuric chloride, releasing in the process an equivalent amount of thiocyanate ion. This reacts with ferric ions derived from the ferric nitrate to produce reddish-brown ferric thiocyanate, which is measured colorimetrically. The instrument is calibrated with a standard sodium chloride solution of 100 mmol/L, and

*Hynson, Westcott and Dunning, Inc., Baltimore, Md. 21201.

†Technicon Instruments Corp., Tarrytown, N.Y. 10591 and Montreal, Que. H4T 1P5.

‡ASTRA 4 and 8, Beckman Instruments, Inc., Brea, Calif. 92621 and Toronto, Ont. M8Z 2G6.

*Instrumentation Laboratory, Lexington, Mass. 02173.

as each sample is aspirated by a peristaltic pump plus mixer system, the absorbance of the color produced is determined in a flow cell and compared with the reading for the standard; the result is displayed on a digital read-out.

In addition to the continuous flow method mentioned above using the Zall color reaction, chloride assays have been automated using the same principle as the Cotlove titrator, except that instead of measuring the time required for the silver ions to react with all the chloride ions present, the total current flowing in the coulometric silver ion generator is electronically integrated. The result of this summation process is directly proportional to the quantity of silver ions and hence to the amount of chloride with which they have reacted.* The most recent method of chloride assay makes use of a special ion-selective electrode in a discrete-type automated analyzer.†

Mercuric Nitrate Titration Method of Schales and Schales (1941)

Principle

The chloride ions of the plasma combine with the mercury ions of the mercuric nitrate to form soluble but virtually undissociated mercuric chloride, which does not affect the indicator. As soon as all the chloride ions are thus combined, the next drop of mercuric nitrate added will release free mercuric ions in the mixture, which will cause the indicator to change from colorless or faint pink to violet. The volume of mercuric nitrate required to produce an end point is, therefore, a measure of the amount of chloride present, and by comparison with the volume of mercuric nitrate solution needed to titrate a standard sodium chloride solution, the chloride of the sample may be calculated.

Procedure

1. In a centrifuge tube place the following:
Serum or plasma—1.0 mL
Deionized water—8.0 mL
10% w/v sodium tungstate solution—0.5 mL
2/3-N sulfuric acid solution—0.5 mL

Mix well, let stand for 5 minutes, and centrifuge. (If only a small amount of serum or plasma is available, dilute 0.2 mL with 1.8 mL of distilled water and substitute for the 2.0 mL of protein-free supernate in step 2.)

2. Pipette accurately 2.0 mL of the protein-free supernate from step 1 into a small porcelain basin. The white background is essential for observation of the indicator change.

3. Add 0.6 mL of diphenylcarbazone indicator.

4. Titrate with standard mercuric nitrate from a microburette readable to 0.01 mL, stirring constantly with a small glass rod bent like a hockey stick, until the appearance of the first faint purple color.

Note: **If the indicator is not fresh, a purple color will appear with the first drop or two of mercuric nitrate added but will disappear as the titration proceeds. Note the volume of mercuric nitrate solution added.**

5. Repeat the titration with a second 2.0 mL of the protein-free supernate. The two titers should not differ by more than 0.02 mL.

Calculation

$$\frac{\text{Test titer}}{\text{Factor}} \times 584.5 = \text{mg/dL (as NaCl)}$$

$$\frac{\text{Test titer}}{\text{Factor}} \times 100 = \text{mmol/L}$$

The factor is determined for each batch of mercuric nitrate solution by titrating 0.2 mL of the standard sodium chloride solution plus 1.8 mL of water as for the test procedure. Perform this titration at least three times, and take the mean of the results, which should not differ by more than 0.02 mL.

Normal Values

See previous method.

Reagents

Mercuric Nitrate Solution. Dissolve 3.0 g of reagent-grade mercuric nitrate monohydrate in 300 mL of distilled water. Immediately add 2.6 mL of concentrated nitric acid, mix, dilute to 1 L, and mix again. This reagent keeps well in a brown glass bottle. Determine the factor for each batch when new and at monthly intervals.

Standard Sodium Chloride Solution. Dry pure sodium chloride in a vacuum desiccator. Weigh out accurately 584.5 mg, dissolve in distilled water in a 100-mL volumetric flask, and make up to volume. Mix.

Diphenylcarbazone Indicator Solution. Dissolve 50 mg of *s*-diphenylcarbazone in 50 mL of ethyl alcohol. Keep in a brown glass bottle in a refrigerator. (Keeps for about a month.)

Notes

1. Mercuric nitrate is difficult to weigh accurately because of its hygroscopic nature, but this is not a source of error, since each batch is standardized as noted.

2. Because of the false end point noted in step 4, it is better to make a small amount of diphenylcarbazone indicator solution fresh for each day's work by dissolving 10 mg (with experience this can be estimated as a spatula-tip full) in 10 mL of ethyl alcohol.

3. If difficulty is experienced in obtaining factor values for the mercuric nitrate solution by titrating 0.2 mL amounts of the sodium chloride standard solution, titrate accurately measured 1.0 mL amounts plus 1.0 mL of distilled water and divide the mean titration value by 5.

Estimation of Chlorides in Other Body Fluids

Chlorides in other body fluids may be estimated by the Cotlove Chloridometer.

*ASTRA 4 and 8, Beckman Instruments, Inc., Fullerton, Calif. 92634 and Toronto, Ont. M8Z 2G6.

†E4A Electrolyte Analyzer, Beckman Instruments, Inc., Fullerton, Calif. 92634 and Toronto, Ont. M8Z 2G6.

The mercuric nitrate method of Schales and Schales may be used for the estimation of chlorides in CSF by diluting 0.2 mL of CSF with 1.8 mL of distilled water and substituting this for the 2.0 mL of protein-free supernate in step 2 of the method. The calculation is the same as for serum or plasma chloride.

For the estimation of urine chlorides, 0.2 mL of urine is diluted with 1.8 mL of distilled water, 0.6 mL of diphenylcarbazone indicator is added, and sufficient 10% acetic acid is used to just dispel the blue color. The mixture is then titrated as in step 4 of the method.

This method illustrates the use of a microburette, a factor to obviate the repeated titration of a standard, and an indicator that is not an acid-base indicator; the influence of proteins on reactions carried out in their presence and absence; and the effect of interfering substances present in urine. It is a simple method using a stable reagent that can still be useful as a "back-up" procedure when the modern electronic analyzers fail to operate.

Estimation of Plasma (or Serum) Sodium and Potassium

As flame photometers are in use in most clinical laboratories, chemical methods for the estimation of these ions are not given.

The general principles of flame photometry as applied to the determination of serum sodium and potassium are given on page 77. The method of operation for each particular instrument is detailed in the manufacturer's instructions, which should be carefully studied, but some general working points are noted here.

1. The purity of the distilled water used in the preparation of standards and serum dilutions is critical, and it is preferable to remove the last traces of ions by passing the distilled water through a mixed-bed ion-exchange column and storing it in a large plastic reservoir. Recent designs of pure water systems using multiple columns (see p. 63) maintain the very high quality of their product by continuously recycling the contents of a relatively small reservoir. If the water contains only one part per million of sodium ion, this will produce a final error in the sodium value of about 8.7 mmol/L if a working dilution of 1:200 of serum is used.

2. The use of manual dilution for sample preparation has been completely replaced by some form of automatic dilutor, employing either peristaltic pumps or pistons. These will provide consistent dilution ratios only if regular attention is paid to the replacement of tubing and piston seals. The intake line for the deionized water should incorporate a fine filter to exclude dust and fibers, and this filter should be cleaned or replaced on a regular basis. If a bench compressed air supply is used it must be fitted with a water and oil trap. Some instruments contain fine sintered metal filters in the air and fuel lines, and these should be replaced on a regular schedule. (The term *sintered* means a filter element made by heating metal or glass powder to the point at which the grains adhere, leaving a maze of tiny channels that create a mechanically strong and, in the case of glass, chemically resistant filter.)

3. In the flame photometer, any optical elements such as filters and collimating lenses must be kept scrupulously clean. If a monochromator is used it is usually in a sealed compartment.

4. If standard solutions are kept as concentrated stock solutions to be diluted for use, it is advisable to inhibit mold formation by including a small amount of reagent-grade formalin.

5. Stock standard solutions are best stored in polypropylene bottles. Working standards are most conveniently dispensed from plastic "squeeze" bottles.

6. The sample introduction system must be kept scrupulously clean. Inspissated serum may accumulate around the fine glass or metal nozzles and on the walls of the chamber where the larger droplets are allowed to settle out and drain away. Such deposits must be removed by regular cleaning according to the manufacturer's instructions. Very thorough flushing of the atomizer system after cleaning is essential.

Range of Normal Values for Serum or Plasma

Potassium: 3.6 to 5.4 mEq/L (3.6 to 5.4 mmol/L).
Sodium: 134 to 148 mEq/L (134 to 148 mmol/L).

Determination of Electrolytes—A New Approach

The introduction in the last few years of ion-selective electrodes of acceptable reliability for sodium, potassium, chloride, and total CO_2 has facilitated the concurrent development of a variety of semi-automated and fully automated analyzers for electrolytes. Two approaches have emerged: one uses whole blood, plasma, or serum and "flow-through" electrodes, for example, the "NOVA" series*; the other employs initial sample dilution and more conventional electrode design, for example, the Beckman E4A.† (Instruments of similar pattern are produced by other manufacturers: there is no intention here to make comparisons or assessments of performance.) There are some arguments in favor of the pattern using whole blood, plasma, or serum, and these are reviewed on p. 113. The "state of the art" is such that reliable results for a set of four electrolytes can be produced at the rate of 100 sets per hour, using sample turntables and microprocessor control. The steady improvement in the reliability of ion-selective electrodes is reflected in the extension of warranty periods from three months to as long as one year. However it would seem prudent to retain the flame photometer as a "back-up" instrument, since it has the virtues of relative electronic simplicity and greater capability for local rectification of failure. Pump tubings, water filters, mixing blocks, and burner heads can be replaced or serviced by the technologist: obscure microprocessor problems require expert attention.

The principles of flame photometry and the factors affecting accuracy and precision have been covered elsewhere in this text (p. 79). In terms of the degree of precision attainable under routine conditions, the assay of sodium and potassium is one of the most reliable determinations.

---

*NOVA Biomedical, Inc., Newton, Mass. 02164; Instrumentation Laboratory, Inc., Lexington, Mass. 02173.

†Beckman Instruments, Inc., Fullerton, Calif. 92634 and Toronto, Ont. M8Z 2G6.

CHAPTER 8—REVIEW QUESTIONS

1. What precautions must be used in obtaining blood samples for determinations of pH and gases?
2. How may a defective P_{O_2} or P_{CO_2} electrode be detected?
3. Discuss the sources of errors in blood gas determinations.
4. Describe the principle of the Cotlove-type titrator for assay of chlorides.
5. What is your interpretation of the following two sets of data?

	A	B
Sodium	142 mmol/L	117 mmol/L
Potassium	3.0 mmol/L	4.4 mmol/L
Chloride	112 mmol/L	79 mmol/L
Bicarbonate	15 mmol/L	25 mmol/L
pH	7.30	7.40
BUN	50 mg/dL	7 mg/dL

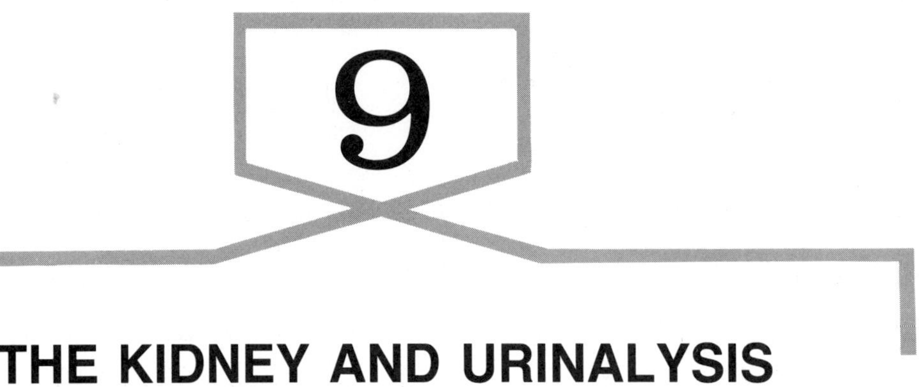

THE KIDNEY AND URINALYSIS

FUNCTIONS OF THE KIDNEY

The functions of the kidney are as follows:

1. Elimination of excess body water.
2. Elimination of waste products of metabolism, e.g., urea and creatinine.
3. Elimination of foreign substances, e.g., drugs.
4. Retention of substances necessary for normal body function, e.g., proteins, amino acids, and glucose.
5. Regulation of electrolyte balance and osmotic pressure of the body fluids.

These apparently varied responsibilities of the kidney are in fact merely different aspects of the overall task—to maintain the critical conditions for the continued metabolic activities of the cells.

THE NEPHRON

This is the functional unit of the kidney (Fig. 9–1). Its two main parts are the renal corpuscle (malpighian body) and the renal tubule. Each kidney contains more than one million nephrons.

The Renal Corpuscle or Glomerulus

This is a tuft of capillary blood vessels invaginated in the expanded blind end of the renal tubule, resembling a golf ball pushed into a punctured, slightly larger, hollow rubber ball. Thus, the glomerulus is surrounded (except for the small area where its blood vessels enter and leave) by two layers of the invaginated blind end of the tubule; these two layers are known as Bowman's capsule, and the space between them is continuous with the lumen of the tubule.

The Renal Tubule

This is divided into three main parts: the first, or proximal, convoluted tubule; the loop of Henle; and the second, or distal, convoluted tubule. Its total length varies from about 30 to 40 mm.

Blood Supply

The blood supply to the kidney is via the renal artery, which runs directly from the aorta. When it reaches the kidney the artery branches repeatedly, ultimately forming the afferent arterioles of the glomeruli. The efferent arteriole leaving the glomerulus is smaller than the afferent vessel and runs in close proximity to the corresponding tubule. In this way the tubules are supplied mainly with blood that has first passed through the glomeruli. The efferent vessels then join together and ultimately flow into the renal vein. At rest, about one-quarter of the heart's output of blood passes through the kidneys.

Effective Filtration Pressure

The function of the glomerulus is filtration. For filtration to occur, the pressure in the glomerular capillaries must be greater than the pressure within the tubule. This pressure difference is termed the effective filtration pressure (E.F.P.) and is the blood pressure within the glomerulus (65 to 75 mm Hg), minus the opposing

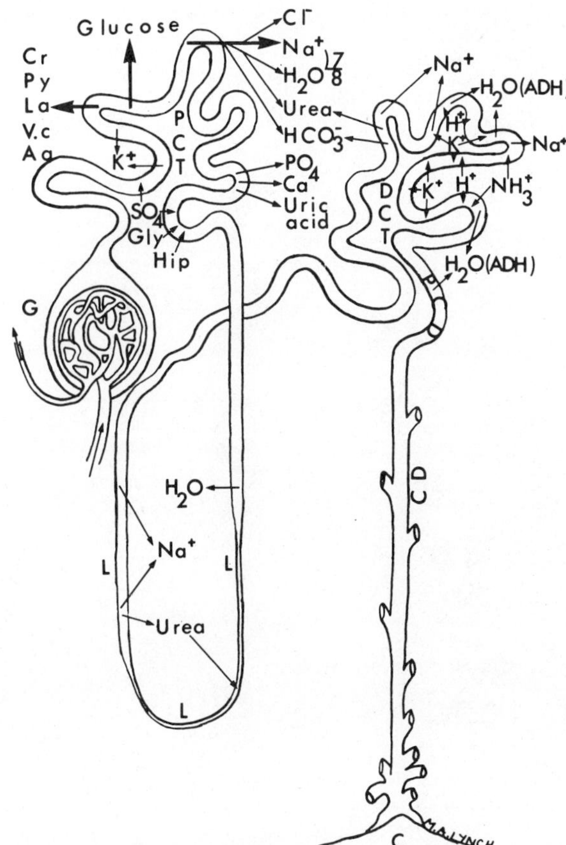

Figure 9–1 The nephron and its functions. Segments of the nephron are, moving distally from the glomerulus *(G)*; proximal convoluted tubule *(PCT)*; loop of Henle *(L)*; distal convoluted tubule *(DCT)*; primary collecting duct *(PCD)*; and collecting duct *(CD)*, emptying into minor calyx *(C)*. *Cr,* creatine; *Py,* pyruvate; *La,* lactate; *Aa,* amino acids; *Gly,* glucuronides; *Hip,* hippurates; *ADH,* antidiuretic hormone. Other symbols are self-explanatory. Arrows indicate movement into and out of tubules.

pressures, which are the osmotic pressure of the plasma proteins (20 to 30 mm Hg; mean, 25 mm Hg) and the pressure within the tubule (5 to 10 mm Hg). Under normal conditions the E.F.P. varies between 20 and 50 mm Hg.

Glomerular Filtration Rate (G.F.R.)

Normally this amounts to about 130 mL per minute (180 liters per 24 hours). It depends on the E.F.P. and the rate of renal blood flow.

TUBULAR FUNCTION

Sequence of Events in Nephron Reabsorption

The combined blood flow through both adult kidneys is about 1200 mL per minute. This corresponds to some 650 mL of plasma; i.e., the renal plasma flow (R.P.F.) is 650 mL per minute. Of this amount, approximately 20%, or 130 mL, passes through the tiny pores of the glomerular capillaries, then through the basement membrane (lamina densa), and finally between the foot processes of the podocytes into Bowman's space (Fig. 9–2). This is an ultrafiltrate and corresponds to the plasma minus all but a small fraction of 1% of the proteins. It has the same osmotic pressure as the plasma (osmolality ≐ 285 mOsm per kilogram of water), and its specific gravity is at the isosmotic point, i.e., 1.010. It contains in solution the same substances as the plasma, and almost in identical concentrations (minor differences are due to Donnan's equilibrium phenomenon).

Proximal Convoluted Tubule. From Bowman's space the filtrate enters the proximal convoluted tubule, a segment of the nephron easily identified in routine kidney sections. Of the tubules seen in cross and oblique section in the cortex, the proximal convoluted are the most numerous, the most eosinophilic, and the only ones having a brush border of microvilli. As the filtrate traverses the 14 mm length of this segment of the nephron, all threshold substances are virtually completely reabsorbed. The threshold substances include glucose, amino acids, creatine, pyruvate, lactate, and ascorbic acid, all of which are absorbed by active transport across the cell membranes.

In the proximal convoluted tubule also, 87.5% of the sodium in the filtrate is reabsorbed by the sodium pump mechanism. Water, HCO_3^-, and Cl^- accompany the sodium passively. In this way 87.5% of the water of the filtrate is removed in the proximal convoluted tubule by obligatory reabsorption in isosmotic proportions, and it takes with it 40 to 50% of the urea in the filtrate.

Loop of Henle. By the time the modified filtrate enters the descending limb of Henle's loop, only 16 mL per minute of the original 130 mL per minute remains in the tubule, but the pH, osmolality, and specific gravity are virtually unchanged. However, in addition to 87.5 per cent of the sodium, all the threshold substances and most of the potassium, calcium, phosphate, chloride, and bicarbonate have been reabsorbed. As this 16 mL of modified filtrate passes down in the descending limb of Henle's loop it loses some water to the increasingly concentrated interstitial fluid, but as it traverses the ascending limb of the loop it loses sodium without water, because this particular segment is relatively impervious to water.

Distal Tubule. When the filtrate enters the distal convoluted tubule (back in the cortex, next to the parent glomerulus), it is actually hypotonic, owing to sodium loss in the distal limb of Henle's loop. In the distal convoluted tubule and first part of the collecting duct all the remaining sodium is reabsorbed (unless the body has an excess of sodium, relative or absolute). Two mechanisms are involved in this: (1) The sodium-retaining hormone, aldosterone. This facultative sodium reabsorption is independent of both water reabsorption and excretion of H^+ or NH_4^+. (2) The cells of the distal segment form and excrete both hydrogen and ammonium ions, and these are exchanged for sodium, which is reabsorbed. Potassium is also actively excreted by this portion of the nephron, and this K^+ participates in the exchange for Na^+. Actually, K^+ excretion here is in competition with H^+ formation and excretion; i.e., when potassium is being excreted, hydrogen ion formation, and therefore acidification of the urine, is proportionately diminished.

Water Reabsorption in Distal Segment. ADH. From the slightly less than 16 mL of modified filtrate entering the distal convoluted tubule per minute, an average of

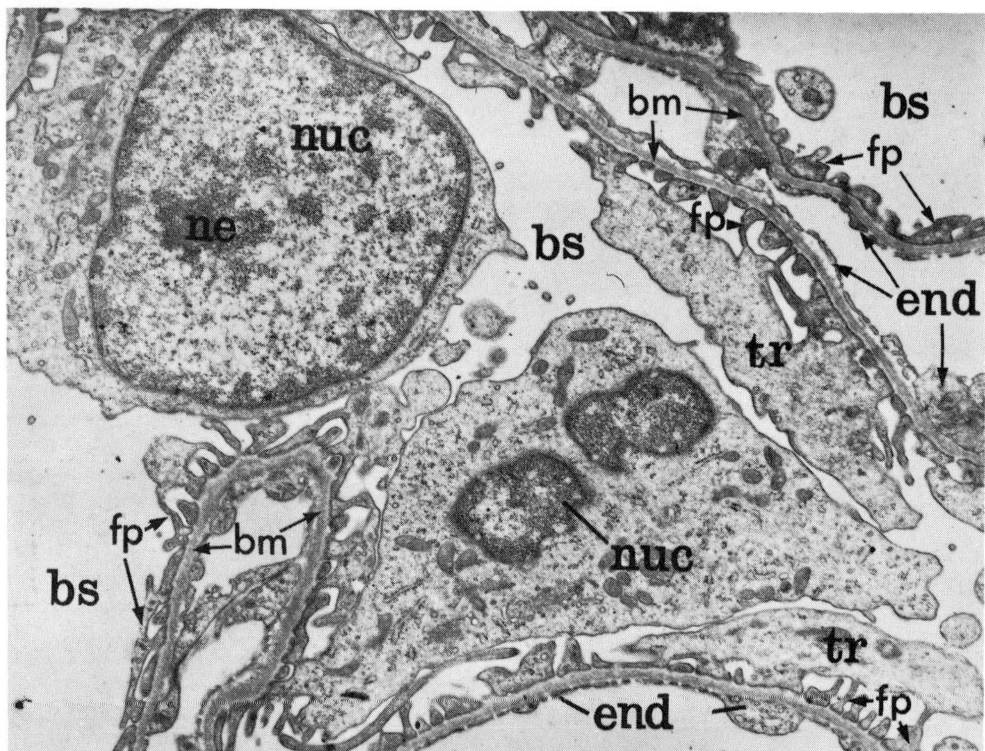

Figure 9–2 Electron micrograph of portion of dog's glomerulus showing two epithelial cells (podocytes) with their trabeculae *(tr)* and foot processes *(fp)*, the latter resting on the outer aspect of the basement membrane *(bm)*, which separates them from the endothelium *(end)* of the glomerular capillaries. *bs,* Bowman's space; *ne,* nucleolus, and *nuc,* nucleus of epithelial cells. Osmium fixation, potassium permanganate stain × 11,200. (From Movat, H. Z., and Steiner, J. W.: Studies of nephrotoxic nephritis. I. The fine structure of the glomerulus of the dog. Am. J. Clin. Path., *36*:289, 1961. Courtesy of the Williams and Wilkins Company, Baltimore, Md.)

almost 15 mL of water is reabsorbed during passage through this segment and the primary collecting duct. This facultative reabsorption of water from the distal segment of the nephron is entirely dependent on the action of the nonapeptide (nine amino acids, eight peptide bonds) antidiuretic hormone (ADH), also known as vasopressin. ADH is secreted by nerve cells in the hypothalamus and stored in the posterior part of the pituitary gland (neurohypophysis). From this store it is released in minute, constant basal amounts, but in larger amounts when osmoreceptor cells in the hypothalamus are stimulated by increased osmotic pressure of the plasma (hemoconcentration). ADH acts here by increasing the size of the pores in the walls of the distal convoluted tubule and primary collecting duct.

Concentration of Urine. Countercurrent Multiplier and Exchange System. The hairpin-like arrangement of the loop of Henle means that the urine in the descending and ascending segments is flowing in opposite directions. This countercurrent arrangement enables a zone of high osmotic pressure to be built up at the tip of the loop because of the fact that sodium, but not water, is extracted from the ascending loop and flows, via the interstitial tissue, to the descending limb. At the same time, water flows out of the descending limb, further increasing the intraluminal concentration. The looped arrangement of the blood vessels accompanying the renal tubule also serves to augment this effect.

Fate of Urea in Filtrate. All movements of urea, both into and out of the nephron, are passive. Some 40 to 50% of the urea filtered is reabsorbed passively with water from the proximal convoluted tubule. Net change of urea in the loop of Henle is small: the amount entering the descending limb is almost balanced by that lost from the ascending arm. From the fluid in the distal convoluted tubule and primary collecting duct the amount of urea reabsorbed varies directly with water reabsorption and ranges from 25 to 75%, approximately. The proportion of filtered urea that is finally excreted in the urine is the algebraic sum of all these various movements; depending on conditions of urine volume, it ranges between 25 and 65%, approximately.

The control of hydrogen ion excretion by the kidney is discussed in the section on acid-base balance.

RENAL FUNCTION TESTS

Renal function tests may be considered as belonging to two major groups:

1. The first of these groups indicates whether disease is present but does not give any indication as to the degree of functional impairment produced by the disease. Under this heading we may consider proteinuria, the presence of casts in urine, hematuria, and the presence of white blood cells in urine.

2. The second group includes those tests that attempt to evaluate the degree of renal impairment produced by disease. Since normal kidneys have a great physiological reserve of function (for example, a person with only one healthy kidney will show no renal dysfunction), such tests, despite their sound physiological and biochemical bases, are limited in their usefulness by the physiological capacity of the kidneys to perform their normal functions although grossly damaged.

Tests for Urinary Tract Involvement

Proteinuria. The normal, healthy glomerular semipermeable membrane passes only substances with molecular weights of less than 70,000. Even if very small amounts of plasma protein are lost, they are reabsorbed almost completely by the proximal tubule. However, the molecular weight of albumin is very close to the "cut-off" value of 70,000, and if the glomerular membrane is diseased, or if tubular reabsorption is inefficient, this protein can gain access to the urine. The larger globulin molecules escape less readily.

Proteinuria may be classified into three groups:

Prerenal. The glomerular membrane damage and tubular reabsorption inefficiency associated with congestive heart failure, certain kinds of cerebral injury, severe infection with high fever, and severe anemia may cause proteinuria. In some types of plasma cell myelomatosis in which the abnormal protein produced has a relatively low molecular weight (Bence Jones protein, or light-chain disease), this protein can pass the healthy glomerular membrane.

Renal. Nephritis, toxemia of pregnancy, renal disease associated with diabetes mellitus and lupus erythematosus, nephrosis, and amyloidosis are examples of renal proteinuria. A brief episode of proteinuria can be produced in a normal person by unusually strenuous exercise.

Postrenal. Inflammation of the urinary tract can release enough exudate from the affected tissues to produce proteinuria.

Presence of Casts. Casts are precipitates of protein formed in the distal convoluted and collecting tubules of the kidney, where conditions of filtrate flow and pH are optimal for protein precipitation. A small number of casts may be found in normal urine (especially hyaline casts after exercise), but a large number is significant indication of active renal disease. Especially significant are blood casts in which the central mass of protein is covered by aggregates of red blood cells, signifying glomerular hemorrhage, and granular casts in which the protein mold is covered by pyknotic and degenerate nuclei, signifying functional standstill of a nephron.

The Nature of Casts. In 1950, Tamm and Horsfall isolated from urine a mucoprotein that displayed unexpected interactions with certain viruses. This Tamm-Horsfall (T-H) protein appears to form a major constituent of hyaline casts.

The T-H mucoprotein is probably formed normally by the tubules; it is not found in plasma. It is a long, rod-like, flexible molecule, M.W. of 28×10^6. As the glomerular filtrate travels down the nephron tubule, the concentrations of salts and hydrogen ion increase. At about pH 4.5, proteins such as albumin (isoelectric point 4.9), hemoglobin (isoelectric point 6.8), and myoglobin (isoelectric point 6.9) change from negatively to positively charged molecules: the Tamm-Horsfall protein (isoelectric point 3.2) is still negatively charged. It has been suggested that this coexistence of proteins of opposite electric charge leads to precipitation and the formation of casts. (The isoelectric point of a protein is the pH at which the numbers of positive and negative electrical charges on the molecule are equal. At its isoelectric point [symbol pI] a protein has its maximum tendency to precipitate.) The presence of T-H mucoprotein explains the periodic acid–Schiff (PAS)–positive reaction of hyaline casts.

Hematuria and Hemoglobinuria. A rare red blood cell may be found in a centrifuged deposit of urine from a normal person, but more than an occasional red cell is considered pathological, indicating bleeding within the urinary tract. In acute glomerulonephritis there is much hemorrhage from the glomeruli; many red cells are ruptured in their passage through the tract, and some hemoglobin is converted to hematin and methemoglobin. These factors combine to give the "smoky" red-brown urine characteristic of the disease. Focal glomerular necrosis, probably on an immunological basis, as in bacterial endocarditis, is another important cause of hematuria. Hemorrhage elsewhere in the urinary tract will be revealed by gross and certainly by microscopic examination, and may indicate disease in the tract or may be a symptom of any of the hemorrhagic diatheses (see hematology section). Hemoglobinuria is usually a manifestation of hemoglobinemia subsequent to a hemolytic episode (see hematology section); occasionally, it is the result of disintegration of red cells within the urinary tract, generally within the bladder.

White Blood Cells. A few white blood cells in a centrifuged deposit of urine are considered normal. In female patients, contamination with white cells from the vulva or vagina must be excluded by obtaining a "clean-catch" or a catheter specimen. An increased number of white blood cells in a correctly collected specimen indicates inflammation in the urinary tract, and it should be noted that leukocytes are also found in considerable numbers in acute glomerulonephritis.

Glitter Cells. These are polymorphonuclear cells whose granules display brownian motion. For a long time they were believed to be pathognomonic of pyelonephritis, but they probably represent toxic or old cells. However, if large glitter cells predominate, a renal origin is likely.

Tests for Degree of Renal Impairment

The tests of renal function are each based on a standardized challenge to a particular renal physiological function.

Tests Based on Water Elimination and Reabsorption. As noted before, about 99% of the water of the glomerular filtrate is reabsorbed normally by the tubules and part of this reabsorption (12.5%) is dependent upon the functional integrity of the tubular lining cells. If this facultative phase of tubular absorption of water is absent, urine having isosmotic pressure will be excreted (sp gr 1.010) regardless of the physiological necessity for the body to conserve or excrete water. Normally, conservation of water is reflected by concentrated urine with a high specific gravity, and excretion of an excess of water (diuresis) is illustrated by urine of low specific gravity. Presenting the body with reduced water intake, followed by an excess of water, tests the physiological response of the tubular epithelium. Generally, concentrating ability is the first to show deficiency, whereas in the later stages of disease, dilution is impaired. In advanced renal disease, urine of fixed specific gravity, i.e., 1.010, is excreted (isosthenuria). The inability of the kidney to regulate water excretion competently also gives rise to an increase in urine secretion at night, and the patient's rest is disturbed by the necessity of micturating; this condition is known as nocturia and is a fairly early symptom in renal dysfunction. By measuring the day and the night urine outputs separately, the severity and significance of nocturia can be assessed.

Impaired Concentrating Power. This occurs (1) in diseases of the kidney, especially those leading to tubular damage, e.g., chronic glomerulonephritis and pyelonephritis, nephrosis, and polycystic disease; (2) temporarily, often in the recovery phase from acute renal shutdown (lower nephron nephrosis); (3) in severe potassium depletion; (4) in hypercalcemia, e.g., due to vitamin D intoxication, hyperparathyroidism, some cases of sarcoidosis, and diffuse osseous metastases with demineralization; (5) in certain inborn defects of tubular function; (6) in organic diabetes insipidus; and (7) in functional diabetes insipidus caused by compulsive water drinking.

Nonprotein Nitrogen Substances in the Blood. One measure of renal function is the excretion of the nonvolatile end products of metabolism, which include urea, uric acid, and creatinine, so that a rise in the serum level of such substances might indicate renal impairment. However, since factors other than renal ones may determine their serum levels, a simple relationship is not possible; nevertheless, the investigation has considerable value.

Nonprotein Nitrogen in Blood. The nonprotein nitrogen of the blood is a heterogeneous collection of substances including urea, creatinine, creatine, uric acid, amino acids, nucleotides, polypeptides, glutathione, and others. Estimation of the "N.P.N." was formerly a common investigation, but it has now been completely replaced by determinations of urea and creatinine. In addition to being more specific indicators of renal condition, these determinations are easily automated.

Blood Urea or Blood Urea Nitrogen (BUN). Urea is the major excretion product of protein catabolism. It is formed in the liver from carbon dioxide and ammonia by a biochemical process known as the ornithine cycle, which may be illustrated as follows:

$$\text{Ornithine} + CO_2 + NH_3 \longrightarrow \text{Citrulline}$$

$$\text{Citrulline} + NH_3 \longrightarrow \text{Arginine}$$

$$\text{Arginine} + H_2O \xrightarrow{\text{Arginase}} \text{Ornithine} + \text{UREA}$$

(Ornithine, citrulline, and arginine are all amino acids.)

After elaboration, urea is passed to the blood and is excreted through the glomeruli and partly reabsorbed in the tubules. Blood urea (or blood urea nitrogen) levels may be raised for several reasons other than inefficient renal excretion and may be considered under the following headings:

Prerenal. Conditions in which circulation through the kidney is less efficient than usual: surgical shock, Addison's disease, congestive cardiac failure, and hemorrhage.

Renal. Renal parenchymal disease, especially glomerular damage.

Postrenal. Obstruction to the urinary tract, such as prostatic hypertrophy.

The term used to describe an increased blood level of urea is *azotemia*; the term *uremia* is correctly applied to the clinical condition of renal failure with azotemia. This distinction is more than academic, as can be seen from the classification, and it also illustrates the fact that urea is not the substance that produces all the manifestations of uremia. Because of the capacity of the kidneys to compensate for damage, there may be a fair degree of renal disease before azotemia is apparent.

Creatinine. Creatine is a nitrogenous substance found almost exclusively in muscle. (98% of the total body content is in muscle). It plays an essential part in muscular contraction and is excreted as its anhydride, creatinine. In adult males, only creatinine appears in the urine, but in adult females, in pregnant and lactating women, and in children of both sexes, some creatine is normally passed in the urine. Creatine is excreted in the urine of adult men only in muscle-wasting disease. The amount of creatinine excreted is fairly constant, roughly proportional to the size of the person, i.e., the muscle mass. The common practice of using the 24-hour excretion of creatinine as a check on the completeness of urine collections should be employed with caution. Various studies have shown variations in single individuals as great as 0.8 g per 24 hours. Since creatinine is derived entirely from endogenous metabolism and is not reabsorbed by the renal tubules, its blood level is a reliable index to renal function. Recent improvements in methods for the assay of creatinine (see p. 220) have led to its increasing clinical use for the assessment of renal function, including the critical monitoring of patients following renal transplants.

BUN/Creatinine Ratio. The ratio of plasma BUN/creatinine in a normal person is approximately 10:1. In most instances of uncomplicated chronic renal insufficiency, the 10:1 ratio is maintained. In certain situations, it is altered:

1. BUN/creatinine ratio more than 10:1:
   a. Excessive turnover of protein (e.g., hemorrhage, burns and infections)
   b. Reduced glomerular perfusion (prerenal uremia)
2. BUN/creatinine ratio less than 10:1 occurs in chronic renal insufficiency, complicated by the following:
   a. Repeated dialysis
   b. Severe vomiting or diarrhea
   c. Liver failure

Dye Excretion Tests. Several dyes are excreted by the kidneys, and their quantitative excretion has been used as a measure of renal function.

Phenolsulfonphthalein (P.S.P.) Excretion Test. P.S.P. is excreted after intravenous injection by both the glomeruli and tubules and thus is dependent on their integrity. In clinical practice, a standard amount of dye is injected, and excretion in timed specimens of urine is measured. Errors due to circulatory disturbances and liver disease diminish the clinical value of this procedure.

Clearance Tests. In order to assign a quantitative measure to the efficiency of the kidney in removing waste substances from the plasma the concept of "plasma clearance" was developed. If the plasma being filtered through the glomeruli contains 100 mg per dL of a substance, and if one minute's production of urine contains 100 mg of the substance, then it follows that in one minute 1 dL of plasma has been purged of its total content of the waste substance. If the amount of the waste substance in the plasma is X mg per dL, the concentration thereof in the urine is U mg per mL (100 U mg/dL), and the rate of urine output is 1 mL per minute, the clearance is given by the expression

$$\frac{100\ \text{U}}{\text{X}}$$

Using the actual values stated earlier, this becomes

$\frac{100 \times 100}{100} =$ 100 mL of plasma theoretically cleared of the waste product per minute. Naturally, the plasma may not be entirely cleared of X, since plasma may leave the kidneys with an appreciable concentration, but the arithmetical expression gives the theoretical amount of plasma that would have been virtually cleared. The clearance values for different substances naturally will differ, since they will vary with the amount of reabsorption by the tubules and the amount of purely tubular excretion. (For example, glucose is not "cleared" at all, since tubular reabsorption is 100%; however, it appears in the glomerular filtrate.) The creatinine clearance rate is often used as a measure of the glomerular filtration rate. However, owing to secretion of creatinine into the glomerular transudate by the renal tubules, it is an imprecise index. The infusion of inulin (to estimate inulin clearance) or the use of various radioisotope methods (such as labeled vitamin B_{12}) is necessary to obtain an accurate estimate of the glomerular filtration rate. In our experience, using an automated method for assay of urine and serum creatinine, creatinine clearance values can be reproduced to within about ± 10%; the limiting factor is the precision of the serum creatinine value.

The clearance principle can be applied to other substances; phosphate clearance determinations have been used in the investigation of parathyroid disease.

GOUT

Metabolism of Uric Acid

The formation of uric acid is set out diagrammatically in Figure 9–3. As already mentioned, most uric acid in humans derives from the metabolism of guanine. The breakdown of adenine appears to be limited, and much of this base seems to be excreted unchanged in the urine. In humans and apes, uric acid is the final product of purine catabolism. All other mammals possess in their livers and kidneys the enzyme uricase, which oxidizes uric acid to allantoin, a much more soluble compound. Approximately 750 mg of uric acid is formed each day (range, 500 to 1100 mg). By isotopic dilution techniques, the average adult male has been shown to have a miscible uric acid pool of 1200 mg (range, 850 to 1600 mg). This is a measure of the amount of accessible uric acid in the various tissues and fluids of the body with which an injected dose of isotopically labeled uric acid mixes promptly.

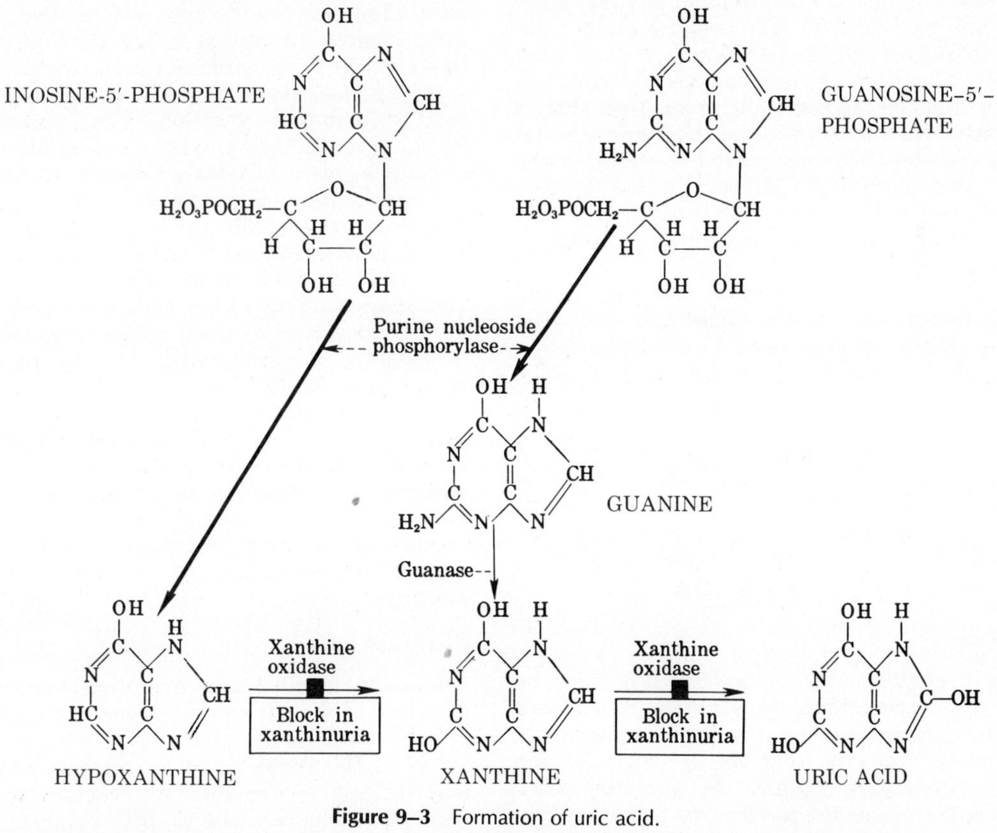

Figure 9–3 Formation of uric acid.

Uric acid is the end product of purine and nucleic acid catabolism and is excreted in the urine. Part of the circulating uric acid is endogenous (from normal breakdown of tissues of the body) and part exogenous (from metabolism of food). An increased level of uric acid in the blood may result from renal impairment or urinary obstruction, but other causes are well-known. Hyperuricemia may be classified as follows: (a) gout; (b) conditions in which there is abnormally rapid nuclear breakdown, e.g., leukemia, some cases of pernicious anemia when treated, hemolytic anemia, polycythemia, and in patients on very severe dietary restriction; and (c) renal disease.

Plasma Levels and Excretion of Uric Acid

By the precise spectrophotometric uricase method, the mean plasma uric acid concentration in normal men is about 5 mg per dL (5.07 ± 0.98 mg per dL), and in women, about 4 mg per dL (4.04 ± 0.96 mg per dL). This mean difference of 1 mg per dL between the sexes has been found consistently in a number of surveys. The lower concentrations in women appear to be owing to the female hormonal milieu. Before puberty the levels in boys and girls are similar, and values rise after the menopause. From 96 to 98% of plasma uric acid is free monosodium urate; i.e., very little is bound to other substances. At a concentration of 6.4 mg per dL plasma is saturated and the extracellular fluids are supersaturated with uric acid.

However, supersaturated solutions of sodium urate in plasma appear to be relatively stable, and plasma uric acid concentrations up to 20 mg per dL can be encountered. Uric acid deposition in connective tissue, with the formation of tophi, generally occurs at these higher concentrations, and indeed dissolution of tophi does not occur until the plasma level falls below 7 mg per dL. Uric acid values from an apparently normal population show a skewed distribution, with occasional values extending up to 10 or 11 mg per dL in males. Most studies have shown that the curve is not bimodal, implying that the skewed distribution is not obviously owing to the presence of two populations. Hyperuricemia is thus difficult to define, but blood levels consistently higher than 7 mg per 100 mL require careful clinical evaluation of the patient.

Some 25 to 30% of the total daily turnover of 750 mg uric acid is excreted in all the juices and secretions entering the gastrointestinal tract. In the large bowel, this is degraded by bacteria. The remainder is excreted in the urine. The renal clearance of plasma uric acid is only 6 to 11 mL per minute (average, 8.7 mL per minute). The total average adult daily urinary excretion of uric acid is 420 ± 80 mg. Modern evidence indicates that practically all the uric acid filtered through the glomerulus is reabsorbed by the proximal convoluted tubule, and that which is finally eliminated in the urine is actually secreted by the renal tubules.

Types of Gout

Gout may be primary or secondary. The latter may be seen in conditions associated with a high rate of cell turnover and destruction, e.g., in pernicious anemia being treated, in hemolytic anemias, in leukemias and other myeloproliferative diseases, in resolving pneumonia, and when there is reduced renal tubular excretion of uric acid, as in chronic renal disease, von Gierke's disease, and acidosis. Most cases of primary gout are familial, but occasional nonfamilial or sporadic cases are seen.

Inheritance

This is complex and rarely amenable to simple analysis. The tendency to hyperuricemia without gout is probably hereditary and may be a dominant trait, but it is not always easy to assess the role of environmental factors such as diet. Hyperuricemia plus the proclivity to gout appears to be governed by a number of genetic factors; i.e., its inheritance is polygenic or multifactorial.

Clinical and Biochemical Features of Gout

Gout is a somewhat heterogeneous disease. For example, some 25 to 30% of gouty patients are habitual overexcretors, i.e., they excrete more than 590 mg of uric acid per day. The remaining 70 to 75% may be divisible into two groups, a larger group that appears to produce uric acid in excess although their urinary excretion does not exceed 590 mg per day, and a smaller group in which, from studies using isotopic dilution techniques, uric acid production does not appear to be excessive. Thus, the majority of gouty patients are overproducers of uric acid.

In gout, despite the increased plasma levels, renal clearance of uric acid is slightly reduced, averaging 7.5 ±2.4 mL per minute (v. normal, 8.7 ± 2.5 mL per minute). This appears to be owing to increased reabsorption by the proximal nephron.

About 95% of gout patients are male, and affected women are almost exclusively postmenopausal. The first attack may appear any time after the age of 20, but most often between the ages of 40 and 50. The pain and inflammation are caused by precipitation of the needle-like crystals of monosodium urate from the supersaturated extracellular fluids. These microcrystals incite a local inflammatory reaction, with great local increase in pain-producing kinins and exudation of leukocytes. Trauma or other physical or mental stress may trigger the attack. Monosodium urate crystals tend to be deposited in microaerophilic, avascular tissues, such as cartilage, joint capsules, ligaments, and tendons. During an attack, the plasma uric acid is generally elevated and averages 9 to 10 mg per dL (range, 7.0 to 16 mg per dL). However, in about 10% of cases the plasma uric acid during an attack may be around the upper limit of normal, i.e., 6.5 to 7.5 mg per dL.

Usually within 2 years of the first acute attack a second one is experienced, and thereafter attacks tend to increase in frequency and to affect more joints. After several years (average about 10), chronic destructive gouty polyarthritis develops, with formation of tophi in about 20% of cases (50% before advent of uricosuric drugs). Gout accounts for about 5% of all cases of chronic arthritis.

Complications

Proteinuria and benign hypertension develop in about one-third of the patients. Deposits of monosodium urate crystals form in the collecting tubules and interstitial tissue of the renal medulla, causing tubular damage and inciting a foreign body reaction with resultant scarring. Glomerulosclerosis also develops.

Urinary Calculi in Gout

These are up to 1000 to 4000 times commoner than in normal persons. Uric acid stones occur in about 40% of overexcretors and in 10 to 20% of normoexcretors of uric acid among gouty patients, as compared with 0.01% of nongouty adults.

ROUTINE URINALYSIS

A SCHEME FOR ROUTINE EXAMINATION OF URINE SAMPLES

Collection of Urine Specimens

Urine should be voided into washed, dried, and, if possible, sterilized containers. Ideally, the specimens should be collected as follows. In the male, the glans and meatal orifice should be wiped with cotton moistened with warm water. The patient is given two urine bottles, labeled 1 and 2; into the first bottle he passes a small amount of urine—this will contain secretions and debris from the urethra and prostate and may be discarded unless disease of these parts is suspected. He then voids the remainder and major portion of the specimen into the second bottle. The female patient is instructed to separate the labia with the fingers of one hand and, using moist cotton, to wipe the urethral orifice from front to back. She then passes a small amount of urine into the first of two clean, suitable receptacles and the remainder into the second receptacle.

For routine urinalysis, first morning samples are preferred, since these are usually the most concentrated. Casts tend to dissolve and are generally less numerous in dilute urine. If the specimen cannot be examined immediately, it should be placed in the refrigerator at 0 to 4° C. If delay before examination is unavoidable, loss of casts may be reduced by acidifying the urine with a few drops of dilute hydrochloric acid.

Procedure

1. Number the urine specimens and their request forms consecutively.

2. Number a series of conical 15 mL centrifuge tubes to correspond with the urine samples.

ROUTINE URINALYSIS

Color	Possible Cause
Straw to amber	Normal (urochrome)
Orange	Concentrated urine
Deep yellow	Riboflavin
Bright orange	"Pyridium" and amidopyrine drugs generally
Orange-brown	Urobilin
Greenish orange	Bilirubin
Smokey	Red blood cells
Wine red or reddish brown	Hemoglobin pigments or uroporphyrins
Brown to black on standing	Melanin or homogentisic acid
Almost colorless	Dilute urine
Reddish orange in alkaline solution	Rhubarb or senna
Dirty green on standing	Excess indican
Red in alkaline solution	Phenolphthalein
Green or blue	Methylene blue
Greenish yellow fluorescence	Flavones in some vitamin preparations

3. Mix each specimen thoroughly and place about 12 mL of the urine in the corresponding centrifuge tube. Note the color and degree of turbidity.

REACTION. A 24-hour urine is normally acid, pH about 6.0. Individual samples will vary between pH 5.0 and 7.5.

SPECIFIC GRAVITY. A 24-hour urine specimen will normally have a specific gravity between 1.010 and 1.025. Individual samples will vary with the intake of food and water. The night urine is usually concentrated, e.g., 1.020 or greater. See tests of kidney function.

Specific Gravity of Small Urine Volumes. The specific gravity of a tiny volume of urine—even 1 to 2 drops—can be determined accurately by means of a refractometer. The process of determining the specific gravity can be expedited by using the combination of a temperature-compensated refractometer and sampling pump (American Optical Flo-Thru; Biovation Digital Urinometer). Even without the addition of the sampling pump, the refractometer is the preferred method for determination of specific gravity.

Temperature and Specific Gravity. Hydrometers are calibrated for a given temperature. Since fluids expand when warmed, their specific gravity falls: an increase of 3°C leads to an 0.001 decrease in specific gravity, and vice versa with a fall in temperature.

Osmolality; Specific Gravity and Solute Concentration. Only *osmolality* (osmotic pressure expressed in osmols or milliosmoles per kilogram of water) expresses accurately and in comparable terms the solute content of various fluids. *Osmolarity* (osmotic pressure in osmols or milliosmols per liter of solution) does not allow for the effects of temperature, nor for the volume occupied by proteins, and is therefore less useful than osmolality. Osmometers measure osmolality by determining the reduction in freezing point of a solution or fluid below that of pure water. The freezing point of water is reduced by 1.86°C for each 1000 mOsm of solute it contains per kilogram. Thus a urine whose freezing point is depressed 1.58°C below that of water has an osmolality of 850:

$$1000 \times \frac{1.58}{1.86} = 850 \text{ mOsm/kg}$$

Specific gravity is affected by the nature and quantity of dissolved constituents but does not accurately reflect the concentrations of these. For example, specific gravity is increased by 0.001 when 1.47 g NaCl, *or* 3.6 g urea, *or* 2.7 g glucose, *or* 3.9 g albumin is added to 1 liter of urine. Between 70 and 90% of the specific gravity of normal urine is due to urea, chlorides, sulfates, phosphates, bicarbonates, and creatinine.

Excretion of diagnostic media used for intravenous pyelography may raise the specific gravity of the urine considerably.

PROTEINS. Detectable amounts of protein are not normally present in urine (except in orthostatic or postural proteinuria). Excretion of plasma proteins occurs in renal disease; the albumins predominate because of their smaller molecular size.

Excretion of abnormal proteins (i.e., Bence Jones protein) occurs in many cases of multiple myeloma and in a few cases of leukemia.

False-positive protein tests may result from tolbutamide medication, massive penicillin dosage, polyvinylpyrrolidone, and a number of diagnostic radiopaque substances.

4. Measure the specific gravity of each urine sample, using a refractometer method.

5. Centrifuge each urine for 5 minutes at 1500 to 2500 rpm. Use the supernatant urine for the tests that follow.

6. Set up two series of 6 × 5/8 inch test tubes; use one set for the sulfosalicylic acid test for protein and the other set for the Benedict qualitative test for reducing substances. Test for acetone if specifically requested or if reducing substances are present (method on p. 209). For the routine processing of large numbers of urine samples, the most convenient method for reaction, protein, glucose, acetone,

TABLE 9–1 COMPOSITION OF NORMAL URINE

The values quoted are for a 70 kg adult with a protein intake of 1.0 g per kg per day. For some substances (e.g., total amino acid nitrogen, creatine, and calcium) there is as yet no general agreement on the normal range; the diversity in values is partly due to dietary influences and differences in methodology.

Substance or Test	Values	Specimen
Addis count	Casts (hyaline): 0–4300 Leukocytes: Up to 2.25 million Red cells: Up to 425,000	12 hour 12 hour 12 hour
Albumin	10–100 mg	24 hour
Amino acids (as N)	Free: 50–200 mg Total: 150–600 mg	24 hour 24 hour
Ammonium	10–105 mEq	24 hour
Bicarbonate	Nil	
Calcium	50–400 mg 2.5–20 mEq	24 hour
Chloride as NaCl	5–20 g (85–340 mEq) Average: 10 g (170 mEq)	24 hour
Creatine	Male: 0–50 mg Female: 0–150 mg Children: 5.4–13.7 mg/kg/day	24 hour 24 hour
Creatinine	Male: 20–28 mg per kg (average 24) Female: 15–21 mg per kg (average 18)	24 hour 24 hour
Nitrogen	Total 7–20 g (average 10) Urea N 5–15 g (average 7.5)	24 hour 24 hour
pH	4.7–7.7 (average 6.0)	Fresh random
Phosphates	0.5–2.2 g (average 1.0)	24 hour
Potassium	25–100 mEq	24 hour
Protein	10–100 mg	24 hour
Sodium	80–290 mEq	24 hour
Solids, total	50–75 g	24 hour
Specific gravity	1.008–1.030 (average 1.018) 1.012–1.025 500–800 mOsm/kg	Random 24 hour 24 hour
Sulfates	Inorganic 0.25–1.25 g Total 0.36–1.44 g	24 hour 24 hour
Titratable acidity	150–400 ml of 0.1 N acid (average 300 mL)	24 hour
Urea	10–35 g (average 15 g)	24 hour
Uric acid	0.3–0.7 g	24 hour
Urobilinogen	0.2–4.0 mg (average 1.0 mg)	24 hour
Volume	Normal range 1200–2000 mL Extreme range 600–3600 mL Average 1400 mL	24 hour

blood, and bilirubin are the "dip and read" impregnated paper strips. It is advisable to check trace reactions for protein by the sulfosalicylic acid test detailed further on and to bear in mind that the stick test is specific for glucose; if the presence of other reducing substances is to be checked, use either Clinitest tablets or Benedict's reagent.

Test for bilirubin and urobilin(ogen) if specifically requested or if the color of the urine suggests the presence of these substances (methods on p. 210).

7. Decant the rest of the urine from the centrifuge tube and examine the deposit as directed on page 210 (see Table 9–1 for the composition of normal urine).

Qualitative Tests for Proteins in Urine

Sulfosalicylic Acid Test

Procedure. **Layer gently onto about 3 mL of urine in a test tube an equal quantity of 10% w/v sulfosalicylic acid in 50% methanol. If proteins are present, a cloudy precipitate will appear at the junction of the two fluids.**

Reducing Substances in Urine

Normally, detectable amounts of reducing substances are not found in urine, except in renal glycosuria. The reducing substance most commonly found in urine is glucose, and its presence there indicates either renal glycosuria, diabetes mellitus, miscellaneous endocrine disorders, intravenous infusion of glucose, or increased intracranial pressure. Other sugars sometimes appear in the urine, e.g., lactose, fructose, pentose, and galactose.

In pregnancy lactosuria occurs at some time in about one-half, glycosuria in about one-fifth, and both sugars together in about one-sixth of the patients, on the average. (See p. 223 for a list of reducing substances occurring in urine.)

Tests for Reducing Substances in Urine

Benedict's Qualitative Test

This test is not specific for sugars and is affected by most reducing substances if they occur in large quantities.

Procedure. **In a Pyrex test tube place 0.5 mL (10 drops) of urine and 5.0 mL of Benedict's qualitative reagent. Mix and place in a boiling water bath for five minutes. Allow to cool to room temperature and read as follows:**

Color	Results	
Blue	Negative	
Greenish blue	Tr.	Trace
Green	+	Approximately 0.5% reducing substance
Greenish brown	+ +	Approximately 1.0% reducing substance
Yellow	+ + +	Approximately 1.5% reducing substance
Brick red	+ + + +	Approximately 2.0% reducing substance or more

This is only a rough test and at best an approximate guide to the amount of sugar (or other reducing substance) present. The presence of glucose or other reducing sugars is determined by specific methods.

Acetone and Acetone Bodies

In conditions in which the metabolism of glucose is impaired, such as untreated diabetes mellitus, fevers, diarrhea and vomiting, and starvation, excessive amounts of intermediate products of fat metabolism, mainly beta-hydroxybutyric acid and acetoacetic acid (diacetic acid), are excreted in the urine. The latter substance is slowly converted to acetone if the urine is left at room temperature.

Tests for Acetone Bodies in Urine

Rothera's Test for Acetone and Acetoacetic (Diacetic) Acid

Principle. Both acetone and diacetic acid give a purple color with alkaline sodium nitroprusside. The test will detect acetone in a dilution of 1 in 10,000 and diacetic acid in a dilution of 1 in 125,000.

Procedure. **In a test tube place a small crystal of sodium nitroprusside; add about 2 g of ammonium sulfate and about 10 mL of the urine under examination. After shaking well, add about 2 mL of concentrated ammonium hydroxide solution (sp gr 0.88). A deep purple color indicates the presence of excessive amounts of acetone, diacetic acid, or both. A pale purple color or no color at all is a negative reaction. It must be remembered that another ketone body, beta-hydroxybutyric acid, does not react with this reagent. For this reason, ketosis may be difficult to detect in hypoxemic states, when more beta-hydroxybutyric acid is produced than either acetone or acetoacetic acid.**

Urobilin and Urobilinogen

Urobilinogen, urobilin, stercobilinogen, and stercobilin are decomposition products of bilirubin, normally present in the feces. In conditions in which there is increased excretion of bile by the liver, e.g., hemolytic jaundice, increased amounts of these substances are absorbed from the intestine and are excreted in the urine. Although it is customary to refer to the substances in the urine as urobilinogen and urobilin, stercobilinogen and stercobilin are usually present in higher concentrations than the former.

Schlesinger's Test for Total Urobilinogen and Urobilin

Principle. Urobilinogen is oxidized with iodine to urobilin. The urobilin is then reacted with an alcoholic solution of zinc acetate, and a green fluorescent complex is formed.

Procedure. **If bilirubin is present, it is removed by adding a few mL of 10% w/v barium chloride solution to about 20 mL of urine and filtering. Place about 10 mL of urine or bilirubin-free filtrate of urine in a test tube and**

add two or three drops of Lugol's iodine solution. In another test tube place about 1 g of solid zinc acetate and add about 10 mL of ethyl alcohol; mix by shaking. Pour the urine into the zinc acetate solution and shake thoroughly. Filter through a Whatman No. 1 filter paper into a clean, dry test tube. Examine the filtrate for green fluorescence, using either daylight or an ultraviolet lamp. Normal urine shows a faint green fluorescence. A definite green fluorescence indicates an increased output of urobilin(ogen).

Bilirubin

Detectable amounts of bilirubin are not normally present in urine. Excretion of bilirubin occurs in obstructive jaundice but not in hemolytic jaundice unless there is secondary liver damage.

Tests for Bilirubin in Urine

Most of the commonly used tests for the detection of bilirubin depend on the oxidation of bilirubin to biliverdin. The following test is probably the most satisfactory one for routine use. (Some commercial "stick" tests incorporate a test square for bilirubin.)

Fouchet's Test

Principle. Barium chloride solution is added to the urine. A precipitate of barium sulfate is produced onto which the bilirubin is adsorbed. The barium sulfate–adsorbed bilirubin is filtered off and a drop of Fouchet's ferric chloride solution added to the precipitate. The ferric chloride oxidizes the bilirubin to biliverdin, producing a greenish blue spot.

Procedure. To about 10 mL of urine in a test tube add a few milliliters of 10% w/v barium chloride. Mix and filter through a Whatman No. 1 filter paper. Spread the filter paper out on another dry filter paper and to the barium sulfate precipitate add one drop of Fouchet's reagent. A greenish blue color indicates the presence of bilirubin.

The filtrate from this test may be used for the Schlesinger's test for urobilin.

Reagents

Benedict's Qualitative Reagent. Dissolve 100 g of anhydrous sodium carbonate and 173 g sodium citrate ($Na_3C_6H_5O_7$. 2 H_2O in about 700 mL of distilled water. Dissolve 17.3 g of copper sulfate ($CuSO_4$. 5 H_2O) in about 100 mL of distilled water and add it to the carbonate-citrate solution, mixing constantly. Make the volume of the solution up to 1 liter with distilled water.

Fouchet's Reagent for the Detection of Bilirubin. Dissolve 25 g of trichloroacetic acid in 100 mL of distilled water and then add 10 mL of a 10% w/v solution of ferric chloride.

Microscopic Examination of Urine

See also the text by Spencer and Pederson (1977). If possible, urine deposits should be examined within 8 hours of collection, preferably within 1 to 2 hours.

Procedure

1. Mix the urine thoroughly and place about 12 mL in a conical centrifuge tube. Centrifuge for 5 minutes at 1500 to 2500 rpm; pour off the supernatant fluid; resuspend the deposit in the few drops of urine that remain by flicking the end of the tube with the finger; then place a drop on a microscope slide and cover with a cover glass.

2. Examine with the low power objective to obtain an overall picture of the deposit. Use the higher power objectives to examine objects more closely. In order not to miss casts the microscope should be set up for critical Kohler illumination, with particular attention to centering of the condenser: the overall intensity of the light should be reduced to obtain maximum contrast.

Substances appearing in the urine deposits are of three main types: cells, casts, and crystals (including amorphous chemical deposits).

Cells

Epithelial Cells (Fig. 9–4)

Squamous Epithelial Cells. These large cells with small round or oval nuclei are derived from the ureters,

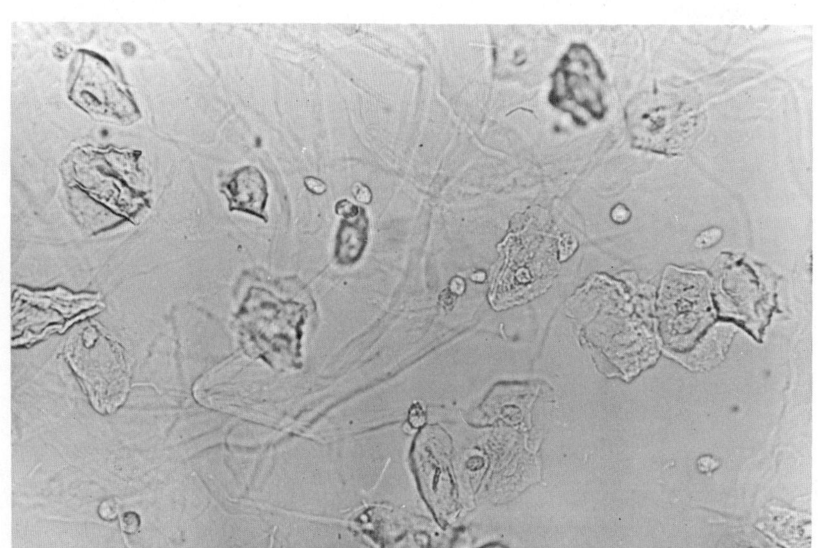

Figure 9–4 Epithelial squames and mucus threads. Print × 300.

bladder, and urethra. In urine from female patients not obtained by catheterization, vaginal epithelial cells may also be present. This is normal and of no significance.

Polyhedral Epithelial Cells. Small, round cells slightly larger than leukocytes, and caudate epithelial cells, which are smaller than the squamous cells and have a tail-like process, may also be present. These derive mainly from the upper tract.

Red Cells. In hypertonic urine the red cells may be crenated and smaller than normal. In hypotonic urine they are swollen and larger than usual, losing their typical "double ring" appearance. The presence of red cells in the urine indicates bleeding in some part of the urinary tract. It is important that contamination from menstrual flow be avoided when urine from females is to be examined.

Leukocytes (Fig. 9–5). The normal excretion rate for leukocytes in the urine is up to 3 per µL, i.e., 3000 per mL, or up to about 200,000 per hour.

Detection of Urinary Tract Infection by Urinalysis. Screening culture of clean-catch, fresh urine specimens for significant bacteriuria is described on page 417. Here we are concerned with the microscopic detection of urinary tract infection. As mentioned, the normal urinary leukocyte rate ranges up to 3 per µL which corresponds approximately to 1 WBC per 3 to 5 high power fields (HPFs) of uncentrifuged urine. It has been shown that leukocyte excretion rates in excess of 400,000 per hour virtually always indicate infection of the urinary tract. This rate corresponds to more than 10 WBCs per µL or more than 1 per HPF. Cases with active upper tract infection frequently show more than 50 WBCs per µL (equivalent to more than 5 per HPF, or a leukocyte excretion rate in excess of 2, or even 3, million per hour).

Spermatozoa. Spermatozoa may be present in the urine of a male after ejaculation or in female urine as a vaginal contaminant after coitus. They are easily recognized.

Bacteria. Bacteria are not normally present in urine. Contamination can easily occur if the urine is not collected by catheterization, however; and if the urine is allowed to stand at room temperature for any length of time, it may be swarming with bacteria. They are of no significance unless the urine has been collected by an aseptic technique and placed in a sterile container.

Casts

Casts are of many types. They are formed by the solidification of protein in the nephron tubule, often with trapped cells, granular debris, and so forth.

Hyaline Casts (Fig. 9–6). Hyaline casts are cylindrical, transparent bodies that are difficult to see unless the illumination is cut to a minimum.

Finely Granular Casts. These casts are similar to hyaline casts but contain fine granules.

Coarsely Granular Casts (Fig. 9–7). These have larger granules than the finely granular casts but are similar in appearance.

Leukocyte Casts (Fig. 9–8). Leukocyte casts are composed mainly of leukocytes.

Blood Casts. These are easily recognized because they are almost entirely composed of red cells and often have a bright orange color.

Fatty Casts. These are any casts that contain fat droplets. Examination by polarized light may show anisotropic lipids, especially in lipid nephrosis.

Waxy Casts (Fig. 9–9). Waxy casts are similar to hyaline casts but are more opaque and often have a curled end or "tail."

Renal Failure Casts. In the late stages of many renal diseases residual nephrons often become dilated. Casts developing in these nephrons tend to have large diameters. If they are numerous they indicate a grave outlook or "end-stage" kidney.

Cylindroids. Cylindroids are long ribbon-like formations that resemble hyaline casts but are much longer and are often tapered.

Mucus Threads. Mucus threads may be mistaken for hyaline casts, but they are usually much longer, less regular, and wavy, and they have tapered ends. Amorphous urates or phosphates may form aggregates on mucus threads which resemble casts but they seldom have the parallel sides and smooth ends of true casts.

The presence of casts in urine, especially if protein is also present, usually indicates kidney disease.

Staining of Urine Sediment

This facilitates recognition of cells, especially for the inexperienced technologist. Wet preparations may be stained in several ways:

1. A drop of resuspended sediment on a slide is mixed with a small drop of a 1:2 to 1:4 dilution of Löffler's methylene blue.
2. Sternheimer-Malbin Stain

Solution A:	
Crystal violet	3.0 g
95% alcohol	20 mL
Ammonium oxalate	0.8 g
Distilled water	80 mL
Solution B:	
Safranin O	0.25 g
95% alcohol	10 mL
Distilled water	100 mL

Working Stain. Mix 3 vol of solution A with 97 vol of solution B and filter. This will last up to three months.

Procedure. To the resuspended sediment in a centrifuge tube add 1 drop of the working stain and let stand 3 minutes after mixing. Then place a drop on a microscope slide, cover, and examine.

Results. Normal polymorphonuclear nuclei take up both dyes and stain orange-purple. Glitter cells tend to take only the crystal violet and appear pale blue or colorless. Hyaline casts are stained pink to purple; RBCs, lavender; cellular casts, dark purple; and *Trichomonas* and nuclei of bladder and vaginal epithelia, light blue, blue, and purple, in that order.

3. Oil Red O. If a drop of sediment is mixed with a drop of saturated solution of oil red O in isopropanol, fatty casts and fat droplets will be stained, but most of the latter, if present, will be found floating on the surface of the urine, especially after centrifugation.

Ova and Parasites in Urine

Trichomonas is occasionally seen, especially in fresh specimens. Ova in urine usually derive from fecal contamination, except in cases of *Schistosoma haematobium* infestation.

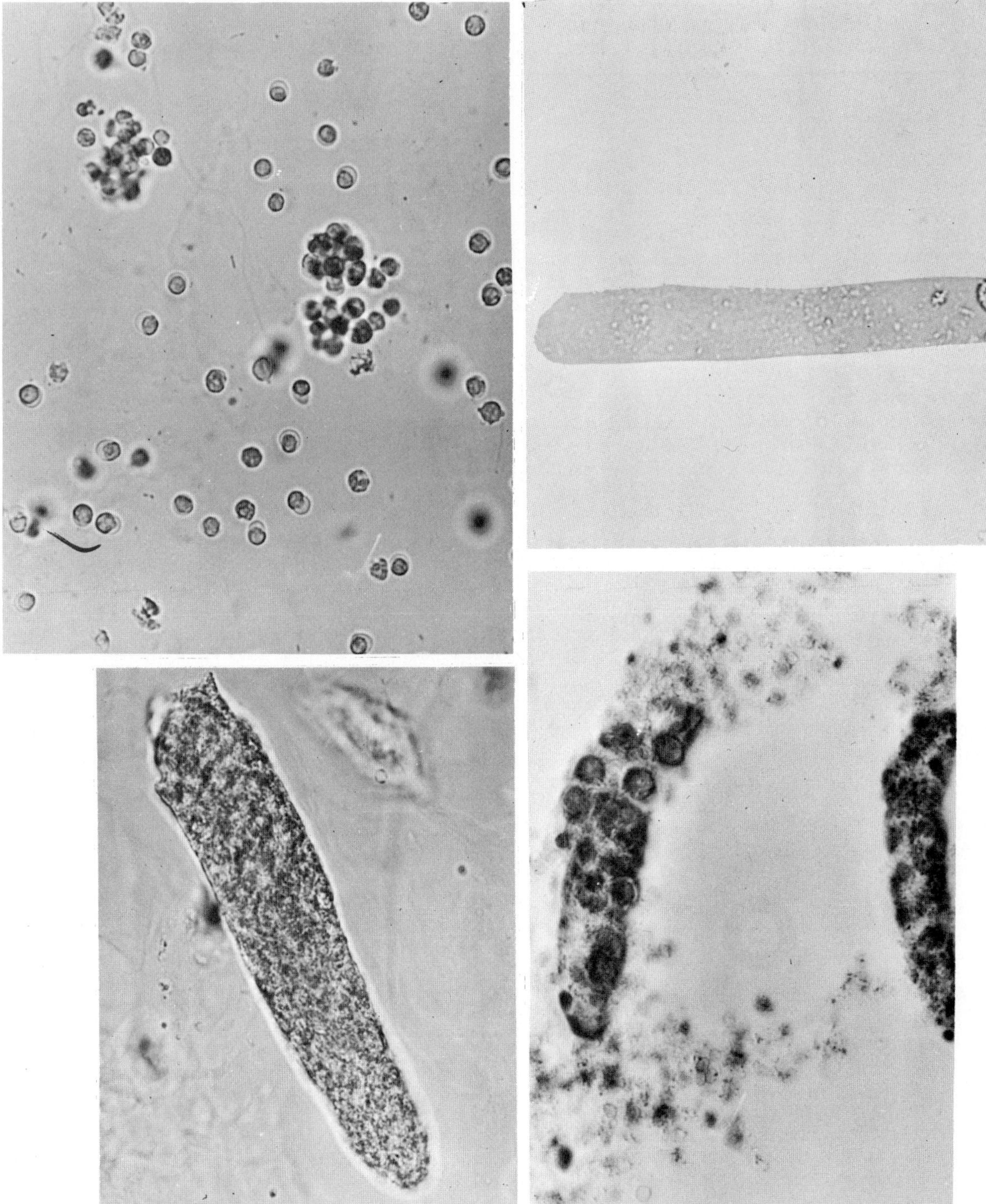

Figure 9–5

Figure 9–6

Figure 9–7

Figure 9–8

Figure 9–5 Pus cells in urine. Print × 300.

Figure 9–6 Hyaline cast with two epithelial cells embedded in its tip. *N.B.* Hyaline casts are so translucent that they are easily missed unless looked for carefully at low illumination. To increase the contrast of this print the background was masked out for one-third of the exposure time. Print × 300.

Figure 9–7 Granular cast. Print × 630.

Figure 9–8 Two cellular cells; phase contrast. Print × 500.

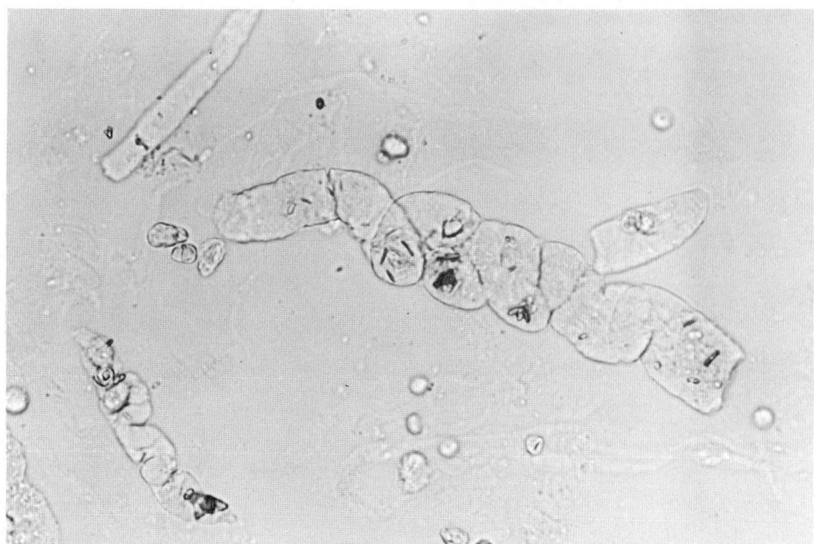

Figure 9–9 Waxy casts, characteristically convoluted. Print × 300.

Crystals

Crystals are not normally present in freshly passed urine and are precipitated from solution as the urine cools. Generally speaking, crystals in the urine are of no significance, except crystals of sulfonamides, cystine, oxalates in persons with a history of ureteral colic or stone formation, and, possibly, urates in those with gout.

Crystals Appearing in Acid Urine

Calcium Oxalate (Fig. 9–10). These are colorless, octahedral crystals and appear as small squares crossed by two diagonal lines. In another form calcium oxalate crystals are dumbbell-shaped. They vary greatly in size.

Uric Acid (Fig. 9–11). Uric acid crystallizes in many forms (e.g., plates, prisms, sheaves, and hexagons). The crystals are usually colored and are easily dissolved by heating. They are soluble in sodium hydroxide but insoluble in hydrochloric acid.

Urate. Urates often appear as an amorphous sediment which dissolves when heated. Sodium urate crystals are often in the form of thorn apples.

Cystine (Fig. 9–12). These crystals are highly refractile hexagonal plates, similar to the plate form of uric acid crystals; however, they may be differentiated from uric acid crystals by their solubility in hydrochloric acid. They are rarely found, but when present are diagnostic of a rare inborn error of metabolism termed cystinuria, in which the patient excretes excessive amounts of the amino acid in the urine. Cystine crystals are soluble in alkali and are not found in alkaline urine.

Tyrosine. Tyrosine is usually in the shape of fine needles or sheaves. They are seldom found except in acute liver failure.

Leucine. The occurrence of leucine crystals in urine is open to question.

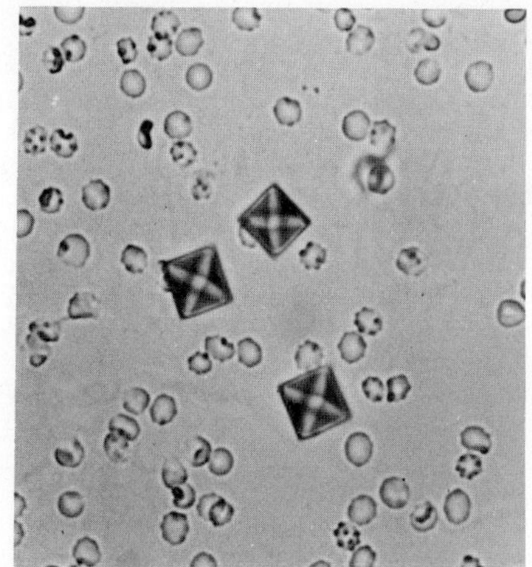

Figure 9–10 Oxalate crystals and red cells. Print × 300.

Crystals Appearing in Alkaline Urine (Figs. 9–13 to 9–15)

Phosphates. Phosphates often appear as an amorphous sediment that is soluble in acetic acid.

Triple Phosphates. The usual forms of these crystals are "prisms" and "coffin lids." They are soluble in acetic acid.

Calcium Carbonate. These crystals can appear as dumbbells, spheres, or amorphous granules. They are soluble in acetic acid.

Ammonium Urate. These crystals can appear in round, oval, or thorn-apple form. They are soluble in acids.

Other Crystals

Sulfonamide (Fig. 9–16). Crystals of the sulfonamides often appear in the urine after administration of these drugs. They are of many forms and may be confused with some of the naturally occurring crystals. If there is any doubt as to the identity of crystals, and if the patient is being treated with sulfonamides, the following test may be applied:

TEST FOR SULFONAMIDES. Deposit the crystals by centrifuging the urine in a Pyrex centrifuge tube. Decant the supernatant urine and add to the deposit 0.5 mL of 50% v/v hydrochloric acid. Mix and place the tube in a boiling water bath for about 30 minutes. Cool the solution and then dilute to 10 mL with distilled water. Apply the color reaction described on page 317 to an aliquot of the solution.

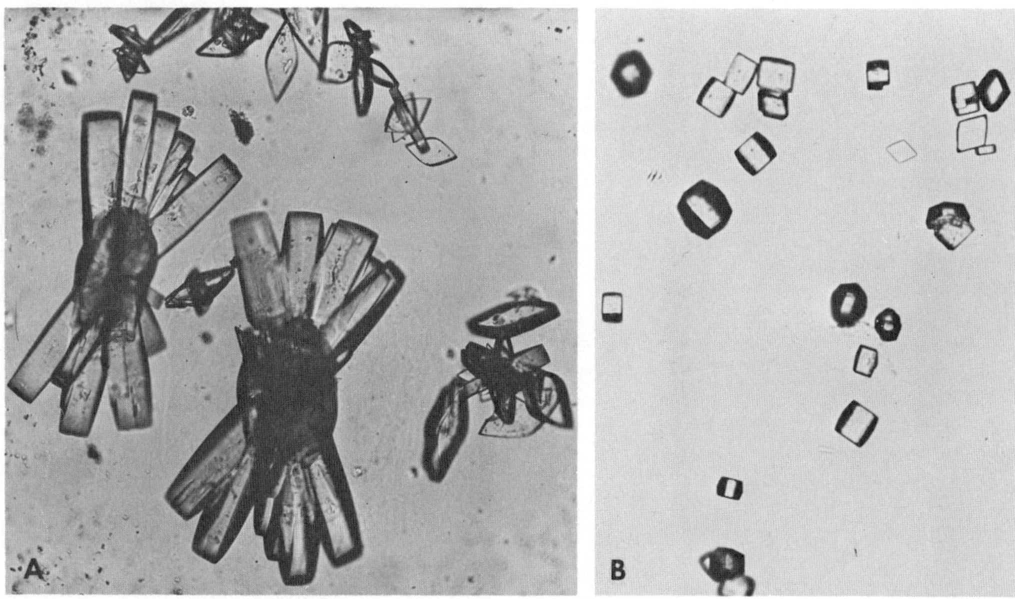

Figure 9–11 *A* and *B*. Uric acid crystals. Print × 300.

The presence in the urine of excreted radiographic contrast media, e.g., iodopyracet (Diodrast), occasionally will produce masses of needle-like crystals, accompanied by a very high specific gravity.

Commercial Reagent Strips and Tablets for Urine Testing

A wide variety of test strips, made of thin plastic and carrying discrete cellulose squares impregnated with reagents, are available, mainly from two companies—Ames Division, Miles Laboratorics, Inc., Elkhart, Ind. 46515 (in Canada, Rexdale, Ontario M9W 1G6) and Bio-Dynamics, Indianapolis, Ind. 46250 (in Canada, Boehringer Mannheim Canada Ltd., Dorval, Quebec H9P 1A9). The selection includes single-test strips for glucose, ketones, protein, and blood and strips with as many as nine tests (N-Multistix-C, with pH, protein, glucose, ketones, bilirubin, blood, nitrite, urobilinogen, and ascorbic acid, made by Ames; Chemstrip 9, with leukocytes, nitrite, pH, protein, glucose, ketones, urobilinogen, bilirubin, and blood, made by Bio-Dynamics). For routine urinalysis, a strip to detect pH, protein, glucose, ketones, and blood is probably the minimum requirement. The main tablet-style test in current use is the Clinitest tablet, made by Ames, used to detect reducing substances in urine and to provide a semi-quantitative measure of glucose in the urine of diabetics. A special single-test strip for the detection of phenylpyruvic acid in suspected cases of phenylketonuria (PKU) is Phenistix, made by Ames.

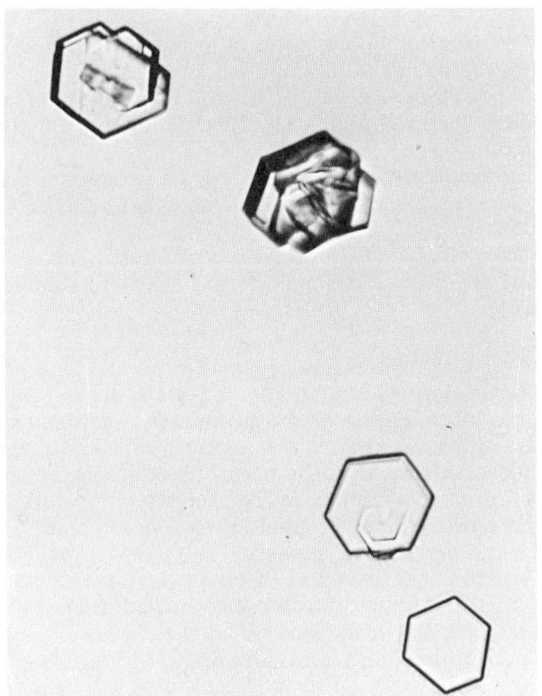

Figure 9–12 Cystine crystals in the urinary deposit from a patient with cystinuria. × 300.

Chemical Principles of "Stick" Tests

Protein. The test square contains the indicator tetrabromphenol blue buffered to pH 3.0, at which it appears yellow. Protein binds selectively to the small fraction of the indicator that is in the ionized form, and this promotes further ionization of the indicator. The ionized form is blue, and the color of the test square at equilibrium of the reaction will change from yellow through shades of green as the protein level increases.

pH. Typically, a mixed indicator is used, such as methyl red and bromthymol blue, providing a spectrum of color change from orange at pH 5.0 to blue at pH 9.0.

Glucose. The test square contains the enzymes glucose oxidase and peroxidase and a chromogen such as potassium iodide. In the presence of glucose and the absence of any other sugar or reducing substance, glucose oxidase converts the glucose to gluconic acid, re-

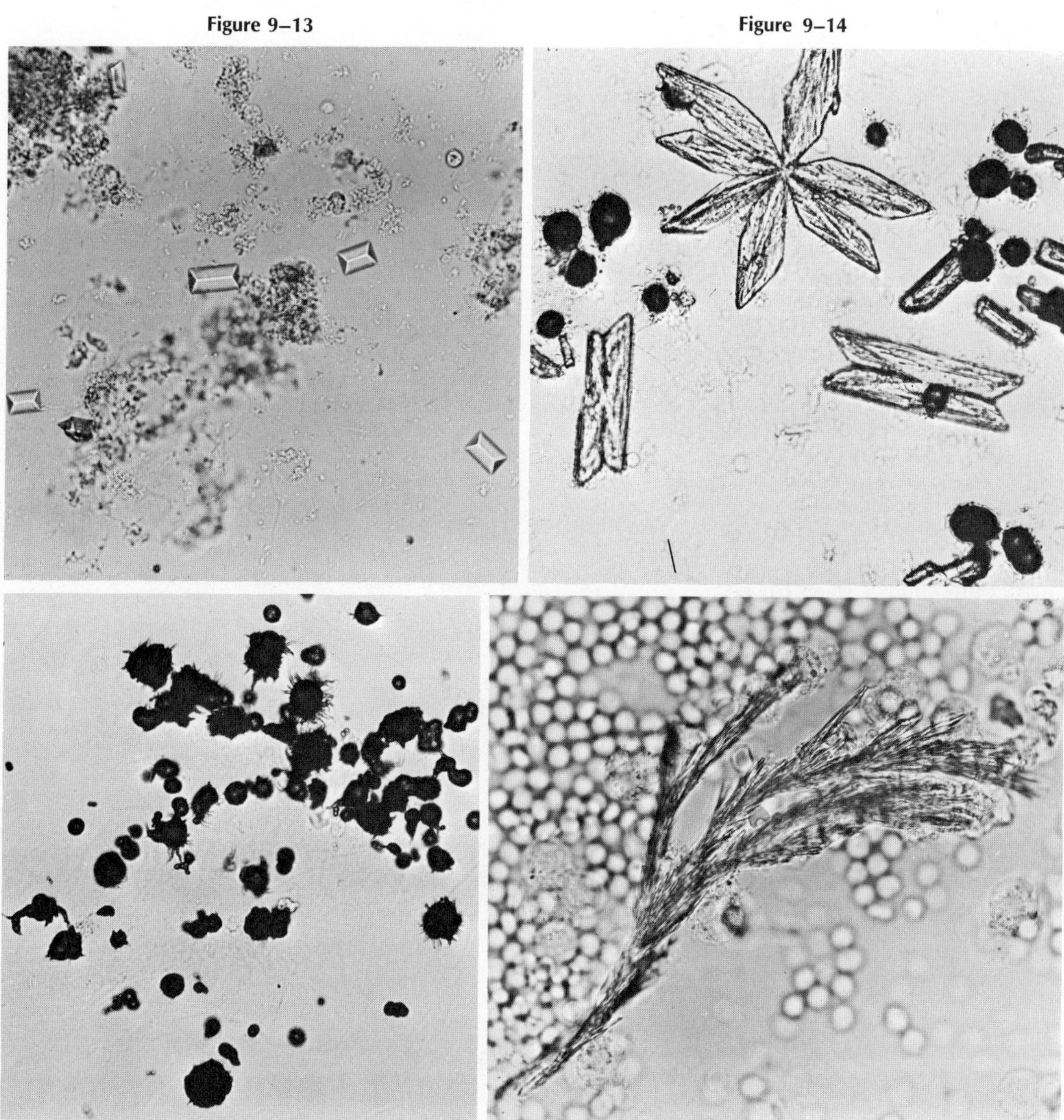

Figure 9–13 "Triple phosphate" crystals and amorphous phosphates. Print × 300.

Figure 9–14 Stellar phosphates and ammonium urate crystals. At this magnification the ammonium urate may be mistaken for some sulfa drug crystals. Print × 300.

Figure 9–15 Characteristic dense, dark, spiny ammonium urate ("thorn-apple") crystals. Print × 300.

Figure 9–16 Sulfadiazine crystal, many red cells and some pus cells. Print × 1050.

leasing hydrogen peroxide; this is in turn decomposed by the peroxidase, releasing oxygen, which oxidizes the iodide to iodine, and changing the color of the square to brown. The reaction will give a color change with as little as 0.1% glucose, and hence will give a positive result when the Clinitest tablet, with a sensitivity limit of 0.25%, shows no reaction.

Ketones. The test square contains sodium nitroprusside, glycine, and a buffer. Acetoacetic acid and, to a lesser extent, acetone give a range of colors with nitroprusside from lavender to purple. Beta-hydroxybutyric acid does not react.

Blood. This reaction detects the heme grouping of hemoglobin and is more sensitive for free hemoglobin than for intact red cells. The heme acts as a catalyst to release oxygen from a peroxide in the square, which then oxidizes *o*-tolidine to produce a blue color.

The reactions for glucose and blood may be inhibited by large amounts of ascorbic acid (vitamin C) in the urine. Highly alkaline urines may give false reactions with the protein test, usually false positives. False reactions for ketones may occur in patients taking certain drugs, such as levodopa. (A complete discussion of the "stick" and tablet tests can be found in the publication "Modern Urine Chemistry," published by the Ames Division, Miles Laboratories, Inc., Elkhart, Ind. 46515.)

QUANTITATIVE ESTIMATION OF URINE GLUCOSE

The plasma glucose method detailed on p. 127 can be used for urine glucose determination with the following changes. Dilute the urine according to the scheme:

	Dilution
Trace reaction with Clinitest	1:5
1+ to 2+ reaction	1:10
3+ to 4+ reaction	1:20

Process 0.1 mL of the dilution exactly as for plasma or serum. The glucose result obtained will have to be multiplied by the reciprocal of the dilution factor used—×5, ×10, or ×20. When using 24-hour urine collections,

$$\frac{\text{Glucose in mg/dL}}{1000} \times \frac{\text{24 hour volume in mL}}{100} = \text{g glucose per 24 hours.}$$

If the final color has a brownish tint instead of clear green, the reason is most probably the presence of xylose from a recent xylose absorption test.

If very small glucose levels are to be measured, the specific hexokinase methods described on p. 000 can be used. The same procedures can be used to assay glucose in the urine in the presence of other sugars.

QUANTITATIVE ESTIMATION OF URINE PROTEINS

Indications. To assess the significance of "trace" proteinuria in random specimens; protein excretion in a 24-hour specimen may be normal.

To quantitate protein loss, e.g., in nephrosis, in which 0.5 to 25 or even 30 g per day may be lost.

In suspected instances of so-called orthostatic or postural proteinuria, separate determinations of urine protein excretion in two 12-hour collections, one made with the patient in bed and the other under conditions of full normal activity, can assist the diagnosis.

DETERMINATION OF PROTEIN IN CEREBROSPINAL FLUID AND URINE (Bradford, 1976; modified by Gadd, 1981)

Principle

The dye Coomassie Brilliant Blue G250 has an absorbance peak in acid solution at 470 nm. Protein forms a soluble blue dye-protein complex with an absorbance maximum at 600 nm. The absorbance of this complex can be compared with that obtained from a suitable protein standard solution. The method is linear to about 300 mg/dL.

Procedure

1. Determine the approximate range of the protein level in the sample—CSF or urine—by applying a drop to the protein test square of the routine urinalysis "stick." If the tint of the test square indicates a protein level above 300 mg/dL, dilute the sample with saline to reduce the level below that limit. (This dilution will have to be taken into account in the final calculation.)
2. Set up 100 by 12 mm tubes for test, standard, and blank. Into each, pipette 2.2 mL of reagent. To test add 0.1 mL of sample, to standard 0.1 mL of protein standard, and to blank 0.1 mL of distilled water.
3. Mix by gentle inversion, using Parafilm. Let stand at room temperature for 5 minutes.
4. Read the absorbances of test and standard at 600 nm in a spectrophotometer with a band pass of 10 nm or less, setting zero absorbance with the blank.

Calculation

$$\frac{\text{Test absorbance}}{\text{Standard absorbance}} \times 100 \text{ (standard value)} \times \text{dilution factor} = \text{Protein in mg/dL}$$

(For SI units, multiply the result by 0.01 to get g/L.)

Reagents

Dye Reagent. In a 1 L volumetric flask place 100 mg of Coomassie Brilliant Blue G250 (N.B. not R250). Dissolve *completely* in 25 mL of methanol. Add 100 mL of 89% orthophosphoric acid, swirl to mix; add 20 mL of concentrated hydrochloric acid with constant mixing. Make to volume with distilled water, and filter through a large Whatman No. 1 filter paper. Filtration to remove impurities is *essential.* The reagent is stable at room temperature. It should be reddish-brown in color.

Standard Protein Solution. Dilute an assayed normal human serum to a level of 100 mg/dL, using a saturated aqueous solution of benzoic acid as the diluent. (This acts as a preservative.) Distribute the diluted serum in small aliquots in tightly stoppered plastic tubes and refrigerate. Do not freeze. Remove aliquot from the refrigerator for use: discard after one day on the bench.

Normal Values (Glasser, 1981)—Lumbar Puncture

Newborn	20–170 mg/dL
Premature newborn	65–150 mg/dL
1 to 3 months	20–100 mg/dL
3 to 6 months	15–50 mg/dL
6 months to 60 years	15–45 mg/dL
Above 60 years	30–60 mg/dL
Adult cisternal fluid	12–24 mg/dL
Adult ventricular	5–15 mg/dL

For SI units, multiply the above values by 0.01 to obtain g/L. (The strict SI unit of g/L yields normal values that are inconvenient: a suggested compromise is mg/L, which would require multiplication of the above values by 10.)

Notes

1. The blue protein-dye complex tends to adhere to glass. It is readily soluble in methanol, but possible contamination of later samples may be avoided by the use of disposable plastic cuvettes.
2. The absorbance of the standard should be recorded when it is first used, and the working solution should be replaced when that absorbance falls below 95% of its original value. A typical value is 0.100 in a 10 mm cuvette. The reagent blank has a typical absorbance against water of about 0.30.
3. The grade of Coomassie Brilliant Blue G250 depends on the source. The best grades are about 70% pure, and although they are more costly, they are to be preferred.
4. Urine samples and CSF specimens if turbid should be cleared by centrifugation. The appropriate safety precautions must be taken with CSF to avoid bacterial or viral infection.
5. The upper limit for 24-hour excretion of protein in urine is uncertain, but values up to about 70 mg/24 hours are not clinically significant.

TESTS OF RENAL FUNCTION—METHODOLOGY

Urine Concentration and Dilution Tests

With the availability of rapid and precise instruments for the measurement of osmolality, the measurement of changes in urine specific gravity in response to variations in water intake, e.g., in such procedures as the Mosenthal and Fishberg tests, has been replaced by determinations of urine osmolality or serum/urine osmolality ratios. This approach reflects the control of water reabsorption in the renal tubule by receptors that are sensitive to changes in plasma solute concentrations.

Modified Fishberg Test

This test determines the ability of the kidneys to maintain excretion of solutes under conditions of reduced water intake plus a high protein diet.

Procedure

1. At 6:00 P.M. give the patient a high-protein meal with less than 200 mL of fluid to drink. No further food or drink is allowed until the test is completed.

2. All the urine passed during the night is discarded.

3. The patient empties his bladder completely at 8:00 A.M., 9:00 A.M., and 10:00 A.M., and each specimen is labeled with the time of collection in a separate container. A sample of venous blood is obtained at the same time as one of the specimens.

4. Determine the osmolalities of the serum and all three urine specimens.

Interpretation

Normal. At least one of the urines will have an osmolality of 850 mOsm per kg or greater. The ratio

$$\frac{\text{Urine osmolality}}{\text{Serum osmolality}}$$ should be at least 3.0.

Abnormal. All the urine specimens will have osmolalities below 850 mOsm per kg, and in severe cases of renal disease the values will approach 300 mOsm per kg, with urine/serum osmolality ratio approaching unity.

Serum Urea Nitrogen Determination (Chaney and Marbach, 1962)

Principle

The urea of the serum is hydrolyzed by the specific enzyme urease and is converted to ammonia and carbon dioxide, with carbamic acid as the probable intermediate stage. The reaction is buffered with ethylenediaminetetraacetic acid (EDTA), which also serves to chelate any heavy metal ions that might otherwise inactive the urease. The ammonia is estimated by the century-old Berthelot reaction, in which it reacts with phenol and alkaline hypochlorite to form *p*-quinone chloroimine.

$$\text{OCl} + \text{C}_6\text{H}_5\text{—OH} + \text{NH}_3 \rightarrow \text{O}{=}\text{C}_6\text{H}_4{=}\text{N—Cl}$$

The *p*-quinone imine reacts with another molecule of phenol to form indophenol, which in alkaline solution dissociates to yield a blue indophenol dye.

$$\text{O}{=}\text{C}_6\text{H}_4{=}\text{N—C}_6\text{H}_4\text{—O}$$

The reaction is catalyzed by sodium nitroprusside. The final dilution of the serum sample is so great that precipitation of proteins is unnecessary.

Procedure

1. Into each of three 150 by 16 mm test tubes, marked test, blank, and standard, pipette 0.2 mL of buffered urease preparation. Using a 20 microliter (20 μL) positive-displacement–type pipette, add 20 microliters of serum to the tube marked test and 20 microliters of working standard solution to the standard tube.

2. Incubate all three tubes for 15 minutes at 37°C.

3. Remove the tubes from the water bath. Pipette 1.0 mL phenol color reagent into each tube, mix by gentle lateral shaking, then add 1.0 mL of alkaline hypochlorite reagent, and mix again. It is essential that these reagents be added in the stated order.

4. Return the tubes to the 37°C water bath for 15 minutes.

5. Remove the tubes from the water bath, and add 10 mL distilled water to all tubes. (See Note 1.) Mix by inversion, covering the mouth of the tube with Parafilm, not with the thumb!

6. Read the absorbance of the test and standard solutions at 630 nm in the spectrophotometer, using the blank solution to set zero absorbance. If a filter-type photometer is used, the filter must have its maximum light transmission close to 630 nm to give a linear relationship between absorbance and concentration.

7. If the absorbance reading of the test solution is above 0.8, dilute both the test and the blank solutions with more distilled water until the absorbance of the test solution falls within the range 0.2 to 0.8. Calculate the test value, and then multiply by the appropriate dilution factor.

Calculation

$$\frac{\text{Absorbance of test}}{\text{Absorbance of standard}} \times 20 =$$

mg urea nitrogen per dL serum

$$\frac{\text{Absorbance of test}}{\text{Absorbance of standard}} \times 7.14 =$$

millimol urea nitrogen per liter

Normal Values

Adults: 8 to 18 mg per dL (2.9 to 6.4 mmol/liter).

Adults over the age of 60 years may have values up to 25 mg per dL. Values as low as 5.0 mg per dL may be found during pregnancy. Full-term infants give values in the lower portion of the adult range. Premature infants may show values somewhat higher than the adult normal range.

Reagents

Buffered Urease. Using good-quality commercial urease with an activity of 800 to 1000 Sumner units per gram, such as Sigma Chemical Type II,* dissolve 150 mg urease and 1.0 g EDTA in about 80 mL deionized or double-distilled water. Using a pH meter, adjust the pH to 6.5. Make up to 100 mL. Store in a plastic bottle in the refrigerator. It will remain stable for one month.

Phenol Color Reagent. Dissolve 25.0 g analytic-grade phenol in about 400 mL distilled water in a 500-mL volumetric flask. Dissolve separately in about 50 mL distilled water 125 mg analytic-grade sodium nitroprusside, and add this to the phenol solution. Make to volume with distilled water. Store in a dark brown bottle in the refrigerator. If kept cold and protected from light, this reagent will keep at least two months.

Alkaline Hypochlorite Reagent. (This reagent may be purchased in a concentrated form from a commercial source.) Dissolve 12.5 g analytic-grade sodium hydroxide in about 400 mL distilled water in a 500-mL volumetric flask. Add a volume of commercial bleach (Clorox) that will contain 1.05 g sodium hypochlorite, usually 20.0 mL. Dilute to volume with distilled water, mix, and store as for the phenol color reagent. Its stability is similar.

Working Standard Solution. Dissolve 215 mg pure dry urea in distilled water in a 500-mL volumetric flask, make to volume, and mix. Transfer to a bottle, add a few drops of chloroform as a preservative, shake well, and store in the refrigerator. This standard contains 20 mg urea nitrogen per dL.

*Sigma Chemical Co., St. Louis, Mo. 63118.

Notes

1. The amount of distilled water to be added to the tubes in step 5 of the procedure will be determined by the spectrophotometer used to make the absorbance readings. The reading of the 20 mg per dL standard should be about 0.2 absorbance, permitting direct reading of test values up to about 80 mg per dL without further dilution. If a high result is anticipated on clinical grounds, it saves time to set up a duplicate test using serum previously diluted 1:5 with saline.

2. Plasma can be used if it is obtained with oxalate, citrate, heparin, or EDTA as the anticoagulant. The use of plasma containing ammonium oxalate is not permissible.

3. The final blue color is stable for at least several hours.

4. If the serum sample is very lipemic, prepare a special blank tube by adding the phenol color reagent to the urease before adding the serum. Set the zero absorbance for the particular sample with this blank.

5. For very urgent determinations, the first incubation time can be reduced to five minutes if a temperature of 55 to 56°C is used, but this must be accurately controlled.

6. Plasma or serum preserved with fluoride cannot be used since this inactivates the enzyme. Urea is stable in frozen serum for months.

7. The quantities of reagents prepared should be designed to last for about one month with a normal laboratory work load. There will then be no problems with deterioration.

8. The method is very sensitive, and contamination of the air of the laboratory with ammonia vapor will cause errors. In this regard it should be noted that some commercial floor cleaners contain ammonia.

9. Urease is inactivated by heavy metal ions, and contamination with mercury salts, e.g., from mercuric nitrate solution used in chloride estimations, on glassware or pipettes will cause errors.

10. For the small laboratory making only a few determinations per day, the reputable commercial kits are the most convenient solution.

11. In emergencies the method can be applied unchanged using cerebrospinal fluid. The clinical significance of results is the same as for serum. Care should be taken during measurement of the sample because of the possibility of bacterial infection.

URINE UREA NITROGEN DETERMINATION

The principle and reagents are the same as for serum urea nitrogen determinations. The procedure is modified to accommodate the higher levels of urea nitrogen present and to allow for the appreciable quantities of ammonia present.

1. Dilute the urine sample 1 to 50 with distilled water and use 20 microliters of this as for serum estimation.

2. Set up a special blank solution using 0.2 mL distilled water in place of the urease reagent. Subtract the absorbance of this special blank solution from the absorbance of

the test before comparing the latter with the absorbance of the standard solution.

3. With a 1 to 50 dilution of the urine, the absorbance of the standard solution will be equivalent to a urea nitrogen value of 50 × 20 = 1000 mg per dL.

4. In a fresh urine sample in which there has not been much bacterial activity, the special blank solution will give an absorbance reading corresponding to about 5.0% of the test result. If the sample is not fresh this value may be considerably higher.

Normal Values

Urea nitrogen range in urine: 0.02 to 4 g per dL (0.7 to 143 mmol).

Urea nitrogen 24-hour output: 4.5 to 16.5 g (161 to 589 mmol).

Other Methods for Determination of Urea Nitrogen

In addition to the urease-Berthelot reaction procedure described previously, the following methods have been used:

1. The urea is condensed with diacetyl (produced by the oxidation of diacetyl monoxime in nitric acid solution) in strongly acidic conditions plus heat to form a pink condensation product. The intensity of the color can be enhanced by the inclusion of thiosemicarbazide. This method requires the precise timing of a continuous flow analytical system to yield consistent results.

2. The ammonia formed from the urea by the action of urease can be determined by a reaction with α-ketoglutarate promoted by the enzyme glutamate dehydrogenase.

$$\alpha\text{-Ketoglutarate} + NH_4^+ + NADH \xrightarrow{\text{Glutamate dehydrogenase}} \text{Glutamate} + NAD$$

The decrease in absorbance at 340 nm associated with the oxidation of the NADH coenzyme to NAD is proportional to the urea concentration. This method has been adapted to continuous flow automated analysis by the use of plastic coils having glutamate dehydrogenase immobilized on their inner surface.

3. In a reaction that is particularly suitable for automation in some discrete-type analyzers, the rate of production of ammonia from urea by the action of urease is determined by the increase in electrical conductivity associated with the ammonium ions. The use of a rate measurement permits very short reaction times.

Note

Some confusion occasionally arises from the use of the terms *urea* and *urea nitrogen.* The use of urea nitrogen to represent the complete urea molecule reflects the physiological role of urea as a carrier of waste nitrogen and is common in America. If the use of the SI units system becomes general, concentrations will be reported in millimoles or micromoles, based on urea with a molecular weight of 60. Urea nitrogen constitutes 28/60 of the urea molecule: thus urea nitrogen multiplied by 60/28 (2.14) equals urea, and urea divided by 2.14 equals urea nitrogen.

Estimation of Plasma or Serum Creatinine

Principle

Serum or plasma is diluted with distilled water, and the proteins are precipitated by tungstic acid. Alkaline picrate, with which creatinine forms a red-colored complex, is added to a portion of the protein-free filtrate (Jaffé reaction). The optical density of the red color is proportional to the amount of creatinine in the filtrate. Unfortunately, the Jaffé reaction is not specific for creatinine, but as most of the interfering substances (mainly ergothionine and glutathione) are confined to the cells, a more accurate measure of the creatinine is obtained using serum or plasma than would be the case if whole blood were used.

Procedure

1. In a clean, dry centrifuge tube place:

Plasma or serum	**2.0 mL**
Distilled water	**2.0 mL**
10% w/v sodium tungstate solution	**1.0 mL**
2/3 *N*-sulfuric acid	**1.0 mL**

Mix thoroughly by inversion (do not shake), and, after a few minutes, centrifuge at about 2500 rpm for five minutes.

2. In clean, dry test tubes place:

	Test	*Standard 1*	*Standard 2*	*Blank*
Supernatant fluid from (1)	3.0 mL	Nil	Nil	Nil
Standard creatinine solution	Nil	1.0 mL	3.0 mL	Nil
Distilled water	Nil	2.0 mL	Nil	3.0 mL
Alkaline picrate solution	1.5 mL	1.5 mL	1.5 mL	1.5 mL

Mix thoroughly and leave at room temperature for 10 minutes.

3. Read the absorbances of the test and standard solutions in a photoelectric colorimeter using a green filter or in a spectrophotometer at 520 nm, setting the zero optical density with the blank solution.

Calculation

Take the standard reading that is nearest the test.

Using Standard 1

$$\frac{\text{Test reading}}{\text{Standard reading}} \times 0.01 \text{ mg} \times \frac{100 \text{ mL}}{1.0 \text{ mL}} = \text{mg creatinine per 100 mL}$$

$$\frac{\text{Test reading}}{\text{Standard reading}} \times 1.0 \text{ mg} = \text{mg creatinine per 100 mL}$$

Using Standard 2

$$\frac{\text{Test reading}}{\text{Standard reading}} \times 0.03 \text{ mg} \times \frac{100 \text{ mL}}{1.0 \text{ mL}} = \text{mg creatinine per 100 mL}$$

$$\frac{\text{Test reading}}{\text{Standard reading}} \times 3.0 \text{ mg} = \text{mg creatinine per 100 mL}$$

Normal Values

0.6 to 1.4 mg per 100 mL of plasma or serum (0.05 to 0.12 mmol per liter).

Reagents

Saturated Picric Acid Solution. Dry picric acid is explosive and must be kept damp at all times. If a high-grade picric acid is used, purification is unnecessary. A saturated solution is best prepared by placing an excess of picric acid in an amber glass bottle containing distilled water, shaking occasionally. After a few days the solution may be decanted into another amber glass bottle. A small amount of the solid chemical should be present to keep the solution saturated.

10% w/v Sodium Hydroxide Solution in Distilled Water. Alkaline Picrate Solution. Prepare just before use as follows: To 10 mL of saturated picric acid solution add 2.0 mL of 10% w/v sodium hydroxide solution and mix. The color of the alkaline picrate should not be more than twice as deep as the color of the picric acid solution alone.

Stock Standard Creatinine Solution. Dissolve 1.602 g of pure creatinine zinc chloride or 1.0 g of pure creatinine in, and make the volume up to 1 liter with, N/10 hydrochloric acid.

Standard Creatinine Solution. Dilute 1.0 mL of the stock standard solution to 100 mL with distilled water. This solution should be renewed each week.

Note. If for a particular purpose the interference from noncreatinine chromogens has to be excluded, the adsorption method can be used. The creatinine from a protein-free filtrate is adsorbed onto Lloyd's reagent—a hydrated aluminum silicate—and then eluted and determined by the picric acid reaction.

ESTIMATION OF URINE CREATININE

Urine creatinine may be estimated by the method for serum or plasma given on page 219 by applying the following modifications:

1. Collect a 24-hour urine sample.

2. Mix the urine thoroughly and measure the total volume.

3. Make a 1 in 100 dilution of the urine with distilled water.

4. Substitute 3.0 mL of the urine dilution for the 3.0 mL of plasma protein-free filtrate in step 2 of the method on page 219.

5. Determine the absorbances of the test and standard solutions as instructed in step 3 of the method.

Calculation

Take the standard reading that is nearest the test.

Using Standard 1

$$\frac{\text{Test reading}}{\text{Standard reading}} \times \frac{0.01}{0.03} \times \frac{\text{24-hr urine volume in mL}}{1000}$$

= g creatinine excreted in 24 hours. (Multiply by 8.85 for mmol.)

Using Standard 2

$$\frac{\text{Test reading}}{\text{Standard reading}} \times \frac{0.03}{0.03} \times \frac{\text{24-hr urine volume in mL}}{1000}$$

= g creatinine excreted in 24 hours. (Multiply by 8.85 for mmol.)

Normal Values

0.4 to 1.8 g per 24 hours (3.5 to 15.9 mmol).

Note. Although manual procedures for serum and urine creatinine are given here, more precise results are obtained by automated methods using a continuous flow–type automatic analyzer, in which the variables inherent in the process can be adequately controlled. A recent development in the assay of creatinine is the measurement of the rate of formation of the creatinine-picrate complex. In one discrete-type automated analyzer,* the rate of reaction is measured at a time when the slow nonspecific reaction has not commenced and a fast nonspecific reaction has gone to completion. In this way the method achieves better specificity for creatinine.

CREATININE CLEARANCE

If the plasma creatinine level is within the normal range, the calculation of the creatinine clearance is a reasonably accurate method of estimating the glomerular filtration rate, i.e, the volume of plasma actually filtered by the glomeruli per minute. When the plasma creatinine level is raised, either in renal disease or by oral administration of creatinine, some of the creatinine is removed from the plasma by tubular excretion. It is not correct, therefore, to compare the glomerular filtration rate, as determined by the creatinine clearance, of a patient with advanced renal disease with normal values based on much lower plasma creatinine levels. Nevertheless, the determination of creatinine clearance is a useful procedure in following the course of progressive renal disease, provided that the results are interpreted in a comparative rather than an absolute fashion.

Procedure

1. The patient is placed on a diet from which meat, tea, and coffee are excluded during the period of urine collection, which should be 24 hours for the best accuracy and in any case not less than eight hours. The patient's water intake should be maintained to ensure a urine output of at least 1.0 mL per minute. Diuretic drugs should be discontinued.

2. The blood sample for creatinine estimation should be taken approximately halfway through the urine collection period, although this is not critical.

3. Determine the urine total creatinine, plasma or serum creatinine, total urine output, and body surface area. (The last value may be determined by the formula on p. 221.)

Calculation

If U = Urine creatinine in mg per dL = 96 mg/dL
V = Urine output in 24 hours = 2160 mL
P = Plasma or serum creatinine in mg per dL = 1.2 mg/dL
A = Body surface area in square meters = 1.73 m^2

*Beckman ASTRA analyzer, Beckman Instruments, Inc., Fullerton, Calif. 92634 and Toronto, Ont. M8Z 2G6.

The creatinine clearance in mL per minute is given by

$$\frac{V}{1440} \times \frac{U}{P} \times \frac{1.73}{A} \quad \text{(1440 is the number of minutes in 24 hours.)}$$

$$= \frac{2160}{1440} \times \frac{96}{1.2} \times \frac{1.73}{1.73} \quad \text{(assuming a body surface area of 1.73 m}^2\text{)}$$

$$= 120 \text{ mL per minute}$$

Normal Range

The normal range is 70 to 157 mL per minute, with a mean value of 120 mL per minute.

Note. As the normal values are based on average adult size (body surface area = 1.73 m^2), it is necessary to correct the values for creatinine clearance for body surface area. The results are multiplied by the factor $\frac{1.73}{\text{Surface area}}$.

Calculation of Body Surface Area. Body surface area is calculated as follows, using the Dubois formula

$$A = H^{0.725} \times W^{0.425} \times 71.84$$

where A = body surface area in cm^2
H = height in cm
W = weight in kg

For example, calculation of the body surface area of a person weighing 60 kg who is 150 cm in height:

1. $A = 150^{0.725} \times 60^{0.425} \times 71.84$
2. $\log A = (0.725 \times \log 150) + (0.425 \times \log 60) + \log 71.84$
3. $\log A = (0.725 \times 2.1761) + (0.425 \times 1.7782) + 1.8563$
4. $\log A = (1.5777 + 0.7557) + (1.8563)$
5. $\log A = 4.1897$
6. A = antilog of 4.1897
7. A = 15,470 cm^2, or 15,470/10,000 m^2 = 1.547 m^2

Determination of Uric Acid

The following are representative of currently used methods for the assay of uric acid in serum and urine.

1. Uric acid will reduce the phosphotungstate ion to tungsten blue in mildly alkaline conditions: the absorbance of the blue product can be compared with that obtained from suitable uric acid standard solutions. The method is simple and easily automatable, but nonspecific.

2. Uric acid is oxidized to allantoin by the specific enzyme uricase. Uric acid has an absorbance peak at 293 nm, which disappears when oxidation to allantoin is complete. Thus the decrease in absorbance at 293 nm is directly proportional to the original level of uric acid. The method is inconvenient for batches because of the difficulty of automation involving absorbance measurements at 293 nm in the ultraviolet range.

3. In the oxidation of uric acid by uricase one of the products is hydrogen peroxide:

$$\text{Uric acid} + 2H_2O + O_2 \xrightarrow{\text{Uricase}} \text{Allantoin} + CO_2 + H_2O_2$$

The peroxide is reacted with the enzyme catalase and methanol to form formaldehyde, which in turn reacts with acetylacetone and ammonium ion to produce a yellow-colored derivative, 3,5-diacetyl-1, 4-dihydrolutidine, the absorbance of which can be determined at 410 nm (Kageyama, 1971). The procedure combines the specificity of uricase with the convenience of a colorimetric reaction, making it suitable for automation.

4. In a variant of the previous method, the hydrogen peroxide is determined by its ability to couple 2,4-dichlorophenol and 4-aminophenazone in the presence of the enzyme peroxidase, forming the complex chromogen 4-*N*-(3,5-dichloro-1,2-benzoquinone-monoimino)-phenazone, with an absorbance peak at 508 nm.

5. For a manual procedure using simple stable reagents (no enzymes), the method of Jung and Parekh, as modified for manual procedures by Kaplan and Szabo, is described below.

Serum Uric Acid Determination (Jung and Parekh, 1970; Kaplan and Szabo, 1979)

Principle

After destruction of the interfering nonurate chromogen ascorbic acid by treatment with trisodium phosphate, the proteins of the serum are precipitated with phosphotungstic acid and removed by centrifugation. Addition of an alkaline carbonate-urea-triethanolamine reagent provides the conditions necessary for reduction of the phosphotungstate by the uric acid to produce a blue complex of uncertain composition, the absorbance of which at 700 nm can be compared with that produced by suitable standards.

Procedure

1. In 100 by 13 mm test tubes labeled test, control, blank, and standard pipette with a positive-displacement piston-type pipettor 0.2 mL of patient's serum, control serum, distilled water, and working standard, respectively.

2. To each tube add 0.2 mL of the trisodium phosphate reagent; mix by gentle lateral shaking. Allow to stand for five minutes.

3. To each tube add 0.6 mL of phosphotungstic acid; mix well on a vortex mixer. Allow to stand two to five minutes to ensure complete precipitation of proteins. Centrifuge for five minutes at 2800 rpm.

4. Into correspondingly labeled spectrophotometer tubes (12 or 13 mm light path) or 10 mm cuvettes transfer 0.5 mL of the clear supernatant.

5. To each tube or cuvette add 0.2 mL of phosphotungstic acid and 1.5 mL of the carbonate-urea-triethanolamine reagent. Mix by inversion, using Parafilm. Let stand at room temperature for 30 minutes.

6. Setting zero absorbance with the blank, read the absorbances of test, control, and standard at 700 nm.

Calculation

$$\frac{\text{Test absorbance}}{\text{Standard absorbance}} \times 5.0 = \text{Uric acid in mg/dL}$$

For SI units mg/dL × 0.06 = mmol/L, or × 59.5 = μmol/L. The latter conversion yields numerical values that are more suitable for reporting.

Normal Values

Males: 3.5 to 7.5 mg/dL (210 to 445 μmol/L).
Females: 2.5 to 6.5 mg/dL (150 to 390 μmol/L).

Reagents

Trisodium Phosphate. Dissolve 1.0 g trisodium phosphate $Na_3PO_4 \cdot 12H_2O$ in, and make up to 100 mL with, distilled water.

Phosphotungstic Acid. Dissolve 50.0 g of molybdenum-free sodium tungstate $Na_2WO_4 \cdot 2H_2O$ (sometimes called "sodium tungstate according to Folin") in 350 mL of distilled water. Add 20.0 mL of 85% orthophosphoric acid H_3PO_4 and reflux gently under a vertical condenser whose rate of flow of cooling water should be adjusted to prevent appreciable loss of fluid from the reflux flask. Reflux for two hours. Add 1 drop of bromine (Use care! Hazardous reagent!), cool to room temperature, and make up to 1 liter with distilled water; mix well.

Carbonate-urea-triethanolamine Reagent. Dissolve 100 g anhydrous sodium carbonate Na_2CO_3, 200 g urea $CO(NH_2)_2$, and 50 g triethanolamine in, and make up to 1 liter with, distilled water.

Stock Uric Acid Standard. In a water bath at about 50 to 55°C dissolve 100 mg lithium carbonate Li_2CO_3 in about 100 mL distilled water in a 200 mL volumetric flask. When this is completely dissolved, add 200.0 mg uric acid and swirl until all is dissolved. Add 4.0 mL of strong formaldehyde (37 to 40% w/v); swirl to mix. Add 1.0 mL of glacial acetic acid slowly with constant swirling. Finally, make up to volume with distilled water; mix.

Working Uric Acid Standard. Make freshly just before use by diluting 5.0 mL of stock up to 100 mL with distilled water. Discard after use.

Notes

1. For improved accuracy with abnormal patient values (in most cases pathological values are elevations), use commercial control sera with "weighed in" values* and plot a calibration curve with uric acid values on the ordinate and absorbances on the abscissa.
2. Turbidity is usually due to precipitation of phosphotungstate if the pH rises above about 10.5: since the pH-controlling agent is the triethanolamine, make that reagent freshly.
3. For assay of urine uric acid, collect a 24-hour urine output with 10 mL of 2 molar sodium hydroxide in the bottle to prevent precipitation of uric acid. Dilute the well-mixed urine with distilled water 1 in 10 and 1 in 20 for analysis, multiplying the result by the reciprocal of the dilution. Normal 24-hour uric acid excretion depends to some extent on diet: typically it is 250 to 750 mg (1.49 to 4.46 mmol).

MELANIN

This substance is the main pigment of the hair and skin and is also found in the choroid layer of the eye. It is a mixture of oxidation products of tyrosine and 3,4-dihydroxyphenylalanine, which are subsequently polymerized to yellow, brown, and black pigments. In patients with tumors arising from the melanin-producing cells, the melanomas, the melanin may be excreted in the urine in large amounts (in the form of a colorless chromogen, melanogen), and its presence is indicative of metastasis of the tumor to the liver or other organ.

*Calibrates," General Diagnostics Division, Warner-Lambert Co., Morris Plains, N.J. 07950 and Scarborough, Ont. M1K 5C9.

Screening Tests

1. Allow the urine sample to stand exposed to the air undisturbed for up to 24 hours. If melanogen is present it will be slowly oxidized to melanin by the air, and the urine will turn dark brown or black from the top downward. Homogentisic acid gives the same effect, but the darkening of melanogen is not accelerated appreciably by alkali.
2. To 5.0 mL urine add 1.0 mL of a 10% w/v solution of ferric chloride in 10% v/v hydrochloric acid. If melanogen is present the urine turns dark brown or black.

Thormahlen's Test

1. Prepare a fresh solution of sodium nitroprusside by shaking a few small crystals in 10 mL distilled water.
2. To 5.0 mL fresh urine add 0.2 mL of sodium nitroprusside solution and 0.5 mL of 40% w/v sodium hydroxide. Mix well.
3. Add 3.0 to 5.0 mL 33% v/v acetic acid and mix again.
4. A dark green or blue color indicates the presence of melanogen. A normal urine should be run as control.

Blackberg and Wanger's Test

1. Evaporate a 24-hour urine specimen to one-fourth its volume.
2. For each 100 mL of concentrate, add 1.0 g potassium persulfate.
3. Mix; let stand two hours.
4. Add an equal volume of methyl alcohol; mix; allow the precipitate to settle.
5. Filter off the precipitate. Wash the precipitate on the filter paper with distilled water until no more color is removed; wash with methyl alcohol and, finally, with ether.
6. A brown to black precipitate remaining on the filter paper which is soluble in 5% w/v sodium hydroxide may be presumed to be melanin.

MYOGLOBIN

Myoglobin (myohemoglobin, muscle hemoglobin) probably functions as a short-term oxygen storage device in the muscles. Because of its relatively small molecular weight (17,500, about one-quarter that of hemoglobin), it is readily excreted in the urine when released into the plasma after muscle destruction as a result of severe crush injuries, dermatomyositis, acute idiopathic rhabdomyolysis of children, or Haff disease (caused by ingestion of fish poisoned by cellulose factory wastes).

Myoglobin imparts a red-brown color to the urine, which does not usually contain red blood cells but may contain brown-stained casts and granules; it gives a positive benzidine reaction. Identification of myohemoglobin and its differentiation from hemoglobin in urine can be done by the following procedures:

Spectroscopic Examination

Examine a 1-inch depth of urine with the reversion spectroscope. (Direct vision instruments do not have sufficient precision). Myoglobin has absorption bands at 582 and 543 nm; oxyhemoglobin, at 577 and 540 nm.

"Salting Out" Test

1. To 1.0 mL urine add 3.0 mL of 3% w/v sulfosalicylic acid; mix and filter. If the pigment is precipitated and remains on the filter paper, and the filtrate is the normal urine color, the pigment is protein in nature. If the filtrate is abnormal in color, the pigment is nonprotein.

2. If a protein pigment is detected in step 1, add 2.8 g solid ammonium sulfate to 5.0 mL urine, mix well to dissolve, and filter. If the protein pigment is myoglobin, it is not "salted out" and will appear as a dark brown color in the filtrate; if hemoglobin is present, it will be precipitated and remain on the filter paper.

Fresh urine at pH 7.0 to 7.5 must be used.

Electrophoresis

When a concentrate of the urine prepared by dialysis is electrophoresed on cellulose acetate by the same technique as is used for serum proteins and a suspension of commercial occult blood testing tablets in water is used as the detection agent, myoglobin will show a faster moving band closer to the cathode than will hemoglobin.

The most sensitive test for myoglobin involves an immunochemical reaction with specific antiserum. Myoglobin detection in serum and urine down to a level of 0.5 μg per mL is achieved; spectroscopic examination requires at least 20 times this amount for a positive result.

IDENTIFICATION OF REDUCING SUBSTANCES IN URINE

Definition

Reducing substances are those compounds that reduce cupric salts in hot solutions, as in Benedict's test. In the urine a number of substances may do this:

Carbohydrates	Noncarbohydrates
Glucose	Glucuronides*
Lactose	Uric acid, urates
Fructose	Phenols
Galactose	Homogentisic acid
Pentose	Ascorbic acid
	Salicyluric acid

Also, urines of patients receiving large doses of penicillin, streptomycin, oxytetracycline, or para-aminosulfones, or of those who have had intravenous dextrans or polyvinylpyrrolidone, may reduce cupric salts.

Normal urine may contain 1.0 to 1.5 g reducing substances per 24 hours, and about one-third of this amount is of carbohydrate origin. Normally, only minute traces of glucose are present in the urine, but greater amounts may occur following ingestion of large quantities of carbohydrates (alimentary glycosuria) and in those persons who have renal glycosuria, a condition that has an incidence of only 1 per 300 cases of melituria and that is the result of a defect in the reabsorption of glucose by the proximal part of the renal tubules. Renal glycosuria is inherited as an autosomal dominant trait and is characterized by the excretion of large amounts of glucose in the urine independent of meals and of the blood glucose level, which is normal, as is the glucose tolerance test. A significant proportion (some claim up to 40%) of otherwise normal women may show glycosuria in the latter half of pregnancy; this has been claimed to be a result of lowering of the renal threshold, but the effects of pregnancy hormone levels on plasma glucose concentrations may be even more important.

*Glucuronides are compounds of glucuronic acid (a derivative of glucose) with an endogenous or exogenous metabolite.

IDENTIFICATION TESTS

The classical methods for identification of sugars—osazone formation, fermentation tests—are not reliable when the amounts of sugars present are small. The tests described below should be regarded largely as preliminary to the chromatographic procedure.

Glucosuria

The most convenient and sensitive test for glucosuria is the enzymatic stick test, in which glucose oxidase in the paper strip promotes the oxidation of glucose by atmospheric oxygen to gluconic acid with the formation of hydrogen peroxide. A peroxidase in the strip catalyzes the transfer of oxygen from the peroxide to an oxygen acceptor, e.g., potassium iodide, to form a brown color. The reaction is both sensitive and specific. The only common interference is from ascorbic acid, which produces false negatives. A positive result can be confirmed by running an assay using the hexokinase method.

Fructosuria

This rare condition (incidence about 1 in 120,000) is inherited as an autosomal recessive character, siblings but not parents being affected. There appears to be an enzymic block in the normal conversion of fructose to glucose in the liver, and this results in excretion of fructose and fructosemia following an oral dose of fructose.

Selivanoff's Test for Fructose

1. In a test tube place 0.5 mL urine and 5.0 mL Selivanoff's reagent (0.05% w/v resorcinol in 33% w/v hydrochloric acid). At the same time set up two controls, one using 0.5 mL normal urine and 5.0 mL reagent, and the other normal urine to which 0.1% fructose has been added.

2. Bring all three tubes just to a boil. It is important that further heating beyond this point be avoided. The presence of fructose is indicated by a red color, and an alcohol-soluble red precipitate may form.

Lactosuria

This tends to occur in pregnant women in the last few days of pregnancy and also during lactation. (Glycosuria is more common in pregnant women than is lactosuria.) It is readily differentiated from glucose by the positive glucose oxidase reaction given by glucose and by chromatography, if necessary (see further below).

Pentosuria

The five-carbon sugars, *l*-arabinose and *l*-xylose may be excreted by normal persons after they have eaten large quantities of berries and fruits. In addition, a rare (incidence 1 in 50,000, or less) "essential pentosuria" exists (mainly among Russian Jews), in which *l*-xylulose is constantly excreted without any ill effects.

Identification of Pentoses

Bial's Test for Pentoses

1. In a test tube place 5.0 mL Bial's reagent (0.4 g pure orcinol dissolved in 200 mL pure concentrated hydrochloric

acid; add 0.5 mL of 10% w/v ferric chloride solution) and 0.5 mL urine.

2. Set up two controls, one with normal urine and one with normal urine to which 0.1% pentose (arabinose or xylose) has been added.

3. Mix well and bring *just* to a boil. Then let stand 5 to 20 minutes. Pentoses give a green color and, if present in large amounts, a bluish-green precipitate. The color can be extracted by shaking with amyl alcohol.

4. If a mixture of glucose and pentose is suspected, perform Bial's test after fermentation with yeast.

Test for Essential Pentosuria

l-Xyloketose (*l*-xylulose) has the ability to reduce Benedict's solution at low temperature. Mix 1.0 mL urine with 5.0 mL Benedict's qualitative reagent and place for 10 minutes in the water bath at 55°C. A yellow precipitate under these conditions is very suggestive of xyloketose.

Galactosuria

Small amounts of galactose may be present in the urine in the latter part of pregnancy and during lactation. Galactose assumes great importance, however, in galactosemia, which is a fairly rare condition inherited as a recessive character (see pp. 8 and 9). In addition to chromatographic identification of galactose in the urine, the primary metabolic defect of deficiency of the enzyme galactose-1-phosphate uridyl transferase can be detected by either an assay method or a qualitative blood spot test.

Other Reducing Substances

If glucose, fructose, lactose, pentoses, and galactose have all been excluded, a slight reduction in Benedict's test is most probably due to glucuronides, uric acid, urates (large amounts), or salicyluric acid. The latter, also known as orthohydroxyhippuric acid, is one of the major forms in which salicylates and acetylsalicylic acid are excreted in the urine (the other being salicyl glucuronide, with smaller amounts excreted as free salicylates). Salicylates are differentiated from other reducing substances by the ferric chloride test.

Because of their unsaturated nature, phenols cause reduction of Benedict's reagent. Phenoluria occurs in cases of phenol poisoning (e.g., carbolic acid) and after excessive exposure to benzene vapor. Urines containing phenols tend to blacken on standing and give a purple color with ferric chloride.

Chromatographic Identification of Reducing Substances in Urine

The chemical tests for reducing substances in urine lack the sensitivity to detect amounts of sugars below about 0.10%. Glucose can be identified by the sensitive and quite specific glucose oxidase test, commercially available as a stick test, but this will not demonstrate if a mixture of sugars is present. In some cases, such as the detection of galactose in urine, the information is of considerable clinical importance. Chromatography pro-

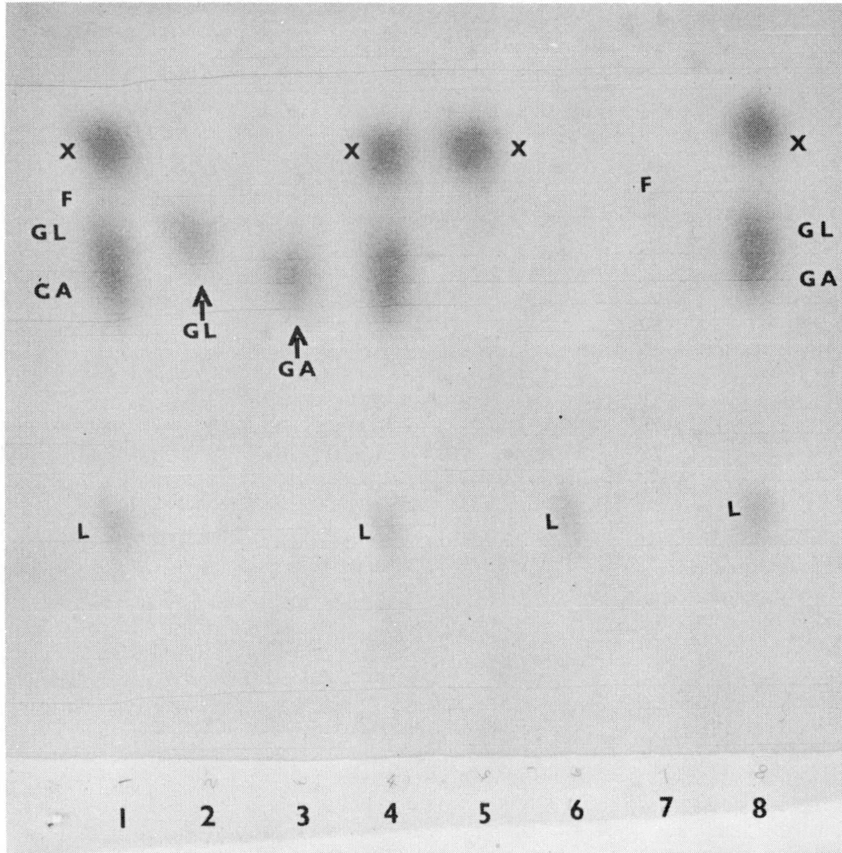

Figure 9–17 Chromatographic separation of sugars on Whatman 3 MM paper, using the "punch disc" technique. Developing solvent—isopropanol/water 16:4. Detecting reagent—aniline phthalate. *X,* xylose; *F,* fructose—this spot is readily seen only with ultraviolet light; *GL,* glucose; *GA,* galactose; *L,* lactose. Col. 1: xylose, glucose, galactose, lactose, and fructose; Col. 2: glucose; Col. 3: galactose; Col. 4: as for col. 1; col. 5: xylose; Col. 6: lactose; Col. 7: fructose; Col. 8: as for Col. 1. The developing solvent was allowed to run 16 hours in order to separate glucose and galactose. The separation was made by the ascending technique in the Gelman chromatographic tank.

vides the necessary combination of sensitivity and identification, provided that close attention is paid to details of technique and the use of controls. For full details see the third edition of this text or standard texts on paper or thin-layer chromatography. Briefly, aliquots of urine and standard solutions of glucose, galactose, xylose, lactose, and fructose are dried as small spots on Whatman 3MM paper and developed with a solvent mixture of four volumes of isopropanol and one volume of distilled water. The separated sugars are located on the dried chromatogram with a freshly made solution containing 1.66 g phthalic acid in 100 mL acetone to which 0.9 mL of pure aniline is added. The sugars appear as brown-to-yellow spots, some of which fluoresce in long-wavelength UV light, after heating at 100°C for 10 to 15 minutes (Fig. 9–17).

CALCULI

Calculi may be divided into four groups:

1. *Urinary Calculi.* These are formed in the renal pelvis or bladder. They may be
   a. Simple, containing one compound.
   b. Mixed, containing two or more compounds.
   c. Foreign body, introduced into the body from outside but forming the nucleus of a true calculus.

The common constituents are calcium oxalate, uric acid and urates, calcium and magnesium phosphates, and magnesium ammonium phosphate; calcium carbonate, cystine, and xanthine are rarely found.

2. *Salivary and Pancreatic Calculi.* These are rare and usually composed of calcium carbonate, calcium phosphate, or mixtures thereof. They are analyzed in the same manner as urinary calculi.
3. *Gallstones.* These are formed in the gallbladder and may be of three types:
   a. Cholesterol stones, usually light in color and smooth.
   b. Bile pigment stones, usually small, very dark, and rough.
   c. Mixtures of cholesterol and pigment plus calcium.

These are rarely analyzed, except as will be noted.

4. *Fecal Concretions.* These are rare in man and may be composed of phosphates deposited around small foreign bodies or of hardened organic material. On rare occasions, they may require analysis to exclude the presence of a gallstone.

Qualitative Analysis of Calculi (Renal) (Simmons and Gentzkow, 1944, Modified)

Reagents

Concentrated Hydrochloric Acid.

Sodium Acetate. Saturated aqueous solution as used in the detection of porphobilinogen in urine.

Ammonium Oxalate. 4.0% w/v aqueous solution.

Concentrated Nitric Acid.

Ammonium Nitrate. 50.0% w/v aqueous solution.

Ammonium Molybdate. Dilute the ammonium molybdate reagent used for the estimation of inorganic phosphate with an equal volume of distilled water.

Phenol Color Reagent and Alkali Hypochlorite Reagent. As used in the estimation of urea nitrogen.

Sodium Carbonate. 14.0% w/v aqueous solution.

Phosphotungstic Acid Reagent. As used in the estimation of uric acid.

Concentrated Ammonia Solution.

Sodium Cyanide. 5.0 w/v aqueous solution.

Sodium Nitroprusside. Dissolve a few small crystals in 5.0 mL distilled water just before use.

Titan Yellow. 0.05% w/v aqueous solution. Make fresh by 1 in 10 dilution of a 0.5% aqueous stock titan yellow solution.

Sodium Hydroxide. 20.0% w/v aqueous solution.

Procedure

The analysis should be carried out in a systematic manner, especially if the limited amount of material does not permit repeat tests.

1. Wash the calculus free of any adherent blood clot or fibrin with distilled water, dry, and describe shape, color, texture of surface, hardness and brittleness, size in millimeters, and weight in milligrams. Oxalate calculi are usually very hard and often show an irregular, crystalline, or faceted surface. Uric acid calculi are moderately hard; phosphate calculi are soft, even friable. Cystine calculi have a soft, waxy texture. A very large calculus of the "staghorn" variety may show distinct differentiation in its external appearance, and separate analyses may have to be done on the different regions.

2. If the calculus is 5 mg or less, powder the whole stone in a small agate or mullite mortar. Small, very hard calculi should be wrapped in a piece of filter paper before the initial crushing to prevent loss by spallation. Larger calculi should be cut with a sharp knife or fine hacksaw blade and a portion crushed. Even when the material is limited in quantity, a small portion should be reserved for checking unusual findings such as cystine or xanthine.

3. Place 5 to 10 mg of the powdered stone in a small (100 by 13 mm) test tube. Add 0.25 mL concentrated HCl slowly. *Vigorous* foaming indicates the presence of *carbonate*. Add 0.7 mL water, mix, and boil to dissolve. Cool; if there is a large amount of undissolved material, centrifuge and use the supernatant for the tests. If the insoluble matter is granular, apply the test for uric acid (see step 8). Transfer 0.2 mL portions after cooling to each of three 100 by 13 mm Pyrex test tubes.

4. (a) Hold one of the small test tubes with the calculus solution at an angle, and carefully run 1.0 mL of saturated sodium acetate solution down the side to form a layer under the extract. Inspect the junction of the two layers under a bright light against a dark background after a gentle tap to produce very slight intermixing. Turbidity at the junction indicates *calcium oxalate*. Cystine may also give the reaction, but the original texture of the stone should have raised this possibility.

(b) Mix the test tube well, allow to stand 10 minutes, and centrifuge. Transfer the supernatant to another small test tube, mix with another portion—0.2 mL—of saturated sodium acetate. Recentrifuge any further precipitate, and test the supernatant with sodium acetate solution again. This process must be repeated until no further precipitation occurs.

(c) Using a Pasteur pipette, carefully layer 0.3 to 0.5 mL of ammonium oxalate reagent on top of the clear solution

from step b. Observe the junction of the fluids as in step a. Turbidity indicates the presence of *calcium combined with an anion other than oxalate.*

5. To another aliquot of extract prepared in step 3, add concentrated ammonia water until the reaction is alkaline as shown by wide range pH paper. A precipitate may form. Add several drops of concentrated nitric acid, which should dissolve the precipitate. Add 2 drops of ammonium nitrate solution, and slightly more than an equal volume of ammonium molybdate reagent. Mix, bring briefly to the boil, and allow to cool. A bright lemon yellow precipitate indicates *phosphates*. This is a sensitive test, and pale yellow tints in the cool solution without any precipitate are usually not significant unless very small amounts of material are being analyzed.

6. To the third aliquot from step 3 add 1 drop of titan yellow solution and 0.5 mL of 20% NaOH. In the presence of *magnesium,* a red precipitate or a definite red color will be produced. Brownish colors are not significant.

7. To about 20 mg of powdered calculus in a large test tube add 3.0 mL distilled water and agitate very vigorously with a vortex mixer. Add 2.0 mL of alkaline phenate, mix vigorously again, then add 2.0 mL of alkaline hypochlorite. (These are the Berthelot reagents as used for the manual estimation of urea nitrogen.) Mix well; place tube in the 37°C water bath for 15 minutes. A definite royal blue color indicates the presence of ammonium ion.

8. Using the end of a small test tube as a pestle, grind a small amount of the original powdered stone with 2 drops of 14.0% sodium carbonate solution. The process can be done in a small porcelain basin, and must be thorough. Add 2 drops phosphotungstic acid reagent. In the presence of *uric acid* or *urates* an intense blue color will be produced.

9. Mix on a porcelain spot plate or small porcelain basin a few milligrams of the original crushed stone, 1 drop of concentrated ammonia water, and 1 drop of 5.0% sodium cyanide solution. Let stand 5 minutes and mix in 2 drops of fresh sodium nitroprusside. A deep magenta red color indicates *cystine*. This should be confirmed by dissolving some of the powdered stone in strong ammonia water, spreading this on a microscope slide, and allowing the ammonia to evaporate spontaneously in the fume hood. If cystine is present the typical regular hexagonal crystals can be seen microscopically.

For each cation detected—calcium, ammonium, or magnesium—a corresponding anion should be found—oxalate, phosphate, or carbonate. If ammonium ion is found, it should be accompanied by magnesium; if not, the analysis should be checked. Carbonate calculi are rare. The most usual combinations are calcium oxalate, ammonium magnesium phosphate, calcium phosphate, and uric acid. The very rare xanthine calculus dissolves in nitric acid, and if evaporated to dryness on a porcelain basin it leaves a yellow residue which becomes orange with alkali and turns red on warming.

CHAPTER 9—REVIEW QUESTIONS

1. A fresh urine sample from a pregnant woman shows a deep yellow color in Benedict's test. What substances might be responsible for the reaction and how may the particular compound present be identified?

2. If the 24-hour urine volume is 2160 mL, the urine creatinine 96 mg per dL, serum creatinine, 1.2 mg/dL, and body surface area 1.73 square meters, calculate the corrected creatinine clearance.

3. List the types of cells that might be seen in the microscopic examination of a centrifuged urine. *Note:* Include *all* types of cells.

4. Summarize the changes in composition of the glomerular filtrate as it travels down the nephron tubule.

5. Explain why plasma or serum urea nitrogen, creatinine, and uric acid are measured in the investigation of possible renal disease. Give the chemical principles of each method.

10

THE GASTROINTESTINAL TRACT: LIVER AND BILIARY SYSTEM

ANATOMY OF THE GASTROINTESTINAL TRACT (Fig. 10–1)

The purpose of digestion is to convert the large, complex molecules of the food into small, simple ones that can be absorbed and utilized by the body. In the case of proteins it also serves to prevent antigenic material from entering the system. Digestion proceeds in two main stages: (1) mechanical fragmentation of the food, so that the largest possible surface may be presented for (2) enzymatic breakdown, in which a large variety of specific enzymes attack the food molecules and break them down by hydrolysis, depolymerization, and so forth, to a size that can be readily absorbed through the intestinal wall. This latter process is also partly enzymatic. After absorption through the intestinal wall the products of digestion enter the blood stream in the radicles of the portal vein, by which they are carried to the liver for further metabolism.

MOUTH

Here the food is comminuted by the action of the teeth and tongue, mixed with saliva from the salivary glands, and formed into boluses of suitable size for swallowing. The saliva contains the enzyme *amylase,* which in the presence of chloride ions attacks the large starch molecule, which is composed of glucose molecules polymerized into branching chains. If this process were allowed to proceed to completion, amylase would break the starch down to the disaccharide maltose, but the action of amylase is stopped by the acid of the stomach. Saliva also serves to lubricate the food bolus and thus facilitates swallowing.

ESOPHAGUS

Each bolus of food is propelled down the esophagus by rhythmic, involuntary action (peristalsis) of the smooth muscle in the wall of the esophagus. Peristalsis is the type of movement characteristic of the entire gastrointestinal (GI) tract and consists of relaxation of the segment of gut in front of, together with contraction (constriction) of the segment immediately behind, the food or waste mass. All parts of the GI tract have two layers of muscle—an inner circular layer (for constriction) and an outer longitudinal layer (for propulsion).

STOMACH

This is a highly distensible sac into which the esophagus opens. It is lined by a loose, thick mucosa arranged in a pleatlike pattern of low ridges or folds. This mucosa contains a very large number of cells of three main types:

1. Chief or peptic cells, producing the protein-splitting enzyme pepsin.
2. Parietal or oxyntic cells, producing hydrochloric acid and intrinsic factor.
3. Goblet or mucus-secreting cells, whose mucus secretion protects the mucosa of the stomach and lubricates the food.

In addition to these substances, the stomach also produces lipase and rennin.

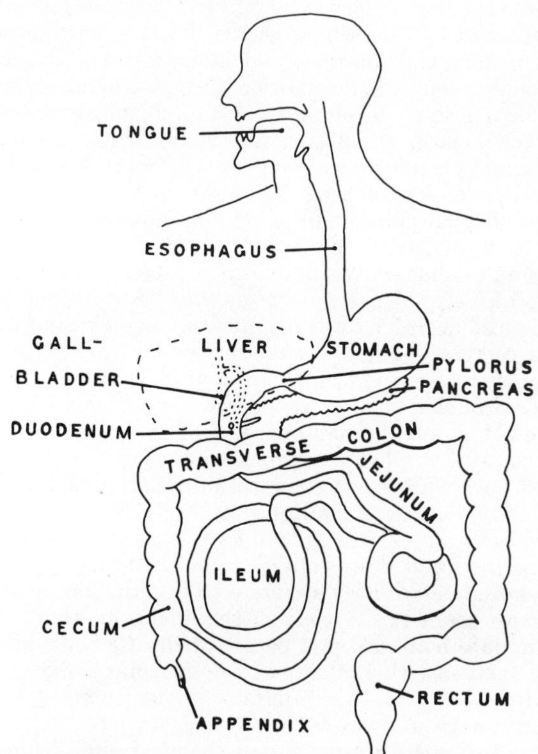

Figure 10–1 Drawing illustrating the gastrointestinal tract.

Lipase. This is a fat-splitting enzyme, but in the acid reaction of the stomach contents it is almost entirely inactive. However, it is not destroyed in the stomach and may be active in the more favorable pH environment of the duodenal contents. It may be active in the stomachs of infants.

Rennin. This enzyme, which is present in young mammals, causes milk to curdle, a process involving partial hydrolysis of the milk protein, caseinogen, to the soluble casein, which in the presence of Ca^{++} forms a coagulum of calcium caseinate that is more easily digested. The existence of rennin in human infants is debatable.

PHYSIOLOGY OF GASTRIC SECRETION

By gastric secretion is meant the release into the lumen of the stomach of all the gastric juice, quantitatively and qualitatively considered, including water, electrolytes, and mucus, in addition to enzymes and hydrochloric acid. However, since hydrochloric acid secretion is the facet most easily studied, it is the best understood and most widely used parameter of gastric secretion.

Mode of Stimulation

The acid- and pepsin-producing cells of the stomach are stimulated to secrete by various mechanisms, most of which potentiate each other or are interrelated.

Psychic and Neural. Pavlov's experiments showed that psychic factors play a large part in gastric secretion. Anticipation of food by sight, smell, and memory stimulates the gastric glands by efferent impulses along the vagus nerve. These impulses act directly, via the neurosecretory cell junction, and indirectly, via the local hormone, gastrin. In addition to psychogenic stimuli, reflexes arising in mechanical and chemical receptors in the mouth, esophagus, and stomach also generate efferent secretory vagal impulses. Stimuli of this type continue as long as food is present in the stomach, i.e., long after psychic stimuli have ceased to operate.

Gastrin. Gastrin is a small peptide containing some 17 amino acids (M.W. 1500). It is produced mainly (90%) by the cells of the gastric antrum. About half that produced during a meal results from vagal stimulation. The secretory stimuli for the remainder are: (a) distension of the antrum by food; (b) contact of antral mucosa with proteins, meat extracts, and alcohol; and (c) alkaline pH of antral contents, e.g., food or duodenal reflux. About 10% of all gastrin produced during a meal results from mechanical and chemical stimulation of the duodenal and upper jejunal mucosae.

Gastrin is secreted as two almost identical peptides. Gastrins I and II are equally potent and more powerful than histamine. They are secreted into the blood, which carries them to the body of the stomach, where they stimulate both acid and pepsin-producing cells; and to the pancreas, where they excite both acinar and ductular cell secretion. Gastrin effects are potentiated by vagal stimulation, and vice versa.

Local Nerve Reflexes. Local chemical and distension effects of food in the stomach also excite gastric secretion.

Role of Histamine. Histamine is a major physiological stimulant of gastric secretion. It was believed to be a specific exciter of hydrochloric acid secretion, but it also promotes pepsin secretion. It may act via nerve endings rather than directly on the cells.

Gastric Inhibition

A number of factors inhibit gastric secretory activity. Sympathetic stimulation (fear, unpleasant taste), secretin, serotonin, and possibly other local hormones have inhibitory effects, whereas rising acid levels specifically inhibit gastrin production.

Parietal Cell Mass and Hydrochloric Acid Secretion

Other factors being equal, the amount of hydrochloric acid secreted in unit time is proportional to the number of parietal cells (parietal cell mass). The normal adult complement of approximately one billion (1×10^9) parietal cells secretes about 12 mEq of hydrochloric acid per half hour when maximally stimulated by histamine (upper limit of normal under these conditions is 30 mEq per 30 minutes). Males generally have a greater parietal cell mass (1.18×10^9) than females (0.84×10^9).

Determinants of Size of Parietal Cell Mass. Although little is known about this, hormonal and genetic factors obviously play a major role; age and diet may also be factors.

Concentration and Functions of Gastric Hydrochloric Acid. Hydrochloric acid in gastric juice is 0.1 to 0.15 N, but as it leaves the parietal cells it is almost 0.5 N. Its functions are:

1. To activate the three pepsinogens (I, II, and III), secreted by the chief cells, by hydrolyzing a polypeptide from them, thus converting them to pepsins (M.W. about 35,000, M.W. of pepsinogens 42,500). This conversion proceeds most rapidly at pH 2.
2. To activate rennin.
3. To combine with food proteins to form acid metaproteins, which are more readily digested by pepsins. Hydrochloric acid also provides the optimum pH for pepsins.
4. To prevent bacterial multiplication.
5. To prevent precipitation of calcium as insoluble calcium phosphate.

Intrinsic Factor

To be absorbed (in the distal small intestine), vitamin B_{12} of the diet must combine with intrinsic factor, which is a glycoprotein or mucoprotein secreted by the parietal cells. In classic adult pernicious anemia there is atrophy of the parietal cells and of the gastric mucosa generally. In about 85% of such cases antibodies against parietal cells are demonstrable in the sera, and antibodies against intrinsic factor are present in 50 to 60%. Whether these are primary, in which case the process would be a true autoimmune one, or secondary (following damage to parietal cells from some other cause, e.g., genetic), is as yet unknown.

Role of the Stomach in Digestion

When it leaves the stomach the food has undergone the following changes:

1. The proteins have been partly broken down to peptides, which have molecular weights on the order of 1000.
2. Starches have been partly broken down to smaller units by the salivary amylase.
3. Fats and simple carbohydrates (mono- and disaccharides) are unchanged.
4. The food has been "homogenized" and passes through the pylorus in regular spurts into the duodenum as "chyme."

GASTRIC ANALYSIS

Normal gastric juice is a colorless watery fluid of low specific gravity. It is about 99% water and contains hydrochloric acid, small amounts of organic acids, sodium and potassium chlorides, pepsin, lipase, and the intrinsic factor. In the newborn infant, rennin, a milk-clotting enzyme, is believed by some to be present.

Tests of Gastric Function

After an overnight fast, a narrow tube is passed into the stomach, and a resting sample of gastric juice is obtained for analysis. Some authors recommend a 12-hour fasting collection, but in practice a one-hour collection appears to be as informative, and is much less uncomfortable for the patient. It is also more reliable, in that a complete collection is more likely to be obtained. Next, some stimulant of gastric function is administered, and further samples are drawn. Such apparent simplicity is complicated in practice by a variety of technical problems that render tests of gastric function at best difficult to interpret, and at worst totally useless. Indeed, the clinical value of such tests is dubious, and gastroenterologists rely increasingly on gastroscopy with biopsy and on serum gastrin estimations. However, many physicians still use these tests; therefore some description will be given.

Pentagastrin (Peptavlon) is an acetylated derivative of the terminal tetrapeptide amide fraction that occurs in all natural gastrins and that is the active portion of the polypeptide. It therefore acts as a physiological gastric acid secretagogue, and given parenterally by any route in a dose of 6 μg per kg body weight, it provides stimulation equivalent to betazole. Mild side effects have been reported, such as nausea, vomiting, headache, dizziness, tachycardia, and sweating, but such reactions have been transient. It appears to be the preferred agent in stimulation of acid secretion.

Even if maximal stimulation is achieved, there is still the problem of adequate sample collection. Rough passage of the tube may produce bleeding, and confuse the interpretation. Constant clearing of the tube is desirable in order to be sure of collecting all the secreted fluid. The presence of succus entericus in the sample, resulting from reflux through the pylorus or passage of the tip of the tube into the duodenum, will neutralize the acid and invalidate the test.

Next comes the problem of analysis of the sample once it is collected. Inspection with the naked eye for bile and blood, with confirmatory chemical testing, is usual. Tests for pepsin and organic acid content have been described, but do not appear to be of value. Lactic and butyric acids accumulate when there is pyloric obstruction (e.g., caused by scarring following healing of a gastric ulcer, or by carcinoma), but obstruction of this type is evident radiologically. Usually, the only estimation made is of the strong acid content (i.e., the free hydrogen ion concentration).

Formerly it was usual to titrate with 0.1M NaOH and Töpfer's reagent (dimethylaminoazobenzene), or with phenol red, and then to continue the titration with phenolphthalein. The first titration gave an estimate of the so-called free HCl, and the second gave the total acidity. Recently there has been a tendency to recommend electrometric titration to pH 7, using a glass electrode and 0.1M NaOH. However, gastric juice contains a number of weak buffer systems, and because of this the titration curve between pH 4 and pH 7 is that of a buffered acid, and an overestimate of the content of strong acid is obtained. Titration to approximately pH 3.5 appears to be the best compromise, using either Töpfer's reagent or a glass electrode.

Interpretation

Formerly it was customary to graph the acid concentration (as mL M/10 HCl/100 mL gastric juice) against time, extending the collections over two to three hours, at 15-minute intervals. It is now usual to report the total strong acid content for (i) the resting sample, (ii) the 60-minute period after stimulation, and (iii) the peak 30-minute period. Specimens are collected at 15-minute periods during the 60 minutes following stimulation.

The normal range of results obtained is wide, and there is divergence between published data. Furthermore, unless the sample collection is made with care, the results will be misleading or meaningless. The normal basal secretion is 1 to 4 mEq (mmol) H^+ per hour. The total maximal acid secretion over one hour is less than 30 mEq in the male and less than 20 mEq in the female, whereas the upper limits of normal for the peak 30-minute period are 20 and 15 mEq in the male and female, respectively.

Peptic Ulcer. A peak 30-minute secretion of 20 mEq H^+ is generally considered to be of confirmatory value in the diagnosis of duodenal ulcer, but in such patients there is a considerable overlap with normal values. Patients with gastric ulcers may exhibit hyperacidity, although again this is variable.

Carcinoma of the Stomach. After stimulation, the total free acid secreted is low, and occasionally achlorhydria is present, depending to some extent on the proportion of mucosa replaced by the tumor. Titration to pH 7 may produce high "combined acid" values, caused by the presence of organic acids formed by fermentation in the stomach. This fermentation occurs when pyloric obstruction is present, with retention of food in the stomach.

Pernicious Anemia. Achlorhydria, even after maximal stimulation, is a characteristic finding in adult pernicious anemia. However, much better tests exist for the diagnosis of this disease, and now the demonstration of achlorhydria is seldom a useful part of the investigation of a megaloblastic anemia. Furthermore, faulty sample collection can give false negative results.

Zollinger-Ellison Syndrome. Patients with this rare syndrome have diarrhea and multiple peptic ulcers, usually in the duodenum but occasionally in the jejunum also. The fasting 12-hour volume of gastric juice is very high (more than 1000 mL), as is the total acid content (100 mEq H^+ or more). Neither histamine nor pentagastrin will produce any further stimulation of acid secretion. The reason is that the parietal cells already are maximally stimulated by high circulating levels of gastrin, which is being secreted by a non–beta cell adenoma the pancreas. Not only do the islets of Langerhans contains alpha cells, which secrete glucagon, and beta cells, which secrete insulin, but other types of cells with individual secretory functions. Some have been shown definitely to contain gastrin, and although the physiological importance of this is unknown, it is thought that gastrin-secreting adenomas arise from these cells. Treatment consists of surgical removal of the tumor.

Normal serum gastrin levels, determined by radioimmunoassay, are less than 200 pg per dL, whereas in the Zollinger-Ellison syndrome they are 600 to 300,000 pg per dL.

Examination of Gastric Juice

Note the color of the specimen:

Clear and colorless—normal.

Yellow or green—bile. Confirm if necessary by applying Fouchet's test as for bilirubin in urine.

Brown flecks—blood. Confirm by the test for occult blood in feces.

Note the consistency of the specimen: mucus causes a stringy appearance. The presence of food particles is confirmed by adding a few drops of iodine to the specimen. A blue color indicates the presence of starch.

Record volume, pH, and time of each sample.

Estimation of Free Hydrochloric Acid

Procedure

The titration of gastric juice samples is conveniently done in small plastic vessels made by cutting off the tops of polyethylene reagent bottles of about 100-mL capacity. This minimizes damage to the delicate glass of the electrodes. A magnetic stirrer should be used, with the pH meter electrodes arranged so that the stirrer bar does not strike them. Titrate 10 mL of fluid if available, adding the titrant—0.1 M sodium hydroxide—from a 50-mL burette mounted above the titration vessel. The addition of titrant should be slow enough to permit continuous thorough mixing.

Calculation (Note that 1.0 mL of 0.1 M = 0.1 mEq.)

Using 10 mL of sample:

Volume of titrant in mL to bring sample to pH 3.5 (or 7.0) divided by 10 = milliequivalents of free HCl in 10 mL of sample. Multiply by $\frac{\text{Complete sample quantity}}{10}$ to get mEq of free HCl in total specimen.

If specimen is less than 10 mL, make up to 10 mL, with distilled water, titrate to pH 3.5 (or 7.0) and $\frac{\text{Titer in mL}}{10}$ = Free HCl in specimen.

With some types of pH meter electrodes it may be necessary to add distilled water to a more convenient volume, but the calculations are unchanged. In some institutions the amounts of free HCl for an hour's collection of samples are totaled for each hour of the test.

If desired, the results can be expressed in mmol/liter by the formula:

$$\frac{\text{mEq per sample} \times 1000}{\text{Sample volume}}$$

since 1 mmol = 1 mEq of a singly ionized acid such as HCl.

If the pH of the specimen is higher than that to which the titration is to be made, a report of no free HCl is made.

PHYSIOLOGY OF THE PANCREAS

The pancreas is a large gland with at least three distinct functions:

1. Its main bulk consists of exocrine secretory tissue, the cells of which are arranged in grapelike clusters about tiny ducts. This acinar tissue produces all the digestive ferments.

2. The endocrine portion of the pancreas consists of the islets of Langerhans, small (0.1 to 0.15 mm diameter) islands of cells that are unrelated to ducts and whose secretions pass directly into the blood stream. Most numerous in these islets are the beta cells, which secrete insulin.

The alpha cells of the islets of Langerhans produce glucagon, a small (M.W. about 3500) protein that raises the blood sugar by activating liver phosphorylase, which breaks down glycogen. Glucagon also reduces the secretory response of the parietal cells to all stimuli except histamine.

The digestive enzymes produced and secreted by the exocrine acinar cells of the pancreas are the following:

Proteolytic Enzymes

Trypsin. This is the main proteolytic enzyme in the pancreatic juice. Secreted as trypsinogen, it is activated by the enzyme enterokinase, which is formed by the duodenal mucosa, and, autocatalytically, by trypsin itself. In both cases activation involves cleavage of a lysine-isoleucine bond. Trypsin hydrolyzes proteins at peptide bonds in which one residue is either L-lysine or L-arginine, and in which the epsilon-amino or guanidino group is free. Proteins are reduced to small polypeptides, but some amino acids are released from those dipeptides containing lysine or arginine.

Chymotrypsin. Two forms of chymotrypsinogen (A and B) are secreted. They are activated by trypsin cleaving an arginylisoleucine bond in their molecules, and possibly also by enterokinase. The action of chymotrypsin on proteins is similar to that of trypsin and, like trypsin, chymotrypsin is most effective on the proteoses and peptones resulting from the action of gastric pepsin.

Collagenase. This enzyme digests collagen and is the one that initiates tissue destruction in necrotizing pancreatitis.

Elastase. This specifically digests elastin, which is the most resistant of all body proteins to lytic agents.

Peptidases

Carboxypeptidase. Procarboxypeptidase is activated by enterokinase. The active enzyme removes amino acids one by one from the carboxyl ends of the peptide chains.

Aminopeptidases. Typified by leucine aminopeptidase, these remove amino acids from the ends of the peptide chains bearing the free amino group.

Nucleases

Ribonuclease and deoxyribonuclease are secreted in probably more than one, or perhaps several, forms; they hydrolyze the respective nucleic acids.

Amylolytic Enzymes

Amylase. Alpha-amylase attacks the alpha-1, 4-glucosidic bonds of starches, breaking them down to the disaccharide maltose.

Lipolytic Enzymes

Lipase. This enzyme partially hydrolyzes neutral fats, splitting off one fatty acid at a time, thus forming diglycerides and monoglycerides along with liberated free fatty acids (stearic, palmitic, oleic, linoleic, linolenic, and others). Strangely, its optimum pH range (7 to 9) differs from that of the duodenum (pH 5.5 to 6.5, because of gastric chyme). Pancreatic lipase is activated by sodium cholate and deoxycholate of the bile, and calcium appears to be necessary for its action also. A peculiarity of pancreatic lipase is that it shows optimal activity when the substrate is in an emulsified form and very little activity in the presence of a substrate in true solution. This is an important consideration in designing methods for its estimation. The action of lipase is greatly facilitated by the bile salts and bile acids, which emulsify the fats to minute droplets, 0.5 to 1 micron in diameter, thus exposing a large surface area for lipolysis. The acid pH range of the intestine prevents the liberated fatty acids from forming soaps.

Lecithinase (Phospholipase). At least two, A and B, are secreted. Phospholipase A hydrolyzes a fatty acid from lecithin or cephalin to yield lysolecithin or lysocephalin. These in turn lose a second fatty acid through the action of phospholipase B, leaving glyceryl-phosphoryl choline, glyceryl-phosphoryl ethanolamine, and glyceryl-phosphoryl serine.

Esterases. These are present in the pancreatic juice but have not been fully categorized. An example is cholesterol esterase, which splits cholesterol from its esters.

Control of Pancreatic Secretion

Enzyme Secretion. Most of the digestive enzymes of the pancreas are contained within the zymogen granules of the acinar cells. The zymogen granules are released by the hormone pancreozymin, which is produced by the duodenal and jejunal mucosae on contact with food substances in the gastric chyme. They are also released by efferent nerve impulses along the vagus nerves. Pancreatic secretion resulting from stimulation by either pancreozymin or vagal impulses is of low volume, viscid, and rich in digestive enzymes.

Fluid and Electrolyte Secretion. Water and electrolytes are secreted by the epithelial cells lining the ducts and ductules of the pancreas, under the stimulus of the protein hormone secretin (M. W. 5000), which is formed by the duodenal and jejunal mucosae when the hydrochloric acid of the gastric chyme comes in contact with them. The volume of pancreatic secretion is reduced by antidiuretic hormone and by serotonin.

Volume and Composition of Pancreatic Juice. Daily volume of the juice varies between 500 and 800 mL, approximately. Its composition, especially as regards enzyme content, shows wide variations, depending mainly on the diet. It is distinctly alkaline (pH 8.5), owing to its high bicarbonate content (80 to 140 mM per liter maximum). About half the bicarbonate is secreted under the influence of carbonic anhydrase, which is abundant in the ductular cells. Its content of chloride varies inversely with that of HCO_3^-, the total of these two anions being constant. Secretin promotes the flow of a large volume of watery juice, high in bicarbonate and low in enzymes. Sodium and potassium are present in amounts similar to their concentrations in the plasma.

PANCREATIC DISEASE AND ITS INVESTIGATION

Because of the inaccessibility of the pancreas, its large reserve capacity of functions that are interrelated with and in part overlapped by those of the stomach, biliary system, and small intestine, and the lack of simple, specific methods for estimating many of its enzymes, functional evaluation of the pancreas has constituted one of the least rewarding, least definitive, and most frustrating aspects of clinical pathology. Diseases to which the pancreas is subject, or in which it may be involved, are classified below.

Congenital

Malformations, e.g., annular pancreas; ectopic pancreatic tissue, e.g., in Meckel's diverticulum or in the wall of the stomach or duodenum. Genetic defect, e.g., mucoviscidosis.

Acquired

Inflammations: viral, e.g., mumps; ascending inflammation of the ducts, acute and chronic, bacterial or chemical (reflux of bile, and so forth); acute necrotizing or hemorrhagic pancreatitis and its sequelae, abscess and pseudocyst; chronic pancreatitis, relapsing and fibrosing; inflammation secondary to peritonitis, perforated ulcer, and so forth.

Degenerative disease: obstruction of ducts by calculi, tumors, strictures, and, rarely, parasites (acinar atrophy results); old age, cirrhosis, and uremia.

Tumors: of ducts and acinar tissue, benign or malignant; of islets, benign or malignant, functioning or nonfunctioning.

Ablation of Pancreatic Function

Malabsorption and Pancreatic Function

Absence of the pancreatic secretions leads to failure to absorb many dietary components. The general clinical picture is described as the malabsorption syndrome, sometimes called steatorrhea. The word *steatorrhea* simply means the excretion of large amounts of fat and refers to the big pale, bulky, fatty, and mephitic stools that are passed by individuals with a severe form of the malabsorption syndrome. However, other dietary components are affected to varying degrees, and the term *malabsorption syndrome* is preferable to steatorrhea.

The malabsorption syndrome can be caused by (i) deficiency of the digestive secretions, of which those from the pancreas are the most important, or (ii) defects of the small bowel mucosa or wall, leading to failure to absorb foodstuffs that have already been acted on by digestive enzymes. Defects of the small bowel are described on p. 238.

Effects on Digestion and Absorption of Fat

Absence of lipase leads to *steatorrhea.* Examination of a loopful of feces emulsified with a drop or two or a saturated solution of oil red O in isopropanol will reveal numerous droplets of neutral fat.

In addition to lack of weight gain, impaired absorption of fats leads to reduced absorption of fat-soluble substances, e.g., vitamins A, D, E, and K, a fact that is used in the vitamin A absorption test and serum carotene levels studies.

Effects on Digestion of Starch

Most of the degradation of starches to maltose is accomplished by pancreatic amylase, although salivary ptyalin effects a variable amyloclasis. Also, variable hydrolysis of starches occurs in cooking and in the intestine itself. Total absence of pancreatic amylase, therefore, does not result in total nondigestion of starches. But generally in such circumstances a substantial though variable amount of starch goes undigested, and this contributes to the bulk of the stools and to the increased bacterial fermentative action in them.

Effects on Digestion of Proteins

Absence of proteolytic enzymes leads to *creatorrhea* (recognizable meat, i.e., muscle fibers, in stool) and *azotorrhea* (nitrogen wastage in feces). In the latter condition much more than the normal minimum of 1 g of nitrogen per day is present in the stool. However, the nitrogen content of the stool is subject to considerable normal variation; also, meat fibers are commonly present in normal feces and are increased with intestinal "hurry." Thus, although microscopic examination of the feces for meat fibers and lipid droplets is still advocated by some as an aid in the investigation or malabsorption, it is without diagnostic value. One should, however, make a careful search for parasites.

Serum and Urinary Enzymes in Pancreatic Disease

In pancreatitis and in obstructive lesions of the pancreatic ducts, provided sufficient acinar function remains, alpha-amylase regurgitates from the pancreas into the bloodstream. In about 50% of cases of acute pancreatitis, enormously increased serum amylase values (more than 500 units per dL) are found within 2 to 12 hours of onset, especially if the onset occurred during or shortly after a meal. The amylase is absorbed first into the venules, but the bulk of it gains access to the bloodstream via the lymphatics; smaller and later absorption takes place from the peritoneum. From the latter, cloudy, dark fluid with very high amylase content may be aspirated and is diagnostic.

The serum amylase in acute pancreatitis usually returns to normal in three to four days, unless persistent or spreading pancreatitis is present or unless a pseudocyst develops. In the latter event, raised serum amylase levels (400 to 1500 units per dL) have been shown to persist for weeks or months, doubtless being absorbed from the pseudocysts, the fluid of which may contain 20,000 or more units per dL. Otherwise, the extent or duration of the rise in serum amylase offers no clue to the extent or severity of the process in the pancreas. Sialadenitis may also lead to increased serum amylase, as may morphine, codeine, a stone in the ampulla of Vater, perforated peptic ulcer, peritonitis, acute intestinal obstruction, and mesenteric thrombosis. Increased intraductal pressure or inflammation or both appear to be responsible in all these conditions. Usually the serum amylase rises above 500 Somogyi units only when the disease process is primarily of pancreatic origin. The estimation of amylase isoenzymes does not appear to be of diagnostic value at present.

Macroamylasemia

This is a rare cause of elevated serum amylase activity, and its recognition is important because of the diagnostic confusion it may engender.

It is characterized by persistent high serum amylase activity in an apparently normal individual. A normal urine amylase activity will generally distinguish it from serum elevations caused by the previously described disease processes. It has been shown that the increased activity is associated with a macromolecular complex in the 7S gamma globulin fraction. This complex does not filter through into the urine, hence the difference in serum and urine activity. The incidence of true macroamylasemia seems to be less than 0.1% in both American and British surveys.

Urinary Amylase

Not everyone would agree that urine amylase determinations are of value; however, the peak of the rise in serum amylase activity may be quite short and easily missed, and for this reason at least, urine amylase determinations can be useful. It has been found that not only is it more convenient to report the amylase activity as units per dL of urine (as this can be determined on a random rather than a timed sample), but this seems to result in a narrower normal range, with 200 Somogyi units per dL as the upper limit.

Amylase Clearance

If urinary amylase determinations are really more sensitive in the detection of pancreatitis, then there must be an alteration in amylase clearance. Briefly, it seems that in pancreatitis the amylase clearance is definitely increased but that this is owing to the fact that the amylase clearance is closely related to the glomerular filtration rate and that an increase in the glomerular filtration rate occurs in the course of pancreatitis. The reason for the alteration in filtration rate is unknown.

The clearance is calculated exactly as for any other compound (creatinine, for example). The normal range for amylase clearance is 1.0 to 3.25 mL per minute in men (slightly less in women), or 2 to 6% of the creatinine clearance.

Serum Lipase

The normal lipase of plasma is probably unrelated to pancreatic lipase and consists mainly of nonspecific esterases. Levels of pancreatic lipase in serum in pancreatic disease parallel almost exactly those of amylase, and for the same reasons. Use of this additional parameter has been discouraged by lack of a precise, specific, or rapid method of assay. Practically all techniques have been unable to differentiate between pancreatic lipase and serum esterases, and it has been difficult to find either suitable substrates or selective activators. Hitherto, the only reliable method has been that of Cherry and Crandall, or some modification thereof; but the long incubation and low values have militated against its clinical usefulness and popularity.

Pancreatic Enzymes in Feces

The simple qualitative test using undeveloped x-ray film is sufficiently sensitive as a screening test, but bacterial trypsin makes this test unreliable and examination of duodenal juice for this purpose is recommended.

Steps in Investigation of Pancreatic Diseases

Congenital Pancreatic Disease

Mucoviscidosis is the main congenital pancreatic disease. Controlled by an autosomal recessive gene, it affects about 1 in 1500 live births of Caucasian parentage. It is very infrequent in Negroes and virtually nonexistent among the Mongolian races. There is a basic dysfunction of mucus-secreting glands and of electrolyte secretion by exocrine sweat glands. Thick, viscid mucus obstructs the ducts of glands, leading to acinar atrophy and cystic fibrosis in the pancreas and to bronchiectasis and recurrent infections in the lungs. Mean sodium and chloride contents of sweat are about 100 and 95 mEq per liter as against mean normal levels of 22 and 18 mEq per liter, respectively.

A sweat chloride concentration of more than 60 mEq per liter is definitely abnormal. This is true whether the value is obtained by chemical estimations on collected sweat or by direct skin testing with an ion-specific electrode. Both methods agree well, but stimulation by pilocarpine iontophoresis always should be employed. Before accepting the diagnosis, abnormal values should be found on several separate estimations obtained at intervals of a week or so. If there is any doubt as to the chloride concentration by the electrode method, it is useful to collect sweat and estimate both sodium and chloride levels. Generally they are close together, with the sodium level slightly higher, whether the values are abnormal or not. Major discrepancies suggest either a faulty technique or some interfering factor. The use of cloxacillin has been found to cause such a discrepancy.

In the Neonatal Period. Owing to the viscid intestinal secretions, meconium ileus is apt to occur and is virtually diagnostic.

Screening of newborn infants has been advocated, using the ion-specific electrode. This is not a reliable procedure, however, the values often tending to be falsely elevated and to show considerable fluctuation during the first few days of life. No definitive data have been published as to the age at which normal and homozygous infants can be reliably distinguished; however, persistently elevated values continuing beyond the age of about six weeks definitely must be considered as abnormal.

In Infancy. Especially during hot weather or in warm environments, the massive salt loss in the sweat may lead to collapse with hyponatremia, dehydration, vomiting, and even death. Children with recurrent lung disease, malabsorption syndrome, or rectal prolapse should always be given a sweat test, apart from any other investigations.

Acquired Pancreatic Disease

Acute Pancreatitis. In the first few days it is preferable to determine the serum amylase at least twice a day, since a high peak value (more than 500 Somogyi units) supports the diagnosis of acute pancreatitis; however, the peak is short and easily missed. Perforation of a duodenal ulcer or peritonitis occasionally may be associated with high serum amylase levels.

Chronic and Relapsing Pancreatitis. Thorough clinical assessment is usually followed by x-ray studies that may reveal calculi in the pancreatic ducts or disease of an associated viscus, e.g., cholelithiasis or peptic ulceration. Routine urinalysis and fasting blood chemistry are carried out as preliminary checks for renal and glucose tolerance impairment, together with measurement of fecal fat.

A useful test uses secretin as the stimulatory agent, followed by measurement of the serum amylase and lipase response with simultaneous aspiration and examination of duodenal contents. Measurement of expired $^{14}CO_2$ in the breath, after the administration of ^{14}C-labeled bile acid (glycocholic acid) appears to be a reliable test for altered bile acid metabolism, which can cause diarrhea and malabsorption. Unfortunately, the test requires liquid scintillation counting equipment.

Tests for Pancreatic Disease

Sweat Chloride Estimation

The simplest procedure to support a tentative diagnosis of mucoviscidosis is to determine the chloride content of sweat. Sweat is obtained by inducing its production in a small area of the skin: this is done by iontophoresis. A small amount of a solution of the cholinergic drug pilocarpine is transmitted through the skin by the application of a small direct current of 2 to 4 mA at low voltage. The sweat is collected on specially cleaned gauze pads and extracted; the chloride is measured by one of the standard methods, such as that of the Cotlove chloridometer. Alternatively, the concentration of chloride ion may be measured directly with a special ion-selective electrode. A result greater than 60 mEq/L of chloride is suggestive of mucoviscidosis.

Estimation of Serum and Urine Amylase

Until recently the only substrate used for the assay of serum and urine amylase was starch, and the various methods differed mainly in the manner of estimating the extent to which the substrate had been hydrolyzed. All such methods were subject to such problems as the inability to prepare a defined solution of starch—that is, a solution in which the molecular weight and extent of internal linkage of the starch polymer were known—and lack of precision in the measurement used for starch breakdown. Another problem was the difficulty in adapting the starch-hydrolysis methods to automation.

These problems have elicited a variety of solutions, which can be summarized as follows:

1. The monosaccharides produced by hydrolysis of a starch substrate (maltose and glucose) are all converted to glucose by the addition of α-glucosidase. The glucose is then measured by the rate of oxygen uptake as it is converted to gluconolactone and hydrogen peroxide by the action of glucose oxidase. Alternatively, the peroxide is broken down by added peroxidase to release oxygen, which then changes a colorless redox compound to a colored chromogen that can be determined spectrophotometrically.

2. Subfractions of the starch polymer, such as amylose and amylopectin, available in the pure state, are linked with various dyes. Under the action of amylase the dye-amylose or dye-amylopectin link is broken and the now soluble dye is released to be measured spectrophotometrically.

3. The defined substrate maltotetraose (maltose is a disaccharide formed by the union of two glucose moieties; maltotetraose is formed by the union of two maltose moieties and can be regarded as a tetrasaccharide of four glucose moieties), when hydrolyzed by amylase, yields two molecules of maltose. In the presence of the added enzyme maltose phosphorylase, the two maltose molecules are split to yield two glucose and two glucose-1-phosphate molecules. The further action of the added enzyme beta-phosphoglucomutase changes the glucose-1-phosphate molecules of glucose-6-phosphate. This in turn is converted to 6-phosphogluconate by the action of glucose-6-phosphate dehydrogenase. This last-added enzyme requires NAD as coenzyme, which is converted to NADH in the process. The associated increase in absorbance at 340 nm is the change actually measured.

4. To simplify the assay method and avoid problems due to various side-reactions in the methods summarized in paragraph 3 above, a new synthetic substrate consisting of a mixture of *p*-nitrophenol-α-maltopentaoside and *p*-nitrophenol-α-maltohexaoside has been produced.* Amylase in the sample splits the pentaosides and hexaosides to produce shorter chain *p*-nitrophenyl oligosaccharides. These are then attacked by added α-glucosidase to release *p*-nitrophenol, the yellow color of which at an alkaline pH can be measured photometrically either as a kinetic or an end-point reaction. Linearity up to a level eight times the upper limit of the normal range is claimed. The procedure is readily adapted to discrete automation, and with a substrate of defined composition results can be stated in International Units.

Although the newer methods summarized above are displacing the starch substrate procedures, one of the latter group is described below as typical of an amyloclastic assay. It has the virtues of simplicity and low cost, since the substrate is locally made.

Sources of Error in Amylase Determinations

1. Serum must be fresh; if it must be stored before analysis, it will keep up to three months in the refrigerator.

2. If plasma is used it must be obtained using heparin; oxalate and citrate cause low results. Fluoride poisons the enzyme.

3. The starch substrate must be prepared and used exactly as specified and must not be used after the stated expiration date.

4. Salivary contamination of pipettes used to measure serum and reagents will cause large errors.

5. The pH must be held within narrow tolerances; the buffer should not vary by more than plus or minus 0.1 pH unit.

6. Errors in timing or incubation temperature will cause false results.

Determination of Amylase in Serum or Plasma (Caraway, 1959)

Principle

The extent of hydrolysis of a starch substrate by the alpha-amylase of serum or urine under standard conditions is measured by the loss of blue color in the test after addition of iodine, compared with a control in which enzymatic hydrolysis is prevented. One unit is that amount of activity which will hydrolyze five mg of starch to the point at which no blue color is given with iodine in 15 minutes at 37°C.

Procedure

1. Pipette accurately into each of two 50-mL volumetric flasks (or large "NPN digestion" tubes marked at 50 mL) 5.0 mL of stable buffered starch substrate. Mark the flasks

*"Pantrak E.K. Amylase," Calbiochem-Behring Corp., La Jolla, Calif. 92037

test and control. Warm the test flask for five minutes in the 37°C water bath.

2. Using washout technique, with a 0.1-mL positive-displacement piston pipette, rapidly add 0.1 mL of fresh serum or plasma to the test flask. Swirl to mix, and incubate *exactly* 7½ minutes in the 37°C water bath. It is not necessary to incubate the control flask.

3. After 7½ minutes remove test flask from bath, and add without delay 5.0 mL of working iodine reagent to both flasks. Swirl briefly, make both flasks to volume with distilled water, and mix well.

4. Read the absorbance of both test and control at 660 nm, setting zero absorbance with water. Readings should be made without delay. Use a cuvette size that results in a control reading of about 0.400.

Calculation

$$\frac{\text{Absorbance of control} - \text{Absorbance of test}}{\text{Absorbance of control}}$$

$\times\ 800 =$ amylase activity in units per dL serum or plasma

If the result is greater than 400 units, repeat the procedure using serum diluted 1 to 5 with normal saline, and multiply the result by 5.

Normal Values

60 to 160 units per dL.

Reagents

Stable Buffered Starch Substrate, pH 7.0. Dissolve 22.6 g reagent-grade anhydrous disodium hydrogen phosphate Na_2HPO_4 and 12.5 g reagent-grade potassium dihydrogen phosphate KH_2PO_4 in about 500 mL of 0.9% w/v sodium chloride solution. Bring this to a boil, and add 0.4 g B.D.H. soluble starch suspended in 10.0 mL of 0.9% sodium chloride solution, rinsing in with 0.9% sodium chloride solution. Let the mixture cool, and add exactly 5.0 mL reagent-grade 37% formaldehyde (HCHO). After diluting the mixture to about 990 mL, check the pH with the pH meter; it should be 7.0 ± 0.1. It must be adjusted if necessary. Then make the solution up to 1 liter with 0.9% sodium chloride solution. This solution will keep at least six months at room temperature (Martinek, 1964).

Stock 0.1 N Iodine Solution. Dissolve 3.567 g potassium iodate (KIO_3) and 45.0 g potassium iodide (KI) in approximately 800 mL distilled water. Add slowly with constant stirring 9.0 mL of concentrated hydrochloric acid (12 M) and dilute to 1 liter. Mix well. Keeps well in a brown bottle.

Working 0.01 N Iodine Solution. Dilute 50.0 mL of the stock iodine solution up to 500 mL with distilled water. Keeps up to one month in the refrigerator. The addition of fluoride as in the original method has been shown to be unnecessary, since enough acid is present to terminate the enzyme activity (Martinek, 1964).

Notes

1. Oxalated and citrated plasma are unsuitable for amylase estimations. Heparinized plasma is suitable.

2. To facilitate running batches of tests, the flasks or tubes can be supported in the water bath by a row of metal tool clips mounted on a wooden or metal bar clamped to one edge of the bath.

3. For estimations of amylase activity in fluids from pancreatic cysts, fistulas, or duodenal intubations, much higher dilutions must be made. As a guide, set up four determinations using undiluted fluid and 1 in 10, 1 in 25, and 1 in 100 dilutions in normal saline. One of these estimations should give a result in the reliable range up to 400 units per dL; the initial dilution will have to be taken into account in the calculation.

4. The unit of amylase activity in this procedure is defined as that amount of enzyme per dL of serum or plasma that will hydrolyze 5.0 mg starch in 15 minutes at 37°C to the point at which it no longer gives a blue color with iodine. In the test 0.1 mL serum is used, 2.0 mg starch, and an incubation time of 7½ minutes. The factor of 800 is derived from the expression $\frac{100}{0.1} \times \frac{2}{5} \times \frac{15}{7\frac{1}{2}}$, in which the first term corrects for the amount of serum actually used, the second term for the actual amount of starch in the test flask, and the third for the reduced incubation time. The expression

$$\frac{\text{Absorbance of control} - \text{Absorbance of test}}{\text{Absorbance of control}}$$

measures the fraction of the original amount of starch hydrolyzed during incubation.

5. The system of reporting the results of enzyme estimations in terms of micromols of substrate transformed per minute (see p. 158) is not applicable to this procedure owing to uncertainty about the molecular weight of starch in the substrate. The alternative method, measuring micromoles of product formed, is applicable only to procedures in which the amount of reducing substances formed is measured. One advantage of the new methods using defined substrates is the concomitant ability to express the results in International Units. The actual ranges are method dependent.

Urine Amylase Determination

The same method may be used for urine, substituting 0.1 mL urine for 0.1 mL serum or plasma. The total 24-hour output of amylase by this method is up to 3000 units.

THE SMALL INTESTINE

In the adult the small intestine measures about 20 feet. Its first part, the duodenum, is U-shaped, about 12 inches in length, and ends at the ligament of Treitz, where it is continuous with the jejunum. The latter measures some eight feet in length and is continuous with the somewhat narrower ileum, which is continuous with the large bowel at the ileocecal sphincter.

To fulfill its functions of digestion and absorption the mucosa of the small intestine is disproportionately large in surface area owing to (1) spiral folds; (2) innumerable, leaflike villi, each 0.5 to 1 mm in length; and (3) microvilli that stud the luminal aspects of the mucosal cells like a stubble. Continuous churning of the fluid chyme over this large surface accelerates the physicochemical processes of digestion and absorption and is brought about by intermittent, segmental contraction and relaxation of the circular and longitudinal layers of smooth muscle in the wall of the gut.

After a variable period (½ to 4 hours) of gastric digestion, during which the pH of the stomach contents falls to about 2, the pyloric sphincter begins to relax intermittently with each longitudinal wave of gastric peristalsis. With each relaxation the chyme is propelled in spurts into the duodenum. There it is mixed with pancreatic juice and with bile ejected by contraction of the gallbladder triggered by contact of the chyme with the duodenal mucosa. The constant admixture of gastric chyme maintains the duodenal contents at pH 6; addition of alkaline juices gradually raises the pH as the chyme progresses onward, until in the distal ileum it approximates pH 8.

Digestion and Absorption of Fats

Churning of the food in the stomach brings about a mixture of liquid triglycerides and phospholipids with other food constituents. This effects a coarse emulsification of the lipids, with particle size about 0.5 to 2 or 3 microns. Admixture of these with bile, plus the action of pancreatic lipase, leads to a reduction of particle size of some one hundredfold—to tiny (1/250 to 1/50 micron) lipid droplets known as micelles. This process is aided by the bile acids, which act as detergents: the hydrophilic end of the bile acid molecule lies on the outside of the micelle spheroid in contact with the aqueous environment, the hydrophobic portion lies on the inside in contact with the lipids. Pancreatic lipase specifically attacks the outer, alpha, alpha′, ester linkages of the triglycerides, producing free fatty acids, beta-monoglycerides, and small amounts of free glycerol.

Evidence to date indicates that fats are absorbed as fatty acids and monoglycerides by direct diffusion across the cell membrane on the luminal aspect of the mucosal cells. The conjugated bile salts act as mobile carriers of the lipid components (as micelles) up to the cell membrane, but they are not absorbed with the lipids; they are absorbed separately in the ileum. Since the fatty acids and monoglycerides are freely soluble in the lipid layer of the cell membrane, no carrier mechanism is required and transport appears to be rapid down the gradient from high luminal concentration to an intracellular concentration that is maintained low by transport of the fat out of the cell at its opposite or serosal aspect.

Virtually all the fatty acids, monoglycerides, and short-chain triglycerides are absorbed, and less than 1% of the dietary triglyceride is excreted. The normal adult excretes approximately 5 g of fat per day. This is derived almost exclusively from desquamated mucosal cells, large numbers of which are shed into the intestine each day.

Fate of Absorbed Lipids. Having gained access to the intestinal mucosal cell, the lipid products are dealt with in two main ways. Short- and medium-chain (fewer than 10 carbons) fatty acids, which are relatively water soluble, appear to diffuse through the cell largely unchanged and are taken up by the portal blood, in which, loosely attached to albumin, they are taken directly to the liver.

Fatty acids with chains longer than 10 C are resynthesized within the mucosal cell to neutral lipids.

Defect of Fat Absorption in Sprue Syndromes. In the sprue syndromes, esterification and resynthesis of absorbed fatty acids are defective—probably as a result of general damage to the mucosal cells rather than an expression of a specific defect.

Formation of Chylomicrons. Within the endoplasmic reticulum of the small intestine's mucosal cells the resynthesized lipid droplets are given a thin membranous coating of protein, cholesterol ester, and phospholipid. Thus encased, they are set free from the Golgi complex and migrate to the serosal pole of the cell, where they are excreted (by reversed phagocytosis) into the intercellular spaces as droplets measuring 0.2 to 0.5 micron. These are the chylomicrons, which are then picked up by the lacteals of the mucosal villi and transported via the thoracic duct into the venous side of the systemic bloodstream. Although their lipoprotein coating is only 1% of their mass, it is essential for their transport out of the mucosal cell.

Digestion and Absorption of Proteins

In the early neonatal period, whole proteins, especially maternal antibodies and colostrum proteins, are absorbed intact by the mucosal cells of the small intestine by pinocytosis. Within a few weeks, owing to maturation of the intestinal cells in an altered hormonal environment, this peculiarly neonatal ability is lost, and thereafter virtually no proteins are absorbed.

In the duodenum and jejunum the polypeptides and residual proteins entering with the gastric chyme continue to be reduced to smaller and smaller fragments by (1) trypsin, chymotrypsin, and carboxypeptidases of the pancreatic juice and by (2) polypeptidases of the intestinal juices. By the time the chyme reaches the distal half of the jejunum all the protein of the food has been reduced to amino acids and dipeptides.

The vast bulk of dietary protein is absorbed as amino acids, which are transported across the cell membrane by carrier proteins.

Digestion and Absorption of Starches and Sugars

As we have seen, the alpha-amylase of saliva effects only a small but variable (probably increased in achlorhydria) hydrolysis of starch. Pancreatic amylase accounts for the hydrolysis of the vast bulk of dietary starches. Approximately 97% of the average starch on hydrolysis yields maltose (two glucose molecules joined by a 1,4-alpha link) and about 3% (from the amylopectin) yields isomaltose (two glucose molecules joined by 1,6-alpha linkage, as in the branches of glycogen). Almost all dietary carbohydrate, therefore, is presented for absorption to the small intestine as disaccharides, i.e., maltose and isomaltose from starch, sucrose, or cane sugar (glucose + fructose) and lactose (glucose + galactose). The splitting of these disaccharides takes place not in the lumen of the intestine, but just within the brush border of the mucosal epithelial cells. There, in the microvilli, the disaccharidases have been located in particulate form by several means. The disaccharide sugars undergo hydrolysis to monosaccharides by the action of disaccharidases. These are located in the superficial part of the membrane covering the brush border

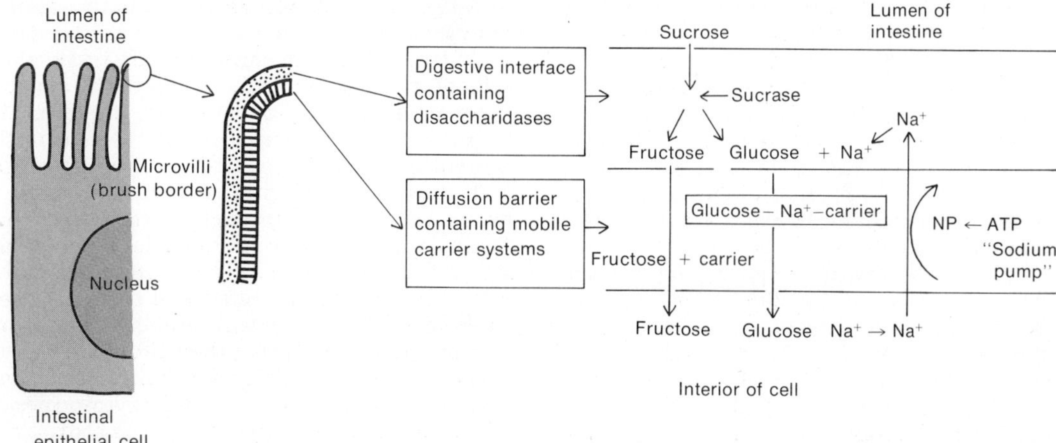

Figure 10–2 Schematic representation of the absorption of sucrose at the surface of the intestinal epithelial cell.

(or microvilli) of the lumenal surface of the intestinal epithelial cell (see Fig. 10–2).

The monosaccharides so produced next are transported into the cytoplasm of the cell by specific transport systems (carrier proteins). Once the monosaccharides have reached the cytoplasm of the cell, they appear to pass into the portal blood by diffusion.

Defects in Absorption of Sugars

Deficiency of Disaccharidases

Lack or deficiency of one or more disaccharidases leads to defective hydrolysis of disaccharides, and therefore, to reduced absorption of their component monosaccharides.

General Effects of Failure to Absorb or Digest Sugars. Unabsorbed sugars act as hydragogues, retaining and drawing water osmotically into the bowel, and thus leading to osmotic diarrhea. Bacterial fermentation of the unabsorbed sugars leads to gas formation (feelings of fullness, distention, or bloatedness) and to acidity of the stool (pH below 6, and often pH 4.5 to 5.5, as against the normal small spread around neutrality). The feces may be watery, frothy, and greenish to yellowish, and they often contain significant amounts of unsplit disaccharide (or unabsorbed monosaccharide).

Lactase Deficit. Lactose Intolerance. This may be congenital or acquired, and the latter may be primary or secondary.

Note. Enzyme activity is rarely found to be completely absent by the usual methods of assay.

Congenital. Congenital absence of the lactase normally present in the brush border has been described in a few cases. The affected infants develop chronic watery diarrhea shortly after birth, which ceases within 24 hours of withdrawing milk and milk products from the diet.

Acquired. By this is meant a lactose intolerance not present during neonatal life, but appearing later in life. Two types may be distinguished.

(a) Primary Form. In man and most mammals, intestinal lactase activity is present during the suckling period, but after weaning it declines rapidly to low levels. The continued ingestion of milk after weaning is, in an evolutionary perspective, an abnormal state of affairs, and in some individuals the decline of intestinal lactase activity is such that they are unable to digest lactose. This state of acquired lactose intolerance is more common in certain ethnic groups, e.g., among Greek Cypriots. Again, the symptoms are watery diarrhea, disappearing on withdrawal of lactose.

(b) Secondary Form. Acquired lactase deficiency may develop as a result of many and varied disease processes that affect the functional integrity of the small intestine. Foremost among these are nontropical and tropical sprue; gluten-sensitive enteropathy probably represents the commonest etiology in Europe and North America.

Defect of Monosaccharide Absorption

Failure to absorb monosaccharides is rare. A defect of the glucose-galactose carrier has been described, producing a flat glucose tolerance curve. Xylose absorption is normal, however. Monosaccharide malabsorption more commonly is secondary to the mucosal abnormalities described under lactase deficiency.

Diagnosis of Disaccharidase Deficiency

Clinical History. A history of intolerance, abdominal distention, cramps, diarrhea, or a combination of all four associated with ingestion of a particular disaccharide, e.g., milk or cane sugar, is suggestive.

Stool. In children especially, chronic diarrhea with watery, foamy, greenish to yellowish, acid (pH 4.5 to 6) feces is suggestive.

Tolerance Tests. The principle of these tests is that, in the presence of a deficiency of a specific disaccharidase, oral administration of a test dose of 100 g (adults) of the appropriate disaccharide will not be followed by the usual or normal rise in plasma glucose. Subsequent testing with 50 g each of the component monosaccharides gives a normal plasma glucose response.

The Lactose Tolerance Test (Dunphy et al., 1965, modified).

1. After an overnight fast (six to nine hours for infants), a sample of blood is taken for fasting glucose

level. The adult patient is then given 100 g lactose suspended in 75 mL water to drink, followed immediately by a rinse of 175 mL water.

Note. 500 mL water would be required to dissolve this amount of lactose readily, but this volume is too large for many patients, though it has been used. The dose for infants and children is 2.0 to 3.5 g lactose per kg body weight, usually given as a 10 to 20% solution in water; stronger solutions may be used if volume is a factor in administration.

2. In addition to the fasting level, plasma glucose determinations are made at 15, 30, 60, 90, and 120 minutes after the lactose is given.

3. In interpreting the results, a peak rise in plasma glucose of more than 20 mg per dL in the lactose tolerance test is considered normal. Peak plasma glucose rises in normal subjects range from 20 to 90 mg (diabetics with normal lactase activity give even higher peaks). Those with deficient or significantly reduced intestinal lactase activity show peak elevations of plasma glucose in the lactose tolerance test of 0 to 18 mg per dL (means range from 7 to 10, ±5 mg per dL).

Symptoms should be sought in every patient given the lactose tolerance test; also, any stools passed within 12 hours of the test should be inspected.

4. All those showing a peak response in the lactose tolerance test of less than 20 mg per dL rise in plasma glucose are given a repeat tolerance test on a subsequent day with 50 g glucose plus 50 g galactose substituted for the lactose. In uncomplicated lactase deficit a normal plasma glucose response should result. If the response is below normal, a malabsorption state is indicated.

Disaccharidase Assay of Mucosal Biopsies. This is the only definitive means for proving the existence and estimating the degree of intestinal disaccharidase deficiency. However, it is best carried out in laboratories with considerable experience with the assay.

ABSORPTION OF IRON

Gastric Acidity

In alkaline media iron is readily oxidized to the ferric (Fe^{+++}) state, in which it tends to form unabsorbable complexes with phytic acid and phosphate compounds in the food. During digestion, by counteracting the alkalinizing effect of pancreatic juice and bile, gastric hydrochloric acid maintains the duodenal contents at about pH6. At this pH iron tends to remain in the ferrous (Fe^{++}) state, in which it does not tend to form complexes and is, therefore, more readily absorbed.

Site of Absorption

The vast majority of iron abosrption takes place in the duodenum and jejunum.

Mucosal Control of Iron Absorption

The mucosal epithelial cells of the intestine are constantly being shed from the tips of the villi. Other cells move up to take their place, and these in turn are replaced by new cells formed by mitotic division of cells near the bases of the villi, i.e., down in the crypts. Experimental studies suggest that in the small intestine mucosal cells are replaced about every 1½ days.

Under conditions of normal dietary intake the mucosal cells of the small intestine regulate the amount of iron absorbed. Evidence to date indicates that iron absorption by the mucosal cells is inversely related to their own content of ferric iron, which is stored in a rather fixed state, possibly as ferritin. This fixed mucosal cell iron varies very slightly throughout the life of the cell. If, for instance, the body has abundant iron, plasma iron will reflect this, and newly forming intestinal mucosal cells will have incorporated into them a large store of fixed, ferric iron. This will inhibit active absorption of iron by these cells during their life span.

On the other hand, if a significant loss of blood occurs, four to five days later increased erythropoietic activity of the bone marrow will draw on the body stores of iron and directly on the plasma iron. As a result, intestinal mucosal cells being formed during this phase will receive a smaller than normal complement of fixed iron and their absorption of iron from the diet will be increased correspondingly. This increased absorption will continue until the body stores have been replenished and new mucosal cells receive a normal complement of fixed iron.

In like manner, a large increase in the dietary intake of iron will reduce iron absorption during the subsequent one to two days. In this case, the mucosal cells absorb more iron by virtue of the increased iron content of the food. However, a large part of this absorbed iron is not transferred to the plasma but is diverted to increase the mucosal cells' store of fixed iron and thereby reduces the iron-absorptive capacity of these cells for the remainder of their life span. Thus iron absorption is self-inhibitory.

ABSORPTION OF VITAMIN B_{12}

Vitamin B_{12} is absorbed very slowly (several hours) in the terminal ileum, in the presence of divalent cations and a pH greater than 6. Combination with gastric intrinsic factor (IF, probably a glycoprotein) results in a macromolecular complex necessary for absorption.

INTESTINAL MALABSORPTION

In the broadest sense intestinal malabsorption means disordered net absorption of any substance ingested or secreted into (or otherwise gaining access to) the gastrointestinal tract. In the usual sense the term connotes a defect of absorption in the small intestine. A very wide range of conditions can give rise to this condition; they are set out in Table 10–1. The great majority of cases of malabsorption syndrome are the result of a relatively limited number of causes, notably pancreatic disease, celiac disease, sequelae of gastrointestinal surgery, and regional enteritis.

Defect of Digestion

Gastrectomy. Malabsorption is common after gastric resection, especially if gastrojejunal anastomosis is involved. Defects in iron, calcium, and fat absorption may occur; a small number of patients develop vitamin B_{12} deficiency, and megaloblastic anemia may appear six

TABLE 10–1 MALABSORPTION SYNDROMES

Defect	Disease or Condition
Defect of digestion	Gastrectomies Pancreatic insufficiency Diseases of liver and biliary tract
Biochemical or genetic	Disaccharidase lack Amino acid transport disorders Abetalipoproteinemia
Mucosal abnormalities	Celiac disease Tropical sprue Regional enteritis (Crohn's disease) Parasitic infestation Lymphomas and malignancies Radiation injury Amyloidosis Neomycin and other drugs
Loss of absorptive area	Resection and short-circuiting operations Fistulas
Altered bacterial flora	Blind loop syndrome Jejunal diverticula
Lymphatic abnormalities and obstruction	Intestinal lymphangiectasia Granulomatous inflammations Malignancies
Endocrine	Adrenal insufficiency Hypothyroidism Carcinoid syndrome Hypoparathyroidism
Cardiovascular disease	Congestive heart failure Constrictive pericarditis Mesenteric artery insufficiency
Miscellaneous	Diabetes mellitus Immunodeficiency syndromes

months to two years after operation. Too rapid gastric emptying, bypass of the duodenum, and, in some, bacterial overgrowth in the afferent loop may contribute to the malabsorption.

Pancreatic Insufficiency. This usually results from chronic relapsing pancreatitis or duct obstruction, but may develop in a matter of months as a result of cancer. In children, mucoviscidosis is by far the commonest cause. In adults, the association of diabetes mellitus with evidence of pancreatic insufficiency or calcification, or both, is strongly suggestive of advanced destructive pancreatitis. In such cases, chemical demonstration of steatorrhea and serum, urinary, and duodenal enzyme assays, together with determination of volume and bicarbonate concentration of duodenal juice, after secretin stimulation, may indicate the diagnosis. This will be strengthened by a normal D-xylose absorption test.

Diseases of Liver and Biliary Tract. Any condition leading to obstruction to the entry of bile into the duodenum or causing diminished or abnormal bile salt secretion is likely to lead to steatorrhea. The resulting deficit in conjugated bile salts has two effects: (1) lack of activation of pancreatic lipase; (2) improper micelle formation. Obviously, both factors result in poor digestion and absorption of fat and of the fat-soluble vitamins, A, D, E, and K. Also, calcium is lost in the formation of soaps in the gut.

Mucosal Abnormalities

Celiac Disease (Gluten Enteropathy; Nontropical Sprue). This mysterious disease is undoubtedly associated with ingestion of gluten, a protein of wheat and rye flour. Specifically, gliadin, obtained by alcoholic extraction of gluten, is held responsible as the toxic agent that damages the mucosal lining of the small bowel, causing malabsorption.

The change in mucosal structure affects the absorption of all dietary components, although fat absorption shows the earliest and most severe defect. Among the factors contributing to malabsorption are: (1) loss of absorptive surface, (2) damage to the mucosal cells with a marked reduction in the capacity of the transport systems and the activity of disaccharidases and fatty acid thiokinases, and (3) disturbance of the lacteal pattern.

Strict adherence to a gluten-free diet usually leads to improvement in the mucosa, beginning within a few days.

Acute enteritis may cause malabsorption, which is usually temporary. The more chronic enteritides, e.g., Crohn's disease, may be associated with partial villous atrophy, but other factors, such as inflammation, fibrosis, and lymphatic obstruction, must also be operative. Mucosal damage always follows therapeutic doses of radiation to the abdomen; heavier radiation may give rise to strictures and fibrosis several years afterward. Several instances of malabsorption have been documented in association with intestinal lymphomas.

Parasites. Heavy parasitic infestation of the upper small intestine, e.g., by *Giardia lamblia*, hookworms, or *Strongyloides stercoralis*, may cause malabsorption. Mucosal inflammation appears to play a part, but other factors may be involved.

Altered Bacterial Flora

Normally the upper small intestine is maintained in a sterile state by the acidity of gastric chyme and especially by the fact that its contents are moved onward with relative rapidity. Conditions leading to delay, stasis, or obstruction permit bacteria to gain a foothold. Malabsorption and steatorrhea have been well documented in states such as blind loops, strictures, fistulas, and diverticula.

Cardiovascular Diseases

In chronic congestive heart failure, congestion, anoxia, and edema of the intestinal mucosa often cause a degree of malabsorption.

Diabetes Mellitus

Malabsorption and steatorrhea in diabetes mellitus may be based on three separate and distinct etiologies. In some adults, both the diabetes and the steatorrhea result from chronic pancreatitis. Some cases represent the association of celiac disease and diabetes mellitus—probably fortuitously, although an increased coincidence has been postulated. In a small number of cases malabsorption and steatorrhea seem to be caused by visceral diabetic neuropathy.

Immunodeficiency Syndromes

Hypogammaglobulinemia is associated with malabsorption. In some instances this may be a result of loss of protein into the bowel. However, 20% of patients with primary acquired hypogammaglobulinemia have a malabsorption syndrome that apparently is secondary to the immune defect.

Diagnosis of Malabsorption

Although the number of conditions that may give rise to malabsorption seems bewildering, relatively few simple and worthwhile tests serve for the diagnosis in most cases. The methods by which diagnosis is made, and the value of the various procedures will become apparent from the following discussion.

Tests Based on Effects on Blood Constituents

Anemia is often present and may be of iron-deficiency or megaloblastic type, and sometimes of both types. Radioactive iron absorption studies are rarely called for; the reduced hemoglobin and plasma iron with correspondingly increased iron-binding capacity, in the presence of a normal diet and gastric secretion, are suggestive. Megaloblastic anemia may be caused by vitamin B_{12} or folic acid deficiency, or both may be operative. Bone marrow examination may be followed by a Schilling test or microbiological assay of serum cyanocobalamin, or both.

Hypoproteinemia of some degree is usually present and may be severe; albumin is most severely affected. Hypocalcemia may be partly owing to the low plasma proteins, but a true calcium deficit is often present, and serum magnesium also may be reduced. Potassium deficit is common. In the absence of biliary tract and liver disease, serum lipids, especially cholesterol and lipoproteins, are generally low in malabsorptive conditions, and also serum carotene and vitamin A, and the prothrombin time is frequently prolonged, though rarely to a marked degree.

Tests of Intestinal Absorption

Two of these tests are the most useful and the most used—fecal fat and D-xylose absorption.

Fecal Fat. Even when no fat is present in the diet, up to 3 g lipid per day may be present in the stools—as triglycerides, free fatty acids, and soaps. These derive from bacteria, desquamated epithelial cells, secretions, and transudates. Normally, less than 25% of the dry weight of the stool consists of fat, and less than one-third of this is unsplit or neutral fat.

In malabsorptive states resulting from biliary, pancreatic, or intestinal disease, the amount of fat in the stools exceeds 10% of the intake and may reach 75% or more. Furthermore, gas-liquid chromatography has shown that this fat derives from the diet, although bacterial action modifies the fatty acids considerably.

Chemical analysis of fecal fat over a three- to six-day period of controlled fat intake remains the best and most accurate index of steatorrhea.

D-Xylose Absorption. The pentose D-xylose is absorbed from the upper small intestine by active transport. Of an oral dose of 25 g, 60 to 70% is absorbed in the first five hours; total 24-hour absorption amounts to about 75% of this dose. During the first five hours after such a dose, normal persons excrete 4 to 8 g in the urine. Abnormally low excretions are obtained in intestinal malabsorption and in renal disease. In this context, intestinal malabsorption includes primary steatorrhea (sprue) and secondary steatorrhea resulting from many diseases of the small intestine (e.g., regional enteritis, diverticulosis, strictures, and fistulas) but, for the purposes of this discussion, excludes that resulting from gastric resections and pancreatic and hepatobiliary disease, almost all of which give normal D-xylose responses.

There is some debate as to whether a 5 g or 25 g dose should be used in adults. Although the 25 g dose is more expensive and more likely to cause nausea and vomiting, the larger dose is recommended: otherwise mild degrees of malabsorption will be missed.

In infants and children it is best to administer 500 mg xylose per kg body weight. The mean 5-hour excretion may then be calculated: Mean 5-hour urinary xylose excretion = [(0.2 × age in months) + 12]%. However, in infants especially, we prefer to measure blood xylose levels and not to collect a urine sample at all.

Glucose Absorption. A flat plasma glucose response after oral glucose is characteristically found in sprue and in other malabsorptive states arising from pathological lesions of the small intestine mucosa.

Beta-Carotene. This natural precursor of vitamin A (a dimer of vitamin A) is also absorbed along with fats, and its absorption and blood levels give information somewhat similar to that derived from vitamin A studies. Its estimation, however, is much simpler. Values in serum vary with diet, but normal persons have a range of 50 to 200 μg per dl. Low values are found in dietary deficiency and in many cases of steatorrhea.

Prothrombin Time. This simple test is usually employed as a screening measure. Since vitamin K absorption is dependent on that of fats, there is some (usually slight) prolongation of the prothrombin time in steatorrhea.

Peroral Biopsy. Since the advent of suitable biopsy capsules and tubes, this technique has become one of the mainstays in the definitive diagnosis of small-bowel lesions.

D-Xylose Excretion Test

Determination of Urine Xylose (Harris, 1969)

Principle

The o-toluidine reagent used for the determination of glucose (see Appendix H) also reacts with pentoses to produce a colored complex. The wavelength of maximum absorbance, however, is at 475 nm instead of at 625 nm, so that the final color with xylose is brown in contrast to the green color obtained with glucose.

Procedure

1. Measure and record the total volume of the test (five-hour) urine collection. Dilute 1.0 mL of the test and control urine collections up to 10 mL with distilled water, making 1:10 dilutions. Mix 5.0 mL of each dilution with 5.0 distilled water to make 1:20 dilutions. Prepare the working xylose standard by diluting 1.0 mL of stock up to 10 mL with distilled water.

2. Set up six 150 × 16 or 125 × 16 mm test tubes labeled test 1:10, test 1:20, control 1:10, control 1:20, standard, and blank. Into each pipette 0.1 mL of the correspondingly marked dilutions, of working xylose standard, and of distilled water for the blank.

3. Add 7.0 mL of *o*-toluidine reagent to all tubes, mix on the Vortex mixer. Heat for *exactly* ten minutes in the boiling water bath. Cool immediately in cold water for two minutes.

4. Setting zero absorbance with the blank tube, measure the absorbancies of tests and standard and controls at 475 nm using cuvettes or spectrophotometer tubes of 10 mm or 13 mm light path. See calculation below.

Calculation

The calculation appears at the bottom of this page.

If the depth of final color obtained with the 1:10 dilution was too high for accurate spectrophotometry, use the values obtained for the 1:20 dilutions and multiply the final result by two.

Normal Values

4 to 8 g per 5-hour collection (26.7 to 53.3 mM).

Reagents

Toluidine Reagent. For plasma glucose determination, see Appendix H.

Xylose Stock Standard. Dissolve 1.0 g xylose in, and make up to 100 mL with, a saturated aqueous solution of benzoic acid.

Notes

1. If the patient has not taken adequate fluid during the course of the xylose excretion test, the concentration of the five-hour collection may necessitate using further dilutions of both test and control urines. If 1:30 dilutions yield absorbancies in the practical spectrophotometric range, multiply the final result obtained from the formula by 3; if 1:40 dilution is used, by 4.

2. If *small* amounts of hexose-type sugars are present in the urine samples, the absorbance of the control urine dilution will correct for this. In most instances the absorbance of the control urine tube is very low—less than 0.03.

SERUM AND PLASMA CAROTENES DETERMINATION

Principle

The carotenoid pigments of the serum or plasma (beta-carotene, lutein, and lycopene) are split from their lipoprotein carriers by ethanol and extracted into petroleum ether. The absorbance of the yellow extract is compared with that of a pure solution of beta-carotene.

Procedure

1. Pipette 3.0 mL of serum or heparinized plasma into a 15-mL glass-stoppered centrifuge tube. Add 3.0 mL absolute ethanol drop by drop with continuous side-to-side agitation; the precipitated protein must be in a finely divided form.

2. Add exactly 6.0 mL petroleum ether; stopper and shake well for 10 minutes on a mechanical shaker. The stopper may be secured with a wide rubber band stretched around the tube tip.

3. Centrifuge for five minutes at 1500 rpm.

4. Carefully pipette off the supernatant petroleum ether layer into a *dry* cuvette, and measure its absorbance at 450 nm, setting zero absorbance with petroleum ether. Use at least a 1.0 cm light path.

Calculation

Dilute 1.0 mL of the 1.0 mg per dL working standard solution (see *Reagents*) with 9.0 dL petroleum ether. Read the absorbance of this dilution as for the test extract. Record the value obtained. The serum carotenes are found from the expression shown below.

$$\frac{\text{Absorbance of test}}{\text{Absorbance of standard dilution}} \times 200 = \mu\text{g per dL}$$

Reagents

Petroleum Ether. This should be analytic-grade, boiling point range 45 to 60°C.

Ethanol. Pure absolute ethyl alcohol, dried over anhydrous sodium sulfate.

Standard Carotene Solution. Using pure beta-carotene, weigh out, from a freshly opened ampule, 50.0 mg and dissolve in petroleum ether in a 100-mL dry volumetric flask. Make to volume and mix. Transfer 2.0 mL of this solution to another 100-mL volumetric flask and dilute to the mark with petroleum ether and mix. This second solution—1.0 mg per dL—is used to prepare the final 1 in 10 dilution as detailed in *Calculation.* The ampule should be flushed out with inert gas, nitrogen, or helium before being resealed (see *Notes*).

Normal Values

The normal value is greatly influenced by diet. A predominantly vegetarian diet may elevate the serum carotenes as high as 500 μg per dL; a normal diet gives values from 50 to 200 μg per dL. Infants have much lower levels, up to 60 μg per dL, except in carotenemia, in which the serum level may reach 350 μg per dL.

Notes

1. Carotene is unstable when exposed to the air; since only large changes in serum carotenes level are clinically significant, it is permissible to prepare the standard dilution as described in *Calculation* and use the absorbance thereof in future calculations, with occasional checking.

2. Serum or heparinized plasma for estimation of carotenes can be stored for two to three days in the freezer; its stability thereafter is questionable.

$$\frac{\text{Test Absorbance (1:10 dilution)} - \text{Control Absorbance (1:10 dilution)}}{\text{Standard Absorbance}}$$

$$\times \frac{\text{Total Urine 5-hour volume}}{100} = \text{Xylose excretion in grams per 5 hours}$$

EXAMINATION OF FECES

Chemical examination of feces is commonly employed in two major instances, in investigation of gastrointestinal bleeding and in investigation of steatorrhea (fatty stools).

Normal Composition of Feces

Normally, about 100 to 250 g of feces are excreted per day, but there is wide variation in the amount, depending on the intake of indigestible cellulose. About 60 to 80% of the fecal volume is water; the solid components are made up as follows: bacteria 30%, remains of intestinal secretions and food residue 50 to 60%, and ether-soluble substances (see further on) 10 to 20%.

Color of Feces

The normal color of the feces results from the presence of stercobilin (urobilin), which is a reduction product of bilirubin. Fecal color changes in different conditions, and gross examination may be diagnostically helpful. The dark-green meconium passed by newborn infants is caused by excretion of biliverdin and porphyrins; the yellow-colored stool of the milk-fed infant results from the normal excretion of bilirubin. Clay-colored stools lacking bile pigment are characteristic of obstructive jaundice. Excessive excretion of urobilin, as occurs in hemolytic anemia, may make the stools a very dark brown. Bulky pale and even "foamy" stools are seen in steatorrhea. Gastrointestinal bleeding will be indicated by melena (passage of black stools) if the bleeding has occurred high in the alimentary tract and the blood has subsequently been partially digested and converted to acid hematin (50 mL of blood or more is necessary to produce melena). Bleeding in the lower intestinal tract (lower colon, rectum, or anus) is usually apparent from the red streaking of the stools. Black stools also occur after the ingestion of iron or bismuth preparations.

BLOOD IN FECES

Blood in the stool may be grossly visible as just described or it may be in small amounts and revealed only by specific tests (occult blood). The presence of blood in the feces is always abnormal and denotes hemorrhage into the alimentary tract. The examination is of considerable value, particularly in investigation of gastrointestinal neoplasms and in obscure iron-deficiency anemias.

Methods for the Detection of Occult Blood in Feces

Principle. Heme compounds (from hemoglobin) catalyze the oxidation of organic substances such as guaiacum and orthotolidine by hydrogen peroxide. The reaction is similar to that catalyzed by true peroxidases, but the tests are made specific by boiling the feces, which destroys the true peroxidases, leaving only the heme compounds, which are thermostable.

Preparation of Patient. The patient should be on a meat-free diet for three days before the examination in order to eliminate the possibility of false results caused by ingested hemoglobin products. Iron does not interfere with these tests.

Extraction of Heme Compounds from Feces

1. Place a portion of feces, about the size of a small walnut, in a Pyrex test tube and add about 3.0 mL of 30% v/v acetic acid. Emulsify, using a glass rod, and then boil over a low flame for two minutes or heat in a boiling water bath for ten minutes. This destroys the true peroxidases.
2. After it cools to room temperature, add about 3.0 mL of diethyl ether and extract the heme compounds by inverting the tube gently several times.
3. Apply the following reaction to the ether extract:

GUAIACUM REACTION. Layer onto about 5.0 mL of guaiacum reagent, prepared as will be described, a few milliliters of ether extract of feces. A positive reaction is shown by the appearance of a deep blue ring at the junction of the two fluids.

GUAIACUM REAGENT. (Prepare just before use.) In a test tube place 5.0 mL of 3% (10 volumes) hydrogen peroxide and a few drops of an alcoholic solution of guaiacum resin (the natural product is often better than the purified substance). The solution will be slightly opalescent and should not turn blue. Alcoholic guaiacum solution must be freshly prepared by shaking a knife point of the powdered resin with a few milliliters of 95% v/v ethyl alcohol.

Hemoccult.* This system for detection of occult blood (that is, blood not visible to the naked eye) in feces uses the same basic reaction as the guaiacum method just described, but it is packaged in a dual-sided paper slide. Small applications of feces are made onto two rectangular areas on one side, which is then sealed. In the laboratory an alcohol/peroxide developing reagent is dropped onto the other side of the paper slide, and positive results are shown by a spreading navy blue stain, which appears within a minute. The system is esthetic, quick, and simple, and the slides can be mailed in the special envelope provided. For the most reliable results (that is, when positive reactions justify further medical investigation) the patient is placed on a meat-free, high-residue diet to reduce the incidence of false positive results and to provoke bleeding from any lesions of the lower gastrointestinal tract. The method can be used for any solid or semisolid material—for example, vomitus; for liquid specimens the routine urinalysis "stick" test is the most convenient method.

FECAL LIPIDS (FAT ABSORPTION COEFFICIENT) DETERMINATION (Sobel, 1964)

Fecal lipid determination is most valuable when expressed as a percentage of dietary fat intake (coefficient of fat absorption). This necessitates controlled intake of known lipid content. A typical regimen for this purpose provides for 75 to 105 g protein, 50 to 135 g lipid, and 180 g carbohydrate per day for five or six successive days. Feces passed on the first two days of the diet are discarded; *all* feces passed on the remaining three to four days are saved in a preweighed container (an unused 1-gallon paint can is best). The collected feces should be kept refrigerated until analysis to minimize hydrolysis of fatty acid esters.

---

*SmithKline Diagnostics, Sunnyvale, Calif. 94086.

Principle

The total lipids in an aliquot of emulsified feces are extracted with petroleum ether after acidification and addition of alcohol. The lipids are estimated gravimetrically after evaporation of the solvent.

Procedure

1. Weigh feces plus container and subtract predetermined weight of empty container to obtain weight of feces. The feces must then be thoroughly mixed; the best method, with the metal paint can, is to mix on a mechanical paint mixer. A large-capacity blender may also be used.

2. Transfer a portion of mixed feces, about 10 g, to a weighed 100-mL beaker. Determine the actual weight of the sample; transfer to the cup of a blender, using a volume of distilled water equal to twice the weight of the aliquot taken. Thus, for a feces sample of 9.8 g, 19.6 mL water would be used. Emulsify thoroughly.

3. Using a 5.0-mL serological pipette with a wide-bore tip, transfer 3.0 mL of the fecal emulsion to a glass-stoppered or screw-capped 50-mL centrifuge tube. Add 2 drops concentrated hydrochloric acid, mix, and check pH with wide-range pH paper. It must be pH 3.0 or lower.

4. Add 5.0 mL ethanol and 20.0 mL petroleum ether, stopper, and shake for 10 minutes, preferably on a shaking machine. Centrifuge for five minutes at 2500 rpm.

5. Using a 10-mL pipette and a Propipette bulb, transfer as much as possible of the yellow supernatant petroleum ether layer to a previously weighed 125-mL Erlenmeyer flask.

6. Evaporate off the solvent on a steam bath in the fume hood. The vapor is extremely flammable. The last traces of solvent can be removed with a jet of air.

7. Repeat the extraction with petroleum ether twice more, adding the extracts after centrifuging to the flask and evaporating off the solvent.

8. Place the flask plus lipid residue in a vacuum desiccator overnight. Weigh, and subtract the weight of the flask. The weight of lipid represents the lipids from 1 g of feces. Multiply by the total weight of feces to obtain the total fecal lipids in 72 hours.

Normal Values

Total lipids per 24 hours, adults: 7% or less of intake, with 10% as absolute upper limit of normal.

Notes

1. The presence of mineral oil in the feces will cause gross errors in both the total lipid and unsplit lipid results.

2. If the feces are liquid, use about 10 mL for emulsification and take a 1.0-mL aliquot for the extraction procedure from step 3.

3. The results of these procedures are reproducible to about ±10%. A clinically significant result would differ from the normal range to a much greater degree than this.

THE LIVER

Anatomy and Physiology

The liver is the largest organ in the body, in the adult amounting to about one-fiftieth of the body weight (1400 to 1800 g in men; some 200 g less, on average, in women). It is situated in the uppermost part of the abdominal cavity, immediately beneath the diaphragm and protected by the lower part of the rib cage. Its superior aspect is convex and smooth; its lower surface is irregularly flat with a slight concavity near the central hilum, through which its blood vessels, nerves, and bile ducts enter and leave. The right and left bile ducts, each draining the corresponding lobe of the liver, join in the hilum to form the common bile duct. At a variable distance from this junction, the common bile duct is joined at an oblique angle by the cystic duct, which connects with the gallbladder, situated beneath the anterior edge of the liver about midway between the midline and the right lateral aspect anteriorly. The common duct then proceeds downward on the posteromedial aspect of the second part of the duodenum, at about the middle of which it is joined by the pancreatic duct; the short remaining portion beyond this junction is dilated to form the ampulla of Vater. This opens on the duodenal papilla, the opening being protected by the sphincter of Oddi.

Liver Lobule

The structural unit of the liver is the lobule (Fig. 10–3), which is roughly pentagonal or hexagonal in cross-sectional outline. At the center is the central vein, which drains blood away from the lobule and eventually empties into the hepatic veins, which join the inferior vena cava on the posteroinferior aspect of the liver near the midline. From the central vein, cords or plates of liver cells extend radially to the periphery of the lobule, separated from each other by blood sinusoids, which also run radially. Around the periphery of the lobule are five or six portal tracts or "triads," so named because each contains a branch of the portal vein, a branch of the hepatic artery, and a bile duct, i.e., three main structures. Nerves and lymphatic vessels are also present in the portal tracts.

Blood Supply and Physiology of Liver Lobule. The liver receives a double blood supply. Of its 1500 mL per minute blood flow, 80% comes from the portal vein, which drains the entire small intestine and most of the large bowel. This portal blood is delivered at a pressure

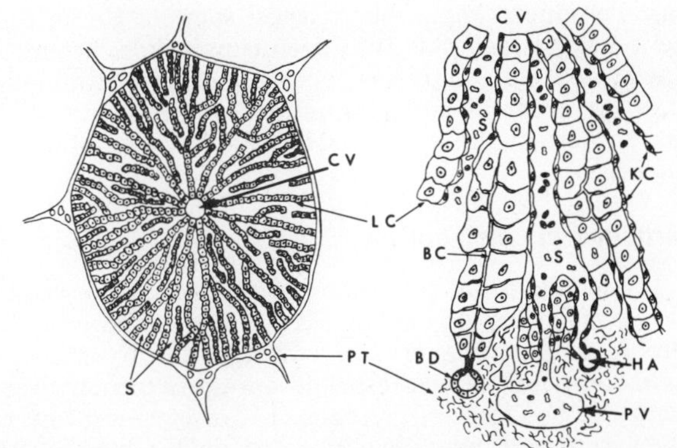

Figure 10–3 Diagram of a liver lobule *(left)* and of a sector of a lobule enlarged *(right)*. *CV*, Central vein; *LC*, liver cell cords or plates; *S*, sinusoids; *PT*, portal tract; *Ha*, branch of hepatic artery; *PV*, branch of portal vein; *BD*, bile duct; *BC*, bile canaliculus; *KC*, Kupffer cells; *L*, lymphatic.

of 7 mm Hg, and its oxygen content is much higher than that of systemic venous blood but lower than that of arterial blood. The hepatic artery supplies 20% of the liver's blood supply.

At the periphery of the liver lobule each radially arranged sinusoid receives two twigs of supply, one from a branch of the portal vein and one from a branch of the hepatic artery. The mixed portal and arterial blood then flows slowly toward the center of the lobule. The sinusoids in which it flows are lined by large (Kupffer) and small endothelial cells. Evidence suggests that this endothelial lining is not complete but has many interruptions. It rests on tiny microvilli that project from the surfaces of the underlying liver cells. This arrangement forms a space between the endothelium and the liver cells, the space of Disse. The interruptions in the sinusoidal endothelium allow the plasma to enter the spaces of Disse and therefore to come in direct contact with the liver cells. Finally, the blood is drained away by the central veins to the hepatic veins, in which the pressure is 5 mm Hg.

The liver cell cords or plates form a complicated system of anastomosing, perforated sheets at least two hepatic cells thick. Between the two layers of hepatocytes forming each plate are the tiny ramifying bile canaliculi. These are merely 5 to 25 nm dilatations of the intercellular spaces, sealed to form microchannels by "zippering" together the contiguous portions of the hepatocytes at their periphery by means of desmosomes. At the periphery of the liver lobule the bile canaliculi connect with the bile ducts in the portal tracts by means of small branches that extend inward from the latter for a short distance (Hering's canals).

FUNCTIONS OF THE LIVER

The liver is the largest and most important biosynthetic, catabolic, and detoxifying organ in the body. All substances (except those transported by the lymph in the thoracic duct) absorbed from the diet pass first through it, and most are modified by it or used to synthesize essential substances, which are then distributed by the circulation for use by the tissues. Other dietary materials are either stored by the liver or prepared by it for storage by peripheral tissues. Arterial blood brings to the liver many biological substances and waste products from other tissues: some of these, e.g., lactic acid, it rebuilds into useful materials; others it inactivates (e.g., many hormones), detoxifies, eliminates itself, or prepares for elimination by the kidneys. Its many functions may be considered under the following headings.

Carbohydrate Metabolism

Besides the usual catabolism of glucose via the anaerobic glycolytic pathway to pyruvic acid, and via the aerobic Krebs cycle to CO_2 and H_2O, the liver is the main organ for the synthesis and storage of carbohydrate energy in the form of glycogen. It can store up to 6 to 7% of its weight as glycogen, and it readily breaks this down to glucose on demand by the tissues.

Interconversion of foodstuffs is accomplished by the liver. Thus, it can manufacture glycogen from glucose and pyruvate and also from lactate, which comes mainly from the anaerobic cycle of muscle work but also derives from glycerol of lipids. In addition, it effects glycogenesis from certain glucogenic amino acids, e.g., alanine, aspartic, and glutamic acids. From two-carbon fragments (acetate), derived from carbohydrates, it can synthesize lipids.

Lipid Metabolism

The liver synthesizes fatty acids and cholesterol from acetyl-CoA. By this means it converts surplus dietary energy into the most economic, long-term storage form of energy—fat. It also synthesizes phospholipids, lipoproteins, and bile acids and esterifies cholesterol. When required, e.g., in a fasting state or in starvation, depot fat is mobilized and transported to the liver as free fatty acids and glycerides. These it degrades for energy production, and in the process produces ketone bodies. Normally, the liver itself stores little if any gross fat, but excess fat may accumulate in it in starvation, excessive carbohydrate feeding, and deficiency of choline or as a result of the action of hepatotoxins such as alcohol, carbon tetrachloride, and phosphorus.

Protein Metabolism

In addition to manufacturing the large variety of enzymes and other proteins required by its own cells, the liver synthesizes a large amount of proteins "for export." It makes most of the clotting factors and virtually all the plasma proteins, with the exception of the gamma globulins.

Detoxification

In many instances this broad term is not truly descriptive since, in addition to the disarming of noxious substances, it includes the inactivation of physiological compounds and, in some cases, the product of the liver's action may actually be more toxic than the original substance. The main chemical reactions involved are:

Oxidation. Examples are the conversion of alcohols to acids (e.g., methanol to formic acid) and the oxidation of aromatic hydrocarbons to phenols (e.g., benzene to phenol, to catechol, to muconic acid; also, the conversion of methyl to carboxyl groups).

Reduction. This is one process that may produce more rather than fewer toxic products. Examples of reduction are: (1) conversion of aldehydes to alcohols, e.g., chloral to trichloroethanol, which is then coupled with glucuronic acid; and (2) conversion of aromatic nitro compounds to amines, e.g., para-nitrobenzaldehyde to para-amino benzoic acid.

Hydrolysis. This is one method that the liver employs in dealing with drugs, e.g., acetylsalicylic acid to acetic and salicylic acids; also, the splitting of glucosides into sugars and aglucones.

Conjugation. This consists of the combination of a substance with a compound readily available in the cells to form a new compound with properties more suitable for excretion. The general effect is to mask the active groups of the original substance and frequently also to make it more soluble, thus facilitating its transport and excretion. In man there are eight main agents used for conjugation. Glucuronic acid is the most important; other groups are glycine, sulfate, cysteine, glutamine, acetate, thiosulphate, and methyl radicals.

BILIRUBIN

FORMATION AND EXCRETION

The process is summarized in Figure 10–4. Approximately 80% of the bilirubin excreted is derived from the hemoglobin of effete red cells that have reached the end of their 120-day life span. The degradation of this hemoglobin takes place in the reticuloendothelial cells throughout the body. These cells are most numerous in the spleen, liver (Kupffer cells), bone marrow, and lymph nodes. Although not yet fully resolved, it is believed that the first step consists of the splitting off of globin, leaving the heme or iron porphyrin. The heme is converted into biliverdin by the action of heme oxygenase, a microsomal enzyme that occurs in many tissues. Biliverdin is converted to bilirubin by the enzyme biliverdin reductase. Some 20% of excreted bilirubin is not derived from old red cells but may come from enzymes containing heme (e.g., cytochromes) and from red cells with an abnormally short life span.

TRANSPORT, CONJUGATION, AND EXCRETION OF BILIRUBIN

Van den Bergh and associates (1916) distinguished between two main types of bilirubin in the sera of jaundiced patients according to their ability to react with diazo reagent either immediately or after the addition of alcohol. The explanation of this phenomenon came in 1957, when Billing and associates showed that bilirubin is excreted as the water-soluble diglucuronide, which gives the direct van den Bergh reaction.

Transport of Bilirubin in the Blood. From its site of production in the reticuloendothelial cells, bilirubin is transported in the plasma in firm combination with albumin, one mole of which can bind two moles of bilirubin. This is the normal unconjugated or indirect-reacting bilirubin; it is insoluble in water and must be separated from albumin by, and dispersed in, alcohol before it will react with the diazo reagent. On arrival at the sinusoidal surface of the liver cell, it is thought that the albumin-bilirubin complex becomes attached to

1.

M V
HC α CH
N
M M
N — Fe^{++} — N → $Fe^{+++}[Fe(OH)_3]$
P V
N
HC CH
P M

M V M P P M M V
HO N C N C N C N OH
H H H_2 H H

Globin → amino acid pool

Hemoglobin

Unconjugated or free bilirubin (M.W. 584)

2. $$\text{UDPG} + 2\ \text{DPN} \xrightarrow{+\ \text{UDPG dehydrogenase}} \text{UDPGA} + 2\ \text{DPNH} + 2\ \text{H}^+$$

$$2\ \text{UDPGA} + \text{Bilirubin} \xrightarrow[\text{transferase}]{\text{Glucuronyl}} \text{Bilirubin diglucuronide} + 2\ \text{UDP}$$

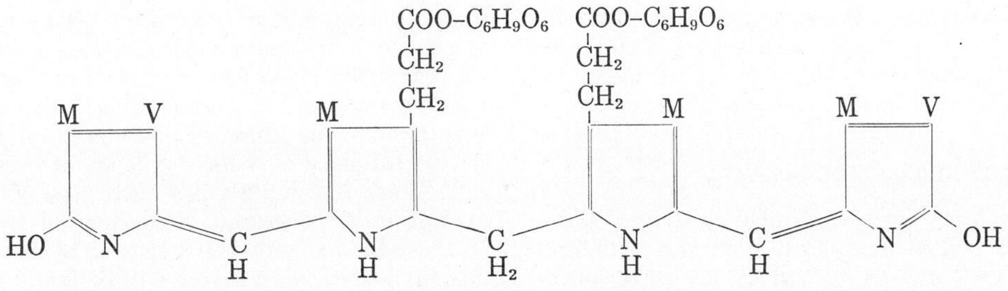

Bilirubin diglucuronide (conjugated or "direct-reacting" bilirubin) (M.W. 925).

Figure 10–4 Formation and conjugation of bilirubin. *M*, methyl; *V*, vinyl; *P*, propionic acid.

the cell membrane. At some unknown point, the bilirubin is separated from the albumin and is bound to a carrier or transport protein, which transfers it to the microsomes for conjugation.

Conjugation of Bilirubin. Within the liver cells, the microsomal enzyme, glucuronyl transferase, transfers glucuronic acid molecules from uridine diphosphate glucuronic acid (UDPGA) to bilirubin, which it attaches to the carboxyl groups of the propionic acid side chains. UDPGA is elaborated by formation of uridine diphosphate glucose (UDPG) from glucose-1-phosphate. Oxidation of the UDPG by UDPG-dehydrogenase then forms UDPGA.

Bilirubin monoglucuronide may be formed first as an intermediate, but the diglucuronide is the form excreted from the cell. This is the direct-reacting or conjugated water-soluble pigment. It is preferable now to discard the van den Bergh terminology and talk of unconjugated and conjugated bilirubin.

Excretion of Bile from Liver Cell. This occurs on the aspect of the hepatocyte opposite to that on which the free bilirubin entered. Its conjugation with glucuronic acid converts the bilirubin molecule from an entirely nonpolar to a mixed polar-nonpolar one that can (1) negotiate the lipid layer of the cell membrane and (2) disperse freely in aqueous media. The excreted bile first lies in tiny channels (bile canaliculi) between the antisinusoidal surfaces of contiguous hepatocytes in the liver lobule plates. At the periphery of the lobules these canaliculi communicate with small offshoots from the perilobular bile ducts.

Fate of Excreted Bilirubin Glucuronide. While it is still in the bile canaliculi, bilirubin glucuronide can be reabsorbed by the liver cells, but once it has entered the bile ducts it cannot negotiate the mucosal barrier. Unconjugated bilirubin is freely absorbed from the gastrointestinal tract, but the conjugated form cannot be reabsorbed.

In the average adult some 300 mg bilirubin a day is discharged into the duodenum. When this reaches the large intestine a series of reductions resulting from bacterial action leads to the formation of many closely related urobilinogens.

The urobilinogens are colorless chromogens that are changed by light and air to orange urobilin. A portion of the urobilinogen formed is absorbed from the large intestine; most of this is excreted in the bile by the liver (enterohepatic circulation of urobilinogen), and a much smaller fraction (0 to 4 mg per 24 hours) is excreted in the urine. The amount of urobilinogen excreted in the urine is increased (1) when there is increased bilirubin formation; (2) in constipation (more time for urobilinogen formation in, and absorption from, the gut); (3) if the small intestine becomes extensively colonized by bacteria; and (4) in the presence of diseases of the liver that curtail the biliary excretion of absorbed urobilinogen, e.g., in the early stages of viral hepatitis.

The Etiology and Pathology of Jaundice

Jaundice is a term used in clinical medicine to describe a visible yellow discoloration of the skin and sclera. It is almost always caused by an elevation of levels of serum bilirubin, and the sudden onset of jaundice may be the first indication of acute or chronic liver disease, of a hemolytic anemia, or of other disease processes. The mode of bilirubin formation and excretion and the nature of the various diseases that can affect it therefore are topics of importance in clinical chemistry.

Total serum bilirubin levels of more than 1 mg per dL are significantly elevated, and overt jaundice appears once the level rises above 2 mg per dL. The measurement of the unconjugated and conjugated fractions is also of some help in distinguishing the nature of the underlying lesion. Many classifications of the causes of jaundice have been proposed: the most useful still seems to be a broad grouping into prehepatic, hepatic, and posthepatic causes. These are given in Table 10–2, which is not intended to be an exhaustive list but simply to provide a framework for the subsequent discussion.

Prehepatic Jaundice

Prehepatic jaundice is caused by the production of excessive amounts of bilirubin, and this is almost always because of an abnormal rate of red cell hemolysis. The numerous causes of hemolytic jaundice are discussed in more detail elsewhere (Chap. 29). What should be understood here is that bilirubin is produced in quantities that overload the transport and conjugating mechanisms of the liver cells, and therefore the excess bilirubin in the serum is of the unconjugated type. As the formation of conjugated bilirubin and its excretion into the gut proceeds normally, without any retention of conjugated bilirubin within the bile duct system, there is no overflow of bile or bile salts into the urine, and the jaundice is thus acholuric. This is an older term applied to the jaundice of hemolytic anemia, especially in hereditary spherocytosis.

The excess unconjugated bilirubin is bound by albumin, and because of its water insolubility it tends to be deposited in those body tissues that contain much fat. Generally, the hemolytic process is not rapid, and it is unusual for total serum bilirubin levels to rise above 5 mg per dL. The demonstration of a hemolytic process by the usual test is not generally difficult. Liver function tests are most often normal; occasionally the formation of pure pigment stones may occur in the bile ducts and may complicate the picture by causing obstruction. High levels of serum lactate dehydrogenase occur in hemolytic anemia, owing to the release of enzyme from the red cells, not the liver, and isoenzyme studies will help to establish this fact.

Hepatic Jaundice

Unconjugated Hyperbilirubinemia. An unconjugated hyperbilirubinemia occurs in association with several rare defects of the transport of bilirubin *into* the microsomal system, and of conjugation. These may be familial or acquired. Two inherited varieties of bilirubin glucuronyl transferase deficiency have been described.

The syndrome known as Gilbert's disease is probably a heterogeneous group of disorders, but many patients in this category may have a defect of transport into the cell. These individuals are quite free of symptoms but exhibit mild persistent unconjugated hyperbilirubinemia, with levels in the range of 2 to 3 mg per dL, although the higher levels will be found on fasting and these fall with repletion. The BSP excretion curve is often abnormal, showing prolonged retention of the dye.

TABLE 10–2 A CLASSIFICATION OF THE CAUSES OF JAUNDICE

Unconjugated Bilirubin

A–Prehepatic (hemolytic retention jaundice)

(i) *Excessive red cell hemolysis*

(a) Familial: e.g., spherocytosis, enzyme defects in red cell

(b) Acquired:

Traumatic, e.g., from hematomas
Toxic, e.g., phenylhydrazine
Infective, e.g., malaria
Neoplastic, e.g., Hodgkin's disease

(ii) *Excessive "shunt" production*

B—Hepatic

(i) *Nonhemolytic retention jaundice* (defect of transport into cell or microsomes)

(a) Familial:

UDP glucuronyl transferase deficiency (Types I and II)
Gilbert's disease
Crigler-Najjar syndrome

(b) Acquired or uncertain inheritance:

Neonatal jaundice, e.g., physiological, breast milk, or serum factor

Conjugated Bilirubin

(ii) *Intrahepatic cholestasis* (regurgitation jaundice)

(a) Hepatocellular injury:

Toxic, e.g., carbon tetrachloride necrosis
Infective, e.g., viral hepatitis
Neoplastic, e.g., primary or secondary carcinoma of the liver
Cirrhosis, e.g., familial or acquired

(b) Bile duct injury:

Familial, e.g., Dubin-Johnson syndrome, Rotor syndrome, recurrent familial cholestasis
Toxic, e.g., drugs (phenothiazines, steroids)
Inflammatory, e.g., sclerosing cholangitis
Neoplastic, e.g., cholangiocarcinoma
Other, e.g., primary biliary cirrhosis, pregnancy, intrahepatic atresias

C-Posthepatic (extrahepatic cholestasis)

(i) *Intramural:* e.g., stones, parasites

(ii) *Mural:*
Congenital, e.g., extrahepatic biliary atresia
Inflammatory, e.g., acute cholangitis
Neoplastic, e.g., cholangiocarcinoma, carcinoma of ampulla of Vater

(iii) *Extramural:*
Inflammatory, e.g., acute pancreatitis
Neoplastic, e.g., carcinoma of pancreas, lymphoma

Occasionally, a moderate unconjugated hyperbilirubinemia in infants may be caused either by some unidentified maternal serum factor that has crossed the placental barrier or by the presence of large amounts of pregnane-3α, 20β-diol in the maternal milk. Both factors inhibit glucuronyl transferase activity. The former appears early and is transient; the latter produces jaundice by the fifth day or so and continues until breast feeding is stopped.

Intrahepatic Cholestasis. The term *cholestasis* is used to indicate the presence of a partial or complete block in the excretion of bile. This may be due to hepatic disease (with failure of excretion from the liver cell or blockage of the small intrahepatic ducts) or to disease affecting the extrahepatic biliary ducts (posthepatic jaundice, see further below).

Primary hepatocellular injury may be acute or chronic. Acute damage to the liver parenchymal cells is most commonly a result of virus hepatitis. The infected liver cells swell and undergo necrosis, the extent of the damage to the cells being quite variable in different individuals. Despite the often considerable damage to the cells, the conjugated and unconjugated bilirubin fractions are present in approximately equal amounts. Swelling of the infected cells may compress the bile canaliculi and contribute to the cholestasis.

Chronic hepatocellular disease, or cirrhosis, has a varied etiology. Slow but continuous loss of liver cells occurs, with foci of regenerating cells forming nodules of varying size. These are separated by sheets of fibrous tissue that at first generally are confined to the portal triads, but that in severe disease eventually seriously distort the hepatic architecture, although seldom producing bile duct obstruction. The disease follows a prolonged course: jaundice is a late event, and is severe only in the terminal stages. The biochemical changes in virus hepatitis and cirrhosis are described in more detail on pp. 253 and 254.

Bile duct injury within the liver, with cholestasis, is relatively uncommon. It can occur in inflammatory disease such as ascending cholangitis, in lupoid hepatitis, or with diffuse neoplasms such as lymphatic leukemia. In primary biliary cirrhosis, an apparently autoimmune disease affecting middle-aged women, marked loss of bile ducts occurs. Occasionally drugs may cause it: C-17 alkyl-substituted steroids such as methyl testosterone appear to affect transport of conjugated bilirubin across the canalicular membrane, whereas drugs of the phenothiazine group (e.g., chlorpromazine) occasionally induce a periportal inflammatory change, apparently an abnormal hypersensitivity reaction.

Familial disorders in this group are rare. Patients with the Dubin-Johnson syndrome have a chronic intermittent conjugated hyperbilirubinemia. The liver contains deposits of a black melanin-like pigment, and the defect appears to lie at some point in the transport of conjugated bilirubin into the bile canaliculi. Affected individuals show abnormal BSP excretion; the plasma level of BSP is normal at 45 minutes, but shows a secondary rise at two hours.

Posthepatic Jaundice

This follows obstructive lesions of the extrahepatic ducts, the common bile duct, or the ampulla of Vater. Gallstones and neoplastic lesions of the bile ducts, ampulla, or pancreas are the most common. Characteristically, the rise in serum bilirubin is almost entirely in the conjugated fraction. However, hepatocellular injury may occur with prolonged cholestasis. The biochemical changes are further discussed on p. 254.

In conclusion, it should be emphasized that acquired hemolytic anemia, virus hepatitis, and obstruction of the common bile duct by stones or tumor are by far the most common causes of jaundice in adults.

Neonatal Jaundice

In the few days immediately following birth, infants normally exhibit a variable elevation of total serum bilirubin levels, up to 15 mg per dL; more than 15 mg per dL, or levels higher than 10 mg per dL persisting beyond the 14th day, suggest the presence of some pathological process.

It is not clear why some babies are affected more severely than others, although the rate of hemolysis undoubtedly is an influencing factor. In some infants there appears to be a transient deficiency in glucuronyl transferase activity, with failure to conjugate and excrete bilirubin adequately. For this reason, phenobarbitone has been administered to babies with high unconjugated bilirubin levels, in an effort to induce enzyme activity. However, reabsorption of *unconjugated* bilirubin from the gut may be a significant factor. It is thought that the unusual levels of beta-glucuronidase activity found in the gut in infants can hydrolyze the bilirubin diglucuronide to unconjugated bilirubin, and that reabsorption of the pigment then occurs.

Other causes of persistent jaundice in infants will briefly be touched on here.

Unconjugated Hyperbilirubinemia. Pathological hemolysis, especially owing to ABO or rhesus incompatibility, can produce very high levels of unconjugated bilirubin in the blood; when the concentration rises above 20 mg per dL, the infant is liable to develop kernicterus. In this condition bilirubin is deposited in nuclei in the brain, notably the subthalamic nuclei, globus pallidus, substantia nigra, and hippocampus; convulsions and spasticity occur, and permanent damage may be a sequel.

The serum albumin in infants appears to have less affinity for bilirubin than that in adults. Thus in infants the bilirubin can be displaced more easily into the tissues by drugs (e.g., sulfonamides) that bind to the serum albumin. The development of kernicterus is therefore really the result of a combination of factors—hemolysis, insufficient conjugating capacity in the liver, and possibly less than optimal binding of unconjugated bilirubin to the serum albumin.

Depression of glucuronyl transferase activity can also be caused by a serum factor or by the presence of pregnanediol in the breast milk, as described already.

Conjugated Hyperbilirubinemia. Complete atresia of the extrahepatic ducts may produce an elevation that is largely of the conjugated bilirubin fraction; however, the diagnosis must be established radiologically.

ESTIMATION OF SERUM BILIRUBIN

The analytical problems associated with the accurate determination of bilirubin in serum include the following:

1. The normal level is less than 10 micrograms per mL and in some cases, e.g., hemolytic anemias, significant changes may be of the same order.
2. For complete clinical information, separate values for the two serum or plasma states of bilirubin—protein-bound and glucuronide-conjugated—are required.
3. The light sensitivity of bilirubin introduces an error-producing factor that is difficult to quantitate.
4. The bilirubin of standards must react in the assay system in the same manner as that of the serum or plasma sample.
5. For the potentially critical determination of plasma bilirubin in neonates, the sample volume is necessarily restricted.

The almost universal answer to problem 1 is the sensitive diazotization reaction, in which the highly chromogenic reaction between water-soluble bilirubin and the unstable but reactive diazonium salt of a primary amine is utilized. The problem of separation is covered by using the latter fact—that only water-soluble conjugated bilirubin, largely as the monoglucuronides and diglucuronides, will react with the diazo reagent; the protein-bound component subsequently can be made reactive by various so-called coupling reagents. Examples are ethanol, methanol, dyphylline, caffeine with or without sodium benzoate, acetamide, antipyrine, and urea. The light-sensitivity of bilirubin is often overlooked as a source of error; merely leaving the serum or plasma samples exposed to light in automatic analyzer cups can reduce the apparent values by 10% in 30 minutes. The only valid standards are those in which known amounts of bilirubin of assured purity are incorporated in a protein-containing base (see later on). For bilirubin assays with limited sample size, direct spectrophotometry and differential spectrophotometry provide valid approaches. Two manual methods are presented here based on several years of experience. They are not the only recommended techniques.

Standardization of Serum or Plasma Bilirubin Determinations

Even with the availability of bilirubin from commercial sources that satisfies the purity criteria of the College of American Pathologists (chiefly that its molar absorptivity in chloroform must be between 59,100 and 62,300 at 453 nm), the preparation of reliable standards requires care and attention to detail. The procedure detailed here is based on recommendations of the IFCC Expert Panel on Bilirubin, 1972, and of Doumas et al., 1973.

Source of Pure Bilirubin. The official bilirubin standard is available from the Office of Standard Reference Materials, National Bureau of Standards, Washington, D.C. 20234, but the cost is high. The bilirubin standard materials from J. T. Baker Chemical Co., Phillipsburg, N.J. 08865; Pfanstiehl Laboratories Inc., Waukegan, Ill. 60085; Harleco, Division of American Hospital Supply Corp., Philadelphia, Pa. 19143; or Fisher Scientific Co., Pittsburgh, Pa. 15219 are suggested.

Protein-based Diluent. The absorptivity of azobilirubin, the final colored product of the diazo reaction on water-soluble bilirubin, is reduced in the presence of protein, which must therefore be incorporated into bilirubin primary standards. To avoid the risk of transfer of hepatitis, the use of pooled patients' sera has been replaced by solutions of bovine serum albumin. The use of human crystalline serum albumin involves greater cost for little practical advantage.

The protein diluent is prepared by dissolving 8.0 g bovine serum albumin* in about 180 mL of deionized water containing 1.8 g sodium chloride and 0.1 g sodium azide (NaN_3). Adjust the pH to 7.4 by careful addition of 1-molar sodium hydroxide and make up to 200 mL with deionized water. Mix by gentle inversion.

Preparation of Initial Standard Solution. *Note.* From this point on all manipulations should be carried out in as dim a light level as possible to minimize loss resulting from sensitivity of bilirubin to light. Weigh out 20.0 mg of bilirubin on a balance sensitive to at least ± 0.1 mg, and preferably to ± 0.01 mg. In a 100 mL volumetric flask suspend the bilirubin in 1.0 mL of dimethyl sulfoxide. Do not shake violently. Add 2.0 mL of 0.1-molar sodium carbonate; swirl to dissolve. Add about 80 mL of the protein-based diluent, and then 4.0 mL of 0.1-molar hydrochloric acid that has been titrated previously against the 0.1-molar sodium carbonate to check their equivalence. The additions should be made with gentle swirling. Finally, make up to 100 mL with the protein-based diluent. Set aside enough of the standard bilirubin solutions for immediate use in standardizing current methods; the rest will keep deep frozen (−20°C) in the dark for 30 days. From this stock solution additional standards can be made quickly by dilution with protein-based diluent, and their use is detailed in the procedures that follow. If methods for serum bilirubin estimation other than those described are used, the range of standards used for calibration should cover the range of values over which the particular procedure gives a linear relationship between absorbance readings and bilirubin levels. This will depend on the chemistry of the procedure, the type of spectrophotometer, and the size of tube or cuvette.

With the availability of pure bilirubin, the older methods of standardization using artificial standards of various dyes and colored compounds are no longer acceptable.

Determination of Serum Bilirubin (Jendrassik and Grof, 1938)

Principle

Sulfanilic acid is converted to its highly reactive diazonium salt by treatment with nitrous acid produced from the reaction between sodium nitrite and hydrochloric acid. Water-soluble bilirubin diglucuronide (conjugated bilirubin) couples with the diazotized sulfanilic acid in a reaction that involves the splitting of the conjugated bilirubin into two moieties, producing a pair of isomeric azobilirubins. The addition of the alkaline Fehling II reagent converts the red azobilirubins to more absorptive blue forms that are determined spectrophotometrically. The protein-bound bilirubin (free bilirubin) is made water soluble and therefore reactive by treatment with caffeine–sodium benzoate; the isomeric azobilirubins produced are slightly different structurally from those produced with conjugated bilirubin, but the difference is not analytically significant.

*BSA Cohn Fraction V, Metrix Clinical Diagnostics, Division of Armour Pharmaceutical Co., Chicago, Ill. 60616.

Procedure

1. Prepare the diazo reagent by mixing 0.1 mL sodium nitrite solution and 15.0 mL sulfanilic acid. The general belief that this reagent is so unstable that immediate use is mandatory has been shown to be untrue.

2. Set up four test tubes marked total, conjugated, reagent blank, and check standard. Add serum and reagents as follows:

	Total	Conjugated	Reagent Blank	Standard
Catalyst	4.0 mL	—	4.0	4.0
M/20 HCl	—	4.0	—	—
Serum	0.5	0.5	—	—
Standard	—	—	—	0.5

Mix all tubes on vortex mixer. To all tubes add 0.4 mL diazo reagent, mix on vortex, let stand two minutes. To all tubes add 0.2 mL hydroxylamine stabilizer, mix. To all tubes add 2.5 mL Fehling II, mix by inversion, and let stand at least five minutes.

3. Determine the absorbances of total, conjugated, and check standard in 19 mm or ¾ inch cuvettes at 600 nm, setting zero absorbance with the reagent blank.

4. Refer the absorbance of the check standard to the calibration curve (see further on); if the value obtained agrees with the curve, refer the absorbances of the total and conjugated tubes to the curve to obtain their bilirubin values. Otherwise use the expression shown at the top of the opposite page.

With turbid or lipemic sera, prepare a mixture containing 0.5 mL serum, 4.6 mL saline, and 2.5 mL Fehling II, determine its absorbance against that of the reagent blank, and subtract this value from the total and conjugated absorbances before referral to the calibration curve.

The final blue-green color is stable for 20 minutes. The results are linear up to at least 6.0 mg/dL; sera that gives values above this should be rerun after dilution with saline. Total bilirubin − Conjugated bilirubin = Unconjugated bilirubin.

Calibration Procedure

Make the following dilutions of the 20-mg/dL bilirubin standard (see earlier for preparation), using the same protein-based diluent for the dilutions: 1:20, 1:16, 1:10, 1:8, 1:4, and 3:10. These will give serum bilirubins of 1.0, 1.25, 2.0, 2.5, 5.0, and 6.0 mg per dL. 0.5-mL volumes of these are processed as for total bilirubin in the preceding method, and the values plotted against their absorbances in the usual manner. The plot should be a straight line passing through or very close to zero, depending on the spectrophotometer used. If the rest of the 3:10 dilution is dispensed in 1.0-mL aliquots in small vials and stored in the freezer immediately, this will serve as the check standard for routine determinations.

Reagents

Catalyst–Caffeine–Sodium Benzoate. In a large beaker on a magnetic mixer dissolve 123.0 g anhydrous sodium acetate ($CH_3 \cdot COONa$) in 200 mL distilled water. Add a further 250 mL water and dissolve 50.0 g caffeine (1,3,7-trimethylxanthine, $C_8H_{10}O_2N_4$) and 75.0 g sodium benzoate, adding more water if necessary. Make up to 1 liter. This solution keeps well at room temperature.

Sulfanilic Acid. Put about 200 mL distilled water into a 500-mL volumetric flask and add 69.0 mL 1 M hydrochloric acid; dissolve therein 2.25 g sulfanilic acid ($C_6H_4 \cdot NH_2 \cdot SO_3H$), and make up to 500 mL. This solution keeps well at room temperature.

Hydroxylamine Stabilizer. Dissolve 3.48 g hydroxylamine hydrochloride in about 6.0 mL distilled water and make up to 10 mL. Keep in the refrigerator and make freshly each week.

Fehling II. In a 1-liter volumetric flask on a magnetic mixer put 500 mL distilled water; dissolve therein 100.0 g sodium hydroxide pellets. Cool under cold running water, and dissolve therein 350.0 g sodium potassium tartrate. Make up to 1 liter, mix well. This solution keeps well in a plastic bottle.

M/20 Hydrochloric Acid. Make by 1:20 dilution of a stock 1 M solution.

Sodium Nitrite. Dissolve 2.6 g sodium nitrite ($NaNO_2$) in 100 mL distilled water. Keep in the refrigerator; make freshly each week.

Normal Range

Total serum or plasma bilirubin—up to 1.2 mg/dL (20.5 μmol/L). Conjugated bilirubin—up to 0.3 mg/dL (5.1 μmol/L).

Notes

1. The automated version of this method using a continuous flow–type instrument and 4.0% w/v ascorbic acid in place of hydroxylamine has proved an excellent way of handling large numbers of tests; it is sensitive to small degrees of turbidity in the serum samples, and it is advisable to run a serum blank set of determinations in which the sodium nitrite is omitted from the diazo reagent. The "bilirubin" value of this set is subtracted from the results of both total and conjugated assay sets.

2. In place of the locally prepared check standard, it is convenient to use a set of commercial controls with weighed-in bilirubin values.

3. When diluting sera with values above 6.0 mg per dL, it is theoretically preferable to use the same protein-based diluent as that employed for the calibration process; in practice the error involved in diluting with saline is negligible.

4. If quality control of both total and conjugated serum bilirubin values is desired, a preparation is available with weighed-in levels of both components.* For routine use, dilution would be required to yield total bilirubin values of about 5.0 mg/dL and conjugated bilirubin values of about 1.2 mg/dL, assuming a 1-in-4 dilution.

5. The manual method can be used for determination of total, unconjugated, and conjugated bilirubin on samples of plasma from infants, but even with the elevated values usually present at least 0.2 mL is required to provide the needed 1.0 mL if a 1:5 dilution is used. (See further on for alternative methods.)

6. In severe obstructive jaundice with the formation of biliverdin, low results for the degree of jaundice will be obtained, since biliverdin does not react with the diazo reagent and cannot be determined.

---

*Elevated Bilirubin Control Serum, Ortho Diagnostics, Inc., Raritan, N.J. 08869 and Don Mills, Ont. M3C 1L9.

$$\frac{\text{Total or Conjugated Absorbance}}{\text{Standard Absorbance}} \times \text{Standard value} = \text{Bilirubin in mg/dL}$$

mg/dL × 17.1 = micromol/liter. (The unit of mmol/L yields inconvenient values.)

TOTAL BILIRUBIN: MICRO METHOD

Collection of Blood Sample

See under *Ultramicro Analysis*, p. 29.

An alternative technique is to collect the blood drops directly from a heel puncture (after smearing the heel lightly with sterile petroleum jelly) into a 6 by 50 mm thin-walled tube in which 2 to 3 drops of heparin (1000 units/mL) have previously been dried in the incubator (available in a commercial form as Microtainer 5963).*

General Considerations of Micro Estimation of Bilirubin

For routine purposes, when the requirements of clinical formation are satisfied by knowledge of the total plasma bilirubin of the neonate, the method that will be described, that of White et al., is reliable and practical. The absorbance values encountered—about 0.26 in a 1-cm cell for a bilirubin of 20.0 mg per dL—permit use of a smaller sample if necessary (see p. 99). In instances when the partition of the bilirubin between free and conjugated fractions is required, the most economical method is to determine the total by the micro modification referred to earlier and to measure the conjugated fraction only on 0.5 mL of a 1:5 dilution of the plasma by the Jendrassik and Grof technique. The most convenient method for rapid processing of micro bilirubin determinations is an instrument such as the Bilirubin Stat-Analyzer, Model BR II.† Thirty microliters of plasma or serum is diluted in 1.0 mL of a buffer in a plastic disposable cuvette with a 1-cm light path. Two simultaneous absorbance readings are made, one at 454 nm, which is the sum of the bilirubin absorbance and that of hemoglobin, the other at 540 nm, which is the absorbance of hemoglobin alone. The instrument subtracts the latter absorbance from the former and compares the difference with that derived from a suitable standard, most conveniently a commercial stable liquid control preparation such as the C8 "Ultimate."‡ If a value for conjugated bilirubin is required, this can be determined by the addition of diazo reagent to the same diluted sample in the same cuvette, with an absorbance reading taken at 540 nm after a set time interval. A suitable control is one with a weighed-in bilirubin value.§ Because of the different wavelength used to correct for the presence of hemoglobin, the Bilirubin Stat-Analyzer gives slightly higher results than White's manual method, to the extent of about 5%.

*Becton-Dickinson and Co., Rutherford, N.J. 07070 and Mississauga, Ont. L5J 2M8.

†Advanced Instruments, Inc., Needham Heights, Mass. 02194.

‡Beckman Instruments, Inc., Fullerton, Calif. 92634 and Toronto, Ont. M8Z 2G6.

§General Diagnostics, Division, Warner-Lambert Co., Morris Plains, N.J. 07950 and Scarborough, Ont. M1K 5C9.

Plasma Bilirubin Determination: Micro Method (White et al., 1958)

Principle

Total bilirubin in plasma is estimated by measuring the absorbance of a dilution in pH 7.4 buffer at the wavelength of peak absorption, 455 nm, and correcting for any hemoglobin present by subtracting the absorbance at 575 nm. The corrected absorbance is converted to a bilirubin value by reference to a factor obtained by making the same measurements on a pure bilirubin standard.

Procedure

1. With a positive-displacement micropipette add 0.05 mL cell-free plasma to 3.0 mL pH 7.4 buffer in a test tube. Mix by gentle inversion.

2. Read the absorbance of the diluted plasma at 455 and 575 nm in a high-resolution spectrophotometer, setting zero absorbance with buffer. (See notes for setting of wavelength.) Use a 1.0-cm cell.

3. Multiply the corrected absorbance (absorbance at 455 nm minus absorbance at 575 nm) by the factor. (See *Calibration.*)

Calibration

1. Use the 20-mg/dL standard bilirubin solution as described under *Standardization of Serum or Plasma Bilirubin Determinations*. Prepare a 1:1 dilution of this with protein-based diluent.

2. Using freshly made and checked pH 7.4 buffer (see under *Reagents*), prepare 0.05 mL plus 3.0 mL buffer dilutions as described under *Procedure*. Make five dilutions of the 20-mg/dL standard, five of the 10-mg/dL standard, and five of the diluent alone. Mix by inversion.

3. Measure the absorbances of the dilutions at 455 and 575 nm without delay, setting zero absorbance with pH 7.4 buffer. For each set of five, determine the mean corrected absorbance.

4. Subtract the mean corrected absorbance for the diluent alone from the mean corrected absorbances for the 20 mg and 10 mg standards. This is the final absorbance.

5. Calculate the factors for both standards as follows:

For the 20 mg standard:

$$\text{Factor} = \frac{20}{\text{Final absorbance}}$$

For the 10 mg standard:

$$\text{Factor} = \frac{10}{\text{Final absorbance}}$$

The factors so obtained should agree to within plus or minus 3.0%. A typical value for a narrow band-pass instrument is 76, using 1.0-cm cells.

6. The factor may also be determined using a com-

mercial control serum with a high bilirubin value, but it should be noted that the peak absorption wavelength of some samples shows a rapid shift from the typical region of 455 nm toward 460 nm within a few hours of reconstitution, even if refrigerated in the dark.

Reagent

pH 7.4 Buffer. Dissolve 4.06 g disodium hydrogen phosphate (Na_2HPO_4) and 1.74 g potassium dihydrogen phosphate (KH_2PO_4) in, and make up to 1 liter with, carbon dioxide–free distilled water. Mix and keep in a plastic bottle in the refrigerator. The pH should be within the range of 7.3 to 7.5.

Notes and Normal Values

1. The ranges of normal values by this and other methods are still a matter for some argument and appear to be method related. For premature infants the levels compatible with the premature state depend on the degree of prematurity: values as high as 27.0 mg/dL have been suggested at 4 to 5 days. The assessment of results largely depends on clinical factors, assisted by successive determinations at daily or shorter intervals. The values that follow should be regarded as guidelines only.

Full-term neonates: Cord blood — up to 3.0 mg/dL
24 hr — up to 6.0 mg/dL
48 hr — up to 8.0 mg/dL
72 hr — up to 12.0 mg/dL

Premature neonates: Cord blood — up to 3.0 mg/dL
24 hr — up to 9.0 mg/dL
48 hr — up to 15.0 mg/dL
72 hr — up to 22.0 mg/dL

2. The spectrophotometer must be a high-resolution type, capable of being set to zero absorbance or balance with a small slit setting corresponding to a band pass of 2.0 nm or less.
3. The wavelength of peak absorption for bilirubin should be checked by running a spectral transmission curve with a solution of pure bilirubin in protein-based diluent at 1 nm intervals from 450 to 465 nm. The peak should be within plus or minus 2 nm of the theoretical value of 455.
4. The plasma should be clear and should not have more than a trace of visible hemolysis. The procedure described (p. 99) for obtaining the samples from newborns will usually yield enough plasma for duplicate determinations if required.
5. The procedure will give acceptable precision and accuracy with bilirubin levels above 4.0 mg per dL. The method is *not* suitable for adult sera or plasmas because of the presence therein of carotenes and other compounds that absorb at or near 455 nm.
6. Exposure of the plasma to strong light and delays in analysis must be avoided.
7. If mold growth in the phosphate buffer is a problem, add a spatula tip of sodium azide, NaN_3.
8. A suitable control is Versatol Pediatric.*

*General Diagnostics Division, Warner-Lambert Co., Morris Plains, N.J. 07950 and Scarborough, Ont. M1K 5C9.

UROBILINOGEN

Increased destruction of red blood cells within the system leads to increased formation and excretion of bilirubin and urobilinogen. When the rate of hemolysis is only slightly increased, the serum bilirubin level may not be significantly raised. In such cases demonstration of increased urobilinogen excretion may be helpful in establishing the existence of a hemolytic process. The use of semiquantitative determinations of fecal and urinary urobilinogen to indicate the presence and extent of a hemolytic process has now been largely discontinued. In cases of clinical difficulty, in which the usual hematological methods yield indecisive results, resort can be made to determination of actual red cell survival time using radioisotope-labeling techniques. (See p. 95). Studies of urobilinogen excretion are invalidated if the patient is, or has recently been, taking antibiotics, since these interfere with the intestinal bacteria that degrade bile pigments to stercobilinogen and urobilinogen. Urobilinogen is diminished in proportion to the degree of obstruction in obstructive jaundice. See also pp. 254 and 256.

BLOOD AMMONIA LEVELS IN HEPATIC DISEASE

Large amounts of ammonia are produced within the body by the deamination of amino acids, both in the tissues and by bacterial action in the gut. Most of this ammonia is taken up by the liver and used in the synthesis of urea. The urea synthesis cycle (Krebs-Henseleit cycle) is shown in simplified form (Chapter 9) on p. 204. The blood ammonia content is normally less than 70 μg per dL, but in certain liver diseases considerable elevations of blood ammonia levels may occur and be associated with bizarre neurological symptoms or coma. These disorders may be inherited or acquired.

Primary Liver Disease. Primary or inherited deficiency of the various enzymes in the urea synthesis cycle is associated with hyperammonemia: these defects are extremely rare. Affected children all show severe mental retardation and characteristically have frequent screaming fits and convulsions. Blood ammonia levels vary from 150 to 800 μg per dL; higher values tend to occur after a protein meal. Indeed, protein intolerance is a common symptom. Chromatography of the serum may show elevated glutamine levels, and this may first arouse suspicion of the diagnosis. Curiously, for unknown reasons blood urea levels are usually normal.

Acquired Liver Disease. By far the most common cause of elevated, usually fluctuating, blood ammonia levels is advanced cirrhosis, in which there is a considerable reduction in functioning liver tissue. Overall liver function is barely adequate for the body's metabolic needs, and some stress such as a high protein intake or alcohol will impair it further. Such patients show moderate elevation of blood ammonia levels and eventually may pass into hepatic coma. The cause of the coma is unknown but may be related to the ammonia levels and to other constituents such as mercaptans and aromatic amino acids. Coma and hyperammonemia are more common in patients who have had portacaval shunts, bypassing the liver in an effort to reduce the portal venous pressure. In these circumstances the liver is unable to exert its detoxifying action directly on the ammonia absorbed from the gut. Reduction of the intestinal flora by giving antibiotics therefore sometimes helps these patients.

Acute Fatty Liver with Encephalopathy in Children (Reye's Syndrome; White Liver Disease)

In 1963, Reye et al. from Australia described this entity and thereby drew attention to what appears to be a worldwide and not excessively rare condition that affects mainly children under two years of age, although some as old as 11 years have been affected. In most instances the disorder begins with an unremarkable upper respiratory tract infection. This improves after two to four days, but within a few days fever recurs and is associated with vomiting; there may also be diarrhea. Hyperpnea commonly develops, and other central nervous system signs usually make their appearance within 24 hours, including lethargy, delirium, convulsions, hypertonic reflexes, coma, and terminal respiratory arrest.

Laboratory Findings. Leukocytosis may be present. Hypoglycemia, hypernatremia, and low glucose level in the cerebrospinal fluid are usual. Serum AST and ALT are generally elevated, and the prothrombin time tends to be prolonged. Ketonuria is present, and the blood urea nitrogen becomes slightly to moderately elevated. Marked elevations of blood ammonia may occur; although this is generally transient, cerebral damage may occur and have serious long-term effects if the child recovers from the acute illness. Many of the patients die, and of those who recover a number have permanent cerebral damage.

Autopsy findings consist of severe fatty infiltration of the liver ("white liver") and of the renal tubules, especially of the proximal convoluted tubules. The brain shows edema and variable but nonspecific neuronal degenerations. The condition appears to represent an acute metabolic disorder of liver and brain, possibly precipitated by a virus infection. The cause is still obscure, and the condition may have a multiple etiology. However, many well-documented cases have been associated with a generalized viral infection, caused by chickenpox, viral hepatitis, Coxsackie B, and certain adenoviruses; vegetable toxins and aspirin have also been implicated.

Serum Cellular Enzymes in Hepatic Disease

There are a number of enzymes whose estimation in serum is of value in the differential diagnosis of liver disease. Of these the more important are: the aminotransferases, alkaline phosphatase, 5′-nucleotidase, gamma-glutamyl transpeptidase, and lactate dehydrogenase. These are discussed in detail in Chapter 7.

REVIEW AND APPRAISAL OF LIVER FUNCTION TESTS

In the present chapter an attempt has been made to collate certain tests commonly used in the investigation of actual or suspected liver dysfunction. Since the functions of the liver are almost innumerable, its reserve capacity enormous, and its ability to recover and regenerate quite phenomenal, no one test is capable of measuring the degree or nature of its dysfunction. For this reason multiple tests are commonly employed, though the good clinician will often be judicious in his selection of investigations. A comparatively few good tests chosen on the basis of sound clinical evaluation and performed with care and accuracy cannot be equaled by any quantity of investigations lacking these essential qualities. It will be noted that a number of tests commonly used in liver function studies are to be found elsewhere than in this chapter—largely because they have major application in the investigation of other systems and conditions or because they are more conveniently grouped in other categories.

Indications for Liver Function Studies

Broadly speaking, candidates for liver function studies fall into two main categories, those who are icteric or jaundiced, and those who are nonicteric.

The causes of jaundice have already been discussed (see p. 246). Most patients with liver disease who are not jaundiced are cirrhotics, convalescent posthepatitis patients, chronic alcoholics, and smaller numbers of patients with rarer conditions, e.g., hemochromatosis, amyloidosis, and glycogen storage disease. Also in this group are those with secondary involvement of the liver from primary disease of other organs or systems, e.g., cases of congestive heart failure and cancer deposits in the liver.

Classification of Liver Function Tests

Although precise categorization is difficult and overlapping occurs, the following is a more or less rational classification of liver function tests:

Metabolic Tests

Primary Enzymic. ALT, AST, LDH, OCT, ICD, LAP, gamma GTP, and serum alkaline phosphatase; depression of blood coagulation factors and of serum proteins manufactured by the liver, especially albumin.

Secondary Enzymic. Alkaline phosphatase, 5′nucleotidase, pseudocholinesterase.

Chemical. Cholesterol esters, hippuric acid synthesis, galactose tolerance, glucose tolerance, blood urea and amino acid levels, and blood ammonia.

Excretory Tests. Bilirubin in serum, feces, and urine, urinary urobilinogen and serum cholesterol levels, serum alkaline phosphatase.

Miscellaneous. Liver biopsy.

Radioisotope Scanning

Application of Liver Function Tests

In Acute Liver Cell Damage

Acute viral hepatitits may be taken as an example. The first tests to show abnormality are the primary enzymic tests. Increases, often enormous, occur in serum alanine aminotransferase (ALT) and serum aspartate aminotransferase (AST); moderate but specific elevations in serum isocitric dehydrogenase (ICD) and ornithine carbamyl transferase (OCT); and relatively minor increases in serum lactate dehydrogenase (LDH) (see Chapter 7, p. 178). Serum alkaline phosphatase becomes elevated more slowly and usually to levels between 5 and 10 Bodansky units per dL (rarely above 15 units), or between 13 and 25 King-Armstrong units (rarely above 30 to 35 K-A units). In cases that progress to necrosis of liver, e.g., acute yellow atrophy, normal liver functions will be almost in abeyance; blood urea nitrogen falls, serum amino acids become elevated, aminoaciduria occurs, and leucine and tyrosine crystals may be found in the urine. Spontaneous bruising may occur as a result of depression of blood clotting factors. Prolonged elevation of serum aminotransferase levels may be found in some individuals, occasionally for many months following infection, but this does not appear to be of any clinical significance.

Portal Cirrhosis

During the early phase of cirrhosis, or between periods of decompensation, affected individuals may appear clinically normal. Borderline elevations of the aminotransferases and alkaline phosphatase and total bilirubin levels may occur. The alkaline phosphatase may show a disproportionate increase compared to the bilirubin levels.

In advanced cirrhosis, or during periods of functional decompensation (such as occur following a period of high alcohol intake), jaundice occurs, with variable elevation of the serum alkaline phosphatase activity, of 5′-nucleotidase (depending on the degree of cholestasis), and of the aminotransferases and gamma-glutamyl transpeptidase (depending on the degree of active cell destruction). When present, β-γ fusion on protein electrophoresis is pathognomonic. Estimation of lactate dehydrogenase alone is not generally a useful test, the isoenzyme pattern giving more information. Total bilirubin levels are seldom high, unless there is some complicating factor, and conjugated and unconjugated fractions are present in approximately equal proportions.

Obstructive Jaundice

The site of the obstruction may be intrahepatic or extrahepatic, and the distinction may be difficult (see further below). In extrahepatic obstruction (e.g., due to gallstones), a marked rise in serum levels of conjugated bilirubin, alkaline phosphatases and 5′-nucleotidase occurs. The aminotransferases show only a modest elevation. Urobilinogen may appear briefly in the urine at the beginning, but soon disappears, and instead large amounts of bilirubin are excreted in the urine, together with bile acids. The presence of bile acids (which have detergent properties) is responsible for the frothing of such urine when it is shaken.

In cases of prolonged cholestasis, the prothrombin time increases considerably (caused by failure to absorb vitamin K), and there is a marked elevation of serum cholesterol levels after several weeks, associated with the formation of xanthomatous nodules in the skin, especially on the palms and extensor surfaces.

DIFFERENTIATION OF INTRAHEPATIC ("MEDICAL") JAUNDICE FROM POSTHEPATIC ("SURGICAL") JAUNDICE

As the alternative names imply, this distinction is frequently of great importance. Generally, accurate differentiation is possible only in the earlier phases by means of the tests under discussion, since prolongation of posthepatic obstruction will ultimately lead to liver cell damage. It is important also to remember that the jaundice is obstructive in both types, and obstruction may be partial or complete in either variety. Greatly elevated ALT, AST, and ICD levels in the early stages strongly suggest diffuse hepatocellular damage (hepatitis). LDH isoenzyme separation by electrophoresis can be very valuable; the interpretative scheme devised by Dito (1973) is recommended. The alkaline phosphatase activity of the serum tends to reach higher values in posthepatic than in intrahepatic jaundice, but borderline and overlapping findings are common, so that the test may be of little help in the individual case. In cases of jaundice with cancer deposits in the liver, the alkaline phosphatase tends to be disproportionately high relative to the serum bilirubin level and some impairment of BSP excretion is usually present.

In summary, the biochemical tests should be done early in the course of jaundice and repeated at intervals, and they should be interpreted only in association with all of the available clinical and radiological data. The actual range of tests used need not be extensive; much can be deduced from the alkaline phosphatase and AST levels alone. Needle liver biopsy is sometimes a satisfactory way of resolving a diagnostic problem.

CHRONIC ACTIVE HEPATITIS

This condition is characterized by acute episodes resembling attacks of viral hepatitis, with progression toward a macronodular cirrhosis. Histologically the liver shows both active cell necrosis, and cirrhotic changes with periportal fibrosis and inflammatory cells in the portal triads and extending into the lobules. The disease pursues a relentless course: survival from the time of onset is rarely more than ten years and is often much less.

Active chronic hepatitis appears to have a multiple etiology. Some patients have recurrent fever, arthralgia, skin rashes, and hyperglobulinemia, and virtually only women are affected. This form has been called lupoid hepatitis, and is of particular interest in that many such patients have antibodies to thyroid and smooth muscle and may have positive R.A. latex fixation and positive lupus erythematosus tests. The etiology of this type is unknown, but is thought to have some autoimmune basis.

Active chronic hepatitis may occur as a sequel to an acute attack of viral hepatitis; such patients do not have the systemic or immunological changes of lupoid hepatitis, but most can be shown to have HB_sAg present in the serum. The sexes are affected equally.

Patients in both groups show variable, though often marked, elevation of serum aminotransferase levels, and fluctuating bilirubin levels. Serum alkaline phosphatase may also be elevated, especially later on in the course of the disease. The definitive diagnosis requires a liver biopsy.

CHAPTER 10—REVIEW QUESTIONS

1. Explain how the newer methods of serum amylase assay have overcome the drawbacks of the older amyloclastic procedures.
2. Give the principle of the lactose tolerance test. How may an abnormal result be checked?
3. Give the chemical principle of the guaiacum test for occult blood. What precautions are recommended to make the test more reliable?
4. Describe two methods for the determination of serum bilirubin based on differing principles. Explain the requirement for protein-based standards and for exclusion of light from samples and the analytical problems in determination of serum bilirubin.
5. Describe the formation and excretion of bilirubin and the relationship between its two forms and its estimation.

11 GENERAL CHEMICAL PATHOLOGY

ORGAN PANELS

The main functions of the hospital laboratory can still be summarized as: (i) assistance in making a diagnosis, (ii) confirmation of a diagnosis, (iii) assessment of clinical progress, (iv) assistance with prognosis, (v) assistance with control of therapy.*

Few laboratory tests are pathognomonic, that is, specific for one disease to the exclusion of all other diagnoses. Since the diagnostic method remains unchanged, from a general impression based on the patient's appearance, history, and physical signs to localization of the field of inquiry to a particular organ or body system, there is an increasing tendency to group laboratory tests into operational sets or "panels." The availability of multichannel or multitest automated analyzers has facilitated the use of these panels, and if they are used responsibly and intelligently they can expedite diagnosis by more rapid exclusion of alternatives. A typical set of tests for the detection of liver disease might include measurements for serum total and conjugated bilirubin, aspartate aminotransferase, alkaline phosphatase, serum protein and electrophoresis, gamma-glutamyltranspeptidase, and urine for bile pigments. For the detection of renal disease a panel might include tests for blood urea nitrogen, creatinine, creatinine clearance, routine urinalysis and urine culture, serum protein and electrophoresis, and urine and serum osmolality.

*The performance of tests on a large number of ostensibly normal people with the object of detecting a particular metabolic disorder, or defect (for example, Tay-Sachs disease or phenylketonuria) should be regarded as a separate operation, usually labeled "screening."

SERUM ACETONE—SEMI-QUANTITATIVE TEST

For clinical purposes, an approximate estimate of the serum level of ketones—largely acetoacetic acid and acetone—can be obtained by adding a drop of serum to a crushed Acetest* tablet. A definite pale lavender tint indicates about 5 to 10 mg per dL of serum ketones: this is shown on the color chart that accompanies the tablets as a 1+ reaction. A tint similar to that of the 4+ reaction corresponds to a serum ketones level of about 40 to 50 mg per dL. If a strong 4+ reaction is obtained with neat serum, repeat the process using saline dilutions of the serum: 1:2, 1:4, 1:8. Multiply 40 by the reciprocal of the serum dilution that gives the 4+ color reaction to obtain an *approximate* measure of the serum ketones level.

ASCORBIC ACID

Ascorbic acid (vitamin C) is an essential vitamin. Although its precise metabolic functions are uncertain, there is evidence that it is necessary for tyrosine metabolism and for the biosynthesis of folic-folinic acids. It is

*Ames Co., Division Miles Laboratory, Inc., Elkhart, Ind. 46514 and Rexdale, Ont. M9W 1G6.

necessary for the normal formation of connective tissue fibrils and of intercellular cement substance (hence the increased capillary fragility in scurvy). Many of these functions may be attributable to the reversible oxidation-reduction (redox) properties of the vitamin (ascorbic acid ⇌ dehydroascorbic acid).

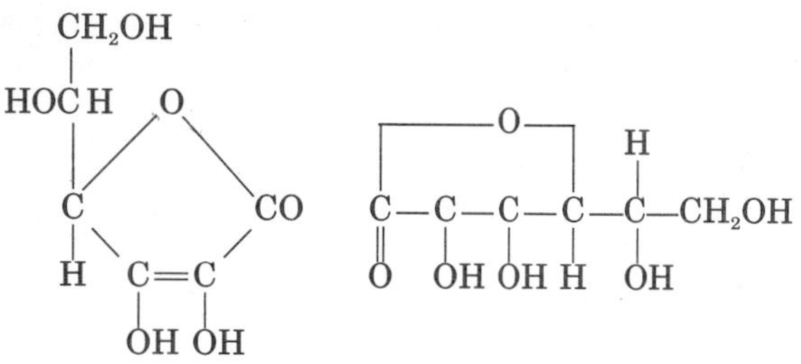

```
  CH2OH
   |
 HOCH   O                 ┌──────O──┐
   |   / \                |         |  H
   |  /   \               |         |  |
   C        CO            C—C—C—C—C—CH2OH
   | \     /              ‖ |  |  |  |
   H  C=C                 O OH OH H  OH
      |  |
      OH OH
```

Ascorbic acid ($C_6H_8O_6$)

The minimal daily requirement of vitamin C is 10 mg, and 30 mg per day is desirable. To ensure this, the diet, before cooking, should contain 70 mg. Plasma levels in a well-nourished population range from 0.5 to 1.2 mg per dL. The concentration in leukocytes is much higher than in plasma (15 mg per 100 g of buffy coat). The adrenal cortex, pituitary gland, and eye are especially rich in ascorbic acid.

The vitamin is quickly destroyed by heat, e.g., cooking and pasteurization. In North America, sporadic deficiency is seen mainly at both extremes of life, in babies aged 8 to 20 months who have been kept for too long on a milk diet, and in elderly persons living alone. Development of clinical scurvy requires about 6 months on a deficient diet. In untreated scurvy the plasma level of ascorbic acid is less than 0.1 mg per dL and the WBC level is below 2 mg per 100 g. Surgical operations cause a 17% and 20% decline in plasma and buffy coat levels, respectively. In patients for surgery, plasma levels below 0.2 mg per dL and WBC levels under 8 mg per 100 g indicate serious deficiency, which may lead to delayed healing or wound dehiscence. Where still performed, assays of ascorbic acid are based on one of the following principles:

(i) The ascorbic acid of a protein-free filtrate of plasma is oxidized to dehydroascorbic acid by the action of Norit (activated charcoal). The dehydroascorbic acid rapidly changes at the acid pH into diketogulonic acid, which is then coupled with 2,4-dinitrophenylhydrazine to form a brown hydrazone: this undergoes a molecular rearrangement (tautomeric change) in strong acid to a soluble red compound whose absorbance is compared with that produced by suitable standards of ascorbic acid similarly treated.

(ii) The ascorbic acid in a protein-free filtrate of plasma will reduce the indicator dye 2,6-dichlorophenol-indophenol (which is pink in acid solution) to a colorless form. The volume of indicator dye required to react with the ascorbic acid in a fixed volume of filtrate is proportional to the amount of ascorbic acid present.

It has been shown that plasma levels of ascorbic acid do not reflect the body status as accurately as those in the leukocytes, and the decline in ascorbic acid determinations is due to the greater technical difficulties of leukocyte assays. For the demonstration of vitamin C deficiency the most convenient procedure is to determine the ascorbic acid level in a 5-hour urine collection by the 2, 6-dichlorophenol-indophenol method after a test dose of ascorbic acid at the rate of 20 mg per kg of body weight. In the presence of severe deficiency less than 1% of the administered dose will be excreted.

CALCIUM, PHOSPHORUS, AND MAGNESIUM

Calcium Metabolism

Dietary Intake and Absorption of Calcium. The daily intake of calcium in the human adult on an average Western diet is some 800 to 1000 mg. This may be considerably higher if much milk is drunk, as milk contains 1.2 g calcium/L; cheese, butter, and hard water are also important sources of calcium. Only 10 to 20% of this ingested calcium is actually absorbed into the body.

Some calcium is present in the digestive secretions and in intestinal epithelial cells that are shed into the digestive tract: about 400 mg per day of endogenous calcium passes into the gut from these sources. This probably pools with the calcium in the food, and from this a total of 600 mg calcium per day is absorbed into the body. Thus the *net* absorption of calcium from the diet is about 200 mg per day.

Calcium is absorbed from the duodenum and upper jejunum by an active carrier-mediated and energy-dependent process, and from the distal small bowel by a process of passive (or possibly facilitated) diffusion.

The rate of absorption of calcium from the gut depends on a number of factors. Normally, humans ingest much more calcium than is absorbed, but, on a low calcium diet, the active intestinal transport is increased. Increased absorption also occurs when there is a greater metabolic requirement for calcium, for example, in children and during lactation. A lactating woman absorbs an extra 300 mg per day, and thus a normal diet containing dairy products usually will provide this without extra supplements. Calcium absorption appears to decrease with age, in both sexes.

The availability of calcium in the diet varies, since it must be present in an ionized form in order to be absorbed. The presence of phytic and oxalic acid, and also of phosphate and fatty acids, can reduce absorption because these substances form insoluble complexes with calcium. However, the effect of these is difficult to assess, since both the ileal mucosa and some cereals contain a phytase that can hydrolyze phytic acid, releasing calcium and phosphate. The presence of some phosphate also appears to be necessary for optimal calcium absorption; only large amounts of phosphate reduce available calcium significantly. Bile and bile salts appear to be of some importance, by increasing the solubility of calcium salts, possibly by the formation of mixed micelles with bile salts and lecithin.

Vitamin D. The name "vitamin D" has been given to a group of steroid compounds that have antirachitic properties and that play a major role in the intestinal absorption of calcium. The naturally occurring compound in man is cholecalciferol (vitamin D_3), which is formed in the skin by the action of ultraviolet rays (295 to 310 nm) on the compound 7-dehydrocholesterol. Only small amounts of cholecalciferol normally are present in the diet; however, milk and butter usually are fortified with the vitamin, and fish liver oils also are a rich source.

Cholecalciferol does not in itself possess biological activity but is transformed in the *liver* to 25-hydroxycholecalciferol, a reaction catalyzed by a specific hydroxylase. This metabolite then is transformed in the *kidney* to 1α, 25-dihydroxycholecalciferol (1,25-DHCC), again by a specific hydroxylase, distinct from the liver enzyme. This second hydroxylation is stimulated by parathyroid hormone. Since the secretion rate of parathyroid hormone itself is directly affected by changes in serum calcium levels, this appears to form the mechanism by which the body adapts to diets of differing calcium content and to varying body requirements for calcium.

1,25-DHCC is the active compound, acting directly on the intestinal mucosal cells to influence calcium transport. Calcium is absorbed into the intestinal mucosal cell initially by a process of faciliated diffusion that is in some way dependent on the presence of 1,25-DHCC. Once in the cell (or in the cell membrane), the calcium ions are bound to a specific transport protein that carries the calcium across the cell to be extruded into the portal blood stream. This second stage is energy dependent and appears to constitute the major point of action of 1,25-DHCC, which probably acts by directly inducing the synthesis of carrier protein. Apart from its effects on the mucosal cells, 1,25-DHCC also has a direct action on bone, mobilizing deposited calcium.

Vitamin D is fat soluble, and its absorption depends on the presence of bile; small amounts are stored in the body fat. Excess vitamin D in the diet is toxic and can cause abdominal pain and vomiting: more serious, however, is the fact that deposition of calcium salts occurs in the kidney, resulting in permanent renal damage. The basic and clinical concepts of vitamin D metabolism are discussed in more detail by Haussler (1977).

Calcium Excretion. The kidney forms the major route for the excretion of calcium. Some 80 to 90% of the daily filtered load of 550 to 700 mg is reabsorbed, leaving a net excretion of 50 to 200 mg, thus balancing the intestinal absorption under normal conditions. When bone is being actively formed, and also during lactation and pregnancy, the total dietary intake is greater than the combined urinary and fecal excretion, that is, there is a positive calcium balance. If the plasma calcium falls below about 7 mg per dL, calcium virtually disappears from the urine.

Plasma (Serum) Calcium. Of the normal total serum calcium, 55 to 60% is ionized; 5 to 10% is complexed (nonionized but diffusible) in combination with citrate, bicarbonate, and phosphate; and about 35% is nondiffusible and nonionized, that is, bound to protein, mainly albumin. Because of this, serum proteins and calcium should always be estimated in parallel.

Distribution of Body Calcium. The concentration of calcium in the extracellular fluids is approximately 65 to 70% of that in the plasma, the difference being caused by the great disparity of protein content. Total plasma calcium in a 70-kg adult is 280 to 300 mg, and the total in extracellular fluids is about 600 mg (exclusive of that in plasma). The bulk of the body's calcium is in bones, in the form of hexagonal, platelike crystals of hydroxyapatite $[Ca_3(PO_4)_2]_3 \cdot Ca(OH)_2$ that measure 50 nm by 25 by 10 nm and are deposited on and parallel to the matrix of collagen fibers. Surrounding these crystals is an extremely thin fluid film (hydration shell), so that bones behave physicochemically as ion-exchange columns. This and the vast area of bone crystals (100 acres) account for the fact that some 20 g of the total 1000 g of calcium in the skeleton is exchanged each day.

Functions of Calcium. Calcium is essential for: (1) the formation, maintenance, and repair of bone; (2) the maintenance of the correct degree of neuromuscular excitability and tone; (3) the proper action of many enzymes, including those involved in the coagulation of blood; and (4) the maintenance of physiological permeability of cell membranes and their pores.

Tetany. If the concentration of ionized calcium in the plasma falls rapidly by 2 to 3 mg per dL (i.e., total serum calcium of 6 to 7.5 mg per dL, provided serum proteins are normal), the patient experiences numbness and tingling in the extremities, together with a feeling of tightness or stiffness or actual cramps in the limb muscles. If the serum calcium declines further, these symptoms are followed by painful carpopedal spasms. In children, spasm of the larynx (laryngismus stridulus) is also liable to occur, and generalized convulsions may ensue at any age. When the fall in serum calcium is gradual, the system usually adapts to the lower levels and mild paresthesia and irritability may be the only signs, although Chvostek's sign (facial spasm when the seventh nerve is tapped) and Trousseau's sign (spasm of limb muscles distal to a constricting tourniquet or blood pressure cuff) usually can be elicited. However, the commonest form of tetany, that caused by alkalosis, is not associated with any decline in the concentration of total serum calcium. This is explainable by the fact that ionization of calcium is depressed by alkali excess, and only ionized calcium affects the neuromuscular junctions.

Phosphorus Metabolism

Phosphate from the food is absorbed in the upper part of the small intestine, and this process is influenced to some extent by the calcium:phosphate ratio in the diet. Phosphate deficiency is practically unknown, since most foodstuffs contain it in abundance. Normally, about one-third of the dietary intake is not absorbed and is excreted in the feces; two-thirds are absorbed and ultimately excreted in the urine. Phosphorus in cereals is largely present as inositol hexaphosphate (phytate). This cannot be absorbed without prior hydrolysis by intestinal phytase, the activity of which is directly proportional to the vitamin D content of the diet. Normally more than 90% of the phosphate in the glomerular filtrate is reabsorbed by the proximal nephron, and when the plasma concentration falls to 2 mg per dL or less, all the phosphate in the glomerular filtrate is reabsorbed and none appears in the urine.

Phosphorus is a very important element in the body. In the bones it constitutes, as phosphate, some 12% of the dry weight, mainly as a calcium phosphate complex of hydroxyapatite type. It is an essential component of many metabolic energizers, for example, the nucleotides adenosine triphosphate and adenosine diphosphate, phosphocreatine of muscle, and glucose-6-phosphate. In the plasma, monohydrogen phosphate ($HPO_4^{=}$) and dihydrogen phosphate ($H_2PO_4^{=}$) constitute part of the buffering system, the plasma phosphate buffer ratio being 0.2 of the monovalent (dihydrogen) salts to 0.8 of the divalent (monohydrogen) phosphates. In urine the opposite ratio obtains, for example, at pH 6.0 the ratio of BH_2PO_4 to B_2HPO_4 is 6.31 to 1.0. Phospholipids form essential structural and metabolic components of most cells and tissues, e.g., cell membranes and myelin sheaths, and also phospholipids and lipoproteins of the plasma.

Total phosphate of the plasma is composed of inorganic phosphate, ester phosphate, lipid phosphate, and nucleotide phosphate. In routine pathological chemistry, however, only the inorganic phosphate is estimated, since the significance of changes in the other fractions is not readily related to clinical problems. There is a general tendency to a reciprocal relationship between plasma phosphate and calcium concentrations. However, because of the multiplicity of controlling influences, this relationship is not simple or uniform, and it is frequently upset in pathological states. Nevertheless, it is mainly because of this relationship that the two are so often concurrently estimated. In uremia and in chronic renal diseases, phosphate estimation is frequently undertaken, since phosphate retention occurs in these conditions (as does hypocalcemia) and contributes to the acidosis. In a normal person serial estimations of plasma inorganic phosphate will show a fall (of 0.5 to 1.5 mg per dL) during a glucose tolerance test; this is evidence of normal glucose utilization, since an essential step in this process is the formation of glucose phosphate. Examples of abnormal calcium and phosphate blood levels are given in Table 11–1. It may be mentioned that in rickets, the fall in serum phosphate is more constant than the decline in calcium. Plasma phosphate also varies with the time of day, rising in the morning; therefore it is preferable to take blood for calcium and phosphate determination from a fasting patient at a definite time of day. The blood should be taken without a tourniquet, since even a short period of venous stasis causes a spurious increase in total plasma calcium; even slight hemolysis should be avoided, since the red cells are rich in phosphate.

TABLE 11–1 Serum Calcium and Phosphorus in Selected Conditions

Condition	Serum Calcium (mg/dL)	Serum Inorganic Phosphate (mg/dL)
Normal — Adult	8.8–10.5	2.5–4.8
Normal — Infant	8.8–12	4.0–6.5
Hypercalcemia:		
Hyperparathyroidism	12–16	1.5–3
Hypervitaminosis D	12–16	4–7
Alkalosis (peptic ulcer diet)	11–14	4–6
Cancer metastases in bones	10–13	3.5–5
Sarcoidosis (generalized)	11–16	3.5–6
Multiple myeloma	10–15	Normal if kidney unaffected
Hypocalcemia:		
Hypoparathyroidism	4.5–8.5	5–8
Chronic glomerulonephritis (advanced to terminal)	4.5–7.5	5–10 (or higher)
Nephrosis (hypoproteinemia)	6.5–10	Normal or slightly elevated
Rickets	7–9	2–4
Malabsorption syndromes (celiac disease, sprue, etc.)	5.5–10	2.2–4.5
Acute pancreatitis (day 2–7)	6–9	Normal or slightly elevated
After multiple ACD blood transfusions	5–9	Normal or slightly elevated

Hormonal Homeostasis of Calcium and Phosphorus

Parathormone. Parathormone is a substance secreted by the parathyroid glands in response to hypocalcemia. It is a single-chain polypeptide of 83 amino acid residues and has a molecular weight of 8500. Unlike many hormones it is not stored in the cell of origin, but is synthesized and secreted continuously. Parathormone has actions both on bone and kidney. In bone it not only has a rapid effect on osteocytes, leading to release of calcium from bone crystal into the plasma, but during phases of pathological hypersecretion it also has a prolonged effect on bone remodeling and calcium turnover.

In the kidney it acts to reduce calcium clearance and enhance phosphate excretion, apparently through the cyclic adenosine 5′-monophosphate (AMP) "second messenger" system within the tubular cells. As outlined earlier, it also plays a critical role in the kidney in controlling the rate of formation of active vitamin D (1α,25-dihydroxy cholecalciferol).

Calcitonin. Calcitonin is a linear peptide of 32 amino acid residues, with a molecular weight of approximately 3600. It is secreted by the C-cells, or parafollicular cells, of the thyroid gland; these are inconspicuous cells that lie in the stroma between the thyroid follicles proper. It is secreted continuously in normal animals, and the secretion rate shows a reciprocal relationship with parathormone secretion, blood calcitonin levels rising during hypercalcemic phases. When injected, calcitonin causes a rapid fall in serum calcium levels, apparently by inhibiting bone resorption and calcium release; it affects calcium levels much more rapidly than does parathormone.

Very high calcitonin levels are found in association with the rare medullary carcinoma of the thyroid gland, which is derived from the parafollicular cells; there is also an increase in circulating calcitonin levels in patients with the Zollinger-Ellison syndrome.

Disorders of Calcium and Phosphate Metabolism

Serum calcium and phosphate levels are closely related in a more or less reciprocal fashion. In most clinical conditions, however, the calcium values are the more important.

Hypocalcemic Conditions

These are frequently, although not necessarily, associated with tetany.

Alkalosis. Generally, acidosis increases the ionization of calcium salts and alkalosis has the reverse effect. These changes are not reflected in the total serum calcium.

The commonest cause of alkalosis is perhaps hyperventilation, which may be hysterical, secondary to disease of the central nervous system, or associated with rarified atmospheric conditions, such as at high altitudes. The mechanism is excessive loss of carbonic acid with diminution of the carbon dioxide content of the blood and consequent elevation of blood pH. Overt or latent tetany commonly develops. Alkalotic tetany also may result from the loss of chloride ions through severe vomiting, prolonged gastric lavage, or acute dilatation of the stomach. In such conditions serum chloride is diminished, and carbon dioxide content, bicarbonate, and pH all are elevated.

Hypocalcemia Caused by Malabsorption. Hypocalcemia and latent tetany are common in severe celiac disease and sprue, since dietary calcium is lost by formation of soaps with unabsorbed fatty acids. The same results are seen in severe pancreatic acinar insufficiency.

Rickets. This condition is caused in the vast majority of cases by deficiency of vitamin D, which leads to inadequate absorption of dietary calcium. The action of vitamin D has already been discussed. In rickets, there is deficient mineralization of the skeleton generally caused by inadequate calcium absorption. Occasionally, rickets follows excessive loss of calcium and phosphate by the kidney (renal rickets). The reduced absorption of calcium usually follows primary deficiency of vitamin D, either because of an inadequate diet or insufficient sunlight. Secondary deficiency of the fat-soluble vitamin D tends to occur in malabsorptive states, for example, obstructive jaundice, celiac disease, and fibrocystic disease of the pancreas (mucoviscidosis).

Bone changes in rickets consist of excessive preparation for, but inadequate accomplishment of, mineralization. Cartilage cells proliferate but fail to undergo normal degeneration, provisional calcification, vascularization, and ossification. This results in thickened, soft, easily deformed, and therefore irregular, epiphyseal plates (e.g., "rickety rosary" of the costochondral junctions). Similarly, osteoid tissue forming beneath periosteum fails to mineralize, and this gives rise to bowing of long bones if the children are walking, and accounts for soft areas in the skull bones (craniotabes). Not infrequently, vitamin C deficiency coexists.

BIOCHEMICAL CHANGES IN RICKETS. The commonest biochemical pattern seen in well-developed rickets is that of serum inorganic phosphate below 3 mg per dL, with serum calcium ranging from 7.5 to 9 mg per dL, typical values being serum phosphate, 2.5 to 3 mg per dL, and serum calcium, 8 to 8.5 mg per dL. When rickets begins to heal, both the serum calcium and phosphate tend to rise. As the serum calcium reaches normal levels, the excessive secretion of parathormone is abolished. The healing bones then take up calcium and phosphate at such a rate that tetany is likely to develop. A marked elevation of alkaline phosphatase also occurs.

Osteomalacia. After completion of growth and union of epiphyses, rachitogenic conditions give rise not to rickets but to osteomalacia. This consists of the deposition of uncalcified osteoid on existing bone trabeculae, plus variable degrees of demineralization of the trabeculae. The softened bones tend to bend at points of stress, thus causing pelvic and other deformities. The condition used to be common in countries in which diets with inadequate or borderline levels of vitamin D and calcium were prevalent. Osteomalacia occurs most often in childbearing women, because they require greater amounts of vitamin D and calcium.

Biochemically, the sequence of events in osteomalacia is the same as in rickets: as serum calcium tends to fall below normal, parathormone secretion is stimulated; this mobilizes calcium from the bones and increases phosphate excretion in the urine. As a result, most patients show only slight depression of serum calcium (7.5 to 8.5 mg per dL) but considerable lowering of serum inorganic phosphate (2.5 to 3.5 mg per dL). Serum alkaline phosphatase is moderately raised but never attains the high values seen in rickets.

Hypoparathyroidism

SURGICAL HYPOPARATHYROIDISM. The commonest cause of hypoparathyroidism is surgical interference with these glands in the course of thyroidectomy. Most often the condition is temporary and caused by trauma to the parathyroids or interference with their blood supply. Permanent hypoparathyroidism is probably a less common result and is the result of inadvertent removal of the glands or their atrophy because of obliteration of their blood supply. In surgical hypoparathyroidism, depending on the severity of damage to or degree of ablation of the parathyroids, signs of latent or overt tetany may be elicited within a few hours of the operation or not until 1 to 4 or more days thereafter. If all parathyroid glands have been destroyed or removed, the serum calcium will fall to 5.0 to 6.0 mg per dL. In the commoner, temporary forms, the serum calcium usually ranges from 7.5 to 6.0 mg per dL, and the serum inorganic phosphate displays a reciprocal increase to values between 5 and 7.5 mg per dL, in adults.

IDIOPATHIC HYPOPARATHYROIDISM. This very rare condition may occur at any age.

Hypercalcemic Conditions

In these, the serum calcium is usually above normal and the serum inorganic phosphate is proportionately reduced. However, just as rickets is an exception to the reciprocal calcium:phosphate relationship in hypocalcemic conditions, exceptions are also seen in hypercalcemic states, notably in hypervitaminosis D, sarcoidosis, metastatic cancers affecting bone, and advanced hyperparathyroidism when renal failure develops.

Elevation of serum calcium depresses neuromuscular excitability. Hence, sluggish weakness of muscles and constipation are prominent in hypercalcemia, as are irritability, mental torpor, and anorexia; polyuria is usual. Death is liable to occur when the serum calcium rises above 17 mg per dL. Hypercalcemia of more than a few weeks' duration is apt to lead to metastatic calcification, especially in sites that are relatively alkaline owing to excretion of acidic ions, for example, lungs, kidneys, and stomach; but calcification also may develop in the walls of blood vessels.

Hypercalcemia in Sarcoidosis. Extensive sarcoidosis may produce hypercalcemia even in the absence of bone involvement. This appears to be caused by excessive intestinal absorption of calcium. The metabolic changes resemble those caused by vitamin D excess; whether this is due to an increased sensitivity to vitamin D, to the presence of some substance resembling vitamin D, or to other factors, is still unresolved at present.

Osseous Metastases. Widespread osteolytic metastases of neoplasms usually are associated with mild to moderate hypercalcemia, normal or slightly elevated serum inorganic phosphate, hypercalciuria, and increased output of hydroxyproline in the urine, the latter reflecting the breakdown of the collagenous osteoid bone matrix. More often than not the alkaline phosphatase is not elevated in such osteolytic lesions, but it is elevated if there is osteoblastic activity or liver metastases. Elevation of serum calcium in multiple myeloma usually is caused by the increased calcium-binding of the raised serum globulins, but rapid and extensive bone destruction undoubtedly contributes. With the onset of renal impairment, the serum calcium falls and inorganic phosphate rises.

Administration of estrogens in the treatment of breast cancer has caused hypercalcemia that has occasionally been fatal. Such hypercalcemia has occurred in the absence as well as in the presence of osseous metastases. Monitoring of serum calcium during such therapy is necessary. It is important to remember that malignancy is by far the commonest cause of hypercalcemia.

Hyperparathyroidism. Hypersecretion of parathormone may be a primary or secondary condition. The secondary form is a feedback response to hypocalcemia, which itself can occur in malabsorption states, uremia, rickets, and osteomalacia. The primary form is usually caused by a functioning adenoma in one parathyroid gland; occasionally, multiple adenomas may be present. Rarely either carcinoma or hyperplasia of all 4 glands may occur.

Excessive parathormone produces a number of serious pathological changes: (1) Withdrawal of calcium from the bones, producing cystic lesions, with giant cell tumors, bone pain, and pathological fractures. (2) Hypercalcemia, with vague symptoms of malaise, anorexia, vomiting, and weight loss. Thirst and polyuria occur as a consequence of the osmotic diuresis required to excrete the abnormal calcium load. (3) Metastatic calcification, most commonly in the tissues of the kidney. Stones also form in the renal pelvis, and produce secondary effects such as pyelonephritis and hydronephrosis. The disease has, in fact, been called one of "stones, bones, and abdominal groans." There is a higher incidence of pancreatitis and peptic ulcer in these patients, but severe abdominal pain can occur without any demonstrable lesion.

All patients with a history of renal stones should have several serum calcium estimations. Occasionally, the hypercalcemia may be the only feature and may have been discovered unexpectedly. The disease is slightly more common in women.

DIAGNOSIS OF HYPERPARATHYROIDISM. The definitive diagnosis of hyperparathyroidism requires the estimation of serum parathormone levels by radioimmunoassay. This particular assay has posed a number of difficult technical problems. However, highly specific assays for the C-terminal of the peptide are now commercially available.

In the absence of parathormone assays, the diagnosis is not easy, and considerable reliance must be placed on accurate serial calcium estimations, preferably measuring ionized calcium. In a patient with primary hyperparathyroidism, such a series will not only give a mean value higher than normal (occasionally close to the upper limit of normal), but will show greater variance than normal. In the few patients who have bone disease, an elevated serum alkaline phosphatase activity is found.

Estimation of Serum Calcium

The multiplicity of published methods for determination of serum calcium is an indication of the analytical problems involved. The normal range is very narrow—8.8 to 10.5 mg per dL, 2.2 to 2.63 mmol per L—and it would be desirable to achieve a precision of about ±1.0%, permitting results for clinical purposes reliable to about ±0.1 mg per dL (±0.025 mmol per L). The methods can be divided into the following groups:

(i) Precipitation of the calcium as an insoluble compound with such reagents as oxalate, chloranilic acid, and picrolonic acid, with subsequent determination of the precipitate by titration or colorimetric methods.

(ii) Formation of colored complexes between calcium and a variety of dyes, such as alizarin, *o*-cresolphthalein complexone, calcein, ammonium purpurate (murexide), nuclear fast red, and others, followed by colorimetric determination of the complex.

(iii) A variant of (ii) involving removal of the calcium from a colored complex by titration with a chelating agent such as EDTA or EGTA (EDTA is ethylene diamine tetraacetic acid or one of its salts; EGTA is ethyleneglycol-bis (2-aminoethyl ether)-*N, N, N′, N′*-tetraacetic acid). The end point of the titration is detected by the recovery of the original color of the dye or the disappearance of the fluorescence of the calcium-dye complex. (A chelating agent is a compound that can trap in its molecular structure certain ions, usually cations, rendering them unavailable for chemical reactions.)

(iv) Flame photometry.

(v) Atomic absorption spectrophotometry.

In practice, the most accurate method is atomic absorption spectrophotometry, but even with automation of sample pick-up and calculation of results it tends to be slow and inconvenient for large batches. It is best used as a reference method. For large numbers of tests, a continuous flow analyzer using the reaction with *o*-cresolphthalein complexone has acceptable precision and accuracy. For small numbers of determinations, a micro titration technique as described below can provide clinically useful results. (This method is given here both as a calcium assay procedure and as a good example of the use of microtitration.) In our experience group (ii) methods on discrete-type automated analyzers cannot reliably give standard deviations better than 0.2 mg/dL, although some recent results on a particular instrument may provide a level of precision approaching that of atomic absorption spectrophotometry.* Group (ii) methods performed manually do not yield precision to the expected extent: factors in this area are variations in dye quality, matrix effects from the presence of protein, interference from other ions (such as magnesium), and, in some methods, very high reagent blank readings that preclude the necessary high-precision spectrophotometry.

Flame photometric methods have been handicapped by the low energy emission of the calcium atom in the usual types of flame—propane-air, natural gas–air, or propane-oxygen.

Determination of Ionized Calcium

The serum calcium is distributed between three states: (i) ionized calcium Ca^{2+}; (ii) protein-bound calcium; and (iii) calcium complexed with citrate, phosphate, bicarbonate, and sulfate: these complexes are diffusible and ultrafiltrable. The protein binding of calcium is complex, with varying affinities of the protein fractions for calcium and different binding proportions in disease states as compared with normals. Normally about 80% of the protein-bound calcium is carried by albumin and 20% by globulins. The proportion of the total serum calcium in the diffusible state (the sum of ionized calcium and the small amount of calcium complexes) depends on a number of factors, the most important of which probably are serum protein level, pH, and temperature. An average value is about 60% of the total serum calcium. The true ionized calcium forms about 47% of the total.

Methods of Determination of Ionized Calcium

By filtration or pressure through a membrane of suitable pore size, the diffusible fraction of the serum calcium (the sum of the ionized fraction and the calcium complexes listed in [iii] above) can be separated from the protein-bound fraction and determined by the usual method. A convenient system for preparation of the diffusible fraction consists of a small circular membrane

*ASTRA 8 analyzer, Beckman Instruments, Inc., Fullerton, Calif. 92634 and Toronto, Ont. M8Z 2G6.

in a plastic holder to which is attached a plastic syringe in a spring-loaded holder. The serum sample in the syringe is forced through the membrane by spring pressure, and the filtrate containing the diffusible fraction is collected in a small cup for analysis.*

For determination of the ionized fraction of serum calcium alone the most practical method is the ion-selective electrode. (For principle see p. 67.) The practical problems of pH and temperature control, which affect the level of diffusible calcium, have been met by the design of anaerobic thermostatted flow-through electrodes, with digital read-out of the result.† The most recent instrument of this type incorporates simultaneous determination of the blood pH and correction of the ionized calcium result based thereon.‡ The reference range for ionized calcium is 4.2-5.2 mg/dL (1.05-1.30 mmol/L).

In view of the practical problems it might be argued that use of the Zeisler formula (Zeisler, 1954) may provide information of clinical usefulness, since some investigators have concluded that the values for the ionized fraction derived therefrom do not differ significantly from actual measurements made with the ion-selective electrode. The formula is:

$$\text{Ionized calcium in mg per dL} = \frac{(\text{Total serum calcium in mg/dL} \times 6) - (\text{Protein}/3)}{\text{Protein} + 6}$$

$$\text{Protein} = \text{serum protein in g per dL}$$

For example, for a serum calcium = 9.0 mg per dL, serum protein = 6.6 g per dL, the ionized calcium would be:

$$\frac{(9 \times 6) - (6.6/3)}{6.6 + 6} = 4.1 \text{ mg/dL } (1.03 \text{ mmol/L}).$$

A number of other formulae have been published for "correcting" for total protein concentration or for calculating ionized calcium. However, it has been our personal experience and that of other authors that ionized calcium measured by a modern ion-selective electrode technique correlates better with the total (uncorrected) calcium level than with any mathematically derived figure. Further studies are needed, but it is probable that such calculations (including the example above) are likely to provide misleading results and be of doubtful value.

Serum Calcium Estimation (Diehl and Ellingboe, 1956)

Principle

In strongly alkaline solution calcium forms a complex with calcein, which exhibits a strong yellow-green fluorescence under long wavelength ultraviolet light. The volume of an EDTA solution required to chelate the calcium, destroying the calcium-calcein complex, is determined using the disappearance of the fluorescence to detect the end-point. The volume required by the test is compared with that required for a standard solution of calcium.

Procedure

1. The microburette (see *Notes*) is filled with EDTA solution. Prepare three plastic titration cups containing the following:

Blank. 20 μL deionized water
100 μL 1.25 M KOH solution
10 μL calcein solution

Standard. As for blank, substituting 20μL calcium standard solution for the water.

Test. As for blank, substituting 20μL of serum for the water.

2. The three cups are titrated in turn, under a 100-watt, long wavelength ultraviolet lamp, in a darkened area if possible. The end-point is signaled by the sudden disappearance of the fluorescence. For the best accuracy the test and standard titrations should be done in triplicate. The small sample size and rapidity of the method facilitate this. The use of Polaroid-type sunglasses has been suggested as an aid to detection of the end-point.

Calculation

$$\frac{\text{Test titer} - \text{Blank titer}}{\text{Standard titer} - \text{Blank titer}} \times 10 = \text{mg calcium}$$

per dL. Mg/dL × 0.25 = mmol/L.

Normal Values

The variations in the range of normal values reflect differences in methodology to some extent. For the procedure described, a normal range of 8.8 to 10.5 mg per dL (4.4 to 5.3 mEq per liter) is suggested. Taking into account the difficulty in obtaining the desirable degree of precision, it would seem reasonable to regard as abnormal results below 8.5 mg per dL or above 11.0 mg per dL.

Reagents

Potassium Hydroxide. Dissolve 50 mg pure potassium cyanide, KCN, in 100 mL accurately standardized 1.25 M potassium hydroxide, KOH. Store in a small brown plastic bottle.

Calcein. Dissolve 25.0 mg calcein in, and make up to 100 mL with, 0.25 M sodium hydroxide solution, NaOH. Store in a brown plastic bottle.

EDTA Solution. Spread out in a clean Petri dish about a gram of pure disodium dihydrogen ethylenediaminetetraacetate, $Na_2C_{10}H_{14}O_8N_2 \cdot 2H_2O$, and dry for 4 hours at 110°C. (This temperature must not be exceeded.) Transfer immediately to a desiccator and dry under vacuum for 12 hours. Remove from the desiccator and immediately weigh out 0.372 g. Dissolve in and make up to 100 mL with deionized or double distilled water. Store in a small plastic bottle.

Calcium Standard Solution. In a clean, dry 50 mL beaker weigh out exactly 250 mg of the highest purity reagent-grade calcium carbonate. Add 6.0 mL of 1 M HCl and heat slowly to boiling on a small electric hot plate. Allow to boil very gently until no more acid fumes

---

*"Ultra-free" calcium filter, Worthington Diagnostics Division, Millipore Corp., Freehold, N. J. 07728.

†Orion Research, Inc., Cambridge, Mass. 02139; NOVA Biomedical, Inc., Neutron, Mass. 02164.

‡Instrumentation Laboratory, Inc., Lexington, Mass. 02173.

are evolved. (Test with a moist blue litmus paper held over the beaker.) Allow to cool. With the most precise technique wash out the contents of the beaker into a 1-L volumetric flask with deionized water. Make to volume with the same; store in a polypropylene bottle. This standard contains 10.0 mg calcium per dL. (This standard can be made in smaller lots—e.g., 100 mL—but difficulty may be experienced in boiling off the excess HCl without evaporating to dryness.)

Notes

1. A suitable pattern of ultra-micro burette for the precise addition of very small volumes employs a mercury column controlled by a piston driven by a micrometer screw.* The contents of the plastic cup are conveniently mixed with a very small magnetic stirrer.
2. It is strongly recommended that tests be done in duplicate as a routine, and any results outside the normal range should be rechecked.
3. Serum samples should be separated from the clot without delay to obviate the possibility of calcium transfer into the cells as their permeability changes. Since the red cells contain only traces of calcium, slight hemolysis does not interfere.
4. The ultraviolet lamp used must be the long-wavelength type, with its energy concentrated in the 354 nm region. The short-wavelength type, with emission around 254 nm, is not only unsuitable but dangerous to the eyes.
5. The measurement of the microliter volumes employed in this procedure is facilitated greatly by the use of the positive-displacement–type piston pipettors with disposable capillary tips.
6. It is advantageous to run a parallel determination using a commercial control serum as a check on reagents.
7. A commercially available instrument using the same principle as this manual method, but employing EGTA as the titrant and photometric detection of the end point, is convenient for small numbers of tests or for pediatric use with restricted sample sizes as low as 5 μL.†
8. A variable source of error with all fluorimetric end-point calcium assay methods is the presence of elevated bilirubin levels. If the best analytical accuracy is essential, rather than just an indication of the presence of hypocalcemia or hypercalcemia, recourse should be made to an automated cresolphthalein complexone or atomic absorption method.

Urine Calcium Estimation

Determinations of urine calcium are best made using atomic absorption spectrophotometry.

Normal Values. Since urine calcium excretion is affected by a variety of factors, including calcium intake, skeletal weight, and endocrine status, the results of determinations are meaningful only if considered in relation to these factors. It has been shown that there is an exponential relationship between the calcium intake per kilogram of body weight and the urine calcium expressed as a percentage of the intake. In adults on a calcium intake of 800 to 1000 mg per day, urine outputs above 300 mg for men and above 250 mg per day for women are excessive.

*Arthur H. Thomas Co., Philadelphia, Pa. 19105; Canlab, Toronto, Ontario, Canada M8Z 9Z9.

†"Calcette," Precision Systems, Inc., Sudbury, Mass. 01776.

Serum Inorganic Phosphate Determination (Dryer et al., 1957, Modified by Henry, 1974)

Principle

After precipitation of proteins with trichloroacetic acid, the inorganic phosphate is combined with ammonium molybdate to form ammonium molybdophosphate $(NH_4)_3[P(Mo_3O_{10})_4]$. This compound is then reduced by *p*-semidine (*N*-phenyl-*p*-phenylenediamine hydrochloride) to form the blue complex molybdenum blue. The amount of blue color produced is enhanced by the simultaneous and stoichiometric oxidation of the *p*-semidine to a blue compound. Under the conditions used, the molybdate reagent is not itself reduced. The absorbance of the blue color is compared photometrically with that produced with suitable standards.

Procedure

1. In a test tube mix: 0.5 mL serum, 4.5 mL distilled water, 1.0 mL 30% trichloroacetic acid. Let stand 5 minutes at least. Filter using a 9.0 cm Whatman No. 41 paper. (This yields a clearer fluid than centrifuging.)

2. Set up three test tubes, marked test, standard, and blank. (If the spectrophotometer uses selected round tubes, these can be used directly.) Into the tube labeled test pipette 2.0 mL of filtrate from step 1. Into blank pipette 2.0 mL of 5.0% trichloroacetic acid. Into standard pipette 2.0 mL of the working standard solution.

3. To all tubes add 0.4 mL of ammonium molybdate reagent and mix. Add 4.0 mL *p*-semidine reagent, and mix well. Allow to stand 10 minutes.

4. Read the absorbance of test and standard at 770 nm, setting zero absorbance with the blank, which should be practically colorless.

Calculation

$$\frac{\text{Test absorbance}}{\text{Standard absorbance}} \times 4.0 = \text{mg inorganic phosphate,}$$

expressed as phosphorus, per dL serum.

$$\frac{\text{Test absorbance}}{\text{Standard absorbance}} \times 1.29 = \text{mmol/L}$$

Normal Values

Adults: 2.5 to 4.8 mg per dL (0.81 to 1.55 mmol/L).

Newborns: 4.2 to 8.5 mg per dL (1.36 to 2.75 mmol/L).

Children: 4.0 to 6.5 per dL (1.29 to 2.10 mmol/L), decreasing to adult levels by about 20 years of age.

Reagents

Trichloroacetic Acid, 30.0% w/v. This should be prepared using an unopened bottle of the solid, and all weighing and mixing should be done with a ceramic or plastic spatula, not a metal one. Weigh out 75.0 g pure trichloroacetic acid, $CCl_3{\cdot}COOH$, in a beaker. Dissolve in about 150 mL distilled water; transfer to a 250-mL volumetric flask, rinsing out the beaker. Make to volume, and mix well.

Trichloroacetic Acid, 5.0% w/v. Dilute 16.6 mL of 30.0% w/v trichloroacetic acid up to 100 mL with distilled water and mix.

Ammonium Molybdate Reagent. Dissolve 25.0 g reagent-grade ammonium molybdate $(NH_4)_6MO_7O_{24}\cdot 4H_2O$ in about 700 mL distilled water in a 1 L beaker. With constant stirring, add 84.0 mL of concentrated sulfuric acid in a thin stream. Allow to cool; transfer to a 1 L volumetric flask. Make up the volume with distilled water and mix. Store in a plastic bottle. This reagent keeps well.

p-Semidine Reagent. Weigh out 125 mg of *p*-semidine (*N*-phenyl-*p*-phenylenediamine hydrochloride—the highest purity obtainable) and place in the bottom of a dry 250-mL volumetric flask; tap the flask so that the solid collects in a small heap. Using a long Pasteur pipette, drip 0.5 mL of 95% ethyl alcohol directly onto the heap of *p*-semidine, wetting it thoroughly. Make up to volume with a previously prepared 1.0% w/v aqueous solution of sodium bisulfite, $NaHSO_3$; shake vigorously until as much as possible of the solid has gone into solution. With a good grade of *p*-semidine, solution is almost complete. Filter into a plastic bottle, and store in the refrigerator. Provided the reagent is not left on the bench for long periods, it is stable up to 1 month. It should be returned to the refrigerator as soon as it has been used.

Stock Phosphorus Standard. Dry a small amount of reagent-grade potassium dihydrogen phosphate, KH_2PO_4, in a vacuum desiccator overnight. Weigh out very accurately 146.3 mg and transfer volumetrically to a 100-mL volumetric flask. Dissolve in, and make up to volume with, distilled water. Add a few drops of chloroform, and shake well.

Working Phosphorus Standard. Pipette 1.0 mL of the stock standard accurately into a 100-mL volumetric flask. Add 16.0 mL of 30.0% trichloroacetic acid, make to volume with distilled water, and mix well. This working standard will keep a few days in the refrigerator.

Notes

1. For urine, mix a 24-hour collection thoroughly. Immediately dilute 1.0 mL urine up to 100 mL with distilled water. Mix 5.0 mL of this dilution with 1.0 mL of 30.0% trichloroacetic acid and centrifuge to clear if necessary. Process 2.0 mL of this mixture as for the 2.0 mL of protein-free filtrate in step 2 of the serum method. Prepare a special working standard by diluting 3.0 mL of the stock plus 16.0 mL of 30.0% trichloroacetic acid up to 100 mL with distilled water. The final calculation becomes:

$$\frac{\text{Test absorbance}}{\text{Standard absorbance}} \times 120 = \text{mg inorganic phosphate,}$$

expressed as phosphorus, per dL urine. The range of normal values is from 0.700 to 1.050 g per 24 hours (22.6 to 33.9 mmol/24 hr).

2. The distilled water used for all reagents must be of high purity; if the blank shows any blue color, one source of the contamination may be checked by substituting deionized for distilled water in reagents.

3. For filter photometers use a filter with a maximum transmission at about 660 nm.

4. To avoid increase in the organic phosphate level of serum, after removal of blood from the vein, by the action of phosphatases, the serum must be separated from the clot as soon as possible. Urine samples may be preserved by addition of about 5.0 mL concentrated HC1 per liter.

5. Heparinized plasma is not suitable for estimation of inorganic phosphate because of the presence of this ion in commercial preparations of heparin.

6. The expression of inorganic phosphate in milliequivalents per liter is complicated by the occurrence of this ion in the serum in two forms—HPO_4^{--} and $H_2PO_4^-$. At physiological pH, about 80% is present in the former mode and 20% in the latter. To convert mg per 100 mL to mEq per liter, a weighted factor has to be used, viz., $10\ (0.8 \times 2/31) + 10\ (0.2 \times 1/31) = 0.58$. This factor is accurate only at the normal blood pH of 7.4, since the ratio of HPO_4^{--} to $H_2PO_4^-$ will vary with pH.

7. The majority of routine methods for determination of inorganic phosphate involve the initial formation of a compound such as molybdophosphate; the chief variations are in the nature of the reducing agent employed to convert this to molybdenum blue. Stannous chloride and aminonaphthol sulfonic acid have the disadvantage of instability, although they both give good color yields. The *p*-semidine reagent is easily and quickly prepared and keeps for a reasonable time.

8. For processing small to medium batches of serum inorganic phosphate assays a number of kits of reagents have been marketed. The general principles are similar: a single reagent incorporates molybdate, a reducing agent, a surfactant, and in some instances a catalyst. When serum is added, the phosphate thereof reacts with the molybdate to form phosphomolybdate, which is simultaneously reduced by a ferrous salt or other reductant, the reaction being accelerated by a catalyst. The reagent is strongly acid, but the precipitation of serum protein, which would otherwise take place, is prevented by the relatively high concentration of surfactant. The blue-green color produced is compared in the spectrophotometer with that developed by a suitable standard. The method is quick, simple, and cheap: errors may be caused by hemolysis, elevated bilirubin levels, lipemia, and, with some reagents, high glucose levels. The amount of surfactant is adequate for normal protein levels and nature: if an abnormal protein is present, as in multiple myeloma, severe turbidity will develop. This is obvious with substantial amounts of the abnormal protein: smaller amounts will produce enough turbidity to give errors but not to be obvious to the naked eye. In our experience the standard must be a protein-containing formulation.

MAGNESIUM

Magnesium Metabolism

Dietary magnesium is absorbed from the upper small intestine and is excreted in the urine. Fecal magnesium represents only that which has not been absorbed from the diet. The Mg^{++} ion is essential as an activator for a great number of enzymes, for example, all the phosphatases and phosphorylases and enolase, and as a cofactor for leucine aminopeptidase and some decarboxylases. Possibly in some cases the magnesium ion may act as a link between enzyme and substrate. The manganese ion can substitute for magnesium in the activation of some enzymes. Magnesium appears to be necessary for oxidative phosphorylation by mitochondria.

As an intracellular cation it is second only to potassium. About 35% of serum magnesium is bound to protein. In general, serum magnesium concentration tends to vary reciprocally with that of calcium. Both have a similar effect on neuromuscular excitability:

$$\text{Neuromuscular excitability} \propto \frac{Na^{+} + K^{+}}{Ca^{++} + Mg^{++} + H^{+}}$$

In other words, increased concentrations of calcium and magnesium tend to depress neuromuscular excitability. (Clinically, hypercalcemia and hypermagnesemia tend to produce drowsiness and atonia.) On the other hand, hypocalcemia and hypomagnesemia tend to produce increased excitability, tremors, and even tetany. It should be clearly understood, however, that this is not a mathematically useful formula, but rather a mnemonic for some of the factors influencing neuromuscular excitability.

After calcium, sodium, and potassium, magnesium is the fourth most abundant cation in the body. As with sodium, about half the total body content is in bones and is not readily mobilizable. Almost all of the remainder is within cells (approximately 20 mEq per liter of intracellular fluid in liver and muscle, 17 mEq per liter in kidney, 13 mEq per liter in brain, and only 6 mEq per liter in red cells). Within cells, only about one-third of the magnesium is free, because of its great tendency to form complexes with many substances, especially ATP, with which it is virtually always associated as a 1:1 complex.

The average adult intake of magnesium is about 300 mg per day, largely from chlorophyll. The daily requirement appears to lie between 200 and 250 mg. Although no single factor controls magnesium absorption, it appears that the magnesium and calcium ions share the same transport system during absorption by both intestinal mucosa and renal tubules, i.e., they compete with each other for absorption at these sites.

Magnesium Deficiency (Table 11–2)

Magnesium depletion probably occurs with some frequency in states of vomiting, diarrhea, and continuous gastric or bowel aspirations and in the course of potassium depletion. The symptoms of magnesium depletion are minor, consisting largely of weakness and general apathy. In severe depletion states, the serum level may fall below about 1.3 mEq per liter, and tremors, muscle weakness, and irritability appear.

Hypermagnesemia

Therapeutically, serum magnesium levels between 4 and 7 mEq per liter are optimum for sedation in eclampsia. Similar or higher values may be found in severe chronic renal failure, and the signs of uremia may be due in part to hypermagnesemia. Values of 5 to 9 mEq per liter may be found in severe diabetic coma. In untreated Addison's disease there are elevated plasma levels and reduced renal excretion of magnesium. In uremia there is an increase in total body magnesium, which is stored chiefly in bone.

TABLE 11–2 CONDITIONS ASSOCIATED WITH ALTERED SERUM MAGNESIUM LEVELS

Hypomagnesemia	Hypermagnesemia
Hyperaldosteronism	Addison's disease and adrenalectomy
Acidosis	Acute and chronic renal failure
Treated diabetic coma	Untreated diabetic coma
Acute pancreatitis	
Delirium tremens	
Hyperparathyroidism	
Prolonged gastric suction	
Prolonged fluid therapy	
Diuresis, pathological or therapeutic	
Malabsorption syndromes	
Hypercalcemia	

Determination of Serum Magnesium

With the availability of practical atomic absorption spectrophotometry, this is the preferred method, since it combines simplicity with precision. Before this, the most common technique involved the use of a dye-lake method, in which titan yellow (also called Clayton yellow and thiazole yellow) is adsorbed on to colloidal particles of magnesium hydroxide ($Mg[OH]_2$) produced when the magnesium in the serum encounters strongly alkaline conditions. (About 70% of the serum magnesium is in the form of free ions; the rest is bound to proteins.) The dye-lake produced is magenta in color, and its absorbance is enhanced and the lake stabilized by polyvinyl alcohol in some published methods. Flame photometry has been used, as well as the formation of a fluorescent complex with 8-hydroxyquinoline. These varying approaches to the assay, plus the influence of the magnesium compound used to prepare standards, have produced a variety of normal ranges in the literature. The value quoted in the method below is therefore somewhat of a compromise. One unusual observation is that magnesium levels in CSF are about 30% higher than in the corresponding serum, in contrast to calcium, whose CSF level closely follows that of the ionized fraction in the serum.

Procedure

For the principles of atomic absorption spectrophotometry, see p. 81. Operational details will vary with the particular instrument used, and therefore cannot be given in detail here. A typical method uses the magnesium emission line at 285.21 nm, with dilution of test sera, controls, and standards in the proportion of 0.2 mL serum in 10.0 mL of lanthanum-perchloric acid diluent. The magnesium hollow cathode lamp is run at a current of 2.5 mA. Sensitivity is excellent, and no scale expansion is needed. For microwork sample volumes as low as 50 microliters can be used.

Normal Values

Adult and infant values are similar.

Serum: 1.6 to 2.6 mg/dL (0.65 to 1.05 mmol/L) (1.3 to 2.1 mEq/L).

Adult urine: Males, 35 to 224 mg/day (1.44 to 9.22 mmol/day); females, 55 to 213 mg/day (2.26 to 8.77 mmol/day).

Notes

1. Hemolyzed serum should not be used—erythrocyte magnesium content is higher than that of serum.
2. Serum magnesium levels may be erroneously low if the blood is obtained shortly after administration of intravenous calcium gluconate.
3. If the urine collection has a deposit of phosphates, redissolve this with a few mL of hydrochloric acid, mix, and then take the aliquot for assay. If the addition of acid is incompatible with other determinations, warm a small aliquot of the well-mixed urine before removing the assay sample.
4. Elevated levels of serum magnesium may be encountered in women treated with magnesium salts in eclampsia and in their neonates.
5. For urine samples, make an initial 1:5 dilution of the well-mixed urine with distilled water before processing as for serum, and multiply the final answer by 5.

Plasma Hemoglobin Determination (Harboe, 1959)

Principle

The absorbance of the Soret band of hemoglobin at 414 nm is determined and compared with the extinction coefficient of hemoglobin after application of an Allen-type correction for background absorbance.

Procedure

1. The blood sample collection must be made with the minimum amount of mechanical damage to the red cells. Avoid a tourniquet if possible, and use a deft and gentle technique for entry into the vein. Heparin is the preferred anticoagulant, and the quantity in the syringe should be just enough to wet the walls and fill the dead-space. After obtaining the sample, remove the needle from the syringe and allow the blood to flow under the unassisted pressure of the piston alone into a clean tube. Centrifuge and transfer the plasma to a clean tube immediately.

2. Set the spectrophotometer—which must be a high-resolution narrow band-pass instrument—to zero with distilled water at 414 nm. Since the best precision of readings is required, a double-beam instrument is preferable.

3. Add 0.4 mL of plasma to 3.6 mL of distilled water, and mix by gentle inversion. Determine the absorbance of the mixture in a 1-cm light path precision square cuvette at 398, 414, and 429 nm. If the instrument has a per cent transmittance scale, record the readings to ± 0.5% T, convert to absorbance by the formula Abs = 2 − log%T, and use as a check on the readings from the absorbance scale.

Calculation

$$\text{Corrected Abs} = \text{Abs at 414 nm} - \frac{\text{Abs at 398} + \text{Abs at 429}}{2}$$

Corrected Abs × 266 = mg hemoglobin per dL of plasma.

Normal Range

Up to 10 mg per dL.

Notes

1. The above procedure should be regarded as only semiquantitative; if maximum accuracy is required, a method using the catalytic action of hemoglobin on the oxidation of benzidine or one of its homologs by peroxide should be used (Naumann, 1970).
2. The plasma must not have an elevated bilirubin level, since this will interfere because of its absorption at 410 nm.
3. If the plasma is grossly hemolyzed, use 0.2 mL plasma plus 3.8 mL distilled water, and multiply the final result by two.
4. Elevated values are found in paroxysmal nocturnal hemoglobinuria, in the acute phases of malignant tertian malaria (the excretion of hemoglobin in the urine in this disease gives it its common name of "blackwater fever"), in severe transfusion reaction, in the acute phase of sickle cell anemia, and to a lesser degree in acquired hemolytic anemia. In view of the care needed to exclude damage to red cells during blood sampling, great weight should not be attached to small elevations.

CEREBROSPINAL FLUID

Formation of Cerebrospinal Fluid and the Blood-Brain Barrier

The cerebrospinal fluid (CSF) is formed by the choroid plexuses, which are tufts of capillary blood vessels in the cerebral ventricles. Basically, the fluid is a filtrate of plasma, similar to interstitial fluid and glomerular filtrate, but with certain important differences. Unlike a similar blood filtrate, in which the crystalloids are in the same concentration as in the original plasma, in CSF many of the crystalloids are in different concentrations. For example, sodium and chloride levels are higher, whereas those of potassium, calcium, bicarbonate, phosphate, sulfate, and glucose are lower. This difference in ionic and crystalloid distribution between the blood in the vessels of the choroid plexuses and the CSF is one reason for the theory that the lining cells of the plexuses (between the two fluids) actively regulate passage of these substances across the capillary walls.

Although many substances cross capillary walls from the blood to the tissues elsewhere in the body, some are prevented from crossing the walls of the choroid plexus capillaries by the vital action of the lining cells. Among such substances are bile pigments and many drugs, such as penicillin. This phenomenon generally is referred to as the blood-brain barrier and arises from the fact that the endothelial cells of the cerebral vessels are all united by continuous "tight" junctions, unlike the endothelial cells in other organs. Under pathological conditions, especially in inflammatory processes, the blood-brain barrier is destroyed.

Pathway of the Cerebrospinal Fluid

From the choroid plexuses in the lateral cerebral ventricles, the fluid passes through the ventricular system and emerges through three minute apertures over the fourth ventricle to the subarachnoid space. The latter covers the brain and spinal cord, and prolongations surround the tiny blood vessels that enter the brain substance. CSF is returned from the subarachnoid space through arachnoid villi to the blood in the dural sinuses. Obstruction to the pathway will give rise to varied clinical pictures, and one of the commonest varieties is congenital hydrocephalus, in which the intracerebral pathway is blocked.

Functions of the Cerebrospinal Fluid

Protection. CSF acts as a fluid cushion around the brain, preventing injury to the relatively soft cerebral substance by such forces as inertia and gravity. The effective weight of the brain is reduced in the surrounding fluid (Archimedes' principle), and this reduction of weight is further protection against these forces.

Volume Regulation. Variations in the amount of CSF permit the brain volume to remain undisturbed, despite changes in blood volume in cerebral vessels within the rigid bony cranium.

Nutrition. CSF may serve as an agent in the exchange of metabolites between blood and brain.

Composition of the Cerebrospinal Fluid

The chemical substances within the CSF that are of clinical interest include proteins and glucose. Although changes in the content of these substances may be the result of intracranial disease, it should be appreciated that they may also reflect metabolic disturbances elsewhere. For example, in uncontrolled diabetes mellitus, there may be a raised glucose level.

Normal Values for CSF (lumbar puncture unless indicated otherwise) (Glasser and Finley, 1981)

Total proteins	*Lumbar puncture*	
	Adult: 15 to 45 mg/dL	
	Full-term neonate: 20 to 170 mg/dL	
	Premature neonate: 65 to 150 mg/dL	
	Cisternal puncture	
	Adult: 12 to 24 mg/dL	
	Ventricular fluid	
	Adult: 5 to 15 mg/dL	
Glucose	Adult: 50 to 80 mg/dL (2.75 to 4.4 mmol/L)	
	Full-term neonate: 34 to 119 mg/dL (1.87 to 6.55 mmol/L)	
	Premature neonate: 24 to 63 mg/dL (1.32 to 3.47 mmol/L)	
Chloride	118 to 127 mEq/L	
Sodium	144 to 154 mEq/L	
Calcium	4.2 to 5.4 mg/dL (1.05 to 1.35 mmol/L)	
Electrophoresis		**% of total protein**
	Prealbumin:	2 to 7%
	Albumin:	56 to 76%
	α_1-Globulin:	2 to 7%
	α_2-Globulin:	4 to 12%
	β-Globulin:	8 to 18%
	γ-Globulin:	3 to 12%

Changes of Composition of the Cerebrospinal Fluid in Intracranial or Spinal Disease (See also Section on Microbiology)

Proteins. The total protein content of the CSF is 15 to 45 mg/dL; upon electrophoresis, this can be shown to comprise prealbumin, albumin, alpha, $beta_1$, $beta_2$, and gamma globulin bands, with an albumin/globulin ratio of 2:1. Formerly, changes in the globulin content were monitored by nonspecific protein precipitation procedures: the Pandy test (using phenol), the Nonne-Apelt test (using saturated ammonium sulfate solution), and the Lange reaction, in which a colloidal gold solution was added to 10 tubes containing successive dilutions of the CSF. These tests are outmoded and should be replaced by protein electrophoresis performed on concentrated CSF. It is true that this technique is a little more demanding of time and money and generally requires a slightly larger sample than the simpler tests, but on the other hand CSF is more difficult and expensive to obtain than, for instance, serum, and it would seem reasonable to use the more informative technique.

Protein electrophoresis generally does not allow a specific diagnosis to be made, having the same limitations as serum in this respect, but several patterns can be recognized.

1. Alterations can occur in the CSF pattern secondarily to changes in the plasma protein pattern. For example, a myeloma protein can be seen in both CSF and serum. For this reason it is preferable to collate CSF and serum patterns.

2. Capillary permeability pattern. This is found in the course of inflammatory lesions of the meninges, neoplasms, arterial disease, and in the Guillain-Barré syndrome. It is marked by an elevation in the gamma, alpha, and $beta_1$ globulin and albumin. The prealbumin band, normally well-marked, and the $beta_2$ band are diminished.

3. A "degenerative" pattern is marked by an increase in $beta_2$ globulin, and is seen in cerebral atrophy, syringomyelia, and ischemic conditions.

4. The "immunoglobulin" pattern consists of an elevation in one or all of the immunoglobulin components, without a corresponding elevation in the plasma levels. It appears as a diffuse band or a series of bands ("oligoclonal pattern") in the gamma region, and is seen, for example, in multiple sclerosis (with an increase of the IgG class only) and in neurosyphilis (IgM elevation).

In blocking lesions of the spinal cord, the fluid beneath the obstruction is often xanthochromic and has a greatly increased content of protein as a result of leakage of albumins from the blood plasma (Froin's syndrome).

Glucose. Glucose in CSF is characteristically reduced in pyogenic and tuberculous meningitis, and the reduction is the result of the metabolic requirements of the infecting organisms and of the inflammatory cells. CSF glucose also is reduced in disseminated leptomeningeal malignancies, for example, meningeal sarcomatosis, caused by utilization of the sugar by the tumor cells. In infections caused by viruses, the glucose level is normal or may be raised because of impairment of the blood-brain barrier. If there is to be any delay (more than 1 hour) in examining a specimen of CSF for glucose (for example, if the lumbar puncture is to be done in the patient's home, or if the specimen is to be mailed), it should be collected in a bottle to which sodium fluoride has been added. It is usual to use 1 mg fluoride for each milliliter of the specimen. The sodium fluoride prevents glycolysis by inhibiting enzymatic activity.

Chloride. The estimation of chloride in the CSF is outmoded and of historical interest only. It does not provide any additional information of value.

AMYLOIDOSIS

Congo Red Test

Principle. The dye Congo red is a derivative of benzidine and naphthionic acid and has an unexplained affinity for amyloid. When a measured amount of the dye is injected intravenously, a greater proportion of the dose is removed from the blood in a given time by patients with amyloidosis than by normal persons. However, the occurrence of false positive results in nephrosis because of excretion of the dye with albumin and the unreliability of the test in some cases of primary amyloidosis have reduced the clinical value of the procedure to the point where its routine use is questionable. Severe reactions to the dye have also occurred in sensitive individuals, and the test cannot be recommended. The diagnosis should be established by tissue biopsy—a simple rectal biopsy can be positive in many individuals.

CERULOPLASMIN

Copper Metabolism

The adult dietary intake of copper ranges from about 2.5 to 5 mg per day. Foodstuffs rich in copper are liver, shellfish, nuts, and chocolate. Absorption takes place in the upper small intestine and amounts to some 25% of that ingested. Studies with the isotope ^{64}Cu have shown that absorbed dietary copper is carried in the blood in loose combination with albumin. It is thus transported in cupric form mainly to the liver, in which it is transferred to a liver protein, hepatocuprein. The postprandial rise in plasma copper is followed within 2 hours by a rather steep decline, which marks the uptake by the liver. This is succeeded by a second and more sustained elevation caused by the release from the liver of ceruloplasmin-bound metal.

Properties of Ceruloplasmin. This blue protein is an $alpha_2$ globulin and a glycoprotein (7.5% carbohydrate) of M.W. 151,000 that is made by the liver. Normally, ceruloplasmin accounts for 95% of total plasma copper (100 μg per dL). Each molecule of ceruloplasmin contains eight atoms of copper (0.32 to 0.34% by weight), four of which are in the cupric form.

Role of Ceruloplasmin. The role of ceruloplasmin is not known; it does not appear to be that of transport, but there is some evidence that it may have anti-oxidant and anti–free radical properties.

Normal Ceruloplasmin Levels. By the common oxidase methods usually employed, with purified ceruloplasmin as standard, normal values in serum are about 36.0 ± 5.6 mg per dL for men, and 40.9 ± 6.8 mg per dL for women. Mg/dL × 0.06623 = μmol/L.

Conditions Associated with Hyperceruloplasminemia. Elevated serum ceruloplasmin levels tend to occur in the latter half of pregnancy and in acute and chronic infections, myocardial infarction, cancers and leukemias, thyrotoxicosis, and cirrhosis of the liver.

Wilson's Disease *(Hepatolenticular Degeneration)*. This rare condition is inherited as an autosomal recessive abnormality, affecting mainly adolescents and young adults of both sexes. The classic form consists of increasing rigidity, spasticity, and difficulty in speaking and swallowing.

In Wilson's disease, the copper content of all tissues is increased, especially liver and brain tissues. In the liver the concentration of the metal may range from 5 to 30 times normal. However, plasma ceruloplasmin levels are much reduced. Because of the deposition of copper in the liver, cirrhosis develops in most patients.

Serum Ceruloplasmin Determination

Ceruloplasmin can function in vitro as an oxidase. (There is a parallel in the pseudoperoxidatic activity of heme used in tests for occult blood). The extent of the conversion of the substrate, *p*-phenylenediamine hydrochloride, into a purple oxidation product, Wurster's red, is measured spectrophotometrically, and the absorbance reading is converted to milligrams of ceruloplasmin per dL by a conversion factor derived from a highly purified preparation of ceruloplasmin.

Normal Values

Males: 36.0 ± 5.6 mg per dL (2.38 ± 0.37 μmol/L)
Females: 40.9 ± 6.8 mg per dL (2.71 ± 0.45 μmol/L)

PIGMENTS

Spectroscopy of Pigments in Blood and Urine (Table 11–3)

Blood and urine samples for spectroscopy should be fresh and examined immediately. Dry potassium and lithium oxalate are suitable anticoagulants for obtaining plasma, but it is essential to avoid hemolysis as a result of overoxalation. If methemoglobin is being sought, heparin, which does not alter plasma pH, is preferable to oxalate. The plasma should be separated from the red cells immediately, especially if extracorpuscular hemoglobin is to be identified.

The direct-vision spectroscope has only low dispersion, and precise measurement of the wavelengths of absorption bands is not possible. The following procedures are suitable for use with the Hartridge reversion spectroscope if desired. (See Fig. 11–1.)

The instrument iris diaphragm setting, the dilution of the sample, and the amount of extraneous light all affect the certainty with which absorption bands may be detected and their wavelength measured. A range of dilutions of the blood sample from 1 in 50 to 1 in 300 should be examined before the presence or absence of an intracorpuscular pigment is reported, and suitable controls containing the suspected pigments should be prepared and examined in parallel. Plasma and urine are examined without dilution; if they are very densely colored, use a cell with a shorter path length. A negative report should not be made unless at least a 3-inch depth of urine or a 1-inch depth of plasma has been examined. The effect of the reducing agent sodium dithionite, $Na_2S_2O_4$, is determined by adding about 5 mg to the cell,

TABLE 11–3 PIGMENTS IN BLOOD AND URINE

Compound	Where Found	Wavelength (nanometers)	How Produced	Effect of Dithionite
Oxyhemoglobin	1. RBCs	578, 540	Normal	Changed to Hb with band at 556
	2. Plasma		Paroxysmal hemoglobinuria, blackwater fever, pernicious anemia	
	3. Urine		March hemoglobinuria and as for plasma	
Reduced hemoglobin	RBCs	556	Cyanosis	
Carboxyhemoglobin	RBCs	572, 535	CO poisoning	Bands persist
Methemoglobin	1. RBCs	630 (578, 540) 500	Poisoning by coal-tar derivatives, drugs, etc. (familial)	630 band disappears immediately
	2. Plasma 3. Urine		Phenylhydrazine, severe sepsis, esp. with *Cl. perfringens*	
Sulfhemoglobin	1. RBCs	618 (578, 540)	Drugs, sulfonamides	618 band resists action of dithionite
	2. Plasma			
	3. Urine	Not detected		
Methemalbumin (see Schumm's test, p. 280)	Plasma	623, 540, 500	Intravascular hemolysis, incompatible blood transfusion	623 band disappears
Nitric oxide hemoglobin	RBCs	578.5, 541.8	Nitrite poisoning	
Myoglobin	Urine	582, 543	Crush injuries, myositides	

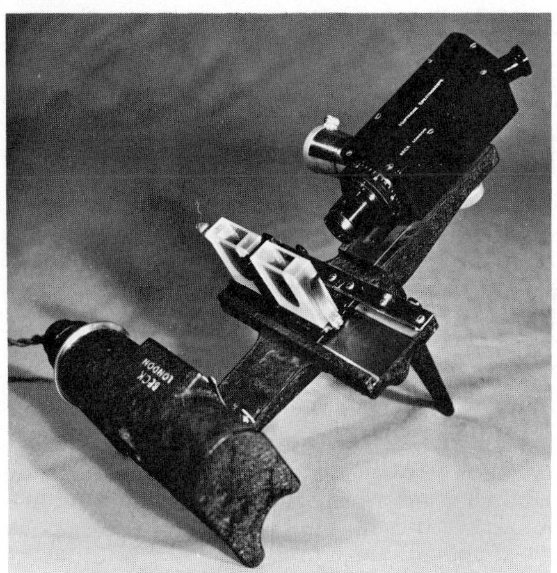

Figure 11–1 Hartridge reversion spectroscope.

inverting several times to mix, and immediately repeating the observation.

The first group of compounds that may be identified in red cells, plasma, and urine are the derivatives of hemoglobin and the related compound myoglobin.

The second group of compounds detectable by spectroscopy are the porphyrins.

The third group comprises substances occasionally responsible for abnormal colors in urine whose identity can be confirmed by spectroscopy. Examples are eosin with an absorption band at 515 nm, phenolphthalein with a band at 560 nm in alkaline urine, and methylene blue with a band at 670 nm (Fig. 11–2).

Preparation of Controls (Levinson and MacFate, 1961)

Carboxyhemoglobin	See under Blood Carbon Monoxide, page 315.
Reduced hemoglobin	To 10 mL of a 1 in 50 dilution of blood add 5.0 mg of sodium dithionite; mix.
Sulfhemoglobin	To 5.0 mL of 1 in 50 blood dilution add 0.9 mL of 0.1% phenylhydrazine hydrochloride and 0.1 mL of water saturated with H_2S or 0.9 mL of strong ammonium sulfide solution. Mix and use immediately (unstable).
Methemoglobin (neutral)	Dilute blood 1 in 50, add a small crystal of potassium ferricyanide, and mix.
Methemalbumin	Incubate 1 volume oxyhemoglobin solution with 4 volumes sterile plasma at 40°C.
Acid porphyrin	Add 0.1 mL whole blood dropwise to 9.9 mL concentrated sulfuric acid, shaking throughout. This solution will also show typical salmon-pink fluorescence under ultraviolet light.

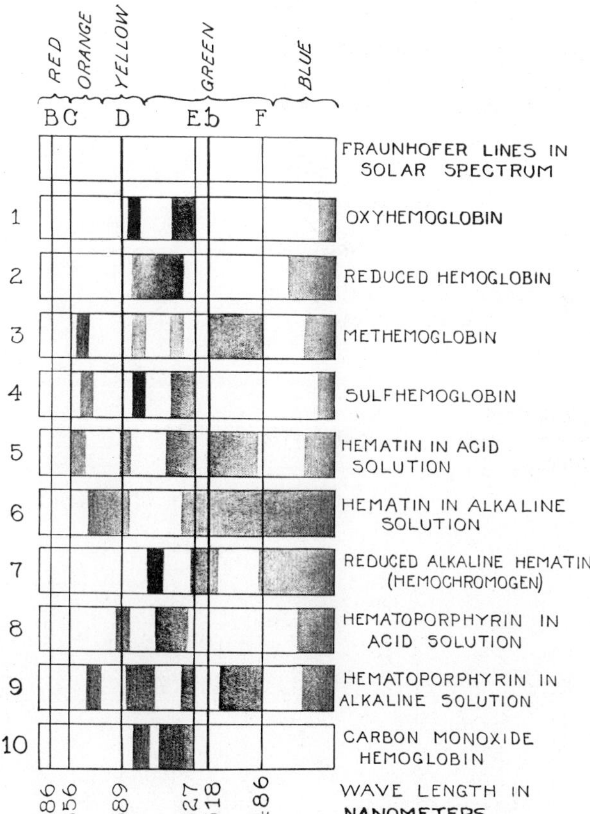

Figure 11–2 Absorption spectra of hemoglobin and its derivatives. (From Todd, J. C., Sanford, A. H., and Wells, B. B.: Clinical Diagnosis by Laboratory Methods. 12th ed., Philadelphia, W. B. Saunders Co., 1953, p. 329.)

Alkaline porphyrins	Add 1.0 mL whole blood to 10 mL concentrated sulfuric acid, mix well, and pour cautiously into 350 mL cold distilled water. Treat the resultant precipitate with about 4.0 mL strong ammonia and filter. Dilute with strong ammonia if necessary.

METABOLISM OF PORPHYRINS

As seen from Figure 11–3, porphyrins are cyclic compounds consisting of four pyrroles joined by methene (-CH=) bridges. This tetrapyrrole structure is characteristic of the nonprotein portion of the oxidative systems of the body, i.e., hemoglobin, myoglobin, the cytochromes, catalases, and peroxidases, all of whose oxidative or oxygen-transferring powers lie in their iron porphyrin structure. It will be obvious that the main porphyrin turnover is concerned with the synthesis of hemoglobin.

As discussed elsewhere, the catabolism of hemoglobin gives rise to bile pigments; i.e., porphyrins are not produced by the degradation of hemoglobin or other heme compounds but arise as by-products during the synthesis of heme. Since practically all cells in the body use and make some heme compounds, almost every cell can manufacture porphyrins. Two tissues, however, are outstanding in this regard: the erythron, because of its continuous and considerable production of hemoglobin (6 g per day); and the liver, because of its mass and the extent and diversity of its metabolic processes.

Synthesis of Porphyrins and Heme

As shown in Figure 11–3, porphyrins are manufactured during heme production from two precursors, glycine and succinate. In the presence of the B complex vitamin, pantothenic acid, succinate (from the Krebs cycle) is activated to succinyl-CoA. It is then condensed with glycine to form deltaaminolevulinic acid (ALA) by the mitochondrial enzyme ALA synthetase which requires pyridoxal phosphate (vitamin B_6) as cofactor. The diagram shows alpha-amino-beta-ketoadipic acid as an intermediate that undergoes spontaneous decarboxylation in this condensation. However, the entire process of condensation and decarboxylation may proceed simultaneously without the formation of this intermediate.

Next, two molecules of ALA are condensed by ALA dehydrase to form one molecule of porphobilinogen (PBG), four molecules of which are then condensed by PBG deaminase to form uroporphyrinogen I. For the production of uroporphyrinogen III, combined action of PBG deaminase and uroporphyrinogen isomerase is required. A decarboxylase now converts uroporphyrinogen (type I or III) to the respective coproporphyrinogen. Next, simultaneous action of a mitochondrial oxidase and decarboxylase converts coproporphyrinogen III to protoporphyrinogen III, which then undergoes enzymatic or spontaneous oxidation to protoporphyrin III. Finally, the enzyme ferroprotoporphyrin chelatase incorporates iron into the protoporphyrin to give protoheme. The various porphyrinogens mentioned are all colorless chromogens and are maintained in this form in the tissues by a variety of reducing agents such as glutathione, cysteine, and ascorbic acid. Also, many of the enzymes involved after the formation of PBG require reduced sulfhydryl groups for their action.

Control of Heme Synthesis

From the foregoing it will be evident that the major rate-limiting reaction or factor in the synthesis of heme is the formation of ALA. Nature's familiar negative feedback control is used to regulate this. The end product (heme) inhibits the formation of the rate-limiting substrate, ALA, by reducing either the activity or the manufacture of ALA synthetase.

Origins of Types I and III Porphyrins

In 1925, the German chemist Hans Fischer reported his success in synthesizing the four isomeric basic or parent etioporphyrins and proposed that derivatives of each parent type be identified by addition of a Roman numeral I, II, III, or IV. Of these four classes, only types I and III have been found to occur in nature. The porphyrins can be regarded theoretically as derived from a parent compound called porphin, which can in turn give rise to 15 different isomers containing varying arrangements of three different types of substitutent

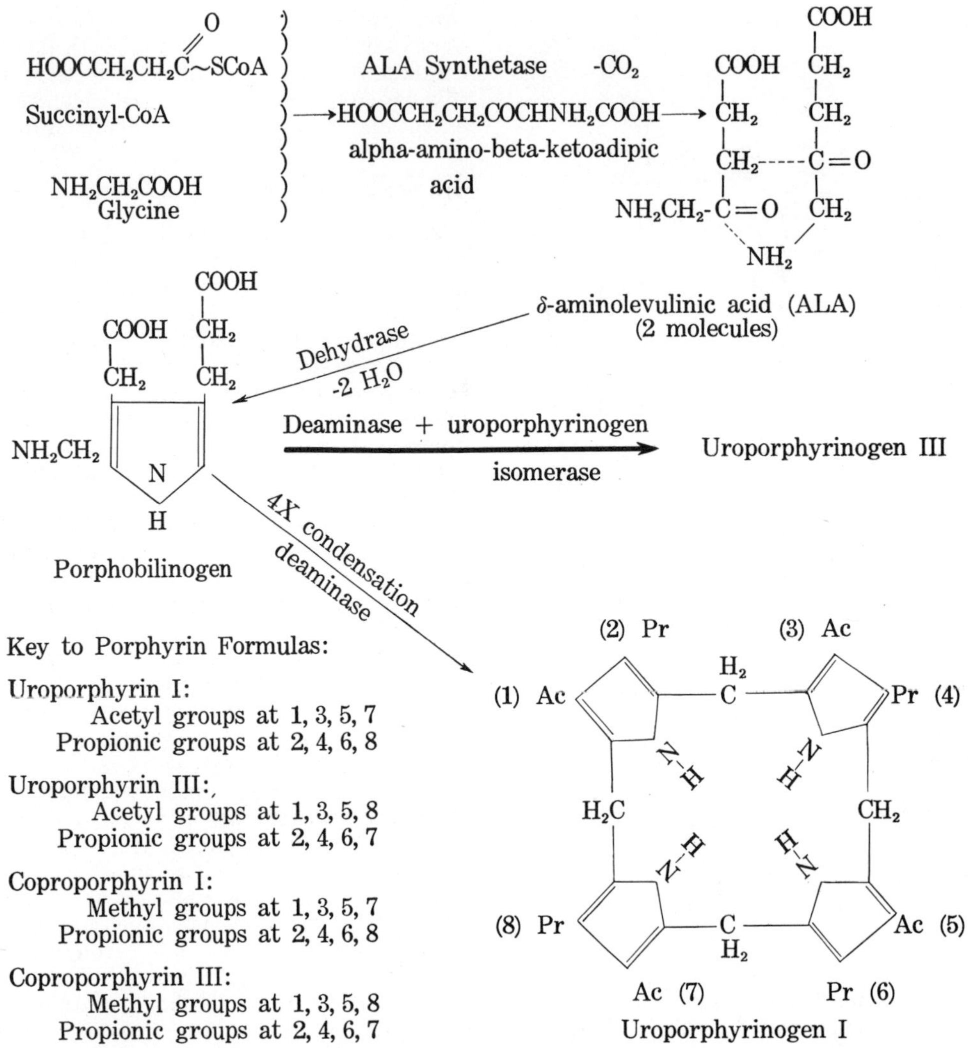

$HOOCCH_2CH_2C(=O){\sim}SCoA$ (Succinyl-CoA) + NH_2CH_2COOH (Glycine) —ALA Synthetase→ $HOOCCH_2CH_2COCHNH_2COOH$ (alpha-amino-beta-ketoadipic acid) —$-CO_2$→ δ-aminolevulinic acid (ALA) (2 molecules)

δ-aminolevulinic acid (ALA) (2 molecules) —Dehydrase, $-2\ H_2O$→ Porphobilinogen

Porphobilinogen —Deaminase + uroporphyrinogen isomerase→ Uroporphyrinogen III

Porphobilinogen —4X condensation deaminase→ Uroporphyrinogen I

Uroporphyrinogen I: (1) Ac, (2) Pr, (3) Ac, Pr (4), Ac (5), Pr (6), Ac (7), (8) Pr

Key to Porphyrin Formulas:

Uroporphyrin I:
Acetyl groups at 1, 3, 5, 7
Propionic groups at 2, 4, 6, 8

Uroporphyrin III:
Acetyl groups at 1, 3, 5, 8
Propionic groups at 2, 4, 6, 7

Coproporphyrin I:
Methyl groups at 1, 3, 5, 7
Propionic groups at 2, 4, 6, 8

Coproporphyrin III:
Methyl groups at 1, 3, 5, 8
Propionic groups at 2, 4, 6, 7

Heme: Methyl groups at 1, 3, 5, 8; Vinyl groups at 2, 4; Propionic groups at 6, 7; and 1 atom of Fe at center.

Figure 11–3 Porphyrinuria: the porphyrias.

groups—methyl, vinyl, or propionic. The most important protoporphyrin, type III, can be regarded as derived from the ninth member of the family, and can thus be described as type 9. All hemes belong to type III and contain only protoporphyrin III(9). This is due to the fact that the enzyme that converts coproporphyrinogen to protoporphyrinogen is specific for type III isomers. The utilization of type III precursors in the synthesis of hemes is very efficient, and only very tiny fractions are wasted by being irreversibly oxidized. On the other hand, type I isomers are incidental by-products that arise in the course of heme synthesis and for which the organism has no use. They arise presumably through the unilateral action of the deaminase on PBG (see the discussion of synthesis).

Normal Porphyrin Excretion

ALA and PBG are excreted in the urine. The urine also is the vehicle for the great majority of uroporphyrin excretion, only a small fraction being excreted in the feces. Most coproporphyrin (mean of about 400 to 500 μg per day) is eliminated via the feces and a smaller amount in the urine. However, because this small amount is, relatively speaking, considerable, coproporphyrin constitutes the great bulk of urinary porphyrin excretion. Protoporphyrin is eliminated only through the bile, the average fecal content being about 1 mg per day.

Urinary excretion of coproporphyrin is increased in obstructive jaundice, liver disease, lead poisoning, and hemolytic anemias.

Etiology of Manifestations of Porphyria

Only two aspects are at all well understood. Photosensitivity is directly connected with the fluorescence of porphyrins. Either this fluorescence or compounds produced by it, such as histamine, or both, damage the epidermal and dermal cells, in which porphyrins probably are produced in some varieties and into which they are absorbed from interstitial fluid in others. Most deleterious is long-wave ultraviolet light (wavelength greater than 320 nm).

The Porphyrias

First, a distinction must be made between porphyrinuria and porphyria. Porphyrinuria is a general term indicating the presence of porphyrins in the urine. This may occur in the course of certain primary diseases, called collectively the porphyrias, but may also be an acquired state, occurring in association with a number of diseases, of which viral hepatitis, hemolytic anemia, lead poisoning, and alcoholism are of importance.

In lead poisoning there is a diminished activity of ALA dehydratase and an increased excretion both of its substrate ALA and of coproporphyrin type III in the urine. These effects occur even at blood levels below which clinical symptoms of lead poisoning occur (that is, in the range of 20 to 80 μg per dL).

The porphyrias comprise a group of rare or uncommon familial disorders, in which some defect of heme synthesis is present, either in the red cells (erythropoietic porphyria) or in the liver (hepatic porphyria).

Erythropoietic Porphyria

Congenital Erythropoietic Porphyria *(Günther's Disease).* This is an extremely rare disorder, in which there is a maturation defect of the erythroid cells in the bone marrow, leading to overproduction of the series I isomers. These accumulate in the skin, and result in extreme sensitivity to sunlight; the initial reaction is burning and blistering, but if the skin is exposed repeatedly to sunlight, severe scarring and mutilation occur. The urine is colored red, of varying intensity, sometimes of the classical "port-wine" color, and large amounts of coproporphyrin I and uroporphyrin I are excreted. The red cells contain excess porphyrins, and the demonstration of this is valuable in diagnosis. The marrow cells, red cells, teeth, and urine show a reddish fluorescence under ultraviolet light.

Erythropoietic Protoporphyria. This is a mild, not uncommon familial disorder characterized by acute urticaria or eczema, developing rapidly on exposure to sunlight. The clinical picture can be very variable; biliary disease often seems to be associated. The urinary excretion of ALA, PBG, uroporphyrins, and coproporphyrins is within normal limits, but large amounts of protoporphyrin III and coproporphyrin III are present in the erythrocytes and also are excreted in the stools. The feces may show a red fluorescence.

Hepatic Porphyrias

To this group belong those conditions in which the liver is solely or primarily the site of abnormal porphyrin production or metabolism and has an obviously increased content of porphyrins.

Acute Intermittent Porphyria. This, although an uncommon disorder, is the most frequently encountered of the familial porphyrias. It is usually seen in people of northern European origin and is inherited recessively. It is the only one of the porphyrias without any skin manifestations; instead, affected individuals have bouts of abdominal pain, peripheral neuropathy, hypertension, and psychosis. It has been proposed, on strong evidence, that this disease was the cause of the madness of King George III, and thus indirectly of the American War of Independence.

Barbiturates are especially prone to precipitate acute attacks, apparently acting in part by inducing ALA synthetase, and may indeed be lethal in affected individuals. The pathogenesis of the symptoms is still unknown.

In acute attacks, excessive amounts of ALA, PBG, and uroporphyrin I are excreted. The urine is usually colorless when passed but darkens on standing to give a reddish-brown color. The most characteristic finding is the enhanced excretion of ALA and PBG during attacks (up to 180 mg per 24 hours and up to 300 mg per 24 hours, respectively.) During quiescent periods, PBG excretion may be normal, but ALA levels are often above normal, although several determinations may be necessary to demonstrate this.

This form is sometimes called Swedish porphyria, to distinguish it from the following disorder.

South African Porphyria *(Hereditary Protocoproporphyria; Variegate Porphyria).* Acute attacks occur, similar to those described above, with enhanced excretion of ALA and PBG. However, this form of porphyria differs from the preceding form in that the excretion of ALA and PBG is normal between attacks, and photosensitivity to sunlight occurs. The disease is inherited dominantly and affects some 10,000 South Africans, who are apparently all descended from two 18th century Dutch settlers.

Hereditary Coproporphyria. This syndrome resembles variegate porphyria, but with only mild abdominal symptoms and skin sensitivity. Drugs can precipitate acute attacks. The distinguishing feature is the excretion of large amounts of coproporphyrin in the feces.

Porphyria Cutanea Tarda. This syndrome is characterized clinically by dermal photosensitivity appearing in later life, with scarring and hyperpigmentation. It probably comprises a heterogeneous group of acquired disorders, of which parenchymal liver disease is probably commonest. Whether there is a genetic predisposition is uncertain. Acute attacks do not occur, nor do ALA or PBG appear in the urine, but large amounts of uroporphyrin are excreted.

General Considerations in Detection of Porphyrinuria

As noted earlier, in some cases the substance excreted is not a porphyrin but a simpler substance—the precursor compound porphobilinogen, for example, in acute intermittent porphyria. Therefore, both porphyrins and porphobilinogen must be sought in any suspected cases. Urine samples must be fresh, especially if one is searching for porphobilinogen, since this is converted on standing to a substance resembling porphyrin. It is important to remember also that fresh urine from porphyrinuric subjects does not necessarily show any marked abnormality of color, though it may do so on standing. Generally, however, if large amounts of porphyrins are present, the urine has a rich burgundy-red color, which deepens on exposure to light, becoming dark mahogany in some cases. The salmon-pink fluorescence that porphyrin-containing urines give when exposed to ultraviolet light provides a simple and useful screening procedure, but if the porphyrins are present as zinc complexes (in hepatic porphyrias), especially in smaller quantities, this test may be unreliable. If the screening tests show porphyrins to be present, an attempt at identification and separation in relative amounts, e.g., porphobilinogen, uroporphyrins, and coproporphyrins, should be made, since this may be of diagnostic significance.

If it is impossible to examine urine for porphyrins while it is still fresh, the specimen should be stored in a dark cold place, e.g., the refrigerator. Slight alkalinization of the urine by addition of approximately 0.5 g sodium carbonate per 100 mL will further reduce porphyrin loss. Porphyrins may be preserved in urine, plasma, or stool by storing in the dark below $-10°C$.

Screening Procedures for Porphyrinuria

Procedure

1. Note the color of freshly voided urine. Large amounts of porphyrins will confer a reddish-brown to mahogany color.

2. In a completely dark room examine the urine in a 15 by 2.5 cm glass test tube using long-wavelength (354 nm) ultraviolet light. A salmon-pink fluorescence is almost proof of high levels of porphyrins. Normal urine shows only a bluish fluorescence.

3. To 5.0 mL of fresh urine add 3.0 mL of a 1:4 mixture of glacial acetic acid and ethyl acetate. Shake vigorously and centrifuge. Examine the supernatant ethyl acetate layer by long-wavelength ultraviolet light in a dark room for salmon-pink fluorescence, indicating an increased level of porphyrins. Normal urines are uniformly negative in this test. The UV light examination should be made immediately: continued exposure to the UV light tends to enhance the fluorescence and may result in a false positive result with some concentrated normal urines. The sensitivity of the test is about 0.5 μg of porphyrin per mL, corresponding approximately to about 500 to 600 μg per 24-hour excretion. This value is about two to three times the upper limit of normal.

4. A convenient alternative method uses a plastic column containing a special ion-exchange resin.* After a packing buffer is drained off, 4.0 mL of fresh urine is passed through the column, followed by 10 mL of deionized water to wash through interfering materials. Any porphyrins remain adsorbed to the resin and are subsequently eluted with two successive 2.0-mL aliquots of 3 M hydrochloric acid. The eluate is examined with long-wavelength UV light in a dark room for any signs of salmon-pink fluorescence. The acid eluate from a normal urine shows a bluish fluorescence. We have obtained definite positive results with urines containing 0.6 to 0.8 μg per mL of porphyrins, but occasionally the results are masked by the bluish fluorescence mentioned previously. In some instances an intense blue fluorescence, probably from a quinine-type drug, has masked the salmon-pink fluorescence of known elevated level urines, so the method should be used with some caution. The columns are stored in the refrigerator but must be allowed to come to room temperature before use.

To differentiate between the relatively common occurrence of increased coproporphyrins and the less common but more clinically significant uroporphyrins, a quick and simple thin-layer chromatographic test can be used. Shake 3.0 g silica gel-G† with 6.5 mL distilled water. With a wide-bore pipette transfer 1.0 mL of the slurry onto a 75 × 25 mm microscope slide, which is tilted and gently agitated until the slurry is evenly spread over the slide. Lay the slide flat until the gel has set, and then dry for a few minutes in a warm oven. A supply of slides can be made and stored in a place protected from dust. Using a Micro-cap‡ apply 10 microliters of the ethyl acetate extract showing an increased pink fluorescence in repeated small aliquots about 2 cm from one end of the slide, keeping the final spot below 3 mm in diameter. Using a Coplin jar as a tank, run a chromatogram of the slide using a mixture of chloroform:methanol:concentrated ammonia water: water in the proportions by volume 12:12:3:2. In about ten minutes the solvent front will have advanced about 4 cm from the starting spot. Remove the slide and examine immediately with long wave-length ultraviolet light. (The chromatogram is seen more easily if the lamp is placed behind the slide.) Coproporphyrins produce a brightly fluorescent band about two-thirds of the distance between the application point and the solvent front, whereas increased uroporphyrins fluoresce at the origin. A normal urine will not show fluorescence at the origin. The fluorescence fades slowly.

5. Porphobilinogen. In a 100 by 16 mm test tube mix 2.0 mL *fresh* urine and 2.0 mL modified Ehrlich's reagent. Shake for 30 seconds. (The immediate appearance of a red color at this stage is suggestive of the presence of porphobilinogen.) Add 4.0 mL of a saturated aqueous solution of sodium acetate and mix again. (The red color that develops at this stage is largely due to urobilinogen; the presence of sodium acetate suppresses to some extent colors produced with other substances, such as indole derivatives and skatole.) Add 4.0 mL of amyl-benzyl alcohol mixture, shake vigorously, and allow to stand for 5 minutes. The red compound formed with urobilinogen is transferred to the amylbenzyl alcohol upper layer. A red color remaining in the lower, aqueous, layer indicates the presence of porphobilinogen. This should be confirmed by pipetting off and discarding the upper (alcohol) layer and replacing it with 4.0 mL of *n*-butanol. Shake well, and allow the layers to separate. A pink or red color that persists in the aqueous (lower) layer is regarded as specific for porphobilinogen. (Urine from patients taking methyldopa (Aldomet) contains metabolites, probably indoles, that give a red color with Ehrlich's reagent. This reaction may be distinguished from that given by porphobilinogen because the red product is distributed equally between the aqueous and solvent layers after the extraction step.) For quantitative determination of urine porphobilinogen, see Henry, 1974. In the procedure described there, the porphobilinogen is adsorbed onto alumina in a small column, eluted with dilute acetic acid, and determined by the red color it produces with a modified Ehrlich's reagent. Normal daily output is up to 2.0 mg.

*Bio-Rad Laboratories, Richmond, Calif. 94804 and Mississauga, Ont. L4X 2C8.

†Brinkmann Instruments, Inc., Westbury, N.Y. 11590 and Rexdale, Ont M9W 4Y5.

‡Drummond Scientific Co., Broomall, Pa., 19008.

Reagents

Glacial Acetic Acid. Reagent-grade.

Ehrlich's Reagent, Modified. Dissolve 0.7 g of reagent-grade *p*-dimethylaminobenzaldehyde $(CH_3)_2NC_6H_4CHO$ in 150 mL concentrated hydrochloric acid; add 100 mL distilled water and mix. Keep in a dark-brown glass bottle.

Sodium Acetate CH_3COONa. Saturated aqueous solution. The bottle should always contain a layer of undissolved acetate in the bottom.

Amyl-Benzyl Alcohol Mixture. Mix 3 volumes of iso-amyl alcohol, $(CH_3)_2CHCH_2CH_2OH$, with 1 volume of benzyl alcohol, $C_6H_5CH_2OH$.

Quantitative Determination of Urinary Coproporphyrins and Uroporphyrins

In the frank porphyrias the detection of the increased amounts of porphyrins in the urine is a relatively simple matter. In some conditions, such as chronic lead poisoning, drug-induced liver damage, hemolytic anemias, and some types of photosensitive dermatitis, the increased excretion of porphyrins may not be readily detectable by the screening tests described earlier. However, two main approaches to quantitation have been made.

(i) Coproporphyrins are extracted from urine buffered to pH 4.8 into ethyl acetate, treated with dilute iodine to convert porphyrinogens to porphyrins, and re-extracted into 1.5 M hydrochloric acid. They are quantitated by measuring the peak absorbance at 401 to 403 nm and correcting for interfering substances by using the Allen principle, which employs absorbance measurements at 430 and 380 nm. The corrected absorbance is referred to the known molecular absorptivity of coproporphyrin.

The remaining urine aliquot is buffered to pH 3.0, at which point uroporphyrins can be extracted using *n*-butanol, and, after suitable washing procedures, are re-extracted into acid using petroleum spirit as the nonpolar separation agent. Quantitation is made in a manner similar to that for coproporphyrins, with a peak absorbance at 406 nm.

(ii) By use of a special ion-exchange resin to which the porphyrins become strongly adsorbed, and after the column is washed free of interfering substances, the porphyrins are eluted separately, using acids of different strengths, and determined fluorimetrically. (The screening test described on p. 272 is a simplified version of this procedure.)

Method (i) requires 100 mL of urine and is somewhat time consuming, although it has proven very reliable in our hands. Method (ii) requires a much smaller sample size and is quicker, but it is liable to errors from interfering fluorescent substances in the urine, including drugs.

Urine specimens for quantitative porphyrin analyses should be collected in a dark-brown bottle containing 10 g of sodium carbonate and kept refrigerated until assayed. In our experience the lability of porphyrins as a source of analytical errors is often not appreciated.

Normal Values. Total coproporphyrins (including coproporphyrinogens) per 24 hours: 0 to 161 μg (0 to 246 nmol). In our experience the majority of normal values fall in the range of 20 to 140 μg.

Total uroporphyrins per 24 hours: 0 to 26 μg (0 to 31 nmol). In our experience the majority of normal values fall in the lower half of this range.

Urinary δ-Aminolevulinic Acid Determination (Tomokuni and Ogata, 1972)

The δ-aminolevulinic acid (*d*-ALA) of the urine is reacted with ethyl acetoacetate to produce 2-methyl-3-carbethoxy-4-(3-propionic acid) pyrrole (ALA-pyrrole). This product is extracted with ethyl acetate and the ALA-pyrrole determined by its reaction with a modified Ehrlich's reagent.

Normal Range. Adults: 0.4 to 3.3 mg per liter (3.05 to 25.18 μmol/L). Children: Average 2.2 mg per liter (16.8 μmol/L).

Notes

1. The 24-hour collection of urine should be made using 10 mL of concentrated hydrochloric acid as preservative; the pH must stay <7.0.
2. An alternative method of urine collection that avoids the use of concentrated acid is the addition to the collection bottle of 8 to 10 g tartaric acid and protection of the specimen from light.

Fecal Coproporphyrin and Protoporphyrin Determination

The porphyrins and porphyrinogens of feces are extracted with ether acidified with acetic acid. After conversion of the porphyrinogens to porphyrins with a dilute iodine reagent, the coproporphyrins are extracted with 0.1 M hydrochloric acid and the protoporphyrins with 5.0% hydrochloric acid. The final quantitations are made by absorbance readings at the Soret-band wavelengths typical of the pigments, with corrections for interfering absorbances as in the urine procedure. Ideally the subject should be on a diet free of meat and green vegetables for 3 days before the specimens are collected.

Normal Values. Coproporphyrins. Estimates of the upper limit of normal daily excretion vary from 900 to 1100 μg per day (1374 to 1680 nmol). An average value is about 300 μg (458 nmol) per day.

Protoporphyrins. Up to 2000 μg (3054 nmol) per day.

Protoporphyrin in Red Cells

For estimation of red cell protoporphyrin content, the more sensitive fluorimetric method is recommended and may also be used for plasma and fecal protoporphyrin determination.

Spectroscopy of Urinary Porphyrins

Urine that contains sufficient porphyrins to be colored will show the characteristic absorption bands of these compounds. The position of the bands depends on the pH of the urine and whether the porphyrins are present in the free state or as metallic complexes (zinc). Generally speaking, free porphyrins occur in the urine of erythropoietic (congenital) porphyria, whereas in the hepatic porphyrias, zinc porphyrin complexes are found. Acidification of the urine liberates the zinc-bound porphyrins and also provides optimum conditions for spectroscopy of the various porphyrins. In a urine made acid with concentrated hydrochloric acid, porphyrins, if present, may be recognized by absorption bands as follows:

Compound	Position of Absorption Bands
Uroporphyrins	554, 577, and 597 nm
Coproporphyrins	550, 575, and 594 nm
Zinc-porphyrins in fresh unacidified urine (rarely distinguishable in practice by spectroscopy)	537 and 578 nm

ANALYSIS OF AMNIOTIC FLUID

Investigation of the state of maturation and viability of the fetus is made almost entirely from analyses on the amniotic fluid. In addition to its mechanical functions of protection and maintenance of relative weightlessness and constant temperature, the amniotic fluid changes in chemical and cellular composition in step with the increasing ability of the fetus to assume an independent existence. The assay of bilirubin levels in amniotic fluid in following the course of a pregnancy in an Rh-sensitized mother is now a well-established procedure (see p. 275). The predelivery diagnosis of inborn errors of metabolism by study of cells cultured from the amniotic fluid has become a more widely used procedure in specialized laboratories. In this section we are concerned with chemical methods of assessment of fetal maturity, particularly of the fetal lung, and assays of bilirubin levels in amniotic fluid. A useful reference source is the text edited by Natelson et al. (1974).

Assessment of Gestational Age

Knowledge of the true gestational age of a fetus, particularly when there is apparent discrepancy between the state of development and the projected time in utero based on the date of the last menstrual period, assumes particular importance if induction of labor or elective cesarean section is contemplated. A variety of amniotic fluid constituents have been studied in this connection, and the consensus favors creatinine levels as the best available guide. For maturity, the creatinine level in amniotic fluid should be above 1.5 mg per dL at the 34th or 35th week, with a rapid rise to 2.0 mg per dL close to term. The source of the creatinine appears to be an increasing efficiency of creatinine clearance by the maturing fetal kidney. There is some correlation between gestational age and decreasing bilirubin levels in the amniotic fluid, but the scatter of the values is too wide. Protein levels slowly decrease with advancing fetal maturity, but the change is not sufficiently marked to be useful.

The elevation of creatinine levels in amniotic fluid with increasing gestational age is accompanied, not surprisingly, by concurrent increases in uric acid. It has been suggested that simultaneous assays of both constituents may provide better information, and since in many laboratories creatinine-uric acid determinations are made by simultaneous continuous flow automation, the suggestion is a practical one. It has been found that the uric acid level rises from a mean of 3.75 mg per dL (SD 0.956) in the second trimester to a mean of 9.9 mg per dL (SD 2.23) at term. Urea nitrogen levels do not provide useful data because of a wide scatter of values at term.

Assessment of Fetal Lung Maturity

It is well known that lecithin plays an essential role in lowering surface tension in the lining of the alveoli of the lung and thus in preventing alveolar collapse during expiration; its correlation with the respiratory distress syndrome in the newborn infant also is well established. Since during intrauterine life the fetal lung exchanges substances from the developing alveolar lining with the amniotic fluid, examination of the fluid for its lecithin content or the ratio of lecithin to sphingomyelin can provide advance warning of development of the respiratory distress syndrome. In many cases the lack of lecithin is caused by the timing of a changeover in the pathways of lecithin synthesis. The methyl transferase pathway, in which phosphatidyl ethanolamine is methylated with methyl groups from methionine to form lecithin, can be detected as early as the 22nd week of gestation. It produces palmitoylmyristoyllecithin, but it is inhibited easily by acidosis, hypothermia, and hypoxia, conditions frequently attendant on premature delivery. The second pathway, in which phosphocholine transferase promotes the union of cytidine diphosphate choline and D-alpha,beta-diglycerides to produce dipalmitoyllecithin, does not begin operating until later in fetal life (about 35 weeks). Thus the aim of treatment of a premature infant with the respiratory distress syndrome (RDS) is to assist pulmonary ventilation and control the acidosis until the second synthetic pathway comes into action to maintain alveolar lining surfactant state.

The initial method for the assessment of the probable degree of maturity of the fetal lung rested on the determination by thin-layer chromatography of the *relative* levels of lecithin and sphingomyelin in fluid obtained by amniocentesis. (Amniocentesis involves the passage of a needle through the abdominal and uterine wall of the mother into the pool of amniotic fluid in the amniotic sac and the withdrawal of a sample of the fluid.) If the ratio of lecithin to sphingomyelin (the "L/S" ratio) was 2:1 or greater, the production of surfactant by the fetal lung was judged adequate. (Sets of reagents are commercially available for the technique.*) Further experience with the method showed that it could be unreliable in some cases, such as diabetic pregnancy: the results were shown to be dependent on the handling of the sample and subject to interference from such contaminants as red cells. The newer methods of investigation are designed to make actual quantitative determinations of the active phospholipids. A typical assay is that for phosphatidyl glycerol (PG): its appearance in the amniotic fluid normally correlates closely with gestational age and fetal maturity and indicates full biochemical maturity of the phospholipid surfactants necessary for rapid and complete expansion of the fetal lung at birth. A typical technique for PG assay uses two-dimensional thin-layer chromatography. (For a full discussion see Freer and Statland, 1981.)

Another approach to the problem involves the direct evaluation of the prime function of the surfactant com-

*Gelman Instrument Co., Ann Arbor, Mich. 48106 and Montreal, Que. H4S 1M7.

pounds—their ability to lower surface tension at the alveolar surface, facilitating lung expansion and aeration. The tests used depend on the ability of the active phospholipids to prolong bubble formation after addition to a sample of amniotic fluid of an amount of ethyl alcohol sufficient to prevent stable foam formation by other substances such as proteins and free fatty acids. The procedure is simple but involves rigid technique and a somewhat subjective estimate of bubble stability.

Determination of Unconjugated Bilirubin in Amniotic Fluid (Brazie et al., 1969)

Principle

The unconjugated bilirubin is extracted selectively from amniotic fluid with chloroform and quantitated by its absorbance at 453 nm.

Procedure

***Note.* The specimen and the chloroform extract must be protected from light *at all stages* of the procedure, particularly from direct sunlight.**

1. In a 150 × 16 mm glass-stoppered tube, mix 3.0 mL of centrifuged amniotic fluid and 3.0 mL chloroform. Shake vigorously by hand for 30 seconds. Immediately place tube in an ice bath for 5 minutes.

2. Centrifuge the tube for 1 to 2 minutes; the minimum time necessary for good separation of the layers and protein mass should be determined by experiment. Briefly inspect the tube, and if some protein strands remain in the lower chloroform layer, gently stir them loose with a fine glass rod and recentrifuge.

3. Stand the tube at room temperature for ten minutes. (If the next step is carried out on a chilled extract, condensation of moisture on the cuvette may cause photometric error.)

4. Using a fine-tipped Pasteur pipette, introduced carefully past the protein layer into the lower chloroform layer, remove enough of the latter to fill a 10-mm cuvette to a level adequate for spectrophotometry. Determine the absorbance at 453 nm against a chloroform blank, preferably in a precision spectrophotometer.

5. If the validity of such a procedure has been previously checked (see further on), the absorbance reading equals the unconjugated bilirubin level in mg per dL. Mg per dL × 17.1 = μmol per liter.

Reagents

Phosphate Buffer, pH 6.0, 0.05 M. Dissolve 3.0 g of sodium dihydrogen phosphate NaH_2PO_4 in about 400 mL distilled water. Adjust the pH to 6.0 by careful addition of 5 M sodium hydroxide with thorough mixing. Make up to 500 mL. Preserve with 50 mg sodium azide NaN_3.

Chloroform. Shake about 200 mL analytical-grade chloroform $CHCl_3$ with about 100 mL of pH 6.0 phosphate buffer in a separating funnel; store the equilibriated chloroform in the funnel.

Stock Bilirubin Standard. Working rapidly in subdued light, weigh out 20.0 mg of pure bilirubin (molar absorptivity 60,700 ± 800) and dissolve in 100 mL chloroform.

Working Standard. Dilute 1.0 mL of the stock standard up to 100 mL with chloroform, mix well, and immediately determine its absorbance at 453 nm against a chloroform blank in the spectrophotometer to be used for the test. The theoretical absorbance value, obtained from the expression (Henry, 1974):

$$\frac{10 \text{ mg/L} \times 60{,}700}{584.7 \text{ (MW of bilirubin)} \times 1000} = 1.04$$

If the absorbance obtained is within the range of 0.99 to 1.09, the simple calculation given in step 5 can be used. If the photometer to be used does not have the degree of precision to reproduce this value, prepare a calibration curve as follows:

Working Standard	Chloroform	Bilirubin Value mg/dL
10 mL	0	1.0
7.5	2.5	0.75
5.0	5.0	0.50
2.5	7.5	0.25

Determine the absorbances against a chloroform blank, and draw a calibration curve, which should be a straight line. This curve will have to be redetermined if the photometer lamp is changed. With a filter-type instrument, use a 450 nm filter.

Interpretation of Results

Generally speaking, a level below 0.06 mg per dL at or before 35 to 36 weeks indicates a normal or only mildly affected fetus, but complete assessment should rest on the total evidence.

Serum Haptoglobins Determination

A variety of analytical approaches have been used for assay of serum haptoglobins. The procedure used will be related to the level of equipment of the laboratory to some extent. The method in which the haptoglobins are combined with methemoglobin to form a complex that is determined by its catalytic effect (peroxidase-like activity) on the oxidation of guiacol to tetraguiacol by hydrogen peroxide requires only a good spectrophotometer. We have found the method using the dextran gel Sephadex G. 100 to adsorb the hemoglobin-haptoglobin complex with subsequent fractional elution using a fraction collector, followed by direct spectrophotometry of those fractions corresponding to both the complex and the excess free hemoglobin, reliable and having the added advantage of linearity over a very wide range of values. The normal ranges reported vary somewhat with the method of assay used; with the above technique, males range from 60 to 150 mg hemoglobin-binding capacity per dL, and females from 46 to 127 mg per dL.

METHEMOGLOBIN AND METHEMOGLOBINEMIA

In the presence of air or oxygen hemoglobin is gradually oxidized to methemoglobin. This involves a change in the heme iron from the ferrous (Fe^{++}) to the ferric (Fe^{+++}) form, with addition of a hydroxyl group, the formula then being written as (Por-Fe-OH) globin. In the test tube, hemoglobin is converted to methemoglobin by oxidizing agents such as potassium ferricyanide or by treating RBCs with nitrite. Within the RBCs in the body, peroxidases and other factors promote the formation of methemoglobin, but four reducing systems combat this tendency, so that the methemoglobin content of normal blood rarely rises above 0.5% of the total hemoglobin.

Hereditary Methemoglobinemia Caused by Hemoglobin M

In common with other hemoglobinopathies, the M hemoglobins differ from normal adult hemoglobin (HbA) in having one amino acid substituted on either the alpha or beta chains. In the HbM hemoglobins the substituent amino acid appears to be close to and capable of reacting with the iron of the associated heme group when this iron is oxidized to the ferric form. This interferes with the normal function of NADH diaphorase in reducing methemoglobin. Also, in the conversion of methemoglobin to cyanmethemoglobin, the association between the polypeptide chain and the iron has to be disrupted. In the alpha chain-substituted types of HbM (HbM_{Boston}, HbM_B, and HbM_{Iwate}, HbM_T), the attachment of the substituted amino acid to the oxidized iron appears to be unusually strong, with the result that the reaction with cyanide is incomplete and unusually slow, and the absorption spectrum of the cyanmethemoglobin is abnormal. In the case of those varieties of HbM in which amino acid substitution has occurred on the beta chains, e.g., $HbM_{Saskatoon}$ (HbM_S) and $HbM_{Milwaukee-1}$ (HbM_{M-1}), the ferric iron–amino acid attachment does not appear to be as strong, and the spectra of their cyanmethemoglobins in the visible region are normal.

Hemoglobin Type	Amino Acid Substituted Chain	Cyanmethemoglobin Spectrum (Visible Region)	Methemoglobin Absorption Maxima (Visible Region) pH6-7
HbA	—	Normal	502 and 632 nm
HbM_B	$alpha_2$	Abnormal	495 and 602 nm
HbM_I	$alpha_2$	Abnormal	490 and 590 nm
HbM_S	$beta_2$	Normal	492 and 602 nm
HbM_{M-1}	$beta_2$	Normal	500 and 622 nm

Because of the complexing of the substituent amino acid with the ferric iron, estimation of the concentration of methemoglobin in HbM cases by the cyanmethemoglobin method is not reliable: indeed, some HbM types fail to react with cyanide at all. The same mechanism explains the relative to absolute ineffectiveness of vitamin C or methylene blue in dispelling the cyanosis in these cases.

Acquired Methemoglobinemia

This may be acute or chronic. Most cases result from the use of drugs or from the absorption or ingestion of chemicals such as acetanilid, anilines, chlorates, nitrites, nitrates, certain phenols, sulfonamide drugs, and phenacetin (rarely). Ingestion of crayon pigments or absorption of anilines from laundry markings on underwear may cause methemoglobinemia in infants or young children. The chemicals mentioned behave as oxidants or are converted to oxidants in the body. Infants fed formulas made up with well water rich in nitrites or nitrates are liable to develop methemoglobinemia.

Blood Methemoglobin and Sulfhemoglobin Determination (Evelyn and Malloy, 1938)

Principle

Methemoglobin is determined by measurement of the absorbance of diluted blood at the wavelength of maximum absorbance for this pigment, 630 nm, before and after its conversion to cyanmethemoglobin. The difference in absorbance values is proportional to the amount of methemoglobin and is compared with the known molecular absorptivity for this substance. Sulfhemoglobin is determined by measurement of its absorbance at 619 nm, which is unaffected by the cyanide used to remove the methemoglobin peak at 630 nm.

Procedure

1. Pipette accurately, using washout technique, 0.2 mL well-mixed heparinized blood into 10.0 mL M/60 phosphate buffer. Let stand for 5 minutes, and centrifuge for 10 minutes at 3000 rpm. Transfer the supernatant to a clean test tube. Measure the absorbance of a portion in a 1.0-cm cell at 630 nm, setting zero absorbance with phosphate buffer. This is reading A_1.

2. Return the contents of the cell to the test tube: add one drop of the neutralized cyanide solution. Mix by inversion, and let stand for 2 minutes. Again read the absorbance at 630 nm, in a 1.0-cm cell as in step 1. This is reading A_2.

3. Return the contents of the cell to the test tube; add one drop of concentrated ammonia solution; let stand for 2 minutes. Measure the absorbance in a 1.0-cm cell at 613, 616, 619, 622, and 625 nm. The presence of a peak value in the readings in the region 617 to 621 nm confirms the presence of sulfhemoglobin. The absorbance value at 619 nm is used for the calculations. This is value A_3.

4. Transfer 2.0 mL of the solution from step 3 into a clean tube. Add 8.0 mL M/15 phosphate buffer to which has been added one drop of a 20.0 w/v solution of potassium ferricyanide. Mix by inversion, and let stand for 2 minutes. Add one drop of 10.0% w/v potassium cyanide solution, mix by inversion, and let stand for 2 minutes; measure the absorbance in a 1.0-cm cell at 540 nm, setting zero absorbance with water. This is reading A_4.

Calculations

Total hemoglobin in g per dL = value $A_4 \times 37.4$. Total methemoglobin in g per dL = (value A_1 − value A_2) × 23.4. Total sulfhemoglobin in g per dL = 6.5 ×

$$\left(\text{value } A_3 - \frac{\text{total Hb} - \text{metHb}}{205} - \frac{\text{metHb}}{84}\right)$$

Normal Values

Total hemoglobin in adult males ranges from 14 to 18 g per dL; in adult females, from 12 to 16 g per dL. Normal values for total methemoglobin are up to about 3.0% of the total hemoglobin, or up to about 0.5 g per dL. Sulfhemoglobin is not normally present.

Reagents

M/15 Phosphate Buffer, pH 6.6. Dissolve 1.9 g anhydrous disodium hydrogen phosphate, Na_2HPO_4, and 2.72 g anhydrous potassium dihydrogen phosphate,

KH_2PO_4, in about 300 mL fresh distilled water. Make up to 500 mL with distilled water; store in the refrigerator. Allow to warm to room temperature before use.

M/60 Phosphate Buffer. Mix 1 volume of M/15 buffer with 3 volumes of distilled water.

20.0% w/v Potassium Ferricyanide. Dissolve 2.0 g pure potassium ferricyanide, $K_3Fe(CN)_6$, in 10.0 mL distilled water.

Neutralized Cyanide Solution. Prepare just before use by mixing equal volumes of a 10.0% w/v aqueous solution of sodium cyanide, NaCN, and 12.0% v/v acetic acid.

Potassium Cyanide, 10.0% w/v. Dissolve 1.0 g potassium cyanide, KCN, in 10.0 mL distilled water.

Notes

1. The spectrophotometer must be a high-resolution instrument that can be set to zero or balanced with a slit setting corresponding to a band pass of 2.0 nm or less. The cells or cuvettes must be precision-made 1.0-cm path length, and must be scrupulously clean.
2. Turbidity will cause errors in total hemoglobin and sulfhemoglobin determinations; methemoglobin values will not be affected. If the original blood sample was lipemic, the cells from a very accurately measured volume of it should be centrifuged down and washed with saline and the washed cells resuspended in saline to give the original volume of blood taken.
3. The procedure is not accurate for low values of methemoglobin, since a result of 0.2 g per dL corresponds to an absorbance difference of only about 0.009.
4. The factor of 37.4 used to calculate total hemoglobin can be verified using blood samples whose hemoglobin values have been determined using the standard cyanmethemoglobin method. For derivation of the other factors used, the original reference should be consulted.

Iron Metabolism

The absorption of dietary iron has already been considered (p. 238). The ferric iron in combination with apoferritin of the mucosal cells is fixed (except under hypoxic conditions) and is ultimately lost when these cells are shed. Probably, dietary iron that is absorbed and transferred to the plasma remains in the ferrous state and may be loosely complexed with amino acids, from which it is picked up by plasma transferrin and carried to the liver.

Absorption of iron normally amounts to 7 to 10% of that in the diet and averages 1 mg per day (range 0.3 to 2 mg per day). Absorption is increased when plasma or body stores of iron are reduced, relatively or absolutely—e.g., in iron deficiency anemia, growth, pregnancy, lactation, and within 3 to 6 days of significant acute blood loss—and when hypoxic conditions prevail. These appear to act by promoting the reduction of the ferric iron of intestinal mucosal cell ferritin to the ferrous form, which can pass into the blood. The resultant decrease in fixed mucosal cell iron leads to increased absorption of dietary iron. Conditions in which this mechanism may be operative are pernicious anemia, hemolytic anemias, and refractory anemias associated with erythron hyperplasia—in all of which hemoglobin may be low without the plasma or body stores of iron being reduced. Increased absorption also occurs in polycythemia vera and primary hemochromatosis.

Iron Requirements

These total about 1 mg per day in an adult man. Urinary excretion accounts for approximately 0.2 mg per day, and 0.7 to 0.8 mg per day is lost by desquamation of cutaneous and gastrointestinal cells, via the sweat and in the bile. Over and above the basic daily requirement, growth, menstruation, and lactation require an additional 0.8 to 1 mg per day, and an extra 2 to 3 mg per day is necessary in the latter half of pregnancy.

Distribution of Body Iron

Total iron in the normal adult ranges from 3.5 to 5 g. Of this, 65 to 70% is in hemoglobin, 20 to 25% is in storage iron, 3% is in myoglobin, 1% is in heme enzymes and transferrin, and the remainder is unaccounted for.

Storage Iron

This is about equally divided between ferritin and hemosiderin. Ferritin is a finely dispersed form consisting of ferric hydroxide bound to the special iron-binding protein, apoferritin (M.W. 460,000). Ferritin contains 20 to 23% iron, which is readily mobilizable, being converted to the ferrous form before complexing with transferrin for transport. Hemosiderin is a coarser form of storage iron and appears to be formed when deposition of iron is too massive for the amount of apoferritin available. In keeping with this, hemosiderin contains 25 to 33% iron. The iron of hemosiderin is mobilized slowly and with difficulty. Within reticuloendothelial cells, which phagocytose it, hemosiderin is harmless, but if deposited in any quantity within parenchymal cells or in stroma, it causes cell damage and fibrosis.

Transferrin

This iron-carrying beta globulin is a glycoprotein of about 90,000 M.W., containing 5.5% carbohydrate (galactose, mannose, hexosamine, and sialic acid). Each molecule of transferrin binds two atoms of iron, and changes from colorless to pink in the process. Ferrous iron is bound more rapidly than ferric iron. Copper, manganous, and zinc ions can be loosely bound.

Genetic Variants of Transferrin. At least 19 variants of transferrin have been identified, but they appear to differ only in electrophoretic mobility on starch gel, ranging from the slowest D type in the $beta_1$ region (close to haptoglobin–2), to the fastest B type in the $alpha_1$ region (next to ceruloplasmin, after postalbumin).

Functions of Transferrin. These are, in order, transport of iron, regulation of iron absorption, and protection against the toxic effects of iron. In the matter of transport, transferrin appears to be especially adapted for the transfer of iron to immature erythrocytes, where it is temporarily stored as ferritin while awaiting incorporation into hemoglobin.

Normal Plasma Transferrin and Iron Values

In the normal person the plasma concentration of transferrin ranges from 0.24 to 0.28 g per dL (mean 0.27 g per dL). Thus there are about 7 to 8 g in the entire plasma. A similar concentration and total amount of transferrin is present in extracellular fluids. Normally, only about one-third of transferrin's iron-carrying capacity is used, and this gives a plasma iron ranging from 65 to 175 μg per dL; in men the mean is about 120 μg per dL, and in women about 100 to 110 μg per dL. It exhibits a diurnal variation, the morning level in day workers being some 30 μg higher than the evening level. The total iron-binding capacity (TIBC) of normal plasma transferrin, however, ranges from 250 to 420 μg per dL; i.e., transferrin is normally 66% unsaturated.

Serum iron is low in iron-deficiency anemias (values of 50 μg per dL are common). Whenever erythropoiesis becomes suddenly active plasma iron concentration declines, e.g., within a few days of significant blood loss or of inception of vitamin B_{12} therapy for pernicious anemia. Increased demands for iron, such as in growth and pregnancy, also tend to reduce serum iron. Acute and chronic infections and malignancy are associated with reduced serum iron levels.

Plasma iron is elevated in hypoplastic and aplastic anemias, untreated megaloblastic anemias (depressed erythropoiesis), hemolytic anemias (increased breakdown of hemoglobin), acute hepatocellular damage (e.g., in hepatitis, owing to release of stored iron from damaged liver cells), and hemochromatosis and siderosis (increased storage).

Hemosiderosis

This consists of the deposition of hemosiderin in excessive amounts. Significant alteration of function does not develop until the deposits are very considerable. Generalized siderosis regularly develops when 100 or more units of blood have been transfused without loss of hemoglobin from the body, e.g., in hypoplastic and aplastic anemias and in thalassemia. Each 500-mL unit of blood contains approximately 250 mg iron, and in an adult of average size a minimum of 20 to 25 g excess iron is necessary to produce the symptoms and signs of iron storage disease. In transfusional siderosis, during the latent period iron is deposited almost exclusively in the reticuloendothelial system, but when the reticuloendothelial cells become saturated, increasing deposition in the parenchymal and stromal cells of many organs takes place, most notably in the liver, myocardium, pancreas, and endocrine glands. Cardiac failure usually develops before cirrhosis of the liver becomes significant in such cases.

Hemochromatosis

This is usually taken as connoting a more harmful deposition of hemosiderin than in hemosiderosis; however, as already shown, the difference is largely one of degree together with peculiarities associated with the route of entry and the nature of the iron entering the body. Hemochromatosis may be primary or secondary. The secondary variety is common in the African Bantu who, by virtue of their cooking utensils and a high consumption of Kaffir beer, may ingest more than 100 mg of iron a day. Secondary hemochromatosis also tends to develop, together with hepatic cirrhosis, in habitually heavy wine drinkers, since wines contain 5 to 22 mg of iron per liter.

Primary Hemochromatosis. This not excessively rare disease results from the accumulation of iron caused by a positive iron balance on the order of 1.5 to 3 mg per day from birth. Accumulation at the rate of 2 mg per day would require 27 years to amass 20 g; at 3 mg per day, 20 g would accumulate in 18 years. Because of this, 95% of the patients do not develop signs of the disease until after the age of 30 years. Also, since an average woman loses 10 to 30 g of iron through menstruation and childbirth, the disease is at least 10 times commoner in men than in women, in whom it rarely develops until after the menopause.

In hemochromatosis, there is increased absorption of dietary iron. Plasma iron becomes obviously elevated after puberty, and after 15 years of age it usually exceeds 170 μg per dL and practically always is above 150 μg per dL at that time. When manifestations of the disease set in, the plasma iron is usually above 200 μg per dL and may reach 275 μg per dL. At the same time, the total iron-binding capacity (TIBC) is diminished and is generally 300 μg or less per dL, so that the percentage saturation of transferrin is commonly 60 to 80% instead of the normal 30 to 40%. (In transfusional siderosis, the plasma iron may be equally high, but the TIBC is usually not reduced.)

This excessive saturation of transferrin appears to favor transfer of iron to storage in parenchymal cells. For many years (20 to 30) the liver bears the brunt of this, but in time iron also is deposited in the pancreas, myocardium, endocrine and salivary glands, and other organs. The accumulation of iron in the parenchymal liver cells and in the stroma of the portal triads leads to cirrhosis.

In hemochromatosis, the major cause of death is myocardial failure owing to heavy iron deposition in the myocardium. In about 15% of cases primary liver cell carcinoma develops.

*Serum Iron Determination and Total Iron-Binding Capacity—TIBC**
(Stookey, 1970)

Principle

The iron-protein complex of serum, transferrin, is split to free the iron by acetic acid in the presence of a nonionic detergent to prevent protein precipitation. The iron is reduced to the ferrous Fe^{2+} state with ascorbic acid and forms a stable magenta complex with ferrozine, 3-(2-pyridyl)-5,6-bis(4-phenylsulfonic acid)-1,2,4-triazine.† Initial color or turbidity, or both, of the serum sample are determined by measuring the absorbance before and after addition of the ferrozine. For the TIBC, a known excess of ferrous iron is added to the serum, using ascorbic acid to maintain the ferrous state and a buffer to promote saturation of the unsaturated binding sites of the serum transferrin. The remaining unbound iron is determined with ferrozine, and the difference between the original amount added and this value equals the unsaturated binding capacity of the serum (UIBC). Serum iron value plus UIBC = TIBC.

---

*Ferro-Chek II, using the color reagent Ferrozine; Hyland Division, Travenol Laboratories, Inc., Costa Mesa, Calif. 92626.

†Hach Chemical Co., Ames, Iowa 50010.

Procedure

1. Prepare the working iron standard by diluting the stock 1:100 with 0.01 M hydrochloric acid. (See *Notes* on purity of solutions and equipment.) Mix; this working standard is good for a week if kept refrigerated.

2. Prepare the ascorbic acid by addition of 5.0 mL iron-free distilled water to each vial. The number of vials reconstituted will depend on the number of tests to be run. Each test, control, standard, and blank requires 1.0 mL; each TIBC assay requires 0.5 mL for each test and control. The combined ascorbic acid-ferrous iron reagent should be made at this time for the TIBC assay, since this reagent has to stand for at least 15 minutes before use. It is made by mixing equal volumes of the ascorbic acid solution and the 800 μg per dL iron reagent.

3. Serum iron assay. Set up a specially cleaned (see *Notes*) 10 mm or ½″ spectrophotometer tube cuvette for each test, for standard, for control serum, and for blank. To test add 1.0 mL serum, to standard 1.0 mL working iron standard, to control 1.0 mL of a control serum, to blank 1.0 mL distilled water.

4. To all tubes add 1.0 mL ascorbic acid solution and 1.0 mL acetic acid-detergent dissociating reagent. Mix by inversion, using Parafilm. Allow to stand for one minute for bubbles to rise.

5. Determine the absorbances of tests, control, and standard at 560 nm setting zero absorbance with the blank tube. Record the values as Abs 1.

6. To all tubes add 0.1 mL ferrozine, and mix well by inversion (do not shake violently), making sure that any initial precipitate redissolves. Let stand five minutes at room temperature.

7. Determine the absorbances as in step 5. Record the values as Abs 2.

Calculation

Abs 2 − Abs 1 = Corrected Abs

$$\frac{\text{Corrected Abs Test (or control)}}{\text{Corrected Abs Standard}} \times 200 = \text{Serum iron } \mu\text{g/dL}$$

Serum iron in μg/dL × 0.179 = μmol/L

Normal Values

65 to 175 μg per dL (11.6 to 31.3 μmol/L). In view of the known large diurnal variation in serum iron levels (up to 50 μg per dL, with high values in the early morning and lower values in the evening), there seems little point in attempting to set different normal ranges for males and females. It is much more important to obtain serum samples for iron assays at the same time each day, particularly if they are being used to monitor the effect of treatment of an iron-deficient state.

Reagents

These are obtained commercially as Ferro-Chek II.*

Serum Total Iron-Binding Capacity Determination

1. Set up a specially cleaned 10 mm or ½″ spectrophotometer cuvette for each test, for control and for blank. (The standard corrected absorbance obtained during assay of serum iron above is used in calculation of the UIBC and TIBC). To test add 1.0 mL serum, to control 1.0 mL of a control serum, to blank add 2.0 mL distilled water.

2. To test and control *only* add 1.0 mL ascorbic acid–iron reagent prepared in step 2 of the serum iron assay.

3. To *all* tubes add 1.0 mL binding buffer. Mix by inversion, using Parafilm.

4. Determine the absorbances of test and control at 560 nm setting zero absorbance with the blank tube. Record the values as Abs 1. Stand the tubes at room temperature for a minimum of 20 minutes (to permit complete binding of added iron by the transferrin) and a maximum of 30 minutes to prevent inactivation of the ascorbic acid at the alkaline pH, with consequent conversion of ferrous iron to the ferric state, which will not react with the ferrozine color reagent.

5. Add 0.1 mL ferrozine to all tubes, and mix well by inversion, using Parafilm (do not shake violently), making sure that any initial precipitate redissolves. Let stand five minutes at room temperature.

6. Determine the absorbances of test and control as in step 4. Record the values as Abs 2.

Calculation

Abs 2 − Abs 1 = Corrected Abs.

$$\frac{\text{Corrected Abs Test (or control)}}{\text{Corrected Abs Standard}} \times 200 = \text{Remaining free iron}$$

400 μg/dL − Remaining free iron = Unsaturated iron-binding capacity (UIBC) Serum iron + UIBC = Total iron-binding capacity (TIBC) TIBC in μg/dL × 0.179 = μmol/L

$$\frac{\text{Serum iron}}{\text{TIBC}} \times 100 = \text{Per cent saturation}$$

Normal Values

250 to 420 μg/dL (44.8 to 75.2 μmol/L).

Reagents

As for serum iron assay above.

Notes

1. In our experience, the plastic reaction tubes provided with the reagent kit are not suitable for use as spectrophotometer cuvettes. A supply of new 10 mm or ½″ tube-type cuvettes should be set aside for iron assays. They should be soaked overnight in 25% v/v hydrochloric acid, rinsed repeatedly in distilled water, and dried inverted in a large glass beaker covered to prevent contamination from dust, especially in the drying oven. After use they should be well-rinsed with tap water, then processed as for new tubes.

2. As many measurements as possible should be made with hand-type pipettors using disposable plastic tips to minimize contamination.

3. Moderate hemolysis and lipemia, and bilirubin levels up to 20 mg per dL do not cause errors.

4. Since the TIBC assay depends on determining the unbound fraction of an added excess of iron, the preparation of the ascorbic acid-iron reagent and its pipetting into the reaction tubes are critical and must be made with volumetric accuracy.

*Hyland Division, Travenol Laboratories, Inc., Costa Mesa, Calif. 92626.

5. The distilled water used must be iron-free.

6. The final magenta color is stable for at least two hours.

7. The absorbance of the 200 mg per dL standard in a 10-mm cuvette at 560 nm should be about 0.310.

8. If the serum available is limited, 0.5 mL serum plus 0.5 mL distilled water can be used for both iron and TIBC assays. The serum iron value will have to be multiplied by two, and the TIBC calculation modified as follows:

TIBC = Serum iron value corrected for dilution plus (UIBC × 2)

9. Blood samples should be collected into iron-free tubes; the plastic tubes provided with the reagent kit are suitable for storing the serum before analysis. The serum can be refrigerated up to one week if necessary and stored frozen up to three months.

10. Serum iron assays have been automated using the ferrozine reaction on a discrete-type analyzer, using the color reagent 5-pyridyl-benzodiazepin-2-one (full name: 7 - bromo - 1,3 - dihydro - 1 - (3 - dimethylamino-propyl) - 5 - (2 -pyridyl) - 2H - 1,4 - benzodiazepine - 2 - one dihydrochloride) on a continuous flow-type analyzer, and using bathophenanthroline on a continuous flow analyzer. Full automation of TIBC assays is difficult because of the requirement for presaturation of the UIBC and separation of the excess iron, except with the discrete analyzer already noted.

11. Determination of serum iron by atomic absorption would appear to be the method of choice, but it is complicated by the need to precipitate protein and liberate the bound iron, plus the high degree of sensitivity required. The development of higher intensity hollow cathode lamps and Boling-type burner heads and the greater stability of double-beam atomic absorption spectrophotometers have improved this situation. A typical method uses hot trichloroacetic acid to precipitate protein and liberate the ferric ion.

Determination of Zinc

The availability of relatively simple and adequately precise atomic absorption methods for the assay of metallic ions, whose metabolic importance could not be readily assessed owing to their very low concentrations, is opening up a new field of analytical interest. Previously, the essential role of zinc in the functions of a variety of enzymes—carbonic anhydrase, lactate dehydrogenase, alcohol dehydrogenase, glutamate dehydrogenase—and its importance in insulin and porphyrin metabolism were largely of academic interest. The main stimulus to routine assays of serum zinc levels was the observation that they had an important influence on the processes of tissue healing and that detection and correction of zinc deficiency could play a major role in healing problems.

Methodology. The sensitivity of atomic absorption for zinc makes this the method of choice for assay. Plasma obtained with heparin is preferable to serum; the latter contains variable amounts of zinc released from platelets and leucocytes. The protein precipitant of choice is perchloric acid.

Procedure. This will depend to some extent on the particular model of atomic absorption spectrophotometer; the method has been used successfully on a single-beam instrument.

Normal Values. 89 to 107 μg per dL (13.6 – 16.4 μmol/L.

Determination of Nickel

The current interest in trace element analysis extends to assays of nickel in serum. With the advent of reliable methods, significant changes in serum nickel levels have been detected in a variety of pathological states. Elevations above the normal range of 1.0 to 4.2 μg per L have been found in acute myocardial infarction, acute strokes, and acute burns. Decreased levels have been encountered in hepatic cirrhosis and chronic uremia. From the point of view of diagnostic usefulness, the changes in acute myocardial infarction, along with the similar changes in serum zinc levels, make further development of these techniques a possible feature of routine clinical chemistry.

Lithium

Lithium is a highly reactive monovalent cation of the same group as sodium and potassium. It is present in normal tissues in trace amounts, but the levels are too small to affect its use as an internal reference in flame photometry of serum sodium and potassium (see p. 78). After oral administration it is rapidly absorbed from the GI tract and apparently interferes with electrolyte distribution across the neuronal membrane and alters the excitability of the central nervous system. These and related effects have led to its use in the treatment of acute manic episodes in patients with manic-depressive psychosis. The effective serum concentration—about 1.0 to 1.5 mEq per liter, 1.0 to 1.5 mmol per liter—is close to the toxic level—about 1.8 to 2.0 mEq per liter. Use of the drug therefore must be controlled with determinations of serum lithium.

Serum lithium can be determined by flame photometry, and some models of flame photometers incorporate circuits for this purpose, using potassium as an internal reference. The best method is atomic absorption spectrophotometry. Exact details will depend on the particular instrument used.

DETECTION OF METHEMALBUMINEMIA (Schumm, 1912)

If the concentration of free hemoglobin in the plasma is too great to be completely bound by haptoglobin, the excess breaks down to hematin and forms a combination with plasma albumin called methemalbumin (ferrihemalbumin). Methemalbumin is identified by the hemochromogen it forms with ammonium sulfide.

Procedure

1. Place 3.0 mL fresh plasma in a test tube and cover with a 1-cm layer of ether.

2. Add 0.3 mL of concentrated ammonium sulfide, $(NH_4)_2S$, solution and 3 drops of concentrated ammonia solution. Shake, and allow to separate. Examine with the spectroscope for the strong absorption band of the ammonium hemochromogen of methemalbumin, which is seen at 558 nm, in the yellow-green area of the spectrum.

UROBILINOGEN EXCRETION IN URINE

Principle. Urobilinogen and certain other substances, such as indoles and skatoles, react with Ehrlich's aldehyde reagent (paradimethylaminobenzaldehyde) to give a cherry-red color. Porphobilinogen gives the same color reaction but can be differentiated by differential solubility extraction of the color complex (p. 272). Fresh urine must be used, since urobilinogen is converted to urobilin on standing or by very brief exposure to light. The Schlesinger reaction takes place with both substances.

Precautions. Urine specimens must be fresh and must be protected from light. The test must be performed within 30 minutes after the urine is voided. If more than a small amount of bilirubin is present, this is removed by mixing 1 volume of urine with 1 volume of 10% aqueous barium chloride and filtering; however, the filtrate represents a 1:2 dilution of urine. The test has no value in patients receiving many antibiotics, since these may inhibit the intestinal bacteria that form urobilinogen. Urine from patients receiving para-aminosalicylic acid gives a yellow color with Ehrlich's reagent, and urine from patients taking methyldopa (Aldomet) gives a red color that is distributed equally between the aqueous and solvent layers in the screening test for porphobilinogen (See p. 272.)

Reagents

Ehrlich's Aldehyde Reagent. Dissolve 0.7 g paradimethylaminobenzaldehyde in a mixture of 150 mL concentrated hydrochloric acid and 100 mL distilled water. This is stable in a dark-brown bottle.

Saturated Sodium Acetate Solution. Add about 1000 g sodium acetate ($CH_3COONa \cdot 3H_2O$), reagent grade, to 1 liter distilled water; shake well, and heat to 60°C with occasional agitation. On cooling to room temperature there should be a large excess of crystals.

Semiquantitative Procedure (Wallace and Diamond, 1925)

1. Set up eight test tubes. In each of tubes 2 to 8, inclusive, place 5.0 mL water. In each of tubes 1 and 2 place 5.0 mL of fresh urine. Mix contents of tube 2 and transfer 5 mL to tube 3, and so on, to give doubling dilutions from 1:1 to 1:128.

2. To each tube add 0.5 mL Ehrlich's aldehyde reagent. Mix well, and let stand 5 minutes to allow color development.

3. Read in good daylight or its equivalent by inspecting vertically through the fluid in the tubes on a white background. The urobilinogen "titer" is the dilution in the last tube showing a faint pink color.

Results. Normal urines give a pink color in dilutions ranging from 1:2 to 1:16. A positive 1:32 dilution is borderline, whereas a positive in 1:64 or greater indicates increased urobilinogen excretion.

The actual clinical usefulness of even semiquantitative assays of urobilinogen in urine is open to serious doubt. The original reasons for such specifications as collection of the sample between the hours of 2 PM and 4 PM have been challenged, and the occurrence of false reactions has been emphasized. It has been shown that urobilinogen added to urines is recovered only to the extent of, at best, about 68%. The detection of increased levels of substances that react with Ehrlich's reagent in a fresh urine may therefore be significant only in early hepatitis, hemolytic diseases, and the presence of porphobilinogen in acute intermittent porphyria.

CHAPTER 11—REVIEW QUESTIONS

1. Discuss the principles of methods used to determine serum calcium.
2. Describe two methods for screening urine samples for increased levels of porphyrins.
3. What chemical changes in the amniotic fluid indicate the readiness of the fetus for an independent existence?
4. Describe the metabolism and actions of vitamin D in its role as a hormone.
5. What information can be gained from an analysis of the proteins in cerebropsinal fluid?

12

THE ENDOCRINE SYSTEM

THE CELLULAR ACTION OF HORMONES

Hormones are chemical substances released by specific cells within the body, which transmit a message to target cells. The specific cells may be grouped into a single organ (e.g., the thyroid gland) or distributed more diffusely (e.g., islet cells). The target cells may be close to the hormone-producing cells, but generally are situated at some distance from them. The amount of hormone released and subsequently picked up by the target cells determines the quantitative response of the target tissue. The hormonal message generally is amplified considerably by the target cells. Hormones circulate in the bloodstream or occasionally in tissue spaces; they may be intermediate messengers (e.g., ACTH) or a final chemical message (e.g., cortisol). By definition, they travel in the extracellular fluid; other messengers are known that operate only within the cell.

The term *endocrine gland* simply means that the secretion of the gland passes into the body tissues, as opposed to *exocrine glands*, whose secretion passes out of the body, even if only into the lumen of the gut.

Hormones are broadly classifiable into steroid hormones, polypeptide hormones, and others, e.g., prostaglandins. Hormones react only with specific target tissues and have very definite effects on these tissues. Sometimes the mode of action is relatively simple (e.g., corticotrophin releasing factor stimulates only the release of ACTH), but generally the actions are complex, although the overall cellular reaction follows a remarkably coordinated pattern. The precise way in which hormones interact with target tissues is still under intensive investigation; much remains to be discovered, and only the broadest outline will be presented here. Hormones act within the cell in a variety of ways, generally having stimulatory effects, but sometimes inhibitory ones. They can affect (i) membrane permeability, (ii) carbohydrate metabolism, (iii) enzyme induction, and (iv) allosteric regulation of enzymes.

(1) The first model of hormone action to be discussed has been called the *mobile receptor model*. This is characterized by specific binding of the hormone to a receptor, probably in the cytoplasm, with subsequent transport of the complex into the nucleus of the cell, where it appears to have direct effects on the various processes of transcription, translation, and protein synthesis. Highly specific receptor sites exist within the nucleus to bind the hormone-receptor complex. Steroid hormones, including the active derivatives of vitamin D, appear to function in this way (Fig. 12–1).

(2) The *fixed receptor model* is applicable to many polypeptide hormones. This model centers on the immensely important discovery of 3′,5′ cyclic adenosine monophosphate (cAMP) by Sutherland in the early 1960s. Cyclic AMP (Fig. 12–2) is derived from ATP by the action of the enzyme adenyl cyclase in the presence of magnesium ions:

$$\text{ATP} + \text{Mg}^{++} \xrightarrow{\text{Adenyl cyclase}} \text{cAMp} + \text{Pyrophosphate}$$

This enzyme is found in the cell membrane of many different tissues, and it appears that specificity or response is achieved by the presence of highly specific receptor sites at the surface of the cell. These are thought to "recognize" or interact with only the precise molecular configuration of the particular hormone to which the cell will respond. It is thought that the receptors and the molecules of the enzyme adenyl cyclase are combined in the cell membrane and that when the hormone is bound by the receptor, the enzyme is activated, perhaps by some allosteric effect.

Cyclic AMP is split by the enzyme phosphodiesterase to form 5′ AMP; this enzyme may have some modulating effect within the cell by controlling the rate of breakdown of cAMP.

Cyclic AMP accumulates within the cell, and acts on various parts of the cellular machinery. Since it transmits the hormonal message onward *within* the cell, it has been called the "second messenger." At least one way in which cAMP operates within the cell has been identified: it stimulates the conversion of inactive phosphorylase kinase (now called cyclic AMP–dependent protein kinase E.C. 2.7.1.37) to an active form and, through a cascade system of enzymes, stimulates the conversion of glycogen to glucose-1-PO_4 (Fig. 12–3). Protein kinase also has an inhibitory action on glycogen synthetase. The net result is to make more energy-producing substrates available for the cell metabolism.

However, active protein kinase appears to have other specific effects within the cell by phosphorylating certain responsive proteins, probably those associated with the internal membranes of the cell. Such phosphorylation alters the tertiary structure of the protein, thus changing its enzymatic or other properties.

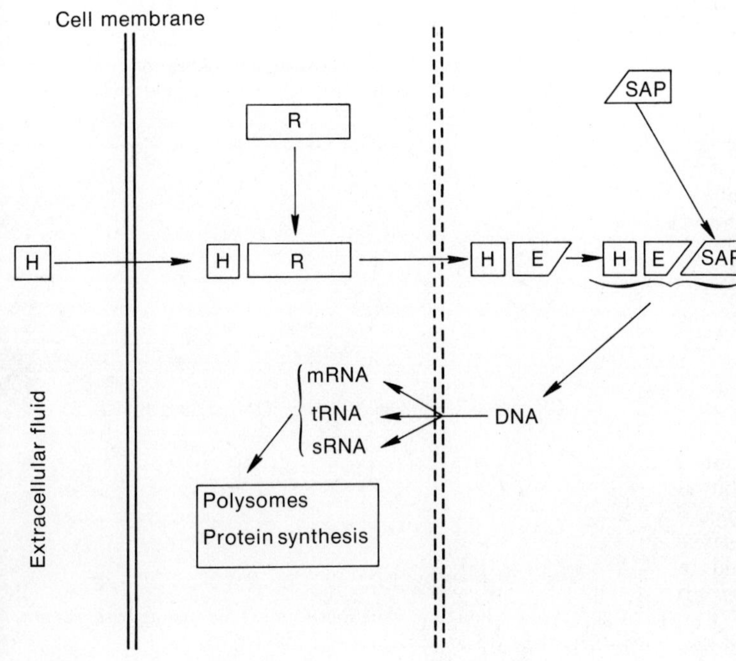

Figure 12–1 The mobile receptor model of hormone action. *H*, hormone; *R*, receptor; *HE*, hormone-effector complex; *SAP*, specific acidic protein.

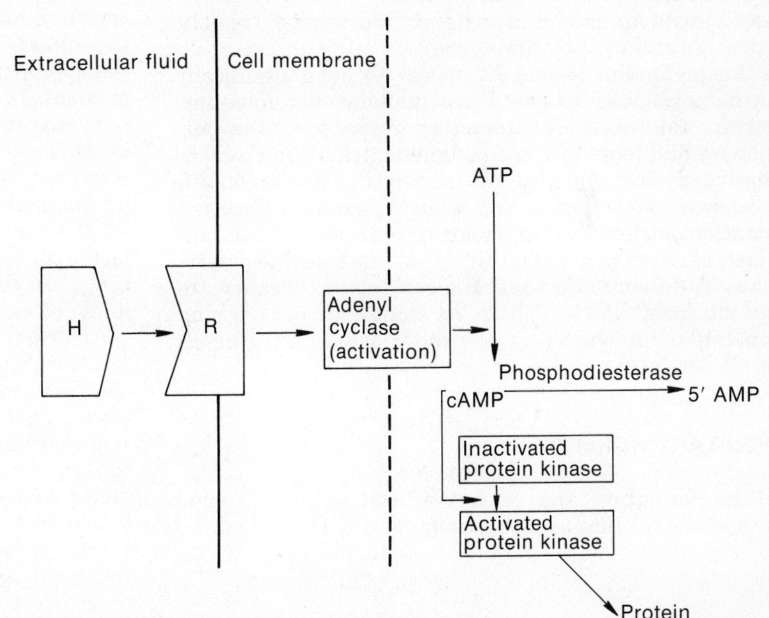

Figure 12–2 The fixed receptor model of hormonal action. *H*, hormone; *R*, receptor.

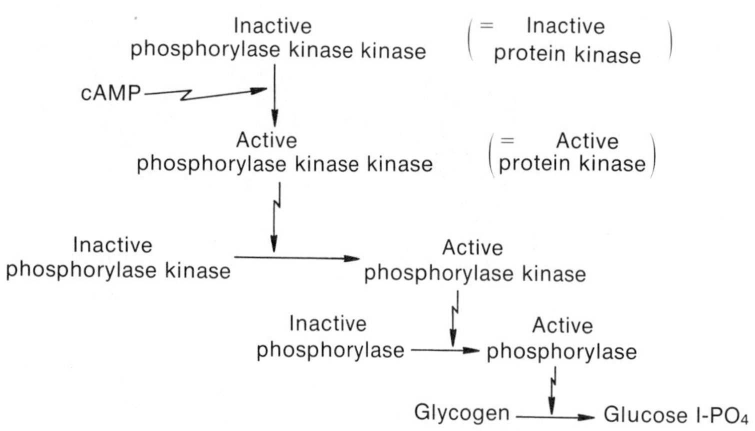

Figure 12–3 The cascade system of enzymes by which cyclic AMP activates liver and muscle phosphorylase.

PROSTAGLANDINS

The term *prostaglandin* is the generic name for a large family of closely related lipids that are distributed ubiquitously in mammalian tissues and that produce a wide variety of physiological effects. The name derives from the fact that they were originally identified in prostatic secretions. Chemically the structure of all these compounds is based on that of prostanoic acid (Fig. 12–4). The principal naturally occurring prostaglandins are designated by Roman letters, according to the functional groups attached to the 5-member ring (Fig. 12–5). Substitutions on the side chains produce many variants; some of the synthetic derivatives are more potent than the parent compounds.

Prostaglandin A is a true hormone; the remainder apparently act intracellularly (within the cell that synthesized them) or within a tissue. Most are extremely active, even in nanogram amounts.

Prostaglandins A and E_2 appear to have significant antihypertensive actions. Prostaglandins also have important roles in the inflammatory response and in pulmonary and reproductive functions. Intrauterine contraceptive devices function by stimulating prostaglandin release in the endometrium, which apparently prevents nidation. Ingestion of salicylate (a prostaglandin antagonist) can be a cause of failure of an intrauterine device. The anti-inflammatory and analgesic effects of salicylate are at least partly due to its action in suppressing prostaglandin synthesis. (For other details see Russell et al., 1975.)

Figure 12–5 Structural variations forming the major prostaglandin subdivisions.

Figure 12–4 The structure of prostanoic acid.

PITUITARY HORMONES

The formation and release of the various trophic hormones of the adenohypophysis are controlled by "neurohumors" elaborated in the hypothalamus and carried to the pituitary gland by the hypophyseal portal system of the tuberal hypothalamus and pituitary stalk. These neurohumors have been called "releasing factors" because this was the action first and most dramatically shown when they were added to adenohypophyseal transplants or cultures. However, they also stimulate the appropriate anterior pituitary cells to synthesize the particular trophic hormone. Generally, secretion of the releasing factors is subject to negative feedback control by the end product of the target organ, e.g., thyroid hormones, cortisol, and estrogens. Some of these end products also exert a direct negative feedback control on the anterior pituitary cells that make the trophic factor concerned, but this action is generally less important than that inhibiting the production of the hypothalamic releasing factors.

At least six trophic hormones are formed by the pituitary gland: thyrotropic (TSH), adrenocorticotropic (ACTH), two gonadotropins (follicle-stimulating hormone, FSH, and luteinizing hormone, LH), growth or somatotrophic hormone (GH or STH), and prolactin. In the case of each of the first five, a hypothalamic releasing factor exerts a major controlling influence on the synthesis and secretion of its respective trophic hormone. Prolactin is an exception in that its hypothalamic neurohumor actually inhibits release of prolactin, and therefore is called the prolactin-inhibiting factor. Because of this, prolactin is the only anterior pituitary hormone secreted in increased amounts after section or destruction of the pituitary stalk—this despite the fact that in humans up to 90% of the gland is infarcted by severance of the stalk. Lesions of the pituitary stalk, e.g., owing to surgery or conditions such as sarcoidosis, therefore may lead to galactorrhea (excessive inappropriate milk secretion), as also may large doses of reserpine or chlorpromazine, which prevent the release of prolactin-inhibiting factor.

Thyroid-Stimulating Hormone (TSH)

The normal plasma level of this glycoprotein hormone is less than 3 ng per mL. Its blood concentration is increased above 10 ng per mL in myxedema and after surgical removal or radioisotope destruction of the thyroid without hormonal substitution therapy. In hyperthyroidism, plasma TSH is usually low but may be normal, and it is low also in patients receiving exogenous thyroid hormones in relatively large doses. The hypothalamic releasing factor for TSH (thyrotropin releasing hormone, TRH) is a tripeptide that has been synthesized.

Adrenocorticotropic Hormone (ACTH)

This single-chain polypeptide (M.W. 4567) is composed of 39 amino acids, the sequence of the first 13 of which is identical to that of MSH (melanocyte stimulating hormone). The normal adenohypophysis contains an average of 15 units (range, 0 to 30 units) of ACTH (potency of ACTH = 100 to 140 units per mg). Although this amount may seem very small, a secretion rate of 4 units per hour produces and maintains maximal adrenocortical stimulation, despite the fact that the half-life of ACTH is only about 20 minutes.

Growth Hormone (GH)

Growth hormone is the most abundant hormone in the pituitary, amounting to a remarkable 5 to 10% of the dry weight of the gland. It is a polypeptide (M.W. about 20,000). Surprisingly, only in the neonatal period does the plasma GH level bear any relationship to growth rate. After this period it shows no relationship to growth or growth spurts but is remarkably responsive to metabolic and activity changes, and especially to hypoglycemia. Patients with hypopituitarism exhibit a greatly diminished or absent GH response to hypoglycemia, and this forms a useful screening test for growth hormone deficiency in dwarfism.

Pituitary Gonadotropins

Follicle-Stimulating Hormone (FSH)

This is a glycoprotein (M.W. 25,000 to 30,000) containing 8% carbohydrate, in which sialic acid is an essential component, since the hormone is inactivated by neuraminidase. In the female, FSH promotes the growth and maturation of the Graafian follicle, but does not act as a primary or potent stimulator of estrogen secretion or synthesis. In the male, FSH stimulates spermatogenesis.

Luteinizing Hormone (LH)

This also is a glycoprotein, whose half-life is about 1 hour. In the female, it stimulates the synthesis of estrogens by granulosa cells already prepared by FSH. At the time of ovulation it appears that a rhythmically determined surge of LH secretion brings about follicle rupture, after which it promotes transformation of the granulosa cells of the ruptured follicle to progesterone-secreting corpus luteum cells (see Fig. 12–19). In the male, LH stimulates secretion of testosterone by the interstitial (Leydig) cells of the testis.

The interplay of FSH/LH releasing factor, of FSH and LH, and of estradiol and progesterone in the estrous cycle is described elsewhere (p. 304).

Menopausal Gonadotropin

After the menopause normal ovaries involute and cease to manufacture estrogens. With this negative feedback control no longer operative, FSH and LH are secreted in large amounts. Most of the LH is metabolized and inactivated, so that less than 0.5% of it is excreted in active form in the urine. A much greater proportion (12%) of FSH is excreted unchanged. Hence, human menopausal urinary gonadotropin consists predominantly of FSH. However, *plasma* levels of LH are markedly elevated in postmenopausal women, whereas a gradual rise occurs in men in the later decades of life.

THE THYROID GLAND

The normal adult thyroid gland weighs 15 to 35 g and is composed of two lobes joined by an isthmus, which lies in front of the first two or three tracheal rings. The lobes lie on either side of the trachea (first 4 to 5 rings) and extend up on the sides of the larynx as far as the oblique line of the thyroid cartilage.

Histologically, the thyroid is composed of more or less round follicles or vesicles, which normally range from 50 to 250 μm in diameter. Each follicle is surrounded by a basement membrane and is lined by cuboidal to low-cuboidal cells. The lumen of the follicle is filled with colloid, seen in hematoxylin-eosin sections as a homogeneous pinkish red coagulum. Occasionally, groups of cells may be found scattered among the cells lining the vesicles. These are the C-cells, which secrete calcitonin.

Synthesis of Thyroid Hormones

Here we are concerned with the formation of the iodothyronines, thyroxine (tetraiodothyronine; T_4) and triiodothyronine (T_3), which are the physiologically important secretions of the gland. This process involves the absorption and concentration of iodide by the gland, conversion of the iodide to an active form that is used to iodinate tyrosine residues, and the secretion and storage of the hormones as thyroglobulin into the follicular lumen, where they remain until required.

Absorption and Concentration (Trapping) of Iodide by the Thyroid

An adult on an average normal diet absorbs some 150 to 200 μg of iodide per day. This is absorbed almost exclusively as inorganic iodide, although T_4 and T_3 are absorbed unchanged. Of the absorbed dietary iodide, about two-thirds is excreted by the kidney and one-third is taken up by the thyroid, which can clear 10 to 35 mL of plasma of iodide per minute, depending on its activity.

The thyroid transport system for iodide is both rapid and efficient and establishes in the normal person a thyroid-serum (T/S) iodide concentration ratio ranging from about 10:1 to 40:1. Thyrotropin (thyroid-stimulating hormone; TSH), which is secreted by basophil cells of the anterior pituitary, is the main stimulatory regulator of iodide transport into the gland. Iodide is also transported by the cells of the salivary gland, placenta, and breast and by the mucoid cells in the necks of the gastric gland crypts. In none of the sites is transport nearly so rapid as in the thyroid, in which labeled iodide appears in the colloid within minutes or even seconds of intravenous injection of the isotope dose.

Within the thyroid gland the iodine is oxidized (that is, loses an electron), in which form it is attached to the benzene ring of tyrosine to form monoiodotyrosine (MIT) and diiodotyrosine (DIT) (Fig. 12–6). The next stage is the coupling of one molecule of MIT with one of DIT to form triiodothyronine, and of two molecules of DIT to form tetraiodothyronine (T_4). All of these steps are under the control of thyroid-stimulating hormone (TSH). The thyroid hormones are stored attached to a large glycoprotein molecule called thyroglobulin, within the follicles of the gland.

The hormones are released from the thyroglobulin molecule by the action of proteases and peptidases, under the stimulating influence of TSH. MIT and DIT are also released at the same time, but their iodine content is salvaged by a deiodinating enzyme in the acinar cells, and the iodine is recycled.

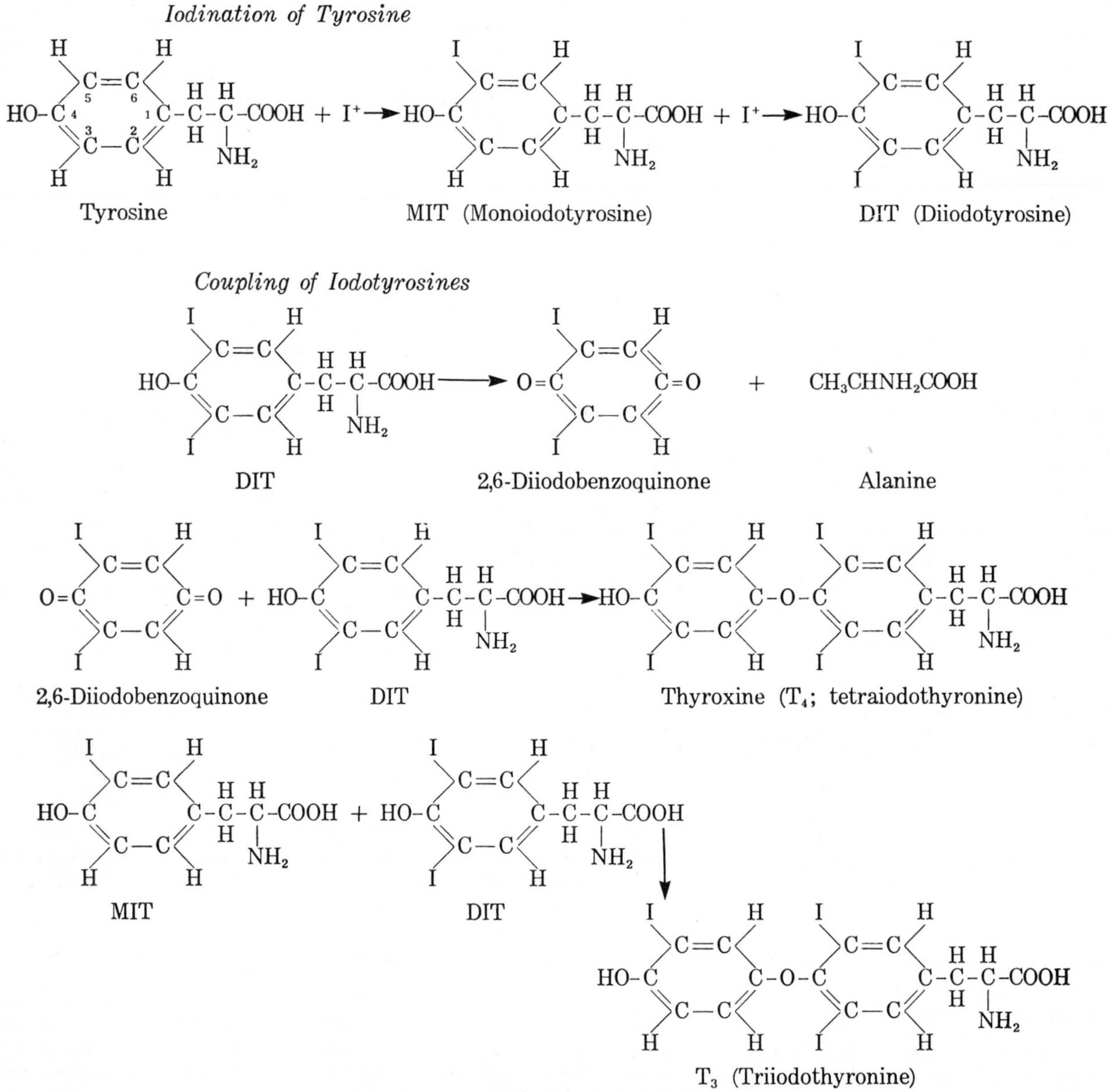

Iodination of Tyrosine

Tyrosine + I^+ → MIT (Monoiodotyrosine) + I^+ → DIT (Diiodotyrosine)

Coupling of Iodotyrosines

DIT → 2,6-Diiodobenzoquinone + CH_3CHNH_2COOH (Alanine)

2,6-Diiodobenzoquinone + DIT → Thyroxine (T_4; tetraiodothyronine)

MIT + DIT → T_3 (Triiodothyronine)

Figure 12–6 Synthesis of thyroid hormones.

Transport and Function of Thyroid Hormones

Normally, more than 80 to 90% of total thyroid hormones in the blood consists of T_4. Over 99% of this is bound to a special globulin, TBG (thyroxine-binding globulin), which is a glycoprotein with electrophoretic mobility close to that of the alpha$_2$ globulins. A very small amount of T_4 is also carried by albumin and by prealbumin (TBPA). The amount of free T_4 in normal plasma is about 1.8 ng per dL, or approximately 0.1% of the bound hormone.

T_3 is also bound by TBG, but the affinity of TBG for T_4 is three times greater than for T_3. T_3 is also carried by albumin but not by prealbumin.

Although the concentrations of free T_4 and free T_3 in the plasma are very small, it is just these fractions that are of paramount importance in establishing the thyroid status of an individual and that, at present, are still very difficult to estimate accurately.

The thyroid secretes, quantitatively, more T_4 than T_3. However, T_3 is the more potent hormone, probably because of its greater binding affinity for the receptor sites in the target cells. Also, it is most important to remember that *T_4 is converted to T_3 in the peripheral tissues*, that this conversion is probably by some enzymatic process, and that it is inhibited by severe nonthyroidal illness, malnutrition, and starvation. Approximately 60% of the daily production of T_3 arises from peripheral monodeiodination of T_4.

Once the thyroid hormones reach the target cell, they bind to a cytosol receptor and pass into the nucleus, where they appear to bind to and act on specific segments of the nuclear DNA. However, there are probably other sites of action within the cell, such as the mitochondria.

The effects of thyroid hormones are complex, and there is good evidence that both T_4 and T_3 are needed for the full expression of the hormone action. Essentially, they appear to stimulate the basal metabolic rate, oxygen consumption, and heat production. They are also very important in the development of the child: lack of thyroid hormone secretions during infancy causes severe mental retardation (cretinism); consequently many health authorities have established neonatal screening programs for thyroid deficiency.

The plasma levels of the free hormones (and consequently of the total) are controlled within relatively narrow limits by a system of negative feedback. As already stated, the synthesis, storage, and release of the hormones in the thyroid gland are largely under the control of TSH. TSH is secreted by specific cells in the anterior lobe of the pituitary gland. These in turn are stimulated by the tripeptide hormone, thyrotropin releasing hormone (TRH), which is secreted by specific neurones in the hypothalamus and travels down the pituitary stalk to the anterior lobe of the pituitary gland.

The release of TRH by the hypothalamus and of TSH by the pituitary are both modulated by the level of free T_4 and T_3 in the plasma. As these rise, so TSH secretion falls. Even a small excess of T_4 or T_3 will effectively inhibit the release of TRH and TSH. These are essential facts in the interpretation of thyroid function tests.

Disorders of Function of Thyroid in Disease

The word *goiter* is applied to any persistent enlargement of the thyroid gland; the enlargement may be diffuse or nodular. The term is not generally applied to a single nodule in one lobe. The goiter may be *endemic*, occurring in many people in a particular geographic area, or *sporadic*, occurring rarely as a familial defect or more commonly as an isolated case. Endemic goiter owing to iodide deficiency was a common disorder in many areas of the world until the introduction of iodized table salt. These areas were mainly inland or mountainous, or other localities, where the iodine has been leached out of the soil, e.g., Himalayas, the Great Lakes region of North America, and Derbyshire in England. Sporadic goiter in younger people is generally diffuse, and may occur physiologically at puberty or during pregnancy. Goiter also occurs in Graves' disease, Hashimoto's disease, de Quervain's thyroiditis, and in thyroid carcinoma. Multinodular goiter tends to occur in older people and may or may not be associated with thyrotoxicosis.

Thyrotoxicosis

Thyrotoxicosis is a condition in which there is excessive secretion of thyroxine and triiodothyronine by the thyroid gland. Graves' disease is the term applied to a diffuse hyperplasia of the gland (a goiter) associated with exophthalmos. It is the commonest form of thyrotoxicosis and occurs far more frequently in females than in males. Single and multiple adenomas of the thyroid gland occur, as do carcinomas, but only a small proportion of these exhibit autonomous endocrine activity and thyrotoxicosis.

The symptoms of thyrotoxicosis are nervousness, tremor, tachycardia, sweating, fatigue, weight loss, and extreme dislike of hot weather.

The cause of Graves' disease is obscure. The diffuse hyperplasia and overactivity of the gland do not seem to be owing to excessive secretion of TSH by the pituitary, in that circulating TSH levels generally are below normal, and the glandular function appears to be autonomous, since it is generally not suppressible by T_3 administration.

The problem of the pathogenesis of Graves' disease appeared to have been solved in 1956 when a long-acting thyroid stimulator (LATS) was discovered in the plasma of patients with thyrotoxicosis. TSH produces a peak secretion of T_4 by the thyroid gland 2 hours after injection, whereas LATS gives a maximum response 16 hours after. LATS was shown to be a gamma globulin, suggesting that Graves' disease was an autoimmune disease. However, although LATS may be an important factor in the pathogenesis of Graves' disease, its discovery does not solve all of the problems, and it appears that other factors must be involved. Furthermore, it seems fairly certain that the exophthalmos is not owing to LATS, and its cause is still unknown.

The laboratory findings are the reverse of those described for myxedema. Both total T_4 and T_3 are usually elevated, although in about 5-10% of cases the T_3 alone is high, a condition referred to as T_3-thyrotoxicosis. Measurement of total T_3 is the best single test at present for the detection of thyrotoxicosis. The assay of free T_4 is probably a superior test but, although some commercial methods for its measurement are available, we feel they require further evaluation. The most sensitive test for the determination of marginal or early thyrotoxicosis, when the available in vitro tests are equivocal, is the TRH stimulation test, described later.

Myxedema

This is an acquired hypothyroid state in a person who previously had been euthyroid. Partial hypothyroidism is most commonly seen in the late phase of a destructive thyroiditis. Myxedema can occur as a side effect of lithium therapy. Primary or idiopathic myxedema usually is seen in the last few decades of life and is associated with complete or virtually complete atrophy and disappearance of the gland without residual fibrosis. The cause is rarely if ever apparent.

Affected patients are characteristically very intolerant of cold weather and show coarsening of the face, thickening of the skin, deepening of the voice, and increasing loss of memory. They gradually become slower in thought and action, and their tendon reflexes exhibit not only rather slow contraction, but an abnormally prolonged relaxation phase. The term *myxedema* is derived from the myxomatous histological appearance of the areas of pseudoedema that occur in the skin.

The basal metabolic rate is low and the total serum thyroxine (T_4), the free thyroxine index, and the true free (dialyzable) thyroxine are all lower than normal, whereas the T_3 resin uptake shows increased binding sites. The neck uptake of iodine is reduced. The most reliable single index of primary hypothyroidism is the measurement of plasma TSH, which will be discussed later. The fall in T_4 and T_3 production causes an elevation of plasma TSH levels by way of the hypothalamic-pituitary feedback mechanism.

Multinodular Goiter

This condition is characterized by the formation of numerous adenomas in the gland. These are benign tumors derived from the thyroid acinar cells; the etiology is unknown. Although these adenomas usually remain under TSH control, for unknown reasons occasionally one or more become autonomous and secrete excessive amounts of thyroid hormones, producing a hyperthyroid (thyrotoxic) state. They may also undergo necrosis, hemorrhage, and calcification.

Hashimoto's Disease

Hashimoto's disease is an autoimmune disease characterized by a diffuse enlargement of the gland and microscopically by extensive destruction of the acini, the presence of a marked lymphocytic infiltration, and the formation of numerous germinal centers. The disease is much commoner in women.

In the early phase the patient usually presents with thyrotoxic symptoms, but eventually, as the destruction of the gland proceeds, the patient passes into an irreversible state of hypothyroidism. The plasma contains thyroglobulin and microsomal antibodies, usually in very high titer. However, it appears that these are only one facet of the disease process and that they arise from a complex and poorly understood derangement of the patient's immune system rather than as a reaction to thyroglobulin released from the gland into the bloodstream.

Thyroid Cancer

The majority of cancers of the thyroid are "cold," i.e., they do not actively take up ^{131}I. The neoplastic cells probably have lost the capacity to produce one or all of the hormonogenic enzymes.

INVESTIGATION OF THYROID FUNCTION

The thyroid and adrenal cortex, both of which are controlled by the hypothalamopituitary system, are, together with the islands of Langerhans, the most important endocrine glands in the body. As already briefly mentioned, the thyroid hormones have a widespread influence, affecting almost every cell and many of the cellular enzymes of the body. Assessment of thyroid function is obviously important; this can be accomplished by: (1) measuring its net effect, (2) estimating the concentration of its hormones in the blood, (3) measuring the proportion of plasma thyroid hormones available for uptake by the cells, and (4) investigating particular aspects of the gland's hormonogenic function and control.

Theoretically, the best test of thyroid function is one that measures overall or net effect on metabolism—in particular, basal metabolism.

Basal Metabolism

The term *basal metabolic rate* refers to the minimal rate of overall energy production in the body. Energy is derived from the oxidation of foodstuffs; some of the energy is stored in various forms such as *energy-rich compounds,* whereas some appears as heat. The energy turnover in the body therefore may be measured indirectly either by estimating heat production or oxygen consumption. Formerly the only way of measuring the thyroid status was by measuring the basal metabolic rate, usually by some respirometer method.

The test is now seldom used, since it is technically difficult to carry out and is unreliable in general use. It is possible, given sufficient care and technical expertise, to estimate the basal metabolic rate accurately, but this is normally so difficult in routine hospital practice that alternative tests are preferred. A detailed description of the technique of measuring the basal metabolic rate will be found in the second edition of this text.

LABORATORY TESTS OF THYROID FUNCTION

The measurement of circulating thyronines can be accomplished by (1) techniques that estimate the iodine content or (2) radioligand assays.

Iodine Content Estimation Techniques

The measurement of basal metabolic rate in the assessment of thyroid function was displaced by the determination of protein-bound iodine (PBI), which once held a major position in such investigations. However, in the face of the alternative techniques available, it cannot be recommended as a satisfactory routine procedure; nor can methods using column chromatography.

Thyroid Hormones Ligand Assay

The principles of ligand assays are discussed elsewhere (p. 91). At present these are the methods of choice for measuring T_3, T_4, T_3-resin uptake, and TSH, using either a radioisotope or an enzyme as the label. A number of commercial methods are available in kit form, most of which have adequate sensitivity and precision. However, bad batches can occur, and a rigorous quality control system must be used.

The method chosen for use by a particular laboratory depends on many local factors, including the number of tests to be done and the available instrumentation. Cost alone must not be the sole factor governing the choice of a particular method or kit: its reliability and performance in terms of accuracy, precision, and other factors are paramount considerations. Some methods are easier to use in automated counting equipment for large batches, whereas others work well in small numbers in the thyrometers that calculate each test as it is inserted into the counter.

Free Thyroxine Estimation

As already described, the important determinant of thyroid status is the unbound fraction of thyroxine present in the plasma, since this is related directly to the tissue dose. By adding some radioactive thyroxine to a serum sample and dialysing the serum across a semipermeable membrane, it is possible to estimate the unbound fraction. The method can be made quite reliable, but it is not a suitable routine procedure; calculation of the free thyroxine index is a more practical method (see further on). Several commercial methods are available: our experience with these so far has not been very satisfactory, and we still rely on calculating a free thyroxine index.

T_3-Uptake Methods

These methods measure the free binding sites available on the carrier proteins of the test sera. The principle is that triiodothyronine (T_3) labeled with ^{131}I or ^{125}I is added to the test serum; this binds to free carrier sites that are not already occupied by nonradioactive T_4 and T_3. The radioactive T_3 that has not been bound is then picked up by adding a carrier; originally erythrocytes were used, but later resins were introduced and were found to give more reproducible results. T_3 was chosen originally, since it binds more firmly to the natural carrier sites, and then is less easily detached from these when the carrier resin is added. The test is usually called the T_3-resin uptake test. It should be understood that it does *not* measure serum T_3 levels, nor does it have anything to do with the measurement of neck uptake of radioiodine in the body. It is purely an in vitro test.

The results are usually expressed as the percentage of the added T_3 that is taken up by the added resin. Thus, in thyrotoxicosis, more T_4 than usual is present in the serum, but because the total binding power remains the same, fewer free binding sites are present. Therefore less added T_3 will be bound to them, and more will be available to be taken up by the resin. Thus a high percentage of resin uptake is found in thyrotoxicosis. However, some tests work inversely to this (e.g., the Thyopac–3 procedure), and the exact method of expressing the test results, and the normal range, vary from method to method, although any particular method should give consistent results. It is recommended that one reliable method be adopted, carefully tested, and evaluated in each laboratory. The various firms supplying T_4 test kits also supply kits for T_3-uptake studies. Because of the variety of units for T_3-uptake, authorities both in North America and Europe recommend reporting a normalized value, so that the median value of the reference range is expressed as 100 (see Solomon, 1976).

TRH Stimulation Test

This is a very sensitive test for the detection of early thyrotoxicosis; it is especially useful when the total T_4, T_3, and FTI are at, or only slightly above, the upper limit of the reference range. It can also be used in suspected hypothyroidism, although it is less useful for this purpose.

Thyrotropin releasing hormone (TRH) is a tripeptide: the diagnostic material is available as a synthetic compound chemically identical to the natural hormone. The detailed instructions supplied with the material should be followed when using it. Briefly, a fasting blood sample is taken, and the patient is then given an intravenous injection of 0.2 mg of TRH as a bolus. Blood samples are taken at 15 and 30 minutes (some take a 60-min sample also). TSH assays are performed on the samples; the responses in hypothyroid, hyperthyroid, and euthyroid individuals are shown in Figure 12–7.

For a normal response the fasting TSH level should be less than 10 μU/mL and should show an incremental rise of 5 to 30 μU. A low fasting TSH with no apparent rise (taking into account the assay error on a single estimate) is indicative of thyrotoxicosis.

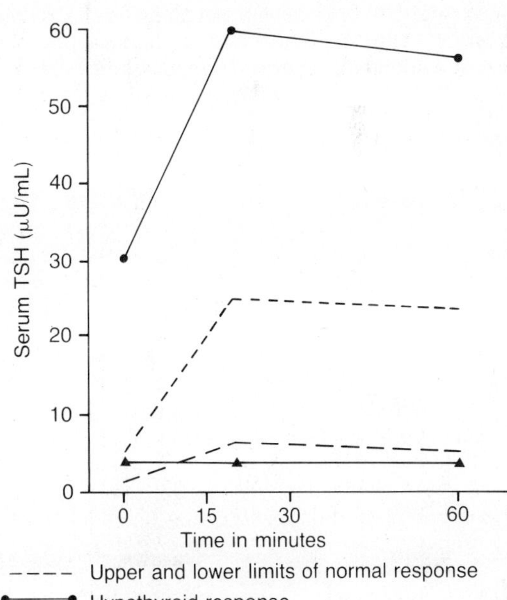

Figure 12–7 The TRH stimulation test.

The Interpretation of in vitro Thyroid Function Tests

The reference range for serum thyroxine depends to some extent on the method and the population samples. Obviously a method with low precision will give a wider reference range than one with higher precision. However, a representative value is 2.8 to 7.5 μg thyroxine iodine per dL (or 55 to 148 nmol thyroxine per liter, or 4.5 to 11.5 μg thyroxine per dL).

The T_4- and T_3-uptake values can be combined to give a figure called the Free Thyroxine Index (FTI). This sometimes has been called the T_7 value, but this use should be discontinued. The FTI shows a very close correlation with the free dialyzable thyroxine levels. It is obtained by multiplying the T_4- and T_3-uptake values together: $\frac{T_3\text{-uptake}}{100} \times T_4$. Again, it is preferable for each laboratory to obtain its normal FTI range for the particular methods used. This can be done simply by analyzing at least 50 normal sera. There does not appear to be any sex difference. The upper and lower limits of the FTI range should *not* be obtained by multiplying the upper and lower limits, respectively, of the T_4- and T_3-uptake ranges.

To understand the way in which the FTI can give a better assessment of thyroid status than the T_4- and T_3-uptake tests alone, consider Figure 12–8. The height of the column *(a)* represents the total thyroxine-binding capacity of the serum carrier proteins, the hatched area represents the proportion of binding sites occupied by T_4, and the blank area represents unoccupied binding sites. Bound and free T_4 are in equilibrium, and the proportion of free T_4 present in the plasma is determined by the ratio of bound T_4 to the free binding sites, *not* by the absolute amount of bound T_4 present. Thus in Figure 12–8 *(b)*, the total binding capacity is the same as in *(a)*, the bound T_4 is increased, the free binding sites are reduced, and the T_3-resin uptake therefore is increased. Multiplying the T_3-uptake and T_4 test values gives a high value outside the normal range, which is indicative of a high free serum T_4 level and thus of thyrotoxicosis. Exactly the opposite reasoning holds for thyroid hypofunction (myxedema), as shown in *(c)*.

To see the real value of the FTI, look at column *(d)*. The total binding capacity is increased, and the bound T_4 is increased also, but the number of free binding sites is also higher. Thus, although the total T_4 will be increased, the T_3 uptake will be reduced, and multiplying the two together will cancel out the two effects and give a value in the normal range. This situation is one in which there is an increase only in the total number of binding sites, and it occurs most commonly in pregnancy and in women who are taking some types of contraceptive pill. The effect is caused by estrogen and is not seen in women taking a pill with a low estrogen potency (mini-pill) or containing only a progestogenic agent. Occasionally increased binding protein is found as a harmless congenital anomaly.

The FTI generally provides a good assessment of thyroid function; a few problems of interpretation occasionally are encountered and will be discussed briefly here. The decision-tree schema shown in Figure 12–9 may be found to be of some help in interpretation.

(1) These in vitro tests are more sensitive in the diagnosis of thyrotoxicosis than of myxedema. If the latter condition is suspected clinically, and the FTI is normal or equivocal, the serum TSH level should be estimated. This will be high in myxedema, provided pituitary function is normal (i.e., in primary myxedema).

(2) In patients who are receiving thyroxine replacement therapy and are euthyroid, the T_4 and FTI tend to be higher than normal. It is usually better to assess the replacement dose in such patients by their clinical status and also by adjusting the dose until the TSH level comes just into the normal range. The reason for the high values is not clear, but T_3 (triidothyronine) is much more potent than T_4, and loss of the normal secretion by the thyroid must represent a significant loss of T_3 to the tissues. It may be, therefore, that the peripheral conversion of T_4 to T_3 must proceed at a higher rate than normal, and higher serum T_4 levels are required to supply this reaction.

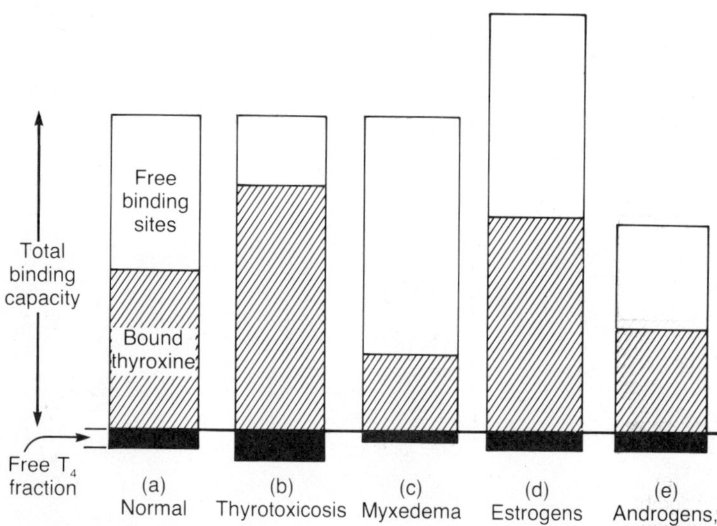

Figure 12–8 Total binding capacity, bound thyroxine, and free thyroxine in various clinical states. (See text for explanation.)

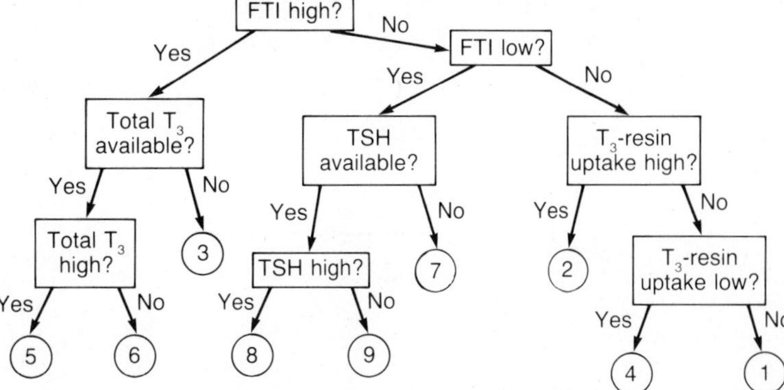

Figure 12–9 Schema for interpretation of in vitro thyroid function tests. *FTI*, free thyroxine index (T_7); *TSH*, thyroid stimulating hormone.

Interpretations

1. Patient is probably euthyroid; obtain total T_3 if thyrotoxicosis is still suspected.
2. Patient is euthyroid, but the elevated T_3-uptake may be due to nonthyroidal illness or to drugs such as salicylates or phenytoin.
3. Patient has approximately 10% chance of hyperthyroidism. Obtain total T_3.
4. Patient is euthyroid, but the low T_3-uptake may be due to estrogen therapy, for example "the pill."
5. Patient is thyrotoxic or is receiving excessive thyroxine therapy.
6. The combination of high FTI with normal or low total T_3 can occur in nonthyroidal illness, thyroiditis, and so forth. Obtain TSH or discuss with pathologist.
7. Patient has approximately 30% chance of hypothyroidism. Obtain TSH.
8. Patient is hypothyroid with normal pituitary function.
9. Patient is probably euthyroid. Secondary hypothyroidism is possible but rare. Obtain total T_3 or discuss with pathologist.

(3) Occasionally an obviously thyrotoxic patient is encountered in whom the serum T_4 and FTI are normal or even low. In such cases a serum T_3 level should be obtained, since the overactive gland can be producing T_3 and not T_4, and the radioligand tests are specific for T_4 only and will not measure T_3.

(4) In rare cases unusually low serum T_4 levels may be found, but the FTI is in the normal range (Fig. 12–7 *[e]*). This is owing to a reduction in the total number of available binding sites and is seen (a) in the course of androgen and phenytoin (Dilantin) therapy; (b) when there is an excessive loss of carrier protein (e.g., nephrotic syndrome, protein-losing enteropathy); and (c) occasionally as a harmless inherited disorder.

THE ADRENAL GLANDS

The adrenal glands are paired organs, one being situated at the upper pole of each kidney. They lie in close apposition to the kidneys, but are separated by fascia, and there is no direct functional relationship between them. They are very vascular organs, and receive a rich blood supply from three suprarenal arteries. Venous drainage is by a large central vein, which on the left side drains via the inferior phrenic vein into the left renal vein and on the right side directly into the inferior vena cava.

The average weight of a normal adult adrenal gland is 4 g, but it is greater (6 to 7 g) in individuals dying after a stressful illness. The adrenal glands possess a pale yellow cortex and a dark brown medulla. The cortex is recognized as being composed of three layers: from the surface inward these are the zona glomerulosa, the zona fasciculata, and the zona reticularis, which secrete aldosterone, cortisol, and sex hormones, respectively. In humans the functional and histological distinction, while present, is not so clear as in some mammals, and the zona glomerulosa does not, in the normal gland, form a continuous layer.

The medulla is a neuroectodermal derivative; its cells store and secrete epinephrine (adrenaline), for which it is the major source, and norepinephrine (noradrenaline).

GENERAL CHEMISTRY AND NOMENCLATURE OF THE STEROID HORMONES

The steroid hormones constitute the largest group of chemically related hormones in the body and comprise the endocrine secretions of the ovaries, testes, and suprarenal cortices. They share—along with cholesterol, bile acids, ergosterol, vitamin D, and cardiac glycosides (digoxin and others)—a similar basic structure, i.e., the cyclopentano-perhydrophenanthrene nucleus. Minor chemical differences in the groups attached to the carbon atoms of this basic ring, as well as changes in the side chain attached to the C-17, lead to profound differences in physiological function, and because of this the numbering of the carbon atoms is of great importance (Fig. 12–10).

The nomenclature of the steroid hormones is somewhat confusing, many having four names: (1) an alphabetical letter used when the compound was first isolated or recognized by its effects and before it was chemically identified, e.g., compounds E, F, and S; (2) a common chemical name, e.g., cortisone, corticosterone, aldosterone, progesterone, estrone, and testosterone; (3) a systematic chemical name, e.g., 17 α-21-dihydroxy-Δ^4-pregnene-3, 11, 20-trione (compound E, cortisone); and (4) commercial names.

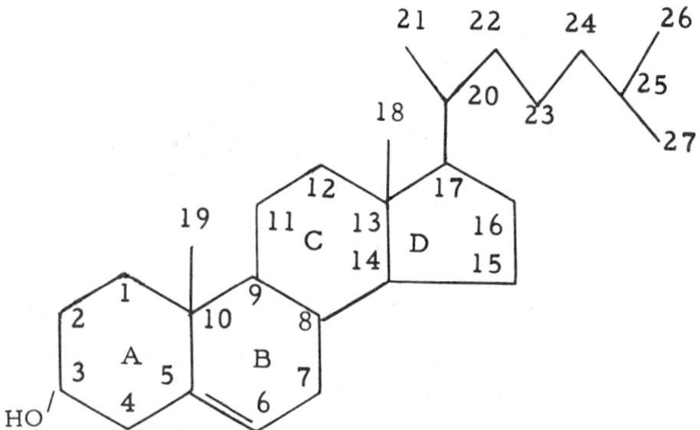

Figure 12–10 Cholesterol: methyl groups are present on carbons 18, 19, 21, 26, and 27.

STEREOISOMERISM OF STEROID HORMONES

Isomerism in the steroids may be of two types. The first is nuclear, depending on the spatial arrangement at the junctions of the rings A, B, C, and D, two configurations being possible—cis and trans. The normal steroids are trans at the junctions of rings B and C, and C and D, and usually cis at A-B (in estrogens there are no A-B isomers because ring A is aromatic). The second type of isomerism in the steroids is based on the methyl group(s) attached to carbon 10 or 13 or both. These serve as reference points to describe the location of other substituent or side groups in relation to the plane of the molecule. By convention, the methyl groups at C-10 and C-13 are regarded as projecting above the plane of the four carbon rings, and any groups on the same side of the molecule are described as being in the cis ("this side of") or beta position (e.g., the side chain attached at C-17) and are shown as solid valence bonds in molecular formulae. Groups on the other side of the molecule from the methyl groups are described as being in the trans or alpha position and are shown in structural formulae as broken-line bonds.

In addition to the methyl groups, hydroxyl (—OH) and keto (=O) groups are frequently attached to the ring nucleus; their location is given by stating the number of the carbon atom to which they are attached, together with the prefix *alpha-* or *beta-* to indicate the orientation relative to the methyl groups, e.g., 11 β-hydroxy or 17 β-hydroxy (in practice, the prefix beta is usually omitted). When unsaturated valences (double bonds) are present between carbon atoms of the ring nucleus, these are indicated by the symbol Δ, followed by the number of the first unsaturated carbon atom; Δ^4, for instance, indicates a double bond between C-4 and C-5. The suffix -ene is used in the systematic chemical name to indicate such unsaturation, e.g., Δ^4-androstene-17-ol-3-one is testosterone. On the other hand, the suffix -ane denotes a saturated ring. The prefix hydroxy- (also oxy-) is used to denote the presence of a hydroxyl (—OH) group, the same being conveyed by the suffix -ol, whereas -diol and -triol indicate possession of two and three hydroxyl groups, respectively. Presence of a ketone (=O) group may be shown by the prefix keto- or by the suffix -one; two and three ketone groups are denoted by -dione and -trione, respectively. An example of the general usefulness and application of this chemically descriptive nomenclature may be seen in the case of testosterone, 17 β-hydroxyandrost-4-en-3-one, the written systematic formula of which tells us that the valence between C-4 and C-5 is unsaturated and that a hydroxyl group is attached to C-17 and a ketone group at C-3.

The prefix deoxy- indicates loss of an oxygen atom (either as =O, or —OH). Dehydro- denotes loss of a hydrogen atom, e.g., loss of H from the —OH group at C-11 leaves the ketone group, =O, and the resultant substance is known as a 11-dehydro compound. The systematic nomenclature of the steroids is governed by rules laid down by the International Union of Pure and Applied Chemistry, and these should be consulted for all details of nomenclature.

ADRENOCORTICAL HORMONES

More than 50 steroids have been isolated from the adrenal cortex, but most of these are intermediates in the synthesis of the steroid hormones actually secreted. These latter fall into four main groups: (1) the largest group, the corticoids, which have 21 carbon atoms and are the adrenocortical hormones proper; (2) estrogens, which have 18 carbon atoms; (3) progesterone (21 carbon atoms); and (4) androgens, which have 19 carbon atoms. Groups 2, 3, and 4 are formed mainly by the gonads.

Essential Structural Features of Corticoids

These are:

1. Unsaturation (double bond) at C-4-5.
2. Ketone (=O) group at C-3.
3. Ketone group at C-20.

Correlation of Chemical Structure and Metabolic Activity of Corticoids

Hormones Affecting Carbohydrate Metabolism ***(Glucocorticoids).*** The presence of an -OH group at C-17 enhances carbohydrate activity but is not essential for it. The presence of an -OH group at C-21 is a requisite for activity in carbohydrate metabolism. (It also promotes retention of sodium.) Most important, however, for activity in carbohydrate metabolism is the presence of the oxygen atom, either as -OH or =O, at the C-11 position; this type of compound has little effect on water and electrolytes, apart from a slight tendency to reduce sodium retention. As a group, those hormones with oxygen at C-11 are known as 11-oxysteroids or 11-oxygenated corticosteroids and include cortisone (11-dehydro-17-hydroxy-corticosterone, compound E), hydrocortisone (17-hydroxycorticosterone, cortisol, compound F), corticosterone (compound B), and 11-dehydrocorticosterone (compound A).

Corticoids Affecting Electrolytes ***(Mineralocorticoids).*** These are of two types: (1) Compounds lacking an oxygen atom at C-11 have a powerful effect on water and electrolytes but little or no effect on carbohydrate metabolism. Examples are 11-deoxy-corticosterone and 17-hydroxy-11-deoxycorticosterone (compound S). (2) Replacement of the methyl group at C-18 by an aldehyde (-CHO) group gives the most powerful mineralocorticoid hormone, i.e., aldosterone, which, because of the spatial

Figure 12–11 Examples of a glucocorticoid *(left)* and a mineralocorticoid *(right)*.

Corticosterone

11-Deoxycorticosterone

proximity of the -CHO at C-18 and an -OH at C-11, exists in the body both as the aldehyde and hemiacetal (OHCH-O) forms. (Aldosterone is an 11-hydroxy compound.)

Biosynthesis of Adrenal Steroids (Fig. 12–12)

Adrenocortical steroids are synthesized from cholesterol, the accumulation of which in the rested healthy gland accounts for the appearance of lipid vacuolation, especially in the cells of the zona fasciculata.

Pregnenolone may be metabolized in at least two ways. The main, or dual-purpose, pathway appears to be oxidation of the C-3 hydroxyl group by 3 β-hydroxysteroid dehydrogenase. The resultant pregn-5-ene-3,20-dione is then isomerized (double bond changed from C-5-6 to C-4-5) to progesterone, which is the immediate precursor of the mineralocorticoids and the main one for glucocorticoids. Alternatively, pregnenolone may be hydroxylated at the C-17 position to give 17α-hydroxypregnenolone, which is then oxidized and isomerized to 17α-hydroxyprogesterone. The latter is the immediate precursor of the glucocorticoids. As shown in Figure 12–12, for elaboration to glucocorticoids, progesterone must first be converted to 17α-hydroxyprogesterone by hydroxylation at the C-17 position.

Hydroxylases of Adrenal Cortex. It will be seen from Figure 12–12 that formation of cortisol from progesterone requires hydroxylation at C-17, C-21, and C-11, in that order. In each case, reduced nicotinamide-adenine dinucleotide phosphate (NADPH) is a necessary cofactor. The cationic oxygen (O^+) required is probably produced

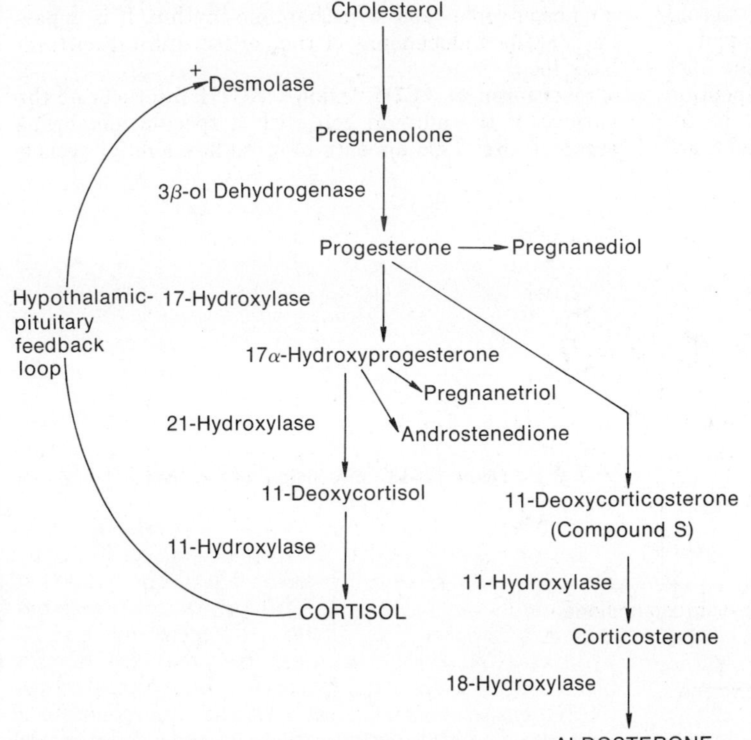

Figure 12–12 Major pathways of cortisol and aldosterone synthesis in the adrenal gland.

from molecular oxygen by a hemoprotein, and one function of the NADPH could be that of regenerating the oxidized metal in the latter. Hydroxylation at each separate carbon position requires a specific enzyme. Furthermore, each of these steroids requiring hydroxylation at C-11 appears to have available its own specific hydroxylase.

Biosynthesis of Mineralocorticoids

See Figure 12–12. For description, see under Aldosterone (p. 299).

Biosynthesis of Adrenal Androgens and Estrogens

The major compounds with androgenic activity formed by the adrenal cortex are testosterone, androstenedione, and dehydroepiandrosterone. Their metabolic interrelationships are shown in Figure 12–13. Testosterone is produced in large amounts by the Leydig cells of the testis, the contribution from the adrenal cortex being very small by comparison in males. Testosterone is not itself biologically active, but it is converted in the tissues to dihydrotestosterone, which appears to be the active molecule.

The major pathway for estrogen formation is the synthesis of estradiol from testosterone (Fig. 12–13); the ovary is the major source of estrogens, and the metabolic pathways are essentially similar to those in the adrenal.

Control and Mechanism of Adrenocortical Steroidogenesis

Adrenocorticotropic Hormone (ACTH)

Chemistry. Production of all adrenocortical steroid hormones (except aldosterone) is under the control of ACTH, which is produced by basophil cells in the adenohypophysis. The ACTH molecule is a polypeptide composed of 39 amino acids. The N-terminal of sequences 1 to 24 is common to cow, pig, sheep, and man, at least; it possesses full biological activity in stimulating the adrenal cortex, and it also possesses weak MSH (melanocyte-stimulating hormone) activity. Synthetic ACTH (tetracosactide or Synacthen, and cosyntropin or Cortrosyn) reproduces this sequence and is of value in adrenal stimulation tests.

Under normal basal conditions, the release of ACTH from the pituitary is under the control of a polypeptide hormone, corticotrophin releasing factor (CRF), which is formed in specific cells in the hypothalamus. These cells are sensitive to the level of circulating free cortisol (i.e., the fraction not bound to transport protein). A negative feedback loop is established: thus if cortisol levels fall, more CRF is secreted; this reaches the anterior lobe of the pituitary by way of a microscopic venous portal system and there stimulates the synthesis and release of ACTH. This in turn stimulates the adrenal gland, and cortisol levels rise. This homeostatic system apparently can be overridden by acute stress (such as trauma or infection), which stimulates cortisol production. Analogues of cortisol, such as prednisone or dexamethasone, will inhibit CRF release; no other compounds have this effect, apart from antidiuretic hormone.

Diurnal ACTH-Cortisol Variations. In normal persons the secretion of ACTH begins to rise gradually after midnight and reaches its maximum between 6:00 and 9:00 A.M. Thereafter, there is a gradual decline throughout the day, and the nadir is reached between 4:00 P.M. and midnight. Since there is little delay in the response of the normal adrenal cortex to ACTH, the plasma concentration of cortisol follows the same time pattern; i.e., highest levels are found at 7 to 9 A.M. and those found at 4 to 6 P.M. are 50% or more lower than the morning values. This diurnal rhythm follows rhythmic changes in CRF production and is probably a consequence of some basic hypothalamic rhythm. It is apparently quite independent of the cortisol inhibition feedback loop.

Mechanism of ACTH Action. ACTH interacts at the surface of the adrenal cell with a specific membrane receptor site. This appears to stimulate adenyl cyclase

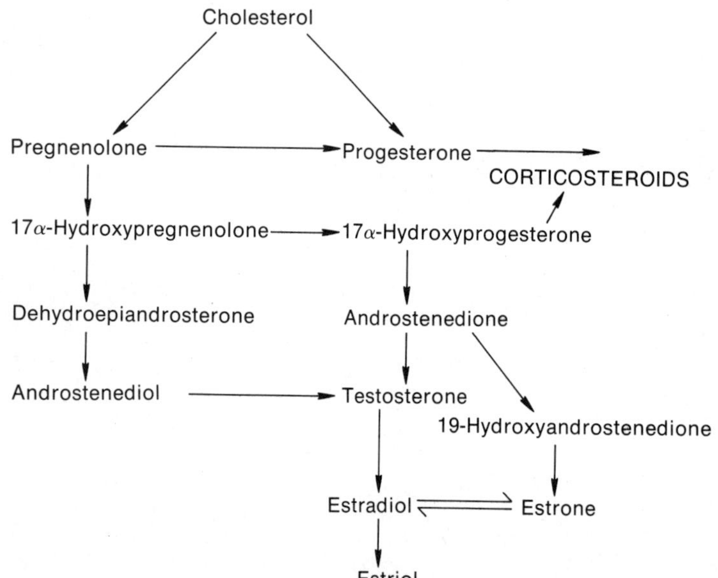

Figure 12–13 Biosynthesis of androgen and estrogens.

activity, leading to the production of cyclic AMP within the cell. This nucleotide acts upon mRNA to modulate the synthesis of a specific regulator protein that, in some fashion not yet clear, increases cholesterol utilization for steroid synthesis.

The action of ACTH on the adrenal cortex exhibits a double pattern: (1) a rapid action consisting of the release of the small amounts of preformed steroids and stimulation of hormone synthesis over the ensuing hours and (2) a slow response to continued ACTH stimulation leading to hypertrophy and hyperplasia of the adrenal cortex.

Metabolism of Adrenocortical Hormones

Glucocorticoids. Cortisol (hydrocortisone) is the main glucocorticoid, comprising more than 30% of the total plasma 17-hydroxycorticoids. From 15 to 30 mg of cortisol (average, 20 mg) is secreted per day by the adrenal cortices in an adult, and 60 to 70% of this is secreted between midnight and 8:00 A.M. This activity represents only about 10% of the potential of the normal glands, which, under maximal stimulation, can secrete 250 mg per day. The only other significant glucocorticoid is corticosterone, of which 2 to 5 mg (average, 3 mg) are secreted per day. Because of the diurnal variation already referred to, normal plasma cortisol values (as free 11-hydroxycorticoids, which consist mainly of cortisol) in the same person may be 25 μg per dL at 7 to 8 A.M. and 6 to 10 μg per dL after 4 P.M.

The half-life of cortisol in the plasma is about 2 hours. One passage through the liver will inactivate about one-third of the free hormone in the plasma. The liver inactivates cortisol and corticosterone by reducing them to the dihydro- and tetrahydro- forms, which it then conjugates at the C-3 position with glucuronic acid. At any one time about one-half the total glucocorticoids in the plasma are in this inactive glucuronide form, and they are excreted as such in the urine. Only a very minor fraction of glucocorticoids is conjugated with sulfate.

Transcortin. The remaining 50% is present in the plasma in unchanged chemical state, but most of this is bound to a special globulin, called transcortin. Transcortin binds the glucocorticoids in a biologically inert but chemically unchanged form, and this bound steroid is in equilibrium with the small amount (about 10% of total cortisol) of free, active hormone in the plasma.

Estrogens cause a considerable increase in transcortin levels, and this accounts for the greatly elevated plasma cortisol values in the later stages of pregnancy, when the bound cortisol may be three times normal. Transcortin is also elevated in patients receiving estrogens. However, since this bound hormone is inactive, signs of hypercortisolism are absent or minimal. This elevation also occurs in women taking contraceptive pills having a high estrogenic component (in terms of potency). This can cause an overlap of plasma cortisol values with Cushing's disease. However, measurement of the urinary free cortisol may allow a differentiation to be made (Fig. 12–14). Urinary free cortisol excretion is directly proportional to the daily tissue exposure to free plasma cortisol.

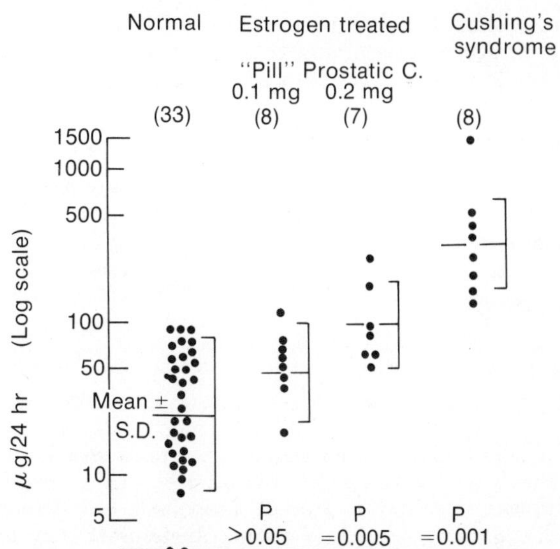

Figure 12–14 Daily urinary free cortisol excretion in normal and estrogen-treated subjects and patients with Cushing's syndrome. (From Burke, C. W.: The effect of oral contraception on cortisol metabolism. J. Clin. Pathol. 23: Suppl. 3, 11, 1970.)

Urinary Excretion Products of Cortisol: 17-Hydroxycorticoids

Only a very small amount of cortisol is excreted unchanged in the urine, the vast majority being degraded by the liver to the dihydro- and tetrahydro-forms. Some cortisol also is converted to cortisone, and, either via this route or directly, is hydrogenated by the liver to tetrahydrocortisone. All of these compounds are included in the estimation of 17-hydroxycorticoids by the Porter-Silber method.

Urinary 17-Ketogenic Steroids. Some 20% of cortisol produced is not metabolized to 17-hydroxycorticoids but is excreted as cortols and cortolones, which are not estimated by the Porter-Silber method. However, these, along with all the 17-hydroxycorticoids and also pregnanetriol and allopregnanetriol, are estimated by the 17-ketogenic steroid technique of Norymberski.

Metabolism of Androgens (Neutral 17-Ketosteroids)

The main adrenocortical androgen is dehydroepiandrosterone, some 25 to 30 mg of which is secreted per day, constituting 75% of the total output of 17-ketosteroids by the adrenal cortex. Androstenedione, androsterone, and etiocholanolone are secreted in much smaller amounts. The quantity of testosterone produced by the adrenal cortex is quite small: women excrete about 50 μg of the free hormone per day, and the bulk of this comes from the adrenals. Most of the dehydroepiandrosterone secreted is converted by the liver to androsterone and etiocholanolone, which are then conjugated at the C-3 position with glucuronic acid and excreted as glucuronides. The dehydroepiandrosterone that is not degraded is excreted as the C-3 sulfate. The net excretory result of the metabolism of the androgens is that androsterone and etiocholanolone together constitute 50 to 60% of the total daily urinary excretion of neutral 17-

ketosteroids. The designation "neutral" is used to differentiate adrenocortical and gonadal androgens from the acidic steroids of bile acids and estrogens.

Metabolic Effects of Corticoids

Obviously, in physiological amounts adrenocortical hormones serve to maintain a state of health and homeostasis.

Glucocorticoids

These are *cortisol,* which is physiologically and quantitatively by far the most important, *corticosterone,* which is of much lesser importance, and *cortisone,* which is of minor importance. Their many effects are best considered under the following separate headings.

Effects on Proteins and Carbohydrates. In excess, the glucocorticoids induce protein catabolism. Partly by increasing the activities of aminotransferases, they promote increased deamination of amino acids and diversion of these to glucose formation. This augmented gluconeogenesis, together with diminished utilization of glucose by muscle and adipose tissue, leads to increased formation of liver glycogen and elevation of blood glucose. The hyperglycemia may be sufficient to cause glucosuria, and this may be facilitated by a lowering of the renal threshold for glucose. Glucocorticoids are insulin antagonists and cause a state of secondary diabetes mellitus. Increased catabolism and diminished formation of the protein matrix of bone, i.e., osteoid, results in demineralization of the skeleton and increased excretion of calcium in the urine.

Effects on Lipid Metabolism. Long-continued hypercortisolism causes a moderate hypercholesterolemia and hyperlipemia, and these may contribute to acceleration of atherosclerosis.

Effects on Hemopoietic System. Because of enhanced sequestration in the lungs and spleen, as well as increased destruction in the blood, cortisol, cortisone, and aldosterone reduce the circulating eosinophils and basophils. Lymphopenia likewise is induced, and widespread lymphocytolysis and reduction in numbers of plasma cells leading to obvious hypocellularity of lymphoid tissues, including the cortex of the thymus, tend to result when large doses of glucocorticoids are given or when these hormones are secreted in excess for any length of time.

In some poorly understood fashion the glucocorticoids also reduce the intensity of antigen-antibody interactions on target cells. These effects account for their successful use as immunosuppressive agents in organ transplantation, in autoimmune disease, and in sensitivity states. Pharmacological, rather than physiological, doses are required to produce anti-inflammatory and immunosuppressive actions, however.

Effects on Renal Function. By increasing glomerular filtration, and less significantly, by opposing slightly the action of ADH, the glucocorticoids promote water diuresis.

Adrenal Androgens

With the exception of testosterone, which is produced in quite small amounts, adrenal 17-keto-steroids are weak masculinizing hormones, having only one-twentieth to one-fortieth the effect of testosterone in this regard. The action of the adrenal androgens is mainly an anabolic one.

Mineralocorticoids

In general, these hormones promote the retention of sodium, chloride, and water and the excretion of potassium, but differences exist between the various hormones. The major hormone is aldosterone, whose secretion and presence in the body is vital for life.

Mixed Metabolic Effects of Corticoids

The classification into glucocorticosteroids and mineralocorticoids conveys the impression of a rigid division of activities and functions. This is not strictly so, however, as the actions of these two classes of hormones overlap to some extent.

Disease States Resulting from Reduced Adrenocortical Function

Adrenocortical insufficiency may be acute or chronic, and the latter may be primary or secondary.

Acute Adrenocortical Insufficiency

The classic type is seen in the Waterhouse-Friderichsen syndrome, which is caused by acute hemorrhagic destruction of the adrenal glands in the course of an acute bacteremia, most commonly meningococcic, although it may be caused by other organisms, e.g., *Haemophilus influenzae.*

The commonest form of acute adrenal insufficiency seen nowadays is that following stress in patients who have been on replacement glucocorticoid therapy or who have inadequate adrenocortical reserve for some other reason, e.g., destructive disease or surgery of adrenal glands. In a patient who has been receiving glucocorticoids or exogenous ACTH, production of endogenous ACTH is suppressed, and in times of severe stress, e.g., acute illness, infection, trauma, or surgery, the atrophic adrenal cortices (in the first example) or the hypothalamopituitary system (in a second example) are unable to respond adequately. As a result, within some 6 to 18 hours of the onset of the stress, weakness, fever, vascular collapse, and shock appear and may go on to coma and death.

Laboratory Tests in Acute Adrenocortical Insufficiency. True acute adrenal insufficiency is rare and must not be presumed to be present in every shock state. When this diagnosis is entertained, it is simplest first to take samples for subsequent determination of sodium, potassium, and cortisol and then to give intravenous cortisol immediately. The sodium-potassium ratio will show a fall to 20:1 (from the normal of 30:1) in true adrenal insufficiency. The cortisol level should provide additional evidence, a low or normal level being confirmatory, but subsequent investigation of the adrenal status is required after recovery from the acute illness.

Chronic Primary Adrenocortical Insufficiency (Addison's Disease)

Until the late 1930s tuberculosis was probably the commonest cause of Addison's disease. Nowadays, about half or slightly more than half of all cases seen in the northern hemisphere are caused by "idiopathic atrophy of the glands." Probably most of these are on the basis of autoimmunity. Rarer definitive causes are fungal infections, e.g., histoplasmosis, metastatic neoplasia (which is neither very rare nor very chronic), amyloidosis, hemochromatosis, and vascular accidents.

Manifestations. The onset is insidious, with fatiguability, especially toward the end of the day, and imperceptibly increasing weakness. In some cases the first sign may be inexplicable prostration or unduly slow recovery from some illness, infection, or stressful experience. Manifestations of hypoglycemia may be seen early in the mornings or 4 to 8 hours after a large carbohydrate meal. Hyperpigmentation is almost invariable and, in addition to areas already pigmented, it may be seen in the mucosae of the inside of the lips and gums, over the points of the elbows, and in skin creases and scars. Loss of weight is usual, and dehydration may be obvious.

Laboratory Tests and Diagnosis in Addison's disease

INDIRECT TESTS. Indirect tests of adrenal function measure the secondary effects on the body of steroid deprivation and at one time were the only basis for establishing the diagnosis. Patients with hypoadrenalism display delayed water diuresis, an altered serum sodium-potassium ratio, a flat glucose tolerance curve, and increased sensitivity to insulin. They also fail to show a fall in the circulating eosinophil count after ACTH (Thorn eosinophil test). With the present ready availability of steroid assays, these indirect tests no longer have a place in the laboratory diagnosis of adrenal cortical dysfunction.

DIRECT TESTS FOR ADRENOCORTICAL INSUFFICIENCY

Basal 24-Hour Urinary Steroids. In full-blown cases of disease the 24-hour urinary excretion of 17-hydroxycorticoids will be less than 2 mg, and values for 17-ketosteroid excretion are similarly reduced. However, the 17-ketosteroid excretion is less specific and may be reduced in any severe illness. In cases of partial adrenal insufficiency, the values for both parameters may be in the low normal range, so that caution is required in interpretation. With more specific hormone assays becoming available, these urine estimations are diminishing in value.

Plasma Cortisol. This usually is estimated by the fluorimetric method of Mattingly; however, the commercial immunoassay methods possess superior specificity and sensitivity and are recommended. In patients with complete adrenal insufficiency, the plasma cortisol levels are low or undetectable.

Response to ACTH Stimulation. The most useful test in the investigation of adrenal cortical failure is the response to ACTH stimulation. This may be carried out in two different ways.

(i) One technique uses natural ACTH (i.e., the whole molecule), and the response is measured by estimation of the 17-hydroxycorticosteroid excretion in the urine and of cortisol levels in the plasma.

(ii) Synthetic ACTH has been introduced as a convenient rapid screening test suitable for outpatient use. The substance originally introduced for the test under the trade name of Synacthen is β 1-24 corticotrophin; a comparable compound is available in Canada under the name of Cortrosyn (α 1-24 corticotrophin). The standard technique is as described by Grieg et al. (1966). A sample of venous blood is withdrawn from the resting patient, and 0.25 mg of Synacthen is injected intramuscularly. After 30 minutes a further venous sample is taken. Plasma cortisol estimations are performed on both samples. Grieg found a mean initial value of 17.4 μg per dL (S.D. ± 4.6); after 30 minutes the mean value in the normal person was 33.7 (S.D. ± 7). The criteria for a normal response are: (1) the initial level should be more than 8 μg per dL (sample taken between 9 and 10 A.M.), (2) the 30-minute increment should be more than 7 μg per dL and (3) the final level should always be greater than 18 μg per dL, irrespective of the initial value.

Plasma ACTH. This measurement, now readily available as an immunoassay, differentiates primary from secondary hypoadrenalism, being high in the former and low in the latter (because of pituitary insufficiency).

Secondary Adrenocortical Insufficiency

This is seen in cases of panhypopituitarism, which may follow ischemic postpartum necrosis of the hypophysis caused by severe hemorrhage at childbirth (Sheehan's syndrome), puerperal septic infarction of the pituitary (Simmonds' disease), or destruction of the adenohypophysis by tumor (e.g., craniopharyngioma or chromophobe adenoma), granulomatous process, or surgery. The extent of the pituitary necrosis varies considerably from case to case, even when the etiology is the same.

DISEASES ASSOCIATED WITH INCREASED ADRENOCORTICAL ACTIVITY

Adrenogenital Syndrome (Congenital Adrenal Hyperplasia)

This name is given to a group of syndromes in which there is a congenital absence from the cells of the adrenal cortex of the enzymes involved in the synthesis of cortisol (or occasionally of aldosterone).

21-Hydroxylase Deficiency. Deficient 21-hydroxylase activity is the most common form of the disease; the incidence varies with the population group, but it may be as high as 1:5000 for the homozygous form.

Reference to Figure 12–12 will show that 21-hydroxylation is the penultimate step in the synthesis of cortisol and that a block at this point results in a failure of cortisol synthesis. The normal feedback suppression of the release of CRF (corticotrophin release factor) by the hypothalamus does not occur, and thus excessive amounts of ACTH are released by the anterior pituitary. This does not result in Cushing's disease, of course, since cortisol is not formed because of the enzyme block. However, the earlier stages of steroid synthesis are stimulated markedly in the cortisol cells, and the products of the side pathways of metabolism are formed instead, in increased amounts. Thus, progesterone and

17-hydroxyprogesterone accumulate and are excreted in the urine as the metabolites pregnanediol and pregnanetriol, respectively.

The excessive amounts of androstenedione and testosterone have a marked virilizing effect. Affected females are often virilized from birth, with fusion of the labioscrotal folds and enlargement of the clitoris; indeed, they may be reared as males if the correct diagnosis is not made. Affected males have the "infant Hercules" habitus, with abnormally advanced development of muscles, height, bone age, and secondary sexual characteristics in relation to their chronological age.

BIOCHEMICAL DIAGNOSIS. The urinary 17-ketosteroid excretion is elevated, but the total excretion of 17-hydroxysteroids is usually low. Urinary pregnanetriol excretion is increased considerably, often to five to ten times normal levels, and this forms a useful diagnostic test for both 17- and 11-hydroxylase block. Plasma cortisol levels are generally low and show little or no rise with ACTH stimulation. Deficiency of 11-hydroxylase, 17-hydroxylase, and 3 β-hydroxylase has also been described. The biochemical and clinical effects of these enzyme defects are reversible by the administration of cortisone or prednisone, which suppresses the excessive release of CRF from the hypothalamus.

Cushing's Syndrome

Cushing's syndrome is rare; although exact incidence figures are difficult to obtain for a general population, it is said to occur in something like 1:5000 of a hospital population. It is about four times commoner in women than in men. On pathogenetic and partly on morphological grounds, it may be divided into three broad types:

(1) Excessive secretion of ACTH by the pituitary.

(2) Secretion of cortisol by benign or malignant tumors of the adrenal cortex.

(3) Ectopic secretion of ACTH by tumors not of either pituitary or adrenal origin (e.g., bronchogenic carcinoma).

Manifestations of Cushing's Syndrome. Most of the manifestations are attributable to excess cortisol secretion. These include the redistribution of fat, with thin limbs contrasting with the moon face, buffalo-hump, supraclavicular fat pads, and pendulous abdomen. Thin skin and polycythemia account for the reddish complexion. Atrophy of the dermis and of elastic fibers causes striae to appear when excess fat is deposited and accounts also for the increased susceptibility to bruising and abrasions in response to minor trauma.

Excess of glucocorticoids accounts also for the muscle wasting and weakness and for the loss of osteoid with resultant demineralization of bone. The latter gives rise to back pain, kyphosis, and stress fractures of vertebrae and ribs. In Cushing's syndrome, demineralization commonly affects the skull, and this feature may help to differentiate it from senile or postmenopausal osteoporosis.

There is a negative nitrogen balance, and the increased gluconeogenesis from amino acids causes elevation of the blood glucose, so that 55 to 80% of the patients have latent diabetes and in 20% clinical diabetes mellitus develops. Mild to moderate hyperlipemia is present and contributes to the fairly rapidly progressive arteriosclerosis. Psychic changes may range from lability of mood to severe depression, psychoses, e.g., mania, may occur. Androgenic signs, e.g., hirsutism and acne, may be present and are due to increased 17-ketosteroid production. Hypertension and increased susceptibility to infections also occur.

Laboratory Diagnosis of Cushing's Syndrome

Urinary 17-Hydroxycorticoids (or 17-Ketogenic Steroids). Values for 24-hour urinary 17-hydroxycorticoids in excess of 10 mg are suggestive. Most patients with Cushing's syndrome show values ranging from 12 to as high as 60 mg per day (and some even higher), whereas normal persons excrete 3 to 10 mg of 17-hydroxysteroids per day. Likewise, the 24-hour urinary 17-ketogenic steroid excretion in Cushing's syndrome ranges from about 20 to 70 mg or more (normal: 5 to 25 mg per day). It will be apparent, however, that some patients with Cushing's syndrome have urinary 17 hydroxycorticosteroid and 17-ketogenic steroid excretions that overlap with the upper ranges of normality.

In obese persons there is an increase in both the rate of production and excretion of cortisol and of its derivatives in the urine. In doubtful or borderline cases, the presence of a normal diurnal rhythm of plasma cortisol levels favors obesity rather than Cushing's syndrome.

Urinary 17-Ketosteroids. Although often elevated, by themselves the 17-ketosteroid excretion values are not used in the diagnosis of Cushing's syndrome. Particularly high levels may be found in some cases of adrenocortical carcinoma.

Plasma Cortisol: Absence of Diurnal Variation in Cushing's Syndrome. Although significantly elevated plasma cortisol concentrations are demonstrable in most cases of Cushing's syndrome, enough patients give values that overlap with those within the upper limits of normal (6.5 to 26 μg per dL as 17-hydroxycorticosteroids) to detract from the value of this estimation. A significant finding in all but a few cases is complete absence or virtual obliteration of the normal diurnal variation in cortisol secretion. As a result, very little if any difference will be found between plasma 17-hydroxycorticosteroid values in samples taken from 6 to 8 A.M. and those taken from 4 to 6 P.M. However, the circadian rhythm of plasma cortisol may be absent in normal persons who are under considerable emotional or other stress, and in severe depression.

Urinary Free Cortisol Excretion. As the concentration of total cortisol rises in the plasma, more is present in the free, unbound form, and this readily spills over in the urine. Consequently, in Cushing's syndrome, the urinary free cortisol ranges from about 300 to 4000 μg per day, whereas the normal range is 0 to 200 μg, with an average of about 70 μg per 24 hours. This is by far the most useful single test in the detection and diagnosis of Cushing's syndrome.

Plasma ACTH. Elevated values are found when the disease is due to excessive ACTH production by the pituitary gland or from ectopic sources. Low or undetectable levels occur when the high cortisol levels are due to an autonomously functioning tumor of the adrenal cortex, caused by negative feedback suppression of ACTH secretion from the pituitary.

Differentiation of Adrenocortical Hyperplasia from Tumor

DEXAMETHASONE SUPPRESSION TEST. This most useful procedure was introduced by Liddle in 1960. The great virtue of dexamethasone lies in the fact that it is 30 to 35 times more potent than cortisol in suppressing ACTH secretion and is therefore effective in doses that do not contribute significantly to the values of plasma or urinary 17-hydroxycorticosteroids.

Procedure. During the suppression test the patient is kept in bed and is protected from any stressing factors.

Day 1: Collect 24-hour urine for measurement of basal 17-hydroxycorticosteroid excretion.

Days 2 and 3: The patient receives 0.5 mg dexamethasone orally every 6 hours.

Day 3: Second 24-hour urine is collected for 17-hydroxycorticosteroid measurement.

Day 5: Third (and last) 24-hour urine is collected for 17-hydroxycorticosteroid measurement.

Results and Interpretation. (1) In normal persons, including those with uncomplicated obesity, the second urine collection (day 3), will show a 50% or greater reduction in 24-hour excretion of 17-hydroxycorticosteroids (or 17-ketogenic steroids), as compared with the first or control urine. After the 0.5 mg dose, patients with Cushing's syndrome, regardless of its etiology, will show little or no suppression of ACTH secretion.

(2) After the 2-mg dose, most patients with Cushing's syndrome caused by bilateral adrenocortical hyperplasia will show a 50% or greater reduction in ACTH secretion, as shown by the 17-hydroxycorticosteroids or 17-ketogenic steroid excretion in the third 24-hour urine collection (day 5).

(3) In cases of Cushing's syndrome caused by adrenocortical adenoma or carcinoma or by tumor of nonendocrine or nonpituitary tissues, there is no evidence of suppression, as shown by 17-hydroxycorticoid excretions or plasma levels. Actually, in such cases, normal ACTH secretion by the pituitary is already completely suppressed. Pituitary adenomas are likely to be insensitive to dexamethasone suppression.

MINERALOCORTICOIDS: ALDOSTERONE

Chemistry and Biosynthesis of Aldosterone

The name *aldosterone* was adopted because of the aldehyde group in its structure. Its systematic chemical designation is 11β,21-dihydroxy-pregn-4-ene-3,20-dione-18-al. Its biosynthesis is illustrated in simplified form in Figure 12–15. It has extremely potent sodium-retaining properties.

Aldosterone Secretion and Its Control

Aldosterone is secreted by the zona glomerulosa of the adrenal cortex, which is largely independent of ACTH. In hypophysectomized animals, cortisol secretion is abolished, but 20 to 40% of normal aldosterone-secreting capacity remains. A potent stimulus to aldosterone secretion is a fall in blood volume, which may raise plasma levels of the hormone as much as 10 to 20 or 30 times and which is mediated through the renin-angiotensin mechanism. By a similar method, sodium deprivation may increase aldosterone formation and secretion five- to tenfold or more.

Renin-Angiotensin Mechanism and Aldosterone Secretion. Renin is a proteolytic enzyme produced by the epithelioid cells of the juxtaglomerular complex in the kidneys. Its substrate is a plasma alpha$_2$-globulin, the glycoprotein angiotensinogen, which is manufactured by the liver. Within seconds, or at most a minute or two, renin hydrolyzes angiotensinogen to yield the decapeptide angiotensin I. Plasma "angiotensin-converting enzyme" then acts on angiotensin I, splitting two amino acids from it, to form the octapeptide angiotensin II. Apart from being a potent vasopressor agent, angiotensin II is the main physiological stimulant of aldosterone secretion. Angiotensin II is rather rapidly destroyed by a number of plasma enzymes, which are collectively referred to as "angiotensinase." Because of this, it persists in the blood for only 5 to 20 minutes.

THE JUXTAGLOMERULAR APPARATUS. The juxtaglomerular apparatus (JGA) is a structural complex at the hilum of the renal glomerulus. It consists of the terminal 50 to 125 μm of the afferent arteriole and the macula densa of the distal convoluted tubule. At this point, the end of the ascending limb of Henle returns to its parent glomerulus and nestles in the space between the afferent and efferent arterioles. Here it continues into the distal convoluted tubule, the beginning of which is marked by a condensation of tubular epithelial cell nuclei on the glomerular side of the tubule, i.e., the macula densa.

The structure and location of the juxtaglomerular apparatus offers several possibilities. Its main function is believed to be that of a stretch receptor. On this basis, a fall in pressure of the blood in the afferent arteriole is believed to stimulate the juxtaglomerular cells to produce and release more renin. The latter generates

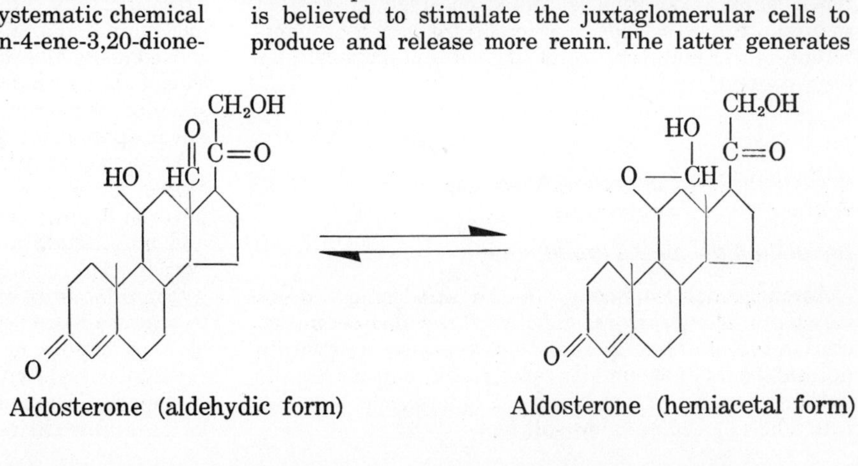

CH_2OH C=O HO HC O — Aldosterone (aldehydic form)

CH_2OH HO C=O O—CH O — Aldosterone (hemiacetal form)

Figure 12–15 Alternate chemical forms of aldosterone.

angiotensin II, which raises the blood pressure by its direct vasopressor action and also stimulates the formation and secretion of aldosterone. By retaining more sodium and water, the aldosterone increases the blood volume, and therefore counteracts the fall in blood pressure that initiated the entire chain of events. The opposite obtains when the blood pressure is raised or the blood volume is increased, i.e., renin production by the juxtaglomerular cells is diminished or suppressed.

There is good evidence that the macula densa is also affected by the sodium concentration in the distal tubule. Increased sodium concentration at the macula densa causes renin to be liberated from the adjacent juxtaglomerular cells, and this renin activates angiotensin locally to produce constriction of the afferent (and/or efferent) arteriole, diminishing sodium resorption in the ascending limb of Henle's loop.

Measurement of Renin Activity. Several methods are available, and almost all measure the final product of renin's activity, i.e., angiotensin II. The techniques are complicated and involve a final bioassay, usually in rats. At present renin activity generally is measured indirectly by the concentration of angiotensin in the plasma. Angiotensin I and angiotensin II can be estimated by radioimmunoassay techniques, and these procedures are becoming more widely available.

Metabolism of Aldosterone

Understandably, since the normal secretion of aldosterone is only 70 to 210 μg per day, its concentration in the plasma is extremely small, i.e., of the order of 0.01 μg per dL. Its half-life in the plasma is very brief—about 10 to 15 minutes. Aldosterone is almost completely removed from blood during one passage through the liver, and the longer half-life it enjoys in conditions such as hemorrhage, shock, and low-output heart failure is probably attributable to reduced hepatic blood flow.

Action of Aldosterone

The main action of aldosterone is the conservation of sodium. This is accomplished mainly in the distal convoluted tubule, in which K^+ and H^+ are exchanged for the Na^+ that is reabsorbed. A similar effect is seen in the gut, where sodium absorption is enhanced and K^+ excretion promoted. Aldosterone reduces the sodium content and increases the potassium content of saliva. Since water absorption is linked passively to that of sodium, an indirect but very important action of aldosterone is the maintenance of plasma and extracellular fluid volume.

Conditions Associated with Abnormal Production of Aldosterone

Reduced Aldosterone Production

Adrenogenital Syndrome. In the salt-losing variety (complete 21-hydroxylase deficiency) the aldosterone secretion rate is subnormal in the severe cases and within normal limits in the milder cases, but in neither are the patients capable of increasing the aldosterone secretion rate when placed on a low salt diet.

Addison's Disease. The major, life-threatening aspects of this disease are caused by diminished or absent aldosterone production.

Adrenocortical Insufficiency Secondary to Pituitary Disease. Here, the manifestations are mainly those of glucocorticoid deficiency. Since the zona glomerulosa is in significant degree independent of pituitary ACTH, it is largely preserved and produces enough aldosterone for normal function. However, its capacity may be taxed in times of unusual or severe stress.

Increased Aldosterone Production

Primary Aldosteronism (Conn's Syndrome). In 1955, Conn introduced the term *aldosteronism* and subdivided the conditions into primary and secondary varieties. In all but a few cases primary aldosteronism is caused by an adenoma of the adrenal cortex, and it is about two and a half times commoner in women than in men. It occurs mainly between the ages of 25 and 60 years. The adenomas measure from about 0.75 to 3.5 cm in size, and are encapsulated, bright yellow, and composed of highly vacuolated cells.

Classically, these patients show the triad of hypertension, hypokalemia, and polyuria. The hypertension is almost always of the benign "essential" type and is mainly owing to the retention of sodium and consequent increase in plasma volume.

Hypokalemia underlies the common complaints of easy fatigability, weakness, and paresthesias, and may rarely cause paralysis.

It must be emphasized that the association of hypertension and hypokalemia, even if intermittent, should arouse suspicion of the presence of primary aldosteronism. Excessive formation of urine (polyuria) and abnormal thirst (polydipsia) are constant features and are based on an impaired ability to concentrate the urine.

Diagnosis of Primary Aldosteronism. The constellation of "essential" hypertension, hypokalemia, alkalosis (usually hypochloremic), polyuria, nocturia, polydipsia, hyposthenuria, hyperkaluria, and alkaline urine is virtually diagnostic of Conn's syndrome. In primary aldosteronism the autonomous secretion of large amounts of aldosterone by the cortical adenoma results in *suppression* of the renin-angiotensin system, with low or undetectable plasma renin and angiotensin levels. In secondary hyperaldosteronism, not only is there an increase in the aldosterone secretion rate and urinary excretion, but the renin-angiotensin system is active, and renin and angiotensin levels in the plasma are high.

Secondary Aldosteronism. In all the conditions mentioned under this heading, the amount of aldosterone secreted or excreted is only slightly above normal and never approaches the values found in Conn's syndrome.

Aldosteronism Associated with Edematous Conditions. Secondary hyperaldosteronism is present in nephrosis, hepatic cirrhosis, and congestive heart failure, and may create a vicious cycle, especially in the first two. In nephrosis and cirrhosis, hypovolemia caused by hypoproteinemia excites the juxtaglomerular apparatus to produce more renin. In cirrhosis, an additional cause of hypovolemia is loss of protein in ascitic fluid as a result of portal hypertension and intrahepatic hindrance to the circulation of both blood and lymph. In congestive heart failure, the renin-angiotensin system is stimulated both by diminished renal blood flow and by hypovolemia owing to increased exudation of fluid as a result of elevated venous pressure. Serum electrolytes are usually normal in all three conditions.

Secondary Aldosteronism in Hypertension. Increased aldosterone secretion is always present in malignant hypertension and in most, but not all, cases of renovascular hypertension.

Steroid Analysis

In recent years the analysis of 17-ketosteroids and other related compounds by chemical methods has been declining, their place being taken by chromatography and immunoassays. Gas chromatography or high-pressure liquid chromatography can provide a simultaneous separation and quantitation of several constituents. However, such methods are time consuming and may lack specificity.

Extensive use is now made of ligand assays, usually radioimmunoassays, which can be made to give high specificity and sensitivity. It is now possible to assay most hormones of interest by such methods: such assays form the mainstay of endocrinological diagnosis, especially for disorders of sexual function. Because of this change and the nature of the present text, no description of the chemical methods will be given here. Detailed bench methods can be found in such sources as Tietz (1976).

CATECHOLAMINES. ADRENAL MEDULLA. SYMPATHETIC NERVOUS SYSTEM

The adrenal medulla is primarily an endocrine gland, its cells producing the hormone epinephrine (adrenaline), which they secrete directly into the blood on receipt of efferent impulses via the splanchnic nerves, as a result of stressful stimuli such as fear or hunger (hypoglycemia), or in response to direct stimulation by insulin, histamine, or angiotensin. As mentioned elsewhere, epinephrine has a number of metabolic effects. By activating the enzyme cyclase, it increases the synthesis of cyclic 3′5′-AMP in a number of tissues. In the liver, this leads to activation of phosphorylase, which breaks down glycogen and leads to elevation of blood glucose levels. By increasing glycogenolysis in skeletal muscle, it raises the blood lactate level. In adipose tissue, it promotes lipolysis and thus mobilizes free fatty acids.

By contrast, norepinephrine is primarily a neurohumor. It is manufactured in the adrenal medulla, in all sympathetic nerve endings, and in the brain. In the latter, it probably acts as a trans-synaptic mediator. Norepinephrine is the final effector substance in peripheral sympathetic nervous action, although epinephrine acts similarly. Although the actions of the two catecholamines are quite similar, important differences exist between them. Thus norepinephrine is more potent in raising blood pressure but is much less effective than epinephrine as a metabolic agent or smooth muscle relaxant. Epinephrine dilates the arteries supplying skeletal muscles; norepinephrine does not, but both agents dilate the coronary arteries.

Biosynthesis of Catecholamines

Norepinephrine is manufactured in the adrenal medulla, brain, and peripheral sympathetic nerve endings. Cardiac muscle is the only other tissue that contains *N*-methyl transferase, and is thus capable of synthesizing epinephrine from norepinephrine. More norepinephrine than epinephrine is synthesized within the cells of the adrenal medulla.

The catechol nucleus (so named because it is obtained by distillation of gum catechu) is dihydroxybenzene (or a phenol with an extra hydroxyl group; Fig. 12–16). It is present in such substances as guaiacol and pyrogallol. Attachment of an amine side chain yields a catecholamine.

The catecholamines are synthesized from tyrosine, which is taken up actively by the cells concerned (Fig. 12–17). Within these, the tyrosine migrates to the mitochondria, where it is hydroxylated in the C-3 position by the enzyme tyrosine hydroxylase to yield L-dihydroxyphenylalanine (dopa).

Dopa leaves the mitochondria to enter the cytoplasm, where the carboxyl group attached to its alpha-carbon (next to the amino group) is removed by the enzyme dopa decarboxylase (aromatic amino acid decarboxylase), to yield L-dihydroxyphenylethylamine (dopamine).

Dopamine then enters the chromaffin granules of adrenal medullary cells or the granulated vesicles of brain cells and nerve endings. Within these, the beta-carbon of dopamine's side chain is hydroxylated by the copper-containing enzyme dopamine beta-oxidase, to yield L-norepinephrine.

The last enzymatic step concerns the elaboration of epinephrine and occurs only in the cells of the adrenal medulla, midbrain, and heart. In these, norepinephrine, on leaving the chromaffin granules, is acted on by the cytoplasmic enzyme phenylethanolamine *N*-methyl transferase, which transfers a methyl group to it from *S*-adenosylmethionine. The resultant L-epinephrine moves back into the chromaffin granule, in which it is stored.

Metabolism of Catecholamines

The catecholamines are liberated from their storage granules or vesicles by sympathetic nervous stimulation

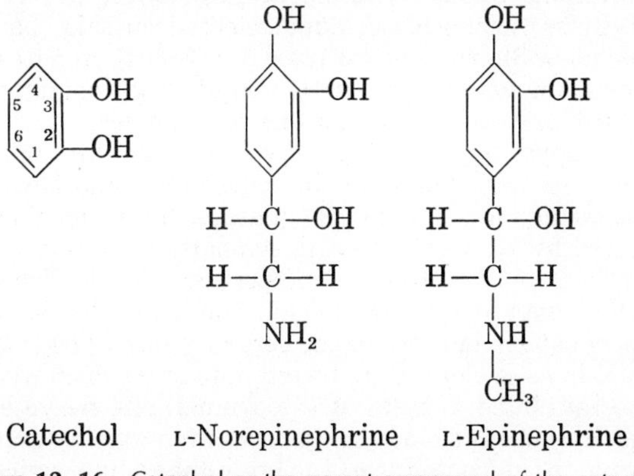

Catechol L-Norepinephrine L-Epinephrine

Figure 12–16 Catechol as the parent compound of the catecholamines.

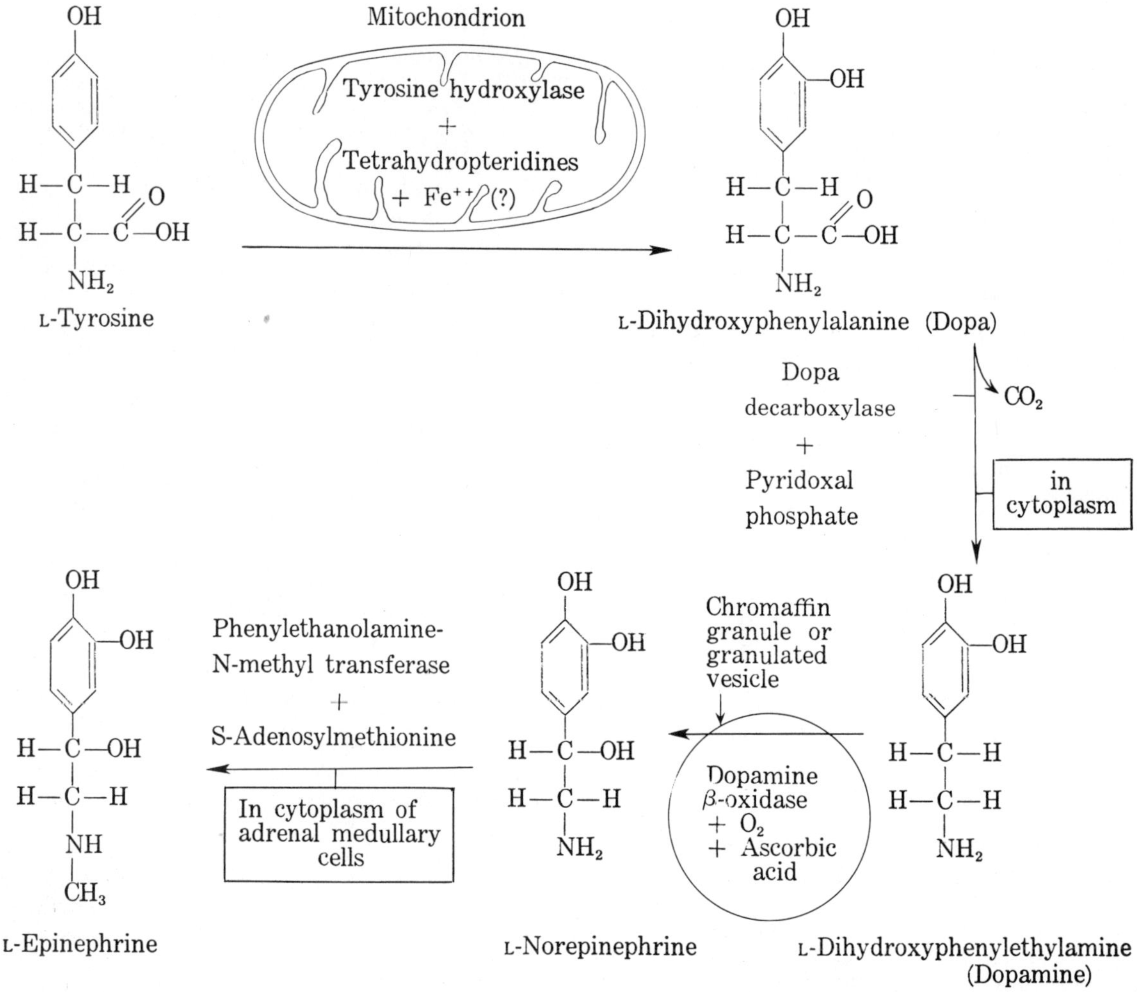

Mitochondrion

Tyrosine hydroxylase + Tetrahydropteridines + Fe^{++} (?)

L-Tyrosine → L-Dihydroxyphenylalanine (Dopa)

Dopa decarboxylase + Pyridoxal phosphate → CO_2

in cytoplasm

L-Dihydroxyphenylethylamine (Dopamine)

Chromaffin granule or granulated vesicle

Dopamine β-oxidase + O_2 + Ascorbic acid

L-Norepinephrine

Phenylethanolamine-N-methyl transferase + S-Adenosylmethionine

In cytoplasm of adrenal medullary cells

L-Epinephrine

Synthesis of catecholamines.

Figure 12–7 Synthesis of catecholamines.

or by histamine. Catecholamine liberation probably proceeds continuously at a low rate as a result of tonic sympathetic activity. This accounts for the small amounts of norepinephrine normally present in the circulation—about 30 ng per dL in arterial, and 40 ng per dL in venous blood. Superimposed on this "basal" catecholamine release are irregular "spurt" releases as a result of many and varied stimuli, e.g., changes in posture, exercise, cold, emotions, and hunger.

The physiological effects of these spurts last only a minute or two because of the extremely rapid clearing of catecholamines from the plasma. This clearing is effected by all organs having sympathetic innervation, and the rate of clearance is proportional to the richness of the sympathetic supply. Thus the heart clears 70 to 80% of catecholamines in the coronary blood flow. Catecholamines so cleared are bound in inactive form within the granulated vesicles of the sympathetic nerve endings. Because the blood-brain barrier is virtually impenetrable to catecholamines, the brain takes up practically none of these from the blood. During the "spurt" releases, the kidneys excrete unchanged a small fraction of catecholamines in the blood perfusing them.

Catabolism and Excretion of Catecholamines

Next to the widespread clearing mechanism of the sympathetic nerve endings, the liver is the most important organ in the removal of catecholamines from the blood, clearing as it does as much as 85% in one passage of blood through it. Although the catecholamines cleared by the sympathetic nerve endings may be used and released in active form again, those cleared by the liver are irreversibly inactivated. This is accomplished by the enzyme catechol-*O*-methyl transferase, which is present in most tissues but is especially abundant in liver and kidney. This cytoplasmic enzyme orthomethylates the hydroxyl group attached to the C-3 position, using *S*-adenosylmethionine as the methyl donor. In the case of norepinephrine and epinephrine, this results in the formation of normetanephrine and metanephrine, respectively (Fig. 12–18). These may be excreted as such or as conjugate sulfates and glucuronides, or they may be converted, through oxidative deamination, to 3-methoxy-4-hydroxy-mandelic aldehyde by the ubiquitous and relatively nonspecific mitochondrial monoamine oxidase. Oxidation of the resultant 3-methoxy-4-hydroxy-

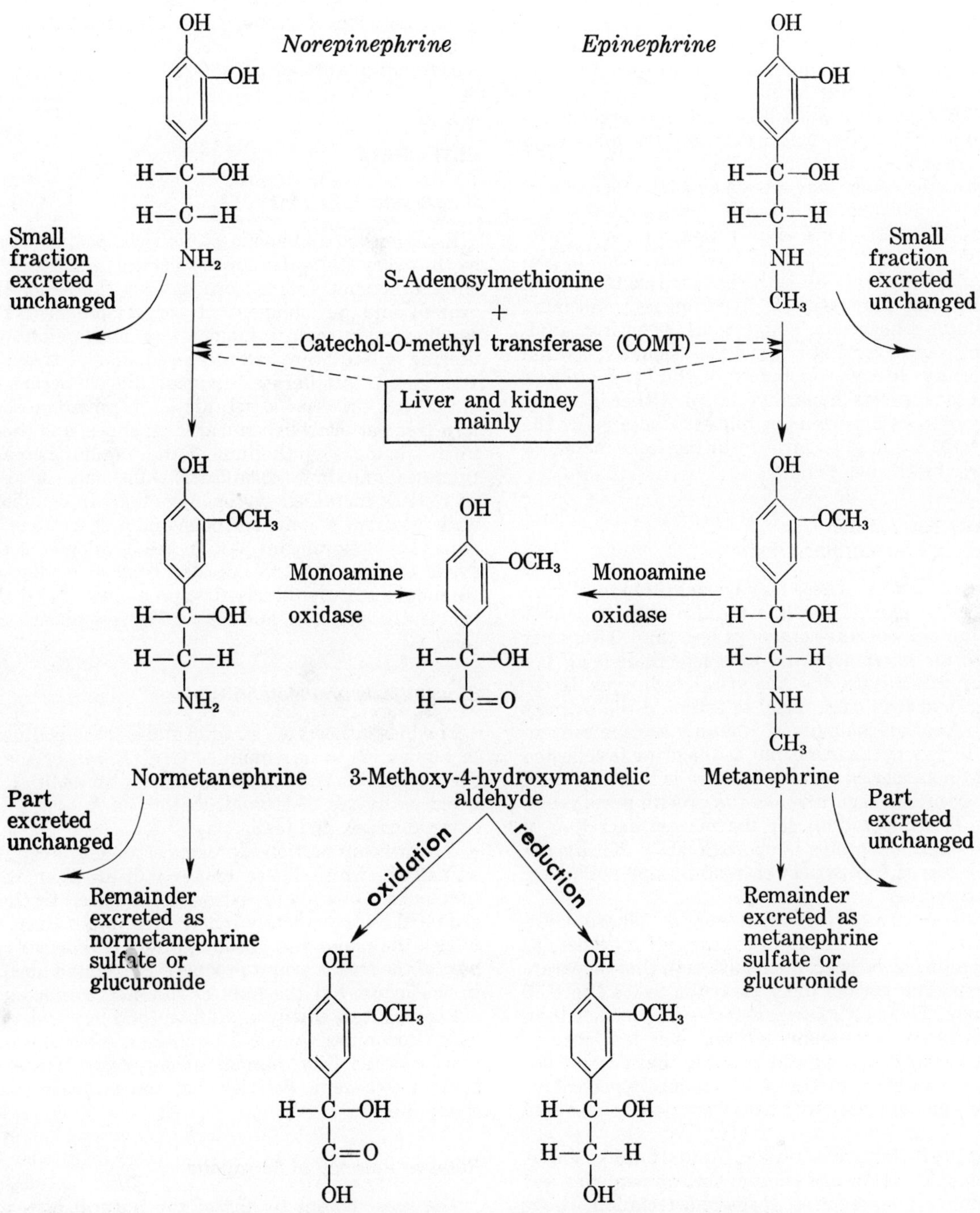

Figure 12–18 Catabolism and excretion of epinephrine and norepinephrine.

mandelic aldehyde yields vanilmandelic acid (VMA); reduction gives methoxyhydroxyphenylglycol.

PHEOCHROMOCYTOMA

This is a relatively uncommon tumor arising in chromaffin tissue. It has been found in 0.5% of patients with persistent hypertension. In approximately 90% of all cases the tumor arises from the adrenal medulla, and in some 10% of these it is bilateral. Although no age group is exempt, most pheochromocytomas present between 20 and 50 years of age. Probably not more than 5 to 8% are malignant.

Pheochromocytomas may secrete epinephrine and norepinephrine continuously, usually with superimposed paroxysmal exacerbations, or only intermittently. Probably about 60% of the patients have persistent hypertension and about 30 to 40% have primarily intermittent symptoms with paroxysms of hypertension associated with pounding headache, palpitations, sweating, anxiety, pallor, hyperventilation, and, occasionally, nausea and vomiting. In some instances, a thin and anxious appearance suggests hyperthyroidism. Other patients are diagnosed as hypertensive diabetics because of the hyperglycemia and glucosuria resulting from increased epinephrine secretion.

Laboratory Tests in the Diagnosis of Pheochromocytoma

CATECHOLAMINES. These may be measured in plasma or urine. The plasma levels are quite low; in venous plasma the epinephrine content is less than 0.5 μg per liter, and for norepinephrine it is less than 5 μg per liter. For this reason the analytical technique is demanding, and it is more usual to estimate the urinary output of free catecholamines. Not only are the concentrations higher in the urine, but as the urine is collected over a 24-hour period or longer, there is less chance of missing a hormone spurt from a tumor with paroxysmal activity. The upper limit for the normal excretion of total free catecholamines is approximately 200 μg per day, and less if the patient is resting and not under emotional stress.

METANEPHRINE AND NORMETANEPHRINE. These methylated catabolites generally are measured together, as there seems to be no special advantage in their separate estimation. The normal daily excretion is 0.12 to 0.55 mg per day. Their estimation is technically easier than for quantitative catecholamines, and it is less open to interference by drugs, especially those that exhibit fluorescence. However, methyldopa, an antihypertensive agent in common use, will cause spuriously elevated values.

4-HYDROXY,3-METHOXYMANDELIC ACID (HMMA, VMA). This metabolite is the end point of both epinephrine and norepinephrine degradation. Numerous techniques have been published for its estimation, both as quantitative assays and as semiquantitative or qualitative screening methods. The normal daily excretion is 2 to 8 mg. The estimation is open to interference by vanillin in the diet (e.g., in bananas and coffee), and by drugs such as methyldopa.

It is probably unwise to place too much reliance on the simpler screening procedures, and it is preferable to perform a quantitative determination of any two of the three groups mentioned above, in the investigation of a patient suspected of having a pheochromocytoma. Total catecholamines + VMA, or total metanephrines + VMA are the usual combinations; if doubtful or equivocal results are obtained, then estimation of the remaining group may be of value, since the metabolism of the catecholamines within tumor tissue varies from one individual to another.

ESTROGENS

Nature and Functions

Estrogens are phenolic steroid compounds produced by the ovary, placenta, adrenal cortices and testes. Their chief functions are concerned with the promotion of growth and development of the female reproductive canal. Under their influence size and weight of the uterine musculature are increased, endometrial stroma and glands proliferate, cervical mucus becomes less viscid and dries or "crystallizes" in an arborescent or fern-tree pattern when smeared on slides, and the stratified squamous epithelium of the vagina increases in thickness and shows cornification of its superficial layers as well as increased glycogen content. In collaboration with pituitary trophic hormone and progesterone, estrogens play a significant part in the development of, and cyclic changes in, the breasts. They also affect other secondary sex characteristics, promote mineral deposition in the skeleton, and tend to depress plasma cholesterol.

Biosynthesis and Metabolism

The biosynthesis of estradiol and estrone is illustrated in Figure 12–13 in simplified form. It will be seen that their synthesis is, so to speak, merely an addition to the basic pathways of steroidogenesis as it occurs in the adrenal cortex and testis.

A significant portion of plasma estrogens is conjugated as sulfate, which has a longer half-life than the free hormones. Most of the estrogens produced in the body are partly or completely inactivated in the liver, which is also the major site of conjugation. A relatively small part of the total amount produced is excreted unchanged in the urine, but the bulk of the metabolites excreted are conjugated, chiefly as sulfates, and to a lesser extent as glucuronides. About 20 estrogen metabolites have been isolated from human urine. Many of these still possess estrogenic activity, but the majority are relatively inert.

Relative Potency of Estrogens

The most potent by far of the natural estrogens is estradiol, which is about 20 times more powerful than estrone. Least potent is estriol, which is only about half as active as estrone.

Cyclic Changes in Ovary

A complex series of hormonal and metabolic changes occurs in the female as part of the estrus cycle; not all facets of this are understood yet, but the broad outlines have been firmly established, especially since the advent of assays for plasma follicle stimulating hormone (FSH) and luteinizing hormone (LH). These changes are shown in composite form in Figure 12–19, which should be read in conjunction with the following description.

In the female, the hypothalamus exhibits an inherent rhythmic activity, with approximately a 28-day periodicity in the human. Specific hypothalamic cells produce a single releasing factor, which passes through the portal venous system in the stalk of the pituitary gland and stimulates specific cells in the anterior lobe of the gland to release both FSH and LH. It has been shown experimentally in rats that this rhythm is present in both sexes, until exposure to testosterone in utero in the developing male fetus permanently abolishes the rhythm.

In the first part of the human menstrual cycle, FSH, together with a little LH, stimulates a primordial follicle in the ovary to hypertrophy, and to form a granulosa cell layer, the cells of which secrete estradiol.

The estradiol levels rise sharply in the late follicular phase immediately before ovulation; they also stimulate LH secretion in turn, and it seems that a positive feedback loop is formed. The result is an explosive rise to very high estradiol levels, with rising LH levels and falling FSH levels. Immediately after the estradiol peak, both FSH and LH show abrupt peaks that coincide temporally, but the peak for LH is much higher. This LH peak causes ovulation to occur and initiates the process of luteinization. By this is meant the stimulation of the thecal cells external to the granulosa layer to the synthesis of progesterone. From mid-cycle onward, the progesterone levels rise and apparently suppress FSH and LH secretion, with an accompanying fall in their plasma levels. However, there is a small secondary rise in plasma estradiol levels at this time. Toward the end of the cycle, luteal involution begins (if conception and implantation of the fertilized ovum have not occurred), together with a fall in plasma steroid levels. At the time of menstruation, FSH levels begin to rise, initiating the next follicular phase.

During the follicular phase, before ovulation, the endometrial glands and stroma exhibit marked cell division and growth (hyperplasia), under the influence of estradiol. After ovulation, the rising progesterone levels stimulate the glands to secretory activity and produce hypertrophy of the superficial stromal cells, in readiness for implantation. If implantation does not occur, the falling steroid levels induce changes in the endometrium that lead to its being shed (menstruation).

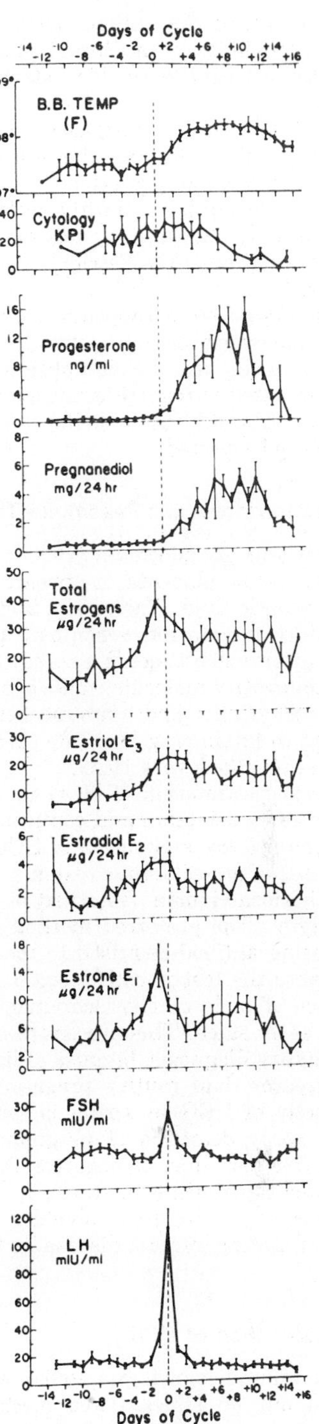

Figure 12–19 Composite profile of serum gonadotropins and progesterone, urinary estrogens and pregnanediol, BBT and KPI of vaginal cytology, throughout the menstrual cycle in 10 normal women. Day 0 = day of LH peak. Vertical bars represent one standard error of the mean. *BBT,* basal body temperature; *KPI,* karyopyknotic index. (From Moghissi, K. S., Syner, F. N., and Evans, T. N.: A composite picture of the menstrual cycle. Am. J. Obstet. Gynecol., *114*:405, 1972. Reprinted with permission.)

Sites of Hormonogenesis in the Ovary

Estrogens are produced primarily by the granulosa cells. However, close association with the theca cells appears to be necessary for this. Ovarian stroma appears to have a wide steroidogenic capability and can manufacture estrogens, progesterone, androstenedione, dehydroepiandrosterone, and testosterone. The cells of the corpus luteum manufacture progesterone primarily, and possibly small amounts of estrogens also.

In women, estrogens are made chiefly in the ovaries and to a much smaller but still significant extent in the adrenal cortices. In men, the small amount normally produced derives from the adrenal cortices and from the Sertoli cells of the seminiferous tubules of the testes. Individual variations in estrogen excretion are quite wide, especially during the estrogen peaks of the cycles, i.e., during the ovulatory and luteal phases. For this reason, isolated estrogen excretion determinations are of little value.

Estrogen Excretion During Pregnancy. Urinary estrogens rise slowly but steadily for the first 4 or 5 weeks, until, by the fifth week of gestation, the levels surpass those found in the normal monthly cycle. Thereafter, the rise becomes more steep but tends to plateau in the last two months of pregnancy. Estriol is the predominant urinary estrogen.

Estrogen Excretion After Menopause. After the menopause the normal ovaries produce virtually no estrogens. Frequently, however, the deficit appears to be partly made up by increased estrogen production by the adrenal cortices, so that the decline in urinary excretion may not be as great as expected.

Chorionic Gonadotropin and Pregnancy Tests

Human chorionic gonadotropin (HCG) is secreted in large amounts by the placenta. It appears in the urine, blood, and amniotic fluid. The serum and urine levels rise rapidly during gestation, reaching a peak at six to eight weeks, after which there is a steady decline. HCG is a glycoprotein with a molecular mass of approximately 30,000. Physiologically and immunochemically it is closely related to luteinizing hormone (LH): antisera to LH show cross-reactions with HCG.

The *qualitative* estimation of HCG in urine is used solely for the early detection and confirmation of pregnancy. The *quantitative* estimation of HCG in serum is of value in cases of pre-eclamptic toxemia, hydatidiform mole, and choriocarcinoma (whether of placental or testicular origin). The preferred method is a radioimmunoassay using antibodies raised to the beta subunit of HCG; because the test is both specific and sensitive, the recurrence of mole or choriocarcinoma can be detected at an early stage. This procedure is not used in routine pregnancy diagnosis, because of its costs (about four times greater than routine pregnancy tests). Radioimmunoassay of HCG in serum is sometimes used for the very early detection of pregnancy, when the usual qualitative tests may be negative. Although more expensive than the routine methods, it is valuable if early decisions, especially about abortion or amniocentesis for investigating genetic disease in the fetus, are necessary.

Qualitative Estimation of HCG

This is an immunological procedure, most conveniently carried out on slides. Tube methods are also available. They are a little more sensitive and sometimes easier to read than the slide tests. Indeed if a slide test gives an equivocal result, a tube test may resolve the problem. On the other hand, slide tests have the advantage of speed. Most commercial methods from the major companies are satisfactory: a comparison of eight kits is given by Porres et al. (1975).

The most widely used methods are agglutination inhibition procedures using red cells or, more usually, latex particles. The principle of the methods is essentially similar: the latex particles are coated with HCG; when they are mixed with a drop of *normal* urine and an antiserum to HCG, their agglutination occurs. This agglutination is visible to the naked eye. However, if the antiserum is mixed with the urine from a *pregnant* woman, the HCG in the urine competes for the antiserum binding sites and *no* agglutination occurs (in other words, the agglutination reaction is inhibited). Instead of this indirect agglutination technique, some methods use direct agglutination: the latex particles are coated with an antibody to HCG.

Although essentially simple in principle, careful attention to details of technique is essential for reliable results. The manufacturer's instructions should be read with great care and adhered to meticulously. For example, use of a fresh specimen of urine free of turbidity and attention to the cleanliness of the slides and the presence of proteinuria are all important considerations. The use of positive and negative controls at least once a day is mandatory.

It should be clearly understood that these tests may not detect a pregnancy in the early weeks, but by six to eight weeks about 98% of pregnancies will give a positive result. The two to three per cent of false negative results are usually due to interfering factors such as protein or drugs or to anomalies such as extrauterine pregnancy.

CHAPTER 12—REVIEW QUESTIONS

1. What is thyrotoxicosis and what laboratory tests can be used to establish the diagnosis?
2. Write about the clinical nature and etiology of Cushing's disease.
3. How do hormones act on the cell?
4. What hormonal effects are produced by a pheochromocytoma?
5. Describe the function of the pituitary gland.

13

ELEMENTARY TOXICOLOGY

Toxicology is the study of poisons and their effects on living tissues: pharmacology is that of drugs and their actions. Since all drugs may be regarded as poisons, the two disciplines necessarily show considerable overlap.

From the point of view of the clinical laboratory, it is useful to think of two major groups of drugs: drugs of abuse and drugs used in long-term therapy. Again, the division is not sharp, and tests for drugs in both categories may be requested as stat. determinations or processed in a routine manner. Methods are given here for rapid assays of the more frequent drugs of abuse, together with a brief discussion of therapeutic drug monitoring.

THERAPEUTIC DRUG MONITORING

Many drugs used in modern clinical practice are usually both specific and potent in their actions, often with a relatively small margin of safety between therapeutic and toxic levels. Consequently, there has been an increasing demand from clinicians for some better way of assessing drug concentrations at the target sites than by a consideration of the administered dose. Although measurement of the plasma concentration is theoretically not ideal, plasma levels generally show a much closer correlation with toxic or therapeutic effects than does the administered dose.

Most drugs are given orally. The plasma levels attained by a given dose regimen in any particular patient show some variation (occasionally considerable) resulting from one or more of the following factors:

A. Absorption
   1. Failure to take medication
   2. Variable bioavailability of different preparations of the same drug
   3. Malabsorption due to gastrointestinal disease

B. Metabolism
   1. Lean body mass, sex, and age
   2. Variations in plasma protein binding (quantity and affinity)
   3. Variations in the rate of hepatic metabolism and in the activity of the metabolites

C. Excretion
   1. Renal disease
   2. Liver disease

Clearly, the plasma concentration of a drug is related to a large number of interacting factors. Pharmacokinetics is the name given to the study of the dynamics of drug absorption, metabolism, and excretion. Some knowledge of the kinetics of a particular drug is essential both in determining the optimal time for taking a blood sample and for interpreting the results. Therefore, an introduction to the terminology will be given here.

Kinetics

When a drug enters the bloodstream, most of it is bound to the plasma proteins, chiefly to albumin. A small fraction remains unbound or free. The free drug passes into the tissues and interacts with tissue receptor sites, transport systems, and catabolic enzymes.

As the administered dose is increased, the resulting plasma concentration rises in a linear response (Fig. 13–1). This is called first-order kinetics (compare enzyme activity terminology). For most drugs the first-order kinetics are maintained over the therapeutic range. However, for some drugs (notably aspirin and phenytoin) the tissue receptor mechanisms are easily saturated and, as the dose is increased, the plasma concentration rises abruptly. This situation of zero-order kinetics (Fig. 13–1) means that toxic levels may be reached rapidly and unexpectedly. Competition and interaction by other drugs given simultaneously may also occur occasionally, producing zero-order kinetics in the drug of interest.

Half-life

After the administration of a single dose of a drug, the plasma concentration shows a rapid rise, followed by a slow exponential decay (Fig. 13–2). The peak concentration is dose related, the time to peak being dependent on the rate of absorption. The fall in plasma concentration is related to the processes of metabolism and excretion.

Because the decay is not linear, the concept of half-life is used. The half-life (T½) is the time taken for the plasma concentration to fall by 50%. In Figure 13–2 the concentration falls from 2 to 1 μg/mL in 2 hours. Therefore, T½ = 2 hours. The half-life for a given drug may vary in different individuals: the values given in Table 13–1 are average values. Some clinical pharmacologists recommend determining the T½ for a patient from the plasma concentrations obtained during the rise to the plateau (steady state).

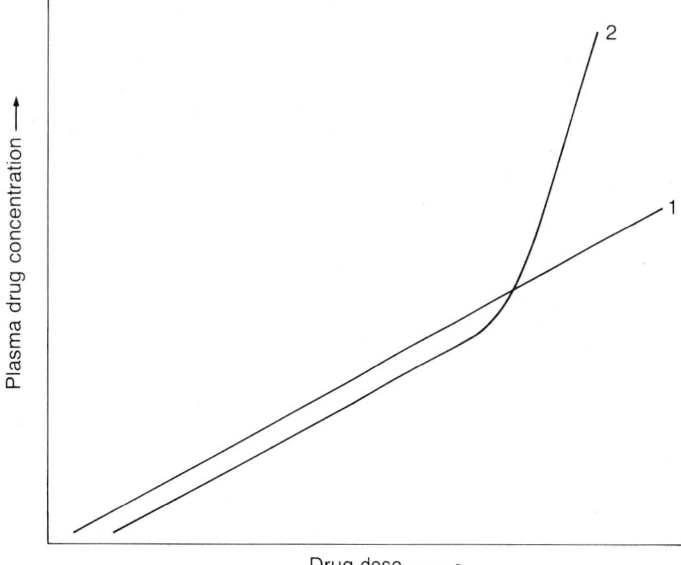

Figure 13–1 Dose-response curve in *(1)* first-order and *(2)* zero-order kinetics.

Steady State

If the drug is given in equal divided doses, the plasma concentrations follow the curve shown in Figure 13–3. Each sequential dose elevates the plasma concentration until the rate of absorption equals the rate of metabolism and excretion. This plateau is the steady-state concentration for that drug and dose, and it is usually reached after five half-lives (5 × T½).

Notice that, because the drug is given in divided doses, high and low concentrations alternate (these are also called peak and trough levels). After the drug is stopped, plasma concentrations fall to low or undetectable levels after 5 × T½.

Sampling Time

Choice of correct sampling time for a particular drug is of great importance. For the majority of drugs the trough time is the most useful, as this shows the minimum effective concentration that is being sustained in the steady state. Therefore it is usual to obtain a blood sample immediately before the next dose, if this is possible.

However, with some drugs, such as the aminoglycosides (gentamicin and tobramycin), both peak and trough values are essential. The peak value indicates that an effective but not toxic level has been achieved; the trough value indicates whether tissue accumulation, with prolonged toxic levels, is occurring.

It is essential for the laboratory report to show (1) the time the sample was drawn and (2) the time the last dose was taken or given. Without this information, the interpretation of the plasma level is made extremely difficult.

It should be clear from the foregoing that the interpretation of a given plasma concentration lies ultimately with the clinician, who has the relevant information about the patient (based on the clinical history and examination, together with a knowledge of previous plasma levels) needed to make the appropriate decisions with regard to dose.

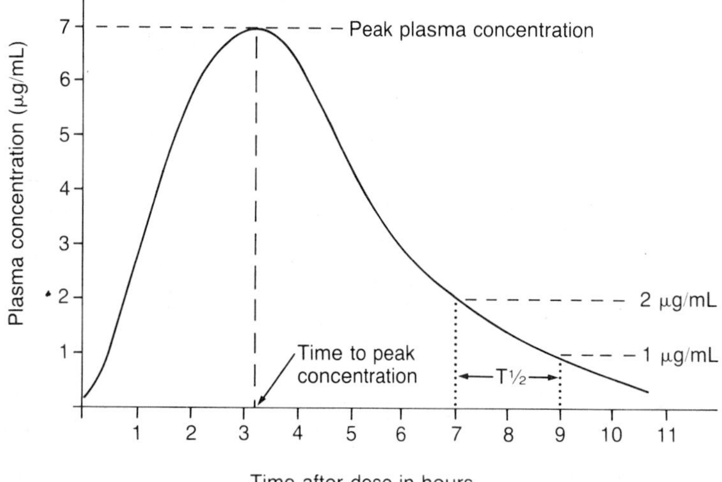

Figure 13–2 Plasma drug levels following a single oral dose.

TABLE 13–1 Reference Data for Monitoring of Plasma Levels of Some Common Therapeutic Drugs

Drug					
Generic Name	*Trade Name*	**Optimal Sampling Time**	**Time to Peak Plasma Value (Hrs)**	**Therapeutic Range (μg/mL)***	**Toxic Range (μg/mL)**
Acetaminophen	Tylenol	Predose	½–1	10–20	>250
Carbamazepine	Tegretol	Predose	6–18	8–12	>15
Digoxin	—	>8 hr	1.5–5.0	0/8–2.2 ng/mL	>2.4 ng/mL
Ethosuximide	Zarontin	Predose	1–2	40–100	>150
Gentamicin	Garamycin	1 hr or predose	Variable	5–10	>12
Lidocaine	Xylocaine	1–2 hr	0.25–0.5	1.5–5.0	>7
Lithium	—	Predose	1–3	0.8–1.4 mmol/L	>2.0 mmol/L
Phenobarbitone	—	>4 hr	6–18	15–40	>50
Phenytoin	Dilantin	>8 hr	4–8	10–20	>20
Primidone	Mysoline	Predose	2–4	5–12	>15
Procainamide	Pronestyl	2 hr or predose	1–2	4–10	>16
Quinidine	—	Predose	1.5–2.0	2–5	>10
Salicylate	—	>4 hr	1–2	100–250	>300
Theophylline	—	1 hr or predose	2–3	10–20	>20
Tobramycin	Nebcin	1 hr. or predose	Variable	5–10	>12
Valproic acid	Depakane	Predose	0.5–1.5	50–100	>200

*Therapeutic ranges in children are generally identical to adult levels.

The accompanying table (Table 13–1) gives suggested therapeutic and toxic levels taken from a number of sources: these are for guidance only and should not be regarded as graven in stone. Different methods for the estimation of drugs may show a constant bias one from the other, and thus the decision value for therapeutic or toxic levels may vary somewhat. The table lists the major therapeutic drugs currently of interest, although more will no doubt be added in the near future.

One further point for consideration is that some drugs are metabolized in the body to forms that are pharmacologically active but that may not be detected if a specific immunoassay is being used for the parent drug. For example, *N*-acetyl procainamide is an active metabolite of procainamide, whereas acetaminophen is derived in the body from phenacetin, and, likewise, phenobarbitone is derived from primidone. It is important in such instances to assay routinely for, the metabolite as well as the parent drug. Conversely, inactive metabolites may be measured by a method with inferior specificity; e.g., quinidine metabolites may be measured by a fluorometric method but not by an immunoassay.

A more extended discussion of this whole topic is given in the text by Richens and Marks (1981).

ANALYTICAL METHODS

The very large number of different drugs and poisons that have been ingested, accidentally or otherwise, by

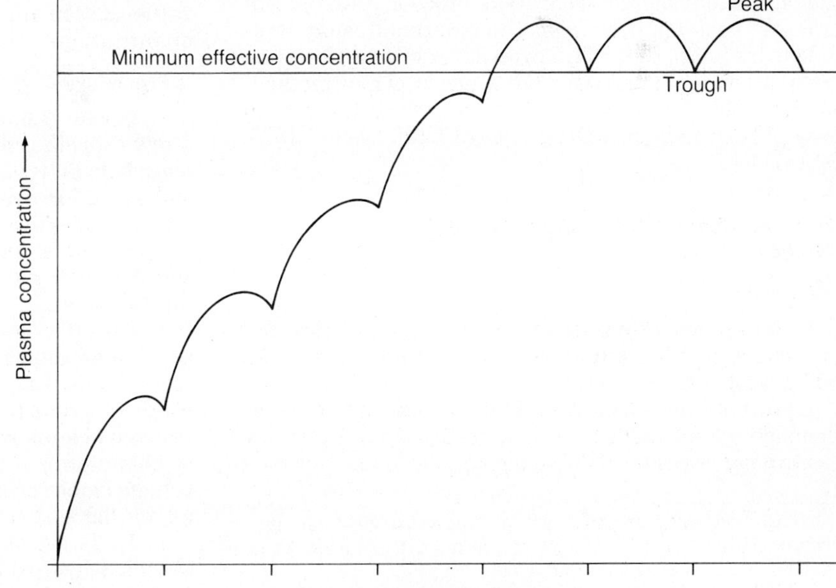

Figure 13–3 Plasma drug levels during repeated oral administration.

patients of all ages presents an analytical problem requiring the most sophisticated instrumentation and methodology for its complete solution. Although it is true that one of the most powerful methods for detection and identification of drugs in body fluids, gas-liquid chromatography (GLC), is now employed in an increasing number of laboratories, it should be noted that the reliability of the results obtained is heavily dependent on the experience and expertise of the operators of the equipment. The necessary level of expertise can be obtained only by frequent use of the method, and in the absence of such constant application of GLC the technologist should perhaps limit toxicological investigations to those tests urgently required for the diagnosis and treatment of life-threatening situations. Improvements in thin-layer chromatographic methods from commercial sources* and the availability of sets of reagents intended for rapid semiqualitative drug assays by the EMIT† technique should facilitate the provision of the important analyses in the average-sized general hospital. In the following sections procedures for the most common drugs and poisons are given that can be set up in the majority of laboratories without special equipment, and the more sophisticated methods are described by principles only. A word of caution: the technologist is strongly urged to become familiar with these methods, including both positive and negative controls, before having to rely on them in an emergency situation. Reliable results by thin-layer chromatography entail meticulous technique that cannot be learned from a textbook or kit insert, only by actual practical experience. The availability of urine and serum control materials facilitates the acquisition of the essential skills. (For more detailed schemes for detection and identification of drugs in blood, urine, and other fluids see Street, 1970; Weissman et al., 1971; and Eastman Kodak Publications JJ-37 and JJ-180.) One approach to providing as complete a drug screening as possible with minimum effort is the QDS-3 plate, which incorporates a preadsorbent layer that concentrates the compounds of interest into a sharp, narrow zone before they commence the chromatographic separation process, plus precut lanes for each application spot to reduce diffusion. Suitable urine controls for TLC procedures of drug detection are available commercially. For a survey of new methods in this field, the technologist is referred to the special issue, "Toxicology and Drug Assay," Clin. Chem., 1974; *20*:111–316.

Urine Amphetamines—Screening Test (Golbey, 1971)

Procedure

1. Set up two 15-mL glass-stoppered tubes, marked test (T) and reagent blank (RB). To T add 2.0 mL urine, to RB add 2.0 mL distilled water.

2. To both tubes add 0.5 mL 2.5 M sodium hydroxide, then add 5.0 mL methylene chloride. Shake for 3 minutes. Centrifuge; aspirate off and discard the upper aqueous layer. Filter the lower solvent layers into correspondingly marked tubes.

3. To the clear solvent filtrate add 1.0 mL metanil yellow reagent, stopper, and shake well for 30 seconds. Centrifuge, aspirate off, and discard the upper aqueous layer.

4. Taking great care not to carry over any residual dye solution, transfer 3.0 mL of each solvent layer into clean tubes. Shake with 3.0 mL 1 M hydrochloric acid.

5. Measure the absorbance of the T acid extract at 540 nm, setting zero absorbance with the RB acid extract.

6. An absorbance in a 1-cm cell greater than 0.2 indicates the probable presence of amphetamines in the urine. A concentration of 0.75 mg per dL of amphetamine gives an absorbance of about 0.6.

***Note:* A positive result must be checked by more specific methods, such as thin-layer chromatography.**

Reagents

Sodium Hydroxide, 2.5 M. Use a commercial concentrate intended to provide 1 liter of 1 M (1 N) sodium hydroxide, and dilute up to 400 mL.

Metanil Yellow Reagent. Dissolve 0.1 g metanil yellow in a solution of 0.5 g potassium dihydrogen phosphate KH_2PO_4 in 100 mL distilled water. Filter if not clear.

Methylene Chloride. Highest purity.

Hydrochloric Acid, 1 M. Dilute concentrated hydrochloric acid 1:10 with distilled water.

Serum Barbiturate Determination (Jatlow, 1973; Goldbaum, 1952; Guzak and Caraway, 1963)

Principle

The barbiturates are extracted from serum or plasma, buffered to pH 7.4, with chloroform. After removal of water by treatment with anhydrous sodium sulfate, the barbiturates are reextracted into 0.45 M sodium hydroxide, and the spectral absorbance of one aliquot of this extract is compared against that of another aliquot whose pH has been adjusted to 10.0 (differential spectrophotometry). The increment of absorbance from the value at 240 nm to the value at 260 nm is used for quantitation.

Procedure

1. Pipette 3.0 mL of serum or plasma into a 50-mL screw-capped centrifuge tube. Add 2.0 mL of pH 7.4 phosphate buffer and 30 mL of chloroform. Secure the cap and shake for five minutes. Add 2.0 g *anhydrous* sodium sulfate, shake five minutes. Add a further 2.0 g anhydrous sodium sulfate, and shake another three minutes. Finally, add a further 4.0 g anhydrous sodium sulfate and shake three minutes.

2. Filter the chloroform through a 9-cm Whatman #1 paper into another 50-mL centrifuge tube. Break up the semisolid mass of sodium sulfate with its trapped water (as water of crystallization) with a glass rod, and pour the released chloroform through the filter. Measure the volume of chloroform; if it is less than 25 mL, record the actual volume before proceeding. If it is more than 25 mL, use 25 mL for the next step.

3. To 25 mL of chloroform extract add 5.0 mL of 0.45 M sodium hydroxide. Secure the cap, shake for five minutes, centrifuge. Using a fine-tipped Pasteur pipette, transfer the

---

*"Toxi-Lab" drug analysis system, Analytical Systems, Inc., Laguna Hills, Calif. 92653. (Now marketed by Marion Laboratories, Inc., Kansas City, Mo. 64114.)

†EMIT-st system, Syva Company, Palo Alto, Calif. 94303.

upper layer into a clean tube. If any chloroform is inadvertently transferred, recentrifuge and retransfer.

4. Pipette 2.0-mL aliquots of the sodium hydroxide extract into each of two 10-mm light path *quartz* cuvettes. To one cuvette, add 0.5 mL of 10.7% w/v ammonium chloride solution, mix by *gentle* inversion, and place in the *reference* beam cell holder of the spectrophotometer. (Overvigorous mixing will produce many small stable bubbles on the inner surfaces of the cuvette.) To the other cuvette, add 0.5 mL of 0.45 M sodium hydroxide, and mix by gentle inversion. Place this cuvette in the *sample* beam holder of the spectrophotometer.

5. With the recorder set to a speed of 60 mm per minute or similar, scan the spectral absorbance curve of the sample cuvette from 230 to 300 nm, using deuterium or hydrogen lamp source. (If a double-beam scanning spectrophotometer is not available, determine the absorbances of the pH 13 aliquot and the pH 10 aliquot at 5-nm intervals over the range 230 to 300 nm, resetting zero absorbance with water at each step. Plot the pH 13 absorbance minus the pH 10 absorbance against wavelength on graph paper. The pH 10 aliquot is the one with added ammonium chloride.)

6. Examine the recorder tracing for the characteristic difference spectrum (Fig. 13–4). In the absence of barbiturate, the tracing will resemble that shown in Figure 13–4 (Right-hand graph). If barbiturate is present, subtract the absorbance at 240 nm from that at 260 nm, and refer this value to the calibration curve.

Calibration Curve

1. Prepare a stock solution containing 25 mg of sodium phenobarbital in 25 mL methanol. Set up 5 test tubes and pipette into each 5.0 mL of a pool of fresh serum obtained by mixing surplus routine specimens from patients not taking barbiturate or from a commercial unassayed serum. Label them blank, A, B, C, and D.

2. To A add 50 microliters of the stock barbiturate solution, using a micropipette and rapid washout technique to achieve rapid dilution of the methanol solution by the serum. To B add 100 microliters, to C add 200 microliters, and to D add 300 microliters. Allowing for the added volumes of methanol, these correspond to serum levels of 0.99 mg per dL, 1.96 mg per dL, 3.85 mg per dL, and 5.66 mg per dL.

3. Perform the assay procedure on 3.0-mL aliquots of the blank serum and the standards. Plot the differences between absorbance at 260 nm and at 240 nm against the standard values. The recorder tracings should be mounted in transparent covers—they serve as useful guides to the typical features of the differential scan for technologists unfamiliar with the procedure. The plot of the absorbance differences against values should be linear.

Note. The calibration curve thus prepared compensates for the incomplete recovery of phenobarbital from serum—about 80% (Jatlow, 1973). If the barbiturate in the patient's serum is one of the short-acting type, recovery is almost complete and the result of the assay will be too high; the error involved is not usually of clinical significance, but if necessary a special calibration curve can be prepared from the particular barbiturate in question. For a laboratory performing such assays fairly frequently, a series of calibration curves from the most common barbiturates could be produced; it is doubtful if the labor involved is justified.

Normal Values

Most barbiturate-free sera give an absorbance at 260 nm that is smaller than that at 240 nm. It has been shown (Jatlow, 1973) that the following drugs do not interfere with this procedure: phenylbutazone, sulfinpyrazone, phenytoin, salicylic acid, nicotinic acid, sulfisoxazole, sulfamethoxazole, theophylline, theobromine, warfarin, dicumarol, phenindione, acetaminophen, *p*-aminophenol, chlorothiazide, hydrochlorothiazide, chlorpropamide, and tolbutamide. The extraction at pH 7.4 prevents interference from salicylates. The occurrence of isosbestic points as an indicator of the presence of barbiturates is not reliable (Jatlow, 1973).

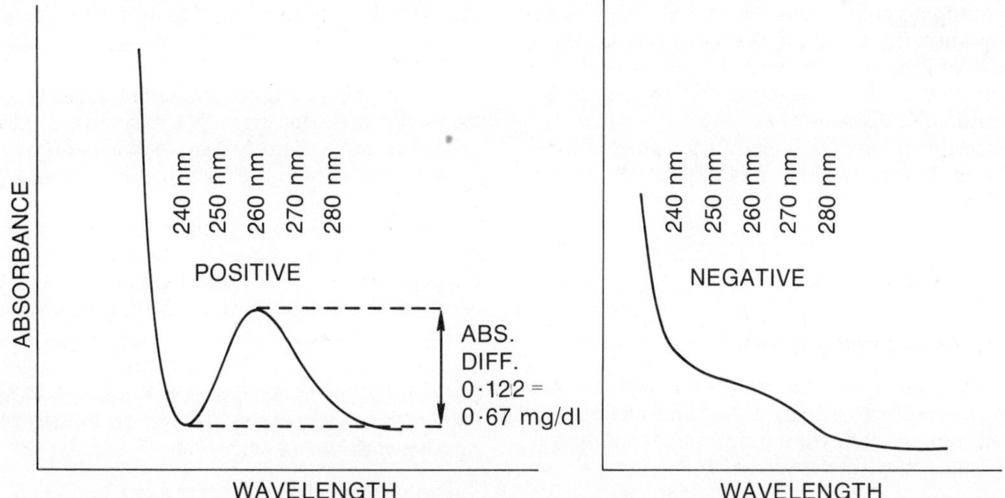

Figure 13–4 The left-hand graph shows the plot of absorbance versus wavelength for the extract from a serum sample containing 0.67 mg/dL of barbiturate. The right-hand graph shows the plot for the extract from a serum negative for barbiturate.

Reagents

Chloroform. Highest quality reagent grade.

Phosphate Buffer pH 7.4, 0.5 M. Dissolve 5.44 g disodium hydrogen phosphate Na_2HPO_4 and 1.36 g potassium dihydrogen phosphate KH_2PO_4 in about 80 mL distilled water. When dissolved, transfer to a 100-mL volumetric flask, make to volume, and mix well. Keep in a polypropylene bottle, adding a spatula tip of sodium azide NaN_3 to prevent mold growth.

Sodium Hydroxide, 0.45 M. Dilute 45 mL of M sodium hydroxide up to 100 mL with distilled water, mix.

Ammonium Chloride, 10.7% w/v. Dissolve 10.7 g ammonium chloride NH_4Cl in about 80 mL distilled water; make up to 100 mL, mix. Keep in a polypropylene bottle.

Notes

1. The removal of water with anhydrous sodium sulfate effectively removes the usual problem with emulsions. If the final volume of chloroform extract after filtration is less than 25 mL, the result will have to be multiplied by the factor:

$$\frac{25}{\text{Vol. of chloroform extract}}$$

2. The method is sensitive enough to permit using smaller volumes of plasma or serum if necessary; a typical absorbance difference between 260 and 240 nm for a serum containing 2.0 mg per dL of barbiturate is 0.25. The final result will have to be multiplied by the factor:

$$\frac{3}{\text{Actual volume of sample}}$$

3. It is convenient to set the recorder pen to about 0.2 absorbance with the zero control before commencing the scan; since the quantitation is based on an absorbance difference, no error results from the offset.

4. In SI units, the A, B, C, and D standard solutions used to make the calibration curve are equivalent to 0.039, 0.077, 0.152, and 0.222 mM per liter.

5. The spectrophotometer used must be a high-resolution instrument with a narrow slit setting equivalent to a band pass of 2 nm or less, and the accuracy of the wavelength scale must have been verified by one of the methods detailed elsewhere (p. 74).

6. If the recorder tracing is "noisy," the cause may be small bubbles on the inner surface of the cuvette. Scrupulous cleanliness of the cuvettes is necessary; soaking in a good detergent or a 10% w/v solution of urea in 0.02 M sodium hydroxide will remove the protein film that is the usual source of the problem.

Urine Barbiturates—Screening Test

The determination of plasma or serum barbiturates provides the most reliable evidence that an overdose has been ingested, but the following quick screening test is useful in an emergency (Helman, 1970).

Principle

The barbiturates are complexed with mercuric ions after extraction into chloroform, and detected by the orange color produced with dithizone.

Procedure

1. Pipette 4.0 mL of urine or gastric contents into a 50-mL Erlenmeyer flask containing a Teflon-coated stirrer bar. Add 5.0 mL of pH 6.95 phosphate buffer, mix, and add 20 mL chloroform. Stir on a magnetic stirrer for four minutes.

2. Aspirate and discard the upper layer, using a Pasteur pipette connected to a vacuum aspirator. Add 2.0 mL of mercuric chloride reagent, stir vigorously for four minutes, and aspirate off and discard the upper mercury reagent layer.

3. Add 20 mL distilled water, stir vigorously, and aspirate off and discard the upper, aqueous layer as completely as possible. In making certain that all the upper layer has been aspirated, it is preferable to take off a little of the chloroform lower layer rather than to leave some of the aqueous layer.

4. Using a 2.0 mL volumetric pipette with a fine tip, *slowly* run 2.0 mL of dithizone solution *below the surface* of the chloroform layer; the flask may be very gently rotated by hand but must on no account be mixed with any force.

5. The immediate appearance of an orange color indicates the presence of barbiturate in a concentration of at least 1 mg per dL. If the test is negative, a blue color will persist.

Reagents

Phosphate Buffer, pH 6.95, 0.066 Molar. Dissolve 0.831 g hydrated disodium hydrogen phosphate $Na_2HPO_4 \cdot 7H_2O$ and 0.363 g of potassium dihydrogen phosphate KH_2PO_4 in about 80 mL distilled water; make up to 100 mL, mix. Keep refrigerated.

Mercuric Chloride Reagent. Dissolve 0.5 g of mercuric chloride $HgCl_2$ in a mixture of 50 mL distilled water and 3 drops of concentrated nitric acid. For use, dilute 1.0 mL up to 50 mL with distilled water and dissolve therein 0.42 g of sodium bicarbonate $NaHCO_3$.

Dithizone (Diphenylthiocarbazone). Dissolve 1 mg of dithizone in 100 mL chloroform. Take out 2.0 mL, dilute with 2.0 mL chloroform, mix, determine the absorbance at 605 nm in a 1-cm cell against a chloroform blank. The absorbance of this dilution should be about 1.0, corresponding to a value of about 2.0 for the actual solution. This reagent will keep for two weeks.

Notes

1. The procedure *must* be done exactly as described; excessive agitation in step 4 may give a false positive.

2. It is convenient to keep a stock of preweighed 0.42-g aliquots of sodium bicarbonate in small stoppered vials.

3. Salicylates do not interfere; glutethimide gives a reaction at 5 mg per dL, phenytoin at 8 mg per dL. Chlorpheniramine and methyprylon react at their toxic levels of 4 mg per dL and 150 mg per dL, respectively (Helman, 1970).

Determination of Barbiturate Type with Thin-Layer Chromatography (Based on Smith, 1960; Aggarwal et al., 1974)

The quantitative method described on p. 310 can be adequate for clinical assessment and treatment of barbiturate overdose, provided the exact type of barbiturate ingested is known. Without this information the significance of a plasma barbiturate level of, say, 3 mg per dL may be difficult to determine, since this amount of a long-acting (8 to 12 hours) drug such as phenobarbital is probably much less dangerous than the same quantity of a medium-acting (6 to 8 hours) drug such as amobarbital (Amytal) or a short-acting (2 to 3 hours) drug such as secobarbital (Seconal). The following procedure will give some indication of the probable duration of action of the barbiturate but cannot provide the exact data on drug identity furnished by gas-liquid chromatography.

Procedure

1. Cut a piece of K301R Chromagram* 20 × 5 cm and activate for 30 minutes at 100°C while the extraction is being made. Mix 6 mL *n*-butanol with 2 mL concentrated ammonia solution SG 0.88, place in the bottom of a tall pattern 300-mL beaker or a screw-cap jar of similar size. Cover the beaker with Parafilm, or secure the jar cap and leave to saturate the atmosphere.

2. Dilute the plasma with an equal volume of distilled water. The volume of plasma required will depend on the total barbiturate level: as a guide, the method will detect 5 μg of barbiturate in the applied spot, and this amount of barbiturate will be recovered by the procedure described further on from 2.0 mL plasma with a barbiturate level of 2 mg per dL. If the plasma barbiturate level is greater than this, use less plasma but make the volume up to 4 mL with water.

3. Add enough of the solid buffer (see *Reagents*) to saturate the plasma-water mixture; about 2 g will be required. Shake well for two minutes. Centrifuge and transfer the supernatant into a 15-mL centrifuge tube with a fine tip.

4. While vigorously mixing the fluid on a vortex-type mixer, add 100 microliters of a 4:1 mixture of chloroform and isopropanol, dropwise. Continue to mix for 20 seconds after completion of the solvent addition, then centrifuge. Aspirate off most of the supernatant with a fine-tip Pasteur pipette. With a fresh Pasteur pipette drawn out to a fine tip, remove about 50 to 60 microliters of the solvent extract and transfer to a small (6 × 50 mm) tube.

5. Remove the activated Chromagram sheet from the oven and, with a very soft pencil, mark four light spots at 1-cm intervals along a line parallel to, and 2 cm from, one end. Using a fresh 25-microliter capillary pipette for each solution, and assisting drying with a gentle stream of warm air, apply 25 microliters of the plasma extract on one of the pencil spots, using repeated small applications to obtain a final spot no larger than 4 mm diameter. Similarly apply 2 microliters of the standard solutions to the other pencil marks. Avoid marring the silica gel layer as much as possible.

6. Remove the cover from the beaker or jar, and insert the spotted Chromagram sheet with the end dipping in the solvent layer, making sure the solvent level is below the spot line. Replace the cover and allow the solvent front to rise to within 1 cm of the top edge. This takes about 1 hour.

7. Remove the Chromagram sheet from the jar, and *without delay* examine with a short-wavelength (254 nm) ultraviolet lamp. The barbiturates appear as dark purple spots against a lightly fluorescent background. The probable type of the plasma barbiturate can be determined by comparison with the standard spots. The long-acting phenobarbital has the lowest R_f value, the short-acting the highest, and the intermediate-acting is between them. Caution! Ultraviolet light of this wavelength is dangerous to the eyes; avoid direct exposure.

8. For the clearest separations the amount of barbiturate in the test spot should not be too great; the method will detect as little as 2 to 3 micrograms.

9. The procedure can be used for urine (Aggarwal et al., 1974) by adding about 5 g of solid buffer to 10 mL urine and proceeding as described.

10. The presence of ammonia is essential for separation. If the beaker or jar atmosphere is not saturated with ammonia, the barbiturates tend to travel too close to the solvent front.

Reagents

Solid Buffer. Make a 3:1 mixture by weight of sodium dihydrogen phosphate NaH_2PO_4 and disodium hydrogen phosphate Na_2HPO_4. The final pH of the plasma-water mixture should be about 9.5.

Standards. Dissolve 0.1 g of each of phenobarbital, amobarbital, and secobarbital separately in 20 mL chloroform. Keep tightly stoppered in the refrigerator. The concentration is 5 μg per μL.

Notes

1. The technologist is strongly advised to obtain working experience with this technique before using it under emergency conditions. In particular the technique of applying the extract and standards so as to obtain compact spots without damage to the silica gel surface requires dexterity.

2. The full systematic names of the reference barbiturates are: phenobarbital: 5-ethyl-5-phenyl barbituric acid; amobarbital: 5-ethyl-5-isoamyl barbituric acid; secobarbital: 5-allyl-5-sec-pentyl barbituric acid.

Borates—Screening Test

Principle

Boric acid transforms the yellow compound curcumin in turmeric into its red isomer rosocyanine, which turns blue or olive green with alkali.

Procedure

Make an aliquot of the urine acid with a small drop of hydrochloric acid. Dip a strip of turmeric indicator paper in the acidified urine. A pink or reddish brown color at the junction of the wet and dry portions of the strip indicates the presence of borates. Dry with a stream of warm air and spot the red area with 1.0% w/v sodium hydroxide solution; it should turn blue, blue-green, or olive green.

Notes

1. A confirmatory test is to mix one drop of a solution of 50 mg of carmine in concentrated sulfuric acid with one drop of urine on a white porcelain test plate. A positive result is shown by a change from red to blue.

2. If intoxication with borate is suspected from the screening tests, and if there is history of possible absorption of boric acid or borates from excoriated or burned skin surfaces, the quantitative technique of Rieders and Frere can be applied (Rieders and Frere, 1963).

---

*Chromagram K301R, Distillation Products Industries Division, Eastman Kodak, Rochester, N.Y. 14650.

Serum Bromide Determination (Torrance, 1973)

Principle

The bromide of a protein-free filtrate reacts with a solution of gold chloride in the presence of an optimum level of chloride ion to produce gold bromide, whose absorbance at 470 nm is compared with that of suitable standards.

Procedure

1. Set up three 125 × 16 mm tubes, marked test, standard, and blank. To test add 1.0 mL serum or plasma, to standard add 1.0 mL working standard solution, to blank add 8.0 mL of 0.9% w/v sodium chloride solution. To test and standard add 7.0 mL of 0.9% sodium chloride.

2. To all tubes add 1.0 mL of zinc sulfate solution, mix, add 1.0 mL sodium hydroxide solution, mix. Heat all tubes for ten minutes in the boiling water bath, remove, and cool to room temperature.

3. Centrifuge at 3000 rpm for ten minutes. The supernatants should be absolutely clear. Transfer 5.0 mL of each supernatant to correspondingly marked tubes, add 0.5 mL of gold chloride solution, mix.

4. Measure the absorbances of test and standard at 470 nm in a spectrophotometer, using 19 mm or ¾″ tubes or cuvettes.

Calculation

$$\frac{\text{Test Absorbance (against zero set with blank)}}{\text{Standard Absorbance (against zero set with blank)}} \times$$

Standard value = Serum bromide in mg per dL

Reagents

Zinc Sulfate, 10% w/v. Dissolve 25.0 g zinc sulfate $ZnSO_4{\cdot}7H_2O$ in about 200 mL distilled water and make up to 250 mL with the same. Mix well.

Sodium Hydroxide, 0.5 M. Prepare by accurate 1:2 dilution of a stock 1 M solution. When equal volumes of the zinc sulfate and sodium hydroxide solutions are mixed, the pH should be close to 7.4.

Gold Chloride, 0.5% w/v. Carefully scratch a 1.0 g ampule of auric chloride ($AuCl_3$) and snap open, taking care to avoid loss of the contents. Drop the two halves of the ampule into about 150 mL of distilled water in a 200-mL volumetric flask. Swirl until all the gold chloride is extracted from the ampule, make to volume, and mix.

Sodium Chloride, 9.0% w/v. Dissolve 45.0 g sodium chloride (NaCl) in distilled water in a 500-mL volumetric flask, make to volume.

Sodium Chloride, 0.9% w/v. Dilute the 9.0% solution 1:10 with distilled water.

Stock Bromide Solution, 1.0% w/v. Dissolve 1.29 g sodium bromide, NaBr, in, and make up to 100 mL with, distilled water; mix.

Working Bromide Standard. For routine purposes, when bromide levels up to about 50 mg per dL are expected, the working standard should be 50 mg per dL. Mix 2.5 mL stock bromide and 5.0 mL 9.0% w/v sodium chloride in a 50-mL volumetric flask, make to volume with distilled water, mix well. If bromide intoxication is suspected or if very high results are obtained with the first assay, prepare further standards of 100, 150, and 200 mg per dL bromide, using 5.0, 7.5, and 10.0 mL of stock bromide plus 5.0 mL 9.0% sodium chloride made up to 50 mL with distilled water. Use the standard whose absorbance is closest to that of the test for the calculation.

Serum bromide levels. Administration of bromides over an extended period of time can produce serum levels up to 100 mg per dL. Toxic symptoms usually appear with levels of 150 mg per dL and above, but they may become manifest at lower levels in susceptible individuals.

Notes

1. The reaction between bromide and gold chloride proceeds via the intermediate products $AuCl_2Br$ and $AuClBr_2$; the level of sodium chloride used in the method is designed to shift the equilibrium of the reaction in favor of the final product, $AuBr_3$.

2. At the wavelengths usually employed for measurement of the gold bromide product, minor degrees of turbidity cause positive errors. The protein precipitation method used is designed to prevent this. The supernatants should be crystal clear.

3. 100 mg Br^+ per dL = 12.5 mM per liter.

Carboxyhemoglobin (Blood Carbon Monoxide)

Owing to the 250-fold stronger affinity of hemoglobin for carbon monoxide (CO) than for oxygen, inhalation of air containing even very small amounts of CO from such sources as automobile exhaust fumes and industrial flue and furnace gases will render a progressively larger proportion of the circulating hemoglobin unavailable for oxygen transport because of the formation of the relatively stable compound carboxyhemoglobin (COHb).

The Determination of Carboxyhemoglobin

Saturation levels of 25% and over are of major clinical significance (see further on). A number of other simple methods, using heat denaturation, tannic acid precipitation, and so forth, have been used in the past but are now outmoded.

Spectrophotometric Methods

When a solution of oxyhemoglobin is examined in a spectroscope, two prominent absorption bands will be seen, with maxima at 577 nm and 541 nm (alpha and beta bands, respectively). A solution of carboxyhemoglobin also will show alpha and beta bands, but these are shifted toward the blue end of the spectrum, with maxima at 570 nm and 535 nm, respectively. This small shift has been used as the basis of several methods of estimation of carboxyhemoglobin.

Methods using a standard grating or prism spectrophotometer with a narrow band pass are to be preferred; most laboratories possess an instrument of this nature, and one such method is chosen for description here. It has the considerable advantage of speed. A direct-reading instrument based on these principles is the IL CO oximeter.

Chemical Methods

Conway described a microdiffusion method using his special diffusion chambers: palladium chloride solution is placed in the central well, and the blood sample in the outer well. The carbon monoxide diffuses into the palladium chloride and reduces it to metallic palladium (which forms a metal "mirror" on the surface of the solution) with the formation of hydrochloric acid. Titration of the HCl with NaOH using a microburette provides an estimate of the CO content of the blood sample. The method works well but is slow and requires a hemoglobin determination.

Gas Chromatography

For accurate determinations, especially at low concentrations, gas chromatography is the method of choice. It is most useful, however, for research and forensic purposes, and, as many hospital laboratories do not have the necessary special equipment, it will not be described further here.

THE SPECTROPHOTOMETRIC DETERMINATION OF CARBOXYHEMOGLOBIN (van Kampen and Zijlstra, 1965; Curry, 1963)

Method. **Dilute approximately 0.1 mL of blood with about 20 mL of 0.1% ammonium hydroxide solution. The precise dilution does not matter, provided that the readings lie between about 0.2 to 0.4 absorbance units, using a 1-cm cell. Add approximately 20 mg of solid sodium dithionate (about enough to cover the tip of a spatula) to convert any oxyhemoglobin to reduced hemoglobin. Read the absorbance immediately in a 1-cm cell against a water blank at 538 nm and 578 nm. The point of maximum absorbance for carboxyhemoglobin is 538 nm, whereas 578 nm is the isosbestic point for CoHb and Hb. The calculation is then:**

$$\text{Saturation of Hb by CO (\%)} = \left[\left(2.44 \cdot \frac{D^{538}}{D^{578}}\right) - 2.68\right] \times 100$$

(D = Absorbance)

Notes. The speed and apparent simplicity of this procedure should not blind the technologist to the fact that a number of pitfalls await the unwary.

1. The handling of the samples of blood containing carboxyhemoglobin is more critical than is commonly appreciated. The sample can be taken into any anticoagulant (although preservation is better with fluoride). At autopsy in cases of death from carbon monoxide poisoning, a striking feature is that the blood fails to clot; however, it is still preferable to preserve a sample with fluoride. The tube should be completely filled, securely stoppered, and kept in the dark. If oxygen is available to the sample, at atmospheric partial pressure, it will exchange with the carbon monoxide in the sample; this process is assisted by light and heat. If there is to be some delay before analysis, it is preferable to keep the sample at 4°C.

2. Some sulfhemoglobin forms on standing after the addition of sodium dithionate; therefore, the absorbance should be read within a few minutes. Never attempt to obtain readings on a turbid solution.

3. The reading at 578 nm is on a steep part of the absorbance curve; slight variations in spectrophotometer settings can make a difference in the results.

It is preferable, for accurate work, to prepare a calibration graph: this is done by making solutions of 0% reduced hemoglobin and 100% carboxyhemoglobin and plotting the ratio D^{538}/D^{578}. The ratio determined for the sample can then be interpolated onto a straight line joining the 0% and 100% values, and the % saturation read off. The method of preparing carbon monoxide is described further on. Note that it is *not* possible to prepare accurate intermediate standards.

Interpretation

The degree of saturation of hemoglobin by carbon monoxide determines the severity of the clinical symptoms. At 5 to 10% saturation the earliest symptoms are slight headache and breathlessness on mild exertion; between 20 to 30% saturation incoordination, drowsiness, and general mental impairment appear; and between 30 to 60% saturation these symptoms become increasingly severe. More than 60% saturation is usually rapidly fatal, and even short periods of exposure at this level can cause irreversible brain damage. The best treatment is removal from the toxic atmosphere and the administration of pure oxygen.

Victims of carbon monoxide poisoning have a unique magenta or cherry-red color, especially noticeable in the lips, face, and mucous membranes. This change is easily observed once the saturation rises above 30%.

Preparation of Carbon Monoxide. Fit a 500-mL flask with a dropping funnel and an exit tube for the gas. Place about 100 mL of 97% formic acid in the flask. Run in concentrated sulfuric acid from the dropping funnel rapidly until the contents of the flask reach about 60°C; then reduce the flow of acid until just sufficient to maintain the reaction. Allow a few minutes for expulsion of air from the flask, and then insert the gas exit tube into the separating funnel containing the diluted blood so that the stream of CO displaces the air from the funnel. Stopper the funnel. Stop the addition of sulfuric acid. Allow the evolution of CO to cease.

Note. It is absolutely essential that this whole procedure be carried out in the ventilating hood with the exhaust fan running throughout. The door of the hood should be lowered as far as possible.

Ethanol Determination

The most convenient method for the assay of ethyl alcohol in blood employs the enzyme alcohol dehydrogenase (ADH) (derived from either yeast or mammalian liver) to convert ethanol to acetaldehyde, with the concurrent reduction of the coenzyme NAD to NADH plus H^+. The increase in absorbance at 340 nm from the NAD reduction is related to ethanol concentration. The reaction conditions are adjusted to drive the process to completion: this is done by using a high pH and incorporating an acetaldehyde acceptor such as semicarbazide in the reaction mixture.

$$C_2H_5OH + NAD \xrightleftharpoons{ADH} CH_3CHO + NADH + H^+$$

Suitable kits of reagents are commercially available.*

---

*Calbiochem, La Jolla, Calif. 92037.

Methanol in Blood (Kaye, 1970)

Principle

The methanol of the blood sample is oxidized to formaldehyde with permanganate, and after the excess permanganate is decolorized with bisulfite the formaldehyde is detected by its reaction with chromotropic acid.

Procedure

1. Mix 2.0 mL oxalated whole blood (do not use heparin or EDTA, since these anticoagulants may give false positives) with 4.0 mL of 20% w/v trichloroacetic acid. Shake well, centrifuge, and clear the supernatant by filtration through a small fast paper.

2. To 1.0 mL of filtrate in a 100 × 12 mm test tube add 4 drops of permanganate reagent. Allow to stand for exactly 2 minutes after a gentle mixing, then add several small crystals of sodium bisulfite. Mix gently until the pink color has gone.

3. Add a spatula tip of chromotropic acid and swirl gently until it has dissolved.

4. With a fine-tipped 2.0-mL volumetric pipette, then run 2.0 mL of concentrated sulfuric acid down the side of the inclined tube to form a sharply delineated layer below the tube contents.

5. Gently return the tube to the upright position and examine the interface against a white background for a dark purple ring.

6. The test will detect 5 mg of methanol per dL of blood.

7. It is advisable to run in parallel a control blood to which has been added 25 microliters of methanol per 5 mL.

8. Large amounts of ethanol may give a brown ring at the interface.

Reagents

Permanganate Reagent. Dissolve 3.0 g potassium permanganate in a mixture of 15 mL concentrated orthophosphoric acid, H_3PO_4, and 85 mL distilled water. Stir on the magnetic mixer for at least an hour to ensure solution.

Sodium Bisulfite and Chromotropic Acid. Reagent grade.

Phenothiazines—Screening Test (Forrest and Forrest, 1960)

FPN Reagent. Mix 5.0 mL of a *freshly made* 5 g per dL aqueous solution of ferric chloride $FeCl_3$ with 45 mL of 14% w/v perchloric acid (made by diluting 20.0 mL of 70% perchloric acid up to 100 mL with distilled water) and 50 mL of 7.5 M nitric acid (made by diluting concentrated nitric acid, 50 mL, up to 100 mL with distilled water). The FPN reagent is stable.

Procedure

1. In a porcelain well spot plate place 1 drop of urine or centrifuged gastric contents. Add 2 drops of FPN reagent and observe any color change that takes place within ten seconds. If a blue, purple, or red color forms within the ten-second time limit, phenothiazines are probably present at overdosage levels.

2. If the test is performed by adding 1.0 mL of FPN reagent to 1.0 mL urine, pink-orange or pink colors indicate drug intakes of up to 70 mg per day (Tietz, 1976).

3. Increased levels of urobilinogen in the urine will give false positives. False negatives after ingestion of excessive amounts of a phenothiazine-type drug do not occur.

Salicylates Determination (Trinder, 1954)

Principle

The sample is treated with Trinder's reagent, which contains mercuric chloride, to precipitate any proteins present, and ferric ions, which produce a purple color with salicylates. The reaction is highly specific; plasma from persons not taking salicylates gives results of less than 1.0 mg per dL.

Procedure

1. Set up two 15 mL centrifuge tubes, marked test and blank. Into test pipette 1.0 mL of specimen—whole blood, plasma, serum, cerebrospinal fluid, urine, or filtered gastric washings. Into blank pipette 1.0 mL distilled water. To both tubes add 5.0 mL of Trinder's reagent, shaking during and after the addition. Let stand 5 minutes.

2. Centrifuge for 10 minutes at 2800 rpm.

3. Prepare standards by mixing 1.0 mL of the 5.0, 10.0, and 20.0 mg per dL working standards with 5.0 mL of Trinder's reagent.

4. Decant the clear supernatants from test and blank into 10-mm spectrophotometer cuvettes; determine the absorbances of test and standards at 540 nm, setting zero absorbance with the blank.

Calculation

$$\frac{\text{Test Absorbance}}{\text{Standard Absorbance nearest to Test}} \times \text{Value of}$$

Standard used = Salicylates in mg/dL. Mg/dL × 0.072 = mmol/liter.

Reagents

Trinder's Reagent. Dissolve 10.0 g mercuric chloride $HgCl_2$ in 200 mL hot distilled water. Cool, add 30 mL 1 M hydrochloric acid. Add 10.0 g ferric nitrate $Fe(NO_3)_3 \cdot 9H_2O$ and shake until dissolved. Make up to 250 mL with distilled water, mix. Keeps well in the refrigerator.

Stock Standard. Dissolve 580 mg sodium salicylate $C_6H_4(OH) \cdot COONa$ in, and make up to 500 mL with, distilled water. Preserve with a few drops of chloroform.

Working Standards. Make 5.0, 10.0, and 20.0 mL of the stock standard up to 100 mL with distilled water, and mix. These correspond to salicylate levels of 5.0, 10.0, and 20.0 mg per dL (0.360, 0.720, and 1.44 mmol/liter).

Notes

1. For urine estimations, it may be necessary to predilute the specimen if large amounts are being excreted; the final result will have to be multiplied by the appropriate factor.

2. If the supernatant obtained with protein-containing specimens is not clear, reshake, let stand an additional five minutes, and recentrifuge.

3. When the assay is being used to monitor intensive therapy with salicylates, as in acute rheumatic conditions, the blood samples should be obtained at some

predetermined time in relationship to the administration of the drug. It should be noted that the blood levels also will be affected by changes in renal function and excretion.

4. Maximum salicylate blood levels usually are reached about 2 hours after ingestion with therapeutic doses; a single dose of 600 mg aspirin produces a blood level of about 5 mg per dL. Toxic symptoms, the earliest of which is tinnitus, start to appear at levels above about 30 mg per dL.

5. If the test is being performed on urine, large amounts of acetoacetic acid therein will interfere. A measured aliquot of sample should be boiled, cooled, and made up to the original volume before analysis if the urine is strongly positive for ketone bodies.

6. The sequence of events in salicylate poisoning is complex: an initial stimulation of respiration leads to hypocapnia (decreased P_{CO_2}) and respiratory alkalosis; later, interference with metabolic pathways, enzyme inhibition, and hypertonic dehydration produce a metabolic acidosis.

BLOOD SULFONAMIDES (Bratton and Marshall, 1939)

NH_2 — Sulfanilamide — SO_2NH_2

NH_2 — para-Aminobenzoic Acid — COOH

Definition

Sulfonamides are synthetic bacteriostatic drugs that exert their effect by metabolic antagonism. Bacteria require para-aminobenzoic acid (PABA) in order to synthesize folic acid but, because of the closely similar structure, they "mistake" sulfa for PABA molecules, and the sulfa blocks their synthesis of folic acid.

Sulfonamides are derivatives of sulfonic acids. In the body they exist (after ingestion) in free and conjugated forms (acetyl sulfonamides).

Estimation

Principle. Free sulfonamide in a protein-free filtrate of whole blood, plasma, or serum is diazotized with nitrous acid and, after destruction of the excess nitrite by ammonium sulfamate, the diazotized sulfonamide is coupled with *N*-(1-naphthyl)ethylenediamine dihydrochloride to form a pink to purplish red azo dye (Bratton-Marshall reaction). The conjugated sulfonamide is converted to the free form by boiling the protein-free filtrate with hydrochloric acid, after which it is estimated as for the free sulfonamide.

TABLE 13–2 CONVERSION FACTORS FOR SULFONAMIDES

Drug Used in Patient	Factor by Which Result Obtained on Sulfanilamide Curve (Standard) Must Be Multiplied
Sulfacetamide	1.24
Sulfadiazine	1.45
Sulfadimethoxime	1.80
Sulfaguanidine	1.24
Sulfamerazine	1.53
Sulfamethizole	1.57
Sulfaphenazole	1.83
Sulfapyridine	1.45
Sulfisomidine	1.62
Sulfisoxazole	1.55

Conversion Factors for Various Sulfonamides. Results are in terms of sulfanilamide and must be converted to the equivalent concentrations of the particular sulfa drug being used in the patient under investigation. The factor for this conversion is derived from the expression:

$$\frac{\text{M W of sulfa drug used}}{\text{M W of sulfanilamide (172)}}$$

See Table 13–2.

Note on Interfering Substances. Under the conditions of the test, arsenical drugs and procaine interfere in the estimation of free sulfonamides; acetanilid and related compounds similarly affect the total sulfonamide estimation.

CHAPTER 13—REVIEW QUESTIONS

1. What factors may influence the plasma level of a drug after oral administration?
2. How do sulfonamide drugs exert their bacteriostatic action?
3. Show with diagrams the meaning of the terms *half-life, first-order kinetics,* and *steady state.*

REFERENCES FOR CHEMISTRY SECTION

Abell LL, Levy BB, Brodie BB, and Kendall FE. A simplified method for the estimation of total cholesterol in serum and demonstration of its specificity. J Biol Chem 1952; *195*:357–366.

Adams AP, and Hahn CEW. Principles and practice of blood-gas analysis. Morris Plains, N.J.: General Diagnostics Division, Warner-Lambert International, 1979.

Advanced Instruments, Inc. Osmometry and cryoscopy school outline. Newton Highlands, Mass., 1967.

Aggarwal V, Bath R, and Sunshine I. Technique for rapidly separating drugs from biological samples. Clin Chem 1974; *20*:307–309.

American Society of Clinical Pathologists. Technical improvement service no. 27. Maintaining optimum spectrophotometer performance. Commission on Continuing Education, Chicago, 1975.

Anderson NG. Analytical techniques for cell fractions. XII. A multiple-cuvette rotor for a new microanalytical system. Anal Biochem 1969; *28*:545–562

Arkin H, and Colton RR. Tables for statisticians, 2nd ed. New York: Harper & Row, 1963.

Babson AL. Phenolphthalein monophosphate, a new substrate for serum alkaline phosphatase. Clin Chem 1965; *11*:789.

Barnett RN. Clinical laboratory statistics. Boston: Little, Brown and Company, 1971.

Barnett RN, and Youden WJ. A revised scheme for the comparison of quantitative methods. Am J Clin Pathol 1970; *54*:454–462.

Bender, GT. Chemical instrumentation: a laboratory manual based on clinical chemistry. Philadelphia: WB Saunders, 1972.

van den Bergh A, Hijmans A, and Mueller P. Ueber eine direkte und indirekte Diazoreaktion auf Bilirubin. Biochem Ztschr 1916; *77*:90.

Bessey OA, Lowry OH, and Brock MJ. Method for rapid determination of alkaline phosphatase with 5 cubic millimetres of serum. J Biol Chem 1946; *164*:321–329.

Bierman EL, and Glomset JA. Disorders of lipid metabolism. *In* Williams RH, ed. Textbook of endocrinology, 6th ed. Philadelphia: WB Saunders, 1981, pp. 875–905.

Billing BH, Cole PG, and Lathe GH. The excretion of bilirubin as a diglucuronide giving the direct van den Bergh reaction. Biochem J 1957; *65*:774–784.

Blackberg SN, and Wanger JO. Melanuria. JAMA 1933; *100*:334–336.

Blondheim SH, Margoliash E, and Shafrir E. A simple test for myohemoglobinuria (myoglobinuria). JAMA 1958; *167*:453–454.

Blumenfeld TA, Turi GK, and Blanc WA. Recommended site and depth of newborn heel skin punctures based on anatomical measurements and histopathology. Lancet 1979; *1*:230–233.

Bodansky O. Serum phosphohexose isomerase in cancer. I. Method of determination and establishment of range of normal values. II. As an index of tumor growth in metastatic carcinoma of the breast. Cancer 1954; 7:1191–1199.

Bradford MM. A rapid and sensitive method for the quantitation of microgram quantities of protein utilizing the principle of protein dye binding. Analyt Biochem 1976; *72*:248–254.

Bratton AC, and Marshall EK Jr. New coupling component for sulfanilamide determination. J Biol Chem 1939; *128*:537–550.

Brazie JV, Bowes WA, and Ibbott FA. An improved, rapid procedure for the determination of amniotic fluid bilirubin and its use in the prediction of the course of Rh-sensitized pregnancies. Am J Obstet Gynecol 1969; *104*:80–86.

Bucolo, G, and David H. Quantitative determination of serum triglycerides by the use of enzymes. Clin Chem 1973; *19*:476–482.

Caraway WT. A stable starch substrate for the determination of amylase in serum and other body fluids. Am J Clin Pathol 1959; *32*:97–99.

Caraway WT and Kammeyer CW. Chemical interference by drugs and other substances with clinical laboratory test procedures. Clin Chim Acta 1972; *41*:395–434.

Castelli WP, Doyle JT, Gordon T, Hames CG, Hjortland MC, Hulley SB, Kagan A, and Zukel WJ. HDL cholesterol and other lipids in coronary heart disease. Circulation 1977; *55*:768–772.

Chaney AL, and Marbach EP. Modified reagents for determination of urea and ammonia. Clin Chem 1962; *8*:130–132.

Cherry IS, and Crandall LA Jr. Specificity of pancreatic lipase. Am J Physiol 1932; *100*:266–273.

Chromy V, and Fischer J. Photometric determination of total protein in lipemic sera. Clin Chem 1977; *23*:754–756.

Collins RD. Illustrated manual of fluid and electrolyte disorders. Philadelphia: JB Lippincott, 1976.

Crymble GG. Quality control seminar notes. Scarborough, Ont.: Warner-Chilcott Diagnostics, 1971.

Curry AS. Poison detection in human organs. Springfield, Ill.: Charles C Thomas, 1963.

Daly JA, and Ertingshausen G. Direct method for determining phosphate in serum with the "Centrifichem." Clin Chem 1972; *18*:263–265.

Davenport HW. The ABC of acid-base chemistry, 6th ed. University of Chicago Press, 1974.

Diehl H, and Ellingboe JL. Indicator for titration of calcium in presence of magnesium using disodium dihydrogen ethylenediamine tetraacetate. Anal Chem 1956; *28*:882–884.

Doumas BT. Standards for total serum protein assays—a collaborative study. Clin Chem 1975; *21*:1159–1166.

Doumas BT, Perry BW, Sasse EA, and Straumfjord JV Jr. Standardization in bilirubin assays: Evaluation of selected methods and stability of bilirubin solutions. Clin Chem 1973; *19*:984–993.

Dryer RL, Tammes AR, and Routh JI. The determination of phosphorus and phosphatase with *N*-phenyl-p-phenylenediamine. J Biol Chem 1957; *225*:177–183.

Dunphy JV, Littman A, Hammond JB, Forstner G, Dahlqvist A, and Crane RK. Intestinal lactase deficit in adults. Gastroenterology 1965; *49*:12–21.

Emmett M, and Narins RG. Clinical use of the anion gap. Medicine 1977; *56*:38–54.

Evelyn KA, and Malloy HT. Microdetermination of oxyhemoglobin, methemoglobin and sulfhemoglobin in a single sample of blood. J Biol Chem 1938; *126*:655–662.

Forrest IS, and Forrest FM. Urine color test for the detection of phenothiazine compounds. Clin Chem 1960; *6*:11–15.

Freer DE, and Statland BE. Measurement of amniotic fluid surfactant. Clin Chem 1981; *27*:1629–1641.

Frings CS, Muscat VI, and Waldrop NT. Convenient method for checking detector response of spectrophotometers at three wave lengths. Clin Chem 1976; *22*:101–102.

Gadd KG. Protein estimation in spinal fluid using Coomassie blue reagent. Med Lab Sci 1981; *38*:61–63.

Gindler EM. Some non-parametric statistical tests for quick evaluation of clinical data. Clin Chem 1975; *21*:309–314.

Glasser L, and Finley PR. Amniotic fluid and the quality of life. Diagn Med 1981; *4*:31–52.

Golbey MJ. A simple screening test for amphetamine in urine. Ann Clin Biochem 1971; *8*:117–118.

Goldbaum LR. Determination of barbiturates. Anal Chem 1952; *24*:1600–1607.

Gordon T, Castell WP, Hjortland MC, Kannel WB, and Dawber TR. High density lipoprotein as a protective factor against coronary heart disease. The Framingham Study. Am J Med 1977; *62*:704–714.

Grieg WR, Browning M, Boyle JA, and Maxwell D. Effect of the synthetic polypeptide Bl-24 (Synacthen) on adrenocortical function. J Endocrinol 1966; *34*:411–412.

Guilbault GG, and Hargis LG. Instrumental analysis manual. New York: Marcel Dekker, 1970.

Guzak R, and Caraway WT. Simultaneous determination of serum barbiturate and salicylate by ultraviolet absorbtion spectrophotometry. Am J Med Technol 1963; *29*:231–239.

Guzak R, and Caraway WT. *In* Bender GT. Chemical instrumentation: a laboratory manual based on clinical chemistry. Philadelphia: WB Saunders, 1972.

Harboe M. A method for determining hemoglobin in plasma by near ultraviolet spectrophotometry. Scand J Clin Lab Invest 1959; *11*:66–70.

Harris AL. Determination of D-xylose in urine for the D-xylose absorption test. Clin Chem 1969; *15*:65–71.

Haussler MR. Basic and clinical concepts related to vitamin D metabolism and action. N Engl J Med 1977; *297*:974–983, 1041–1050.

Helman EZ. Emergency screening of urine, plasma, or gastric contents for barbiturates. Clin Chem 1970; *16*:797–798.

Henry RJ, ed. Clinical chemistry: principles and technics, 2nd ed. New York: Harper & Row, 1974.

Hoffman RG. Statistics in the practice of medicine. JAMA 1963; *185*:865–873. Also, New York: John Wiley and Sons, 1973.

IFCC Expert Panel on Bilirubin. Canadian Society of Clinical Chemists Newsletter No. 4, October 1972.

Itaya K, and Ui M. A new micromethod for the colorimetric determination of inorganic phosphate. Clin Chim Acta 1966; *14*:361–366.

Jatlow P. Ultraviolet spectrophotometric analysis of barbiturates: evaluation of potential interferences. Am J Clin Pathol 1973; *59*:167–173.

Jendrassik L, and Grof P. Vereinfachte photometrische Methoden zur Bestimmung des Blutbilirubins. Biochem Ztschr 1938; *297*:81–89.

Jones RA. An introduction to gas-liquid chromatography. New York: Academic Press, 1970.

Jung DH, and Parekh AC. An improved reagent system for the measurement of serum uric acid. Clin Chem 1970; *16*:247–250.

Kageyama N. A direct colorimetric determination of uric acid in serum and urine with uricase-catalase system. Clin Chim Acta 1971; *31*:421–426.

van Kampen EJ, and Zijlstra WG. Determination of hemoglobin and its derivatives. Adv Clin Chem 1965; *8*:141.

Kaplan A, and Szabo LL. Clinical chemistry: interpretation and techniques. Philadelphia: Lea & Febiger, 1979, pp. 122–124.

Kark RM, Lawrence JR, Pollack VE, Pirani CL, Muehrcke RC, and Silva H. A primer of urinalysis, 2nd ed. New York: Hoeber Medical Division, Harper & Row, 1963.

Kaye S. Emergency toxicology, 3rd ed. Springfield, Ill.: Charles C Thomas, 1970.

King EJ, and Armstrong AR. Convenient method for determining serum and bile phosphatase activity. Canad Med Assoc J 1934; *31*:376–381.

Levinson SA, and MacFate RP. Clinical laboratory diagnosis, 6th ed. Philadelphia: Lea & Febiger, 1961.

Lippman RW. Urine and the urinary sediment: a practical manual and atlas, 2nd ed. Springfield, Ill.: Charles C Thomas, 1964.

Lolekha P, and Charoenpol W. Improved automated method for determining serum albumin with bromcresol green. Clin Chem 1974; *20*:617–624.

Martinek RG. Starch substrate with improved stability for the clinical determination of amylase activity. Clin Chim Acta 1964; *9*:590–592.

McQueen EG. The nature of urinary casts. J Clin Pathol 1962; *15*:367–373.

Meites S, and Faulkner WR. Manual of practical micro and general procedures in clinical chemistry. Springfield, Ill.: Charles-C Thomas, 1962.

Miskiewicz SJ, Arnett BB, and Simon GE. Evaluation of a glucose oxidase-peroxidase method adapted to the singe-channel AutoAnalyzer and SMA 12/60. Clin Chem 1973; *19*:253–257.

Natelson S. Microtechniques of clinical chemistry, 2nd ed. Springfield, Ill.: Charles C Thomas, 1961.

Natelson S, Scommegna A, and Epstein MB, eds. Amniotic fluid, physiology, biochemistry and clinical chemistry. New York: John Wiley and Sons, 1974.

National Diabetes Data Group. Classification and diagnosis of diabetes mellitus and other categories of glucose intolerance. Diabetes 1979; *28*:1039–1057.

Naumann HN. The measurement of hemoglobin in plasma. *In* Tietz NW, ed. Fundamentals of clinical chemistry, 2nd ed. Philadelphia: WB Saunders, 1976.

O'Brien D, and Ibbott FA. Laboratory manual of pediatric micro- and ultramicro-biochemical techniques, 3rd ed. New York: Hoeber Medical Division, Harper & Row, 1962.

Porres JM, D'ambra C, Lord D, and Garrity F. Comparison of eight kits for the diagnosis of pregnancy. Am J Clin Pathol 1975; *64*:452–463.

Posen S. Turnover of circulating enzymes. Clin Chem 1970; *16*:71–84.

Putnam FW, Easly CW, Lynn LT, Ritchie AE, and Phelps RA. The heat precipitation of Bence-Jones proteins. I. Optimum conditions. Arch Biochem 1959; *83*:115.

Raab WP. Diagnostic value of urinary enzyme determinations. Clin Chem 1972; *18*:5–25.

Rand RN. Practical spectrophotometric standards. Clin Chem 1969; *17*:839–863.

Richens A, and Marks M, eds. Therapeutic drug monitoring. New York: Churchill Livingstone (Longman Group Ltd.), 1981.

Rieders F, and Frere FJ. Detection and estimation of toxicologically significant amounts of borate, chlorate and oxalate in biologic material. J Forensic Sci 1963; *8*:46–53.

Roy AV, Brower ME, and Hayden JE. Sodium thymolphthalein monophosphate: a new acid phosphatase substrate with greater specificity for the prostatic enzyme in serum. Clin Chem 1971; *17*:1093–1102.

Russell PT, Eberle AJ, and Cheng HC. The prostaglandins in clinical medicine. A developing role for the clinical chemist. Clin Chem 1975; *21*:653–666.

Schales O, and Schales SS. Simple and accurate method for determination of chloride in biological fluids. J Biol Chem 1941; *140*:879–884.

Schreiner GE. The urinary sediment. Summit, N.J.: Ciba Clinical Symposia; 1962, *14*:35–48.

Schumm OL. Hoppe-Seyler. Z Physiol Chem 1912; *80*:1–5.

Schuurs AHWM, and van Weeman BK. Enzyme immunoassay: a powerful analytical tool. J Immunoassay 1980; *1*:229–249.

Scriver CR, and Rosenberg LE. Amino acid metabolism and its disorders. Philadelphia: WB Saunders, 1973.

Sidbury JB, Smith EK, and Harlan W. An inborn error of short-chain fatty acid metabolism. J Pediatr 1967; *70*:8–15.

Siggaard-Andersen O: The acid-base status of the blood, 3rd ed. Baltimore: Williams & Wilkins, 1965.

Simmons JS, and Gentzkow CJ. Laboratory methods of the United States Army. Philadelphia: Lea & Febiger, 1944.

Skelley DS, Brown LP, and Besch PK. Radioimmunoassay (Review). Clin Chem 1973; *19*:146–186.

Smith I. Chromatographic and electrophoretic techniques, 2nd ed. London: William Heinemann Medical Books Ltd, 1960.

Sobel C. *In* Henry RJ. Clinical chemistry. New York: Harper & Row, 1964, pp. 881–883.

Solomon DH, et al. Revised nomenclature for tests of thyroid hormones in serum. J Clin Endocrinol 1976; *42*:595–598.

Spencer ES, and Pedersen I. Hand atlas of the urinary sediment. Baltimore: University Park Press, 1977.

Stanbury JB, Wyngaarden JB, and Fredrickson DS., eds. The metabolic basis of inherited disease, 4th ed. New York: McGraw Hill, 1977.

Stookey LL. Ferrozine—a new spectrophotometric reagent for iron. Anal Chem 1970; *42*:779–781.

Street HV. Identification of drugs by a combination of gas-liquid, paper and thin-layer chromatography. J Chromatogr 1970; *48*:291–294.

Swinscow TDV. Statistics at square one. London: British Medical Association, 1976.

Szasz G. A kinetic photometric method for serum gamma-glutamyl transpeptidase. Clin Chem 1969; *15*:124–136.

Tamm I, Horsfall FL Jr. Characterization and separation of an inhibitor of viral hemagglutination present in urine. Proc Soc Exp Biol Med 1950; *74*:108–114.

Tietz NW, ed. Fundamentals of clinical chemistry, 2nd ed. Philadelphia: WB Saunders, 1976.

Tomokuni K, and Ogata M. Simple method for determination of urinary *d*-aminolevulinic acid as an index of lead exposure. Clin Chem 1972; *18*:1534–1536.

Torrance FH. An improved method for serum bromide. Med Lab Technol 1973; *30*:255–258.

Trinder P. Rapid determination of salicylates in biological materials. Biochem J 1954; *57*:301–303.

Wallace GB, and Diamond JS. The significance of urobilinogen in the urine as a test for liver function; with a description of a simple quantitative method for its estimation. Arch Intern Med 1925; *35*:698–725.

Walton HF. Principles and methods of chemical analysis, 2nd ed. Englewood Cliffs, N.J.: Prentice-Hall, 1964.

Weissman N, Lowe ML, Beattie JM, and Demetriou JA. Screening method for detection of drugs of abuse in human urine. Clin Chem 1971; *17*:875–881.

White D, Haidar GA, and Reinhold JG. Spectrophotometric measurement of bilirubin concentrations in the serum of the newborn by the use of a microcapillary method. Clin Chem 1958; *4*:211–215.

WHO Memorandum: Classification of hyperlipidemia and hyperlipoproteinemias. Circulation 1972; *45*:501–508.

Wilkinson JH. Isoenzymes, 2nd ed. London: Chapman and Hall, 1970.

Young DS, and Mears TW. Measurement and standard reference materials in clinical chemistry. Clin Chem 1968; *14*:929–943.

Young DS, Pestaner LC, and Gibberman V. Effects of drugs on clinical laboratory tests. Clin Chem 1975; *21*:1D–432D.

Zeisler EB. Determination of diffusible calcium. Am J Clin Pathol 1954; *24*:588–598.

Zettner A. Principles of competitive binding assays (saturation analyses). I. Equilibrium techniques. Clin Chem 1973; *19*:699–705.

Section II

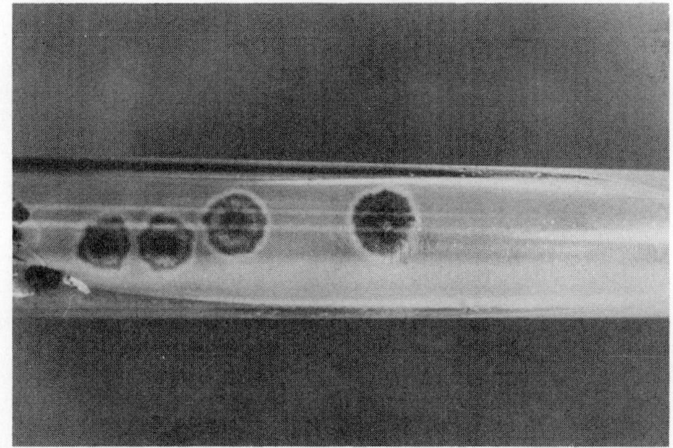

MICROBIOLOGY

14

APPLIED MICROBIOLOGY: SOME BASIC CONCEPTS, TECHNIQUES, AND METHODS

INTRODUCTION

The medical microbiologist is concerned fundamentally with the isolation and identification of those microorganisms causing disease (pathogens) in man. This task, however, is complicated by the ubiquitous distribution of microorganisms throughout the biosphere and, in particular, by the colonization of the skin surfaces of the human body by what constitutes the normal microbial flora existing in a state of commensalism with the host. Hence, in addition to allowing the microbiologist to differentiate between a commensal and a pathogen and providing a controlled environment for the propagation of the microorganism, the techniques employed in microbiology also must provide for the exclusion of contaminants.

This chapter is primarily concerned with the relation between the microorganism and the environment, specifically, microbial nutrition, the influence of environmental factors on microbial growth, and those external factors affecting their viability. Moreover, it examines how knowledge of these factors enables us to culture organisms in vitro and how, with knowledge of the different requirements of differing species, we are able to use such demands to differentiate one species of bacteria from another. This leads into a discussion of culture media and stains and why they show their various reactions and finally to a consideration of quality control in which the laboratory is challenged to show that it provides the facilities for growing bacterial species and the expertise for recognizing them and understanding their significance.

A CONSIDERATION OF SOME EXTERNAL FACTORS AFFECTING THE VIABILITY OF MICROORGANISMS

As we have indicated earlier, it is fundamental to all microbiological procedures, particularly when cultures of organisms are required, that all materials and apparatus utilized must be bacteriologically clean before culture of the material submitted for investigation is attempted. If contaminated media or apparatus are used, the resultant culture will show not only those bacteria resident in the original specimen, but also the presence of any contaminating microorganisms. Furthermore, it is vital that a worker in microbiology be aware of the constant hazard of the spread of infectious agents within a working environment as a result of either poor technique, lack of knowledge of the mechanisms of sterilization, or both.

A fundamental characteristic of a living cell is the property of growth. Bacterial growth is extremely rapid—in fact, the generation time of a microbe such as *Escherichia coli* is on the order of 20 minutes (although *M. tuberculosis* requires 10 to 20 hours). During this time there is a processual exchange between the cell and the environment, namely, the absorption of food molecules and their subsequent transformation into cellular components so that the organism will exhibit a positive addition to its existing body material, and anabolism will exceed catabolism.

Microorganisms are able to grow only within certain limits of pH, temperature, and other specific environmental criteria. And although an organism may survive outside of those limits delineated by it species, it will of necessity be unable to grow and reproduce; indeed, it is predictable that further departure from the so-called optimal conditions will lead to the organism's death. From this it is clear that an intimate knowledge on the part of the microbiologist of a microorganism's physiology is a necessary prerequisite to ensure: (i) the successful establishment of a microbial culture and (ii) its ultimate destruction once the necessary studies have been completed. The viability of a microorganism is dependent on the existence of a balance between a number of environmental factors. Some of these variables will now be characterized.

Influence of Oxygen and Redox Potential

The natural environment of a microorganism is determined by its oxygen and redox potential requirements. Furthermore, the ability of an organism to thrive when transferred to a fresh medium is largely dependent on the status of the oxidation-reduction potential of that medium. This is controlled by the oxidizing and reducing agents present in the medium. Strongly oxidative substances yield positive potentials, whereas strongly reducing ones produce negative potentials.

Obligate aerobic microorganisms use molecular oxygen as their terminal electron acceptor. By contrast, obligate anaerobes use some alternative substances. However, it is important to remember that although an anaerobe fails to grow in the presence of oxygen, it may survive. Facultative anaerobes are capable of growing in the presence or absence of oxygen. The microaerophilics require low concentrations of oxygen. It is now generally recognized that all bacteria require the presence of a small amount of carbon dioxide for growth.

Each medium has an oxidation-reduction potential (redox), which is a measure of whether it will accept or donate electrons. The substances that donate electrons are considered reducing agents, and those that accept electrons are oxidizing agents. The redox potential is affected by the pH of the medium and by the presence of oxygen, hydrogen, or other substances. It can be measured by using a calomel half-cell electrode and measuring the electrical flow between the electrode and the medium in millivolts (mV). The resultant measurement is the Eh. Anaerobes grow best at an Eh of −150 to −400 mV, but there is much variation. To place this measurement in perspective, body tissues are between +125 and +250 mV, depending on the nature and adequacy of the blood supply.

Thioglycollate medium may contain resazurin (0.001 g/L) or methylene blue (0.002 g/L) as an indicator of Eh. At the correct pH, the medium will become, respectively, pink or green if the Eh is not sufficiently negative.

Influence of Temperature

Four temperatures are important for microbial viability: the thermal death point, and the minimum, optimum, and maximum temperatures. In the clinical laboratory, microorganisms are grown at their optimum temperatures; that is, the temperature at which growth is most rapid, in a thermostatically controlled incubator. In fact, this optimum temperature approximates that of the microorganism's natural habitat—which in the case of those organisms that are parasites in mammals, is in the region of 37°C. The majority of these organisms and the soil saprophytes are mesophiles and have a wide growth temperature range of between 25 to 40°C. However, those organisms known as psychrophiles and thermophiles grow best outside of the mesophilic range. In the case of psychrophilic organisms, they have an optima of approximately 15°C and a range from −5 to 30°C. By contrast, thermophiles require elevated temperatures, growing best at temperatures between 55 to 80°C.

The thermal death point of an organism may be defined as the lowest temperature that will kill it within a given time. However, some workers prefer to use the term *thermal death time,* defined as that time required to kill a culture at a specific temperature; this is considered more practical.

In a moist environment the thermal death time for nonsporing microorganisms ranges from several hours at 47°C, to 1 hour at 60°C, to 5 minutes at 70°C; and very few are capable of survival for more than a few minutes at a temperature of 80°C. The extreme limit of resistance to moist heat is exhibited by some strains of spores of *Bacillus stearothermophilus*, which require an exposure to 121°C for 10 to 35 minutes to bring about death. The resistance of bacterial spores constitutes a major problem in heat sterilization, for although some bacterial endospores are killed by exposure to temperatures of between 86° to 88°C for 30 minutes, the majority require a temperature above that of 100°C for the same period of time.

Most viruses are inactivated by exposure to temperatures between 50 to 60°C for 20 minutes. However, there are a few exceptions, such as the poliovirus and infective hepatitis virus, which are destroyed only at higher temperatures, e.g., 75°C for 30 minutes.

Influence of Moisture

The majority of transit substances entering and leaving a cell do so by using water as a vehicle. Thus the mechanism of osmosis is seen to play an integral role in the maintenance of the living status of an organism.

Osmosis. Osmosis is the passage of solvent molecules through a semipermeable membrane from a region of higher concentration to one of lower concentration. Osmotic pressure is an expression of molecular concentration, and it has been shown experimentally that the laws governing this mechanism are analogous to the laws governing the movement of gases.

Plant and animal cells undergo drastic changes when exposed to environments having a low osmotic pressure (hypotonic); there is a tendency for excessive amounts of fluid to pass into the cell protoplasm, creating a very high intracellular pressure. In fact, those organisms not possessing strong cell walls undergo plasmoptysis (bursting). Plasmolysis (shrinking) occurs when normal cells are placed in solution of very high osmotic pressure (hypertonic). An example of the application of plasmolysis is in the preservation of foodstuffs—a 10 to 15% sodium chloride or 50 to 70% sugar solution is quite an adequate preservation concentration.

Desiccation. By weight four-fifths of the microbial cell consists of water. Hence moisture is an absolute necessity for growth. A change occurring in the environment that leads to desiccation is injurious to many bacteria; different species appear to vary in their ability to survive dehydration when it occurs under natural conditions. Some (e.g., *N. gonorrhoeae*) resist drying very poorly, whereas others (e.g., *M. tuberculosis*) are able to withstand dry conditions for months.

Lyophilization (Freeze-drying). If desiccation is obtained by the removal of water by sublimation under reduced pressure from frozen bacterial suspensions, the dried cells remain viable and may be stored for long periods. Protein-rich materials or sucrose as well as some other substances are cryoprotective agents, and before lyophilization, bacteria are suspended in such solutions. The process avoids intracellular water and salt crystallization, which is lethal.

Lyophilization is a common method of preserving cultures. The preserved organisms are generally made available in glass vials and may be recovered by opening the vial and adding a small quantity of nutrient broth. The latter is then in turn inoculated into a larger quantity of broth, and finally, this suspension is plated on or inoculated into the appropriate media.

Influence of pH

pH is an essential factor influencing the growth and reproduction of microorganisms. Microorganisms grow over a pH range, usually within a well-defined optimum. The minimum pH for growth is about pH 2.5, and maximum about pH 9.0, with an optimum frequently between pH 5.0 to pH 7.5. The majority of the human commensal and pathogenic microorganisms have an optimum hovering around neutral, that is, between a pH of 7.2 to 7.6. However, fungi, e.g., *Penicillium* and *Aspergillus,* are capable of flourishing in the presence of a considerable degree of acid, and therefore are referred to as acidophilic. By contrast, there are those organisms that are tolerant of alkaline conditions (e.g., *Vibrio cholerae,* which has an optimum pH of 8.2). Similarly, some species of *Bacillus* can grow at pH 11.0.

Exposure to strong acids or alkaline solutions is rapidly lethal to the majority of microorganisms.

Ultraviolet Radiation

At wavelengths of 330 nm or less, this type of radiation has a lethal effect on bacteria. Basically the radiation alters DNA and so interferes with its replication. To a lesser extent UV light causes lethal mutation.

Although UV light is employed as a bactericide in laboratory safety hoods and to a lesser extent in operating rooms and areas of food processing, its wider application is, to a large extent, prevented by its deleterious effect on the eyes, in which it causes irritation and even opacities. To prevent these, eyeglasses must be worn, since glass is opaque to UV light.

ASPECTS OF MICROBIAL GROWTH

To ensure successful propagation of an organism, a suitable medium containing all required nutrients must be supplied, and other environmental factors such as pH, temperature, and aeration must be controlled. Other factors that should be considered include the salt concentration and osmotic pressure of the medium.

Under ideal conditions the growth of a cell occurs according to a geometric progression with time. A single bacterium such as *Escherichia coli,* having a generation time of 20 minutes, would produce in 48 hours of exponential growth 2.2×10^{43} cells; if the average weight of a single bacterium was taken as 10^{-12} g, then the total weight of this 48-hour culture would be 2.2×10^{31} g. However, since bacterial growth generally occurs under finite conditions, certain limiting factors come into play which retard and ultimately terminate the growth rate.

The Growth Curve

As mentioned, under ideal conditions the growth of a cell takes place according to a geometric progression with time. Initially, the first generation division will be in synchrony. After an interval of time, because of differences occurring in the new population, the time of division will become randomized. In such a culture the number of cells doubles with each generation. That is, the population increases in direct proportion to time. This is the principle of exponential growth.

The growth rate of a population is expressed in terms of the generation time, which is that period of time required for the doubling of population numbers.

In a closed system, a culture eventually will stop growing as a result of: (i) exhaustion of essential nutrients, (ii) accumulation of toxic products, and/or (iii) development of an unfavorable pH. A typical population growth curve (see Fig. 14–1) can be obtained by counting the bacteria in a culture at specific time intervals after inoculation. The curve may be discussed in terms of four main phases:

I. The Lag Phase. This phase represents a period of adjustment in which enzymes and metabolic intermediates are formed and accumulated until optimal concentrations are reached, permitting a resumption of growth. This period of adaptation varies according to the nature and number of cells present in the inoculum and to differences between the medium, from which the inoculum was derived, and the new medium.

II. The Exponential Phase. This is a period of logarithmic multiplication of the population. The population of a normal culture doubles in each consecutive time interval. As the culture approaches the next phase, there is a short retardation period in which the growth rate decreases.

III. The Maximum Stationary Phase. Here either one or more of a medium's nutrients becomes exhausted, or there is an accumulation of toxic metabolic products, resulting in a transient balance between cell division and cell death.

IV. The Decline or Death Phase. As unfavorable conditions continue to develop, there is complete cessation of bacterial multiplication, such that the death rate in the culture increases progressively—often following an exponential curve.

Liquid and Solid Media. There are two main varieties of culture media, liquid and solid. Bacterial growth in liquid media does not exhibit particular characteristic appearances, hence such media are of limited use in identifying species. Also, organisms cannot be separated from "mixed cultures" by growth in liquid media. However, if liquid media are made semisolid, some of these disadvantages can be overcome, for example, in the use of the Craigie tube in salmonellae studies. By contrast, cultural appearances on solid culture media are extremely useful in initial differentiation of colonial types and indispensable in the isolation of pure cultures.

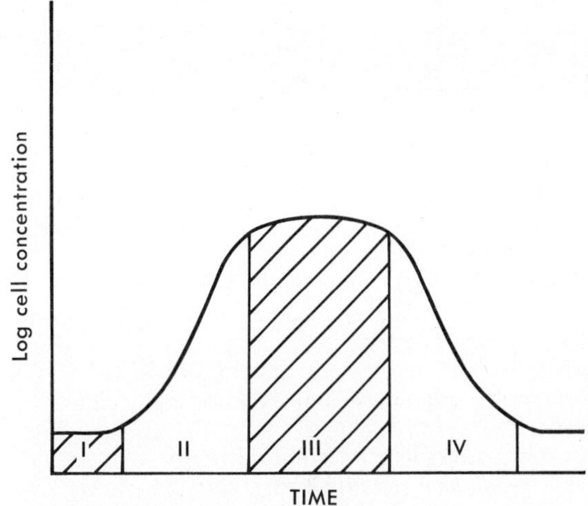

Figure 14–1 Idealized bacterial population curve. *I,* lag phase; *II,* exponential phase; *III,* maximum stationary phase; *IV,* death phase.

Growth of Bacteria on Solid Media. A cross-section of a bacterial colony reveals a stratigraphic record of a population's development, the base representing the present and the superior surface the past. The growth of bacterial colonies on solid media is often characteristic of the species. In the description of colonial appearances the size of the colonies and their color present immediately. They may also produce pigment that diffuses into the medium. Colonies may be glistening, dull, wrinkled, or mucoid and transparent, translucent, or opaque. Their consistency may be tough or viscid, butyrous (like butter), and so forth. Colonial morphology may best be described by reference to Figure 14–2*A*. After some practice, the student will be able to recognize typical appearances but will need the vocabulary of description to explain features to his fellows or instructors. A lens or dissecting microscope is often very useful (Fig. 14–2*B*). The conditions affecting colonial morphology and the rate of growth are multifactorial. For example, (i) limitation of available nutrients diffusing from medium to colony complicated by (a) aqueous surface, (b) atmospheric conditions, and (c) thickness and diameter of colony; (ii) autolysis of organisms in the center of older colonies; (iii) temperature; (iv) pH; and (v) osmotic conditions.

Counting Bacteria and Measuring Bacterial Growth

A *total count* will measure the number of cells, alive or dead, present in a culture. In contrast, a *viable count* measures only those cells capable of growth—and assumes that a visible colony will develop from each organism present in the original culture.

Total Counts

Browne's Opacity Tubes. These tubes are available commercially (see Fig. 14–3). This method requires the comparison of the opacity of an unknown bacterial suspension with that of a series of ten standard tubes containing different dilutions of suspended barium sulfate. A table is provided equating the opacity of each tube with the number of organisms per milliliter.

Turbidimetry. A nephlometer, colorimeter, or spectrophotometer can be used to determine the degree of

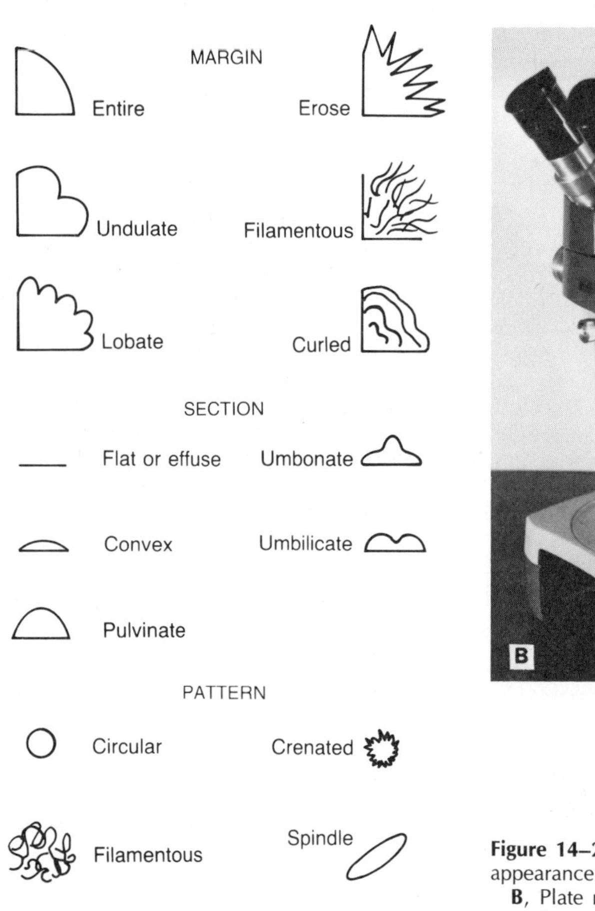

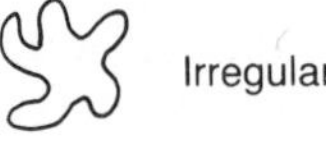

A

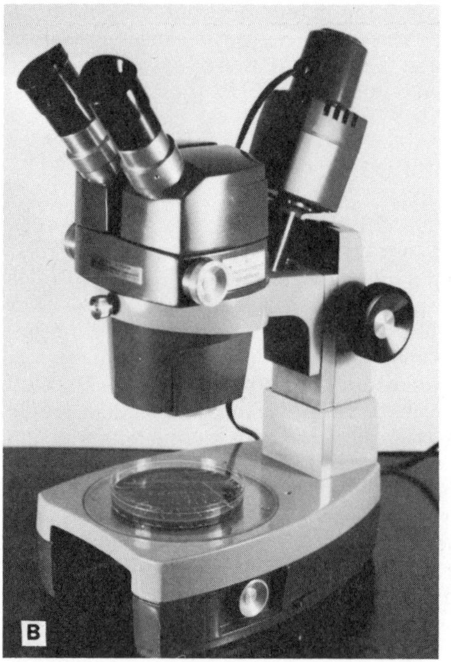

Figure 14–2 **A**, Descriptive terms for colonial appearance.
B, Plate microscope: a useful piece of apparatus for examination of bacterial colonies.

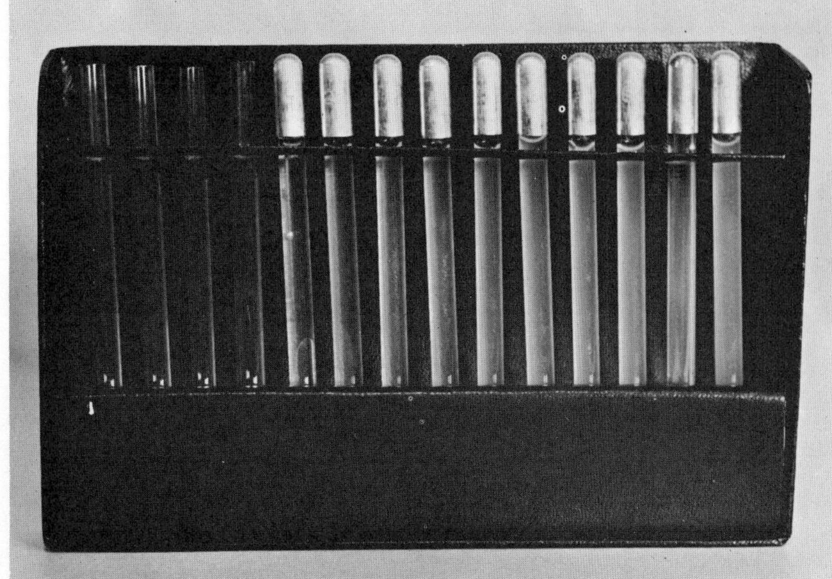

Figure 14–3 Brown's opacity tubes, containing varied concentrations of barium sulfate, with matched tubes for bacterial suspensions.

turbidity of a bacterial suspension. As long as a suspension contains small and evenly distributed particles, its ability to scatter light is seen to be proportional to its concentration. With a spectrophotometer there is an inverse relationship between turbidity (optical density) of a suspension and the amount of light permitted to pass through it. Thus, the optical density (OD) can be determined:

$$OD = \log T$$

Initially, using a blank, the instrument is adjusted to read 100% transmittance. The blank is then replaced by the test suspension and the transmittance value recorded. These arbitrary OD values then can be compared with OD values determined using bacterial suspensions of known cell content.

Viable Counts

Membrane Filter Counts. This method involves passing a liquid containing bacteria through a special filter, available commercially, which will retain the organisms. The filter pad is then placed directly on conventional solid culture media. Following a 24-hour incubation period at 35°C, the number of resultant colonies is counted. A *calibrated loop* may also be used. It removes a known quantity of fluid medium (usually 0.001 mL) with which a plate is inoculated. After adequate incubation, a count of the colonies on the plate will represent the number of viable bacteria in the volume of the calibrated loop inoculum.

Basal Growth Requirements of Bacteria

Bacteria may be divided into lithotrophic (autotrophs) and organotrophic (heterotrophs) varieties. The first category, which includes soil and water bacteria, obtains nitrogen and carbon from the atmosphere and from simple inorganic matter.

The organotrophs require more complex organic compounds as a source of carbon and nitrogen, and thus use proteins, or their derivatives, as well as carbohydrates and fats. Very few are photosynthetic; most are chemoorganotrophs. We are most concerned with chemoorganotrophs in medical microbiology. Such organisms can use a general source of amino acid or transform one amino acid into another; the few that do not have such capabilities and require a particular amino acid are said to be exacting.

As indicated in the opening passages of this chapter, the successful cultivation of microorganisms in the laboratory is dependent upon the provision of a satisfactory nutritional environment. This nutrient environment is divided into (a) the physical environment, embracing such factors as temperature, humidity, and atmosphere, and (b) the chemical environment, consisting of those compounds supplied in a culture medium to permit growth of microorganisms.

Protein Hydrolysates. Proteins are polymers of amino acids and possess high molecular weights. There are a wide variety of protein sources available throughout the animal and plant kingdoms, e.g., meat, fish, casein, gelatin, ground nut meal, yeast, and soya meal. The hydrolysis of protein into peptides and amino acids can be accomplished either by acid or enzyme hydrolysis.

Acid hydrolysis is carried out at high temperatures using mineral acids, such as hydrochloric acid. A compound typical of this procedure is casein hydrolysate. By such a process, some amino acid and vitamin content may be lost. Enzyme hydrolysis of protein can be achieved by a variety of proteolytic enzymes, e.g., pancreatin (trypsin, chymotrypsin), pepsin, and papain, and there is much better preservation of vitamins and amino acids.

Peptone consists of water-soluble products obtained from the digestion of protein materials with proteolytic enzymes. Its important constituents are peptones, proteoses, amino acids, inorganic salts, and certain accessory growth factors. Carbohydrates present in the original meat or yeast survive the enzymatic process, and thus such peptones cannot be used for fermentation studies. Commercial peptones are available.

Meat Extract. A commercial product can be used as a suitable substitute for an infusion of fresh meat. The product is an aqueous solution of peptides, amino acids, nucleotide fractions, mineral salts, organic acids, and accessory growth factors.

Yeast Extract. The U.S. Pharmacopeia describes yeast extract as a peptone-like substance derived from the cells of *Saccharomyces*. Commercial yeast extract is generally prepared from either brewer's or baker's yeast. Basically, the extract contains a mixture of amino acids and peptides, water-soluble vitamins, inorganic salts, and over 10% carbohydrate including glycogen, trehalose, and pentoses.

Gelatin and Agar. As a solidifying agent, gelatin was first used by Koch, who quickly recognized its limitations. A coworker, Hesse, proposed the use of agar, which was rapidly adopted as a more satisfactory solidifying agent.

Gelatin is prepared from bone or hide. As a solidifying agent it has several major disadvantages. It is a protein highly susceptible to microbial digestion and liquefaction. Furthermore, it changes from a gel to a sol at temperatures of about 24°C. Generally a 15% solution of gelatin is employed.

Agar is considered to be a mixture of two polysaccharides, approximately 70% agarose and 30% agarapectin. It is gel-forming polysaccharide extracted from a wide variety of red seaweed (agarophytes).

Agar has the important property of forming a gel with water that becomes a sol at 95°C, remaining so until cooled to approximately 42°C, when it becomes a gel again. Hence, heat-labile supplements such as blood can be added at a temperature of between 45 and 50°C, while the agar is still in the sol phase. Apart from its gel-forming properties agar is also a source of calcium and other organic ions.

Although there are differences encountered between agars harvested and manufactured at various global locations, the refined agars marketed by reliable companies yield satisfactory gels at concentrations between 1 and 2%.

Carbohydrates. The carbohydrates provide carbon for synthesis. In addition, their fermentation liberates energy that is utilizable in metabolism. They are composed of carbon and water and can be divided broadly into two groups: the simple and complex sugars.

SIMPLE SUGARS. *Pentoses*: arabinose, rhamnose, xylose; *Hexoses*: fructose, glucose, galactose, mannose; *Disaccharides*: sucrose, maltose, lactose, trehalose.

COMPLEX SUGARS. *Polysaccharides*: dextrin, glycogen, inulin starch; *Alcohols*: glycerol, erythritol, adonnitol, mannitol, dulcitol, sorbitol; *Glucosides*: salicin, esculin.

Mineral Salts. Some inorganic mineral salts are essential for the growth and metabolism of living organisms. The following are essential trace elements: copper, cobalt, zinc, iron, magnesium, manganese, molybdenum, and calcium. Agar will provide most minerals, but the amount donated will depend on the individual characteristics of the agar. Further, other media constituents supply adequate amounts of mineral salts.

Accessory Growth Factors. These include some of the B complex vitamins (thiamine, niacin, pyridoxine, and biotin). These vitamins provide a necessary cofactor that the microorganism is unable to synthesize.

Other factors necessary for growth of some bacteria include complex substances such as blood, serum, and egg yolk. The trend, as the subject advances, is to replace such empirical nutrients with synthetic or better chemically defined substances.

PREPARATION, DISTRIBUTION, AND STORAGE OF MEDIA

CONTAINERS

Disposable Plastic Containers. Probably the largest single plastic container utilized in the modern microbiology laboratory is the presterilized Petri dish, which can be purchased in a variety of shapes and sizes. A great many laboratories also use presterilized plastic containers for the collection of pathological specimens. With the gradual expansion of laboratory facilities and a resultant increase in work load combined with a disproportionate decrease in budgets, many laboratories now are purchasing prepoured culture plates in an attempt to reduce the amount of valuable time spent in the preparation of routine media by the technologist. Another method to meet this situation is in the automatic plate pouring machines that are available commercially.

Glass Containers for Liquid Media. Liquid media may be distributed in test tubes or bottles with slip-on metal caps, cotton-wool plugs, or colored foam plugs, the tubes being half-filled.

Glass Containers for Solid Media. Solid media also may be distributed in test tubes with slip-on metal caps or other suitable plugs. The usual media form in test tubes is the slope or slant, which provides a large surface area of the media for inoculation. If the medium is to be used as a stab or shake culture, a test tube is half-filled with melted media and then allowed to solidify in an upright position.

When larger surface areas are required, that is, the separation of organisms from mixtures into discrete colonies, the media is allowed to solidify in Petri dishes, which can be purchased in a variety of diameters.

ADJUSTMENT OF pH IN MEDIA

As previously stated, many bacteria will grow only if the medium used is at an optimum pH; others will show vigorous growth within a fairly wide range of acidity or alkalinity. To obtain the best growth, therefore, it is often necessary to adjust the reaction of the medium. This applies not only to media prepared in the laboratory, but also to many media purchased in the dehydrated form from commercial firms.

The procedure for adjusting culture media to a definite pH is comparatively simple, except that in the case of solid media greater care must be exercised.

In preparing media in bulk it is preferable to have the reaction slightly alkaline and to adjust it for use by the addition of acid. This is because addition of alkali to an acid medium causes precipitation of phosphates, which then must be removed by filtration. On the other hand, if acid is added to an alkaline medium, no precipitate forms and the medium remains clear.

pH Meter. This apparatus is extremely useful in checking or correcting the pH media. The pH of a solution is sensed by a special glass membrane situated at the end of the pH electrode, developing electrical potentials that are proportional to the pH of the solution in which it is immersed. Figure 14–4 shows a characteristic example of this type of apparatus.

Various pH Indicators

Bromcresol Purple (Dibromo-*o*-Cresolsulfonphthalein). Dissolve 0.1 g in 9.2 mL of 0.02 M sodium hydroxide. Dilute to 250 mL with distilled water; this gives a 0.4% solution. Color reaction: yellow at pH 5.2 and blue at 6.8.

Bromthymol Blue (Dibromothymolsulfonphthalein). Dissolve 0.1 g in 8 mL of 0.02 M sodium hydroxide. Dilute to 250 mL with distilled water; this gives a 0.49% solution. Color reaction: yellow at pH 6.0 and blue at 7.6.

Methyl Red (4′–Dimethylamino-Azobenzene-*o*-Carboxylic Acid). Dissolve 0.1 g in 300 mL ethanol and dilute to 500 mL with distilled water. Color reaction: red at pH 4.4 and yellow at 6.0.

Phenolphthalein. Dissolve 1.0 g in 60 mL ethanol and make up to 100 mL with ethanol. Color reaction: colorless at pH 8.3 and red at 10.0.

Phenol Red (Phenolsulfonphthalein). Dissolve 0.1 g in 14.1 mL 0.02 M sodium hydroxide. Dilute to 250 mL with distilled water; this gives a 0.4% solution. Color reaction: red at pH 8.4 and yellow at 6.8.

Thymol Blue (Thymolsulfonphthalein). Dissolve 0.1 g in 10.75 mL of 0.02 M sodium hydroxide and dilute to 250 mL. Color reaction: yellow at pH 8.0 and blue at pH 9.6.

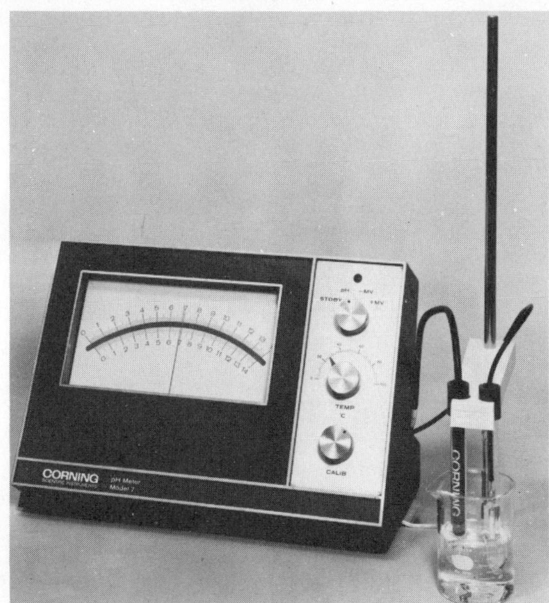

Figure 14–4 Corning pH meter. (Courtesy of Corning Scientific Instruments, Medfield, Mass. 02052.)

Sterilization of Prepared Media

As implied earlier, the method employed to sterilize a medium is dependent on whether or not the ingredients are degraded by heat. Those ingredients known to be heat sensitive, such as egg yolk, serum, or whole blood can, fortunately, be obtained naturally sterile. Hence these are simply added aseptically to the autoclaved, heat-resistant ingredients of the medium. Those ingredients not normally sterile that are known to be heat sensitive must be sterilized by filtration. Figure 14–5 depicts a typical Seitz filtration assembly.

As soon as the culture media has been prepared, it should be sterilized. If a medium is allowed to stand at room temperature or in a refrigerator, organisms inadvertently introduced during its preparation may multiply. Generally speaking, the sterilization times, for instance at a temperature of 121°C, required for the following volumes of media in Erlenmeyer flasks are: 10mL—15 minutes; 100 mL—20 minutes; 500 mL—25 minutes, and 1000 mL—30 minutes. Ideally, media should be autoclaved only once; furthermore, when using commercial dehydrated media care should be taken not to exceed the time and temperatures recommended by the manufacturer.

Following sterility checks, all poured or dispensed media should be stored at 4°C. Tube media with nonscrew caps or snap-on lids may be stored in screw-cap jars to prevent drying. Alternatively, cotton-wool plugs can be dipped in melted paraffin wax. Petri dishes of medium should be kept refrigerated in plastic bags to avoid dehydration. Precautions should be taken to label stored media for identification purposes; some laboratories utilize an arbitrary color code to identify media that look alike.

Inspissation of Serum and Egg Media

Media containing serum (e.g., Löffler's slopes) and egg yolk (Löwenstein-Jensen) are usually solidified in an apparatus called an inspissator. Such material usually coagulates in 50 to 60 minutes at 80°C. Fundamentally, the apparatus consists of a water bath, thermostatically controlled at 75 to 80°C. The tubed media are placed in racks arranged so that they are immersed in the hot water bath at the desired angle for forming slopes. Care must be exercised not to exceed 80°C, otherwise bubbling will occur.

ROUTINE CULTURE METHODS

Plate Method

The aim of using solid media poured into Petri dishes is to inoculate successively smaller quantities of material onto the medium so that at one point organisms are plated so thinly as to allow the growth of individually isolated colonies. Such materials as sputum or feces, both of which often contain a great many bacteria, are best diluted or made homogeneous before inoculation. The material can be spread with either a glass spreader or, preferably, a loop, the loop being charged with the material for examination and successive strokes being made on the medium in a clockwise direction.

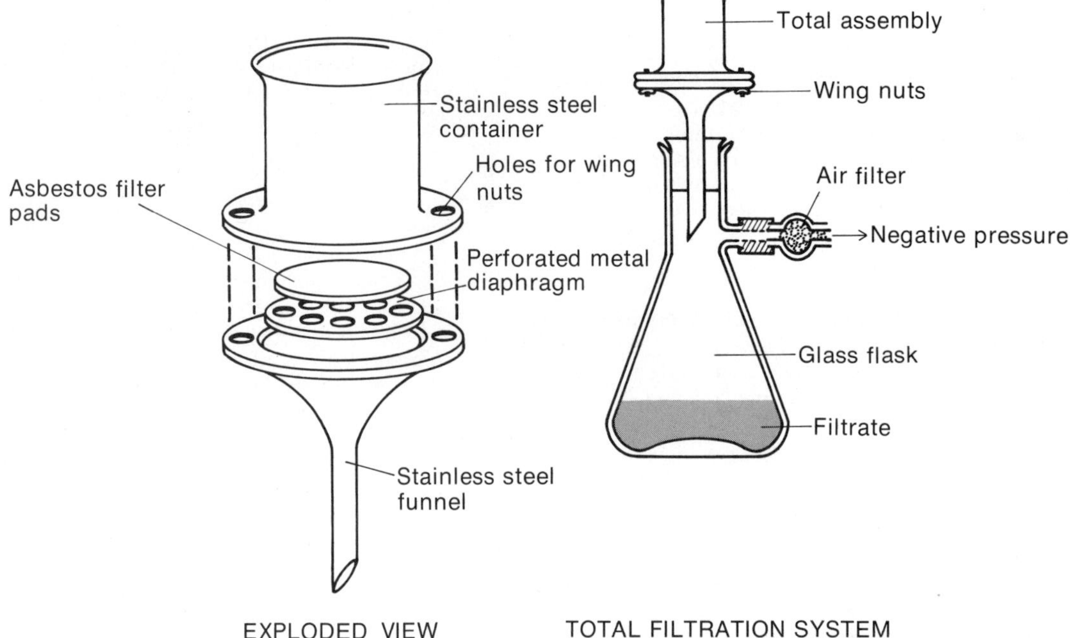

Figure 14–5 A Seitz filter.

Swabs often are submitted for culture. In this case instead of charging the loop, the swab itself is used to make the original inoculation, after which it is spread with a loop as described. Certain important points in the use of the plate method should be stressed. Plates should be perfectly dry before use, or organisms will tend to spread, hindering the formation of discrete colonies. The loop should be flamed properly and cooled before use by touching the inside of the Petri dish. The loop should be held lightly between the fingers, and care should be taken not to dig it into the medium. Moreover, one should always work near the Bunsen flame when inoculating, since the upward surge of air created by the flame carries the dust in the air upward away from the plate and then, as the air cools, down away from the plate. Platinum loops are used for plating and subculturing anaerobic organisms. Nichrome loops should be avoided in anaerobic work.

Colonies that require subculturing should be removed with a straight wire (not a loop) and then transferred to fresh media.

Slope Cultures

This type of culture is used mainly in subculturing isolated strains either for further identification or for stock culture. This method requires practice. Inoculation should always be done close to the Bunsen burner flame, and the neck of the tube or bottle should be flamed before recapping or replacing the cotton-wool plug.

Shake Cultures

This method of culture is of particular use in isolating spore-bearing anaerobes. A tube or bottle of agar or other suitable medium is melted and then cooled to approximately 50°C. The infective material is then added and the tube capped and rolled between the hands to mix its contents. The medium is then placed in an upright position and allowed to set. After incubation at 37°C, colonies that warrant further investigation can be extracted from the bottom of the medium with a wide-bore sterile Pasteur pipette and subcultured to either a slope or a plate.

Stab Cultures

Material for investigation by this method is placed on a straight wire and plunged into the medium. Care should be exercised to make the track of exit the same as that of entry. Certain organisms have a characteristic appearance in stab culture. The method can also be used for preserving stock cultures and in testing for gelatin liquefaction.

Fluid Cultures

In the inoculation of a fluid medium such as peptone water or thioglycollate broth, the tube should be inclined at an angle and the material removed from the loop by rubbing it against the tube wall. When the tube is righted the material is then below the surface of the medium.

STOCK CULTURES

Most microbiology laboratories endeavor to keep stock cultures of certain standard strains of bacteria for use in testing culture media and in checking biochemical tests and immunological sera. There are a variety of ways in which a culture can be maintained or preserved, all of which are variations of the themes of (i) serial subculture, or (ii) lyophilization.

In order to initiate a stock culture collection, or to replace those cultures lost by contamination, etc., species can be obtained from the following sources: United States: American Type Culture Collection, 12301 Parklawn Drive, Rockville, Md., 20852. Canada: Cultures are available from a variety of institutions; see the H.M.S.O. publication, *Directory of Collections and Lists of Species Maintained in Canada.* United Kingdom: National Collection of Type Cultures, Central Public Health Laboratory, London, NW9. 5HT., England. Cultures are also commercially available, and organisms distributed by proficiency testing programs may be maintained.

Maintenance of Common Bacteria

The best technique is that of freeze drying, but it is a method that is beyond the resources of most community hospitals. Organisms can be preserved in glycerol citrate (60 mL glycerol, 5 g tribasic sodium citrate and 100 mL water autoclaved at 20 lbs for 20 minutes) at −70°C.

Available in all microbiology laboratories are the facilities to maintain stock cultures in commonly accessible media at refrigerator or room temperature. All such cultures should be kept moist and thus in screw-cap bottles possibly sealed over with wax and kept in the dark (see Table 14–1).

SUPPLY OF A SUITABLE ATMOSPHERIC ENVIRONMENT

ANAEROBIC TECHNIQUES

The cultivation of anaerobes is undoubtedly more difficult and time consuming than aerobic culture, but the difficulties are greatly exaggerated. If the technologist adopts a routine procedure timed to fit in with the rest of his work, regular anaerobic studies will not be onerous and certainly the effort will be worthwhile.

Pre-Reduced Anaerobically Sterilized (PRAS) Media

These are made essentially by adding the media constituents, boiling off the dissolved air, and then replacing the remaining air in the tube with an oxygen-free gas. Subsequently, air is prevented from returning to the tube by keeping a stopper in the tube and by "gassing out" the tube with a gas such as nitrogen when bacterial culture manipulations are being made. Gassing out is best performed after removing the rubber stopper, by inserting a canula from which flows oxygen-free gas. The inoculation of the medium is by a loop or by a Pasteur pipette, and without allowing air to re-enter the tube, the canula is removed after inoculation and the stopper replaced.

McIntosh and Fildes Jar

This, for many years, was the best available method for plate anaerobiasis in the community hospital. Essentially it combined oxygen and hydrogen in the presence of catalytic palladinized asbestos to form water and thus render the atmosphere anaerobic. Unfortunately, the oxygen and hydrogen were combined by means of an electrical heating current and the procedure was not without risk of explosion. Fortunately, it has now been replaced by safer techniques.

TABLE 14–1 METHODS OF MAINTAINING STOCK CULTURES OF VARIOUS BACTERIA

Organism	Subculture Interval	Medium	Temperature
Actinomyces *Erysipelothrix* *Listeria*	1 month	Blood agar	35°–37°C until growth, then 18°–25°C
M. tuberculosis	6 months	Dorset egg	35°–37°C for 10–20 days or until visible growth, then 15°–25°C
Clostridium and other anaerobes	12 months	Robertson's meat	35°–37°C for 24 hours, then −20°C; some at R°
Salmonella *Shigella*	12 months	Dorset egg	35°–37°C for 24 hours, then 4°–25°C
Enterobacteriaceae *Acinetobacter* *Alcaligenes* Staphylococci	6 months	Nutrient agar	35°–37°C for 24 hours, then 4°–25°C
Streptococci (including anaerobic)	2 months	Robertson's meat	35°–37°C for 24 hours, then at R°
C. diphtheriae	2 months	Robertson's meat	35°–37°C for 24 hours, then at R°
Neisseria } Spp. *Haemophilus* }	1 month	Serum agar (with peptic digest of blood for *Haemophilus*)	35°–37°C, then seal under paraffin at 35°–37°C
Pseudomonas	3 months	Peptone water	35°–37°C for 24 hours, then at 4°C
Brucella } Spp. *Pasteurella* }	Several weeks	Blood agar	35°–37°C until growth, then 18°–25°C

R°, room temperature.

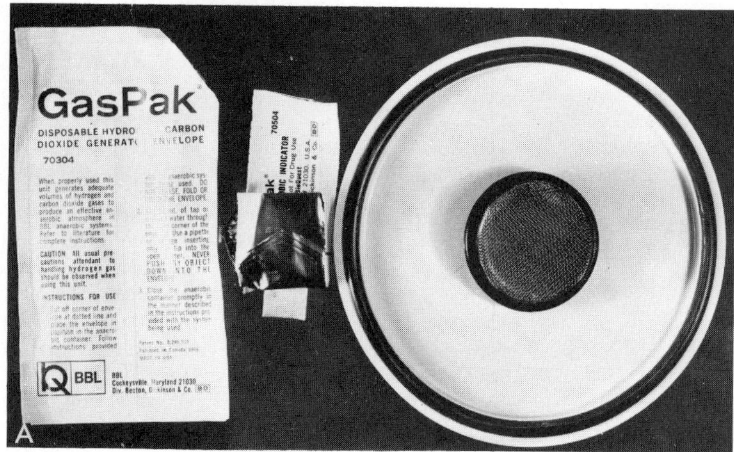

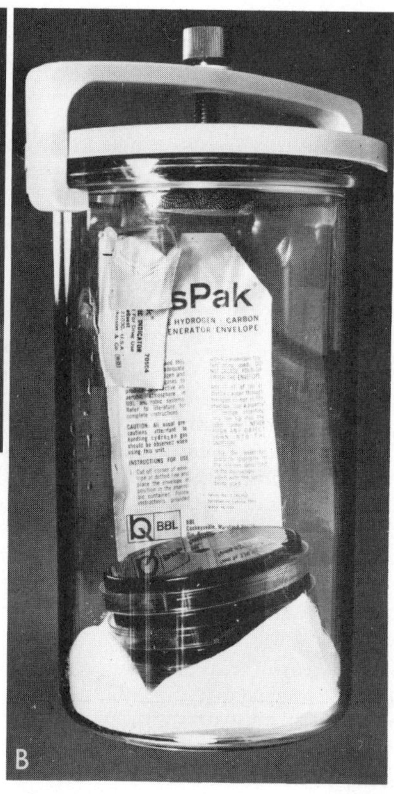

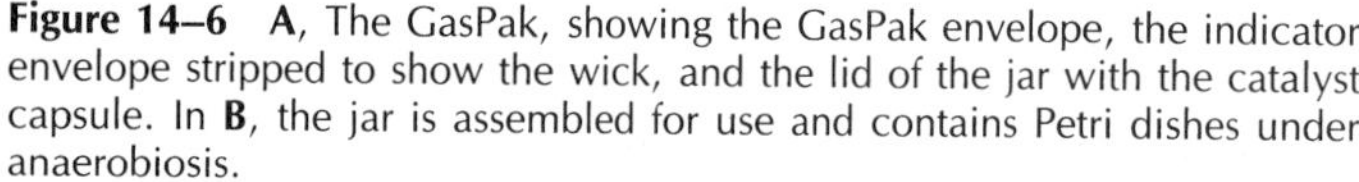
Figure 14–6 **A**, The GasPak, showing the GasPak envelope, the indicator envelope stripped to show the wick, and the lid of the jar with the catalyst capsule. In **B**, the jar is assembled for use and contains Petri dishes under anaerobiosis.

GasPak Anaerobic System

The system as illustrated (Fig. 14–6) has a polycarbonate resin jar with palladium catalyst active at room temperature in its lid. Also available are envelopes that contain reagents that will yield both hydrogen and carbon dioxide when water is added. A disposable anaerobic indicator also is supplied in an envelope, and catalyst replacement cartridges are available. An older indicator, not often used now, is a mixture of 6% glucose, 6% of N/10 NaOH, and 0.015% methylene blue in equal parts. The mixture is freshly prepared from the separate ingredients just before use and then boiled. It becomes colorless on boiling and then is placed in the anaerobic jar before incubation. Provided that anaerobiasis is obtained and maintained the solution will remain colorless. A blue color indicates that the atmosphere in the jar contains oxygen. A biological control such as a culture of *Ps. aeruginosa* or *C. albicans* may be used. Neither of these organisms will grow under adequate anaerobiasis.

The required culture plates or tubes are placed in the jar with one gas-producing envelope and an indicator envelope. Ten mL of water is added to the envelope contents through a cut made in the envelope corner, and the indicator envelope is peeled to reveal the indicator wick. The lid is screwed on firmly. After the gases are produced, water will form and the lid, through catalytic activity, will become warm. If water condensation does not occur, the catalyst should be replaced. This is easily screwed into place. The anaerobic indicator wick is colorless under anaerobiosis. The method is very satisfactory in practice.

If the anaerobic plates can be ready as a batch, a single jar may be used; but obviously, if plates are charged at intervals during the working day, some will be under aerobic conditions for a prolonged period. Such a situation can be prevented by a constant flow CO_2 system (Martin, 1971).

CULTURE OF ORGANISMS IN CARBON DIOXIDE ATMOSPHERE

Several organisms will grow only if there is an increased amount of carbon dioxide in the atmosphere, e.g., *Brucella abortus*. Others will grow more luxuriantly in such an atmosphere, for example, pneumococcus and *Neisseria gonorrhoeae*. Most facultative aerobes grow well in a CO_2 atmosphere.

Methods

1. The simplest way to create an atmosphere rich in carbon dioxide is to place the culture plates in an airtight jar along with a candle which is lit before the lid is replaced. Oxygen is reduced during combustion, and the amount of carbon dioxide is increased to satisfactory proportions.
2. A jar is used in which the air is exchanged with a gas mixture in which the concentration of CO_2 is 3 to 5%. The usual technique is to flush out the jar three times with the CO_2 mixture after partial evacuation.
3. A large test tube containing 8 mL of 25% hydrochloric acid and a small marble chip (0.5 to 1.0 g) are placed in an airtight tin with the inoculated plates. Carbon dioxide is liberated from the mixture, and the

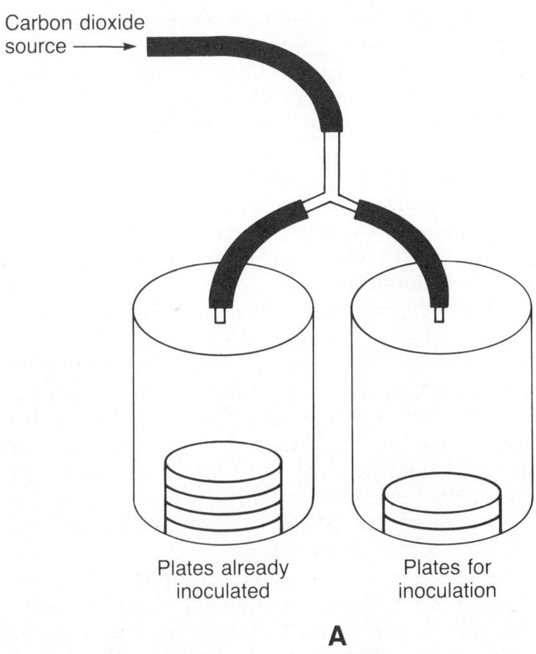

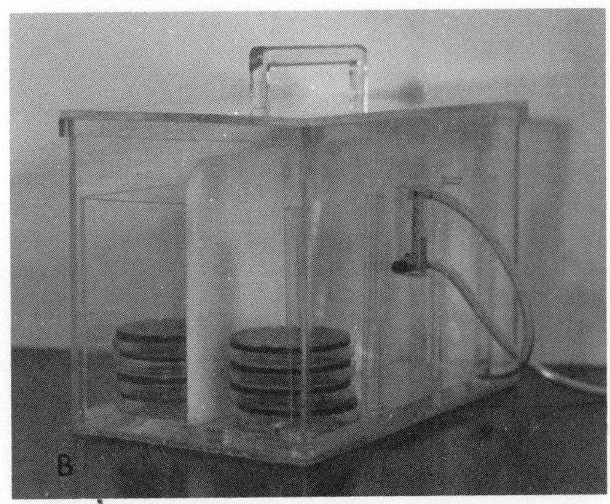

Figure 14–7 **A**, Constant CO_2 or N_2 flow system for anaerobic work.

B, A convenient inert gas flow system made on the principles shown in **A** for anaerobic work. Uninoculated plates are seen on one side of a perforated divider, and inoculated plates ready for incubation on the other. The apparatus is provided with a flow meter that is adjusted to allow a flow of 0.25 $ft^3 N_2$/hour. (Axotec International, Inc., P.O. Box 1024, Station A, Windsor, Ontario N9A 6P4.)

slight increase of atmospheric pressure within the tin is of no practical importance.

4. Incubators that allow an adjustable amount of carbon dioxide with air to enter are available. The atmosphere in the incubator is circulated by a blower and the humidity also may be controlled.

SUPPLY OF SUITABLE NUTRIENT ENVIRONMENT

Since the majority of organisms to be studied in a medical microbiology department are either pathogens or commensals of the human body, it is obvious that an artificial environment should be provided simulating those conditions encountered in the body tissues and fluids, namely, a provision of nutrients and a pH of about 7.2. For routine purposes many of the nutrient requirements are satisfied by *basal media,* such as nutrient broth, peptone water, and nutrient agar. Some fastidious organisms require media with complex additives in order to grow. Such media are called *enriched.* These additives include defibrinated blood, serum, ascitic fluid, egg, and glycerol. *Selective media* owe their importance to the fact that they contain deterrents to the growth of any bacteria other than those under investigation. Different deterrents are employed; for example, bile salts in a medium prohibit the growth of nonenteric organisms; malachite green is inhibitory to organisms not in the group Mycobacteriaceae; acidity permits the growth of fungi, but inhibits most bacteria. Additives are also incorporated in some media to stimulate growth of specific bacteria, e.g., glycerol in Löwenstein-Jensen medium for the growth of mycobacteria. Blood agar, apart from being an enriched medium, is also differential inasmuch as it aids recognition of hemolytic streptococci. A *differential* medium is one permitting the visual differentiation of one colony from another as a result of metabolic activity on some particular substance incorporated in it. To this end, MacConkey medium contains lactose and an indicator. Lactose fermenting colonies are red, and nonlactose fermenters appear as pale pink or colorless colonies. In addition to being a differential medium, MacConkey is also selective. The term *enrichment medium* generally is applied to a liquid medium favoring the growth of a particular species; it contains either enrichments that selectively favor it or inhibitory substances that suppress competitors. An example would be selenite F medium, used to isolate *Salmonella* species from feces. Obviously only a few representative media can be described, but it is hoped they will be sufficient to show the principles on which they depend for their usefulness.

Provision of a Suitable Temperature

Most of the organisms with which we deal in medical microbiology grow optimally at 35°C. A few organisms flourish at room temperature (22° to 28°C), but if rooms are hotter or colder, then a special incubator must be provided for such organisms such as *Yersinia pseudotuberculosis,* which is motile at 22°C but not at 37°C. *Campylobacter jejuni,* an important intestinal pathogen, may also be differentiated by its growth at 42°C.

Basal Media

Peptone Water. This is widely used as a 1 to 2% solution and provides nitrogenous metabolites.

Nutrient Broth. This forms the basis of most media employed in the study of medical pathogenic bacteria. There are three types: meat infusion, meat extract, and digest broths.

Meat Infusion Broths. These consist of a watery extract of meat made by extracting lean meat for 24 hours at 2°C. Any juice remaining is squeezed from the meat. The extract is then simmered for 15 minutes and filtered. Protein is removed in this process and must, therefore, be replaced by adding 1% peptone. Sodium chloride in a 0.5% concentration is added last. Such broths generally contain a high percentage of fermentable sugar, which makes them unsuitable for many purposes, e.g., toxin production.

MEAT EXTRACT BROTHS. These are prepared from peptone and commercial meat extracts, that is, Lab-Lemco. Such broths are easily prepared and widely used. However they are less nutritious than infusion and digest broths. They are most suitable for preservation of stock cultures. A good example is *brain-heart infusion:* this medium is most useful, since it will allow many fastidious organisms to grow. A small amount incorporated into agar will permit the deep areas of the medium to support anaerobic growth.

DIGEST BROTHS. These consist of a watery extract of lean meat digested with a proteolytic enzyme—hence additional peptone need not be added. The proteolytic enzyme employed varies, though generally it is trypsin, obtained in the form of a pancreatic extract. *Hartley's broth* is an example of a digest broth. They are ideal for growth of exacting organisms.

Nutrient Agar. Nutrient agar consists of beef extract, peptone, agar, and water. It is often used as a base in the making of more complex media. For special purposes agar may be added to a medium in concentrations insufficient to solidify it, that is, a semisolid or "sloppy" agar. For example, 0.2 to 0.5% agar concentrations produce an ideal medium through which motile organisms may spread, yet they localize nonmotile bacteria. Concentrations of agar between 0.05 to 0.1% prevent convection currents and thus retard air diffusion into a medium, e.g., transport media. By increasing the agar concentration to between 4 and 6%, swarming bacteria such as *Clostridium tetani* and *Proteus vulgaris* will grow as discrete colonies. Many workers in North America use BBL Columbia agar base, which contains peptones derived from both casein and meat to provide an efficient base for the preparation of more complex media. As a broth it is recommended for use in blood cultures. Also cysteine is added to overcome inhibition of some organisms such as the pneumococci from accumulated oxidation products; furthermore, the presence of magnesium ions is vital to the growth of many pathogenic bacteria.

Another good routine media in this category is *tryptone-soy agar and broth.* Essentially the two peptones (tryptone and soya peptone) incorporated in this medium will support growth of many fastidious organisms that generally would require an enriched medium.

BASIC ENRICHED MEDIA

Blood Agar and Broth. Blood agar consists of 5 to 10% sterile defibrinated blood added to melted nutrient agar that has been cooled to about 45°C. (This is usually tested by placing the bottle against one's cheek—it will feel pleasantly warm). Following the addition of blood to the agar, it is mixed by swirling in a circular fashion; avoid shaking, since this will cause air bubbles. The medium is then dispensed into sterile Petri dishes or containers and allowed to set. Bubbles are removed by "playing" a Bunsen flame across the surface of the still-molten media. Alternatively and preferably, an antibubble additive such as Pourite* is added (¼ to 3 drops per liter of medium) before heating or autoclaving. The method is especially valuable in using automated plate pouring methods and has no deleterious effect on the growth of human pathogens.

The medium is used to encourage the growth of bacteria unable to grow on nutrient agar and to detect hemolytic streptococci. If the medium is too thick it becomes difficult to detect hemolysis, even with the aid of transmitted light. To overcome this problem some workers employ layered plates consisting of an initial thin layer of nutrient agar, which is allowed to set, upon which is poured a layer of blood agar—thereby reducing the density of the blood layer.

Five to 10% blood added to nutrient broth yields an enriched liquid medium.

Fildes' Peptic Digest Agar and Broth. This medium consists of an aqueous solution of 0.85% sodium chloride, hydrochloric acid (analytical grade), defibrinated sheep's blood, pepsin, sodium hydroxide, and chloroform. It can be obtained commercially. The digest is added to nutrient agar or broth in a 2 to 5% concentration, after initially heating it at 55°C for 30 minutes to drive off chloroform preservative. Fildes' digest is used to enrich media for the growth of such organisms as *Clostridium* and the *Haemophilus* group.

Heated Blood Agar—Chocolate Agar. Chocolate agar is used particularly as a supply of factors essential for the growth of *Haemophilus* species, and when incubated with carbon dioxide it is ideal for the isolation and maintenance of *Neisseria meningitidis* and *N. gonorrhoeae.*

It is prepared by heating 10% sterile blood in a sterile nutrient agar. Once the nutrient agar is melted, it is cooled in a water bath or incubator at 75°C, and at this temperature the blood is added and mixed. Leave mixture at 75°C, gently agitating at intervals. The blood slowly becomes chocolate-brown in color. This takes about 10 minutes. Another method uses freshly poured blood agar plates, which are held in an incubator at a temperature of 55°C for 1 to 2 hours.

SPECIFIC MEDIA

Medium for Bordetella Species

Bordet-Gengou Medium. A complex medium used in the primary isolation and growth of *Bordetella pertussis,* this medium basically consists of a potato agar base reinforced with proteose peptone and enriched with 15 to 20% *fresh whole blood.*

Medium for Brucella Species

A Castaneda-type biphasic medium (Fig. 14–8) is used, which has both a slope of trypticase soy agar and a trypticase soy broth in the same bottle. The broth includes the anticoagulant polyanetholsulfonate (SPS), which is also anticomplimentary and antileukocytic. Within the bottle there is an atmosphere of 10% CO_2. The broth-blood mixture should be washed over the agar daily. *Brucella* colonies usually appear on or after the sixth day of incubation. After three weeks of incubation at 35°-37°C, the culture may be discarded as negative.

Medium for Campylobacter

Skirrow's Medium. This medium contains a Columbia or Brucella agar base with 7% lyzed horse blood and antimicrobials. The latter comprise vancomycin (10 μg/mL), trimethoprim (5 μg/mL), and polymyxin B sulfate

*Analytical Products Inc. P.O. Box 845, Belmont, Cal. 94002.

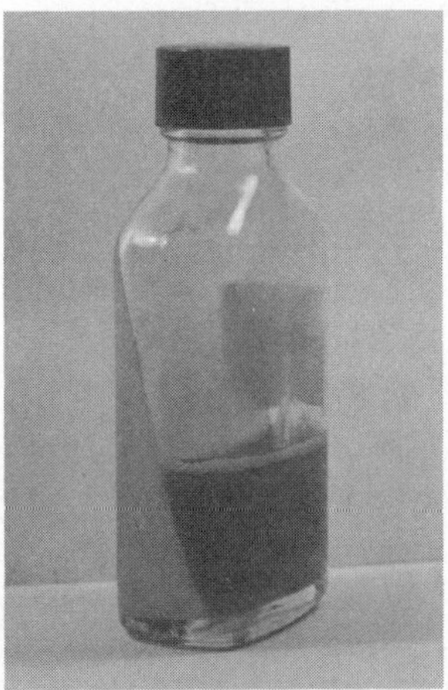

Figure 14–8 Castaneda double medium. The blood culture bottle contains an agar slope and a broth medium. For *Brucella* there is trypticase soy agar and broth. The agar is flooded with the broth every 24 hours during incubation after inoculation with the patient's blood, and the slope is subsequently examined for colonies.

(2.5 IU/mL). The charged plate, as noted above, is incubated at 42°C in an atmosphere of 5% CO_2 in nitrogen and freon. Growth of usual bowel flora is inhibited by the antimicrobials and by the temperature of the incubator.

Medium for Yersinia

Recently a primary medium for *Yersinia* has been introduced*—Schiemann's selective agar. It contains antimicrobials and irgasan for selection and mannitol as a differentiator. Feces are inoculated directly and the plates incubated at 29°C for 48 hours. *Yersinia enterocolitica* and *pseudotuberculosis* appear as red colonies about 1 to 2 mm in diameter.

Media for Clostridium Species

Cooked Meat Medium. This medium can be obtained commercially. It consists essentially of beef particles, peptone, and sodium hydroxide.

In addition to being a general-purpose medium for the growth of both aerobic and anaerobic organisms, it is employed frequently for the primary isolation of anaerobes. If the latter is intended, it is essential that the inoculum be introduced deep into the medium, namely, in contact with the meat particles, since it is here that anaerobic conditions exist. The addition of haemin (5 μg/mL) and vitamin K_1 (0.1 μg/mL) also promotes the growth of anaerobic organisms. Generally the medium is dispensed into 1-oz screw-cap bottles such that there is approximately a 1-inch column of medium, with at least ½ inch of broth above. The medium is also an excellent general stock culture medium.

Thioglycollate Broth. This medium is very useful in the primary isolation of both aerobes and anaerobes. The medium contains yeast extract, casein hydrolysate, dextrose, L-cystine, agar, sodium chloride, sodium thioglycollate, and reazurin. The amount of agar added is just sufficient to prevent convection currents and assist in the maintenance of anaerobic conditions produced by the presence of the reducing agent thioglycollate. Reazurin acts as an indicator of oxidation-reduction potential. At the interface of medium and atmosphere the medium will be oxidized, indicated by the formation of a pink-colored ring. If the ring extends more than one-third down into the medium, then it should be reduced by steaming at 100°C for several minutes before use.

Schaedler's Medium. This medium contains cysteine hydrochloride and glucose. These act as reducing substances, and the former inhibits *E. coli* to some extent. The addition of the antimicrobial nalidixic acid with Tween 80 further enhances the selective value of the medium for anaerobic organisms. The medium includes haemin. It may be further supplemented with lyzed or defibrinated horse blood (50 mL/liter) and vitamin K_1 (1.8 mL/liter). These are added when the Schaedler's agar has cooled to 50°C after preparation.

A large number of enriched and selective anaerobic media are available (Dowell et al., 1980).

Media for Corynebacteria

The addition of potassium tellurite to blood agar medium has an inhibitory effect on most organisms constituting the normal respiratory flora, thus permitting the isolation and growth of *Corynebacterium diphtheriae,* which is unaffected.

Cystine-Tellurite Medium. This is said to be the preferred medium for *C. diphtheriae*. Its formula is as follows:

Heart infusion agar, 2% soln.	500 mL
Agar	25 g

Adjust to pH 7.4 and autoclave at 121°C for 15 minutes. Cool to 56°C, and add

Defibrinated rabbit or sheep blood	25 mL
Sterile potassium tellurite	75 mL
L-Cystine	22 mg

Store at 5°C and use within one month of preparation.

Modified Tinsdale's Medium (of Moore and Parsons). This medium is commercially available. It has cystine and sodium thiosulfate in a nutrient base with tellurite. On it, *C. diphtheriae, C. ulcerans, and C. pseudotuberculosis* appear as black or gray colonies with brown halos of H_2S production. However, the medium has a shelf life of only 4 days and must be rigorously controlled with known positive organisms. If freshly made and controlled it is of value in the laboratory as a medium that will identify pathogenic corynebacteria (p. 395).

Löfflers' Serum Slopes. This medium is heavily enriched by serum: it contains 75% serum and 25% glucose broth. Tubes containing the medium are sloped in an inspissator and kept at a temperature of between 75 to 80°C for several hours, after which they are sterilized at a temperature of 90°C for 20 minutes on each of 3 successive days.

The medium is used mainly for the culture of the corynebacteria, although it can be used to show proteolytic properties of the clostridia, and the lacunae developed by *Moraxella lacunata*. An 18-hour culture of *C. diphtheriae* will produce typical colonial morphology and characteristic staining reaction using Neisser's or Albert's methods.

Media for Enterobacteria

MacConkey Agar. This is a differential and selective media, used for primary plating and subculturing of enteric organisms. The medium contains peptone, sodium taurocholate, sodium chloride, 1% lactose, neutral red, and agar. The bile salt, sodium taurocholate, is

---

*Oxoid, Columbia, Md. 21045 and Nepean, Ont. K2E 7K3.

incorporated to discourage growth of nonintestinal bacteria, though some staphylococci generally grow quite well. It is for this reason that some manufacturers include crystal violet, which will inhibit staphylococci, as well as most yeasts. Colonies of lactose fermenters are pink to red as a result of the action of acid (formed during the fermentation of the lactose) on the indicator, neutral red. Nonlactose fermenters remain colorless.

Levine's Eosin–Methylene Blue Agar. Some workers use this medium routinely in preference to MacConkey agar for the detection and differentiation of enteric bacilli. It can be used for the isolation and identification of *Candida albicans.* The medium's contents are as follows: peptone, lactose, dipotassium phosphate, eosin, methylene blue, and agar. Lactose fermenting organisms produce acid that acts on the two dyes, giving these colonies a blue-black center. Nonlactose fermenting colonies are colorless. Many of the gram-positive organisms are inhibited, although staphylococci, enterococci, and yeasts may grow well.

Hektoen's Medium. This is a differential and selective medium for salmonellae and shigellae. It contains bile salts as well as lactose and sucrose and a bromthymol blue indicator. It is less inhibiting to shigellae than are many similar media; these organisms form green, almost transparent, colonies, whereas the salmonellae are blue-green. *E. coli* and other lactose fermenters are pink or salmon colored. Organisms producing H_2S are identified by the production of a black discoloration due to the reaction with ferric ammonium sulfate in the medium. It loses some of its selective value in the case of Yersiniae. These organisms ferment sucrose, will appear pink or salmon colored, and may go unnoticed.

Salmonella-Shigella Agar. This is a differential and selective media designed specifically for the isolation of pathogenic enteric bacilli belonging to the *Salmonella* and *Shigella* genera. It is fundamentally a modification of the original DCA medium. It contains beef extract, peptone, bile salts, 1% lactose, sodium citrate, sodium thiosulfate, ferric citrate, neutral red, brilliant green, and agar.

Lactose fermenting organisms yield red colonies. Nonlactose fermenting colonies are colorless, and if hydrogen sulfide producers are present they will produce colonies having black centers (ferric citrate being the indicator). The brilliant green inhibits gram-positive organisms.

Selenite F Broth. This is an enrichment medium for salmonellae and some shigellae. The growth of coliforms and gram-positive organisms such as the enterococcus is discouraged by the presence of sodium selenite for 12 to 18 hours, whereupon they begin to grow rapidly. Hence, subcultures should be made within this limited time period. The medium consists essentially of peptone, lactose, sodium phosphate, and sodium acid selenite. Isolation success is greater with salmonellae than with the shigellae. *Tetrathionate broth* is another similar selective enrichment medium for *Salmonella,* but it is not suggested for *Shigella.* It includes peptone, salts, and an iodine solution.

Hajna's Gram-Negative (GN) Broth. GN broth is a selective enrichment medium devised for the cultivation of salmonellae and shigellae. It has been shown that the deficiencies of selenite F, with regard to the isolation of some *Shigella* species, can be avoided by using GN broth. The medium contains peptone, dextrose, D-mannitol, sodium citrate, sodium desoxycholate, phosphate buffers, and sodium chloride. The bile salts and citrates inhibit the growth of gram-positive organisms. The growth of gram-negative organisms such as *Proteus* and *Pseudomonas* spp. is limited by the incorporation of dextrose and mannitol. Coliforms are inhibited up to 6 hours only and may grow after this time. Yersiniae are not inhibited in these enrichment broths.

Media for Haemophilus

Chocolate Agar. See Basic Enriched Media, p. 334.

Horse Blood Agar. Sheep blood agar may contain inhibitors to haemophili, and horse blood agar is to be preferred. To prevent the growth of other organisms from the respiratory tract, a bacitracin disk is used, and the disk also has X and V factors necessary for the growth of haemophili. Thus, around the disk, *Haemophilus* colonies will grow more luxuriantly and possibly in pure culture.

Columbia CNA Medium. This is a selective medium for the organism *Gardnerella vaginalis,* which is regarded as a cause of one type of vaginitis. The medium is essentially lyzed 5% horse blood in Columbia agar together with the antimicrobials colistin and nalidixic acid. The latter inhibit the usual vaginal flora and contaminants, while the lyzed blood, especially if incubation is held under an increased tension of CO_2, encourages the growth of *G. vaginalis.*

Media for Mycobacteria

Löwenstein-Jensen Medium. This is a complex inspissated medium, containing several mineral phosphates, sulfates and citrates, as well as glycerol, starch, and egg fluid. The addition of 1% malachite green acts as an inhibitor of organisms other than the Mycobacteriaceae. The complicated substrate is necessary to support the growth of mycobacteria. The medium is recommended for the primary isolation of human type of tubercle bacillus, whose growth is enhanced by the presence of glycerol. Furthermore, the colonial morphology on this medium permits differentiation of the human and bovine types.

Dorset's Egg Medium. This is essentially a simple egg medium that can be used to maintain growth of strains of tubercle bacilli. For primary isolations, malachite green can be added. The medium is prepared from beaten eggs added to sterile broth, dispensed into suitable containers, and inspissated.

Middlebrook and Cohn 7H-10 Agar. Some workers prefer this to Löwenstein-Jensen as the primary isolation medium. It is available from commercial sources. It consists of a complex agar base, to which enrichments have been added, namely, dextrose and an oleic acid-albumin complex.

Dubos Broth. This medium is often used for the rapid growth of pure cultures of mycobacteria. The medium consists of phosphates, citrates, sulfates, asparagin, polysorbate 80 (Tween 80), and casein or lactalbumin hydrolysate (used as a 20% solution). The pH of solution is adjusted to 7.4, then dispensed in 100 mL quantities in suitable containers and autoclaved. For use, 4 mL of a 9% bovine albumin fraction V is added aseptically to these 100-mL aliquots. Polysorbate 80 (polyoxyethylene sorbitan mono-oleate) is a surface active water-soluble lipid and is employed in this medium to produce a submerged growth of mycobacteria. Dubos broth is also useful as an in vitro virulence test media—that is, to demonstrate "cording."

Media for Neisseria

Chocolate Agar. See Basic Enriched Media, p. 334.

Mueller-Hinton Agar. This medium was devised for the primary isolation of *Neisseria gonorrhoeae* and *Neisseria meningitidis*. It can also be used for determination of antimicrobial sensitivity and in particular with the Kirby-Bauer technique (p. 433). The medium consists essentially of a beef infusion, plus peptone, starch, and agar.

Thayer-Martin Medium. This selective medium has a base of chocolate agar, to which is added a solution including the antimicrobials colistimethate, nystatin, and vancomycin (CNV or VCN). These inhibit contaminating organisms. Also added is an enrichment supplement (Supplement B or Iso-Vitalex) to provide essential nutrients, especially for *Neisseria*.

New York City Medium. This is a translucent medium that is even more enriched and selective and that is currently undergoing further evaluation. A modified Thayer-Martin medium in a plastic dish enclosed in a small plastic bag containing a CO_2-generating tablet is available and is known as a *Jembec plate*. After the medium is inoculated, the tablet is moistened and the containing pouch is sealed, thus creating a closed capneic environment (Fig. 16–9).

Transgrow Medium. This is a further modification of the Thayer-Martin medium, and it includes a further antibiotic, trimethoprim, which prevents swarming and growth of *Proteus* spp. Transgrow medium is especially valuable as a transport medium in cases of suspected gonorrhea. Thayer-Martin plates are serviceable in the laboratory.

Media for Staphylococci

By virtue of the high salt tolerance (halophily) of staphylococci, salt may be incorporated into a medium to inhibit the growth of other organisms. Thus, one can use a variety of media to isolate staphylococci from clinical material.

Salt-Cooked Meat Broth. This is prepared in the same way as cooked meat broth except for an addition of 10% sodium chloride.

Mannitol-Salt Medium. This medium consists of a nutrient agar base to which has been added D-mannitol and 7.5% sodium chloride. *Staphylococcus aureus* ferments mannitol and tolerates the high salt concentration—colonies are surrounded by a yellow zone.

Phenylethyl Alcohol Agar. This contains 2.5 μg/mL of phenylethyl alcohol, which inhibits most gram-negative bacteria, especially species of *Proteus*, and allows growth of streptococci and staphylococci.

Media for Vibrios

Cary and Blair Transport and Holding Medium. This medium contains thioglycollate, phosphate, and sodium chloride in 0.5% agar at a pH of 8.4. It is semisolid and has been shown efficient in maintaining the viability of *V. cholerae* for up to 4 months. It is also of value for the other vibrios. PRAS (see p. 331) Cary and Blair can be used as an anaerobic transport medium.

Thiosulfate Citrate Bile Medium (pH 8.6). This is a commercially available medium in which vibrios grow well, while *E. coli* and related commensals as well as *Proteus* spp. are inhibited. The more routinely used enteric media may be inhibitory to the vibrios.

Monsur Agar. This medium, which contains sodium taurocholate, potassium tellurite, and sodium carbonate, is another preferred selective medium.

Media for Streptococci

Todd-Hewitt Meat-Infusion Broth. This medium is used for typing streptococci (e.g., Lancefield grouping). It contains 0.2% glucose and has a pH of 7.8.

Columbia Starch Agar. This medium, which can be obtained commercially, contains 1 g of starch per liter. Group B streptococcci, when grown on such a medium anaerobically, will produce easily identifiable yellow-orange or brown pigmented colonies.

Transport Media

These media have been devised to protect pathogens present in clinical specimens that might not otherwise survive or that might be overgrown by nonpathogens during the transport of the specimen from the patient to the laboratory. Such a lapse of time may involve either minutes, hours, or days.

Stuart's Transport Medium. This medium is ideal for swabs, e.g., maintaining viability of gonococci on cervical swabs. The medium consists of an anaerobic salt solution (namely, thioglycollic acid), 0.5% agar, and 0.002% methylene blue. Some workers use swabs charged with charcoal, while others incorporate it into the medium. Whichever modification is employed, the charcoal must be purified activated charcoal. Its purpose is to adsorb formed bactericidal and bacteriostatic substances.

Amies Transport Medium. This is not unlike Cary and Blair medium for transport of vibrios (see above), but the pH is adjusted to a more usual 7.3 and charcoal is added.

Glycerol-Saline Transport Medium. When a delay in culturing feces is anticipated, the specimen can be preserved using this medium, which prevents intestinal flora from overgrowing the enteric fever bacilli. The medium consists of glycerol, saline, disodium hydrogen phosphate, 0.02% phenol red, and water. Phenol red acts as an indicator. Thus, if the medium becomes acid, shown by a color change from red to yellow, it should not be used. Because organisms such as *V. parahaemolyticus* and *Campylobacter jejuni* require a more alkaline medium, it is now recommended that Cary-Blair transport medium be used for all stool cultures.

MEDIA EMPLOYED TO TEST CARBOHYDRATE METABOLISM

Simple Carbohydrate Media

Peptone Sugar Water. Simple carbohydrate media are classically of peptone water to which sugar has been added in a concentration of 1%. To demonstrate fermentation or oxidation, an indicator (often phenol red) is added. Change of color indicates acid production. Inverted Durham's tubes trap any gas produced; thus bubbles at the top of these tubes indicate gas production. The metabolism of carbohydrates by bacteria may give rise to numerous products, including acids, gases (CO_2 and H_2), alcohols, and fatty acids.

Litmus Milk Medium. This medium is used to demonstrate an organism's ability to ferment lactose and clot milk. For instance, the formation of acid and strong production of gas is a characteristic of most strains of *Clostridium perfringens.*

The medium consists of skim milk and litmus (indicator). It should be placed in a boiling water bath prior to use, to drive off residual oxygen. It is also recommended that a strip of iron be placed in the medium prior to inoculation; the iron will act as a reducing agent, maintaining anaerobic conditions. Acid production is indicated by coagulation of media and a change in color, i.e., from purple-blue to pink; gas production is seen by gas bubbles in the clot.

Methyl Red (MR) Test. The organism is grown in 5 mL peptone-glucose-phosphate medium and incubated for 5 days at 30°C; if this is not possible, the incubation should be at 35°C for a minimum of 48 hours. Following this incubation period 5 drops of methyl red indicator are added to the medium. A red color indicates a positive (acid) reaction. The principle of the test is that, in the fermentation of glucose, different organisms producing different end products reach differing pH values. Initially, all enteric organisms will give a positive MR reaction; however, with extended incubation times, the truly negative organisms will have time to break down their acid products to carbonates and even to ammonium compounds, thus making the resultant mixture MR negative.

Positive control: *E. coli*

Negative control: *Enterobacter aerogenes*

Voges-Proskauer Test. The medium employed here is identical to that used in the methyl red test. After 18 to 24 hours of incubation at 35°C, to 2.5 mL of the culture add 0.6 mL of 5% α-naphthol (in absolute ethanol) and then 0.2 mL of 40% w/v aqueous KOH. Shake to aerate and wait ten minutes. A positive result is a red color resulting from the formation of acetylmethylcarbinol (plus butylene glycol).

$$\text{Glucose} \longrightarrow CH_3-\underset{H}{\overset{OH}{C}}-\overset{O}{\overset{\|}{C}}-CH_3 \xrightarrow[KOH]{O_2} CH_3-\overset{O}{\overset{\|}{C}}-\overset{O}{\overset{\|}{C}}-CH_3$$

Glucose *Acetylmethylcarbinol (acetoin)* *Diacetyl*

The diacetyl reacts with some fraction of the medium to produce the red color. The appearance of the latter can be hastened by the addition of a tiny amount of creatine after the other reagents.

Positive control: *Enterobacter aerogenes*

Negative control: *E. coli*

ONPG Broth. Lactose is a disaccharide consisting of a molecule of glucose and galactose, joined by a beta-galactoside link. The fermentation of lactose is dependent on the presence of two enzymes: a permease, which controls intracellular penetration of the lactose, and a beta-D-galactosidase, which metabolizes lactose. Delay in lactose fermentation, it appears, is generally caused by lack of permease. Thus, examination for the presence of the galactosidase should give a rapid indication as to whether the organism will ferment lactose. *o*-Nitrophenylbeta-D-galactopyranoside is a colorless substance that, when its galactoside linkage is broken, yields a yellow compound, and this acts as an indicator of galactosidase activity.

The substrate is made as follows:

ONPG	0.6 g
0.01 M Na_2HPO_4 (pH 7.5)	100 mL

One part of the ONPG solution is mixed with 3 parts of peptone water and dispensed in aliquots of 2.5-mL amounts into test tubes of appropriate size. These will remain stable for 1 month at 4°C.

Organisms are inoculated and the solutions incubated. Results often can be seen in 30 minutes, usually in 3 hours, and certainly after overnight incubation, if positive.

Positive control: *E. coli*

Negative control: *Proteus mirabilis*

Differentiation of Aerobic and Anaerobic Breakdown of Carbohydrate

Hugh and Leifson's O–F Medium. This medium aids in the differentiation of those organisms utilizing carbohydrates oxidatively rather than fermentatively. The utilization of glucose by oxidation or fermentation is critically different. Fermentation is anaerobic, and phosphorylation is a first step; oxidation is aerobic, and no phosphorylation occurs. Glucose is generally added, but other carbohydrates may be employed. The tubes are inoculated by stabbing; one is covered with sterile petrolatum and the other is left uncovered. The medium differentiates between oxidation and fermentation of the carbohydrate:

	Open Tube	Petrolatum Tube
Oxidation	Yellow	Green
Fermentation	Yellow	Yellow

The medium of Hugh and Leifson contains a relatively high concentration of carbohydrate and a low level of peptone, which prevents the possibility of digestion of the latter's producing sufficient alkalinity to upset the result. Furthermore, the peptone used is a pancreatic digest of casein, which is said to negate the possibility of excess alkaline production. Bromthymol blue is the indicator.

Controls:

Fermentative: *E. coli*

Oxidative: *Ps. aeruginosa*

Inactive: *Acinetobacter lwoffii*

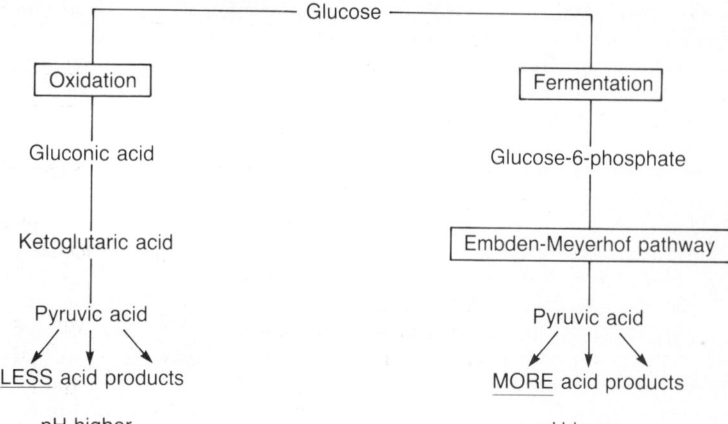

Figure 14–9 Essential differences in the utilization of glucose by oxidative and fermentative organisms.

Beckford Constricted Tube in O–F Studies. This tube has a constricted portion that divides the contained fluid into an upper portion, which is relatively aerated, and a lower part, below the constriction, which is relatively anaerobic. The medium above and below the constriction is inoculated with a single stab by a straight wire. By use of a carbohydrate medium with an indicator, the upper portion will show if oxidation of the carbohydrate occurs, whereas the lower part of the tube will demonstrate fermentation after incubation for at least 18 hours at 37°C.

The tubes that are available ready for use have the advantage of avoiding the need for the use of oil overlay in the fermentation study, and employ one tube instead of two.

The results are as follows:

Oxidation (above the constriction)
- Yellow—positive
- Green or blue—negative

Fermentation (below the constriction)
- Yellow—positive
- Green—negative

Complex Carbohydrate Media

In a preliminary identification of the Enterobacteriaceae, Kligler's iron's agar (KIA) or triple sugar iron (TSI) agar is used. They are similar. In a nutrient base, they contain 1% lactose, 0.1% glucose, and an iron salt. In addition, TSI agar has 1% sucrose. The reactions of each of these media are similar, but for clarity the reactions of KIA will be discussed specifically. The media are poured as slants in tubes and are inoculated from single colonies by smearing the slant and stabbing the butt. It is important in such preparations not to use screw-cap containers, but rather tubes lightly plugged with cotton swabs.

If glucose alone is fermented (i.e., the organism is a nonlactose fermenter), the butt of the tube becomes yellow because of the production of acid from glucose fermentation. In the tube slant, there is an initial yellow change, but, since the glucose is in low concentration, the organism under aerobic conditions here utilizes peptones in the medium and the slant becomes relatively alkaline with catabolites of peptone. In the butt, under anaerobic conditions no such reversal takes place within an 18- to 24-hour period. Thus the reaction of a glucose fermenter and nonlactose fermenter would be an alkaline slant and an acid butt: Alk/A.

If both glucose and lactose are fermented, then both the butt and the slant are acid after 18 to 24 hours. The greater amount of lactose acid end products cannot be reversed by any alkaline catabolites of aerobic peptone digestion in the slant. Thus the reaction is A/A.

If neither glucose nor lactose is fermented, the organism grows by utilization of peptones. If these are metabolized aerobically and anaerobically, both butt and slant will be alkaline (Alk/Alk). If peptone utilization is only aerobic, the reaction will be Alk/no change.

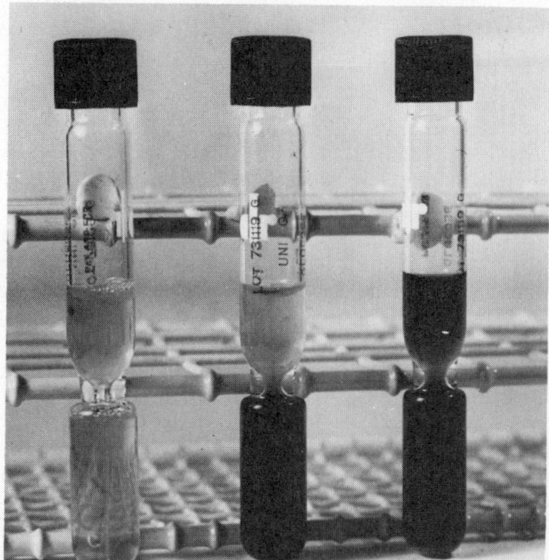

Figure 14–10 The O-F test in the Beckford constricted tube (Uni–OF–Tube, Diagnostic Research, Inc., Roslyn N.Y. 11576). On the left, the entire tube is yellow = fermentation; in the middle, the upper portion of the tube is yellow and the lower part is green = oxidation. In the tube on the right, the entire tube is green, i.e., neither oxidation nor fermentation has occurred.

Gas formation will result in the agar's splitting, or the agar may be forced toward the neck of the tube. H_2S production will in turn change the iron in the medium to be precipitated as a black sulfide.

With TSI agar, the additional sucrose will cause different slant reactions in those organisms that are sucrose fermenters; e.g., *Serratia marcescens* is Alk/A with KIA but A/A with TSI agar.

Controls:

E. coli: A/A gas

Citrobacter freundi: A/A H_2S

Proteus mirabilis: Alk/A gas H_2S

Ps. aeruginosa: Alk/Alk or Alk/no change

By convention, slant reactions are given first, followed by those in the butt.

Use of Discs and Tablets Impregnated with Carbohydrate

Carbohydrate Discs. Single sugar media have been made easier to prepare by the introduction of paper discs impregnated with various carbohydrates.* The discs may be used in semisolid, liquid, or solid media. Semisolid medium cystine trypticase agar (CTA) is poured into 6-inch test tubes, in 15 to 18 mL amounts. The carbohydrate discs are transferred to the tubes after they have been inoculated by stabbing the medium for about one-half its depth. The bottom half of the tube serves as a control. Fermentation is indicated by a change in color of the medium to yellow, occurring first near the disc and then spreading; gas bubbles beneath the disc and in the inoculation track indicate gas production. Control tubes of inoculated and noninoculated medium without carbohydrate are also used. CTA medium supports the growth of such organisms as neisseriae and the pneumococci, which normally require serum enriched environments.

Buffered Substrates

This method is employed to overcome the problem of detecting changes, e.g., acid production, enzyme activity, and so forth, in media that are chemically inadequate to reveal minor but significant biochemical activity, although they may support growth. Buffered specific substrate materials, conveniently available in tablet form in a wide range,** are dissolved in water, and then a massive inoculum of bacteria is added—much larger than that to which the substrate is usually exposed, under optimal conditions of pH, and so forth.

Organisms generally are grown on Kligler iron agar in tubes at least 2 cm in diameter with growth slants 3 to 5 cm long so as to provide an adequate number of bacteria. After 18 to 24 hours incubation, 2 mL of distilled water, not necessarily sterile, are added to the slant and the growth is suspended in liquid with the aid of a paper drinking straw or a wire loop. The substrate tablets are placed in tubes of 12 mm diameter, and 1 to 2 mL of distilled water is added, followed by approximately 0.2 mL of the bacterial suspension. Incubation of the tube may be continued for differing periods of time depending on the substrate used, i.e., on the particular reaction being studied.

MEDIA EMPLOYED TO TEST FOR PROTEOLYSIS

Gelatin Media. Gelatin liquefaction by bacterial gelatinase is determined most readily by the use of charcoal gelatin discs. These are composed of formalin-denatured gelatin, with a large amount of charcoal granules included. The denatured gelatin does not liquefy at 37°C, and thus incubation at 37°C resulting in liquefaction indicates bacterial gelatinase activity. The liquefaction allows the release of the charcoal granules, which on gentle shaking are easily swirled around, blackening the medium. The gelatin-charcoal discs are placed in a small amount (approximately 1 mL) of warmed (37°C) peptone water, which is then inoculated. Liquefaction may take only a few hours.

The use of small strips (3 × 20 mm) covered with a green gelatin inserted into 0.1 mL distilled water previously inoculated with a colony to be tested is said to give fast, accurate results. Gelatinase removes the green gelatin from the strip, revealing the blue transparent base within 2 to 4 hours.

Positive control: *Serratia liquefaciens*

Negative control: *E. coli*

Decarboxylase Media. Further help in the differentiation of the Enterobacteriaceae may be obtained by study of the specific decarboxylase activity on a series of amino acids, viz., lysine, arginine, and ornithine. The media contain a nutrient base as well as dextrose, the specific amino acid, and bromcresol purple, which acts as the indicator. If the amino acid is decarboxylated, the pH of the medium becomes alkaline despite the fermentation of glucose, since the decarboxylation products are alkaline:

$$\underset{\text{Amino Acid}}{\mathrm{H{-}\overset{\displaystyle H}{\underset{\displaystyle H}{C}}{-}\overset{\displaystyle NH_2}{\underset{\displaystyle H}{C}}{-}COOH}} \xrightarrow{} \underset{\text{Decarboxylation}}{} \underset{\text{Amine}}{\mathrm{R{-}\overset{\displaystyle H}{\underset{\displaystyle H}{C}}{-}\overset{\displaystyle H}{\underset{\displaystyle H}{C}}{-}NH_2 + CO_2\uparrow}}$$

However, if there is no decarboxylation, the medium remains acid and thus yellow. During incubation, the medium surface is sealed with paraffin oil to allow the oxygen within the system to be used and to retain CO_2, which adds to the alkalinity. The medium is incubated in screw-cap test tubes and may be read after 24 hours at 37°C.

Positive controls:

Arginine: *Ps. aeruginosa*

Lysine: *E. coli*

Ornithine: *Enterobacter cloacae*

A rapid paper strip test is available. (Other paper test systems are available and include those for oxidase, H_2S, indole, malonate utilization, nitrate reduction, phenylalanine deamination, urease, the Voges-Proskauer test, and more.)

*Carbohydrate Taxo Discs, Baltimore Biological Laboratory, Inc., Cockeysville, Md. 21030.

**Key Scientific Products, P.O. Box 66307, Los Angeles, Cal. 90066.

Phenylalanine Deaminase Medium. This medium tests the ability of an organism to deaminate phenylalanine. The test organism is grown on phenylalanine agar at 37°C for 18 to 24 hours. Five drops of reagent are then applied to the culture slope and shaken, to loosen the growth. Within 1 to 5 minutes, if the reaction is positive, a green color develops in the medium. The color depends on the breakdown of L-phenylalanine by bacterial phenylalanine deaminase, with production of phenylpyruvic acid. The latter reacts with ferric ions in the reagent to produce a green color. The reagent is made as follows:

Ammonium sulfate	2.0 g
10% sulfuric acid	1.0 mL
Half-saturated aqueous ferric ammonium sulfate	5.0 mL

Positive control: *Proteus mirabilis*
Negative control: *E. coli*

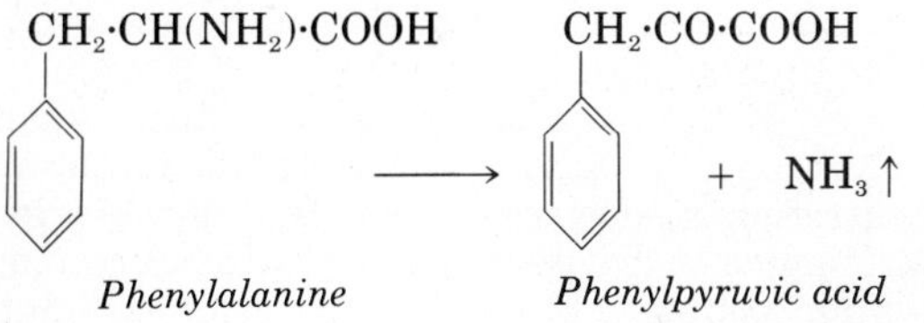

$CH_2{\cdot}CH(NH_2){\cdot}COOH$ → $CH_2{\cdot}CO{\cdot}COOH$ + $NH_3\uparrow$

Phenylalanine *Phenylpyruvic acid*

SIM Medium. This medium is used as an indicator of motility, the production of hydrogen sulfide from thiosulfate, and indole from tryptophan.

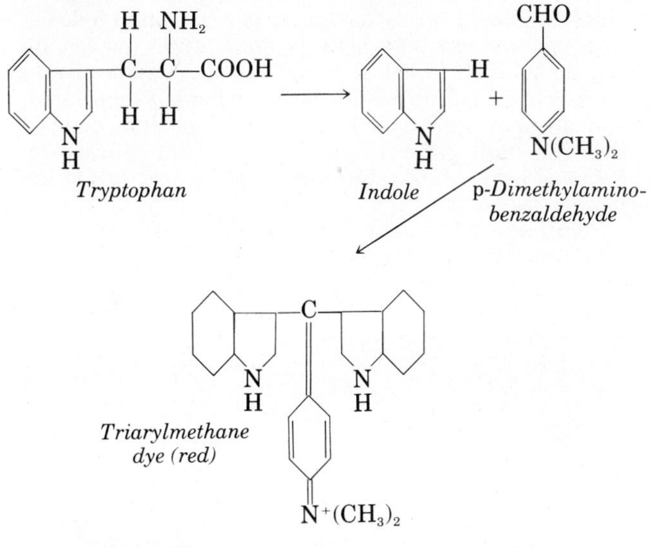

Tryptophan → *Indole* + *p-Dimethylaminobenzaldehyde* → *Triarylmethane dye (red)*

Present in the medium is ferrous iron, which blackens if H_2S is produced. A strip of filter paper, which has been dried after being soaked in saturated oxalic acid, is suspended from the neck of the culture tube by wedging it in with the cotton plug. The strip will become pink if indole is produced. Motility through the semisolid medium can be noted by the spread of bacterial opacity away from the stab line of inoculation.

Alternatively, Ehrlich's or Kovacs' test for indole may be performed. After the motility of the organism and its production of H_2S have been noted, a small amount of ethyl ether is poured down the side of the tube and mixed as much as possible with the medium by shaking. Ehrlich's reagent is made as follows:

Paradimethylaminobenzaldehyde	4 g
Hydrochloric acid (sp gr 1.19)	80 mL
Ethyl alcohol, absolute	380 mL

It is then poured down the side of the tube to form a layer beneath the ether. In the presence of indole (now dissolved in the ether) a rose red ring appears within 5 minutes at the liquid interface. Xylene is probably more convenient than ether for extraction of indole from the medium, since it is nonflammable. It is used in the same fashion as the ether.

Kovacs' Reagent

Paradimethylaminobenzaldehyde	5 g
Hydrochloric acid (sp gr 1.19)	25 mL
Amyl alcohol	75 mL

Add 0.2 to 0.3 mL of Kovacs' reagent to the culture and shake. A red color can be seen between the medium and the reagent if indole is present.

Ehrlich's reagent keeps well indefinitely at room temperature and appears to be more sensitive. Kovacs' reagent should be prepared in small quantities and stored in the refrigerator. Neither Ehrlich's nor Kovacs's reaction is specific for indole, and either may react to α-methylindole. Indole itself is volatile, and thus the oxalic strip method is more specific, although its chemistry is unknown.

Positive control: *E. coli*

Negative control: *Serratia marcescens*

Hydrogen sulfide production in other media may be identified by another paper strip test. These strips are soaked before use in 10% lead acetate and left suspended from the cotton plug over the medium in the manner described. If H_2S is produced, the paper will blacken owing to the production of lead sulfide. Different enzymes are able to liberate sulfur from different substrates. Unless the medium is specified, the results of different tests may not be comparable.

In testing for motility, 0.005% of the dye triphenyl tetrazolium chloride may be added to the motility test medium. The dye may be added before autoclaving, or aseptically to a sterile medium. The medium is inoculated by stabbing. Where growth occurs, the colorless dye will be reduced to insoluble red formazan. Thus in nonmotile growth a thin sharp red line will occur, but motile organisms will produce a diffuse pink cloud.

MISCELLANEOUS MEDIA EMPLOYED IN BACTERIAL IDENTIFICATION

Bile Esculin. The medium, in addition to the usual nutrients, contains bile, esculin, and a ferric salt. Esculin is a glucoside in which glucose is linked to a nonglucose entity known as an aglycone. The connection between the two parts of the molecule is a glycosidic link. The test depends on the ability of some bacteria to produce an enzyme that can sever this link.

A positive test is shown by the appearance of a blackening of the medium following incubation (see over).

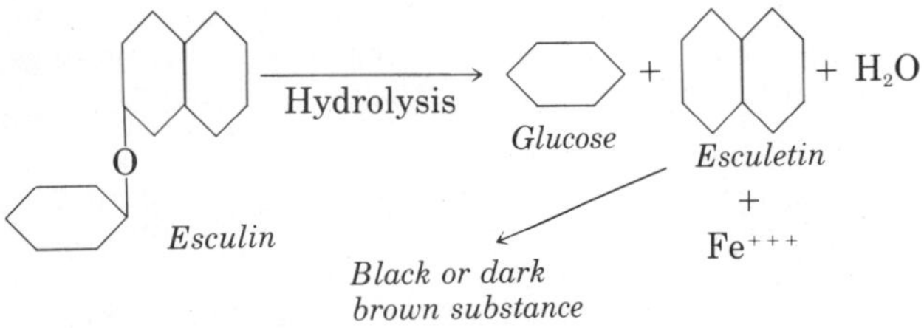

Esculin —Hydrolysis→ Glucose + Esculetin + H_2O

Esculetin + Fe^{+++} → Black or dark brown substance

Group D streptococci are esculin positive, but streptococci in other groups may also be positive and must be differentiated by other tests. *Listeria,* among the gram-positive rods, are notably positive in the esculin test.

Positive control: *Streptococcus faecalis*

Negative control: *Streptococcus agalactiae* (Group B)

Citrate Agar (Citrate Utilization Test). Simmons' modification of Koser's citrate medium contains sodium citrate and bromthymol blue as the indicator. The only source of carbon in the medium is citrate. Those organisms that can use citrate as a sole source of carbon will grow, and the indicator will become blue as the citrate is metabolized to acetoin and CO_2. The milieu of the medium is then changed from acid to alkaline. Those organisms not capable of this metabolic feat will not grow, and thus the medium will preserve its green color. During the inoculation procedure care should be taken not to introduce into the medium traces of carbon, i.e., charred remnants on the loop. To safeguard against this it is recommended that the loop be cleaned with acid and flamed dry prior to use.

Positive control: *Citrobacter freundii*

Negative control: *E. coli*

DNase Test Agar. This medium is used to detect the production of an extracellular deoxyribonuclease. Essentially, the medium contains deoxyribonucleic acid (DNA) and toluidine blue O, in a concentration of 0.01%. DNA degraded by the enzyme deoxyribonuclease results in the formation of a pinkish area in the otherwise blue medium—indicating a positive test. This is due to the paradoxical reaction of bathochrome, or negative metachromasia, in which the metachromatic color of the dye is progressively produced with *dilution* of the reactant rather than with concentration, which is the usual state of affairs. The basis of this reversal of the general rule is unknown. With a negative result, there is growth of the organism, but a failure to produce a pink color. Gram-positive organisms will not grow, since they are inhibited by the presence of toluidine blue.

Positive control: *Serratia marcescens*

Negative control: *E. coli*

Gluconate Test. This medium determines the ability of an organism to oxidize gluconates (nonreducing) to the 2-ketogluconate form, which is a reducing compound.

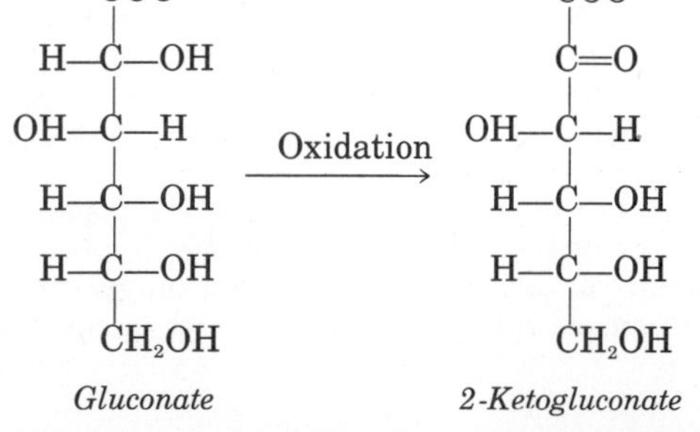

Gluconate		2-Ketogluconate
COO^-		COO^-
H—C—OH		C=O
OH—C—H	Oxidation →	OH—C—H
H—C—OH		H—C—OH
H—C—OH		H—C—OH
CH_2OH		CH_2OH

Gluconate *2-Ketogluconate*

One milliliter of the nutrient medium, containing 4% potassium gluconate, is inoculated and incubated at 37°C for 48 hours. The culture is then tested for the presence of reducing compounds using Benedict's reagent. Production of cuprous oxide precipitate is indicative of a positive result.

Positive control: *Ps. aeruginosa*

Negative control: *E. coli*

Malonate. Like the citrate medium, this medium is used to determine whether an organism can use malonate as a sole source of carbon. In the medium there is a small amount of dextrose, which if fermented alone may cause the bromthymol blue indicator to become yellow from its usual yellow-blue; but often there is no appreciable change. If malonate is metabolized, alkaline products result in the indicator's becoming blue.

Positive control: *Citrobacter diversus*

Negative control: *E. coli*

Potassium Cyanide Broth (KCN). Potassium cyanide is an inhibitor of certain enzymes, in particular those involved with aerobic respiration, and as such is a potent poison to humans. Many aerobic bacteria are also inhibited by this substance, but others are resistant. This difference is the basis of the test in which organisms are challenged to grow in a nutrient broth with a concentration of KCN of 1:13,000. If 0.005% of triphenyl tetrazolium is added, growth, if any, will be accompanied by a pink coloration in the formerly colorless solution.

Positive control: *Citrobacter freundii*

Negative control: *E. coli*

Nitrate Reduction Test. The presence of the enzyme nitrate reductase is detected by inoculating a nitrate broth or a nitrate agar and incubating it for 12 to 24 hours (and only rarely for longer periods, up to 5 days). The medium consists of a peptone water potassium nitrate solution (0.1%) with agar in the case of nitrate agar. A broth culture should be fairly heavily inoculated, and an agar slant should have the inoculum stabbed into the butt. After incubation, 1 mL of solution A, followed by 1 mL of solution B is added to 1 mL of the culture.

Solution A 0.8% sulfanilic acid in 5 M acetic acid

Solution B 0.5% alpha-naphthylamine in 5 M acetic acid

The reduction of nitrate to nitrite is demonstrated by the formation of a red color. The basis of the reaction is as follows:

NO_3 (*Nitrate*) → $NO_2 + H_2O$ (*Nitrite*)

HNO_2 (*Nitrous acid*) + NH_2–C₆H₄–SO_3H (*Sulfanilic acid*) + NH_2 (*α-Naphthylamine*) → —N=N— *Red diazo dye*

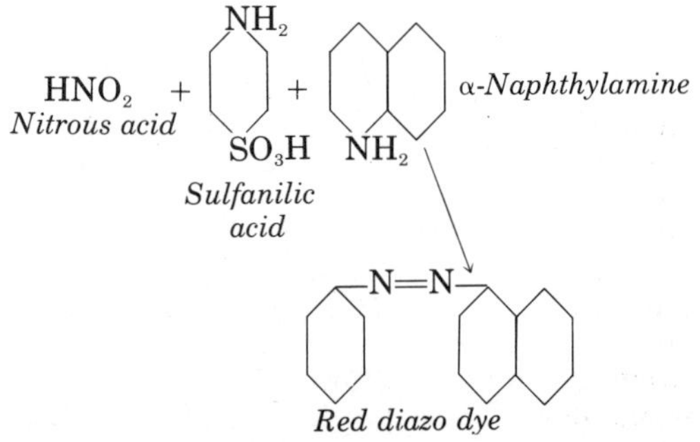

However if the organism splits the nitrate beyond nitrite, it may yield ammonia, nitrous oxide, nitrogen gas, and so forth. In such instances, the test above will be negative. It will not be known whether, indeed, the nitrate remains or has been so degraded. Metallic zinc reduces nitrate to nitrite; thus, a red color following addition of a small quantity of zinc indicates that the organism was unable to reduce nitrate to nitrite. Should the zinc test be negative, the nitrate has been reduced beyond nitrites.

Alpha-naphthylamine is the classic reagent used in this test, but because of the possibility of carcinogenesis, it is recommended that *N,N*-dimethyl-1-naphthylamine be substituted.

Positive control: *E. coli*

Negative control: *Acinetobacter calcoaceticus*

Reduction beyond nitrite (negative with zinc): *Ps. aeruginosa*

Urea Agar. Christensen's medium (pH 6.8) includes dextrose, peptones, and agar (which permits the growth of many types of enteric organisms), as well as urea and phenol red, which acts as an indicator. Those organisms producing urease form ammonium carbonate from urea, and the subsequent change in pH is detected by the indicator, turning the medium red.

$$2H_2O + CO(NH_2)_2 \longrightarrow (NH_4)_2CO_3$$

Positive control: *Proteus vulgaris*

Negative control: *E. coli*

Oxidase. This is an enzyme produced by some aerobic bacteria as a part of their respiratory oxidation mechanism. In vitro, the enzyme is allowed to act on a substrate, producing a color change. In one method, a few drops of a 1% solution of tetramethyl-*p*-phenylenediamine is added to a few colonies growing on the plate. With oxidase added, the colonies become blue in 10 to 15 seconds. The colonies are killed by the reagent after a few minutes, so that they should be quickly selected and picked off for further study if required. Filter paper may be wetted with the reagent and suspicious colonies rubbed thereon with a platinum loop. Nichrome loops per se may initiate a positive test and should not be used here. A blue coloration is positive. The reaction is as follows:

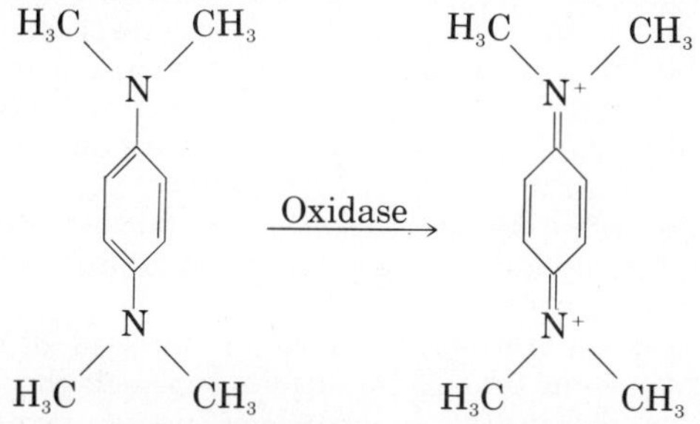

H_3C CH_3 N — N H_3C CH_3 —Oxidase→ H_3C CH_3 N^+ = = N^+ H_3C CH_3

Tetramethyl-p-*phenylenediamine* *Wurster's blue*

A more commonly used reagent is dimethyl-*p*-phenylenediamine impregnated into a paper strip together with alpha-naphthol. The reaction here is as follows:

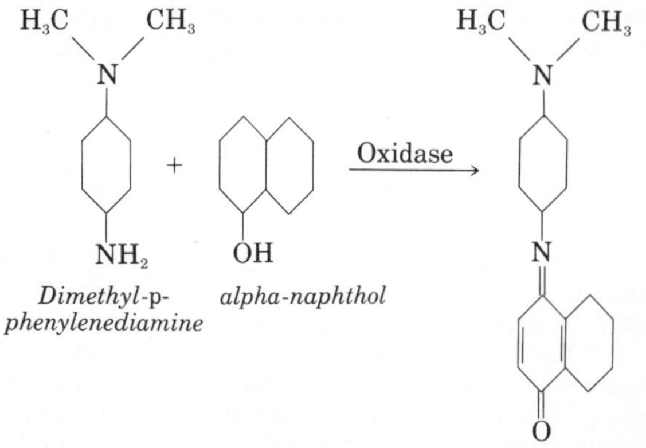

H_3C CH_3 N — NH_2 + OH —Oxidase→ H_3C CH_3 N — N = — O

Dimethyl-p-*phenylenediamine* *alpha-naphthol* *Indophenol blue*

Use of Rapid Identification–Screening Kits

In recent years several kits have been developed to enable the routine diagnostic laboratory to eliminate those delays often encountered in the speciation of the enteric organisms. Examples of such kits are: r/b System, Enterotube, and the API System. In the majority of cases these kits will enable speciation without having to resort to additional tests; however, it is urged that the results obtained from such kits not be considered conclusive, unless they have been confirmed serologically, where applicable, or by other means.

r/b System. This kit consists of four culture tubes in which metabolic tests are performed.

Enterotube. Fundamentally this consists of a multicompartmented plastic tube containing a series of bacteriological media, with a metal inoculating rod passing through the compartments. To use, the rod is inoculated with a single colony at one end and then withdrawn through the entire tube, thereby inoculating all eight compartments. The tube is incubated for 24 hours at 37°C and then read.

API System. This kit is a plastic strip with 20 miniaturized compartments containing specific test reagents. The colony to be identified is suspended in water and then used to inoculate the reagent series. The system thus permits a single organism to be evaluated by 20 biochemical parameters, which include: ONPG, decarboxylases (arginine, lysine, and ornithine), citrate utilization, hydrogen sulfide production, urease activity, tryptophan deaminase, acetoin production (Voges-Proskauer), gelatin liquefaction, and carbohydrate metabolism (glucose, mannitol, inositol, sorbitol, rhamnose, sucrose, melibiose, amygdalin, and arabinose). Nitrate reduction may be performed in the glucose compartment by adding a special reagent (see Figure 14–11*A*). The system is incubated for 18 hours at 35 to 37°C and then read. In our opinion, this system is currently the most complete and accurate means of speciating the Enterobacteriaceae in a kit form. Other API test strips for anaerobes and yeasts are also available.

Automation in Clinical Microbiology

In microbiology, automation has developed less rapidly than elsewhere in the clinical laboratory because until recently, the bacteriological techniques employed and the data gleaned have not easily been grafted onto sophisticated automated machines. Two advances however have aided this process. The first has been the introduction of multitest manual systems (commercial kits) such as the API 20E (Fig. 14–11), the Minitek system, the Enterotube system, and others, which have shown the way to simplification in biochemical differentiation and also brought a wider understanding of the mathematical and statistical basis of bacterial identification. The second advance has been a spin-off of the space program. Initially, McDonnell Douglas Corporation proposed a system for detecting microorganisms in spacecraft; the system then received recognition for its application in clinical microbiology. This, in turn, resulted in the Auto Microbic System (marketed by Vitek Systems, Inc., a subsidiary of McDonnell Douglas). Another impetus to automation has been the increase in the workload in clinical microbiology, which at the usual 10% annual increase will double in 6 to 7 years and often without a concomitant increase in staff.

The AMS (Auto Microbic System). This is currently the most advanced of the automated systems and may be used for urine bacterial counts and identification, Enterobacteriaceae identification, gram-negative bacilli and Group D enterococcal identification, antimicrobial sensitivity, and yeast identification.

The instrument itself is modularized and has seven modules (Fig. 14–12), each of which has a different function. The specimen, either urine or a pure culture of the organism under study, is placed in a transfer tube, where it is diluted according to the manufacturer's specifications in the diluent-dispenser module. It is then drawn into the channels of a test card that has a number of microcuvettes charged with a series of biochemical or antimicrobial agents that are thus simultaneously rehydrated and inoculated. This process occurs in the filling module, and the charged and sealed card is then placed in the reader-incubator (which can hold up to 120 cards) at 35°C. Every 15 minutes, the cards are rotated through 90° to present the card to a reader. The latter, via a computer module, reports changes in light transmission (signifying growth, biochemical activity, and so forth) to the data terminal and printer module. For urine specimens, the results are automatically reported in 13 hours. For antimicrobial sensitivity of gram-negative rods (Fig. 14–13), the results may be available in 4 hours; for identification of fermenting gram-negative rods, the results may be diagnostic in 4 hours, whereas for nonfermenters, 12 hours is necessary.

In use, the automated system saves considerable technician time, simplifies ordering supplies (since no Petri dishes, media discs, and so forth are needed), and saves storage space (since the diagnostic cards are small and thin). The automated print-out prevents clerical errors and human interpretive error, and the results are available in a relatively short time. It has been claimed that the system, in addition, produces a considerable saving in money when compared with traditional methods. There appears to be little doubt that in accuracy it compares well with standard manual methods.

Other Automated Systems. The Bactec system (Fig. 14–14) is produced by Johnston Laboratories, a division of Becton, Dickinson and Company. It is a semiautomated or automated system in which proliferating bacteria liberate radioactive carbon (as $^{14}CO_2$) from ^{14}C isotope–labeled substrates. The amount of radioactivity is very small, and no radioactivity passes out of the vials in which the cultures are maintained.

The system is of particular value in blood cultures, in which 30% of positive cultures are detected within 12 hours, 60 to 70% within 24 hours and 80 to 90% within 48 hours. It has been used similarly with other usually sterile fluids, such as cerebrospinal, pleural, and synovial fluids. Differentiation of *Neisseria* species can be made in 3 hours with this instrument, and the growth of Mycobacteriaceae can be detected more speedily than with the classic methods. Similarly, drug sensitivity results of Mycobacteria may be obtained in a relatively short time. Antimicrobial sensitivity results of rapidly growing organisms may be obtained in as little as 3 hours.

The MS-2 Microbiology System (Abbot) measures bacterial growth by light absorption and scatter. It can identify Enterobacteriaceae, indicate bacterial growth in urine specimens (in 5 hours), and thus eliminate the needless testing of noninfected specimens, and it is available for antimicrobial tests. A light-scattering system is also used by the Pfizer Autobac 1, which determines antimicrobial sensitivities and can be used to identify bacteria by their antibiogram profiles.

The Repliscan System (Cathra International) is based on multiple inoculation (see p. 433). The replicator can inoculate 36 isolates onto a single plate. The plates are charged with a series of biochemical or antimicrobial containing media. After overnight incubation, the plates are read by the technologist and the results are fed into a computer. The latter identifies the organisms from data stored on "floppy" discs and prints the identity of the organism and its antimicrobial sensitivity pattern.

Other systems are also available, and, in view of the reasons given above, there appears to be little reason to doubt that automation will expand into clinical microbiology.

SOME TECHNIQUES FOR STUDYING BACTERIAL MORPHOLOGY

Staining and Allied Methods

Following the isolation of an organism, microscopic examination will yield important information regarding its gross morphology and staining reaction that will enable the investigator to place the organism into one of the major groups. From this, speciation can follow, usually involving the study of the organism's specific biochemical activity. In this section we are concerned only with the demonstration of a cell's gross morphology, that is, its shape, staining reaction, and other morphological features.

Since the refractive index of bacteria differs only slightly from that of the media in which they grow, it is often difficult to discern them in the unstained condition. Thus, diagnostic microbiology usually uses the different stain affinities of bacteria to identify them more accurately. However, there is some merit in unstained preparations to determine motility, and in so-called negative staining, which will be discussed later.

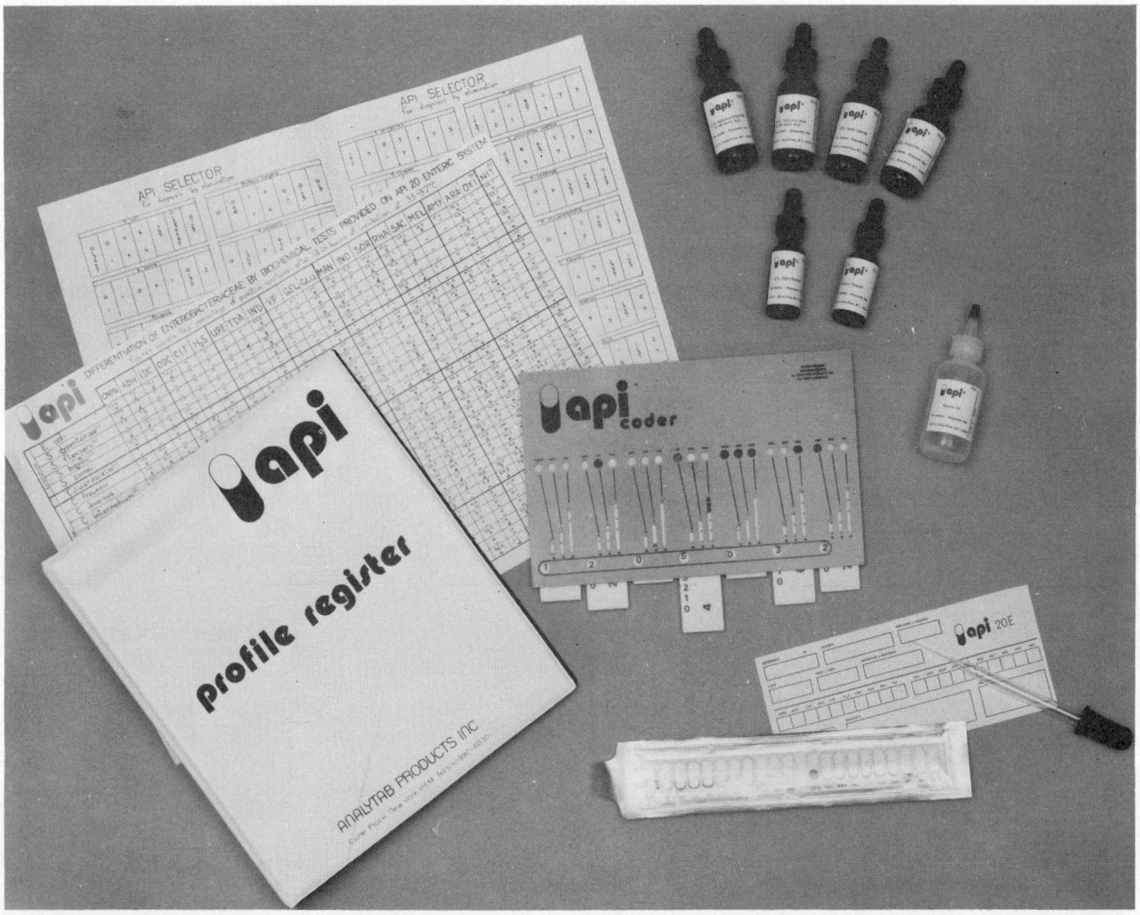

A

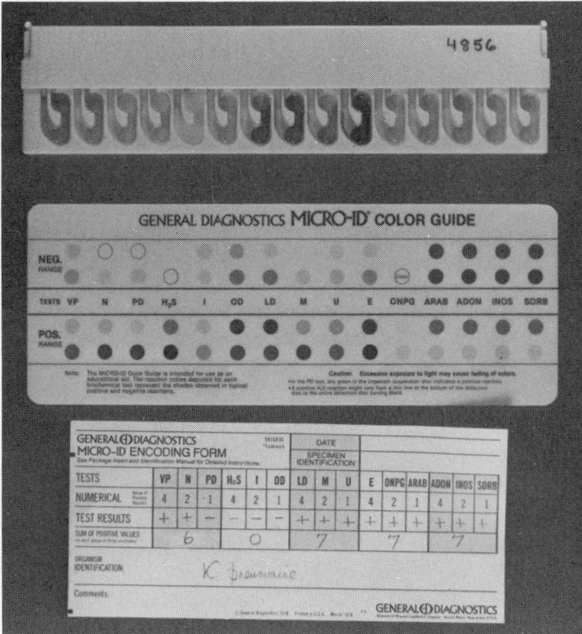

TESTS	VP	N	PD	H_2S	I	OD	LD	M	U	E	ONPG	ARAB	ADON	INOS	SORB
NUMERICAL	4	2	1	4	2	1	4	2	1	4	2	1	4	2	1
TEST RESULTS	+	+	−	−	−	−	+	+	+	+	+	+	+	+	+
SUM OF POSITIVE VALUES	6			0			7			7			7		

B

Figure 14–11 A, The API System. The prepared biochemical media are contained in small plastic tubes in the plastic tray seen in the lower righthand corner of the figure. Each is inoculated with a suspension of the unknown organism in sterile water or saline. The tubes used to test deamination of arginine, ornithine and lysine are also overlayed with sterile mineral oil. After incubation at 37°C for 18 hours, reagents (ferric chloride, Kovacs', and KOH and α-naphthol) are added to the tubes testing tryptophane deamination, indole production, and the Voges-Proskauer (V-P) reaction, respectively. Twenty reactions may then be read and compared with the key. In some cases, the reactions may be recorded on the coder (in the center of the picture). This expresses the reactions in a numerical fashion. In turn, the numeral expressing the reactions of the organism can be found in the profile register (shown on the left), and thus the identity of the organism is revealed.

B, The Micro-ID system for the identification of the Enterobacteriaceae. There are 15 biochemical discs, each in its own plastic compartment, to which is added a small liquid inoculum. V-P, nitrate reduction, deamination of phenylalanine, H_2S production, indole, ornithine, lysine, malonate utilization, urea, esculin hydrolysis, ONPG, arabinose, inositol, and sorbitol are the parameters measured. Only the V-P needs the addition of 20% KOH. The results are ready 4 hours after incubation at 35°C. These results are converted into a 5-digit octal code number, and identification is made from a computer-generated manual of identification.

In the illustration is the plastic chamber tray, beneath which is a color chart to aid in interpretation after incubation. Below this is the encoding form from which the identifying code is calculated. (**A** courtesy of Analytab Products, Inc., Plainview, N.Y. 11803; **B** courtesy of General Diagnostics Division, Warner-Lambert Co., Morris Plains, N.J. 07950.)

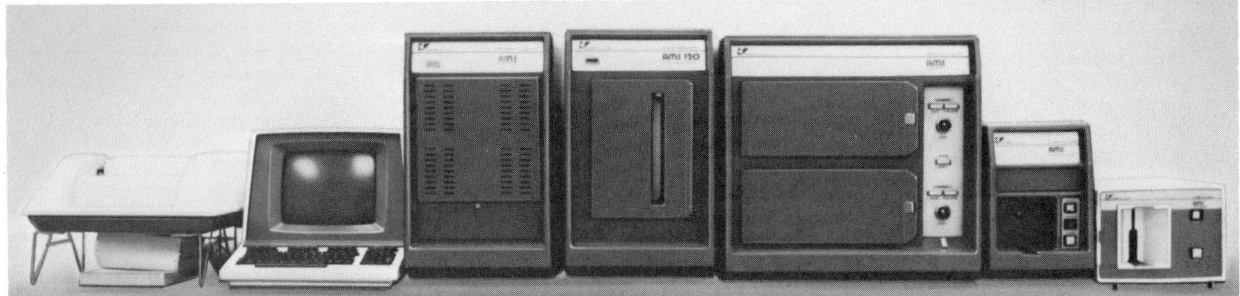

Figure 14–12 The Vitek AutoMicrobic system. The illustration shows the seven modules, from the diluent dispenser on the right to the printer module on the left. (Courtesy of Vitek Systems, Inc., Hazelwood, Mo. 63042.)

It should be noted here that there are those bacteria, such as the spirochetes, that are so feebly refractile that they are not revealed by ordinary light microscope techniques, and it is necessary to employ dark-ground illumination or phase-contrast microscopy for their demonstration (see pp. 36 and 37).

Wet Preparations

Hanging Drop Method for Motility

1. Place either an emulsion of a colony or a drop of (4 to 6 hour) fluid culture on a coverslip.
2. Make a small ring of Plasticine on a standard microscope slide.
3. Lower the slide onto the coverslip so that the drop of fluid is between the two glass surfaces and is prevented from touching the slide's surface by the thickness of the Plasticine.
4. Press gently to form a chamber, and quickly invert the preparation so that the drop hangs from the coverslip into the chamber.
5. Examine under high dry power for motility, making sure not to confuse Brownian movement with true motility. True motility is demonstrated by the bacteria moving in opposite directions and actually crossing; in Brownian movement particles or bacteria oscillate in the same spot.

Figure 14–13 The Vitek plastic card for antimicrobial sensitivity of gram-negative organisms. On the left is the sterilized card in its foil wrapper. On the right it is in position to be filled from a transfer tube of a broth culture. The wells contain 13 antimicrobials, and after adequate incubation the card is automatically scanned. Growth or no growth is detected and printed out as resistant, sensitive, or intermediate. Results are available in between 4 to 10 hours, depending on the rapidity of bacterial growth. (Courtesy of Vitek Systems, Inc., Hazelwood, Mo. 63042.)

Negative Staining

Unstained organisms stand out against a black background. Nigrosin or India ink may be mixed in equal quantities with suspensions of cultures on a slide and spread to an even thickness. The smear is then dried

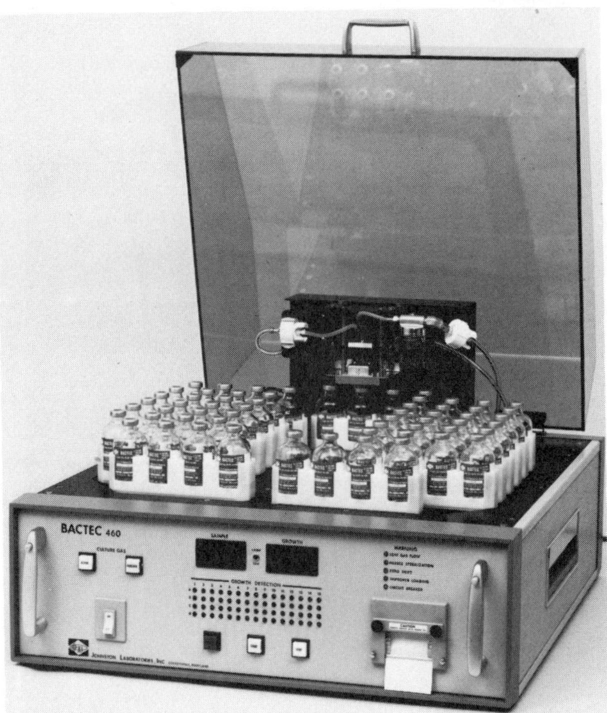

Figure 14–14 The Bactec 460. A semi-automated system that detects radioactive CO_2, which proliferating bacteria generate from an isotope-labeled substrate. (Courtesy of Johnston Laboratories, Cockeysville, Md. 21030.)

and examined microscopically. Organisms with a characteristic morphology, such as *Cryptococcus* and *Clostridium tetani*, are easily recognized.

Fixed Stained Preparations

These preparations are done almost universally both on specimens received and on colonies cultured. A smear from the original specimen is made on the slide directly or with a loop; the preparation must be thin and even. To examine a colony, a thin emulsion is made in a drop of saline and then smeared thinly on a slide with a loop. The air-dried films are fixed by gentle heating above a Bunsen burner flame and then by passing through the flame. Care should be exercised to prevent excessive heat, which would distort bacterial morphology. A reasonable heat is one at which the slide is just too warm to be held when placed on the back of the hand.

Gram's Method

This is the most widely used bacteriological staining method, and most organisms are classified by their reaction to Gram's stain.

Theory of the Gram Stain. An organism that is gram-positive must have an intact cell wall. A similar organism with a wall damaged by any of various means will be gram-negative. This indicates the importance of the wall in the retention of the dye lake. A theory of the mechanism of staining is as follows.

The basic dye diffuses into the organism and subsequently forms a water-insoluble lake with the iodine. The decolorizing alcohol or acetone dehydrates the mordanted walls of gram-positive organisms, forming a barrier through which the dye lake cannot pass. In gram-negative cells, the lipids in the wall (which are proportionately more than in gram-positive cells) may be dissolved, allowing the crystal violet-iodine complex to escape. Some objections to this theory have been raised, but the importance of the cell wall is undeniable.

Solutions

Crystal violet 0.5% in distilled water

Gram's iodine

Iodine	1 g
Potassium iodide	2 g
Distilled water	300 mL

70% ethyl alcohol

Dilute carbolfuchsin

Ziehl-Neelsen carbolfuchsin	1 part
Distilled water	9 parts

Procedure

1. Prepare and fix film as described.

2. Stain with crystal violet for 1 minute and then wash off with iodine.

3. Mordant with additional iodine for 1 minute.

4. Decolorize with alcohol until no more blue washes out.

5. Wash with water.

6. Counterstain in dilute carbolfuchsin for 1 minute.

7. Rinse in water and dry.

Many laboratories use alternative methods for differentiation or counterstaining, some of which are:

Acetone. Acetone, or acetone 1 part with ethyl alcohol 2 parts, is a much more rapid decolorizer than 70% ethyl alcohol. Rapid decolorization may be disadvantageous with certain bacteria on films with scanty organisms or in the hands of inexperienced technologists.

Neutral Red. Neutral red (neutral red 1 g, 1% acetic acid 2 mL, and distilled water 1000 mL) may be used as a counterstain. It is useful in staining intracellular organisms, and it does not mask weakly gram-positive organisms. However, the color given by the stain is somewhat brown-red and is not as clear as dilute carbolfuchsin.

Safranine. Safranine (0.5% in distilled water) is another counterstain, but it has no obvious advantages.

The following common organisms are *gram-positive,* i.e., they are stained blue-black: staphylococci, streptococci, pneumococci, diphtheroids, anthrax and its group, clostridia, and fungi.

Staining of Tubercle and Other Acid-Fast Bacilli

As it is with the Gram stain, an intact cell wall is important in the staining of organisms. The Mycobacteriaceae are difficult to stain because they possess waxy envelopes and special methods must be used. Besides being difficult to stain, once stained the organism is hard to decolorize. It is thought that the phenol-dye complex of carbolfuchsin is more soluble in the mycobacterial lipid than it is in differentiating acid.

Ziehl-Neelsen Method

Solution

Powdered basic fuchsin	5 g
Phenol	25 g
95% alcohol	50 mL
Distilled water	500 mL

Dissolve the fuchsin in phenol with a little water over a boiling water bath; add the alcohol and mix; add the rest of the water, and filter before use.

Procedure

1. Flood the slide with carbolfuchsin solution, and heat until steam rises. Stain for about 20 to 30 minutes. Do not allow to evaporate.

2. Wash with water.

3. Differentiate with 20% sulfuric acid until the film is yellow and then wash in water. If it becomes pink, repeat the process until it remains yellow when washed.

4. Wash well in water.

5. Treat with 95% alcohol for 2 minutes.

6. Wash.

7. Counterstain with methylene blue (Löffler's) for 30 seconds.

8. Rinse and dry.

Results. Acid alcohol-fast organisms—red; other organisms—blue. Although this is a well-accepted method, some modifications are used. These include the use of 3% hydrochloric acid in 95% ethyl alcohol, often followed by 1 to 2 minute treatment with 20% sulfuric acid for differentiation.

Kinyoun's Method

This is a more radical modification of the Ziehl-Neelsen method in which no heating is required.

Solution

Basic fuchsin	4 g
Phenol	8 g
95% ethyl alcohol	20 mL
Distilled water	100 mL

Prepare as for Ziehl-Neelsen carbolfuchsin.

Procedure

1. Flood the slide with stain for 30 minutes at room temperature.

2. Drain, and decolorize with 1% acid alcohol for at least 30 minutes. Decolorization may be continued overnight if convenient without deleterious effect.

3. Rinse in water.

4. Counterstain with methylene blue.

Results. As with Ziehl-Neelsen technique.

Stains for Corynebacteria

Löffler's Methylene Blue

This method is excellent for the demonstration of metachromic granules.

Albert's Stain

Solutions

Albert's I:	
Toluidine blue	0.15 g
Malachite green	0.2 g
95% ethyl alcohol	2 mL
Glacial acetic acid	1 mL
Distilled water	100 mL
Albert's II:	
Iodine	2 g
Potassium iodide	3 g
Distilled water	300 mL

Procedure

1. Fix in the usual way.
2. Stain with Albert's I for 3 to 5 minutes.
3. Wash and blot dry.
4. Stain with Albert's II for 1 minute.
5. Wash and blot dry.

Results. Protoplasm—light green; bars—dark green; granules —black.

Neisser's Method (Modified)

Solutions

Neisser's methylene blue:	
Methylene blue 2% aqueous	10 mL
Ethyl alcohol	4 mL
Glacial acetic acid	10 mL
Distilled water	180 mL
Neisser's crystal violet:	
Crystal violet	1 mg
Ethyl alcohol	10 mL
Distilled water	100 mL
Bismarck brown:	
Bismarck brown	1 g
Distilled water	500 mL

Heat water to 60°C, add the dye, and dissolve.

Procedure

1. Fix the films in the usual way.

2. Stain with 2 parts of solution A and 1 part of solution B for a few seconds.

3. Rinse rapidly in water.

4. Counterstain in solution C for 30 seconds.

5. Wash rapidly in water, blot, and dry.

Results. Protoplasm of bacteria—yellow-brown; granules—blue-black.

Demonstration of Capsules

These can be shown either by a negative method, such as nigrosin, or by Hiss's technique.

Hiss's Method

Procedure

1. After fixing the slide by heat, pour on the following solution:

Saturated alcoholic basic fuchsin	**1 part**
Distilled water	**19 parts**

2. Heat until steam rises and leave 30 seconds.

3. Wash the slide with the following solution.

Copper sulfate	**20 g**
Distilled water	**100 mL**

4. Allow to dry.

Results. Bacteria—red-brown; capsules—pale brown.

Litmus Milk

Litmus milk may be used to emulsify the suspension of bacteria. The film is then stained by Gram's method. Under the microscope the organisms appear stained, surrounded by an unstained capsule on a background of pale blue.

Demonstration of Flagella

Flagella are not easy to stain, but a practical method is that of Leifson.

Leifson Method

Solutions

Tannic acid	0.85 g
Sodium chloride	0.5 g
Pararosaniline acetate	0.35 g
95% ethyl alcohol	35 mL
Distilled water	65 mL

The solid components may be purchased in a powdered form*; 1.9 g is dissolved in 33 mL of 95% alcohol and 67 mL of water. The stain may be used immediately after preparation or stored for several weeks in a tightly stoppered bottle.

Procedure

1. From an agar culture or single colony, emulsify a loopful of bacteria in 5 mL of distilled water to obtain an opalescent suspension.

---

*Difco Laboratories, Detroit, Mich. 48232.

2. Using a new, thoroughly cleaned slide, flame one side and then allow to cool.
3. When the slide is cool, make a continuous line with a wax pencil along its margins, leaving an unmarked area at one end of the slide for handling.
4. Place a large loopful of bacteria at one end of the marked area and tilt the slide to allow the drop to spread over the marked area. Allow it to dry at room temperature.
5. Add 1 mL of stain to the slide, allow to stain for 8 to 10 minutes. The stain should not flow outside the marked area.
6. Flood off the stain with tap water; do not tip the slide until this is done, then drain and allow to dry in the air.
7. Counterstain, if desired, with Löffler's methylene blue, diluted 1:3 in distilled water for 1 to 2 minutes. Flood with tap water and allow to dry in air.

Results. Flagellae—red; body of the organism—blue.

Demonstration of Spores

Spore Stain

Solutions

Ziehl-Neelsen carbolfuchsin
30% aqueous ferric chloride
5% aqueous sodium sulfite
1% aqueous methylene blue

Procedure

Film should be fixed with a minimum of heat.

1. Stain with Ziehl-Neelsen carbolfuchsin for 3 to 5 minutes, heating until steam rises.
2. Wash in water.
3. Treat with ferric chloride solution for 1 to 2 minutes.
4. Without washing, treat with sodium sulfite solution for 30 seconds.
5. Wash in water.
6. Counterstain with methylene blue for 1 minute.
7. Wash, blot, and dry.

Results. Spores—bright red; protoplasm of the bacteria—blue.

Fluorescent Stain for M. tuberculosis

A more detailed discussion of fluorescent microscopy is to be found elsewhere (pp. 37 and 548), but for convenience the following is discussed here.

Solutions

Auramine phenol:	
Aqueous solution of auramine 1:1000	95 mL
Liquefied phenol	5 mL
Acid alcohol:	
Alcohol 70%	97 mL
Hydrochloric acid	3 mL
Potassium permanganate:	
Aqueous solution 1:100	
Löffler's methylene blue	

Procedure

1. Flood smears with auramine phenol, heat until boiling, and leave for 10 minutes.
2. Wash in running water.
3. Differentiate in acid alcohol for 20 seconds.
4. Wash in running water.
5. Rinse in potassium permanganate for 5 seconds.
6. Wash in running water.
7. Counterstain with methylene blue for 1 second.
8. Wash and dry.
9. Examine under ultraviolet light, using standard equipment for fluorescent microscopy. *M. tuberculosis* fluoresces yellow and stands out against a dark background.

This method is more rapid than standard techniques and gives a higher percentage of positive results.

SUMMARY OF QUALITY CONTROL IN MICROBIOLOGY

The quality control program endeavors to check the accuracy and the reproducibility of the isolation and identification of significant organisms. It also examines the adequacy of antimicrobial sensitivity tests and of serological examinations. If quality control shows deficiencies, they may be corrected; if it demonstrates efficiency, a sense of achievement and satisfaction is generated. The program in a large laboratory may be very sophisticated, taking the full time of one or several technologists, but even in a small laboratory, quality control is an absolute necessity and should include the following areas of investigation.

Equipment

The working temperatures of refrigerators, freezers, ovens, incubators, and water baths should be logged at least once a day, and the daily log should be kept close to the individually monitored piece of equipment.

Autoclave efficiency is best tested with spore strips (see p. 26).

Newly activated catalyst should be used each working day in GasPak anaerobic jars. The catalyst is activated for 1½ to 2 hours in a hot-air oven at 160°C and then stored until use in a desiccated container. Each anaerobic jar has a methylene blue–type indicator strip incorporated at the initiation of incubation, and a plate culture of *Ps. aeruginosa* and of *Candida albicans* is included with plates to be examined. These two organisms grow very poorly or not at all under anaerobic conditions.

CO_2 content within incubators can be measured by the commercially available Fyrite Gas Analyzer. The adequacy of capneic conditions in such apparatus as a candle jar can be monitored by the attempted growth of a control organism such as *N. gonorrhoeae,* which demands an atmosphere enriched with CO_2.

pH meters are checked daily using standard solutions.

Glassware, including pipettes, beakers, flasks, and so forth, should be regularly inspected for fractures and if etched or chipped should be discarded.

Ultraviolet light in hoods should be surveyed quarterly for performance. The output of ultraviolet light may be measured by commercially available meters.

Media

All media must be prepared carefully according to the manufacturer's instructions or to the written instructions of the laboratory manual. Each batch of prepared media must be checked for sterility by incubating representative samples (about 5% of the plates) at 35°C or at the temperature at which the medium is intended for use. Selective media do not lend themselves to such methods, and contamination is generally recognized after subculture during diagnostic studies in which an apparently pure colony will prove contaminated on a less inhibitory medium.

Media should be stored so as to avoid dehydration, and plastic bags are very suitable for the storage of plates. Plates in such bags or sealed tube media are kept in the refrigerator. They are removed about 2 hours before use and are allowed to come to room temperature. Plates or slants should be inspected before use for evidence of dehydration, precipitation, or incorrect coloration. In the event of untoward appearance, the plate or batch should be discarded and a new batch prepared avoiding the error.

Finally, each batch of medium should have samples challenged with the organism that they are intended to elucidate. For example, on MacConkey medium, *E. coli* should appear as a pink colony and *Proteus vulgaris* should appear colorless, transparent, and entirely without evidence of spreading. For this purpose, stock cultures are kept, and methods of preserving stock organisms are given elsewhere (see p. 331). Batch numbers for each group of prepared media are assigned, and logs of these with sterility tests and performance grades are kept.

Sera

Sera must be kept carefully according to the instructions of the manufacturer. A log is kept recording the date of receipt of the serum and the date of rehydration in the case of lyophilized material. Appearance is again important; opaque or turbid serum should not be used. Regular checking of sera, at approximately monthly intervals, should be made using known organisms or cells. Hydrated sera should not be exposed to room temperature for longer than necessary. A log should be kept of the titer of the serum when checks are made, and of course the conditions of storage will be available in the control logs of the storing equipment.

Reagents and Stains

Chemical and biological regents as well as stains should be stored under appropriate conditions. For example, X and V disks used in the differential diagnosis of *Haemophilus* spp. should be kept with a dessicant in the refrigerator. Expiry dates on manufacturers' labels must be observed. All reagents and stains must be subject to periodic checks against known organisms with known reactions. Special attention should be given to those stains or reagents that are infrequently used. A log should be kept with dates of preparation or purchase and the results of quality control procedures.

Antimicrobials

Further details are given elsewhere (see p. 434). Suffice to say here that disks should be kept in the freezer compartment of the refrigerator at −14°C or below and with a dessicant if possible. Disks should not be used beyond the allowable expiry date on the manufacturer's label. Monitoring of the sizes of zones of inhibition against control organisms is carried out each day, and a log is kept.

Department Staff

An adequate manual of procedures must be maintained in an up-to-date condition. Methods should be referenced. There is much to be said for including manufacturers' package information as an integral part of the manual.

A good core library should be kept of both texts and journals and such publications as the Cumitech series (published by the American Society for Microbiology), Morbidity and Mortality Weekly Report (published by the U.S. Department of Health and Human Services), and the Canada Diseases Weekly Report (published by Health and Welfare, Canada). Every encouragement should be given to promote staff attendance at courses, seminars, and conventions.

Proficiency Testing

Many sources are available for obtaining samples as "external unknowns" for the laboratory to identify and examine. In some U.S. states and Canadian provinces, such proficiency testing is part of a licensing program, as in the Province of Ontario (Laboratory Proficiency Testing Program). In Ontario, bacteriology participants receive six mailings a year, each with four lyophilized organisms or mixtures. The American Society of Clinical Pathologists has an excellent Check Sample program, which again distributes lyophilized material and critiques written by authorities in the field. The College of American Pathologists has a similar program, and there are others. In general, such samples have been pure lyophilized cultures of one organism but with more difficulty, a mixed culture with significant and nonsignificant bacteria (more closely resembling clinical material) has been distributed. In smaller geographical areas, true or doctored clinical samples have been distributed, but this requires both a great deal of careful subterfuge so that technologists believe the specimen is genuine and an adequate "fail-safe" mechanism so that a floor nurse, an attending physician, or the record room is saved the agitation of looking for a mythical patient with a potentially infectious disease.

"Internal" unknowns, that is, material possibly somewhat doctored but confined in distribution to the producing laboratory, may also be used for quality control. Again the allotment and documentation of such material will require subterfuge, but to a lesser extent.

Proficiency testing must be regarded as a test of all the steps in the examination and identification of bacteria—media, incubation, serological tests, antibiotic sensitivity testing, and so forth—as well as of technical and professional expertise. It is an educational and not a punitive exercise.

Liaison

All community hospitals should have an adequate relationship with some individual in a recognized ref-

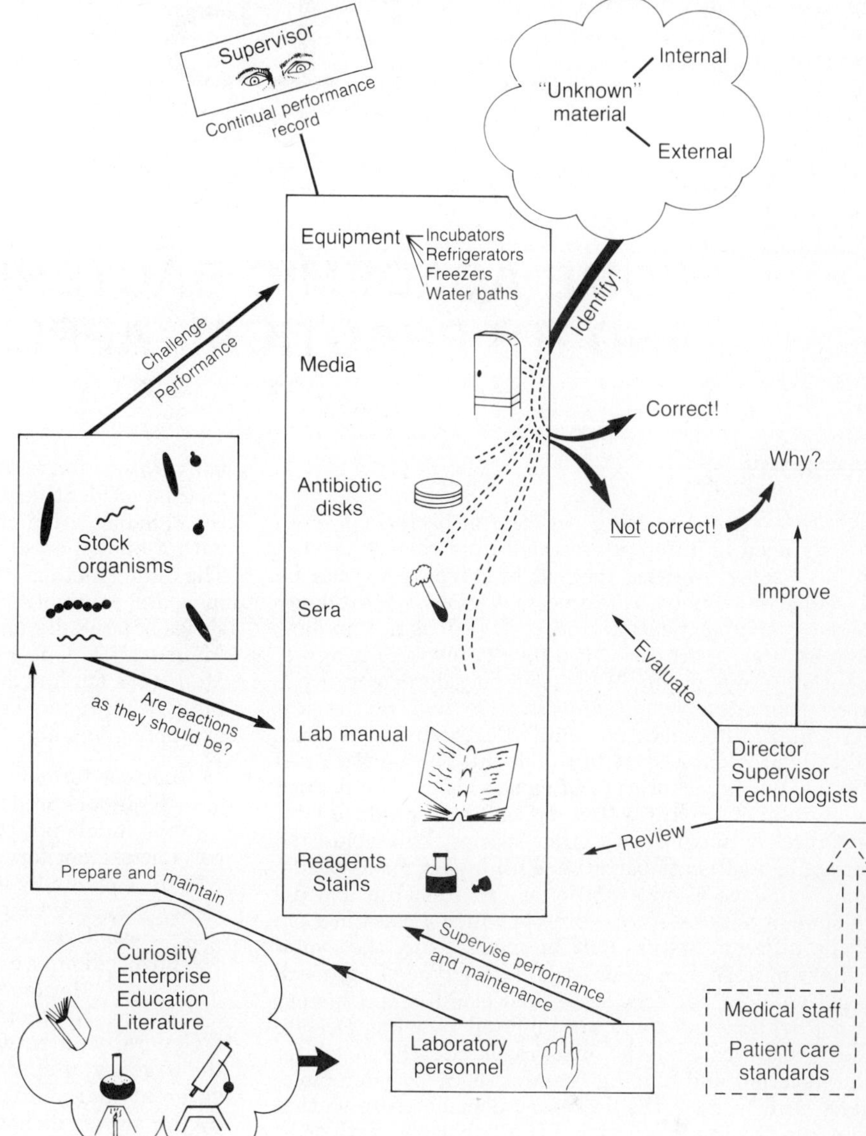

Figure 14–15 The interplay of personnel and equipment performance in microbiological quality control.

erence laboratory. In case of difficulty, such liaison may be invaluable not only in a specific case but also in similar instances in the future.

Review

Generally, in the community hospital, the supervisor of the bacteriology department continually reviews the results of quality control. It is just as important that the staff are aware of the results of their efforts as it is that they participate in the work, so regular meetings of the department are held. At such meetings, the department staff, together with the director or medical microbiologist, evaluate the results of the program.

CHAPTER 14—REVIEW QUESTIONS

1. Define *enriched medium, selective medium,* and *differential medium,* and give an example of each.
2. Describe the changes that occur in Kligler's iron agar when inoculated with a nonlactose fermenting, but glucose fermenting, non-H_2S producing organism.
3. Explain the essential chemical changes that occur with a positive test in (a) citrate agar, (b) urea agar, and (c) phenylalanine deaminase medium.
4. What organism identification is aided by (a) GN broth, (b) Lowenstein-Jensen medium, (c) Thayer-Martin medium, (d) Columbia starch agar, and (e) DNase test agar?

15

SOME ACADEMIC BACTERIOLOGY AND ITS PRACTICAL APPLICATION

TAXONOMY

Since we are discussing varieties of bacteria, we obviously need to differentiate them from each other and to have some accepted method by which they can be classified and named. This process is known as taxonomy (*taxis* = arrangement; *nomos* = law). It is not an easy process, since apart from the difficulty involved in agreement on terms, groups of bacteria may differ very little from each other, and some workers will not regard particular differences as valid. Furthermore, a most difficult problem resides in the definition of a bacterial species. In higher forms of life a species may be defined as a group of creatures that are able to reproduce with one another but not with other species. This definition cannot be applied to bacteria. With higher forms of life, some evidence of an evolutionary relationship and development may exist according to which a classification of the different species may be made, using the evolutionary pattern as a guide. Again, this type of approach is not valid for bacteria, since their evolutionary history is not evident and there are no fossil remains. Despite the difficulties and the disagreements, the need for classification and naming remains, because microbiologists need to have the necessary nomenclature so that they can communicate with one another and with their clinical colleagues.

A generally accepted nomenclature is given in *Bergey's Manual of Determinative Bacteriology,* and the International Committee for Systematic Bacteriology, with taxonomic subcommittees, exists and publishes in order to publicize agreed-upon definitions.

METHODS OF TAXONOMY

Natural

This term is used to describe a phylogenic method based on evolutionary origin. As noted earlier, this method is not applicable to bacteria.

Artificial or Phenetic

This classification is based on easily recognizable characteristics that are weighed in importance. That is, certain features are stressed to indicate groups that are related to one another; for example, motility vs. nonmotility, oxidative vs. fermentative metabolism of carbohydrates, and so forth. This is the basis of the "key" method of identification. Identification, to be precise, is the demonstration of identity of the unknown organism with a known organism already in its taxonomic place. The "key" method of identification often can be shown in a diagrammatic form as a series of dichotomies (a series of pairs distinguished by opposite qualities), as in Figure 15–1. One method of identification in *Bergey's Manual* is similar, but there the choices are given in a tabular form indicated by an alphabetic code for the example given above:

a. Lactose fermented
  b. Indole produced: *E. coli*
  bb. Indole not produced: *Enterobacter aerogenes*
aa. Lactose not fermented
  b. Acid and gas from glucose
    c. Urease produced: *Proteus vulgaris*
    cc. Urease not produced: *Salmonella*
  bb. Acid only from glucose
    c. Motile: *S. typhi*
    cc. Nonmotile: *Shigella dysenteriae*

Generally in medical bacteriology, especially under the urgency of clinical pressures, a battery of tests for different characteristics is done simultaneously and not by the slower dichotomous routes indicated earlier. To accommodate this approach, diagnostic tables are drawn, using identical information, and these give the bacteriologist the identifying pattern of his results. Such diagnostic tables are given in many works (Cowan, 1974; MacFaddin, 1980; Lennette et al., 1980).

A diagnostic table for this same example is shown.

	Lactose	Indole	Glucose	Urease	Motility
E. coli	+	+	AG	–	+
Enterobacter aerogenes	+	–	AG	–	+
P. vulgaris	–	+	AG	+	+
Salmonella	–	–	AG	–	+
S. typhi	–	–	A	–	+
Sh. dysenteriae	–	–	A	–	–

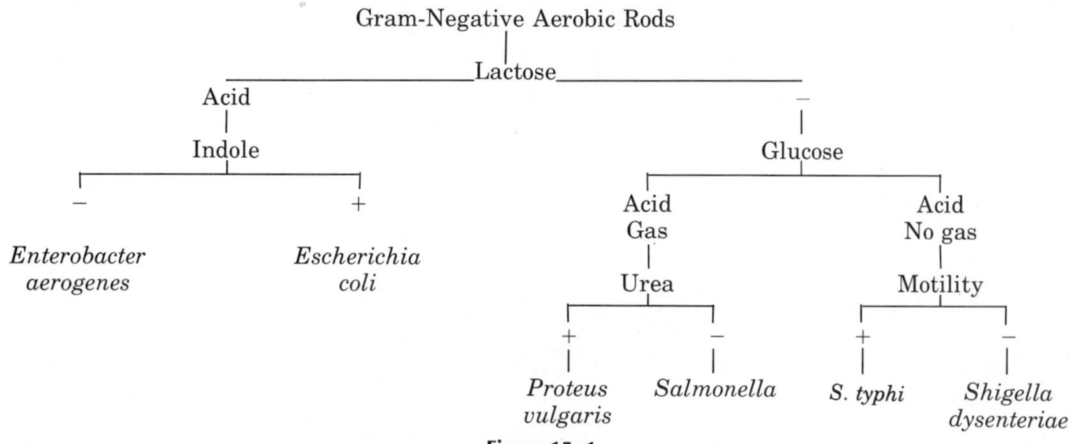

Figure 15–1

It will also be noted that this method gives more items of information than the dichotomous methods above, e.g., *E. coli* does not produce urease, is motile, etc.

DNA Homology

The DNA in the chromosome of the bacterium will contain the bases adenine, guanine, cytosine, and thymine. Members of the same species will have identical cellular DNA and thus a ratio

$$\frac{\text{Guanine} + \text{Cytosine}}{\text{Guanine} + \text{Cytosine} + \text{Adenine} + \text{Thymine}} \times 100$$

will be the same in each cell of each member of the species.

However, it will be remembered that the important feature of the genetic code is the base sequence, and this ratio cannot give information in this regard. Nevertheless, within this limitation it can be suspected that if the $\frac{G + C}{G + C + A + T} \times 100$ ratio is similar, then the organisms may be similar. Further progress in this field may be gained by testing the homology of the DNA sequence by attempting to form molecular hybrids with DNA strands from different organisms. At this time such procedures are not available in the routine hospital laboratory.

Numerical Taxonomy

This is a mathematical approach to taxonomy in which all features are given equal weight. The development of computers has made this Adansonian approach to taxonomy easier to apply. In some cases it has been able to reveal relationships and differences between organisms that were not apparent by other means. The taxonomic implication can be appreciated from the similarity matrix shown. It is recommended that some 50 to 60 features be investigated to make the result mathematically significant. The percentage of similarity of the organisms can be calculated by a formula and entered on the matrix. In the sample given here the strains under investigation are shown initially in the order in which they were investigated, and then in an arrangement that brings out their relationships. Organisms shown to be related by this method are known as phenons.

Strain	A	B	C	D	E	F	G
A	100						
B	15	100					
C	90	0	100				
D	70	10	75	100			
E	10	90	20	35	100		
F	10	75	20	45	90	100	
G	15	80	15	35	85	90	100

The following diagram, after rearrangement, shows two phenons: A, C, and D; and B, E, F, and G.

Strain	A	C	D	B	E	F	G
A	100						
C	90	100					
D	70	75	100				
B	15	0	10	100			
E	10	20	35	90	100		
F	10	20	45	75	90	100	
G	15	15	35	80	85	90	100

If desired, these data may be graphed to show relationships in an even more visually apparent pattern by means of a Sneath diagram (see Fig. 15–2).

Identification by Gas Chromatography

Although as yet gas chromatography has been used mainly for identification, with further development it may alter our ideas on classification and taxonomy. In fact, some progress has been made along these lines. Gas chromatography (p. 85) has been used to analyze the pyrolyzed products of bacterial cells; to analyze the acidified and ether extract of cells or the methyl derivatives of acidified cells; to identify the production by bacteria of alcohols and amines; or to detect the presence of microbial products in urine, cerebrospinal, or possibly other biological fluids. Gas chromatography is an exquisitely sensitive and extremely rapid method of analysis, but it can detect only volatile substances and it does not identify the detected substance. At the moment, at least in the area of bacteriology, it is not a routinely used method. It is, however, becoming increasingly useful.

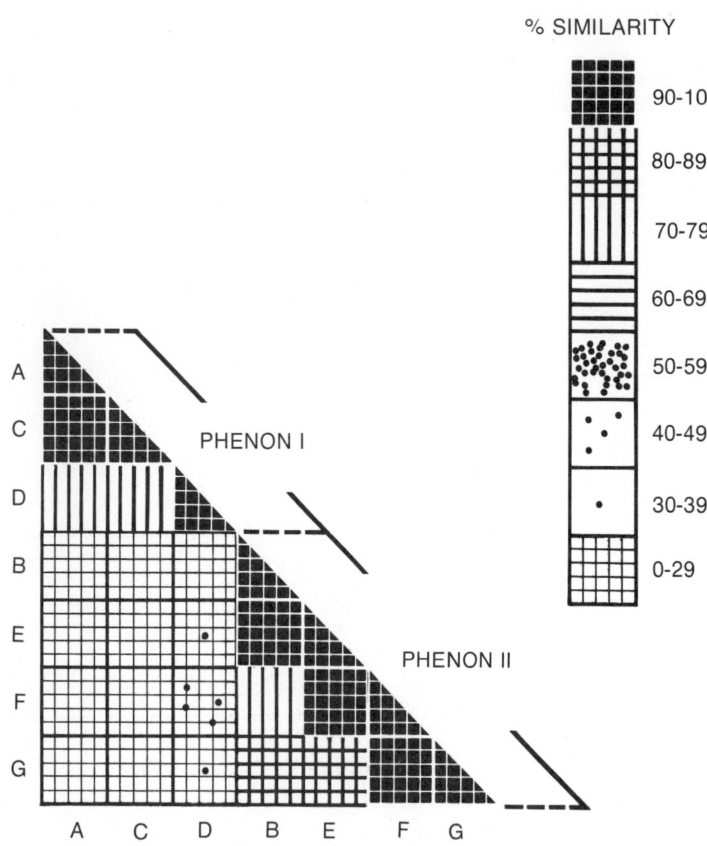

Figure 15–2 Sneath diagram. The data given in the tables above are graphed, and the resultant two distinct phenons are immediately apparent.

The Evolution of Bacterial Taxonomy

Because bacteriology is a progressive and advancing subject, it is continually subject to revision. Such revision is often reflected in nomenclature, since this is the expression of the result of altered thinking and concepts. A good recent example of change in nomenclature reflecting advances in knowledge is in the changes occurring in the genera *Proteus* and *Providencia.* Until recently it was accepted that there were four medically important species of *Proteus—P. mirabilis, P. vulgaris, P. rettgeri,* and *P. morganii*—and two species of *Providencia—Prov. alcalifaciens* and *Prov. stuartii.* However, *P. morganii* by DNA homology is closer to *E. coli* and *Salmonella* and less close to other *Proteus* spp. Hence it has been decided to form a new genus and species—*Morganella morganii.*

With *Proteus rettgeri,* it became apparent that by DNA homology some varieties are merely urea + *Prov. stuartii* and the urease gene may be plasmid borne. Other strains of *P. rettgeri* appear both genetically and biochemically like *Providencia* and are now known as *Providencia rettgeri.* The easy division of *Proteus* from *Providencia* by the presence or absence of urease, respectively, has crumbled.

Thus, in place of the four protei and two providencias we now have, tentatively at least, two protei, three providencias, and a new genus, *Morganella.* Other similar changes are going on in other genera.

Classification in General Use

The commonest nomenclature for bacteria is that given in *Bergey's Manual,* and this classification is kept current by the International Committee for Systematic Bacteriology. In the classification adopted by *Bergey's Manual,* there is a progressive division of the plant kingdom through numerous subdivisions to individual species. The naming of the groups as the classification proceeds is shown here. Following the name of the group are the endings of the words used to describe that group. Thus Eubacteri*ales* is an order, whereas Streptococc*eae* denotes a tribe.

Kingdom
/ | \
Division
/ | \
Class
/ | \
Order (-ales)
/ | \
Suborder (-ineae)
/ | \
Family (-aceae)
/ | \
Subfamily (-oideae)
/ | \
Tribe (-eae)
/ | \
Subtribe (-inae)
/ | \
Genus
/ | \
species

The current edition of *Bergey's Manual* (8th edition, 1974) abandons much of the hierarchial system previously used, "because a complete and meaningful hierarchy is impossible." The kingdom to which the bacteria of medical interest belong is now the Monera (i.e., the prokaryocytes, see p. 442). Division II of this kingdom is divided into 3 classes. Class III (without cell walls) includes the family of Mycoplasmataceae, and Class II (obligate intracellular organisms) includes the Rickettsiaceae, the Bartonellaceae, and the Chlamydiaceae. Class I embraces the vast majority of bacterial organisms of medical interest. A much abbreviated summary of Class I can be constructed as follows:

Order Spirochaetales, incorporates the family Spirochaetaceae, in which are the genera *Treponema, Borrelia,* and *Leptospira.*

Gram-negative aerobic rods and cocci include the family Pseudomonadaceae, in which is the genus *Pseudomonas.* Also in this grouping are the genera *Alcaligenes, Brucella, Bordetella,* and *Francisella.*

Gram-negative facultatively anaerobic rods encompass the family Enterobacteriaceae, in which are placed the genera *Escherichia, Edwardsiella, Citrobacter, Salmonella, Shigella, Klebsiella, Enterobacter, Hafnia, Serratia, Proteus, Yersinia, Erwinia;* and the family Vibrionaceae, containing the genera *Vibrio* and *Aeromonas.*

Gram-negative anaerobic bacteria: *Bacteroides* and *Fusobacterium.*

Gram-negative cocci and coccobacilli have the family Neisseriaceae, in which are the genera *Neisseria, Moraxella,* and *Acinetobacter.*

Gram-negative anaerobic cocci: the genus *Veillonella.*

Gram-positive cocci include the families Micrococcaceae, Streptococcaceae, and Peptococcaceae, in which are the genera *Staphylococcus, Streptococcus, Peptococcus,* and *Sarcina.*

Endospore-forming rods and cocci encompass the family Bacillaceae *(Bacillus* and *Clostridium).*

Gram-positive asporogenous rod-shaped bacteria: *Listeria.*

Actinomycetes and related organisms: *Corynebacterium, Actinomyces, Mycobacterium, Nocardia,* and *Streptomyces.*

Style and Convention

It is usual to use a capital letter for a word indicating a genus or for any group above a genus. A genus is usually printed in italics, and the specific word relating to the species (known as the specific epithet) also is italicized. The first letter of this specific epithet is not capitalized, although it may be derived from a proper noun; for example, *Staphylococcus albus, Salmonella london, Haemophilus ducreyi* (after Augusto Ducrey). When the generic name is used adjectivally, the capital letter is dropped, as are the italics: streptococcal, staphylococcal, and so forth. The capital letters are also omitted when the generic term is used colloquially in the plural: salmonellas or salmonellae, staphylococci, neisseriae, and so forth. The first letters of names of groups above that of genus are capitalized, but apart from that there are no specific conventions. The printed term may be in either roman or italic type: *Enterobacteriaceae* or Enterobacteriaceae.

Common names for bacteria are used in conversation and by long tradition for some organisms. It is easier to say "pneumococci" than *Streptococcus pneumoniae* and "gonococci" than *Neisseria gonorrhoeae.* Some terms are used as an euphemisms to avoid impact on anxious ears or eyes: "acid-fast bacilli" for *M. tuberculosis,* KLB (Klebs-Löffler bacillus) for *C. diphtheriae,* "gram-negative intracellular diplococci" for *N. gonorrhoeae,* and so on.

Prokaryotic and Eukaryotic Cells

As indicated above, the bacteria and blue-green algae are regarded as belonging to the prokaryotes, which are sharply differentiable from the eukaryotes. Eukaryotic cells, which include a wide range of organisms—amebae, algae, mammalian cells, and so forth—have a true nucleus within a nuclear membrane; they possess mitochondria in which respiration takes place; and their walls are thin and of polysaccharide or inorganic substances rather than the chemically complicated thick walls of the bacteria. The differences may be summarized in Table 15–1.

TABLE 15–1 PROKARYOTIC AND EUKARYOTIC CELLS

Cell Structure	Prokaryotic (e.g., *E. coli*)	Eukaryotic (e.g., hepatocyte)
Nucleus	Double helix of DNA unbounded by membrane. Acts as a single chromosome. No histone present.	DNA divided into chromosomes within nuclear membrane. Closely related to histones. Undergoes mitotic division.
Wall	Rigid wall of repeating units of mucopeptide.	Very thin, flexible coat of acid mucopolysaccharide.
Respiration	Occurs in membrane.	Occurs in specialized structure, e.g., mitochondria.
Intracellular membranes	None apparent.	Complex endoplastic reticulum with Golgi apparatus.
Ribosomes	70 S type distributed in cytoplasm.	80 S type situated on the membrane of the endoplasmic reticulum.
Motile structures	Flagella: usually 3 fibrils peripherally.	Cilia, tails of spermatozoa: 9 fibril pairs surround central pair.

THE STRUCTURE OF BACTERIA

There is a basic anatomy of bacteria. Knowledge of the structure is of value in the understanding of bacteriogenic disease and in the identification of bacterial species.

Bacterial cells (Fig. 15–3) are of course essentially prokaryotic. Cell walls are one of the most distinguishing features, with a rigidity and strength that protect the cellular content. The wall consists of repetitive units of peptidoglycan (mucopeptides). Other substances, including teichoic acids, may be present in gram-positive organisms, although not in gram-negative organisms, in which there is also less extensive linking of the peptidoglycan units. Gram-negative units also have an outer microcapsule as part of the wall. The wall contains protein, polysaccharide, and lipid. The relatively high proportion of lipid in the gram-negative bacterial wall and its looser structure underlie the basic theory of the most acceptable explanation of the Gram stain mechanism (see p. 347). Endotoxin, which may cause profound symptoms in gram-negative septicemia, is derived from the outer microcapsule of gram-negative organisms.

Surrounding the cell wall (and the microcapsule if present) is a layer of "loose slime" composed of polymers of polysaccharide or peptide. Bacterial capsules are, in effect, a more compact loose slime. Capsules may be identified by staining or negative staining techniques (see p. 348). They are important in some serological identification, especially in differentiating serotypes of pneumococcus, *Haemophilus influenzae,* and *Klebsiella* spp. Capsules are of immunological significance, since they impart a defense against phagocytosis and thus a measure of virulence. The organism *Streptococcus mutans,* in the presence of sucrose, forms an extracellular polysaccharide glucan that adheres to the surface of teeth. This glucan is the basic component of dental plaque, in which a heterologous group of bacteria are able to live in continual contact with dental enamel, eventually producing dental caries. The glycan binding to dental enamel is an example of a method by which bacteria are able to adhere to vulnerable cells or structures (also see below).

Within the cell wall is the plasma, or cytoplasmic membrane, which has the usual three-layer structure and which acts as a vital membrane guarding over the passage of substances into and out of the cell itself. Unlike eukaryotic cells, bacteria have no mitochondria, and respiratory processes in prokaryotic cells are carried on in the plasma membrane. Mycoplasmatales, which include the mycoplasmas, are bacteria that naturally have no cell wall and are bounded by the plasma membrane. They are thus inherently pleomorphic. Some organisms can be induced to lose their cell walls by the action of antimicrobials such as penicillin, which inhibits cell wall manufacture. If the cell wall–deficient organism is protected against osmotic forces by a slightly hypertonic solution it will survive as a protoplast. If there is loss of only some of the wall material, as for example in gram-negative organisms that retain lipopolysaccharide, the structure is known as a spheroplast.

The plasma membrane has some convoluted invaginations called mesosomes, and these are larger in gram-positive than in gram-negative organisms. They are of importance in cell division and in the secretion by the cell of such substances as penicillinase.

Within the cell wall and cytoplasmic membrane, the cell itself has the nucleus, which has no nuclear membrane and lacks a definitive shape. It is of DNA alone, without histones, and is a single chromosome, which in *E. coli* is about 1.0 to 1.4 mm long and has approximately 3 million base pairs of possibly 1000 genes. Since the chromosome is solitary, it must be considered haploid.

Emerging from some cells are flagella, which are anchored in the plasma membrane by blepharoplasts. These are relatively long and are actively motile, with a nonprotein core surrounded by usually three fibrils of a specific flagellar protein. This contrasts with cilia of eukaryotic cells, which have nine fibrils (or microtubular doublets) around a core of two fibrils (or a central pair). Flagella may be arranged all around the bacterium (peritrichous), or they may be at one or the other pole of the organism (polar) or at both poles. They bestow motility to cells, and this may be of diagnostic importance. Polar flagella are found only in *Pseudomonas, Spirillum, Campylobacter,* and *Vibrio* species among medically important bacteria; other motile species are peritrichous. The differing protein composition of flagella and the body of bacterium adds a second antigenic determinant that is especially helpful in the serological identification of *Salmonella* spp.

Bacterial pili are so named because of their resem-

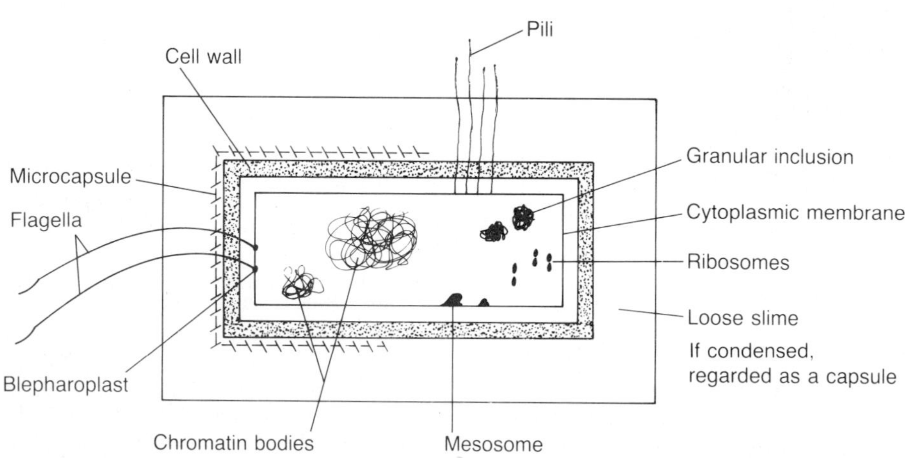

Figure 15–3 Schematic representation of bacterial anatomy.

blance to small hairs; they also arise from the cytoplasmic membrane and project from the bacterial surface. As we shall see they are of considerable importance in the sexual mating of bacteria but are rarely seen on gram-positive organisms. They cannot be seen by ordinary light microscopy. They may have a large part to play in the adherence of bacteria to mucosal cells, which is the major step in the initiation of disease of the respiratory, gastrointestinal, and genitourinary tract. Specific adherence by bacteria to specific cells also explains the pattern of bacterial disease, e.g., why *S. typhi* is a cause of gastrointestinal disease and why *Str. pneumoniae* most often causes primary disease in the upper respiratory tract.

Within the cell are numerous ribosomes, which are the sites of protein synthesis. These are present in all cells and are essential for conveying the genetic code of the nucleus into instructions in the manufacture of cellular components. Their presence is of little significance morphologically, but some antimicrobials, q.v., bind to bacterial ribosomes, disturbing transcription and interfering with peptide chain formation and protein synthesis, thus causing death of the bacteria.

Cytoplasmic inclusions are seen in some bacteria and they appear to be a reserve of food materials. Metachromatic or volutin granules are perhaps the best known of these and are especially associated with *Corynebacterium;* here they have the eponym *Babes-Ernst granules.* In *C. diphtheriae* the granules are most numerous and often more prominent at the polar regions—hence the term *polar bodies.*

Endospores are formed by species of *Clostridium* and *Bacillus.* Teleologically it is tempting to consider endosporulation as a response to environmental adversity, but they are produced by cells growing under optimal conditions just after the maximal growth rate. The spore includes the chromosomal material surrounded by several layers of a wall. Within the wall is dipicolinic acid, which is found only in relation to spores and is not in vegetative cells. The resistant properties of a spore extend to stains that are enabled to enter its substance if they are avid dyes and are heated. The shape of spores and their position in the cell may be of diagnostic assistance; e.g., spores of *C. tetani* are terminal, and their diameter is larger than the parent cell so that they are characteristically of a drumstick appearance (see Fig. 20–10). The heat resistance of spores, especially of the *Clostridium* species, is of paramount significance in operating room sterilization procedures.

BACTERIAL METABOLISM

The bacterial cell has to perform the biological functions that support life and has to replicate itself within a generation time that may be as short as 20 minutes. The cell's achievement of these astounding feats depends on the energy supply of nutrients from its surroundings and on a series of programmed enzymes within its cytoplasm that provide the necessary storage of energy for anabolism. The entire orchestration ultimately is controlled by the cellular DNA.

Nutrients must include water and may be either in a complex form such as protein, fat, sterols, and so forth, or as simple compounds of nitrogen, carbon, or phosphorus. Most of the organisms with which we are concerned require rather complex nutrients. To enter the cell, they must be digested by cell-produced enzymes acting outside the cell (proteinases, lipases, and various carbohydrases). Partially processed nutrients then can enter the cell by passive diffusion; or this may be accelerated by enzyme action producing facilitated diffusion; or they may enter by active transport.

Within the cell, the various substances undergo biological oxidation, i.e., the removal of hydrogen and electrons. This may occur in one of several ways that are described here. Some substances are not oxidized, but partially digested products (such as amino acids) are used in bacterial anabolism.

Fermentation

The Embden-Meyerhof pathway is the best known of the processes of anaerobic glycolysis, yielding pyruvic acid and energy in the form of adenosine triphosphate (ATP). Some bacteria (including *E. coli*) have enzymes for only part of the E-M pathway and may produce lactic acid or ethanol. Others may produce ethanol.

Respiration

Pyruvate from glucose (or amino acids or fatty acids from protein or fat) may enter the Krebs cycle. This may yield energy that is stored as ATP, or released as heat, or used immediately in the biosynthesis of essential substances. In addition, hydrogen and CO_2 are produced. Ionized hydrogen from this process is also oxidized by the cytochromes of the respiratory chain, producing further energy and water in this final respiratory step.

Oxidation

In fermentation, there is initial phosphorylation of glucose followed by anaerobic glycolysis. Oxidation is an aerobic process that does not involve initial glucose phosphorylation, although it, too, finally yields pyruvic acid.

Anaerobic Organisms

Unlike aerobic organisms, in which respiration yields hydrogen to oxygen, these bacteria yield hydrogen to an acceptor other than oxygen. Some organisms use sulfur and make H_2S; others produce methane with carbon. The details of the processes by which they achieve these ends have not yet been elucidated.

The energy given up in these processes generally is stored as high-energy phosphates and then is used to serve the purposes of the cell. The synthesis of protein is conducted by cellular DNA and is from absorbed amino acids or from amino acids synthesized from ammonia or slightly more complex substances, such as indole. Fatty substances are formed from the substrate malonyl coenzyme A, which in turn is made from acetate via acetyl coenzyme A. Polysaccharides, which are especially important for cell walls and capsules, are formed from polymerization of substances derived from acetyl glucosamine. The biosynthesis of the bacterial wall is important, in that differing antimicrobials are able to inhibit specific steps in the building process.

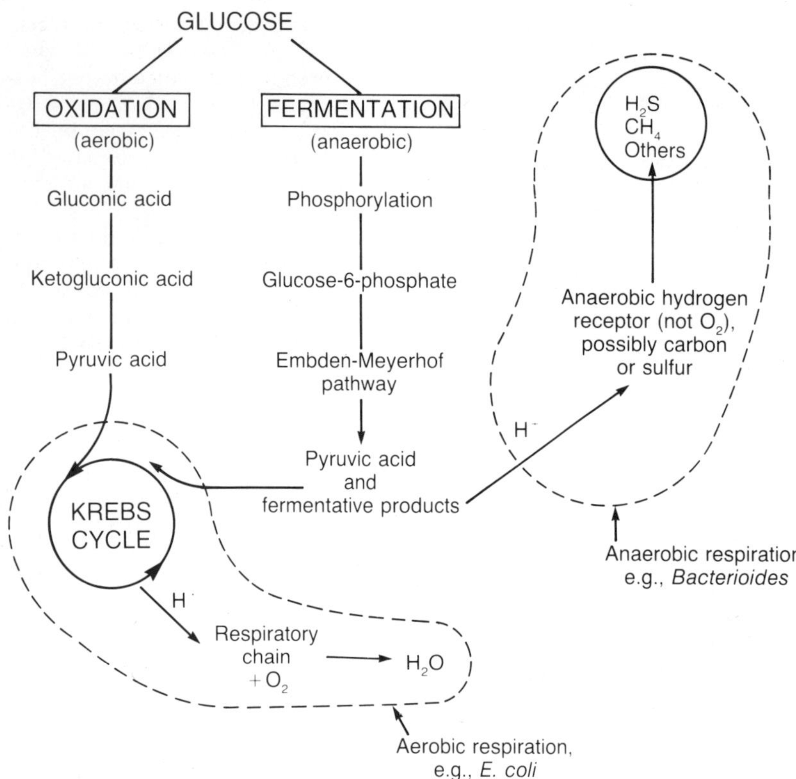

Figure 15–4 Bacterial metabolic systems: their relationship (simplified).

Practical Applications

Bacterial metabolism is a large subject and one not without some fascination, since the parallels between the metabolism of bacteria and that of higher life forms are very close if one excludes some specific and unique adaptations, e.g., nitrogen fixation by azobacteria and carbohydrate formation from CO_2 in photosynthesis. In medical bacteriology, the extracellular enzymes produced by different species are very important in differentiation. Whether an organism can survive in a particular medium may be decided by whether it needs some particular substrate; for example, *Haemophilus* species need X and V factors (hemin and NAD). Assimilation of carbon in the form of citrate is unacceptable to some of the Enterobacteriaceae, such as *E. coli,* but acceptable to others, such as the klebsiellae. A very basic division of organisms is by their mode of respiration—whether aerobic or anaerobic—and whether organisms attack carbohydrates by fermentation or oxidation. Some organisms are so specific in their metabolic requirements that they are unable to accommodate themselves to any artificial environment and can survive only within a parasitized cell—e.g., the viruses, rickettsiae, and chlamydiae.

BACTERIAL GENETICS

Like all other forms of life (with the exception of some viruses, which have RNA as their genetic material), bacteria have DNA as the repository of their inheritance and as the coordinator of their cellular activity. In *E. coli,* a typical prokaryotic organism, the DNA is a singular circular chromosome arranged in a double helix and not confined within a nucleus. Its molecular weight is 2.8×10^{-9} g and it has 4.7×10^{6} nucleotide pairs; it is about 1.2 mm long.

MUTATIONS

The DNA of the bacterial cell is remarkably stable but because of the rapid replication of cells, the incidence of spontaneous mutation is measurable. The mutation rate can be increased by such stimuli as ultraviolet light, x-irradiation, nitrogen mustards, and alkylating agents. The mutations are caused by a substitution in the genetic code of one base pair by another, or by a deletion of a portion of the code carrying some gene(s).

Recognition of Mutation

Morphological. One of the commonest forms of mutation is seen in the change from smooth to rough colonies (S ---→ R), in which the organism loses its capsule. The reverse mutation (R ---→ S) can also occur, but is less frequent. The change S ---→ R is often associated with loss of virulence. Another morphological change that is easily recognizable is change of color or pigmentation.

Antigenicity. Loss of antigen is not uncommon, and is typified by the loss of motility of an organism, accompanied by loss of flagella. With the loss of flagella, flagellar antigen also is lost. Salmonellae (p. 378) often lose one antigenic type of flagellar antigen to gain another.

Loss of Enzymes. Biochemical mutations occur involving loss of enzymes and are revealed by an organism's inability to ferment carbohydrates or to grow on a usual medium.

Resistance to Antimicrobials. By means of the Lederberg replica plating method (Fig. 15–5), it can be shown that mutants resistant to antimicrobials arise spontaneously and not in response to challenge by the inhibitory agent. The organism is grown for a few hours on a simple nutrient agar. Subsequently a metal cylinder, slightly smaller than the Petri dish, wrapped in sterilized velveteen is pressed lightly on the growth. It is then pressed on a plate containing nutrient agar impregnated with antimicrobial. The threads of the cloth of the velveteen carry over organisms that appear in positions in the second plate that are identical to those in which they appeared in the first. Naturally, only resistant organisms will grow on the second plate. If positions coincident with these resistant colonies are subcultured from the first plate, it is found that these areas have a high proportion of resistant strains as compared with other areas of the same plate. Hence, resistant strains arise spontaneously without exposure to the antimicrobial.

Although mutations occur and alter the genetic code of the cell, the process of mutation does not involve exchange of genetic material. Transfer of such material may be accomplished in one of three ways.

TRANSFORMATION

Since this was the first type of genetic transfer to be elucidated in bacteria, it may be of interest to outline the steps in the discovery of the process. In 1928, Griffith injected mice with live nonencapsulated type 2 cells and with capsulated but killed type 3 cells. Some animals died of infection, and the causative organism was an encapsulated type 3 pneumococcus. It was realized at the time, of course, that something had been transferred from the dead type 3 pneumococci to the avirulent live type 2 pneumococci, making the latter virulent and type 3. It was not until 1944 that Avery, MacLeod, and McCarthy demonstrated that the substance responsible for the transformation was DNA. In the early 1950s the genetic importance of DNA was suspected, but not until 1953 did Watson and Crick publish their work on the structure of DNA. This discovery heralded the greatest biological advance since the time of Darwin and Mendel.

Cells able to be transformed are said to be competent. Such cells are able to accept and allow exogenous DNA to pass across the cell membrane. The stage of competence comes only at certain periods in the life of the bacterium. The DNA accepted must be at least 4×10^6 in molecular weight, and double-stranded DNA is accepted preferentially. Part of the donated DNA is incorporated permanently in the chromosome of the host. Only some organisms are capable of transformation, and these include the *Haemophilus, Bacillus, Streptococcus, Staphylococcus,* and *Neisseria* genera. Generally, transformation occurs between strains of the same species, but it also occurs between members of closely related species. The characteristics so transferred may be for capsular polysaccharides, drug resistance, and enzyme properties.

TRANSDUCTION

In this process, a portion of donor chromosome is carried by a temperate bacteriophage (see p. 482) to another organism. Temperate bacteriophage is a virus that usually lives symbiotically as part of host bacterial DNA and that replicates in synchrony with the host cell. When transduction occurs, the bacteriophage frees itself from the host DNA and carries part of the host DNA with it as it infects another bacterial cell. This portion of the donor chromosome may carry various recognizable traits such as carbohydrate fermentative enzymes, antigenic characteristics, and drug resistance. The process of transduction has been described as occurring in numerous gram-negative groups, e.g., *Salmonella, Escherichia, Shigella, Pseudomonas, Vibrio, Proteus,* and also among *Staphylococcus* and *Bacillus.*

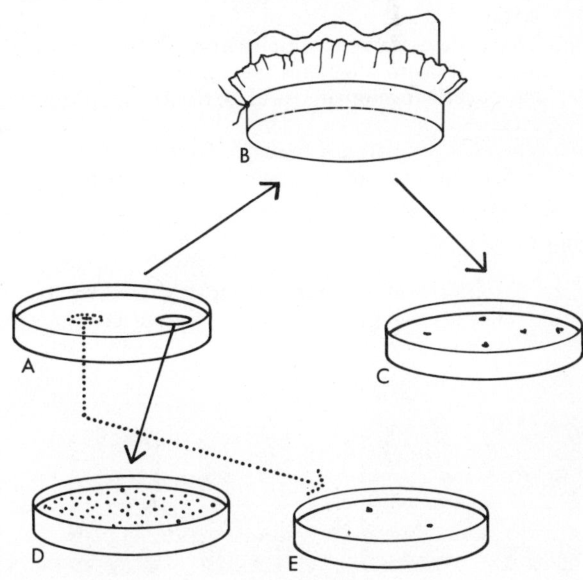

Figure 15–5 The Lederberg replica plating technique. Plate *A* has a growth of organisms on an antibiotic-free medium. In *B*, sterile velveteen is pressed on the growth, and subsequently on plate *C*, which has a medium impregnated with antibiotic. A few antibiotic-resistant colonies are able to grow on this medium. Subcultures from plate *A* in a position coincident with the site of resistant strains (as shown on plate *C*) to an antibiotic-impregnated plate *D* yield a larger number of resistant strains than subcultures from areas not coincident *(E)*.

Lysogeny

Here a temperate phage enters the cell and unites its DNA with that of the bacterial host. The phage may persist in the host DNA for many generations or even permanently, and this "inherited" phage is called prophage. While the phage is in lysogeny, the functions of the phage genes are repressed, although in some instances the presence of the lysogenized phage may be apparent. Such examples include the production of toxin by *C. diphtheriae,* which without the phage is nonpathogenic. The erythrogenic toxin in some strains of Group A streptococci is also produced by lysogenized phage. The otherwise hidden phage may be induced to reappear in its vegetative form by such stimuli as moderate ultraviolet irradiation. Then the phage genes replicate, producing phage packets and lysis of the bacterial cell. Spontaneous, i.e., noninduced, return of the prophage to the vegetative form is said to be a rare event.

Conjugation

This process was first described by Lederberg and Tatum in 1946, and differs from the foregoing genetic exchange mechanisms in several ways.

1. There is a transfer of genetic material across a cellular tube (F-pilus) between the mating bacteria. Bacterial contact or proximity is necessary.
2. Sexual differentiation between the bacteria is apparent, and donor and recipient varieties are identifed.
3. The amount of chromosome transferred is variable, and in some instances the entire genetic code of one bacterium is transported to another.

The donor or male cell has a "sex factor," which is of DNA. This conjugon may be integrated within the circular chromosome or may exist as a separate structure generally replicating in unison with the host DNA. The amount of DNA in the "sex factor" is approximately 2% of that of the host chromosome. If the "sex-factor" is attached to the host chromosome it may be called an episome; if it is free in the cytoplasm it may be called a plasmid. There are several known "sex factors:"

i. The F^+, which is the fertility factor carried by the male cells and the Hfr (high frequency recombinant) strains.
ii. The colicin factors, which carry DNA to code the preparation of colicins. Colicins are toxins produced by enteric organisms and toxic to nonparenteral strains.
iii. The RTF (resistance transfer factor), which carries resistance to antibiotic and chemotherapeutic agents.

The Fertility Factor, F^+

In a mixture of F^+ and F^- (lacking fertility factor) cells, there is passage of F^+ material across a conjugation bridge or F-pilus. The DNA of the plasmid replicates at about the same time as the formation of the conjugal bridge, and then one strand of replicated DNA assumes a linear shape and enters the F^- cell. The F^+ factor alone appears to cross the bridge in most cases, and only rarely does the F^+ take genetic material from the chromosome of the male cell. Within a relatively short period of time, all the cells in the mixture have F^+ material and thus are male. The lack of exchange of other material is illustrated by the fact that only relatively few of the new males (formerly females) involved in the mating will obtain recognizable genetic determinants from the original male cells. The general inability of the F^+ to carry material from the host chromosome may be owing to the fact that it is generally a plasmid and not attached to the chromosome. In those instances when it does carry some of the host chromosome, it may carry any segment of the circular structure. In this it differs from Hfr, to be described next, which is attached to specific segments of the chromosome and transfers certain features with more frequency than others.

The Hfr (High Frequency Recombinant)

These cells are also male, but in these the "sex factor" is attached to the host chromosome as an episome. In the transfer of material across the F-pilus, after replication in the male cell, the "sex factor" and the replicated host chromosome *both* commence to enter the F^- cell. The circular chromosome opens to form a linear structure at the insertion of the F^+, and the broken end furthest from the "sex factor" starts to enter the F^- cell first. Since complete transfer of the entire chromosome strand is unusual, the F^- cell does not generally receive the F^+ portion and thus remains female. However, it does receive replicated male DNA with its genetic message. With Hfr strains, there are about 1000 times as many exchanges of chromosomal material as occur in simple F^+F^- matings. Different Hfr strains have the F^+ factor inserted at different segments of the circular chromosome. Since the chromosome break before conjugation occurs at the insertion of F^+, with this knowledge, and by breaking conjugation bridges at different time lapses, it has been possible to make a genetic analysis of the circular chromosome of one organism, *E. coli*, strain K 12.

RTF (Resistance Transfer Factor)

This striking phenomenon of antimicrobial resistance that is spread by conjugation was first described in Japan in 1958. Like the fertility factor F^+, it is a plasmid and is spread in a manner identical to that of F^+. In addition to its academic interest, it is of great importance in medicine for the reasons outlined here.

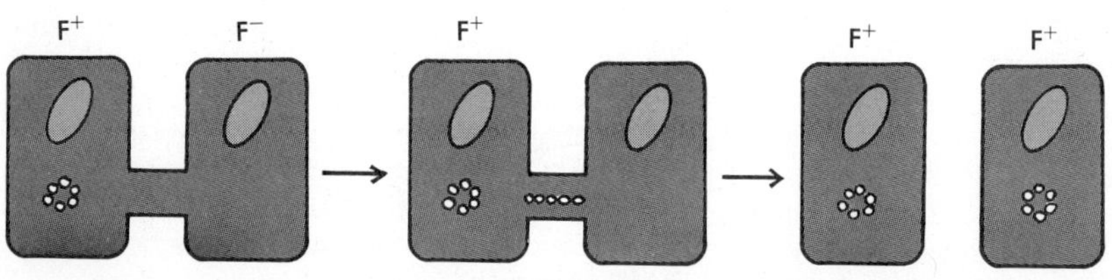

Figure 15–6 Conjugation (F^+, RTF, etc.). Here F^+ (fertility factor), a plasmid, replicates. The replicated material assumes an elongated form to cross the F-pilus. The recipient cell, F^-, receives the F^+ and itself becomes F^+, while the F-pilus involutes. The F^+ rarely carries any of the host chromosome with it. The process is essentially similar for transfer of RTF and colicins.

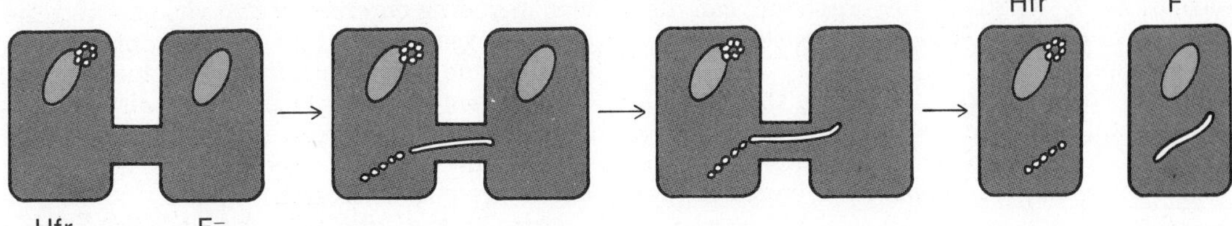

Figure 15–7 Conjugation (Hfr). Here the "sex factor" is Hfr (high frequency recombinant), and is an episome attached to the host chromosome. Replication of Hfr and the host chromosome occurs, and the newly formed strand breaks at the insertion of the Hfr. It subsequently crosses the F-pilus to the F^- cell, with the host chromosome leading. The F-pilus generally breaks before passage is complete, and thus the recipient cell obtains new genetic material but not the Hfr. Thus the recipient cell remains F^-, but its progeny may show varieties of genetic change.

1. The plasmid can be exchanged between members of different genera, e.g., from *E. coli* to salmonellae or shigellae and to other gram-negative bacilli. Antimicrobials have been used for many years in animal husbandry to increase livestock weight, and in these animals the incidence of organisms with RTF is high. It can be spread to humans via milk or meat and can of course be transferred at some point to virulent organisms.

2. Conjugation is an efficient mechanism, and the RTF so transferred may carry many genes of resistance to different antimicrobials. Among these are ampicillin, streptomycin, tetracycline, sulfonamide, chloramphenicol, neomycin, and nalidixic acid. RTF may carry resistance characteristics against one or more of these substances in varied combinations.

A cell carrying F^+ will not accept RTF, and a cell carrying an identical RTF plasmid will not accept further RTF. However, since there are varieties of RTF, these are interchangeable. With *E. coli* as donor, *Klebsiella, Enterobacter, Salmonella,* and *Shigella* are good recipients, whereas *Proteus, Pasteurella,* and *Serratia* are poor ones.

Penicillinase-producing plasmids of *Staphylococcus* differ from RTF in that they are spread by transduction and not by conjugation.

A detailed discussion of the mechanisms of bacterial resistance to antimicrobials will be found on p. 430 ff.

Bacterial Tests for Carcinogens

It does not seem out of place here to illustrate one of the effective practical applications of the knowledge of bacterial genetics. The widespread use of chemical and physical agents in our environment has caused considerable concern, especially as regards their carcinogenic properties. It appears that some of the carcinogens, e.g., asbestos, may take as long as 20 years to show their effect. Hence, the rapidly dividing bacterial cell and the large bacterial population that is easily manageable provide an effective biological amplifier to a process, carcinogenesis, which is essentially initiated by unrepaired damage to the chromosome DNA. Since the basic structure of human and bacterial DNA is identical, the results of bacterial DNA damage by specific agents may indicate their carcinogenicity. Indeed the Ames test has proved positive when used with 90% of known carcinogens.

Briefly, in the classic Ames test, a mutant *Salmonella typhimurium*, which is unable to manufacture an enzyme to manufacture histidine, is incubated with the test material and a rat liver extract. The latter is used in case the suspected carcinogen is actually a metabolite of the test material, in which case the liver will possibly uncover the true carcinogen. Subsequently the organisms are plated on a solid medium lacking histidine, on which normally they would not grow. If colonies appear after adequate incubation, the suspected substance is very likely carcinogenic, since a histidine-producing mutation has occurred.

Another variation of this test is to use lysogenic *E. coli*. If the DNA of the bacterium is prevented from replicating adequately, the dormant phage is induced, reverts to its vegetative form, and lyzes the cell. This accounts for the appearance on the solid medium of colonies that demonstrate lytic plaques if the test material is carcinogenic.

INDIGENOUS BODY FLORA

The primary function of the microbiologist in the clinical laboratory is to identify pathogenic organisms from clinical specimens. Although at times this identification is easy, there are many times when the decision of pathogenicity is by no means easy or clear cut. The problem lies in the fact that relatively few organisms per se are always pathogenic. Such organisms as *M. tuberculosis, N. gonorrhoeae,* and *S. typhi* immediately come to mind. If these are identified in any specimen, they can be regarded as pathogenic, although even among these organisms *S. typhi* may produce no disease in a carrier and may be merely a potential pathogen to persons with whom the carrier may come into contact. If the specimen comes from a normally sterile area, e.g., the cerebrospinal fluid or blood, and an organism is cultured, then it is most likely pathogenic, although even here one must be certain that the specimen was collected and processed properly. The examples of the "permanent pathogen" and the "permanent sterile area" are at the two extremes of the questions posed to the microbiologist. More frequently, his questions concern the specimen from the nonsterile area (throat, vagina, sputum), in which there normally is a population of bacteria. On occasion these bacteria are normal inhabitants, and on other occasions they are disease-producing. In other words, a large proportion of the organisms that we isolate are at best potentially pathogenic, and the line between commensal and pathogen is not always intrinsic to the organism.

The decision as to whether the organism can be considered as part of normal flora or as a pathogen can be helped immeasurably by:

1. An adequate clinical history, including the clinical suggestions of the attending physician.
2. A specimen taken in a manner most likely to yield microbiological information and swiftly delivered to the laboratory.
3. A specimen that, on receipt by the laboratory, is examined expeditiously and in a fashion designed to yield the maximum amount of information directed toward the clinical problem.

Koch's Postulates

Academically, the progress of bacteriology as a clinical science was much aided by the demand that reported putative pathogens meet Koch's postulates. Briefly, these stated that:

1. The organism must be found in every case of the disease.
2. The organism must not be found in a healthy person.
3. It must be isolated and grown in pure culture.
4. Inoculation into an animal should reproduce the disease, and the organism should be recoverable from the animal.

Since Koch's time, it has been found impossible to satisfy these postulates in all microbiological disease. For example, *M. leprae* cannot be artificially cultured; healthy carriers may carry virulent bacteria; and some human disease cannot be reproduced in animals.

A fifth postulate has been added:

5. Infection will produce circulating antibodies specific for the infecting organism.

Even this postulate is not absolute, since cross-reactions do occur, for example, between *Br. abortus* and *Fr. tularensis*, as well as remote reactions such as the stimulation of antibodies to species of *Proteus* by typhus organisms.

With all their exceptions, the postulates remain as a yardstick by which to measure the pathogenicity of an organism. However, in the usual clinical bacteriology situation, we must accept the circumstance as the patient and the physician present it, and we cannot possibly make a decision based on the academic (and lengthy) methods of Koch's postulates. We must depend on education, technique, and experience at nearly every juncture.

Normal Flora

Regions and Specimens That Are Normally Free of Bacteria

These include the cerebrospinal fluid, blood, joints, the body cavities (pleura, peritoneum, pericardium), the lower respiratory tract, and the gallbladder. The stomach and duodenum are sterile except when food recently has been ingested. The kidneys, ureters, urinary bladder, and urethra normally are sterile, as is the middle ear.

Regions and Specimens That Normally Contain Bacteria

The skin normally supports the growth of *Staph. albus;* corynebacteria spp.; some varieties of *Streptococcus*, including enterococci and viridans varieties; as well as some yeast-like fungi. Even *Staph. aureus, Str. pyogenes*, and some dermatophytes have been found on skin without the presence of overt disease. Also present here are anaerobic organisms such as *Propionibacterium acnes* and *Clostridium perfringens*. Species of *Acinetobacter* are not uncommon.

Usually, the external auditory canal has a flora similar to that of the skin, but *Str. pneumoniae* and various gram-negative coliform rods more commonly are noted here. Despite the lysozyme in tears, the conjunctiva has a scanty flora of staphylococci, *Str. viridans,* and corynebacteria. Other organisms, including *H. influenzae*, yeast-like fungi, and coliform organisms, also are found here.

In the mouth, a vast number of organisms are present (calculated as 15×10^7 per mL of saliva). These include staphylococci, streptococci (some of Group A), pneumococci, lactobacilli, actinomyces, coliform gram-negative rods, fusobacteria, *Bacteroides* spp., the genus *Veillonella, Borrelia* spp., and yeast-like fungi. Included among the viridans streptococci here are *Str. mutans* and *Str. sanguis*, which are of great importance in the etiology of dental caries and which are always present in the mouth. Anaerobic streptococci are also very usual. *Actinomyces israelii*, which, when invasive, is the cause of debilitating disease, is commonly present in the mouth as part of the normal flora.

The throat has a flora similar to that of the mouth. The nasal passages generally support staphylococci and occasionally pneumococci and meningococci. The sputum coming from the lower respiratory tract should be sterile, but in its passage through the upper part of the tract and the mouth it becomes contaminated by the normal flora of those areas. *Haemophilus influenzae* and *parainfluenzae* are frequently present here. Viridans streptococci, by their presence, are inhibitory to colonization by Group A streptococci, pneumococci, *Staph. aureus*, and the Enterobacteriaceae.

The large bowel supports the growth of a large number of organisms (approximately 10^{12} per g of wet feces), the majority of which are anaerobes of the genus *Bacteroides*. In addition, enterococci, anaerobic streptococci, lactobacilli, members of the family Enterobacteriaceae, viridans streptococci, corynebacteria, *Clostridia* spp., actinomyces, staphylococci, yeast-like fungi, and a number of protozoa (including *Giardia*) normally live in this area.

The vagina in the biologically mature woman supports the growth of many lactobacilli, as well as staphylococci, enterococci, viridans streptococci, corynebacteria, some of the Enterobacteriaceae, *Acinetobacter* spp., *Clostridia* spp., and yeast-like fungi. Also present are many anaerobic gram-positive cocci. *Bacteroides* species may also be present normally.

The Significance of Normal Flora in Health

It has been possible to raise animals that are germ-free (gnobiotic), and with these it has been proven that the intestinal flora aid in the host's metabolism by the production of various B vitamins and of vitamin K. Some substances normally indigestible by the host, e.g., cellulose, may be digested by the indigenous bacteria.

Lymphoid tissue in germ-free animals is diminished

in bulk, and the serum globulin, in which antibodies generally are found, is decreased in these animals. When challenged with living organisms living commensally in normal animals of the same species, they become severely ill and may die. All this indicates that the indigenous bacteria normally evoke immunity to themselves. In turn, this may play some part in protection against that organism should it become pathogenic: for example *E. coli*, which is generally harmless in the bowel, is a common pathogen in urinary tract infections. Furthermore, the immunity to normal flora may be protective against another organism with which they share some antigenic determinants. An example of this, as shown by the Widal reaction, is the normal presence of antibodies to such organisms as *S. typhi*, with which the patient has not come into contact. Presumably the antibodies are to some antigenic component of normal bacterial flora shared in part by the pathogenic typhoid organism.

An indigenous population may have some method of protection against displacement by another population that may not be so harmless to the host. Colicins are produced by some enteric organisms that are lethal to other varieties of enteric organisms and some to *Candida*. The indiscrete use of antibiotics that kill indigenous organisms often is followed by their replacement by *Candida*. In the bowel, antibiotic-induced changes in the fecal bacterial population encourage the growth of *Clostridium difficile* with the production of an endotoxin that damages the colonic mucosa and clinically gives rise to pseudomembranous enterocolitis. Colonization of an area such as the umbilical stump by *Staph. aureus* has been observed to prevent umbilical sepsis with *Pseudomonas*.

The Significance of Normal Flora in Disease

A glance at the list of organisms that normally are present at various sites will indicate that many of these are potential pathogens. Occasionally, they become obviously pathogenic, although their reasons for doing so are host related rather than owing to any change in the organism. Well-known but poorly understood examples of such a change are seen in actinomycosis, Vincent's angina (caused by *F. necrophorum* and a spirochete), recurrent herpes simplex, and herpes zoster. Meleney's progressive synergistic gangrene is an example of a mixed infection of anaerobic cocci with *Staph. aureus* or *Str. pyogenes*. Neither organism can produce the spreading gangrene that generally occurs postoperatively from an abdominal wound, but together they produce this startlingly aggressive and dangerous rapid necrosis and ulceration of tissue.

Some changes in the host are fairly obvious; in diabetes, *Candida* infections are more common, and in diabetic ketosis the generally nonpathogenic fungi of the Phycomycetes group may invade the palate and tissues at the base of the skull. Subacute bacterial endocarditis owing to *Str. viridans* occurs when this otherwise harmless mouth commensal enters the blood and proliferates on an abnormal cardiac valve or shunt. In cystic fibrosis, among other abnormalities, respiratory mucus is of increased viscosity and causes difficulty in expectoration, with consequent recurrent respiratory infection. This infection is a major cause of death in many patients with cystic fibrosis, and they appear especially liable to infection by *Staph. aureus* and *Ps. aeruginosa*. The example of candidiasis after antibiotic therapy has already been alluded to; perhaps the most dramatic iatrogenic infections are seen with immunosuppressive or steroid therapy when infections with *Aspergillus, Nocardia*, and *Pneumocystis carinii* may arise as well as generalized cytomegalovirus disease. Infections with *Ps. aeruginosa* also are increased with these drugs. Admittedly, some of these organisms are not considered normal commensals of the body; however, the increased incidence of disease caused by these organisms, evoked by immunosuppressive measures, indicates that the normal immunological mechanisms of the body usually prevent pathogenicity by such of these organisms as may be present. Drugs that cause agranulocytosis or neutropenia also may lead to severe infections by organisms that usually are tolerated. Absence of the spleen occurs in some patients either as a simple congenital abnormality or in association with abnormalities in the location of viscera (Ivemark's syndrome). Such a condition may be suspected by the appearance in the peripheral blood of many normoblasts and schistocytes. Some patients with sickle cell anemia have functional asplenia due to numerous splenic infarcts, and others have undergone splenectomy by surgery. All such patients have an increased liability to overwhelming infection by pneumococci or salmonellae. Transplant surgery (kidney, marrow, heart) involves much and lengthy immunosuppression, bringing with it the danger of opportunistic infection. Congenital deficiencies of complement factors C3 and C5 have been reported to produce inability to counter some bacterial infections.

In the course of diseases such as leukemia, lymphoma, and other malignant diseases there is again an increased incidence of aspergillosis, histoplasmosis, cryptococcosis, nocardiosis, and pneumocystosis. Infections with organisms of generally low virulence, e.g., *Serratia, Clostridia* spp., and *Ps. aeruginosa* are increased in frequency, and there is often an abnormal response to otherwise mild viral infections, e.g., measles and varicella.

Similar situations with decreased resistance and thus apparent increased virulence by microorganisms arise in those afflicted with congenital abnormalities of the immune system or granulocyte abnormalities such as Chédiak-Higashi syndrome or chronic granulomatous disease of childhood.

Patients with autoimmune disease such as rheumatoid arthritis, SLE, or Sjögren's disease are more liable to infections with organisms that are generally of low pathogenicity.

A breach of normal defenses, such as is met with following urethral or venous catheterization or in the placement of a cardiac valve prosthesis will allow entry of organisms of low pathogenicity that will cause disease. Obstruction of a duct, channel, or tract, such as in intestinal, bronchial, urinary, or biliary obstruction, will, in time, allow organisms that would normally be kept under control by natural phagocytic and immune mechanisms to proliferate and cause disease. The same situation occurs on the body surface in cases of skin injury, especially by burns.

Age reduces protection against infection, and many elderly patients succumb to bronchopneumonia in which normally commensal upper respiratory flora invade the lower part of the respiratory tract. The newborn also has little resistance to *E. coli* infections, presumably because the maternal IgM antibodies to this organism are unable to cross the placental barrier. In the case of the elderly, the mechanism of breakdown of normal defenses is less clear.

Those diseases that present in persons with some debilitating condition that allows or encourages infections with commensal or uncommonly pathogenic organisms are said to be caused by "opportunistic" organisms.

This admittedly brief survey indicates the difficulty in some instances of assessing the significance of an isolated organism without an adequate knowledge of the clinical status of the patient. It also indicates how narrow and, indeed, nonexistent, the line between pathogenic and nonpathogenic or virulent and nonvirulent can be.

Nosocomial Infections

It is not generally realized that about 5% of the patients admitted to hospitals in North America present an infection during their stay that was not present on admission. Many of these are opportunistic infections or are closely related, e.g., urinary tract infections subsequent to catheterization, or infections related to malignant disease or transplantation that may occur in a host compromised by disease (cancer, diabetes, etc.) or by therapy (steroids, antimicrobials, antineoplastic drugs). Urinary tract infections are commonest in this group (33 to 50% of nosocomial infections), followed by respiratory tract (20 to 25%), skin and wound (20%), and miscellaneous infections, including gastroenteritis, infections associated with intravenous therapy or prosthetic joints or valves, hepatitis, and bacteremia. The cost of such infections in the United States has been put at one billion dollars annually.

To some extent nosocomial infections are preventable, and all hospitals have programs that have prevention as their major function. Besides surveillance of all infections, the programs supervise operating room sterility, isolation of the infectious and the dangerously vulnerable (e.g., transplant patients), pre-employment infection examination for hospital personnel, and other functions. Their work brings them in close relationship with the bacteriology laboratory.

Pathogenicity and Virulence

Having illustrated some of the changes in the host that contribute to disease, it may be worthwhile to consider those features of microorganisms that are known to be instrumental in their disease-producing potential.

Pathogenicity refers to the potential of the group of organisms for causing disease, without any specification of conditions. Hence, *Cl. perfringens* is pathogenic, although in the bowel it generally behaves as a harmless commensal. *Mycobacterium smegmatis* is a nonpathogen, since it does not produce disease under any circumstances. Many organisms can be regarded as showing low-grade pathogenicity, indicating that most often they are not disease producing, but given special conditions they may produce disease, as in the case of *Str. viridans.*

Virulence is defined as the degree of pathogenicity under specified conditions in a given host of a given strain of the organism. The organism owes its virulence to three major factors: invasiveness, production of extracellular enzymes, and toxogenicity.

The terms *virulence* and *pathogenicity* are often used loosely, but it will be appreciated that when used precisely, virulence becomes an almost measurable property, whereas pathogenicity is a much more general description.

Invasiveness

Many of the features of invasion are little understood. It would appear that most organisms enter the body through some breach in the integumentary epithelium, although salmonellae and shigellae have been shown to penetrate the intact bowel mucosa. The spread of organisms is more a host-regulated matter than it is dependent upon the microorganism, but *T. pallidum* spreads very rapidly to regional lymph nodes. Unlike many organisms, *Actinomyces israelii* tends to cross tissue planes. Some organisms, e.g., streptococci and staphylococci, produce leukocidin, which destroys phagocytes and thus weighs the scales in favor of the invading organism. Some organisms use phagocytosis as a means to invasion, e.g., *M. tuberculosis, S. typhi, Brucella* spp., and *L. monocytogenes.* These often remain viable in macrophages and are carried from the site of entry to a distant site to proliferate. Capsules often help the organism to resist phagocytosis, e.g., pneumococci, *Klebsiella* spp., and *H. influenzae*, whereas avirulent strains may be without capsular protection. The M protein of *Str. pyogenes* appears to act like a capsule in this organism in inhibiting phagocytosis.

Extracellular Enzymes

Some bacteria (streptococci, staphylococci, pneumococci, and clostridia) produce hyaluronidase, which depolymerizes hyaluronic acid. Hyaluronic acid is the ground substance of connective tissue. Destruction of the hyaluronic acid theoretically aids the diffusion of the organism in the tissues, but its importance in spontaneous disease is less clearcut than it is in experimental infections. Streptokinase produced by streptococci and staphylococci digests fibrin clots and renders fibrinogen incoagulable, aiding bacterial dissemination. Proteolytic enzymes, including collagenase, are produced by species of *Clostridium* and assist in their spread. It seems unlikely that coagulase contributes to the virulence of staphylococci.

Toxogenicity

Toxic substances formed by bacteria may be considered as exotoxins and endotoxins. Exotoxins usually are associated with gram-positive organisms, and endotoxins with gram-negative bacteria.

Leukocidins, coagulase, hyaluronidase, and so forth can be regarded as exotoxins, but will be considered under other headings, since their actions can best be explained there.

TABLE 15–2 DIFFERENCES BETWEEN BACTERIAL ENDOTOXINS AND EXOTOXINS

	Endotoxins	Exotoxins
Organisms producing	Gram-negative	Gram-positive (but *B. pertussis* and *Sh. dysenteriae*)
Origin	Components of cell wall	Secreted by cell
Effect of heat	Heat stable	Generally heat labile
Effect of antibody	Partial, if any	Neutralized
Toxoids	Not formed	Formed
Pathological effect	All are similar	Specific (i.e., on bowel, skin, etc.)
Toxicity	Relatively weakly toxic	Generally highly toxic
Composition	Liposaccharide and conjugated protein	Protein

The differences between endotoxins and exotoxins can be seen in Table 15–2. The exotoxins produced by various organisms can best be discussed individually. All are protein in nature.

Endotoxins

These are components of the cell wall of many gram-negative organisms (e.g., *E. coli, S. typhi, N. meningitidis*) liberated by cell lysis (see p. 356). The organisms may enter the circulation in a number of ways, but many enter following urinary tract or venous catheterization. Some enter during the course of such disease as diverticulitis or mesenteric artery thrombosis, ascending cholangitis, after septic abortion, following extensive burns, and also in the course of typhoid and meningococcal septicemia. In addition to the signs and symptoms of the primary condition, the toxemia will produce fever with chills, and in a severe case, signs of shock. The patient may have gram-negative sepsis as well as toxemia. The shock is caused by the endotoxin's acting on some intermediary in blood or tissues, resulting in the vascular changes of shock with attendent acidosis, relative hypovolemia, and oliguria. In addition, there is disseminated intravascular coagulation (DIC), with depletion of clotting factors and resulting bleeding into the tissues, including the lung. In DIC, various clotting mechanisms are altered (see Chap. 31), and this has been well shown in meningococcemia. Classically in meningococcemia, but in other forms of gram-negative toxemia as well, there is adrenal cortical hemorrhage and necrosis. This adrenal destruction is part of the Waterhouse-Friderichsen syndrome, and its etiology is possibly the thrombosis of small adrenal blood vessels caused by the toxemic-triggered DIC or by the Shwartzman phenomenon.

RECOGNITION OF ABNORMAL FLORA

After reading this chapter for the first time, the student may well be concerned that, considering the remarkable ubiquity of bacteria, he or she will have difficulty in recognizing pathogens. To a large extent his or her success will depend on careful technique and experience, as well as on knowledge of bacterial disease. However, there are a few generalizations that may be helpful.

1. It is essential to obtain a good specimen from the right site, taken in the correct fashion, and delivered to the laboratory with a minimum of delay.
2. The specimen should be accompanied by some pertinent clinical data and by a note as to the clinical opinion of the attending physician.
3. Gross examination and microscopy often may help. Pus usually means infection (but not in sputum or in material from the vagina). The organism may be seen in a comparatively diagnostic pattern, e.g., *Candida* with pseudohyphae in thrush, or chains of streptococci in pus, or gram-negative rods accompanied by pus cells in freshly passed urine.
4. As noted previously, bacteria grown from a normally sterile site are regarded as pathogens until proven otherwise.
5. Cultures from normally nonsterile sites should be examined as to whether they include unusual bacteria, and many techniques are fashioned to bring these alien bacteria into prominence. A knowledge of the clinical problem may suggest the possible pathogenic organism in these cases. It is far easier to look for some particular organism than to screen in a routine fashion; for example, *H. influenzae* should be diligently searched for in epiglottitis, *N. gonorrhoeae* in many cervical swabs, *S. schenkii* is a possibility in chronic ulceration of the finger with lymphangitis, and so forth.
6. Cultures from nonsterile sites are naturally mixed. Thus, pure primary cultures should be regarded with suspicion. Conversely, mixed cultures from usually sterile sites raise the possibility of contamination. Generally, for example, in urine, a growth of 3 or more varieties of bacteria is accepted as evidence of contamination, and repeat examination is requested.
7. Occasionally, the organism itself is undoubtedly virulent, e.g., *M. tuberculosis, N. gonorrhoeae*, etc.
8. β-Hemolytic colonies should be viewed with suspicion, although they are not necessarily those of disease-producing organisms, e.g., *E. coli* in stool culture. However, the generalization is worthwhile.
9. Bacterial counts may be performed. Because of clinical experience, a certain level, e.g., 10^5 per mL in urine, is regarded as indicative of infection in the genitourinary tract. Such methods are also applied to environmental bacteriology (e.g., bacterial counts in water and milk). Similarly, in sputum, a Gram-stained specimen with a ratio of less than 25 polymorphs to more than 10 epithelial cells, when examined under the $\times 10$ objective, is rejected as having excessive oropharyngeal contamination.

10. When in doubt, the patient's serum can be examined to see if antibodies to the suspected organism are present. A rising titer would be significant. Occasionally, the patient's titer against the organism may be compared with a panel of sera available from patients with dissimilar disease.

11. In patients with inadequate or breached immune defenses, the rules change. Here, many organisms generally regarded as nonpathogenic are viewed with suspicion. For example, coagulase-negative staphylococci may cause endocarditis in those with prosthetic heart valves; aspergillosis is fatal in many patients with acute leukemia; normal anaerobic mouth flora become invasive and dangerous in those with severe leukopenia.

CHAPTER 15—REVIEW QUESTIONS

1. Explain the terms *peritrichous* and *polar flagella*. Name four genera that have polar flagella, four genera with peritrichous flagella, and four genera without flagella.
2. What organisms commonly cause infectious complications in (a) diabetes, (b) cystic fibrosis, (c) asplenia? Where do these infections occur?
3. What are the three major factors in virulence in an organism? Give examples of each factor with reference to a particular microorganism.
4. Describe four criteria that would lead you to believe that the organism you have isolated from a specimen is probably pathogenic.

AN INTRODUCTION TO SYSTEMATIC BACTERIOLOGY: THE GRAM-POSITIVE AND GRAM-NEGATIVE COCCI

INTRODUCTION

There are very few routine methods of investigation in a bacteriology laboratory. Admittedly, specimens such as swabs, feces, or urine may be treated in a routine fashion when received, but the manipulation of bacterial colonies obtained and their exact identification depend to a large extent on the application of the technologist's knowledge of academic bacteriology.

To give a simple example, a wound swab that shows few or rare pus cells and plump, gram-positive rods suggests the possibility of an anaerobic infection and thus indicates the need for particular attention to anaerobic culture. In another instance, although a few colonies of pneumococci in a throat swab culture have little significance, their presence in a culture made from fluid taken from a joint would be very significant. Thus, the bacteriology technologist must have a good knowledge of bacteriology and a basic understanding of disease etiology to guide his use of techniques and to help him to interpret his findings.

There is a great deal of information available on the behavior of bacteria, and much of it is based on observation—for example, whether or not a sugar is fermented. Although the cause of an observed change may be known, the result cannot be deduced but has to be memorized. Fermentation of sugars by bacteria results from the possession by the bacteria of specific enzymes that enable them to decompose the carbohydrate. Other enzymes decompose protein, with production of amino acids and indole. Some bacteria have enzymes with highly specific actions, such as urease, which breaks down urea.

Other facts about groups of bacteria also have to be memorized. However, many of these facts are not necessarily of diagnostic importance. For example, virtually all the organisms in the Enterobacteriaceae family ferment glucose, and thus this observation is of little value diagnostically as compared to observation of lactose media, since lactose is generally not fermented by salmonellae and shigellae. On the other hand, the reaction to Gram's stain and morphology are important diagnostic factors in any bacterial examination.

The Differentiation of Organisms

The bacteriologist is striving to obtain from the specimen a growth of a species of organism that may be responsible for the patient's illness. To that end, employing a knowledge of pathology, specimens are taken in a particular way, transported with necessary care, and inoculated on suitable media to give every advantage to the uncovering of possible pathogens. After suitable incubation, the organism may be recognized or partially identified by its colonial appearance, an odor, its reaction with some component in the medium, an antimicrobial pattern, morphology, serology, and so forth. Much will depend, especially in the Enterobacteriaceae family, on its biochemical reactions. Here, although species are considered homogeneous, there are variations in the biochemical reactions of strains within the same species just as there are some differences in serology, pigmentation, and so forth, but these latter properties are not so easily measurable.

Biochemically, a reaction may usually be regarded as positive or negative. Within a species, perhaps 90% of the strains are positive. If only 50% of the strains are positive for a particular reaction it is not a very useful characteristic, although if less than 10% are positive it is regarded as negative and becomes a more useful parameter. Tables of the percentage of strains of a species that react positively, negatively, or late with a variety of reagents are available in larger works. However, one cannot practice bacteriology entirely by tables, and some facts must be memorized. To help in this regard, it is usual to adopt some convention of signs to indicate biochemical reactions, and the following are used:

+	90% are positive in 1 to 2 days
−	< 10% are positive in 1 to 2 days
(+)	a delayed + reaction occurs in 3 or 4 days
+/−	*most* strains are + and fewer are −
d	differing reactions without specificity
$+^w$	weakly positive

It is worth trying to remember very specific reactions, e.g., the coagulase + reaction of *S. aureus*, or the phenylalanine deaminase reaction of the *Proteeae*, or the nonmotility of *Shigella*. With other and biochemical tests one can try to remember important majority reactions. As an example of the latter, 99% of *E. coli* produce indole, but only 2% *P. mirabilis* do so. Although there is an error in considering *E. coli* + and *P. mirabilis* −, the statement is generally true, and in the small minority of unusual strains the errors are corrected by consideration of other parameters. For example here if an indole + *P. mirabilis* was mistakenly considered as *E. coli*, the production of phenylalanine deaminase (99% + in *P. mirabilis*) would soon correct the misapprehension. Even so, there is a theoretical possibility that 2% of 1% of strains of *P. mirabilis* (= 0.02%) would be indole + and phenylalanine deaminase −. This is a remote possibility and would be further ruled out by mannitol fermentation (97% + *E. coli* and 0% + *P. mirabilis*), in which only a very remarkable strain would remain problematical.

Thus, it can be seen that a knowledge of majority reactions can be extremely useful and that use of a few discriminative tests may easily differentiate between related species.

THE GRAM-POSITIVE AEROBIC COCCI

The family Micrococcaceae are characterized as spherical gram-positive cells that are aerobic (or facultatively anaerobic) and that divide to form regular or irregular clusters or packets. The family includes the medically important genus *Staphylococcus* and a less important family, *Micrococcus*. They are nonmotile, nonspore forming, and nonencapsulated.

MICROCOCCUS

These gram-positive cocci are found in soil and water as well as on the skin. They are nonpathogenic and are generally differentiated from Staphylococci in that they form small pockets of tetrads or cubical arrangements of cocci and fail to ferment glucose anaerobically, whereas staphylococci will ferment this carbohydrate. Colonies appear more slowly than do those of staphylococci.

STAPHYLOCOCCUS

Organisms in this genus include the very important pathogenic species *S. aureus*. Two other species, *S. epidermis* and *S. saprophyticus*, are generally nonpathogens (but see below). Three further species, *S. hominis, S. haemolyticus,* and *S. simulans*, have recently been described in this latter group.

The bacteria grow well on blood agar and on selective media such as phenylethyl alcohol agar, which inhibits gram-negative organisms. Most strains will grow in the presence of 15% NaCl or 40% bile. Colonies on blood appear overnight at 35°C and are 1 to 3 mm, shiny, circular, entire, and convex. They often show pigment, which may be white, gold, or yellow, and they may show hemolysis.

The most important test in their differentiation is the coagulase test. *Coagulase* is an enzyme produced by *S. aureus* that reacts with prothrombin, or with a prothrombin derivative in plasma that is similar to thrombin, and converts fibrinogen to fibrin. Human plasma is often used, but citrated or EDTA-treated rabbit plasma is preferable (lyophilized plasma is commercially available). The coagulase test may be conducted in two ways. A *slide test*, which detects coagulase bound to the bacterial cells, is quick, but false negative results occur, so a negative result must be checked by the more lengthy but more accurate tube test. For the slide test, a heavy suspension of bacteria is made in distilled water on a slide to which a drop of plasma is added. Within 10 seconds, if the test is positive, the bacteria will clump together. False positive results may appear if the reaction is allowed to extend for a period longer than 10 seconds or if the colonies of organisms used are taken from a higher salt concentration medium.

The *tube test* employs 0.1 mL of an overnight culture in brain-heart infusion broth with 0.5 mL of plasma in a tube incubated at 37°C in a water bath for 4 hours. Any degree of clotting within the allotted time is considered positive.

An agar method that incorporates coagulase plasma in an agar base has also been used.* After incubation, which may be up to 72 hours, opaque zones appear around coagulase-producing colonies.

S. aureus usually ferments mannitol, produces phosphatase, and liquefies gelatin, but such tests are not widely employed or necessary. In the differentiation of the important species of *Staphylococcus,* the following may be helpful.

	S. aureus	S. epidermidis	S. saprophyticus
Coagulase	+	−	−
D-Mannitol	+	−	− or $+^{w}$
Phosphatase	+	+	− or $+^{w}$
Novobiocin	S	S	R

S, sensitive; R, resistant.

The novobiocin resistance test may be with a 5 μg susceptibility disc on a P agar plate freshly inoculated with the organism (P agar is a simple nutrient peptone agar with 5 g NaCl/liter). *S. saprophyticus* shows 1 to 5 mm inhibition from the disc margin. The procedure for production of phosphatase is to be found in larger texts.

Often it is desirable to distinguish streptococcal colonies on plates, and this is most easily done by the *catalase* test. Staphylococci are positive, but streptococci are negative. A slide test is convenient, and here a colony is emulsified in one drop of 30% H_2O_2. An immediate effervescence indicates a positive test. Caution is necessary if the colony is taken from blood agar plates, since blood cells, if transferred with the colony, will produce a false positive result. It is also best to use a nichrome loop, since platinum may also produce a false positive reaction. In addition, a very rare streptococcus may produce catalase, and a more specific test is a benzidine test. *Staphylococcus* has the cytochrome oxidase giving a positive result, whereas streptococci are negative.

S. aureus produces other extracellular enzymes that may not be important in diagnostic bacteriology but may be of considerable significance in the pathogenesis of staphylococcal disease. Among these are a number of hemolysins (α, β, γ, and δ), a leukocidin, an exfoliatin, and an enterotoxin.

In epidemiological investigations, it may be desirable to identify a particular type of *Staphylococcus aureus* as the cause of some epidemic, such as staphylococcal wound contamination. This is best done by phage typing (p. 482) and is done by central reference laboratories.

Pathology

Staphylococci cause many skin infections (boils, carbuncles, and furunculosis) and in addition infect wounds and burns. Osteomyelitis and breast abscess are commonly staphylococcal. Staphylococcal food poisoning is due to the enterotoxin. Typically, nausea, vomiting, and diarrhea commence 2 to 6 hours after ingestion of food in which *S. aureus* elaborated the toxin. Typically such

*Baltimore Biological Laboratory, P.O. Box 243, Cockeysville, Md. 21030.

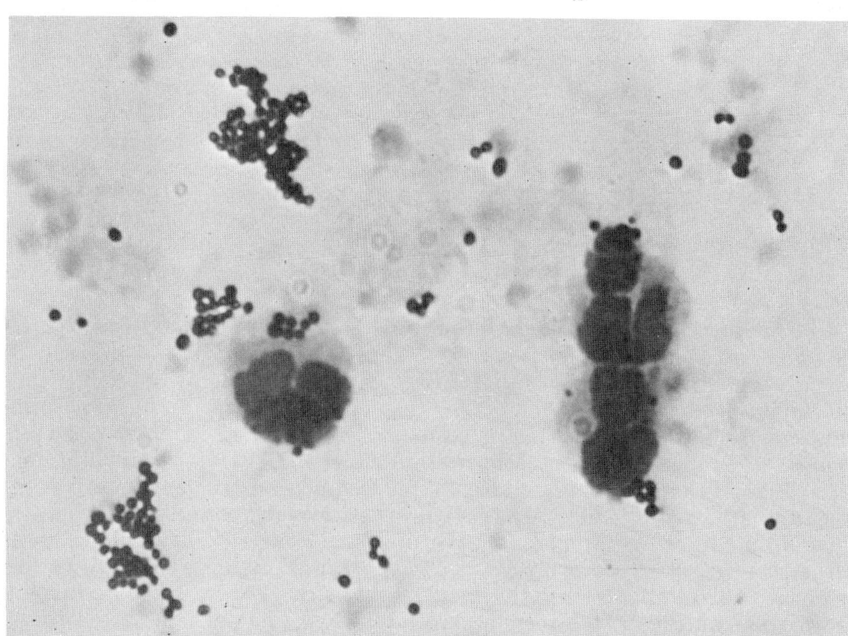

Figure 16–1 Staphylococci in pus. Gram stain × 2250.

foods are dairy foods (pastry, custard, salads, milk, etc.) or cold meats that have been left for several hours at room temperature after preparation by contaminating food handlers. The toxin is heat stable and will resist 100°C for 30 minutes, so mere reheating of nonrefrigerated food will not destroy it.

In the investigation of such an outbreak, the identical phage type organism is found in food leftovers, possibly on the food handler's hands and also in the patients' feces.

The toxic shock syndrome of high fever, vomiting, diarrhea, shock, and a skin rash is a recently recognized disease thought to be caused by the elaboration of a toxin by *S. aureus* contaminating vaginal tampons. It has occurred in women during their menstrual periods, and the condition is serious, with a mortality of about 10%.

In the newborn, a scalded skin syndrome is described. The name is very descriptive, and the infant becomes very ill with perioral crusting, skin erythema, fever, and, later, separation of the epidermis and formation of bullae. Staphylococcal septicemia may occur.

Although coagulase-negative staphylococci are generally nonpathogenic, under certain conditions they may produce disease. They are considered significant in urinary bladder infections and in bacterial endocarditis as well as in infections complicating implanted devices such as are used for ventriculo-atrial shunts in hydrocephalus.

THE STREPTOCOCCACEAE

These are another family of nonmotile, nonsporing, aerobic gram-positive cocci that are benzidine negative. One genus of these, *Streptococcus*, is of considerable medical importance.

The genus *Streptococcus* generally forms pairs or chains of cells in culture and is characteristically catalase negative. Streptococci are divided into several species on the bases of a number of cultural and serological properties.

Hemolysis

Since hemolysis on blood agar plates is so much a pivotal characteristic in the identification of streptococci, it is worth considering this phenomenon in some detail. Sheep blood is best in such plates, particularly for its inhibitory effect on *H. haemolyticus*, which is a normal throat commensal also producing β-hemolysis. Outdated human blood bank blood should not be used, since both citrate and antimicrobial substances may be inhibitory. α-Hemolysis is a green or brown-green area around colonies due to partial lysis of red blood cells in the medium. β-Hemolysis is a clear or colorless zone due to complete lysis of red cells. The Greek letter γ is sometimes used to denote no hemolysis. α′-Hemolysis is a zone of α-hemolysis around the colony within a wider zone of β-hemolysis.

Because there is a streptolysin O (oxygen labile) and a streptolysin S (oxygen stable) responsible for hemolysis, it is possible, unless organisms are studied anaerobically or implanted beneath the agar surface to ensure some degree of anaerobiosis, that only organisms producing streptolysin S will be correctly identified in routine aerobic studies.

Antigenicity and Serology of Streptococci

Within the cell wall of the streptococci is a C-carbohydrate that is extractable. On the basis of the differing structure of the carbohydrate, the β-hemolytic streptococci and some non-β streptococci (in Groups B and D) are separable into Lancefield groups. There are numerous procedures to extract and type the carbohydrate based on general serological principles, e.g., precipitin, agglutinin, and so forth. A recent, simple, commercially available latex test (Streptex)* is simple and reliable.

Methodology of Latex Agglutination Test

1. An extract may be made either from colonies on solid media or from broth culture. In the first instance, make a heavy suspension of the culture in 0.4 mL of the extraction enzyme (protolytic enzyme from *Streptomyces*), incubate 1 hour at 56°C, and then centrifuge at 1200 G for 10 minutes, retaining the clear supernate. Centrifuge an overnight broth culture at 1200 G, keeping the precipitated button of cells, which is then treated in the enzyme exactly as above.

2. With a Pasteur pipette, place 1 drop of clear extract in each of 6 circles on a glass slide.

3. Resuspend by shaking the A, B, C, D, F, and G latex suspensions, and add 1 drop of each to each drop of extract on the slide. Mix with sticks, and rock the slide for 2 minutes or until agglutination occurs. A positive result appears within 2 minutes.

*Burroughs Wellcome Co., Research Triangle Park, N.C. 27709.

TABLE 16–1 DIFFERENTIATION OF STREPTOCOCCI

Type	Hemolysis	Bacitracin Sensitivity	CAMP	Esculin	6.5% NaCl Growth	Optochin Sensitivity: Bile Solubility
Group A	β	+	−	−	−	−
Group B	βγ	−	+	−	+	−
Not A, B, or D	β	−	−	−	−	−
Enterococcal D	αβγ	−	−	+	+	−
Nonenterococcal D	αγ	−	−	+	−	−
Viridans	αγ	+	−	−	−	−
S. pneumoniae	α	±	−	−	−	+

A speedier, simplified Streptex test, recently introduced, is performed as follows:

1. A light loopful of colonies (5 or more) is taken from the plate, or a single drop of a 4-hour to overnight broth culture is used.
2. The loopful or drop is added to 0.4 mL of an extraction enzyme and incubated at 37°C for 1 hour.
3. One drop of latex reagent is placed in each of 6 circles on a glass slide.
4. One drop of extract is added to each circle, and each of the 6 areas is separately spread and mixed.
5. The slide is rocked for *1 minute* at the most. Positive agglutination will occur in the appropriate circle within this time.

False negative results may occur if too few cells are used for extraction. False positive results may be noted if there is bacterial contamination of the latex or, rarely, if organisms containing similar or identical antigens are challenged. *Klebsiella* spp. may possess these but are generally excluded by cultural features.

Lancefield Group A Streptococci, *S. pyogenes*. The organism grows well on blood agar (sheep's blood shows excellent hemolytic zones), yielding a circular, entire, convex, shiny, translucent or white colony about 0.5 mm in diameter after overnight incubation, with a surrounding zone of β-hemolysis two or even four times the size of the colony in diameter. The colony is often hard and can be moved across the plate without rupturing.

Unlike other streptococci, they are sensitive to bacitracin discs containing 0.04 unit (routine sensitivity discs hold 10 units). Any inhibition is considered positive.

Lancefield Group B Streptococci, *S. agalactiae*. These are generally similar but larger than Group A colonies on blood agar. The zone of β-hemolysis is often smaller or may be absent. They are able to grow on MacConkey medium (without crystal violet), unlike Group A organisms, are softer than Group A organisms, and cannot be pushed intact across the plate.

The CAMP (an acronym* from the names of its discoverers) test is used for identification of Group B organisms. A streak of β-hemolytic *S. aureus* is made on a blood agar plate, and another streak of the streptococcus is made at a 90° angle, but the two streaks do not meet, since a 5-mm gap is left. The plate is incubated at 35°C aerobically. Group B organisms enhance the β-hemolysis of the *S. aureus*, forming an "arrow head" or "crescent" of hemolysis at the point at which the two streaks are nearest one another. The test is also positive with γ-hemolytic Group B streptococci.

Another simple test is to grow the suspect organism anaerobically in Islams's (1977) starch serum agar medium. After overnight incubation, the colonies are bright orange in color.

Lancefield Group C Streptococci. These have a colonial appearance similar to that of Group A on blood agar, but they are resistant to bacitracin.

Lancefield Group D Streptococci. Unlike Groups A, B, F, and G streptococci, these are not a single species, but they do have a common antigen. They may be α-, β-, or γ-hemolytic, but all will utilize bile esculin agar (unlike other streptococci) and will also grow on MacConkey medium. The different species will be considered below.

Lancefield Group F Streptococci, *S. anginosus*. These are typically tiny β-hemolytic colonies (about half the size of Group A), which are often better seen when the organisms are grown as facultative anaerobes.

Lancefield Group G Streptococci. These morphologically resemble Group A.

*Christie, Atkins, Munch-Peterson (1944).

Figure 16–2 *Streptococcus pyogenes*, Lancefield group A. The plate demonstrates the colonies surrounded by a zone of β-hemolysis and inhibition of the growth around a bacitracin disc (0.04 unit).

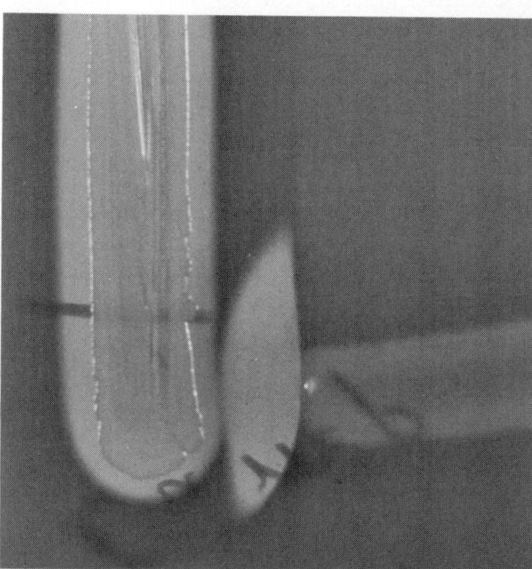

Figure 16–3 The CAMP test. On a blood agar plate, a streak of Group B streptococcus is made at right angles to a hemolytic staphylococcal streak that is separated from it by about 5 mm. At a point at which the organisms are at an optimal distance there is a flame-shaped area of augmented hemolysis.

TABLE 16–2 Differentiation of Group D Streptococci

	Bile Esculin	6.5% NaCl	Lactose	β-Hemolysis	Gelatin Liquefaction	Sorbitol	Arabinose	
S. faecalis	+	+	+	−	−	+	−	Enterococci
S. faecalis var zymogenes	+	+	+	+	d	+	−	Enterococci
S. faecalis var liquefaciens	+	+	+	−	+	+	−	Enterococci
S. faecium	+	+	+	−	−	−	+	Enterococci
S. durans	+	+	+	d	−	−	−	Enterococci
S. avium	+	+	+	−	−	+	+	Enterococci
S. bovis	+	−	+					Non-enterococci
S. equinus	+	−	−					Non-enterococci
Non–Group D	−							Non-D

d, Variable characteristics.

Speciation of Group D Streptococci. The Group D streptococci consist of several species, all of which will hydrolyze bile-esculin medium (p. 341). In addition the subgroup of enterococci will grow in 6.5% NaCl, and these include the species *S. faecalis, S. faecium, S. durans, S. avium,* and their varieties. The nonenterococci are *S. bovis* and *S. equinus*. The 6.5% salt broth (commercially available) is inoculated with the suspect colonies and incubated at 35°C. Growth occurs within 48 hours and is indicated by turbidity or a change of color in a bromocresol purple indicator. Further identification with the group is best appreciated by reference to Table 16–2.

A most important feature in the speciation of Group D streptococci is the fact that penicillin is ineffective against the enterococci but the antimicrobial is valuable against the Group D nonenterococci. Since Group D streptococci cause bacterial endocarditis, this differentiation is important. For epidemiological purposes, speciation of the enterococci is important in the hospital, especially in the monitoring and prevention of urinary tract infections.

Other Extracellular Streptococcal Enzymes of Medical Interest

Streptolysin S and O have been described above. In addition to the importance of these substances in colonial identification, antistreptolysin O titers (p. 545) in the patient's blood are used in the diagnosis of nonsuppurative streptococcal disease (glomerulonephritis, rheumatic fever). Streptolysin S and O may damage cell membranes in vivo, and streptolysin O can cause cardiac arrest in laboratory animals. Erythrogenic toxins produced by Group A (and some Group C and G) streptococci are the cause of the rash in scarlet fever. DNase (see p. 382) is also produced by Group A, and an anti-DNase is also used diagnostically in nonsuppurative streptococcal illness. Streptokinase (from Group A and C organisms) will lyze fibrin. Despite this remarkable property, the enzyme does not play any proven part in disease but has been used therapeutically to treat early thrombotic disease. Hyaluronidase (from Group A strains) is believed to enable streptococci to spread rapidly by lyzing connective material substance, and it plays some part in streptococcal disease.

Group A Streptococcal Disease

Acute streptococcal pharyngotonsillitis with or without tonsillitis is the classical disease caused by this organism. It is also responsible for related otitis media and quinsy. Puerpural sepsis, acute bacterial endocarditis, and various diseases of the skin are also well-known results of such infection. Among the latter, erysipelas, impetigo, and cellulitis are listed.

In addition, Group A streptococci cause nonsuppurative disease. In rheumatic fever, the heart, joints, skin, and even the central nervous system are affected. The onset is generally 2 to 3 weeks subsequent to a streptococcal throat infection, and the exact mechanism is a little obscure, although obviously it demonstrates some unusual immunological features. There are two theories of causation:

1. That the streptococcal infection activates some autoimmune process against the patient's own tissues by a cross-reaction of streptococcal antibodies against cardiac, valvular, and neural tissues.
2. That streptococcal substances (such as streptolysin O and S) are cytotoxic to the patient's tissues.

The first of these theories is currently the most popular, but it does not explain all the features of the disease.

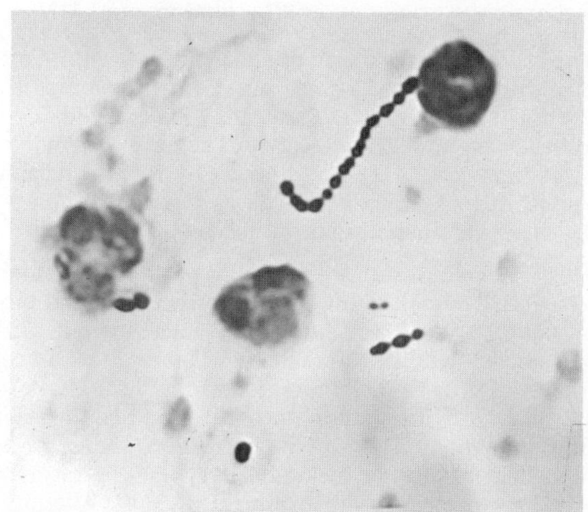

Figure 16–4 Streptococci in pus. Gram stain × 2250.

In the other nonsuppurative disease, acute glomerulonephritis, the initial streptococcal infection may be of the throat or skin. Male patients predominate, and the period between infection and onset of glomerulonephritis is shorter than that in rheumatic fever. In addition circulating C_3 is diminished in glomerulonephritis. This latter finding suggests the formation of antibody-antigen complexes, and indeed C_3 and streptococcal antigens have been demonstrated in the glomerular lesions. On the other hand, cross-reaction between streptococcal antibody and the glomerular basement membrane is possible and would be an autoimmune response.

Streptococci of Other Groups and Disease

Group B streptococci are found without apparent disease in the vagina but cause severe disease in newborns. An early-onset disease in babies occurs within a few hours of birth, whereas a late-onset syndrome occurs at several weeks or months. The early-onset disease is mainly respiratory but may be accompanied by meningitis and septicemia. The late-onset disease is a meningitis possibly accompanied by septicemia. Mortality in early-onset disease is 40 to 80% but is less in the late-onset type. Infection in the early-onset type is probably acquired in the uterus or birth canal and in the other type, from the mother, other infants, or the nursing staff. Group B streptococci also cause other diseases in growing children (e.g., otitis media, arthritis, and urinary tract infections) and similar conditions in adults.

Group C streptococci are found in the pharynx but their etiological role in pharyngitis is debatable. They do cause some cases of impetigo, respiratory disease, and puerperal sepsis.

Group D organisms, which are normal inhabitants of the bowel, cause urinary infections and a fair minority of cases of subacute bacterial endocarditis. *S. equinus* is generally nonpathogenic.

Group F streptococci may be causative of some wound infections, deep abscesses, sinusitis, and meningitis.

Group G streptococci are found in the pharynx, but whether they cause pharyngitis is debatable. They have been involved in cases of bacterial endocarditis, impetigo, wound infection, puerperal sepsis, empyema, and urinary tract disease.

Streptococcus pneumoniae (Pneumococcus)

The organism grows well on blood agar, forming, after overnight incubation, 1-mm round entire colonies that are often transparent or that may be mucoid. Older colonies often appear umbilicate. They are α-hemolytic. They differ from other streptococci by their sensitivity to optochin (ethylhydrocupreine hydrochloride) as well as by other less usually performed tests.

The Optochin Test. **A 6-mm disc with 5 μg optochin (commercially available) is placed on an inoculated blood agar plate. After overnight aerobic incubation at 35°C, pneumococci will show a zone of more than 14 mm diameter of growth inhibition around the disc. The test is better than 90% accurate in pneumococcal identification.**

Bile Solubility. **This test is less often used as a presumptive identification method. Here, the organisms are grown in a nutrient broth overnight at 35°C. Aliquots of 0.5 mL of the broth culture are placed in two tubes with 1 to 2 drops of phenol red indicator and neutralized with M. NaOH. 0.5 mL of 2% sodium deoxycholate is added to one tube and 0.5 mL of saline to the other. The tubes are reincubated at 35°C for 2 hours. If the organism is a pneumococcus, the bile tube will clear and the saline tube will remain turbid. Alternatively, a few drops of 10% sodium deoxycholate are dropped directly on the suspect colony on a blood plate. If positive, the colony appears to dissolve.**

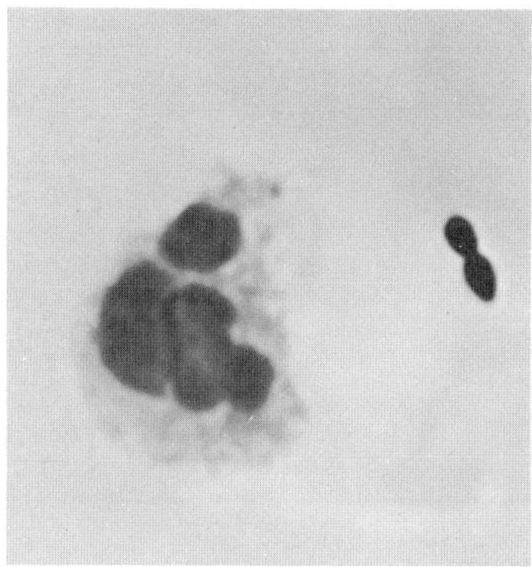

Figure 16–5 Pneumococci in pus. Gram stain × 2250.

The organisms are typically diplococcal and somewhat lanceolate with a distinctive capsule. The capsule possesses a carbohydrate acting as a haptene, and it confers specific antigenicity on the enclosed organisms. By these antigens, pneumococci are divisible into numerous types (about 80), 1, 2, 3, and so forth. Types 1, 2, and 3 are most important in adults, and type 14 in children.

Serologic Typing of Pneumococci (Quellung Test). The organisms present in body fluids (sputum, pleural fluid, and so forth) can be examined directly, or bacteria from a broth culture or emulsified colony can be used.

A drop of the fluid containing the organism is placed on a slide and mixed with a loop of antiserum. Then a drop of

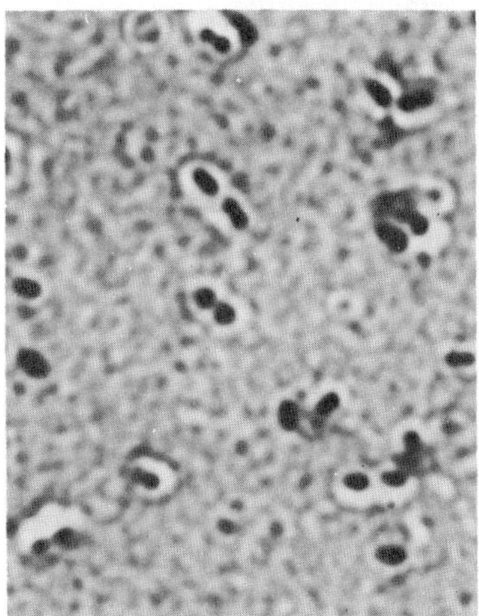

Figure 16–6 Pneumococcal capsules. Capsules appear as unstained areas between diplococci and stained background. Gram preparation × 2250.

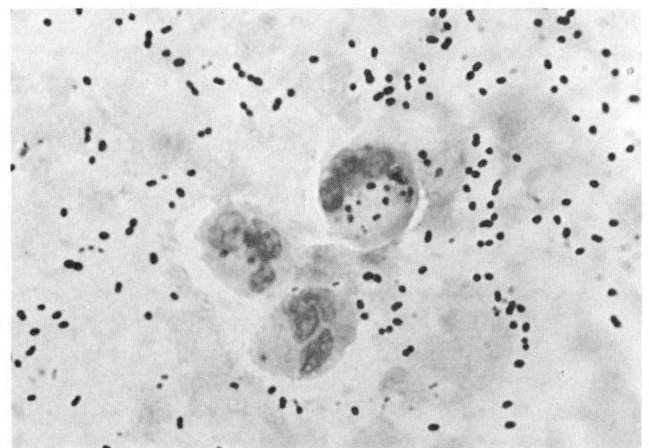

Figure 16–7 Pneumococcal meningitis. A direct smear from the cerebrospinal fluid. The gram-positive cocci are seen in an intracellular and extracellular position. Gram stain × 2300.

saturated aqueous methylene blue is added and mixed again. The slide is cover-slipped and examined microscopically after 10 minutes. If the test is positive, the capsule of the organism appears to swell, but this appearance is due to antigen-antibody combination, which changes the refractive index of the capsule. The contained organisms are stained blue, which helps by heightening the contrast.

Generally, the antiserum used is an omnivalent serum reacting with all pneumococcal types. Monotypic sera are also available, but since knowledge of the type of organism is not necessary for therapeutic purposes but only for epidemiological reasons, they are much less widely used.

Pathology. Pneumococci are normally found in the nasopharynx but are responsible for many cases of pneumonia. In such patients bacteremia is common, and from the blood, organisms may invade the meninges, joints, pericardium, or peritoneum. They also cause otitis media and sinusitis.

Although *S. pneumoniae* responds to antimicrobial therapy (although strains resistant to penicillin are appearing), some prevention against pneumococcal disease can be given to those particularly at risk with a polyvalent vaccine.* The latter contains the polysaccharide antigens against 14 types implicated in 80% of pneumococcal diseases. It is used in the elderly, those with chronic pulmonary disease, and those who were born with no spleen or in whom the spleen has been removed. In patients with sickle cell disease in which the spleen is functionally inadequate the vaccine may also be used.

Figure 16–8 Meningococcal meningitis. Spinal fluid. Note intracellular position of most organisms. Gram stain × 1350.

The Viridans Streptococci

These organisms are separable into numerous species, but separation is not often made in a clinical situation. On blood agar, they form colonies of varied size and appearance and are generally surrounded by a zone of α-hemolysis. The organisms form chains of gram-positive cocci. Their differentiation from other streptococci is best appreciated by reference to Table 16–1.

Pathology. The organisms are normal inhabitants of the mouth. In minor trauma to the gums or even during mastication, especially if there is some degree of dental disease, they may enter the circulation. Normally such transient bacteremia is of little consequence but should heart valves or chambers be altered by previous (usually rheumatic) disease or by congenital abnormality, *S. viridans* may find a lodgment in the damaged area and produce subacute bacterial endocarditis (SBE). Viridans streptococci are responsible for about 80% of cases of SBE and about 50% of all cases of bacterial endocarditis (acute and subacute).

THE GRAM-NEGATIVE AEROBIC COCCI

These organisms include the genera *Neisseria* and *Branhamella* in the family Neisseriaceae. The gram-negative cocci occur in pairs with flattened adjacent sides and are nonmotile. They generally demand complex media on which to grow, and they grow well at 35° to 37°C. All species are oxidase positive.

Neisseria meningitidis

The organisms grow well on enriched media such as chocolate agar and in such media as Thayer-Martin medium in an atmosphere of 5 to 10% CO_2. On blood agar, the colonies are about 1 mm in diameter after overnight incubation and are round, entire, and butyrous. They will metabolize glucose and maltose. Fluorescent methods may also be employed, using fluorescent-tagged antimeningococcal serum, and agglutination techniques are used in grouping meningococci into several types. Some types have a capsule so that a Quellung test may be done.

---

*Pneumovax, Merck, Sharp and Dohme, West Point, Pa. 19486.

Pathology. As noted, the organism often lives commensally in the nasopharynx. For reasons not yet clear, the organism occasionally becomes pathogenic, invading the bloodstream and causing meningococcemia. The latter may be chronic, with fever and cutaneous manifestations, or acutely fatal, with destruction of the adrenals (Waterhouse-Friderichsen syndrome). The organism is most often carried to the meninges, causing meningitis. Characteristically in the polymorphs within the cerebrospinal fluid in meningitis, the organisms are seen as gram-negative intracellular diplococci. Groups B and C are most usually found in meningococcal disease in the United States.

Neisseria gonorrhoeae

Because the organisms are unusually susceptible to drying and variations in temperature and also because only relatively few organisms are found in clinical material, special precautions have to be taken so that viable organisms will reach the laboratory.

Material is best plated directly on to such media as Thayer-Martin medium or New York City medium, which contain both nutritives and antimicrobial inhibitors. The media are incubated in 5 to 10% CO_2 at 35°C for 48 hours. Transportation in a bottled modified Thayer-Martin medium with 10% CO_2 or in a JEMBEC plate (see below) can also be done, and the media incubated further on arrival in the laboratory. Thayer-Martin or New York City agar will allow the growth of pathogenic neisseriae and prevent the growth of most contaminants. The colonies are small (0.5 to 1 mm), gray or white, and mucoid, and they will give a positive oxidase reaction. It is best to perform the oxidase reaction on a representative colony selected on a prepared filter strip rather than to flood the plate with oxidase reagent, since the reagent is bactericidal in 5 to 10 minutes. A platinum loop is preferable to one of nichrome, since the latter may give false positive oxidase reactions. If colonies are not seen, the plate may be flooded with reagent to reveal inapparent colonies, which are removed and dealt with quickly to prevent their demise.

Oxidase-positive colonies are then subjected to Gram staining, and these should show typical gram-negative diplococci. Gonococci will oxidize glucose but not other carbohydrates. Fluorescent techniques may also be used in identification.

Pathology. In the male gonorrhea classically causes an acute urethritis, and a direct smear from this urethral discharge will show typical intracellular gram-negative diplococci in pus cells. Extension from the urethra may involve the prostate and epididymis. In the female there is cervicitis, and this may extend to the uterus and oviducts and even to the peritoneum and perihepatic tissues. Although the disease is often asymptomatic in females and generally symptomatic in males this is not invariable. In both sexes gonococcaemia and joint disease may occur. Infants born to mothers with gonorrhea may develop gonococcal eye disease (ophthalmia neonatorum). Proctitis and pharyngitis are also well documented, and a nonvenereal gonococcal vulvovaginitis conveyed by accidental contamination occurs in prepubertal girls.

N. lactamica is rarely causative of meningitis, septicemia, or pulmonary disease, and it is often present in the nasopharynx. Its major importance is that, along with *N. gonorrhoeae* and *N. meningitidis*, it will grow on modified Thayer-Martin medium and New York City agar and produces acid from glucose and maltose. However, if the latter sugar is not routinely used, *N. lactamica* may be confused with *N. meningitidis*. Further differentiation is that *N. lactamica* is ONPG positive and ferments lactose slowly, and that most strains will grow on nonenriched media.

Figure 16–9 JEMBEC plate (*J. E.* Martin *B*iological *E*nvironment *C*hamber). The plastic plate holding the medium (MTM, chocolate agar, etc.) has a small capsule inserted at the time of inoculation. The capsule is of sodium bicarbonate and citric acid. The plate is then covered with its lid, enclosed in a zip-locked plastic bag, and incubated. Moisture from the medium activates the capsule to produce CO_2, creating the desired atmosphere.

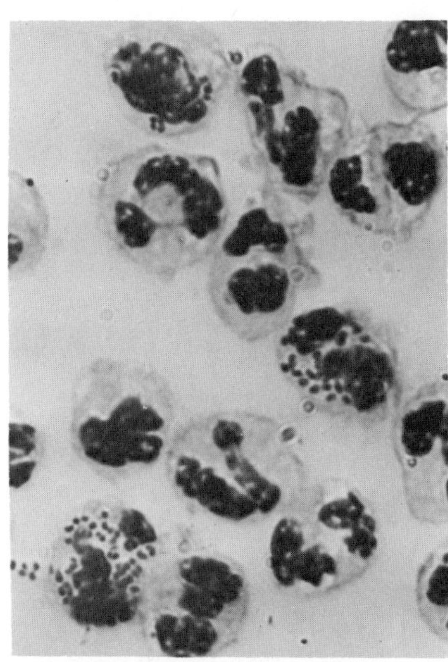

Figure 16–10 *Neisseria gonorrhoeae* in pus from urethral discharge. Note intracellular position of the diplococci. Gram stain × 2250.

TABLE 16–3 Differentiation of *Neisseriae* and *B. Catarrhalis*

	Growth on			Oxidation of			
	MTM Medium	*Blood Agar at 22°C*	*Nutrient Agar at 35°C*	*Glucose*	*Maltose*	*Lactose/ ONPG*	*DNase*
N. meningitidis	+	−	−	+	+	−	−
N. gonorrhoeae	+	−	−	+	−	−	−
N. lactamica	+	d	+	+	+	+	−
B. catarrhalis	−	+	+	−	−	−	+
Other neisseria	−	d	+	d	d	−	−

MTM, Modified Thayer-Martin medium; d, variable characteristics.

Branhamella catarrhalis and Remaining *Neisseria* Species

These are normally found in the nasopharynx and are very rarely pathogenic. They will grow at room temperature (22°C) on enriched media and at 35°C on nonenriched media. *B. catarrhalis* differs from the *Neisseria* genus in that it has a DNase.

Distinction between the species of *Neisseria* and *B. catarrhalis* may be seen best in Table 16–3.

Oxidation of Carbohydrates

Because the reaction of carbohydrate media is so significant in the differentiation of this group of organisms, it is most important that testing be done under optimal conditions. The usual CTA-carbohydrate media are somewhat unreliable, and much more dependable results can be obtained with starch agar media (Flynn and Waitkins, 1972), which are commercially available from Institut Armand-Frappier (Laval-des-Rapides, Quebec, H7V 1B7).

The Minitek system* (Fig. 20–4) can also be used advantageously to differentiate the *Neisseria* species and is said to be very reliable. It uses a special buffered broth and paper discs impregnated with appropriate carbohydrates. A small volume of a heavy suspension of the organism in the broth is incubated at 35°C, without CO_2, together with the discs in the wells of a plastic plate. Only clearcut changes of the indicator system are read as positive. Generally, identification can be made with this method in 4 hours, but incubation may have to be prolonged overnight. The manufacturer's instructions should be strictly followed.

The Bactec radiometric procedure can also be used (p. 344) and is considered extremely dependable in differentiation.

Gonorrhea and Penicillin

Although it is dealt with elsewhere (p. 437) the appearance of penicillinase-producing *N. gonorrhoeae* (PPNG) strains is noted here to stress their growing significance.

*Baltimore Biological Laboratory, Cockeysville, Md. 21030.

CHAPTER 16—REVIEW QUESTIONS

1. What distinguishes the enterococci from other streptococci? What do the enterococci share with *S. bovis* and *S. equinus*? What is the effect of penicillin on the enterococci?
2. What tests distinguish the pneumococci from other streptococci? What is the Quellung test? Name four sites in which pneumococci may cause disease. What is the normal habitat of pneumococci?
3. What test distinguishes *B. catarrhalis* from the neisseriae? Will the pathogenic neisseriae grow at 22°C? Using the three carbohydrates glucose, maltose, and lactose, construct a chart differentiating *N. meningitidis, N. gonorrhoeae,* and *N. lactamica*.
4. What organism does the coagulase test identify? Describe the methodology of the coagulase slide test. What infections may be due to *S. epidermidis*?

17

THE ENTEROBACTERIACEAE

The family Enterobacteriaceae are gram-negative rods that are aerobic and facultatively anaerobic. They ferment glucose and other carbohydrates, reduce nitrates to nitrites, and are catalase positive and oxidase negative. They may or may not be motile (by peritrichate flagella) and may or may not have capsules. Many of the genera and species are normal inhabitants of the intestinal tract. Some of them are pathogens of the intestinal tract, and many cause urinary tract disease and many nosocomial infections. Other organisms, which are not Enterobacteriaceae, are also found normally or abnormally in the bowel, and since as a practical matter they are so closely related, at least in a pathological sense, they will be dealt with in the next chapter. Among such organisms we can include *V. cholerae, Pseudomonas* spp., *Acinetobacter* spp., *Campylobacter,* and others.

ESCHERICHIA COLI

Escherichia coli is the common aerobic organism in the large bowel. It grows well on simple media, and perhaps its most common appearance is on a medium such as MacConkey's, on which after overnight incubation at 35°C it is a pink, lactose-fermenting, shiny, butyrous, round, entire, convex colony about 1 cm in diameter. On blood agar, it may be β-hemolytic. Biochemically, if typical, it ferments lactose and/or is ONPG positive, it produces gas in glucose, forms indole, is VP negative, is citrate negative, and does not produce H_2S. On TSI (triple sugar iron agar) the reaction is A (Alk)/ A gas + (−) H_2S − (occasional reactions are in parentheses).

Pathology

Urinary tract infections are commonly due to *E. coli,* as are other nosocomial infections such as bacteremia. Rupture of the bowel may lead to *E. coli* peritonitis, and surgical wounds may be contaminated with *E. coli.* The organism may also cause meningitis in infancy.

***E. coli* Diarrhea.** Although, as noted, *E. coli* is a normal inhabitant of the bowel, it may produce enteric disease. Such strains include enteroinvasive *E. coli* (EIEC), which, like *Shigella,* infiltrates the bowel, causing colitis. The invasive property is tested in reference laboratories by the organism's ability to cause keratoconjunctivitis in the eye of a guinea pig. Enterotoxic strains of *E. coli* (ETEC) produce a heat-stable and/or heat-labile enterotoxin. Again such strains are detected by a biological test.

The toxin causes dilatation of an isolated loop of rabbit bowel. ETEC strains produce a whole range of bowel diseases from infantile diarrhea to traveler's diarrhea. Formerly it was considered that some serotypes of *E. coli* produced infantile diarrhea, and those were known as enteropathogenic *E. coli* (EPEC). Stools from infants with diarrhea were examined for these serotypes. However, more recent work and the demonstration of toxin-producing *E. coli* strains have put this examination in some disrepute, since it would appear that the relationship of the serotypes to ETEC is not clearcut. In an epidemic situation it appears that the ETEC is of a particular serotype, and serological typing may be useful. The production of the enterotoxin is mediated by a transferable plasmid, and this plasmid may be picked up (and lost) by any serotype. Thus, in a nonepidemic or sporadic case, serotyping is of no value. The pathology of *E. coli* diarrhea is further complicated by the possibility that EPEC organisms cause diarrhea by unknown mechanisms, but our methods for their detection are unreliable and not worthwhile in a sporadic case. In epidemics, as noted, serology is of some value, but, in addition, strains should be referred to a reference center.

The stool in cases caused by EIEC will contain pus cells (as it does in *Shigella* infections), but in diarrhea due to ETEC and EPEC there is no purulent exudate.

Since serological identification *per se* is of dubious value, there is little advantage in serological examination without biological tests for ETEC and EIEC. Thus, suspect organisms should be sent to central reference laboratories with clinical data.

***E. coli* in Extraintestinal Sites.** *E. coli* is a common agent in urinary tract infections and in other extraintestinal sites, as noted above. In cultures of feces, lactose fermenters are generally disregarded as nonpathogens, but in other cultures it is important to speciate such colonies. This may best be done by a small battery of tests to exclude other lactose-fermenting colonies. Any result indicating that the colony is not a typical *E. coli* strain is subject to a more extensive biochemical examination.

Short Set for Typical *E. coli*

Test or substrate	*Typical E. coli result*
H_2S	−
Urease	−
Indole	+
Citrate	−
Oxidase	−

TABLE 17–1 DIFFERENTIATION OF *Citrobacter* SPECIES FROM *Salmonella* AND *Arizona*

	Salmonella	*Arizona*	*C. freundii*	*C. diversus*	*C. amalonaticus*
Urease	–	–	d	d	d
Lactose	–	d	(+)/+	d	d
Sucrose	–	–	d	–/+	d
Malonate	–	+	d	+/–	–
Indole	–	–	–	+	+
Growth in KCN	–	–	+	–	+
Lysine	+	+	–	–	–
H_2S	+	+	+	–	–
Gelatin	–	+/(+)	–	–	d

d, For an explanation of the symbols see p. 367

THE ALKALESCENS-DISPAR TYPES OF *E. coli* (A-D GROUP)

These are a group of anaerogenic and nonmotile biotypes of *E. coli* that may be confused with shigellae in the stool. They may easily be differentiated by agglutination with a polyvalent antiserum. This latter serum is usually included in the set of shigellae antisera so that the likelihood of an error is diminished. The organisms are not enteropathogens (see also p. 381).

EDWARDSIELLA TARDA

This species has been found in various suppurative lesions, in urine, as a cause of meningitis, and in diarrhea. Its important biochemical reactions are that it produces indole but also H_2S and that it fails to ferment lactose or produce phenylalanine deaminase (unlike *E. coli* or *Proteus, respectively*). On TSI its reactions are Alk/A gas+ H_2S+.

THE GENUS *CITROBACTER*

Citrobacter is a genus divided into several species. The organisms grow well on blood agar and on enteric media. Their colonies are not easily distinguishable from *E. coli* on blood agar, but, for example, on Hektoen's agar they will produce a black pigmented colony because of their production of H_2S. They are lactose fermenting, but because they give positive results for citrate and often for H_2S they may be confused with *Salmonella* or *Arizona*. The three species in the genus are *C. freundii*, *C. diversus*, and *C. amalonaticus*, and their important reactions (compared with *Salmonella* and *Arizona*) are given in Table 17–1. The late lactose fermenting *C. freundii* especially may be confused with *Salmonella* on initial examination. On TSI they show as Alk(A)/A gas+ H_2S+(–).

Pathology

Citrobacter organisms cause urinary tract infection and are occasionally responsible for bacteremias. They are often found in nosocomial infections and are opportunistic. Their normal habitat is soil and water.

THE GENUS *SALMONELLA*

Although many agents may be responsible for diarrhea, a large number of bacterial diarrheas are due to *Salmonella* infections, and a suggested flow chart for stool examination is shown here for convenient reference (Fig. 17–1). In essence, from the stool, these organisms are initially recognized as nonlactose fermenters and are identified and confirmed by biochemical and serological examination.

The genus comprises motile organisms that do not ferment lactose or sucrose; nor do they produce urease

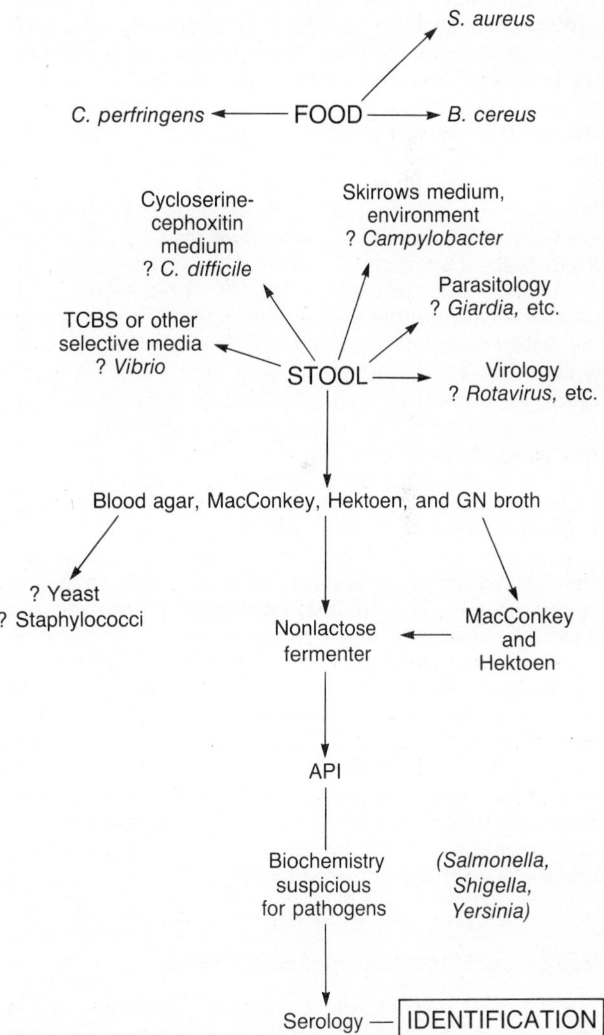

Figure 17–1 Possible investigation of stool in cases of diarrhea (and of food in some cases of gastroenteritis).

TABLE 17–2 DIFFERENTIATION OF *Salmonella* SPECIES

Test	*S. enteritidis*	*S. cholerae-suis*	*S. typhi*
H_2S	+	+/−	$+^w$
Citrate	+	(+)	−
Ornithine	+	+	−
Dulcite	+	d	d
Gas from glucose	+	+	−

or gelatinase or utilize malonate. They generally ferment dulcite and do not grow in KCN medium. They grow easily on blood agar and on MacConkey and Hektoen agars. On the latter two, they are colorless (on MacConkey) or blue-green (on Hektoen) possibly with black centers and, after overnight incubation at 35°C, about 5 mm in diameter, circular, convex, and soft and smooth if the colony is in a smooth phase. With TSI the reaction is Alk/A gas+ H_2S+(−), but *S. typhi* may not produce H_2S (Alk/A gas− H_2S−).

The genus *Salmonella* includes about 1800 serotypes and bioserotypes that are regarded by some as individual species. In North America it is now becoming accepted that there are three species—*S. typhi, S. cholerae-suis,* and *S. enteritidis*—which are separable by biochemical activity and serology. In addition *S. enteritidis* is divisible into several hundred bioserotypes and serotypes, which will be considered below. A serotype indicates a group of organisms having a common antigenicity, whereas a biotype indicates a group with common biochemical reactions. In *S. enteritidis* there are organisms that are designated as serotypes, e.g., *S. enteriditis* ser Typhimurium, whereas other serotypes may be divisible into further biotypes and are serobiotypes, e.g., *S. enteritidis* bioser Paratyphi C. In an older terminology, in which each organism was a species, these were designated *S. typhimurium* and *S. paratyphi C,* respectively. The differentiation of species of *Salmonella* can be seen in Table 17–2.

KCN Broth

The base may be purchased commercially. To 100 mL of the prepared and sterilized broth base, 1.5 mL of freshly prepared 0.5% KCN in sterile water is added. This is dispensed in aliquots of 1 to 2 mL in screw-capped bottles. The KCN is extremely poisonous, and great care should be taken in preparation. After its use, ferrous sulfate and alkali are added to glassware before autoclaving. KCN growth is of value in differentiating *Citrobacter* species (see above) among themselves and from *Salmonella* and may be of value in other differentiations. The test depends upon the fact that iron-containing cytochromes that are vital to aerobic respiration are inactivated by cyanide. Those organisms that survive in KCN broth have nonferrous respiratory enzymes that are not poisoned by KCN.

Serological Identification of Salmonellae

When the biochemical pattern of an organism is suggestive of *Salmonella,* confirmation is made by serological methods.

Antigenic Structure of Salmonellae

O Antigens. (The antigens are present in the body of the organism.) These are of many types and are numbered 1, 2, 3, and so on. The formula for *S. enteritidis* ser London, for example, is 3, 10. The O antigens resist extraction with alcohol and are thermostable, and thus may be preserved by killing the bacteria at 45°C for 30 minutes in absolute alcohol.

Vi Antigen. This is the most superficial of the somatic antigens of *S. typhi* and when fully developed will mask or completely inhibit the O antibody-antigen reaction. Therefore, any organism giving biochemical reactions suggestive of *S. typhi* but no agglutination in tests with the polyvalent and group O antiserum should be checked against *Salmonella* Vi antiserum.

H Antigens. (The antigens are present in the flagella of the organism.) H antigens are of two types, which are interchangeable and are classified as phase 1 or 2. An organism may be in one or the other of these phases, and the entire colony may be a mixture. Phase 1 antigens are denoted by letters a, b, c, and so on, and phase 2 by numerals 1, 2, 3, and so on. However, this is not uncomplicated, since some organisms, e.g., *S. enteritidis* ser Chester, have two phases, but both are of phase 1 type (the H formula for *S. enteritidis* ser Chester may be e,h or e,n,x). This type of phase changing is called the alpha-beta variation. H antigens are thermolabile and are destroyed by alcohol. They are not affected by formalin, which destroys O antigens. Thus, H antigens are preserved exclusively in formalin-killed organisms.

Many organisms share common antigen both somatically and in their flagella. For example, 12 is found in *S. enteritidis* ser Paratyphi B, ser Stanley, and ser Dublin. 1 is found in *S. enteritidis* ser Reading, ser Thompson, ser Eastbourne, and ser Aberdeen. Flagella phase 1 antigens e and h, for example, are found in *S. enteritidis* ser Lomita, ser Norwich, ser Reading, ser Newington, and many others. *Salmonella* antisera are commercially available from several firms.

Procedure for Serological Identification of Salmonellae

1. From an agar slope, take a loop of culture and emulsify on a slide in saline. The suspension is optimally dense. Add a drop of *Salmonella* polyvalent O antiserum. If there is agglutination, it is probable that the organism is a salmonella, although some species of Enterobacteriaceae may include salmonellae antigens.

2. If the organism has given biochemical results suggestive of *S. typhi,* then the O antigen may be masked by its capsular Vi antigen and a false negative result obtained with O antisera. In such cases, a slide agglutination test using antiVi serum must be em-

ployed. Positive agglutination demonstrates the presence of Vi antigen. The combination of a positive test with Vi antiserum and typical biochemical pattern is diagnostic of *S. typhi* or *S. enteritidis* bioser Paratyphi C. However, demonstration of Vi antigen alone is not conclusive, since other "coliform" organisms may have it, including the *Citrobacter* genus. If desired, the Vi antigen may be destroyed by boiling a saline suspension of the organism for 1 hour. The suspension is then washed by centrifugation in saline and the O antigens are unmasked.

3. If polyvalent agglutination is obtained, proceed with group antisera:

Group A	Anti-2
Group B	Anti-4
Group C_1	Anti-7
Group C_2	Anti-8
Group D	Anti-9
Group E_1	Anti-3, 10

depending on the range of antisera provided. Some antisera are supplied as antisera against the entire O component of a particular organism; e.g., Anti-1, 2, 12 would be the antiserum against *S. enteritidis* bioser Paratyphi A. Others, such as those listed, are absorbed out so as to be specific. It will be realized that specific antisera, such as those listed, are preferable because there cannot be cross-reaction.

4. After the group to which the organism belongs has been identified, it is necessary to identify the flagellar antigens. In the Spicer-Edwards tube test seven antisera (which are commercially available) are tested against the bacterial suspension. The pattern of precipitation permits identification of 17 types and groups of H antigens, both phase 1 and 2. The method obviates the necessity of keeping on hand a large collection of individual H antisera.

***Method* (Modified)**

a. Take seven test tubes and label tham 1, 2, 3, 4, 1-7, L, and en.

b. Into each tube place 5 mL of formalized saline.

c. To tube 1 add 2 drops of Spicer-Edwards serum 1, to tube 2 add 2 drops of Spicer-Edwards serum 2, and so on with the other tubes. This is approximately a 1:75 dilution of the serum.

d. From an overnight culture of the organism on a nutrient agar slant, make a heavy suspension of the organism by adding 3 mL of formalized saline, mixing by gentle rotation. Transfer to a sterile tube.

e. Take seven Kahn tubes and label them as the original set of seven tubes. Add 5 drops of formalized suspension of the organism to each. Then add to each tube an equal quantity of each diluted antiserum.

f. Incubate the tubes at 56°C for 3 hours.

g. Remove the tubes from water bath, and allow them to stand at room temperature overnight, keeping them covered with a clean cloth.

h. Read the tubes on the following morning, noting those with typical fluffy H agglutination.

Reagents

Spicer-Edwards Antisera

Formalized Saline

Commercial formalin	6 mL
Sodium chloride	8.5 g
Distilled water	to 1 L

Results. Agglutination may occur in both phase 1 and phase 2 antisera, thus yielding a complete flagella antigen formula as shown in the table:

H Antigen	Spicer-Edwards Antisera 1	2	3	4	
a	+	+	+	−	Phase 1 antigens
b	+	+	−	+	
c	+	+	−	−	
d	+	−	+	+	
e,h	+	−	+	−	
G complex	+	−	−	+	
i	+	−	−	−	
k	−	+	+	+	
r	−	+	−	+	
y	−	+	−	−	
z	−	−	+	+	
z_4 complex	−	−	+	−	
z_{10}	−	−	−	+	
z_{29}	−	+	+	−	
e,n,x, e,n, z_{15}	e,n complex antiserum				Phase 2 antigen
ℓ,v,ℓ,w,ℓ,z_{13},ℓ,z_{28}	L complex antiserum				
1,2 1,5, 1,6, 1,7	1 complex antiserum				

Note: the G complex includes flagellar antigens f,g, f,g,t, g,m, g,m,s, g,m,t, g,p, g,p,u, g,q, g,s,t, m,s, and t. The z_4 complex includes z_4,z_{23}, z_4,z_{24}, and z_4,z_{32}.

If the organism can be found in only one phase and identification requires knowledge of the other phase, Craigie tubes are used. Sloppy (0.2 to 0.5% nutrient) agar is placed in a wide-mouthed short test tube. A narrow glass tube opened at both ends is inserted in the tube to present a separate surface. The organism is seeded in the center of the glass tube, and 2 drops of the agglutinating serum (which has given a positive response in either phase 1 or phase 2) are placed in the medium surrounding the glass tube. Organisms grow down the glass tube, out from the lower open end, and up the test tube. The agglutinating serum inhibits the growth of its phase, allowing the opposite phase to proliferate and reach the surface outside the glass tube. These organisms are inoculated on a nutrient agar slope and allowed to grow overnight. The Spicer-Edwards technique is repeated using the series of antisera to the uninhibited and unknown phase. If no agglutination takes place, the Craigie maneuver must be repeated until the organism changes phase.

5. At this stage it may be possible to state the antigenic formula of the organism and possibly its identity. Usually the possibilities have been narrowed down to a few organisms and more specific antisera are necessary to pinpoint identity. Occasionally further antiO antisera testing is done. For example, if, with the methods described, an organism has been identified as a salmonella in group B with H phase 1 antigen r and phase 2 antigen 1 complex, it could be:

	S. enteritidis ser Heidelberg	1,4,5,12	r	1,2
or	*S. enteritidis* ser Bradford	4,12,27	r	1,5
or	*S. enteritidis* ser Remo	1,4,12,27	r	1,7

Distinction could be made by the use of specific O antisera, or by the use of specific H phase 2 antisera, 2, 5, and 7.

Differentiation of H phase 2 antigens may be the only recourse, viz.,

S. enteritidis ser London	3,10	e,v	1,6
S. enteritidis ser Sinstorf	3,10	e,v	1,5
S. enteritidis ser Nehanga	3,10	e,v	1,2

6. The Kauffman-White tables of antigenic formulas are necessary for intelligent application of the scheme just outlined. Most textbooks show part of the scheme, which is reproduced in extenso in *Bergey's Manual.*

Although an organism may be identified as a *Salmonella* species of a particular group, it is often impossible to speciate the organism with the limited antisera available in most laboratories. The organism should be sent to a reference laboratory on a nutrient agar slope for complete identification.

Pathology and Epidemiology

Salmonella organisms are widespread in nature and are found not only in humans but often in poultry and eggs. Chickens and turkeys become infected by feedstuff including meat obtained from infected hogs and other animals. Humans acquire the infection by ingesting diseased or contaminated meat or contaminated water. Contamination may be caused by a person who has the disease or who is a carrier. Contaminated water may affect shellfish in which organisms live symbiotically but may cause human disease if ingested. Salmonellosis is particularly common in children younger than 10 years of age. After that it is suggested that an acquired immunity prevents a large number of infections. Infections are common. In 1979, more than 33,000 isolations of *Salmonella* were made in the United States, but it has been estimated that only 1% of all infections are reported. During the same period, 8700 isolates of *Salmonella* were reported in Canada.

There are three types of clinical disease, viz., enteric fever, gastroenteritis and septicemia. Enteric fever is due to *S. typhi* or occasionally to *S. enteritidis* ser Paratyphi A or ser Typhimurium. There is an incubation period of 7 to 14 days, followed by fever and other symptoms, including mental torpor and a rash. The patient is severely ill for 7 to 10 days, after which there is slow recovery unless there is some complication. During the illness there is often constipation rather than diarrhea.

Septicemic disease occurs without any sign of intestinal disease. It is often due to *S. cholerae-suis.* During the septicemia, with its accompanying fever and chills, suppurative foci may occur in bone, kidneys, lungs, and so forth.

Gastroenteritis is the common manifestation. The incubation period is 8 to 24 hours and is followed by nausea, vomiting, abdominal pain, and diarrhea with a mild fever. The disease is self-limiting, and recovery is usual within a week.

Laboratory Diagnosis

Blood cultures are often positive during the first two or three weeks of the illness in cases of enteric fever and septicemic disease. Urine cultures may be positive in the third or fourth weeks of enteric disease.

Feces culture is positive in enteric fever and gastroenteritis. In the former syndrome, a positive culture is not usual in the first week of the disease. Serological testing (p. 537) in cases of enteric fever is more likely to be positive in the third week of the disease.

After the disease, some individuals may excrete the organisms for a month or two (convalescent carriers) or for many years (chronic carriers). Some of the latter may excrete the organisms only periodically (intermittent). Chronic carriers often harbor the organisms in the gallbaldder and are often apparently healthy.

Common Serotypes

In Canada and in the United States, during 1979 the five commonest serotypes from human sources were

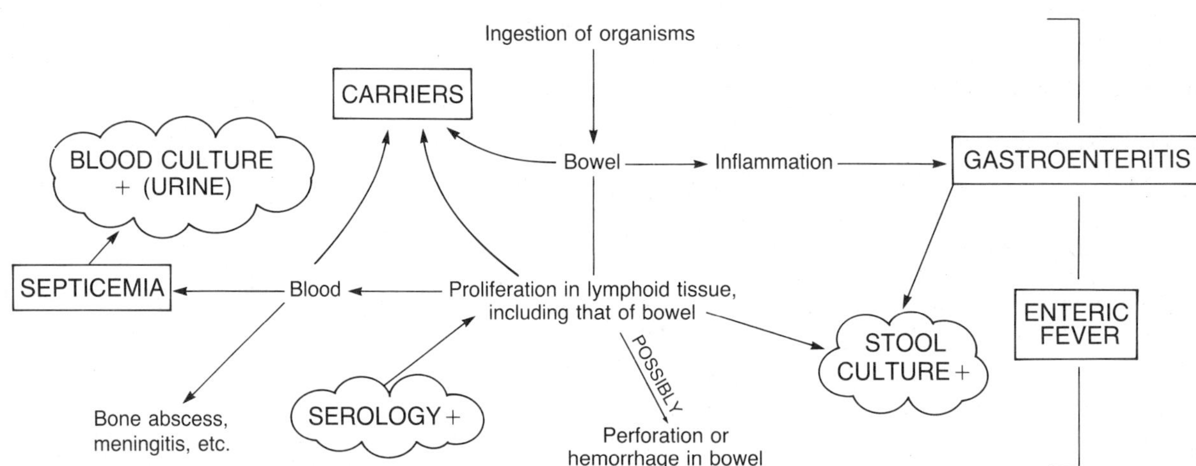

Figure 17–2 Pathology of *Salmonella* infections (simplified). The disease may be limited to a gastroenteritis. Septicemic cases are more serious and may occur in enteric fever which may include gastroenteritis, focal infections, and severe bowel complications. Carriers may occur following each type of disease. The relationship of laboratory investigations to pathological events is also shown.

similar, viz., *S. enteritidis, ser Typhimurium, ser Enteritidis, ser Heidelberg, ser Newport,* and *ser Infantis.*

ARIZONA HINSHAWII

These organisms are not unlike the salmonellae as regards colonial appearances and morphology, but they differ particularly in that many of them are late lactose fermenting or ONPG positive, will ferment malonate, are late liquefiers of gelatin, and (see also table on p. 377) do not ferment dulcitol. On TSI, reactions are like those of *Salmonella enteritidis,* but occasionally the slope may be acid, Alk(A)/A gas+ H_2S+. They have a complicated serology, like salmonellae, but one that is distinctive and separate. A polyvalent *Arizona* serum is available for identification. The organisms were originally recovered from reptiles but are causative of gastroenteritis in humans as well as in some domestic animals.

THE GENUS *SHIGELLA*

This genus causes bacillary dysentery. As a group *Shigella organisms* are gram-negative rods that are nonmotile and generally nonaerogenic. Some shigellae are late lactose fermenters. On enteric media, the colonies are smaller than those of salmonellae, and a few are mucoid, but they are otherwise not notable. On TSI, the reaction is Alk/A gas− H_2S−.

The genus is divisible serologically and chemically into four species, all of which cause dysentery in varied degrees of severity. The species are *S. dysenteriae*[(A)] *S. flexneri,*[(B)] *S. boydii,*[(C)] and *S. sonnei.*[(D)] The last-named is responsible for about 74% of isolates in the United States and *S. flexneri* for about 25% (1979), so that the others are isolated rarely. They may be differentiated biochemically as shown in Table 17–3.

Serology

Differentiation may also be made serologically between the four species, which are also considered as four groups of related serotypes (A, B, C, D) and the A-D group of *E. coli* (see p. 377). The sera are available commercially, and slide agglutination tests are made, using a drop of thick suspension of the organism from an overnight nutrient agar slope, in saline with a drop of antisera. Since some of the organisms may have capsular antigens that render the group antigen inagglutinable, it may be necessary to destroy these in cases in which there is high suspicion but in which agglutination tests are negative. The capsular antigens may be eliminated by boiling a suspension of the organism for one hour and then washing with saline by centrifugation. The slide agglutination test may then be repeated after the specific group antigens have been unmasked.

Pathology

The organisms are ingested in contaminated food or drink. There is an incubation period of 2 to 3 days, followed by fever, abdominal pain, and diarrhea. Stools are watery, possibly bloody with mucus, and microscopically show pus. The organisms invade the mucosa of the distal ileum and colon and produce shallow ulcers. Very rarely, there is bacteremia, and the disease usually subsides in about a week. The patient may pass viable organisms (and remain infectious) for 1 to 3 months.

The disease caused by *S. sonnei* is relatively mild, but that due to *S. dysenteriae* is severe and associated with a measurable mortality. *S. boydii* and *S. flexnerii* are intermediate in severity, with the latter causing a more severe disease than the former.

Antimicrobial treatment is advised only in severe infections. In the usual mild *S. sonnei* disease, antimicrobial therapy may result in prolongation of the carrier state and in transmissible drug resistance.

Laboratory Diagnosis

This is made by culture of feces or from swabs taken from colonic ulcers under sigmoidoscopic control. Serological testing is generally not useful in a clinical setting.

THE K-E-S GROUP (THE TRIBE KLEBSIELLEAE)

These are a group of genera within the Enterobacteriaceae that have certain features in common. They generally utilize citrate, the Voges-Proskauer reaction is often positive, and they ferment lactose. They do not usually produce indole or H_2S but may form urease, which produces a delayed reaction (unlike *Proteus,* which hydrolyses urea rapidly). The major differences in the genera within this tribe can be seen in Table 17–4. *Hafnia* is also represented, since it is very similar to *Enterobacter.*

THE GENUS *Klebsiella*

These nonmotile gram-negative rods have a mucoid capsule. Like the pneumococci, the capsules have a carbohydrate-associated antigen, and, by means of quellung reactions, the genus may be typed into more than 70 varieties. There are three species, of which the most commonly encountered in North America is *K. pneumoniae.* This organism is found in water and soil and is

TABLE 17–3 DIFFERENTIATION OF *Shigella* SPECIES

Test	*S. dysenteriae*	*S. flexneri 1–5*	*S. flexneri 6*	*S. boydii*	*S. sonnei*
Indole	−/+	+/−	−	−/+	−
Ornithine	−	−	−	−	+
Mannitol	−	+	+/−	+	+
Lactose	−	−	−	−	(+)

Note. Serotypes of *S. flexneri* are divisible into two biotypes.

TABLE 17–4 DIFFERENTIATION OF THE K-E-S GROUP

Test	*Klebsiella*	*Enterobacter*	*Serratia*	*Hafnia*
Motility	−	+	+	+
DNase	−	*−	+	−
Ornithine	−	+	+/−	+
Gelatin	−	+/(+)/−	+	−
Sorbitol	+	+/−	+/−	−

*Some strains of *E. agglomerans* may be positive. *E. sakazakii* gives delayed positive (2–6 days) results.

a normal inhabitant of the bowel and upper respiratory tract. It grows easily on blood agar and enteric media, producing after overnight incubation fairly large (1-mm diameter) mucoid colonies that are round, entire, shiny, and lactose fermenting. It is a fairly common cause of urinary tract infections and may cause bacteremia, peritonitis, and wound infection. In addition it may produce a severe type of pneumonia. *K. oxytoca* is a very similar organism but produces indole and may liquefy gelatin. *K. ozaenae* occurs infrequently and *K. rhinoscleromatis* rarely in North America. These latter organisms are responsible for chronic nasal diseases not often seen in the United States or Canada. *K. rhinoscleromatis* produces colonies not unlike *K. pneumoniae* on blood agar but only a small nonlactose fermenting colony on MacConkey agar; *K. ozaenae* is said to be similar.

The TSI reaction for *K. pneumoniae* is A/A gas+ H_2S−. Biochemical differentiation between the species may be made as shown in Table 17–5.

THE GENUS *Enterobacter*

This is a closely related group of gram-negative motile rods that are nonencapsulated. Gelatin is liquefied by the frequently discovered species. Ornithine is decarboxylated. There are several species, the commonest of which is *E. cloacae*. Others are *E. aerogenes, E. agglomerans,* and the newly described species *E. sakazakii* and *E. gergoviae*.

The organisms are again found in soil and water and in the intestinal tract. Colonies on blood agar and enteric media are not unlike those of *E. coli*. The organisms are frequent opportunistic pathogens and are found in wounds, in the urinary tract, and in cases of bacteremia. TSI shows A/A gas+ H_2S−. Differentiation of the species may be made as shown in Table 17–6.

Hafnia alvei

This species is quite similar to those in the genus *Enterobacter* and has been called *E. hafniae*. One of its distinguishing features is that it is a late lactose fermenter or does not ferment lactose at all. Its other characteristics are seen in Table 17–6. TSI features are Alk/A gas+ H_2S−.

THE GENUS *Serratia*

This is a group of motile gram-negative rods that are nonencapsulated. There are three species. The majority of these encountered belong to *S. marcescens,* whereas many fewer are in the species *S. liquefaciens* and *S. rubidaea*. Some strains of *S. marcescens* produce a red pigment, which is better produced at 22°C than at 35°C. All are rapid gelatin liquefiers and produce DNase. On TSI they show Alk(A)/A/gas− H_2S−. The colonies are not particularly noteworthy unless the pigment is produced on MacConkey agar. They are nonlactose fermenters but may show a slight opacity in the surrounding medium. They are found naturally in water and soil but are important opportunistic pathogens and have been responsible for urinary tract, pulmonary, and wound infections as well as septicemia. Biochemically, they may be separated as shown in Table 17–7.

The DNase Test

DNase test medium that contains nucleic acid is commercially available. To 1 liter of the prepared medium add 0.1 g Toluidine blue. Autoclave, cool, and pour into Petri dishes.

Organisms to be examined are either streaked or locally inoculated and incubated at 35°C overnight. A positive result is the production of a rose-pink zone around the streak or colony (this contrasts well with the clear blue medium). The theoretical basis of the test is the degradation of nucleic acid in the substrate by bacterial DNase, causing negative metachromasy (the reversal of usual metachromasy) in the Toluidine blue dye.

THE TRIBE PROTEEAE

This group of organisms has undergone considerable taxonomic change since the last edition of this book.

TABLE 17–5 DIFFERENTIATION OF *Klebsiella* SPECIES

Test	*K. pneumoniae**	*K. ozaenae*	*K. rhinoscleromatis*
Urease	+	d	−
Lactose	+	d	d
VP	+	−	−
Citrate	+	d	−
Lysine	+	−/+	−
Malonate	+	−	+/−

**K. oxytoca* is indole positive and may liquefy gelatin.

TABLE 17–6 THE DIFFERENTIATION OF THE GENUS *Enterobacter* AND *H. alvei*

Test	*E. cloacae*	*E. aerogenes*	*E. agglomerans*	*E. sakazakii*	*E. gergoviae*	*H. alvei*
Urea	+/−	−	d	−	+	−
Gelatin (22°C)	(+)	(+)/−	d	−	−	−
Ornithine	+	+	−	+	+	+
Arginine	+	−	−	+	−	d
Lysine	−	+	−	−	+/(+)	+
DNase	−	−	−	+*	−	−
Pigment	−	−	Yellow	Yellow at 25°C	−	−

*2 to 6 days in Toluidine blue medium.

TABLE 17–7 DIFFERENTIATION OF *Serratia* SPECIES

Test	*S. marcescens*	*S. liquefaciens*	*S. rubidaea*
Sorbitol	+	+	−
Raffinose	−	+	+
Malonate	−	−	+/−
Ornithine	+	+	−

Figure 17–3 Production of DNase; details are in text. On this toluidine blue plate, a colony of *Serratia marcescens* on the left has produced a pink surrounding zone by DNase activity, whereas the colony on the right does not produce this enzyme.

TABLE 17–8 DIFFERENTIATION OF SPECIES OF THE TRIBE PROTEEAE

Test	*P. vulgaris*	*P. mirabilis*	*P. alcalifaciens*	*P. stuartii*	*P. rettgeri*	*M. morganii*
Swarming	+	+	−	−	−	−
Gelatin (22°C)	+	+	−	−	−	−
Indole	+	−	+	+	+	+
Citrate	d	+/(+)	+	+	+	−
H_2S	+	+	−	−	−	−
Mannitol	−	−	−	d	+	−
Adonitol	−	−	+	−	+	−

There are now two species of the genus *Proteus,* i.e., *P. mirabilis* and *P. vulgaris;* three species of *Providencia,* i.e., *P. alcalifaciens, P. stuartii,* and *P. rettgeri;* and another genus with one species, i.e., *Morganella morganii.* The tribe are gram-negative, motile, rather pleomorphic rods without capsules. All of them grow well on blood agar and the usual enteric media, and on the latter they produce nonlactose fermenting colonies. They all elaborate a phenylalanine deaminase. The methyl red test is positive, and, with the exception of a few strains of *P. mirabilis,* all are VP negative.

THE GENUS *Proteus*

The two species here are rapidly urease positive, and on blood or nutrient agar they tend to swarm, producing an appearance of waves of a spreading growth. Swarming is inhibited on MacConkey agar and other enteric media as well as on an agar base if the agar concentration is 5% or more. Addition of sodium azide, chloral hydrate, and phenylethyl alcohol is also preventive. On TSI agar the expected reaction for these two species is as follows: *P. vulgaris,* A(Alk)/A gas+ H_2S+; *P. mirabilis,* Alk(A)/A gas+ H_2S+.

The organisms are not unusually found in the intestinal tract and are also present in the soil. They are pathogens in the urinary tract, in wounds, in the bloodstream in bacteremia, and so forth. An important clinical differentiation between these two species is that *P. mirabilis* is, as a rule, sensitive to penicillin and ampicillin, but *P. vulgaris* is resistant.

THE GENUS *Providencia*

This genus has the general features of the Proteeae: their colonies are similar, but there is no swarming. Unlike *Proteus* they are H_2S negative. Two of the species here are urease negative; *P. rettgeri* is urease positive but is included here on other taxonomic criteria. Reactions in TSI are Alk/A gas+ or − H_2S−.

The organisms have a distribution and pathogenicity similar to those of the *Proteus* species. In addition, *P. stuartii* has a propensity to infect burned areas.

Morganella Morganii

This organism is closely related to the genera *Providencia* and *Proteus.* It fails to utilize citrate, does not produce H_2S, and has been separated into a species by other parameters (see also p. 354). On TSI it gives Alk/A gas− (+) H_2S−.

Differentiation of the species within the tribe Proteeae can best be seen in Table 17–8.

YERSINIA ENTEROCOLITICA AND *PSEUDOTUBERCULOSIS*

These species belong to a genus that has recently been included within the Enterobacteriaceae. They are gram-negative, facultatively anaerobic rods or coccobacilli that are motile at 22 to 25°C by peritrichous flagella but not motile at 35°C. The organism will grow on usual enteric media, but more slowly than other Enterobacteriaceae, and colonies may not be visible for 48 hours. It is advisable that after overnight incubation at 35°C, the plates be allowed to incubate further at room temperature (22°C). The colonies appear as small nonlactose fermenters. A differential agar for *Y. enterocolitica* is now available commercially (see p. 335). On blood agar, colonies will appear at as early as 18 hours. There are four species within the genus, but *Y. pestis,* the cause of plague, and *Y. ruckeri,* which causes disease in fish, will not be considered. The two remaining species that may be found in feces have all the general features of the Enterobacteriaceae, but their unusual motility pat-

TABLE 17–9 DIFFERENTIATION OF YERSINIAE, PROTEEAE, AND SHIGELLAE

Test	*Y. enterocolitica*	*Y. pseudotuberculosis*	*Proteeae*	*Shigella*
Lactose	−	−	−	d
ONPG	+*	+	−	d
Motility at 25°C	+	+		
Motility at 37°C	−	−	+	−
Urease	+	+	+/−	−
Phenylalanine deaminase	−	−	+	−
Ornithine	+	−	d	d
Sucrose	+	−		
Rhamnose	−	+		

*At 25°C.

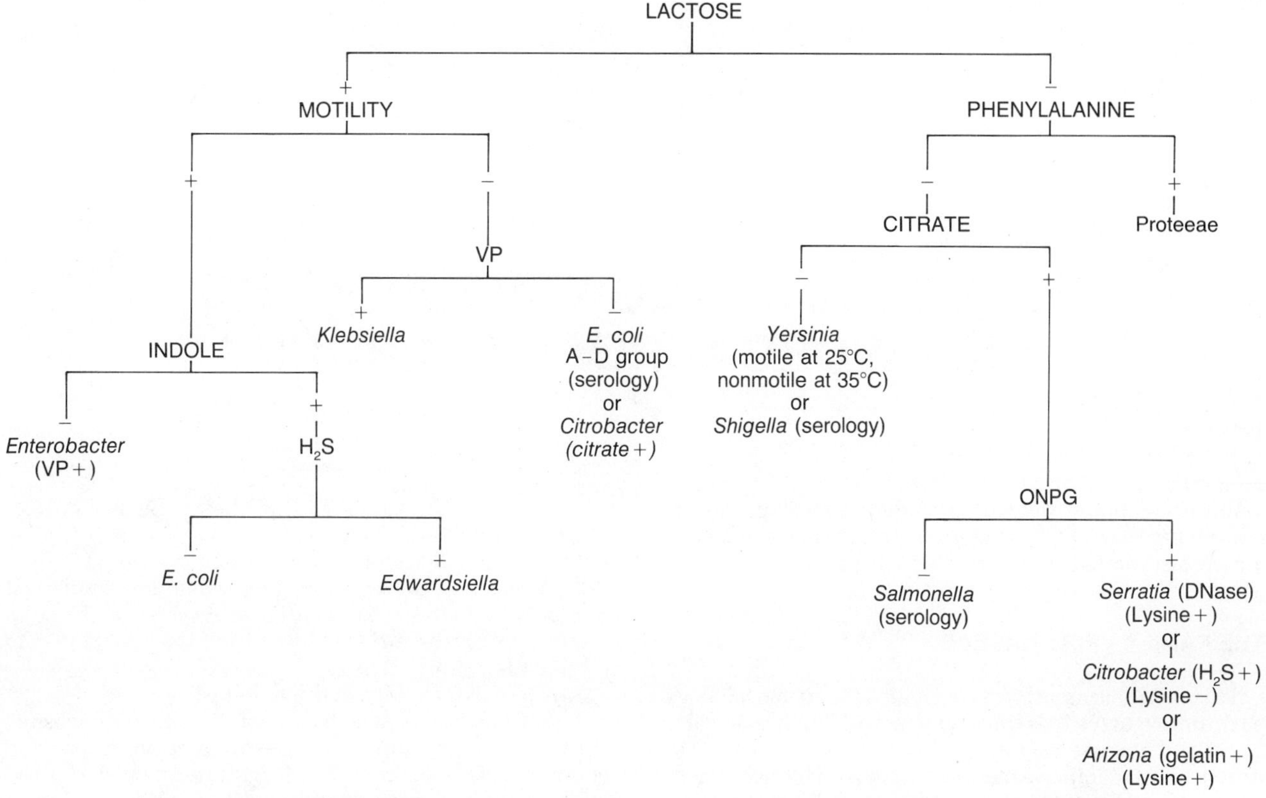

Figure 17–4 A simple dichotomous table for the differentiation of the Enterobacteriaceae. It separates genera and tribes by simple tests. The table is not exhaustive but shows a pattern that the student may imitate in remembering major reactions. Some exceptions will enter simple tables, but as long as these are noted (e.g., here the fact that *S. typhi* is citrate negative is ignored) the advantages of the exercise outweigh the disadvantages.

tern has been noted. In addition they are urease positive (but do not produce phenylalanine deaminase), and this combination should be sufficient to suspect *Yersinia.* A nonmotile organism may be confused with *Shigella,* but serology will rapidly make that exclusion. On TSI, *Y. enterocolitica* appears as A/A gas− H_2S− and *Y. pseudotuberculosis* as Alk(A)/A gas− H_2S−.

Differentiation within the genus and the two species as well as from Proteeae and *Shigella* may be seen from Table 17–9.

Pathology

Y. enterocolitica and *pseudotuberculosis* are found in wild and domestic animals and in their feces, from whence they infect humans. *Y. enterocolitica* commonly infects children of 2 years or younger and causes them to present with diarrhea and fever. Older children may have ileitis or acute lymphadenitis. In adults there may be fever, enteritis, or arthritis. Meningitis and septicemia may occur. *Y. pseudotuberculosis* generally causes mesenteric lymphadenitis.

Laboratory Diagnosis

The organism may be recovered from the feces, blood, or lymph nodes. The infection produces a recognizable histological pattern that may be recognized by the pathologist in surgically excised tissue. Infected patients develop specific antibodies to the organisms, which are of a number of serotypes.

CHAPTER 17—REVIEW QUESTIONS

1. Explain the terms ETEC and EIEC. Can one differentiate the diseases they produce by fecal examination?
2. How can one differentiate *Arizona* and *Salmonella* by production of gelatinase? How can one differentiate *C. freundii* and *Salmonella* by growth on KCN? How can one differentiate *C. freundii* from *Arizona* by indole production? How can one differentiate *S. typhi* from *S. enteritidis* by citrate production?
3. Give the usual reactions of *Salmonella, Shigella,* and *Klebsiella* on TSI slopes.
4. What is a major biochemical difference between:
   - *K. pneumoniae* and *K. oxytoca*
   - *S. sonnei* and other shigellae
   - *E. coli* and *E. tarda*
   - *S. marcescens* and *E. cloacae*
   - *P. vulgaris* and *Y. enterocolitica*
   - *P. vulgaris* and *P. mirabilis?*
5. Describe the antigenic structure of a *Salmonella.*

18

OTHER GRAM-NEGATIVE AEROBIC AND MICROAEROPHILIC RODS

In this chapter we will consider several groups of organisms. Some of these cause enteric disease, whereas others are related simply by their morphology.

THE FAMILY VIBRIONACEAE

This family is associated by virtue of their morphology as gram-negative rods that are generally motile by polar flagella. They are oxidase positive and utilize carbohydrates by fermentative metabolic means. The two genera that are considered here are *Vibrio* and *Aeromonas*.

The Genus *Vibrio*

This genus includes several species that are of importance in the clinical laboratory: *V. cholerae, V. parahaemolyticus,* and *V. alginolyticus.*

V. cholerae

This is the organism responsible for cholera. The disease is usually spread by contaminated water supply and is virtually unknown in the industrialized West. However, besides cases that may arrive in North America from endemic areas, other cases have occurred relatively recently in Florida and Louisiana following ingestion of raw oysters and steamed crabs. The patient is taken with diarrhea and vomiting. The former becomes progressively more watery (rice water stools), and the patient may die unless the great loss of fluid in the stool is replaced. The organism produces diarrhea not by bowel wall invasion but by elaboration of an enterotoxin that affects small-bowel mucosa.

The stool, in a suspected case, should be inoculated on TCBS (thiosulfate citrate bile salt sucrose) agar and incubated at 35°C for 18 to 24 hours. Most strains will also grow on MacConkey medium, producing colorless colonies. If it is decided to transport the material, Cary-Blair should be used (see p. 337). The reaction on TSI is A/A gas– H_2S–, but on KIA it is Alk/A gas– H_2S– (*V. cholerae* ferments sucrose). On TCBS medium, overnight colonies are yellow or green and 2 to 3 mm in diameter.

Since the disease is rare in North America and so potentially dangerous, suspect cultures should be sent to reference laboratories with all haste. Suspicion may be aroused by the following:

1. The clinical history, by signs and symptoms.
2. A positive string test, i.e., when an emulsified colony in aqueous 0.5% sodium deoxycholate clings to the loop when the latter is lifted from the slide for 45 to 60 seconds.
3. A positive oxidase and indole test.
4. A slide test in which a loopful of 2 to 5% washed chicken RBCs in saline is mixed with a heavy suspension of the suspect culture. Rapid agglutination of the red cells occurs within one minute with *V. cholerae* biotype El Tor, which is a common variety.

The Halophilic Vibrios

This is a group of organisms in the same genus as *V. cholerae*. They will not grow in a peptone broth containing less than 3% NaCl, whereas *V. cholerae* will not grow in a broth with more than 3% NaCl. They include *V. parahaemolyticus* and *V. alginolyticus*.

V. parahaemolyticus may cause gastroenteritis that is associated with eating contaminated seafood such as crab and shrimp. The disease is common in Japan but occurs also in North America. If it is suspected, the stool, which is not unlike that of more classic cholera, is plated on TCBS agar and in 1% peptone water with 3% NaCl. It will grow poorly on MacConkey agar. On TCBS agar colonies are large (2 to 5 mm in diameter) blue-green, and on TSI the reaction is Alk/A gas– H_2S–.

V. alginolyticus lives in sea water and most often causes wound infections and septicemias and rarely diarrhea. Its growth requirements are like those of *V. parahaemolyticus,* and appearances are similar, although the colonies are yellow; on TSI it will give an A/A gas– H_2S– reaction.

Differentiation of the vibrios may be best appreciated from Table 18–1.

The Genus *Aeromonas*

This genus is similar to the vibrios, and the differential bacteriological features are minor. They are motile by polar flagella and are oxidase positive and fermentative. On blood agar *A. hydrophilia* is often β-hemo-

TABLE 18–1 DIFFERENTIATION OF VIBRIOS

Test	*V. cholerae*	*V. parahaemolyticus*	*V. alginolyticus*
Oxidase	+	+	+
Indole	+	+	+
Lactose	(+)	−	−
Sucrose	+	−	+
Growth with 0% NaCl*	+	−	−
Growth with 10% NaCl	−	−	+
VP	d	−	+
String test	+	−	−

*One may use CLED (cysteine lactose electrolyte deficient) medium for this test: it will allow the growth of *V. cholerae* but not of halophilic vibrios.

lytic. They are slowly and weakly DNase positive; on TSI they show Alk(A)/A (N) gas−(+)H_2S−. *A. hydrophilia*, which naturally lives in fresh or salt water, has caused wound infection, diarrhea, septicemias, and other infections. Some of the important features can be seen in Table 18–2.

THE GENUS *PSEUDOMONAS*

This is a large group of organisms with many species, several of which are of importance in medical bacteriology. They are gram-negative rods that are motile by means of polar flagella, and they are strictly aerobic, catalase positive, and indole negative. Most important, they are nonfermentative and often oxidative.

Pseudomonas aeruginosa is the commonest species of this group encountered in the medical laboratory. It has the general features of its family and grows easily on blood agar and enteric media. On blood agar it yields, after overnight incubation, a large flat colony with an entire margin that is usually opaque and occasionally mucoid. The colonies tend to spread, and the surrounding medium may be green (less often brown or red) because of pigment production. The pigment is generally fluorescent under ultraviolet light. In addition there is a characteristic odor said to be "grapelike." It metabolizes glucose oxidatively, produces oxidase and arginine dehydrolase, and grows at 42°C. On TSI it gives Alk/Alk gas− H_2S−.

Pathology

Ps. aeruginosa is a normal inhabitant of the soil and is also found in feces. It is a common cause of urinary tract infections and is also found in wounds, burns, infections of the respiratory system, and occasionally septicemia. It acts as an opportunistic organism in patients who have been treated with immunosuppressants or who have had some instrumental procedure (lumbar puncture, tracheostomy, etc.).

There are numerous other species of *Pseudomonas*, and only a few more common varieties will be considered here.

Ps. fluorescens is also found normally in soil or water and is an occasional opportunistic pathogen. Most strains are nonpigment producing, although they may produce a fluorescent substance. It has contaminated blood bank materials, into which it may release an endotoxin that causes fatal reactions.

Ps. maltophilia is found widely in nature and is the second most commonly isolated Pseudomonad in the clinical laboratory. It may be associated with opportunistic infections. Colonies are yellow or tan, and they produce an ammoniacal odor on blood agar. They are oxidase negative and are not pigment producing on routine media.

Ps. cepacia often appears in nosocomial infections. It is found widely in nature but also has been demonstrated in the hospital environment: in distilled water, deter-

TABLE 18–2 DIFFERENTIATION OF *Aeromonas* AND *Vibrio*

	Aeromonas	*Vibrio*
Growth on MacConkey agar	+	d
Oxidase	+	+
Halophilic	−	d
Lysine	−	+
Ornithine	−	+
Growth without NaCl	+	d

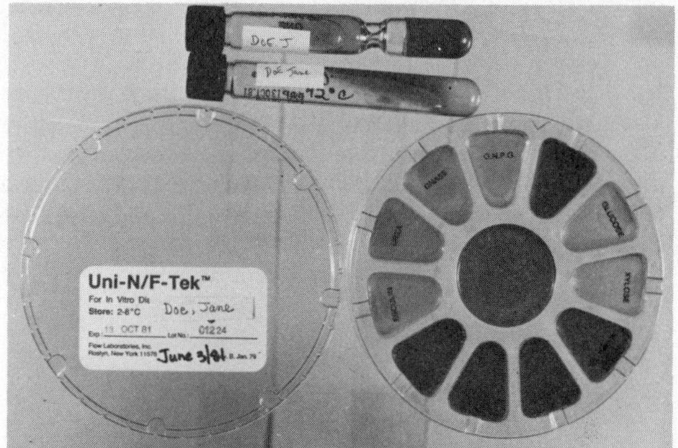

Figure 18–1 The Uni–N/F System (Flow Laboratories, Inc., Roslyn, N.Y. 11576) for the identification of nonfermenters. It consists of a two-tube screen, one of the tubes being incubated at 42°C and the other at 35°C. *Ps. aeruginosa* and *Ps. fluorescens* may be identifiable at this stage on the basis of fluorescence, production of nitrogen gas and pyocyanin, and growth at 42°C. Glucose fermenters are also noted in the tube stage. If necessary, the plate is inoculated, and a further 12 parameters are available. A chart of expected reactions is available delineating the probable results for a large number of nonfermenters.

TABLE 18–3 DIFFERENTIATION OF *Pseudomonas* SPECIES

Test	*Ps. aeruginosa*	*Ps. fluorescens*	*Ps. maltophilia*	*Ps. cepacia*	*Ps. alcaligenes*
Oxidase	+	+	−	+	+
Arginine dehydrolase	+	+	−	−	−
ONPG	−	−	+	+	−
Growth at 42°C	+	−	d	d	d
Maltose	−	−/+	+	+	−
Production of N_2 gas	+/−	−	−	−	−
Polymyxin susceptibility	+	+	+	−	+

A more complete differential table including other *Pseudomonas* species will be found in larger works.

gent solutions, incubators, respirators, and so forth. Some strains produce pigments.

Ps. alcaligenes is again widely found in nature and may be an opportunistic pathogen.

Differentiation of the *Pseudomonas* species may best be seen in Table 18–3.

THE GENUS *ALCALIGENES*

These are gram-negative, aerobic rods that are motile by peritrichous flagella. They are oxidase and citrate positive and urease negative and have no action on carbohydrates. The organisms grow well on blood and MacConkey agar but not on SS agar. On TSI the pattern is Alk/Alk gas− H_2S−. There are three species: *A. faecalis, A. odorans,* and *A. denitrificans. A. odorans* produces a dark green color on blood agar, and the colonies smell like apples. They live widely in nature and may be found in the hospital environment, where they may be involved in opportunistic infections.

THE GENUS *FLAVOBACTERIUM*

This is a group of gram-negative, aerobic, nonmotile, oxidase-positive organisms that are oxidizers or weak fermenters and DNase positive. Colonies are yellow, and the organisms will grow on nutrient agar and generally on MacConkey agar but not on SS medium. *F. meningosepticum* is the species of this group most commonly seen in the nosocomial infections with which the group is associated. *F. meningosepticum* has caused meningitis and septicemia, particularly in premature babies, and is found (like *Ps. cepacia*) in the hospital environment as well as in soil and water. *F. meningosepticum* is indole and ONPG positive and produces gelatinase. On TSI the reaction is Alk/N (A) gas− H_2S−.

THE GENUS *ACINETOBACTER*

These organisms are gram-negative rods that often show bipolar staining so as to appear almost diplococcal. They are aerobic, nonmotile, and oxidase and indole negative; if they use carbohydrates, the metabolism is oxidative. They do not reduce nitrate. They grow well on MacConkey agar but generally not on S.S. agar. Occasionally a colony will produce a pale brown pigment. On blood agar, colonies are usually small, entire, and soft. On TSI the appearance is Alk/N (Alk) gas− H_2S−. Although there is only one accepted species, *A. calcoaceticus*, there are a number of biotypes, of which the most commonly met are bio. anitratus and bio. lwoffii. The major differences between these are best seen in Table 18–4.

The organisms are found as part of the normal flora of the skin and the gastrointestinal and upper respiratory tracts, but they are responsible for opportunistic and nosocomial infections, including meningitis, wound infections, and septicemia following instrumentation.

THE GENUS *MORAXELLA*

This genus has several species that are significant in the clinical laboratory. The organisms are small gram-negative bacilli or coccobacilli that are aerobic, nonmotile, oxidase positive, and nonsaccharolytic (inactive against carbohydrates). They are all sensitive to penicillin. Generally they grow on MacConkey agar and will grow on blood agar. On TSI the reaction depends on the species but is generally Alk/Alk gas− H_2S−; however, either the butt, the slope, or both may show no change. The organisms are found normally on the mucous membranes of animals and humans and can be opportunistic pathogens.

M. lacunata, which may cause conjunctivitis or respiratory tract infections, will not grow on MacConkey agar. It reduces nitrate to nitrite and liquefies gelatin. Differentiation of the several species is detailed in larger reference books.

PASTEURELLA MULTOCIDA

This organism is the commonest *Pasteurella* encountered in the medical laboratory. It is a small, gram-negative, coccobacillary organism that is nonmotile and aerobic and that grows well on blood agar to produce a small colony (1 to 2 mm) after 24 hours with perhaps a green discoloration of the surrounding medium and a characteristic musty odor. It is oxidase positive (but some commercial test strips may be falsely negative), reduces nitrate, and produces indole. It will not grow on

TABLE 18–4 DIFFERENTIATION OF BIOTYPES OF *A. calcoaceticus*

Test	Bio. anitratus	Bio. lwoffii
O/F Glucose	Oxidative	Inactive
10% Lactose	+	−
Xylose	+	−

MacConkey agar and is urease negative. It is fermentative and will ferment glucose and sucrose. On TSI it shows A/A gas− H_2S−.

The organism is a commensal in the mouth and respiratory tract of domestic and wild animals. The common infection in humans is an infected wound following a dog bite or scratch from a cat. Pulmonary infections occur especially in patients with a compromised respiratory tract, such as those with bronchiectasis; septicemia, osteomyelitis, and meningitis are also reported. Any animal bite should be suspect. If the organism fails to grow on MacConkey medium and is oxidase and indole positive, it is very likely *P. multocida*, and confirmatory tests should be performed. The organism is sensitive to penicillin.

TABLE 18–5 Differentiation of *Campylobacter* Species

Test	*C jejuni*	*C. fetus s.s intestinalis*
Growth at 42°C	+	−*
Growth at 35°C	+	+
Growth at 25°C	−	+
Oxidase	+	+
Catalase	+	+
Nalidixic acid 30 μg/disc	S	R
Cephalothin 30 μg/disc	R	S

*A few strains have been reported as growing at 25°C and at 42°C.

R = resistant; S = sensitive.

THE GENUS *CAMPYLOBACTER*

This genus is made up of gram-negative curved rods or spirals that have a polar flagellum by which they are motile in a corkscrew or dashing fashion. Some species are microaerophilic and oxidase positive. *C. fetus s.s. intestinalis* usually causes septicemia in the immunologically suppressed, whereas *C. jejuni* is a common cause of gastroenteritis and is responsible for a large proportion of cases that in some geographic areas has exceeded all other bacterial causes combined.

C. Jejuni

The organism can be transported effectively in a number of transport media, including buffered glycerol-saline or Cary-Blair medium. Inoculation is made onto Skirrow's medium, or some suitable modification (many of which are available commercially), which contains vancomycin, trimethoprim, and polymyxin B sulfate in a nutrient base to prevent the growth of other organisms. The charged plates are incubated at 42°C for 48 hours in an atmosphere of 10% CO_2 and 5% O_2. (BBL's* Campy Pak II contains the required reagents to produce such an atmosphere.)

After incubation, colonies of *C. jejuni* are small (1 to 2 mm) and flat with an irregular margin. They may be slightly pink or pink-gray. A gram film is made of suspicious colonies, and gram-negative curved rods that are oxidase and catalase positive are presumptively identified. This method will not detect *C. fetus s.s. intestinalis*, but this organism is clinically much more important in cases of septicemia in the newborn and immunologically suppressed and will be cultured directly from blood culture or some focal disease. *C. fetus s.s. intestinalis* requires the same atmospheric conditions as *C. jejuni*. For some differential features, see Table 18–5.

Pathology

C. jejuni is responsible for a common and worldwide type of gastroenteritis with fever, bloody diarrhea, and abdominal pain. Because of its common incidence, the organism should be sought, by the means outlined, in all cases of febrile diarrhea.

*Baltimore Biological Laboratories, Cockeysville, Md. 21030.

REVIEW

In the preceeding part of this chapter and in the last chapter are described the numerous types of gram-negative bacilli and coccobacilli that are fairly commonly encountered in the clinical laboratory. To the student, at first reading, their differentiation is bound to be somewhat confusing, but it may be rendered more comprehensible by reference to Table 18–6. It will be seen that with relatively few simple tests the species or family of the index organism can be pinpointed, and further differential tests within that group can then be applied.

A few further organisms are considered here because morphologically they are similar to those discussed previously but these additional organisms are unrelated in a wider bacteriological sense and are associated pathologically with a different part of the spectrum of disease.

THE GENUS *HAEMOPHILUS*

These organisms are gram negative coccobacillary, rod shaped or filamentous, and markedly pleomorphic. They are aerobic and nonmotile and require a supply of growth factors present in blood, particularly X and/or V factors.

X factor is heat-stable hemin, and V factor is heat-labile nicotinamide adenine dinucleotide. Both factors are present in blood cells, but only X is available in blood agar. If the red cells are disrupted by heating, as occurs in the production of chocolate agar or Levinthal's medium, V factor is also made available and the heat treatment concurrently destroys anti-V substances in blood. V factor is also available in the medium around staphylococcal colonies, which secrete this substance. This latter phenomenon is the explanation for the occurrence of satellitism of colonies of some haemophili around staphylococci, in that within the medium near the latter colonies on blood agar both X factor and V factor are present (Fig. 18–2). Sheep blood may contain inhibitors to haemophili, and horse blood is preferable. Generally with spinal fluid, blood cultures, or swabs from lesions suspected of *Haemophilus* etiology, chocolate agar and/or a horse blood agar that, after inocula-

TABLE 18–6 Differentiation of Aerobic and Microaerophilic Gram-Negative Rods

	Growth on MacConkey Agar	Oxidase	O/F Glucose	Polar flagella	Motile
Enterobacteriaceae	+	−	F	−	+
Vibrio	d	+	F	+	+
Aeromonas	+	+	F	+	+
Pseudomonas	+	+*	O	+	+
Alcaligenes	+	+	I	−	+
Flavobacterium	d	+	I or F[w]	−	−
Acinetobacter	+	−	O or I	−	−
Moraxella	d	+	I	−	−
Pasteurella	−	+	F	−	−
Campylobacter	NA	+	I	+	+
Haemophilus	−	+/−	F	−	−
Gardnerella	−	−	F	−	−
Brucella	−	+/−	O	−	−
Bordetella	d	d	O or I	−	d

*Except. *Ps. maltophilia.*
d, Varies between or within species; F, fermentative; O, oxidative; I, inactive; NA, nonapplicable; +/−, most species are positive, fewer are negative; F[w], weak fermenter.

tion, is streaked by a staphylococcal streak may be used. In the differentiation of isolated *Haemophilus* species, the organism is re-inoculated onto trypticase soy agar, and then paper strips or discs impregnated with X, V, and X and V factors are applied to the medium. After overnight incubation at 35°C, a *Haemophilus* species will demonstrate its dependence for growth by growing in proximity to the X and XV disc (if it needs X), the V and XV (if it needs V), or the XV disc (if it needs both factors). It will not grow on the trypticase soy agar remote from the discs, where no factor has diffused. The organisms, of course, will not grow on MacConkey agar. Their action on carbohydrates is fermentative.

Haemophilus Influenzae

H. influenzae requires both X and V factors, so it will show satellitism around staphylococci on blood agar, will grow near a disc with X and V factor on trypticase soy agar, and will flourish on chocolate agar. Colonies are small, convex, and entire. The organisms may be typed, for serotypes a through f, by their capsules. The capsules may be identified with specific antisera by the quellung phenomenon (see p. 372). In the last few years, *H. influenzae*, which had been universally sensitive to ampicillin, has developed strains producing β-lactamase and thus ampicillin resistance.

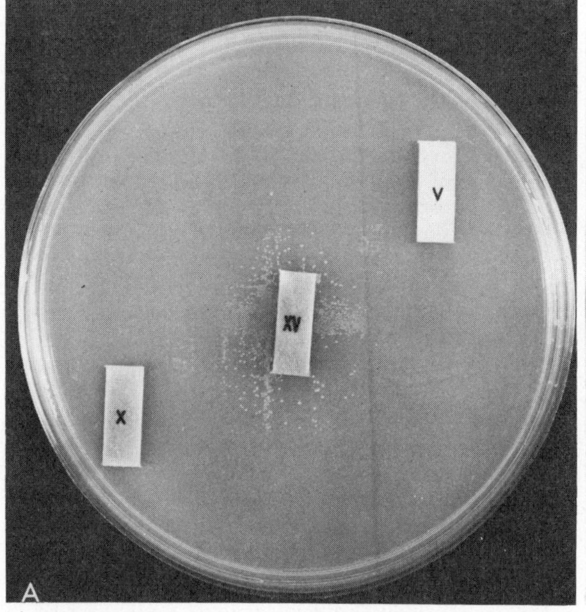

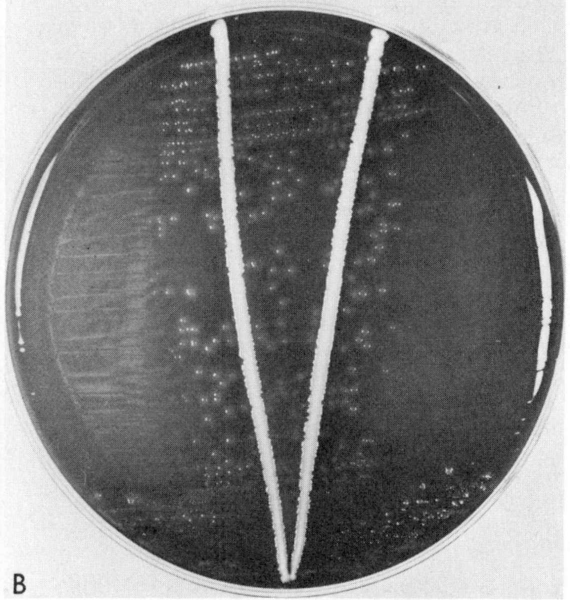

Figure 18–2 **A**, *H. influenzae*. Organisms plated on nutrient agar show growth only around the central strip, which has diffused X and V factors into the medium. X or V factor alone is unable to support growth. **B**, Satellitism. After the blood agar plate was inoculated with a specimen suspected of including a *Haemophilus* organism, it was streaked with *Staph. pyogenes*. After incubation, the *Haemophilus* organism is seen growing well in the neighborhood of the *Staphylococcus*, where V factor has diffused into the medium.

Pathology

H. influenzae, although at times a devastating pathogen, may often be found in the nasopharynx of a normal individual. The factors that transform the symbiotic organism into a disease-producing agent are not understood. If discs containing bacitracin and X and V factors are used on throat swab cultures, the presence of *H. influenzae* and other *Haemophilus* species in the throat will be appreciated.

H. influenzae is a common cause of bacterial meningitis in children and is often caused by serotype b organisms. The gram-negative, pleomorphic, coccobacillus can often be provisionally diagnosed as present on stained cerebrospinal fluid deposits (Fig. 18–3). The clinician should be informed, so that the patient can be treated with chloramphenicol rather than ampicillin. After culture, the colonies should be examined for production of β-lactamase. Also in children, acute epiglottitis, which is a life-threatening condition, is generally due to the same serotype. The tissues of the throat are greatly swollen, especially the epiglottis, so that the child, usually age 2 to 5, is threatened by suffocation. A minority of cases occur in adults. Possibly George Washington's death was due to this condition. The infection in the throat is often accompanied by septicemia. Again chloramphenicol is given, on the assumption that the organism may produce β-lactamase and be ampicillin resistant. Septicemia may lead to arthritis, pericarditis, and other focal lesions. Otitis media is not uncommon and may be the precursor of meningitis. Nonencapsulated *H. influenzae* organisms also cause otitis media and other upper and lower respiratory tract infections.

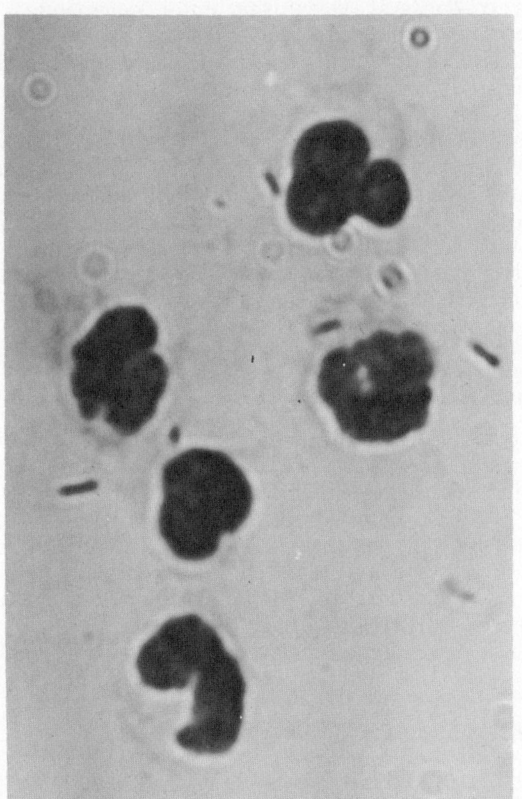

Figure 18–3 *Haemophilus influenzae* meningitis (spinal fluid). Gram stain × 2250.

Other Species of *Haemophilus*

Several of these are nonpathogenic inhabitants of the upper respiratory tract. They include *H. parainfluenzae, H. parahaemolyticus,* and *H. haemolyticus.*

H. aegyptius (Koch-Weeks bacillus), which is very similar to *H. influenzae* in the laboratory, commonly causes conjunctivitis.

H. paraphrophilus, segnis, and *aphrophilus* occur normally in the mouth. Some of these commensals have occasionally been implicated in endocarditis and focal septic disease. *H. ducreyi* is the cause of chancroid, which is an unusual venereal disease in North America. In suspect cases, the lesion is cleaned with saline and then swabbed with a cotton swab moistened with broth. Material from infected lymph nodes may also be available for culture. Culture is as above, but *H. ducreyi* grows optimally at 33°C and needs 5 to 10% CO_2 and a moist atmosphere.

Other species of *Haemophilus* exist but are of little significance in human disease.

Differentiation of the genus *Haemophilus* can be best made and appreciated from Table 18–7.

It should be noted that when testing for X factor, one should take particular care that even minute amounts are not transferred from a primary medium. Traces of X factor in basal media such as Mueller-Hinton may be sufficient to cause incorrect interpretations, particularly in identifying *H. parainfluenzae* (needs V only) instead of *H. influenzae* (needs both X and V).

GARDNERELLA VAGINALIS (*Haemophilus vaginalis, Corynebacterium vaginalis*)

This organism is a bacillus or coccobacillus that is nonmotile and that may appear gram positive in young cultures but is gram negative in older cultures. Electron microscopy demonstrates a wall that has gram-positive features. As the heading above indicates, the organism taxonomically has had a rather uncertain identity. It does not need X or V factor, unlike *Haemophilus*, and is catalase negative, unlike *Corynebacterium*. It is now placed tentatively in its own genus, *Gardnerella*. β-hemolysis occurs on human and rabbit blood agar but not on sheep blood agar. *G. vaginalis* will not grow on MacConkey agar. It is aerobic and facultatively anaerobic. Many strains are ONPG positive.

Pathology

It is now considered that *G. vaginalis* is the cause of nonspecific vaginitis. (Specific vaginitis may be due to gonorrhea, *Candida*, or *T. vaginalis*). The disease is associated with a gray malodorous vaginal discharge in which "clue cells" are often seen. The latter are vaginal epithelial cells with numerous adherent gram-negative rods. There is some possibility that the disease may be the result of synergism between *G. vaginalis* and vaginal anaerobes. Metronidazole is very efficacious therapeutically, and this suggests, since the drug is very effective against anaerobes and only moderately active against *G. vaginalis*, that the anaerobic syngergistic theory may have some merit.

TABLE 18–7 DIFFERENTIATION OF MAJOR *Haemophilus* SPECIES

Test	*H. influenzae* and *aegyptius*	*H. parainfluenzae*	*H. haemolyticus*	*H. parahaemolyticus*	*H. paraphrophilus*	*H. aphrophilus*	*H. ducreyi*
Requires X factor	+	−	+	−	−	−*	+
Requires V factor	+	+	+	+	+	−	−
β-Hemolysis	−	−	+	+	−	−	−
Catalase	+	d	+	+	−	−	−

*On primary culture usually requires X factor, but on subculture may not.

Culture

Swabs are inoculated on Columbia CNA agar, which is commercially available, supplemented by 5% rabbit blood. The medium contains colistin and nalidixic acid, which inhibits commensals. The plates are incubated at 35°C for 48 hours in a 5% CO_2 atmosphere. Subsequently β-hemolytic colonies that are morphologically acceptable and catalase negative are considered presumptively to be *G. vaginalis*. If the organisms are grown on chocolate agar or dextrose starch agar, a zone of inhibition can be obtained adjacent to a dense streak of α-hemolytic streptococci or pneumococci. The inhibition is believed due to production of H_2O_2 by the last-named organisms, and this presumptive test is known as the "reverse satellite" test (Park et al., 1968). Further confirmatory tests are available if desired, but presumptive tests are generally sufficient in a clinical setting.

THE GENUS *BRUCELLA*

These are gram-negative coccobacilli that are aerobic and that often thrive with additional CO_2. They are nonmotile, use carbohydrates oxidatively, are catalase positive, and may be urease positive. They generally will not grow on MacConkey agar and on first isolation are often encapsulated. Important species such as *B. abortus* and *B. suis* are oxidase positive. Several species are known, of which *B. abortus, B. suis, B. melitensis,* and *B. canis* cause disease in humans as well as in cattle, swine, goats or sheep, and dogs, respectively. In addition, these species have numbers of biotypes. Because the disease caused (i.e., brucellosis) has far-reaching epidemiological significance and consequences, and because *Brucella* is seldom seen, detailed bacteriology is best carried out by reference laboratories.

Brucella abortus may be studied as a relatively important member of this group. Besides having the general features of the genus, it reduces nitrates to gas and oxidizes glucose, arabinose, and galactose. *B. abortus* is inhibited by the dyes thionine and basic fuchsin. The inhibitory dilutions of the dyes within media are used to differentiate between brucellae.

Pathology

The organisms are primarily pathogens in different animals, causing, for example, abortion in cattle, but they are spread to humans via milk, urine, vaginal secretions, and so forth. They are also spread from the flesh of animals to humans involved in such occupations as meat processing and packing. Organisms enter the human through the mucous membranes of the oropharynx, through slightly damaged skin, or across the conjunctiva (those who wear spectacles in meat processing plants are more often seronegative to *Brucella* than are their co-workers). Organisms enter macrophages, in which they proliferate and spread. They are obligate intracellular organisms but are released into the blood periodically, causing intermittent septicemia. Located in tissues, they lead to granulomas, occasionally abscesses, meningitis, endocarditis, arthritis, and so forth. There is an incubation period of a few weeks to several months after infection, following which the patient complains of ill-defined symptoms—headache, weakness, etc.—as well as intermittent fever. The disease if untreated may persist for many years. Fortunately it is uncommon. Only 232 cases were reported in 1977 in the United States and only 16 cases in Canada in 1979.

Diagnosis

Blood culture is the usual mode of laboratory diagnosis, and the Castaneda technique (solid and liquid medium) is used (see p. 334). The bottles should contain 5 to 10% CO_2 and medium for *Brucella*. Blood cultures should be kept for three weeks. Other cultures (e.g., from abscesses) are plated on 5% sheep blood medium or on medium with antimicrobials to prevent contaminant growth (Lennette et al., 1980).

Serological diagnosis is described elsewhere (p. 538).

BORDETELLA PERTUSSIS

This is a gram-negative rod that is nonmotile and inactive against carbohydrates. Because of the characteristic pallor of the organisms on the gram film, it is

TABLE 18–8 Differentiation of *Bordetella* Species

Test	*B. pertussis*	*B. parapertussis*	*B. bronchiseptica*
Growth on blood agar on primary isolation	−	+	+
Motility	−	−	+
Urease	−	+ (24 hr.)	+ (4 hr.)
Nitrate → nitrite	−	−	+
Growth on MacConkey agar	−	+	+

advisable to lengthen the time of counterstaining. *B. pertussis* does not require X or V factor and will not utilize urea or reduce nitrates. It is causative of whooping cough.

For successful culture, the technique of collection and growth is very important. Swabs are taken on a pernasal nasopharyngeal swab. Since *B. pertussis* is sensitive to fatty acids, the swabs used are of alginate and are supported on thin, long, flexible wire supports (these are commercially available). After the swabs are taken, they should immediately be inoculated onto Bordet-Gengou agar. The latter is essentially 30% sheep blood in a potato-glycerol agar. Penicillin or methicillin are often added to prevent the growth of commensals. Incubation is at 35°C for 3 to 5 days. If it is necessary to convey swabs to a reference laboratory for culture, special transport media are available, and such advice should be sought from the reference laboratory.

Pathology

Whooping cough has an incubation period of 7 to 10 days, after which there is sneezing and coryza followed by coughing. The latter becomes characteristic when after a paroxysm there is the typical inspiratory "whoop." Vomiting may occur, and complications include bronchopneumonia and encephalitis. There is also a considerable absolute peripheral blood lymphocytosis. The usual length of uncomplicated disease is about six to seven weeks.

Another organism, *B. parapertussis*, also causes a whooping cough–like disease; *B. bronchiseptica* is likewise a cause of a similar disease or may be found in wound infections. It is a normal inhabitant as well as a pathogen in domestic and other animals. A summary of the differentiation of these species of *Bordetella* is given in Table 18–8.

CHAPTER 18—REVIEW QUESTIONS

1. Describe the string test, the action of chicken RBC, the oxidase and the indole test, and the action of 10% NaCl in *V. cholerae*.
2. Check the correct characteristics of *Aeromonas* in the list below:

Polar flagella	Peritrichous flagella
Oxidase negative	Oxidase positive
Fermentative	Oxidative
DNase negative	DNase positive

3. Answer true or false for *Ps. aeruginosa*:
   - Pigment nonfluorescent
   - Will grow at 42°C
   - Fermentative
   - Indole negative
   - Facultative anaerobe
   - Catalase positive
   - Oxidative
   - Sensitive to polymyxins
   - ONPG positive
4. Describe briefly the media and culture requirements for the selective growth of *C. jejuni*. What simple confirmatory tests are available for diagnosis after growth?
5. Describe the media and culture requirements for the selective growth of *G. vaginalis*. What simple confirmatory signs and tests are available for diagnosis after growth?

19

AEROBIC GRAM-POSITIVE RODS, MYCOBACTERIACEAE, AND *TREPONEMA PALLIDUM*

The aerobic gram-positive rods, which include the genera *Bacillus* and *Corynebacterium* as well as *Listeria monocytogenes,* are discussed in this chapter.

THE GENUS *BACILLUS*

These are gram-positive, aerobic, spore-bearing rods that are motile (except for *B. anthracis*) and that may be fermentative, oxidative or both. Most species live in the soil, and some are insect pathogens. There are very many species. One, *B. anthracis,* is the cause of anthrax. *B. cereus* may cause gastroenteritis, whereas other species may be rarely pathogenic under unusual circumstances.

B. anthracis

This organism has the general features of the genus and, unlike others, is nonmotile. The organism grows well on blood agar incubated at 35°C overnight. The colonies are nonhemolytic and are said to have a characteristic viscosity or tenacity: when deranged by an exploring bacterial loop, they retain their disturbed configuration. Spores, when present, are central and do not swell the cell. In direct films from a cutaneous clinical lesion, the rods are arranged singly or in small chains. Although capsules may not be seen, a specific fluorescent antibody can be used to show them. Such a test may be used as a presumptive diagnostic test by reference laboratories in which the antibody is available. A preliminary series of diagnostic tests is shown in Table 19–1, which, if necessary, may be helpful in differentiating *B. anthracis* from *B. cereus* and others.

Because of the highly infective nature of the organism, the rarity of cases of anthrax, and the economic and social consequences of the diagnosis, reference laboratories should be urgently consulted if the diagnosis is considered.

Pathology. *B. anthracis* is primarily a pathogen of herbivores, but it may occur in other animals also. The organism enters wounds or may be ingested or inhaled. Subsequently bacteremia, toxemia, and death may follow.

Fortunately, human anthrax is a rare disease: in 1978 there were six cases reported in the United States; since then only one other case has occurred, in Colorado in 1980. Cutaneous anthrax occurs when a cut or abrasion is contaminated with the organism, generally from animal hide or tissue. It presents as a central eschar or scab surrounded by edematous blebs. The organism may be inhaled from hides and may produce pneumonia, or it may be ingested in contaminated meat. The inhaled and ingested varieties of the disease are progressive, with bacteremia, toxemia, and death, and cutaneous anthrax may pursue the same course.

Blood, sputum, and spinal fluid cultures may be taken, as well as swabs from cutaneous lesions. The organism, as noted, is highly infectious, so aerosols must be avoided and all other safety precautions, such as safety cabinets and decontamination of benches with 5% hypochlorite or 5% phenol, must be employed.

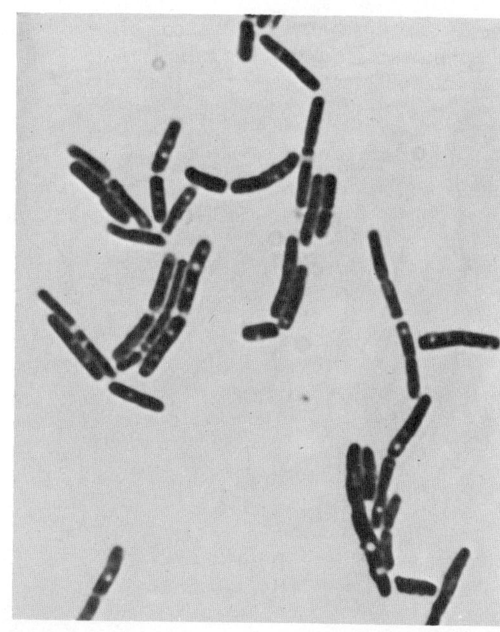

Figure 19–1 *Bacillus anthracis*. Smear from culture. Gram stain × 2250.

TABLE 19–1 Differentiation of *B. anthracis* from *B. cereus* and Other *Bacillus* Species

	B. anthracis	*B. cereus* and others
Hemolysis (sheep cells)	−	+
Motility	−	+
Salicin	−	+
Gelatinase 7 days	−	+
Growth on PEA* medium	−	+
String of pearls† test	+	Resistant to penicillin

*0.3% phenylethyl alcohol in heart infusion agar.

†A Mueller-Hinton plate is inoculated with the growth. A penicillin G disc (10 μ) is applied and incubated for 6 to 8 hours at 35°C. *B. anthracis* is sensitive to penicillin, and under the microscope at ×100, cells in the vicinity of the disc will appear spherical and in chains like a string of pearls.

B. cereus

This organism produces a toxin that is a cause of food poisoning. There is an incubation period of 10 to 12 hours, followed by diarrhea and pain without fever, a period lasting a further 12 to 24 hours. Another variety has a shorter incubation period after which there is vomiting. The diagnosis is accepted if 10^5 *B. cereus* organisms per gram are found in the incriminated food. Recovery of the organism from the feces is not helpful, since it may be a normal inhabitant of the bowel.

The organism grows easily on blood agar, giving hemolytic colonies, but investigations are best carried out by reference laboratories.

Other Organisms of the Bacillus Genus

These are generally seen in the laboratory as contaminants in cultures, but they may cause opportunistic infections in relation to prosthetic devices, e.g., meningitis with a cerebral ventricular catheter or more disseminated disease in patients with immunodeficiency.

Bacteriology of Bacillus Species

Differentiation is somewhat complicated, since there are many species that are similar. *B. anthracis* is the only nonmotile member of the genus. *B. cereus* is β-hemolytic, but others are similar. Differentiation, if required, is essentially the work of a specialized laboratory.

THE GENUS *CORYNEBACTERIUM*

These are gram-positive straight or slightly curved rods that may be club shaped at one pole and may contain metachromatic granules. The method by which they divide often produces an angular or picket-fence arrangement in smears. They are aerobic or facultatively anaerobic, nonmotile, nonencapsulated, and generally catalase positive. Albert's and Neisser's stains (p. 348) are techniques for demonstration of the intrabacillary granules. There are several species, of which one, *C. diphtheriae,* is the cause of diphtheria.

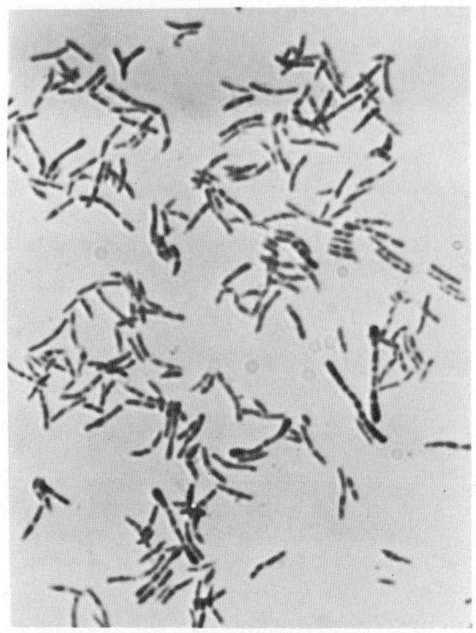

Figure 19–2 *Corynebacterium diphtheriae*. Smear from culture. Note the granules and the pleomorphism and the swollen club-shaped ends of some of the bacilli. Methylene blue × 2250.

C. diphtheriae

The organism has the general features of the genus. In suspect cases and in contacts, swabs of both the throat and nasopharynx should be submitted, since a single specimen may be positive in only 80% of cases. Specimens are inoculated into Loeffler's serum agar, sheep blood agar, and tellurite medium (p. 335). The blood agar and Loeffler's slope are incubated overnight at 35°C, and the tellurite medium can then be incubated a further 24 hours if necessary. Direct films from the patient may be misleading, but if morphologically the smears from the Loeffler's slope resemble *C. diphtheriae* a preliminary report may be issued. Subcultures from Loeffler to tellurite are made after overnight incubation. On tellurite, *C. diphtheriae* has a black or gray colony due to tellurite reduction. Such colonies, which are morphologically suspicious, are subcultured to blood agar for further study. Some diphtheroids (see below), staphylococci, and streptococci may also blacken tellurite, and these must be excluded by morphological examination or by further tests. A few strains of *C. diphtheriae* are inhibited by tellurite but will grow on blood agar, so the latter should be screened. Blood agar will also show β-streptococci, which may be the cause of a patient's sore throat or *Candida,* which may have produced a membrane that has created clinical confusion.

There are three biotypes of *C. diphtheriae,* viz., *gravis, intermedius,* and *mitis*. These were initially named to indicate the severity of the disease produced, but the names are no longer believed to have any clear relation to clinical severity. On blood agar, *mitis* forms large convex colonies, and many types are β-hemolytic; microscopically, these are long pleomorphic rods with well-formed metachromatic granules. Biotype *intermedius* has flat, creamy, transparent colonies on blood agar and morphologically has very pleomorphic forms with irregular bands and large terminal granules. Biotype *gravis* on blood agar forms large convex colonies that may be rarely β-hemolytic. They are very pleomorphic with some coccoid forms, and they tend to stain uniformly.

Biochemically *C. diphtheriae* is catalase and nitrate positive. It forms H_2S. The latter is an important test that is positive in this group only with *C. diphtheriae, C. ulcerans,* and *C. pseudotuberculosis* (see below). This test may be done using modified Tinsdale agar base, which contains cystine and sodium thiosulfate.* The plates are streaked with the organisms and are also stabbed with the inoculating loop. Browning due to H_2S production occurs as halos around *C. diphtheriae* and *C. ulcerans* in 12 to 24 hours. Dextrose, maltose, starch, and glycogen are positive, but only biotype *gravis* ferments the latter two carbohydrates.

Toxin Production. Diphtheria is produced by the toxin of *C. diphtheriae,* so all suspect organisms must be examined for toxin production. Often this is done by a reference laboratory to which the organisms are sent on a Loeffler's slope. The Elek test is the usual method of *in vitro* testing for the toxigenicity of isolated organisms. A strip of filter paper soaked in diphtheria antitoxin (100 μ/mL) is pressed onto Elek's agar. The latter is streaked at right angles to, and across the paper strip with, the suspect organism, as well as with toxigenic and nontoxigenic *C. diphtheriae* control strains. The plate is incubated at 37°C for 18 to 24 hours. A white precipitate line of antigen-antibody complex will be seen running from the junction of the inoculum and the paper outward at 45° if the suspect strain is toxigenic. If the suspect strain is made running parallel to a known toxigenic strain, the two lines will meet, showing a reaction of identity.

Pathology. As noted, diphtheria is a disease produced by the toxin of *C. diphtheriae,* of which man is the only host. Children are the usual victims and present with a sore throat and fever. A gray membrane may be found in the throat. Here the organism lives, secreting its toxin into the damaged underlying tissues. (Streptococcal disease, infectious mononucleosis, Vincent's angina, and candidal pharyngitis may also produce membranes). Diphtheritic membrane may be present in the nose, nasopharynx, trachea, larynx, or conjunctiva and also in wounds and on traumatized skin.

*Baltimore Biological Laboratory, Cockeysville, Md. 21030.

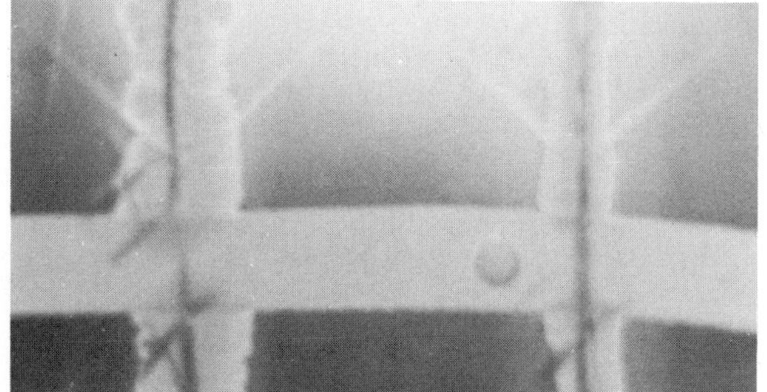

Figure 19–3 The Elek test. Across the plate is a strip of filter paper soaked in diphtheria antitoxin. Running vertically are two streaked inoculates of *C. diphtheriae*. At a point just above the filter paper, radiating into the medium, are 2 V-shaped areas of precipitation of toxin-antitoxin aggregate into the medium, showing the production of toxin by the bacterial streaks. The organisms are therefore toxigenic. (Preparation courtesy of the Public Health Laboratory, Windsor, Ont.)

The exotoxin causes necrosis in the tissues underlying the membrane, and when it enters the circulation, it has a propensity to damage heart muscle and nerve fibers.

The membrane may cause complications by blocking respiratory passages and causing asphyxia. Myocardial damage may result in heart failure, whereas neural damage may appear as peripheral and cranial nerve paralyses.

C. diphtheriae is a normal inhabitant in the throat of rare persons. Whether the person will develop disease will depend on the virulence of the organism and the resistance of the host. The latter has been statistically raised by widespread programs of immunization with diphtheria toxin or a suitable derivative. To attest to the value of immunization, in 1930, 66,576 cases of diphtheria occurred in the United States, but in 1979 only 59 cases were reported. The disease is spread to the susceptible mainly by droplet infection.

Apparently healthy persons may be carriers of diphtheria and may harbor toxin-producing strains of *C. diphtheriae* in the nasopharynx. They are protected against the disease by sufficient circulating antitoxin, but they may infect others. Some nonimmune persons are also carriers, and although, again, they may infect others, they are manifestly healthy. However, they may later show clinical disease. Carriers must be treated with antimicrobials, among which erythromycin and penicillin are most effective. Diphtheria is, as noted, a toxemia, and for this, antitoxin must be administered. It is interesting to note that toxin production by *C. diphtheriae* is due to a viral genome within the organism (i.e., β-prophage) and that nontoxic strains may be made toxic by exposing them to beta phage.

C. ulcerans

This organism is very similar to *C. diphtheriae,* produces a similar toxin, and is responsible for similar disease. As noted, it is H_2S positive on Tinsdale's medium but may be differentiated from *C. diphtheriae,* since it is urease positive and nitrate negative.

Other Corynebacteria

C. haemolyticum is a rare cause of skin ulcers or pharyngitis and, more rarely, other disease. *C. pseudotuberculosis* is a pathogen for sheep and horses but is very unusually a pathogen in man, since it very rarely produces diphtheria toxin. Other corynebacteria are often part of the normal body flora (in the conjunctiva, skin, or throat) but may be opportunistic pathogens in individuals with immunosuppression. These include *C. xerosis, C. hofmannii, C. equi,* and so forth. The basic differentiation is best seen by reference to Table 19–2. The other corynebacteria are often called diphtheroids and are generally recognized in direct smears from areas in which they are found, although of course they may be confused with *C. diphtheriae.* They grow easily on blood agar and on tellurite media but can be differentiated from *C. diphtheriae* by their failure to produce

H_2S on modified Tinsdale's medium. Biochemical differentiation of these is not often required, but details may be found in larger works should the organisms be thought to be the cause of opportunistic disease such as endocarditis.

Diagnosis of C. diphtheriae

Although a rare disease, diphtheria is a potential killer and may spread rapidly in a community in which immunization has been neglected. Awareness of the disease may be maintained in the laboratory by submission of the organism at intervals in control programs. Some laboratories will inoculate each throat swab onto modified Tinsdale's medium as a screening maneuver.

Listeria monocytogenes

This is a gram-positive, *motile,* nonsporing rod that is catalase positive and facultatively anaerobic. The organism is widely present in nature and causes disease in other mammals as well as in fish and birds. It is also found as a part of the flora in some normal human feces. On sheep's blood agar, the colony from inoculated clinical material often takes 48 hours at 35°C to reach a diameter of 0.5 to 2 mm. Colonies are circular, entire, and convex, commencing as translucent but becoming gray and opaque. Around the colony there is a narrow zone of β-hemolysis. The most characteristic feature is motility, which is best judged from a 6-hour broth culture at 25°C, when the organism will show a "head-over-heels" tumbling motion. Another unique feature is the "umbrella effect." When a culture of *L. monocytogenes* is stab inoculated into semisolid agar and cultured at 25°C, the organisms will move to and congregate in areas in which there are optimal conditions for growth. They tend to form a disc-shaped zone 2 to 3 mm beneath the surface of the agar, with a somewhat convex lower surface: hence the term *umbrella.*

Pathology. The organism causes disease, particularly in the newborn and in those with some immunodeficiency. Although possibly humans become infected from animal sources, it is most likely that most infections are from healthy human carriers.

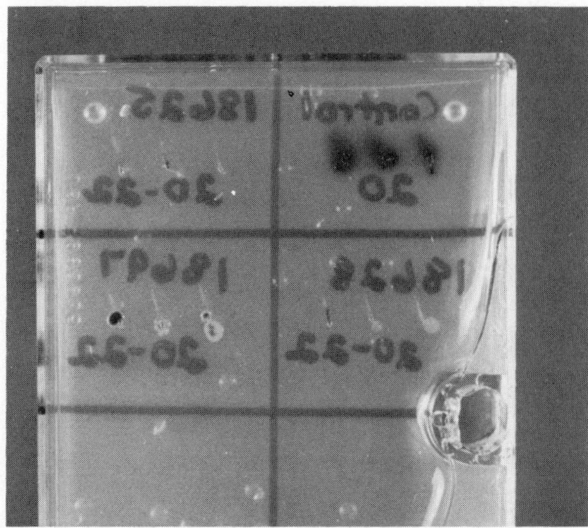

Figure 19–4 *C. diphtheriae* screening. A JEMBEC plastic plate is used for convenience and economy. It is prepared with a modified Tinsdale or cystine-tellurite medium. The organisms under study are stabbed into the medium. In the upper right-hand corner, the positive control organisms show a halo of browning around the stabs, but elsewhere the organisms are negative.

Intrauterine infection may cause abortion or stillbirth, and subclinical infection is possibly a cause of habitual abortion in humans (as it is in animals). A stillborn infant may have generalized "granulomatous sepsis" due to miliary listerial granulomata in all the organs. The infant may be born apparently healthy and in a week or so develop septicemia and meningitis. Vaginal cultures in these cases may reveal *L. monocytogenes,* and the mothers may be considered carriers. Serum tellurite agar* may be used on such specimens as a selective medium on which *L. monocytogenes* will appear as tiny black colonies after 4 to 5 days' incubation. In older patients numerous forms of the disease occur, viz., conjunctivitis, pharyngitis with lymphadenopathy, pneumonitis, meningoencephalitis, and so forth. The

*Baltimore Biological Laboratory, Cockeysville, Md. 21030.

TABLE 19–2 Clinically Essential Difffferentiation of *Corynebacterial* Species

Test	*C. diphtheriae*	*C. ulcerans*	*C. pseudotuberculosis*	Other Corynebacteria
H_2S halo in modified Tinsdale's medium	+	+	+	−
Diphtheria exotoxin production	+	+	rarely*	
Urease	−	+	+/−	
Nitrate reduction	+†	−	d	
Arginine	−	−	+	
Trehalose	−	+	−	
Gelatinase (25°C)	−	+	d	

**C. pseudotuberculosis* produces its own exotoxin but may be infected by beta phage, which may lyse the organism or become lysogenized, after which the host organism will produce diphtheria exotoxin as well as its more usual toxin.

†Some strains of *C. diphtheriae* bio *mitis* are nitrate negative.

TABLE 19–3 Basic Differentiation of *Corynebacterium Listeria*, and *Bacillus* Species

Test	*Corynebacterium*	*Listeria*	*Bacillus*
Motility	−	+*	+/−
Spores	−	−	+
Esculin hydrolysis	−	+	NR
Salicin	−	+	NR
Vosges-Proskauer	−	+	d

*at 25°C more than at 37°C.
NR, no result available.

organism is able to thrive within mononuclear cells, and immunity to the disease is of a cellular type.

Note on Diagnosis. The diagnosis is not difficult to make, provided that the possibility of *L. monocytogenes* is considered and that the organisms are not dismissed as contaminating "diphtheroids." Some differential features of the gram-positive rods discussed here are presented in Table 19–3.

THE GENUS *MYCOBACTERIUM*

This genus consists of slightly curved or straight rods that are not easily stainable by Gram's technique but that are acid-fast. They are nonmotile and without spores. Growth is slow, with the most rapid growers appearing in 2 to 3 days and most of the pathogens taking 6 to 8 weeks. *M. leprae* does not grow on artificial media. Optimal temperature for growth ranges from 24°C for some species to 37°C. There are many species that cause human disease, among which the most important is *M. tuberculosis*.

Recognition of Mycobacterial Disease

Because of the decline in the incidence of tuberculosis and the complexity of differentiating species of often slow-growing and dangerous pathogens, many hospitals restrict their investigations to relatively simple procedures sufficient to fulfill urgent clinical requirements while referring the organism to more specialized laboratories for more detailed investigation. *M. tuberculosis* will be described in some detail here, and methods of differential diagnosis will be given. If work with mycobacteria is contemplated, then avoidance of aerosol formation and inhalation of airborne organisms is most important. Preventative methods are given on p. 425. The mycobacteria may be divided into four groups in addition to *M. tuberculosis* and *M. bovis*. These other four groups are the Runyon groups I to IV. *M. leprae* cannot be cultivated in vitro. *M. tuberculosis* and *M. bovis* will not grow at room temperature. The other groups will grow at 24°C. Group I of Runyon are slow growers (two weeks or more) that are photochromogenic; i.e., they are pigmented after exposure to light. Group II are also slow growers and are scotochromogens; i.e., they are pigmented in the dark. Group III are nonchromogenic and nonphotochromogenic and are slow growers, whereas Group IV are rapid growers, appearing as colonies in less than one week at 25°C or at 37°C. The groups each include several species, and the classification may be sufficient for some laboratories. However, some species are occasionally found in one group, whereas at other times the same species may appear in another group. For example, *M. kansasii* is generally in Group I, but a few strains may be found in Group II or III. *M. szulgai* is in Group I if grown at 25°C and in Group II at 37°C. Some species in Group IV are also scotochromogens (Table 19–4).

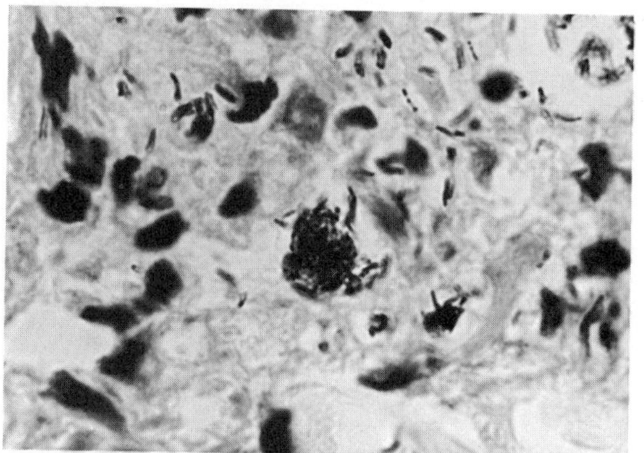

Figure 19–5 Leprosy. Section of a skin nodule stained by Ziehl-Neelsen method. There is a globus (cluster of organisms) in the center and other bacilli are scattered individually and in small groups. Note the beading. × 2300.

Preliminary identification may be aided if two slants of Lowenstein-Jensen (L-J) medium are inoculated with a thin suspension of the primary culture. One tube of each pair is shielded from light by aluminum foil, and a light-shielded and non-shielded tube are incubated at 37°C until growth appears in the unshielded slant. The growth is examined for pigment, and the time of appearance of the growth is noted. The shielded growth is also examined. If no pigment is observed, then half the shielded tube is exposed to a 60-watt bulb at 8 to 10 inches for one hour and re-examined. Such simple maneuvers will differentiate the four Runyon groups.

Useful Tests in Differentiation of Mycobacteria

It is worth emphasizing again that if full and safe facilities are not available, organisms suspected of being mycobacteria by acid-fast properties and cultural appearances should be referred to a more specialized center, and only a provisional report should be issued by the referring laboratory.

Niacin Test

M. tuberculosis produces niacin, which may be extracted from the medium by water and then tested with a commercially available paper strip. The latter will change color if the test is positive. A four-week culture is used in one method and is extracted in water when the slant is covered by the fluid and subjected to 121°C for 15 minutes in an autoclave. An extended period of extraction is said to give strong reactions with *M. tuberculosis* and fewer false positive reactions with other species.

Tellurite Reduction

M. avium-intracellulare complex strains will reduce potassium tellurite to metallic black tellurite. Two drops of 0.2% aqueous potassium tellurite are added to a seven-day fluid culture of the organism in 5 mL of Middlebrook

TABLE 19–4 Primary Differentiation of Mycobacteria

Group	Growth at: 37°C	Growth at: 25°C	Pigment in Light	Pigment in Dark	Rate of Growth
M. tuberculosis / *M. bovis*	+	–	–	–	S
Runyon I	+	+	+	–	M or S
Runyon II	+	+	+	+	M or S
Runyon III	+	+	–	–	S
Runyon IV	+	+	–	d	R

S, slow; M, moderate; R, rapid; d, some species.

7H9 liquid medium, and the culture is then replaced in the incubator at 37°C. In a few days a black precipitate indicates a positive reaction. *M. phlei, M. smegmatis,* and *M. vaccae* (Group IV) are also positive.

Nitrate Reduction

M. tuberculosis, M. kansasii, M. szulgai, and *M. haemophilum* are pathogens for which this test is positive, but some usual nonpathogens *(M. fortuitum)* are also positive. In this test, 0.5 mL of distilled water is added to a clean screw-capped tube (20 × 110 mm), and then growth from a four-week L-J slope is added to make a dense suspension. A nitrate test strip, which is commercially available, is added as directed by the manufacturer. The tube is capped and incubated at 37°C for two hours. It is shaken gently at the end of the first and second hours, but the middle of the strip is not made wet until incubation is complete. Then the tube is tilted six times and left in a horizontal position so that fluid covers the strip. After 10 minutes, the top of the strip is examined for blueness.

Tween Hydrolysis

In this test, 100 mL of M/15 phosphate buffer at pH 7 (Na_2HPO_4, 9.47 g/liter, 61.1 mL; KH_2PO_4, 9.07 g/liter, 39.8 mL) is mixed with 0.5 mL of Tween 80 and 2 mL of a 1 % aqueous solution of neutral red. Four-millimeter aliquots are placed in screw-capped tubes (16 × 125 mm) and autoclaved. The color should become amber. Stored in a refrigerator, the solution will keep for two weeks. A loopful of culture is suspended in the mixture and incubated at 37°C for up to ten days. A pink or red color owing to the formation of oleic acid from the Tween 80 is expected, but this should appear in five days for a positive reaction. If it appears between five and ten days, it is a doubtful positive, and if on or after the tenth day, it is considered negative. *M. kansasii* is positive.

Growth on MacConkey Agar

MacConkey agar *without* crystal violet is used. Subculture to this agar is made from 7- to 10-day-old Tween albumin or 7H9 broth. *M. fortuitum-chelonei* complex will grow to the end of the inoculating streaks. Other mycobacteria may grow if the inoculum is heavy.

Production of Urease

A commercially available urease test disc method is available (Murphy and Hawkins, 1975). It is helpful in differentiation, particularly within the Runyon groups.

Growth Inhibition by Thiophene-2-Carboxylic Acid Hydrazide (T_2H)

For this test, 5 g/mL concentrations of T_2H are incorporated into 7H10 agar. A loopful of a barely turbid broth culture of the organism to be investigated is streaked so as to obtain discrete colonies. The culture is then incubated for 14 to 21 days at 37°C in 5 to 8% CO_2. *M. bovis* is inhibited, but *M. tuberculosis* will thrive.

Optimum Temperature of Growth

M. ulcerans, M. marinum, and *M. haemophilum* rarely grow at 37°C and should be cultured at 32°C or possibly below. They have been reported as causing infection of the skin, and this explains the optimal temperature of growth. *M. ulcerans* will grow only at 32°C and has a very limited range of growth. It causes infections that have been reported mainly from Africa and Australia (buruli ulcer). *M. marinum,* which has a wider range of growth, is the cause of "swimming pool granuloma," another type of skin ulceration, which has been reported in North America. Some of the Group IV organisms as well as *M. xenopi* will grow at 45°C, and a few strains of the *M. avium-intracellulare* complex will also grow at this temperature.

Other tests, such as sodium chloride tolerance, catalase, and iron uptake, are also available. Details of these are available in larger works. The student will be able to see the value of some of these tests in differentiating mycobacteria within the major groups but should realize that much of this work falls correctly within the province of specialized centers. Table 19–5 may better illustrate the value of the tests mentioned in differentiating organisms that have been mentioned.

M. Tuberculosis

This organism has the general features of the genus *Mycobacterium,* and many of its characteristics will be found above. It is slow growing and forms buff, rough colonies on L-J medium in 4 to 6 weeks at 37°C. Smears from the colonies are difficult to make, since the organisms are not easy to spread. The organisms tend to form cords or strands, especially in liquid media. The niacin test is positive.

Pathology of Tuberculosis

There are many types of tuberculosis, which is generally caused by *M. tuberculosis* but also by *M. bovis,*

TABLE 19–5 Differentiation of Some Important Mycocbacterial Species

	Growth at 22–25°C	Growth at 37°C	Rate of Growth	Pigment in Dark	Pigment Photo-activated	Niacin Production	Tellurite Reduction	Nitrate Reduction	Tween Hydrolysis	Growth on MacConkey Agar	Urease	Resistance to T_2H
M. tuberculosis	−	+	S	−	−	+	−	+	d	−	+	+
M. bovis	−	+	S	−	−	−	−	−	−	−	+	−
M. marinum	+	−*	M	+	−	−	−	−	+	−	+	
M. kansasii	+	+	S	+	−	−	−	+	+	−	+	
M. scrofulaceum	+	+	S	+	−	−	−	−	−	−	+	
M. szulgai	+	+	S	+†	−	−	−	+	d	−	+	
M. gordonae	+	+	S	+	−	−	−	−	+	−	−	
M. xenopi	+	+	S	+	−	−	−	−	−	−	−	
M. avium	+	+	S	−	−	−	+	−	−	d	−	
M. intracellulare	+	+	S	−	−	−	+	−	−		−	
M. haemophilum	+	−	S	−	−	−	−	−	−	−	−	
M. ulcerans	31°C‡	−	S	−	−	−	−	−	−			
M. fortuitum	+	+	R	−	−	−	+		d	+	+	
M. smegmatis	+	+	R	−	−	−	+		+	−		

S, growth in 14 days or more; R, growth in less than 7 days. M, growth intermediate
*On primary isolation will grow at 31°C only, but may adapt on subculture at 37°C.
†In Group II if grown at 37°C, i.e., pigmented in dark.
‡Will not grow at 22–25°C or at 37°C. Optimal temperature is 31°C.

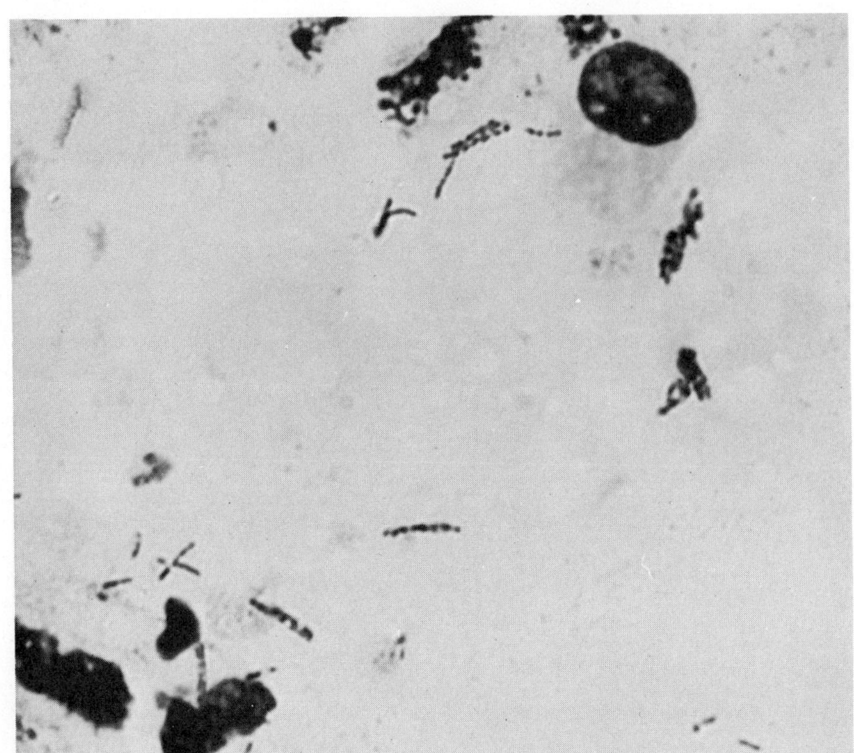

Figure 19–6 *Mycobacterium tuberculosis.* Smear from a lesion from guinea pig inoculated with material from human patient. Note the beading of the organism. Ziehl-Neelsen stain × 1840.

M. kansasii, M. avium, and, more rarely, by other organisms. Ten per cent of tuberculosis is possibly caused by mycobacteria other than *M. tuberculosis.* The organisms usually enter through the respiratory tract and are spread by the infected person when he coughs or expectorates. The entry of the organism may also be via the intestinal tract, but with widespread pasteurization of milk, the dissemination of *M. bovis* in this fashion—from infected cattle—is greatly diminished. In the more usual pulmonary disease, the inhaled organisms form a lesion in the lung with secondary areas of infection in draining lymph nodes. This pulmonary and nodal infection is known as the primary complex; it generally heals to form a Ghon lesion and often occurs in childhood. Later, in early adult life, the lesion may become reactivated and then progress to pneumonitis, in which the necrotic caseous lesions may cavitate. The cavity communicates with the bronchial tree. The patient, in coughing, brings up infected material from the cavity. This material is disseminated in aerosols and in expectorated matter.

At any stage of the disease, hematogenous spread of organisms may occur and cause tuberculosis of the kidney, joints, meninges, endometrium, and so forth. The most devastating type of disseminated disease is miliary tuberculosis, in which the organisms are seeded in all organs, causing a profound and serious illness that until the advent of antimicrobials was universally fatal.

Tuberculosis occurs particularly in poor social conditions and is now relatively uncommon in the affluent North American continent. In the past, it was relatively frequent and was at one time known as the "white plague" or "the captain of the men of death." Better social conditions, medical care, and chemotherapy have reduced the number of new cases in the United States from 101 per 100,000 population in 1930 to 12 per 100,000 in 1979.

M. bovis infections have been rare since widespread pasteurization of milk and control of tuberculosis in cattle began. *M. kansasii* and *M. marinum* (in Group I); *M. scrofulaceum, M. szulgai, M. xenopi,* and *M. gordonae* (Group II); *M. intracellulare* (Battey), *M. avium,* and *M. ulcerans* (Group III); and *M. fortuitum* have all caused disease in man.

Speciation is important, because the chemotherapy of the disease caused by mycobacteria other than *M. tuberculosis* is different from that caused by *M. tuberculosis* and because man-to-man transmission of infection does *not* occur in disease caused by mycobacteria other than *M. tuberculosis.*

Animal Inoculation

In the past, animals, especially guinea pigs, which have little if any resistance to *M. tuberculosis* and *M. bovis,* were inoculated with suspect material. However, in view of modern diagnostic methods, there seems little justification for the maintenance of such animals, to say nothing of the risks of having contaminated animals in the environment. The decontamination-digestion methods (p. 425) followed by culture are just as satisfactory for diagnosis as were animals, and in addition, the latter are naturally immune to some mycobacteria that are pathogenic in humans.

TREPONEMA PALLIDUM

Treponema pallidum is the cause of syphilis. Among other species in the same genus, *T. pertenue* is the

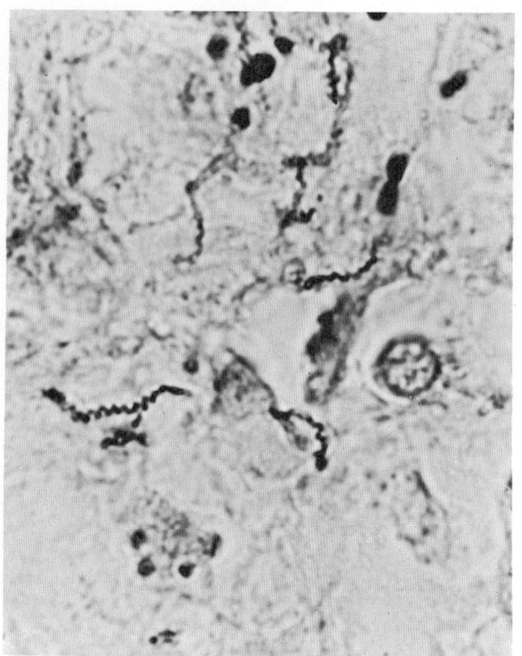

Figure 19–7 *Treponema pallidum*. Section of liver in congenital syphilis. Levaditi × 2250.

etiological agent of yaws and *T. carateum* causes pinta. These latter diseases are seen in the tropics. Treponemes belong to the family Spirochaetaceae, and some other genera in this family also include human pathogens, viz., *Borrelia* and *Leptospira*.

Treponemes are helical rods with a spiral shape. They are gram negative but are generally revealed best with silver stains or are seen by dark-field or phase-contrast microscopy. *T. pallidum* is microaerophilic, but the organism *cannot* be cultured in vitro. The organism is motile, with rotation around its long axis as well as flexion and extension laterally. The genus has immunologically related species, so that a patient with yaws or pinta has the serological responses of a patient with syphilis.

Natural History of Syphilis

T. pallidum survives only in patients with syphilis, and it has no other habitat. The organism passes during sexual intercourse by contact through minute epithelial tears from the infected partner to the new host. After an initial incubation period of two to three weeks, a chancre appears at the site of inoculation, which is generally on the genital organs but may, in 5% of cases, be extragenital. The chancre develops as a shallow, weeping, nonpainful ulcer with enlarged local lymph nodes. Untreated, the chancre will heal in about two weeks. About two months after infection, secondary syphilis, with a skin rash, mucosal ulcers, fever, lymph node enlargement, and other symptoms, appears.

A large minority of infected persons have no recognizable primary or secondary symptoms and so do not present themselves at these curable stages of the disease.

About one-third of infected subjects undergo spontaneous remission after the second stage of the disease and become serologically negative. Another one-third of these individuals have a latent type of disease with positive serological findings but no clinical disease. The rest develop tertiary syphilis, which becomes manifest 2 to 10 years after the individual contracts the disease. The most serious of these tertiary lesions are diseases of the cardiovascular system (aortic aneurysms or aortic valve insufficiency) or of the central nervous system (general paresis or tabes dorsalis).

T. pallidum can cross the placenta and can cause death of the fetus or disabling disease in the newborn. Although the organism can cross the placenta early in pregnancy, early treatment of the mother may prevent congenital syphilis from appearing in the child.

Syphilis is the third most frequently reported communicable disease in the United States, with 24,874 cases of primary and secondary disease reported in 1979. In Canada 1851 cases were reported during that same year. In regard to congenital syphilis, 331 cases were reported in the United States in 1979.

Diagnosis of Syphilis

In the first stage of syphilis, the only method of diagnosis is by the demonstration of typical treponemes in the exudate by dark-field microscopy (see p. 36). Phase-contrast microscopy is less efficient. The organisms are very numerous in the lesions, so gloves must be worn and all precautions taken. Secondary lesions are also rich in treponemes and must be treated with caution.

Serological tests become positive one to two weeks after the appearance of the chancre, i.e., about two to four weeks after infection. After adequate therapy, nontreponemal serological tests should become negative in 6 to 12 months after primary syphilis and 12 to 18 months after secondary syphilis. A falling titer of nontreponemal antibody may occur in tertiary syphilis. Treponemal serological tests tend to remain positive.

CHAPTER 19—REVIEW QUESTIONS

1. What diseases are caused by (a) *B. anthracis* and (b) *B. cereus?* Under the headings of hemolysis, motility, gelatinase, and penicillin sensitivity, differentiate these species.
2. H_2S is produced by three species of corynebacteria. How is this best demonstrated and what is its clinical significance? Describe the major differential feature between *Corynebacterium* and *Listeria*.
3. a. Describe and typify the four Runyon types of mycobacteria.
   b. Under the following headings list the properties of *M. tuberculosis*.
      - Growth at room temperature
      - Pigment in dark
      - Niacin production
      - Growth in less than seven days
4. What are the methods of diagnosis of syphilis in
   a. The primary stage?
   b. The secondary stage?
   c. A case that presents 20 years after possible exposure?

20 OBLIGATE ANAEROBIC BACTERIA

Aerobic respiration combines oxygen with carbon compounds, producing CO_2, H_2O, and energy. Oxidation is a loss of hydrogen or a gain of oxygen. Aerobic respiration may be depicted as follows:

$$C_6H_{12}O_6 + 6\ O_2 \rightarrow 6\ H_2O + \text{Energy}$$

In anaerobic respiration, the process may be shown as follows:

$$C_6H_{12}O_6 + 12\ KNO_3 \rightarrow 6\ CO_2 + 6H_2O + 12\ KNO_2 + \text{Energy}$$

In the second process, the potassium nitrate is reduced and the carbohydrate is oxidized but without the addition of extrinsic oxygen. In such a way do anaerobic bacteria respire, and indeed the presence of free oxygen may be lethal to the organism.

The term *obligate anaerobes* strictly means those organisms that are unable to grow in oxygen. However, the majority of "obligate" anaerobes met in clinical laboratories and associated with disease are capable of growth in a reduced O_2 atmosphere of 2 to 8% but will not grow on the surface of a supportive medium in an ambient atmosphere. *Microaerophilic* or *aerotolerant* organisms are not strictly defined, and the terms may apply to organisms that grow in an atmosphere with reduced oxygen tension, in an aerobic atmosphere with 10% CO_2, or that remain viable for some hours on the surface of a medium in an aerobic atmosphere after having been cultured anaerobically. *Facultative anaerobes* include those organisms that will grow under laboratory anaerobiosis but that will thrive in aerobic atmospheres. Many of the Enterobacteriaceae are in this group.

In this chapter, we shall deal with the more clinically important obligate anaerobic bacteria. These organisms are normally widespread, living on the skin and upper respiratory tract and in large numbers in the mouth, intestine, and genital tract. Because they are so ubiquitous, it is important that specimens submitted for anaerobic studies be taken properly. Therefore specimens such as (a) throat, nose, and mouth swabs; (b) sputum and bronchial aspirates; (c) intestinal contents or feces; (d) vaginal and cervical swabs; and (e) voided urine are unsatisfactory for anaerobic work, since they are naturally contaminated with normal flora that may be mistakenly identified as pathogens. The only specimens that are regarded as satisfactory are as follows:

(a) Blood cultures.

(b) Aspirates from abscesses, pleural or peritoneal fluid, facial sinuses, joints, and so forth taken through needles into glass syringes.

(c) Percutaneous transtracheal aspirates or lung aspirates.

(d) Specimens from the female genital tract obtained by culdocentesis.

(e) Wound and sinus specimens collected by use of a plastic catheter inserted as deeply as possible into the wound or sinus.

(f) Surgically obtained material.

A double catheter is available commercially in which the inner catheter is protected from contamination by the outer. Such an instrument has been used in bronchoscopy and in taking specimens from the uterine cavity.

Transport of the specimen to the laboratory assumes great importance here. The "two-quick-feet" method is best, but if transport media have to be used, then prereduced anaerobically sterilized Cary and Blair medium can be employed or a commercially available anaerobic transport system* can be used. The latter has an inner tube for the specimen and an outer tube that generates an oxygen-free atmosphere. Other methods are also procurable.

When the specimen reaches the laboratory, direct Gram films are made that, if of typical appearance, may help in presumptive diagnosis—clostridia are plump, large, gram-positive rods; fusobacteria are fusiform; and *Bacteroides* are faintly staining gram-negative rods tending to pleomorphism. Preliminary culture techniques are described on pp. 332 and 335. Colonies considered as possible anaerobes are subject to further examination.

THE GRAM-NEGATIVE ANAEROBIC BACILLI

In this group *Bacteroides* and *Fusobacterium* will be considered.

The Genus *Bacteroides*

This genus is divided into numerous species, but classification may be somewhat simplified by considering the *B. fragilis* group (which includes five species), the *B. melaninogenicus-asaccharolyticus* group, and others. The organisms in the genus are gram-negative, nonsporing, generally nonmotile rods that live as normal flora in the mouth, intestinal tract, urethra, and female

*Becton-Dickinson and Co., Rutherford, N.J. 07070 and Mississauga, Ont. L5J 2M8.

genital tract. Infections are often endogenous from these sites.

Identification of Major Bacteroides Groups

The importance of differentiation of this group lies in its significance in antimicrobial sensitivity. *B. fragilis* is the most commonly encountered in infections and is insensitive to penicillin. On Schaedler's blood agar it presents 2 to 3 mm, entire, smooth, shiny, pale gray colonies. Because of the complexity of differentiation, presumptive identification is often made by rapid tests and on a Lombard-Dowell (L-D) Presumpto plate (available commercially). The plate has, in each of its four quadrants, esculin agar, 20% bile agar, egg yolk agar, and a basal medium for indole production. Not all of the reactions of *B. fragilis* will be described here, but it will grow on 20% bile agar, and beneath and around each colony on this medium there will be a precipitate. This precipitate is not seen with other species of *Bacteroides*.

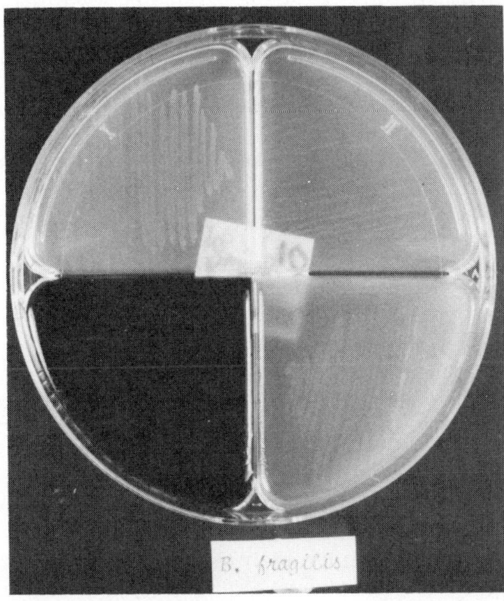

Figure 20–1 The L-D Presumpto Plate* (Anaerobe Systems, Santa Clara, Calif. 95050). The Presumpto quadrant plate contains L-D agar, L-D bile agar, L-D egg yolk agar, and L-D esculin agar. The plate is inoculated and incubated anaerobically for 48 hours at 35°C.

Indole production can be examined with a drop of paradimethylaminocinnamaldehyde reagent on a paper disc on the L-D agar. Growth can be positive or negative on the bile agar. Lecithinase, lipase, and proteolysis can be identified on the egg yolk quadrant (lecithinase = opaque precipitate in the agar, lipase = sheen or oily layer on surface, proteolysis = translucency around colonies). Browning or blackening of the esculin agar indicates esculin hydrolysis; black colonies here indicate H_2S production. The esculin quadrant may be flooded with 3% H_2O_2, and bubbling would indicate catalase production.

In the picture, the example is *B. fragilis*. There is growth in each quadrant with esculin hydrolysis *(left, lower)*. There is no production of lecithinase or lipase or evidence of proteolysis.

*Dowell, V.R., Jr., and Lombard, G. L. Presumptive Identification of Anaerobic Non–spore-forming Gram-negative Bacilli. Atlanta, Centers for Disease Control, 1977.

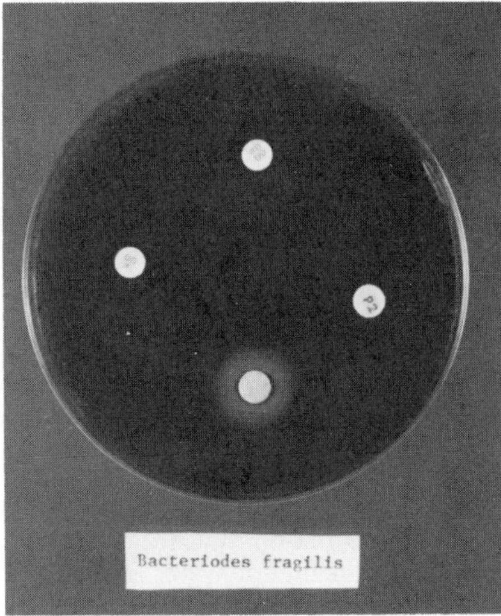

Figure 20–2 *B. fragilis* identification. *B. fragilis* is resistant to kanamicin (1 mg/disc) and to oxgall (25 mg/disc), unlike other *Bacteroides* or *Fusobacterium* species. The bile in this illustration *(lower disc)* is seen to encourage the growth of *B. fragilis*.

(Methodology from Draper, D. L., and Barry, A. L. Rapid identification of *Bacteroides fragilis* with bile and antibiotic disks. J Clin Microbiol 1977, *5*:439–443.)

Differentiation may also be made by the antimicrobial sensitivity pattern. In such testing, a group of antimicrobials on paper discs are used. This group comprises erythromycin, 60 μg/disc; rifampicin, 15 μg/disc; colistin, 10 μg/disc; penicillin, 2 units/disc; kanamycin, 1000 μg/disc; and vancomycin, 5 μg/disc. The organism to be investigated is grown anaerobically on blood agar, with the discs applied after inoculation. Incubation at 35°C is continued for 48 hours. Inhibition zones of ≥ 10 mm in diameter are considered as indicating sensitivity; those < 10 mm are considered insensitive (Leigh and Simmons, 1977; see Table 20–1). *B. fragilis* is uniformly resistant to penicillin, kanamycin, and vancomycin and generally to colistin. The set of antimicrobial discs is available commercially (An-ident disc*). Commonly,

*Oxoid, Columbia, Md. 21045 and Nepean, Ont. K2E 7K3.

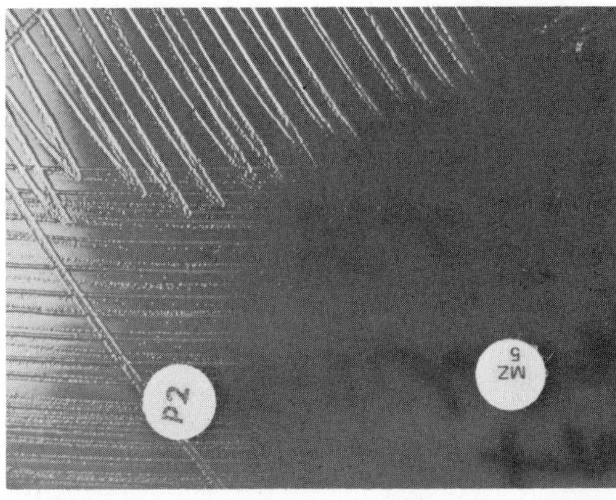

Figure 20–3 *B. fragilis*. Culture on blood agar demonstrating inhibition by metronidazole (MZ5) and insensitivity to penicillin (p2).

TABLE 20–1 Differentiation of *Bacteroides* Species and *Fusobacterium* by Antimicrobial Sensitivity Patterns

	E	Ri	C	P	K	Vn
B. fragilis	S^R	S	R^S	R	R	R
B. melaninogenicus-asaccharolyticus	S	S	V	S	R^S	R
Other *Bacterioides* species	S	S	S	S	V	R
Fusobacterium	R^S	R^S	S	S	S	R

(From Leigh DA, and Simmons K. Identification of nonsporing anaerobic bacteria. J Clin Pathol 1977, *30*:991–992. By permission of the authors and the editor of the Journal of Clinical Pathology.)

E, erythromycin, 60 μg; *Ri,* rifampicin, 15 μg; *C,* colistin, 10 μg; *P,* penicillin, 2 units; *K,* kanamycin, 1000 μg; *Vn,* vancomycin, 5 μg; *S,* sensitive; S^R, occasional strains are resistant; *V,* variable; R^S, occasional strains are sensitive; *R,* resistant.

isolated strains are tested for catalase positivity by adding 30% H_2O_2 to the growth on egg yolk and esculin agar. More extensive biochemical tests are available with an API-20 A strip, which is the anaerobic analog to the API-20 E for the Enterobacteriaceae, or with the Minitek anaerobic system (Fig. 20–4).

B. melaninogenicus-asaccharolyticus Group

This group is sensitive to penicillin and resistant to vancomycin and generally to kanamycin, although some strains are sensitive to the latter antimicrobial. Colonies will fluoresce brick-red under ultraviolet light (365 nm wavelength) and will develop a black or tan pigment in 2 to 10 days.

Other Bacteroides

These are resistant to vancomycin and are sensitive to penicillin and colistin.

Pathology

The *B. fragilis* group are particularly common in infections below the diaphragm, e.g., peritonitis and vic inflammatory disease in women, but may occur in brain abscess, sinusitis, and other head and neck infections as well as in lung and pleural inflammatory disease. The *B. melaninogenicus-asaccharolyticus* group are more generally seen in infections above the diaphragm, as in pleuropulmonary disease and bite infections. Other organisms of the genus *Bacteroides* may be pathogenic.

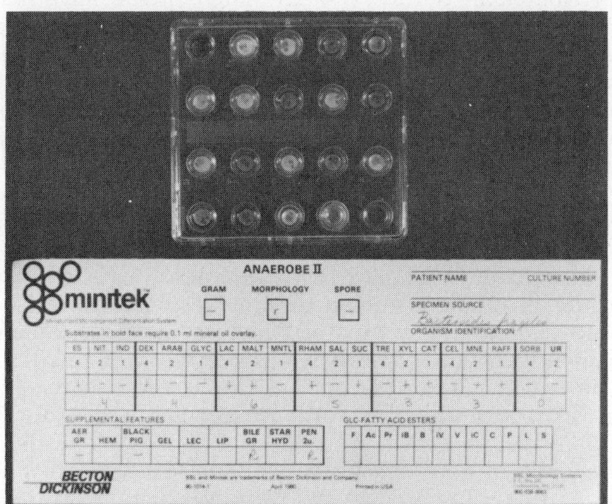

Figure 20–4 Minitek System (Baltimore Biological Laboratory, Cockeysville, Md. 21030) for identification of anaerobes. Paper discs impregnated with biochemicals and carbohydrates are dispensed into wells of a plastic plate. Test organisms in an anaerobic broth are inoculated, and then the plate is incubated anaerobically for 48 hours at 35°C. After incubation, an indicator is added to the carbohydrate substrates and other reagents to determine the reactions. Results may be read from differential tables.

The Genus *Fusobacterium*

These are gram-negative rods with narrowed poles, and they may be pleomorphic or irregularly staining. Some species will show colonial fluorescence. They are sensitive to kanamycin, unlike the majority of *Bacteroides,* but are resistant to vancomycin. Most strains are also resistant to erythromycin and rifampicin (unlike *Bacteroides*).

F. nucleatum is the commonest species encountered. They are normal mouth and bowel inhabitants and are also normally found in the female genital tract. They are found in the same types of infection as *Bacteroides. F. necrophorum* and an as yet unidentified spirochete together cause trench mouth, an acute necrotizing ulcerating gingivitis in which there is acute ulceration of the gums with membrane formation, considerable pain, and distressing halitosis. Diagnosis can be made by the appearance of a direct Gram film from the exudate (Fig. 20–5).

THE ANAEROBIC COCCI

This is a heterogeneous group, most of which are gram positive. The single exception is *Veillonella parvula,* which is gram negative. The other members of the group are *Peptococcus* and *Peptostreptococcus.* The organisms are normally found in the mouth as well as in the intestinal and upper respiratory tracts.

The Genus *Peptococcus*

The organisms occur singly or appear in small packets like micrococci. They grow slowly on Schaedler's medium and are resistant to vancomycin but sensitive to kanamycin and colistin.

The Genus *Peptostreptococcus*

These grow in chains like streptococci and have an antimicrobial pattern similar to that of *Peptococcus.* The chains of growth may be induced by thioglycollate or chopped meat broth. *P. anaerobius* is inhibited by so-

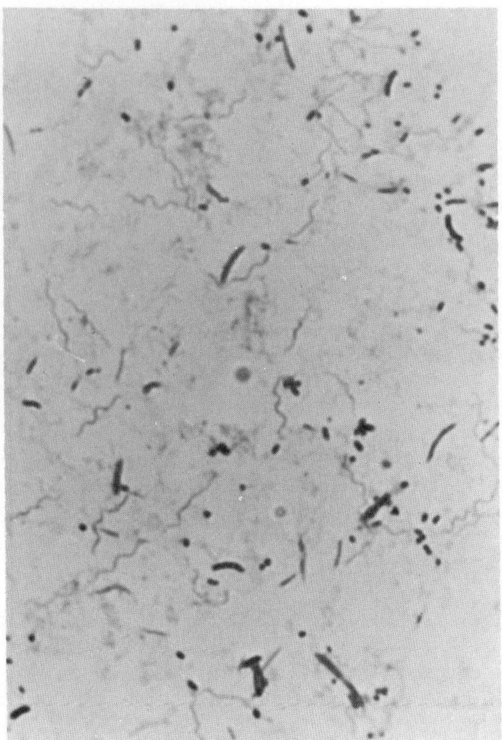

Figure 20–5 Vincent's angina. Smear from a lesion. Note the predominant curved fusiforms and the loosely coiled thin *Treponema*. Giemsa × 2250.

dium polyanethol sulfonate: 20 μL of a 5% solution of SPS is placed on a ¼-inch filter paper disc and dried at room temperature. A zone of more than 12 mm of inhibition around the disc indicates *Peptostreptococcus anaerobius*. More extensive biochemical identification may be made with the Minitek system or with the API 20 A.

Veillonella parvula

The organism is rarely involved in disease, but it is to be remembered so that its presence in direct films is not confused with that of *Neisseria*.

Pathology

Peptococcus and *Peptostreptococcus* have been involved in brain abscesses, gum infections, sinusitis, pleuropulmonary disease, appendicitis, female pelvic inflammatory disease, endocarditis, soft-tissue cellulitis, osteomyelitis, and so forth.

ANAEROBIC, GRAM-POSITIVE, NONSPORING BACILLI

These include several types. One is the family Actinomycetaceae, which is dealt with in the section on mycology (more correctly they are bacteria but by usage are often considered with the fungi). The others in the group are the lactobacilli and *Propionibacterium*.

The Genus *Lactobacillus*

This genus comprises rather pleomorphic gram-positive rods that are facultatively aerobic and generally nonmotile. They are widely dispersed in nature and are normal inhabitants of the intestinal tract and the vagina in humans. They are very rarely pathogenic. By their action on glycogen in desquamated cells, they maintain the adult vagina at an acid pH with lactic acid and thus inhibit colonization by potentially pathogenic organisms.

The Genus *Propionibacterium*

These are also gram-positive rods that are anaerobic, slightly aerotolerant, and nonmotile. *P. acnes* is a normal inhabitant of the skin and may be found in blood culture. It is not possible to dismiss such bacteria as a contaminant, because these organisms have caused bacterial endocarditis superimposed on rheumatic valvular disease or on cardiac prostheses. If cultures have been taken under good aseptic conditions, and if more than one culture is positive, then there is evidence for suspicion that *P. acnes* is clinically significant. It should always be reported so that the clinician may make a final decision. The definitive identification of the organism may be lengthy, but it can be done with API 20 A. An anerobic gram-positive rod that is catalase and indole positive is dependably *P. acnes*.

THE ANAEROBIC, GRAM-POSITIVE, ENDOSPORE-FORMING RODS

This group is essentially the genus *Clostridium*. They are gram-positive rods that bear spores and are anerobic or aerotolerant. There are many species, of which some of the more important will be described. They are widely distributed in nature and are found in the intestinal tract of humans and animals and also on the human skin. They are responsible for a number of diseases that may in turn be due to different types of toxemia or to bacterial invasion. They grow well on standard anaerobic media, and they may be hemolytic or may show swarming.

Clostridium perfringens

On blood agar *Cl. perfringens* produces fair-sized (2 to 5 mm in diameter) colonies, around which there is a zone of hemolysis with a secondary zone of incomplete hemolysis beyond (on rabbit or sheep blood) (Fig. 20–6). The organisms are plump rods (Fig. 20–7). Spores are not usually seen but may be encouraged to appear if the organisms are grown on chopped meat agar (Dowell et al., 1980) at 37°C. They are oval and subterminal. The organisms cause a positive Nagler reaction.

The Nagler Reaction. This test for *Cl. perfringens* is performed as follows:

1. Prepare an egg yolk agar plate (it is one of the Presumpto Quadrant Plate differential media described by Dowell and Lombard) by spreading half the plate with *Cl. perfringens* antitoxin.

2. Inoculate the suspect colony on the prepared plate.

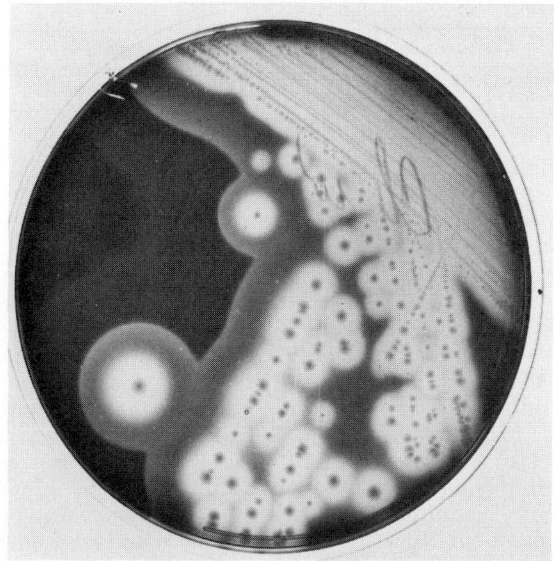

Figure 20–6 *Cl. perfringens*: culture on blood agar showing the characteristic double zone of hemolysis and even, on the left, a faint zone of tertiary hemolysis.

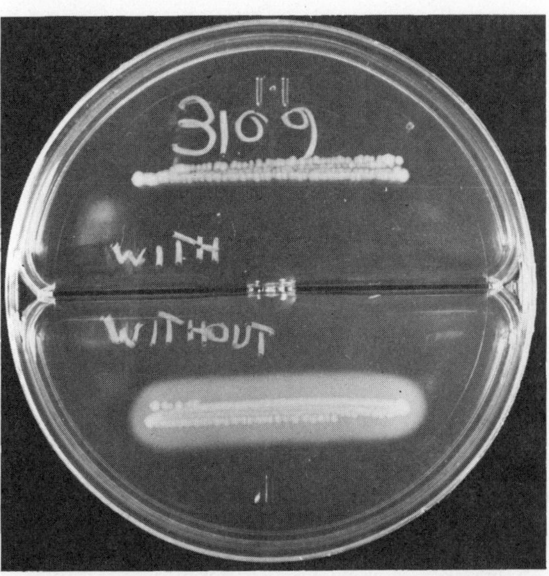

Figure 20–8 Nagler reaction; details in text. The notations "with" and "without" signify addition of or absence of antitoxin in the agar. A zone of precipitation around the colonies growing on the agar without antitoxin indicates lecithinase production by *Cl. perfringens*. This is prevented by antitoxin in the upper inoculum of the same organism.

After 24-hour incubation, *Cl. perfringens* will produce precipitation in the medium around its colonies on the side of the medium *without* antitoxin. On the other side the antitoxin will neutralize the lecithinase that causes the change, and no precipitation will occur (Fig. 20–8).

Cl. bifermentans, Cl. sordellii, and *Cl. paraperfringens* all produce Nagler reactions similar to that of *Cl. perfringens*. However, the last-named organism rarely occurs in clinical material and may safely be ignored. The others may be excluded by testing for motility, indole, lactose fermentation, and urease production (see Table 20–2).

The Reverse CAMP Test. A more specific test than the Nagler reaction has recently been described (Gubash, 1980). It has been referred to as a reverse CAMP test (see also p. 370). It depends on the production of enhanced hemolysis when colonies of Group B streptococci and *Cl. perfringens* are brought together.

Method (modified)

1. **5% sheep blood in tryptose blood agar base is used.**
2. **Streaks of suspected *Cl. perfringens* colonies and of**

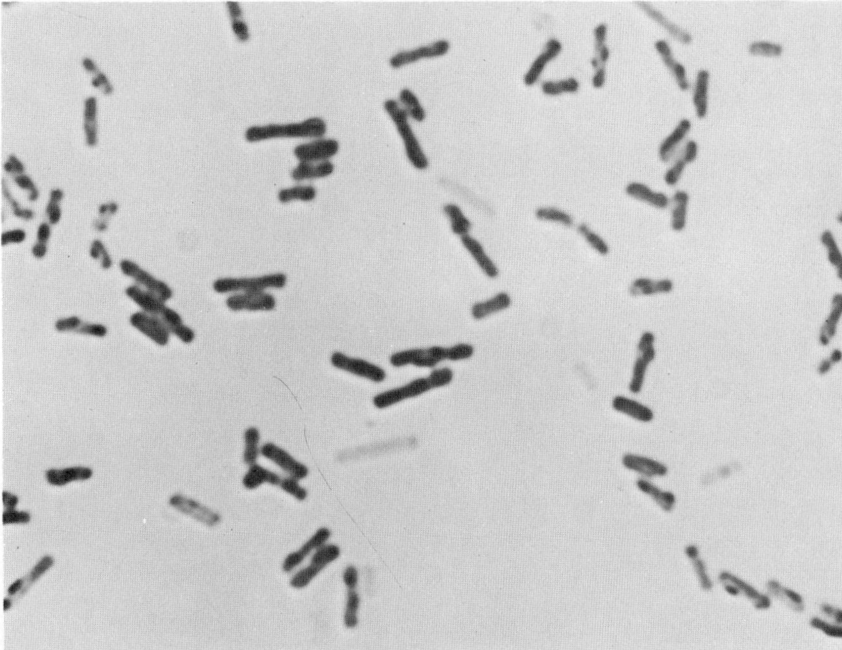

Figure 20–7 *Clostridium perfringens*. Smear from culture. Gram stain × 2250.

TABLE 20–2 DIFFERENTIATION OF NAGLER-POSITIVE CLOSTRIDIA

Test	*Cl. perfringens*	*Cl. bifermentans*	*Cl. sordellii*
Motility	−	+	+
Indole	−	+	+
Lactose	+	−	−
Urease	d	−	+

known Group B streptococci are made at right angles to one another, leaving a gap of about 5 mm at their closest point.

3. The plates are incubated anaerobically at 35°C overnight.

Result

Cl. perfringens will give a crescentic or bullet-shaped zone of enhanced hemolysis at the point at which the bacterial streaks are closest (Fig. 20–9). *Cl. bifermentans* and *Cl. sordellii* show this reaction only on human blood agar, which may need calcium supplementation.

Other Tests. The motility test may be made in SIM medium (p. 341) incubated anaerobically. Indole testing may best be done by growing the organism on SIM medium and then spreading the growth on commercially available test strips or on filter paper previously saturated with 1% paradimethylaminocinnamaldehyde in 10% (v/v) HCl. A blue color indicates the presence of indole. Urease is tested for by using urea semisolid medium (Dowell et al., 1980). The medium is heavily inoculated and incubated at 35°C for 24 hours. A positive result is indicated by a bright red color in the medium. However, the indicator may have become reduced so that a negative result is further questioned by the addition of Nessler's reagent. A brown color with Nessler's reagent shows the presence of ammonia and hence of urease. For carbohydrate fermentation, CHO medium base* is used. It is semisolid and includes thioglycollate, L-cystine, yeast extract, peptone, ascorbic acid, agar, and a bromothymol blue indicator. The carbohydrate is added to form a 0.6% solution. To achieve anaerobiosis in the medium, it is easiest to boil or steam it for 10 minutes before inoculation. The indicator will go from blue to yellow if fermentation occurs, *but* the indicator itself may become reduced. Such medium can be tested by removing a few drops and adding them to an equal quantity of dilute (nonreduced) bromothymol blue indicator. A final decision as to whether the carbohydrate has undergone fermentation may be delayed for seven days, but many isolates show results in 24 hours. The API 20 A set is used in many laboratories, and it saves the expense and effort of preparing special biochemical media. A Minitek system† is another commercially available system for the identification of anaerobes.

Pathology. *Cl. perfringens* is involved in a number of diseases, among which are gas gangrene, gastroenteritis, gangrenous cholecystitis, some cases of puerperal sepsis and septic abortion, and other even more rarely encountered infections.

Gas gangrene is seen as a complication of war wounds and is less frequent in a civilian setting. Infection enters a wound from soil, clothing, or a ruptured bowel. Other

*Difco Laboratories, Detroit, Mich. 48232.

†Baltimore Biological Laboratory, Cockeysville, Md. 21030.

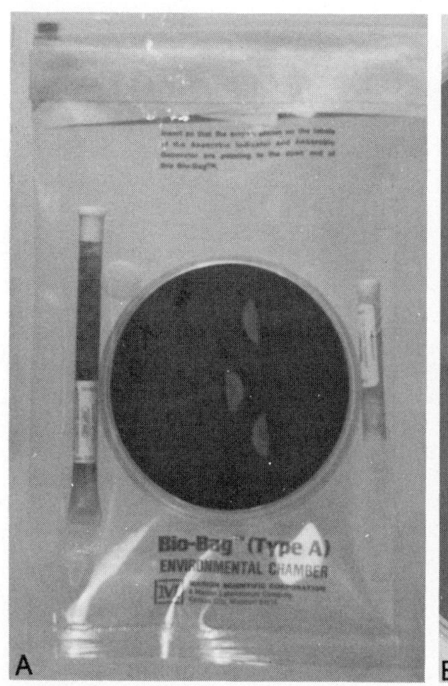

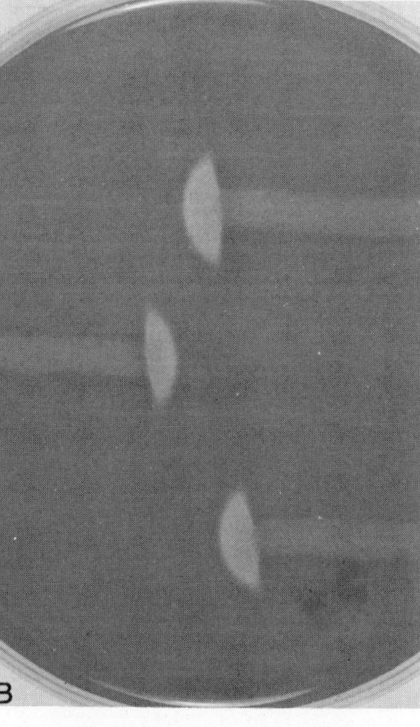

Figure 20–9 The "reverse CAMP" test. In **A**, a sheep blood agar plate has been incubated anaerobically in an anaerobic bag (Bio-bag, Marion Scientific Corp. Kansas City, Mo. 64114). *C. perfringens* has been streaked vertically, and a Group B streptococcus horizontally. Where the streaks are in close proximity, there is a crescentic zone of enhanced hemolysis. In **B**, a closer view of the plate is shown.

clostridia generally participate in the infection and include *Cl. novyi, Cl. septicum, Cl. sordellii,* and *Cl. histolyticum*. True gas gangrene occurs with wound pain, and the patient is obviously ill. The wound has a serosanguinous discharge; bubbles of gas then appear in the tissues, causing crepitation. The wound has a foul odor and becomes discolored. Untreated, the patient deteriorates rapidly and dies. Clostridial postpartum sepsis or septic abortion pursues a similar course. *Simple contamination of wounds* by gas gangrene organisms and perhaps by anaerobic streptococci also occurs. This condition typically remains uncomplicated and heals. *Anaerobic cellulitis* may be an extension of simple contamination or may be clostridial from initiation. Although gas appears in the tissues and the area has a foul odor, there is little pain and there may be little discoloration. Most important, there is no toxemia of the patient, and the condition is very much less serious than gas gangrene. In both anaerobic cellulitis and simple contamination, clostridia may be detected in the laboratory, but the finding has a much less serious import than in gas gangrene, which is essentially a clinical diagnosis. A *spontaneous nontraumatic clostridial bacteremia* with soft tissue localization also occurs, particularly in association with diabetes and malignant disease.

In all these instances, a direct Gram film from the lesion showing the presence of clostridia and the absence of inflammatory cells may be of invaluable assistance to the clinician. It should be noted that even in gas gangrene, inflammatory cells are rare or not seen in the exudate, and again it is worth emphasizing that the clinical significance of the finding of clostridia is a clinical prerogative. *Cl. perfringens* from tissues is typically seen without spores. Gas gangrene is a toxemia caused by the many exotoxins produced by clostridia. Among these, as we have noted, lecithinase is used diagnostically.

Gastroenteritis caused by *Cl. perfringens* has an incubation period of about 12 hours, followed by abdominal pain, diarrhea, and possibly nausea, vomiting, and fever. It is often associated with moderately cooked, refrigerated, and then rewarmed food or with food served cold, and outbreaks involving a group of persons occur. To prove the origin, *Cl. perfringens* of the same serotype should be found in the incriminated food and in the feces of the sufferer. The count of *Cl. perfringens* in the food should be $\geq 10^5$/g, and a possible fourth criterion is that the *Cl. perfringens* count in the stool should be $\geq 10^6$/g. Such investigations obviously can be carried out only with the help of reference laboratories.

Clostridium tetani

Cl. tetani is the causative organism of tetanus, which is due to the toxin elaborated by the bacillus. The organism itself has the usual features of the clostridia, and its spore is typically round and terminal, producing a characteristic "drumstick" appearance (Fig. 20–10). It produces a swarming type of growth on blood agar, so efforts at obtaining a pure culture should be made by subculture from the edge of a spreading colony. Colonies also produce a narrow zone of hemolysis. The organism is inert against carbohydrates; gelatin is slowly liquified, and lecithinase is slowly produced. The organism is a normal soil inhabitant.

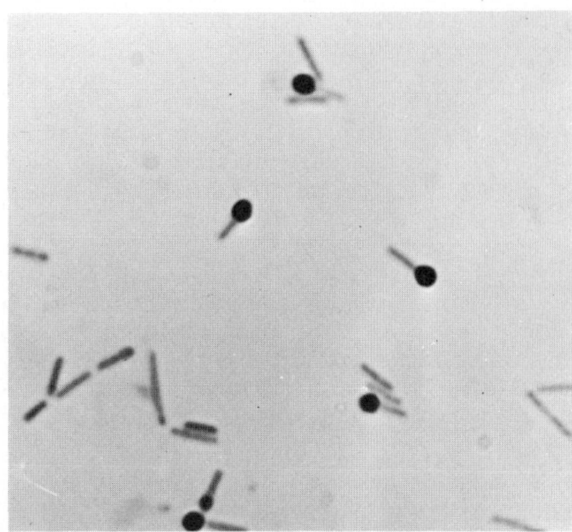

Figure 20–10 *Clostridium tetani*. Smear from culture. Carbolfuchsin and methylene blue stain for spores × 2250.

Pathology. After the inoculation of tetanus into the wound in a nonimmune subject, the incubation period is generally from a few days to three weeks, but periods of up to several months have been recorded. The type of wound liable to tetanic infection is similar to those prone to develop gas gangrene. Tetanus of the newborn may occur in primitive societies when the umbilicus is contaminated as the cord is cut. Tetanus may occur as a complication of burns or cuts. The clinical picture is well known and generally easily recognizable. Widespread prophylaxis is maintained with tetanus toxoid.

Clostridium botulinum

Cl. botulinum is another member of this genus. It forms another and unique type of toxin, probably the most poisonous substance known, which acts on the nervous system, producing paralysis. The organism, which is fortunately clinically rare, is a soil inhabitant and may contaminate canned or bottled food, particularly those incorrectly sterilized in home processing. Nevertheless, commercially prepared canned or bottled food has also carried the toxin, which is elaborated under the anaerobic conditions in which these foodstuffs are maintained. Fish and meat are most frequently implicated.

The organism has the general features of the clostridia. It has subterminal spores and is hemolytic. Glucose and maltose are fermented, and a lipase is produced. Because of its public health implication, identification of *Cl. botulinum* should be made and confirmed by central reference laboratories. In addition, such laboratories are able to identify seven types of neurotoxin, A to G. Types A, B, and E are usually associated with human disease.

Pathology. There are four recognized types of human disease. Classic botulism after ingestion of botulinum toxin has an incubation period of 12 to 24 hours, possibly with gastroenteritis followed by muscle paralysis that may proceed to respiratory paralysis and death. The contaminated food has no visible sign and no odor of spoiling. The toxin is destroyed by heating for 10 minutes at 80°C. Wound botulism is the appearance of the disease after contamination of a wound with *Cl. botulinum,* probably from the soil. The incubation period in this instance may be up to two weeks after the wounding. Infant botulism is more recently described. Here the ingested food does not contain toxin but includes *Cl. botulinum* organisms. These colonize the infant's bowel and elaborate toxin there. The infant becomes weak, cries and swallows with difficulty, and becomes dyspneic and cyanotic because of respiratory paralysis. Toxin is found in the stool. The disease does not appear to be that rare. In the first half of 1980, eleven such cases were admitted to hospitals in California. A fourth type of botulism occurs in patients more than a year old in which no wound or food source is apparent.

Clostridium difficile

Cl. difficile forms a toxin that causes pseudomembranous colitis, a disease that has occurred following antimicrobial therapy. Relatively frequently it follows clindamycin, but almost all antimicrobials have been recorded as having been given before the development of the colitis. It is considered that in such cases the antimicrobial has eliminated many other bacterial flora, allowing the proliferation of *Cl. difficile,* which is an occasional human bowel commensal. The organism may also be isolated from the stool in both normal persons and in those suffering from pseudomembranous colitis. A medium containing D-cycloserine and cefoxitin may be used to inhibit normal bowel flora and other clostridial species, but it allows *Cl. difficile* to grow. The presence of the organism will not *prove* the diagnosis and only measurement of the specific toxin in the stool of a patient with the correct clinical history and picture can be considered diagnostic. At this time, demonstration of the toxin in the feces is beyond the capability of most hospital laboratories.

CHAPTER 20—REVIEW QUESTIONS

1. Define (a) *obligate anaerobe,* (b) *facultative anaerobe,* and (c) *aerotolerant organism*. Give an example of each.
2. Give two diagnostic features of *B. fragilis* and two of *B. melaninogenicus-asaccharolyticus*. Give an example of a disease in which each may be the pathogen.
3. a. Describe the Nagler reaction. What organisms are positive?
   b. Name the tests that may differentiate *Cl. perfringens*.
   c. Give the results of these tests for *Cl. perfringens*.
4. a. In classic botulism where would you expect to find the toxin?
   b. Where do you look for toxin in infantile botulism?
   c. List the properties of *Cl. tetani* and *Cl. perfringens* under the following headings:
      Motility
      Hemolysis
      Position of endospore
      Action on carbohydrates
      Nagler reaction
   d. Does botulinum toxin spoil the taste or appearance of food? Is it heat stable?

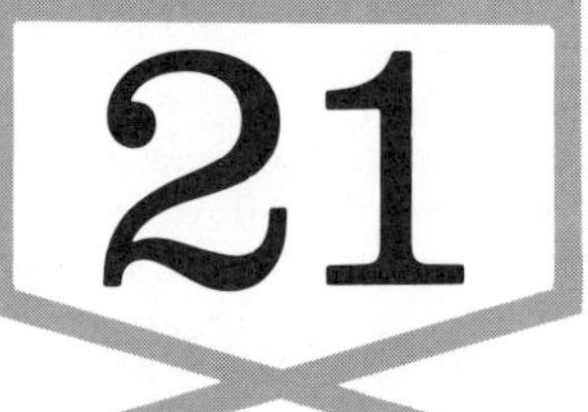

COLLECTION AND EXAMINATION OF SPECIMENS FOR MICROBIOLOGICAL INVESTIGATION

COLLECTION OF SPECIMENS

Some General Considerations

Once they have been collected, specimens should be attended to as soon as possible. A delay in the transmission of a specimen to the laboratory may diminish the success of a diagnostic investigation. The diagnosis of an acute infection becomes more difficult with time, since some pathogens are extremely delicate and sensitive to slight changes in environmental parameters. It is also well known that if left at room temperature, a pathogen present in a specimen containing either normal flora or other organisms inadvertently introduced during collection will most likely be outgrown by these other organisms, thereby reducing the probability of its recovery. Hence the reasons behind the cardinal rule that all specimens should be dealt with expeditiously.

The following procedures are considered essential in the collection of specimens, if reliable results are to be obtained.

1. All specimens should be clearly labeled with the patient's name and the date and time of collection.

2. The specimen should be accompanied by a requisition slip that clearly states: (a) patient's full name and age; (b) origin of requisition, i.e., department or floor; (c) nature of specimen and location of site, e.g., "swab: pus from abscess on left forearm"; (d) patient's antimicrobial history (if any); (3) type of examination requested, e.g., "culture and sensitivity"; and (f) clinical diagnosis if available.

3. It is advisable that a department standardize its specimen containers as much as possible, that is, stock only a limited range (preferably disposable sterile containers), assigning a specific container to a specific range of specimens. Such an arrangement is more economical and less confusing. Furthermore, the design of the specimen containers should permit safe handling of the sample without fear of leaks and should also allow for easy transfer of the specimen.

4. All specimens *must* be sent to the laboratory on the day of collection, with as little delay as possible. Bacteriological specimens referred to the department from external sources should be sent in transport media or in media containing a suitable preservative. When possible, all routine specimens should be sent to the laboratory early in the day. Early reception of specimens will permit adequate time for examination during normal working hours.

Use of Swabs for the Collection of Specimens

Many types of swabs have been available for the collection of specimens. Cotton swabs may possess a small amount of inhibitory lipoprotein, which reduces their usefulness in bacteriology. Survival of bacteria on synthetic fibers such as dacron is said to be higher, although there may be some variation in batches. Calcium alginate, another type of fiber, is reputed to be nontoxic to bacteria and is soluble in sodium hexametaphosphate. The advantage of this solubility is that organisms drawn along the alginate fibers by capillary action are released into the dissolving phosphate and are more easily recoverable on culture. However, this theoretical advantage is offset by the time and the technical maneuvering required to dissolve the fibers.

It is agreed that dry swabs, even if the substance of the swab is nontoxic to the suspected organism, are not advisable, and it is best to obtain swabs on material such as polyester or calcium alginate, which is then placed in transport medium, such as Stuart's or Amies' (see p. 337). Commercial swabs are available in which, after inoculation, the swab is placed within an ampoule of transport medium enclosed in a plastic pouch or tube for easy conveyance to the laboratory (Fig. 21–1).

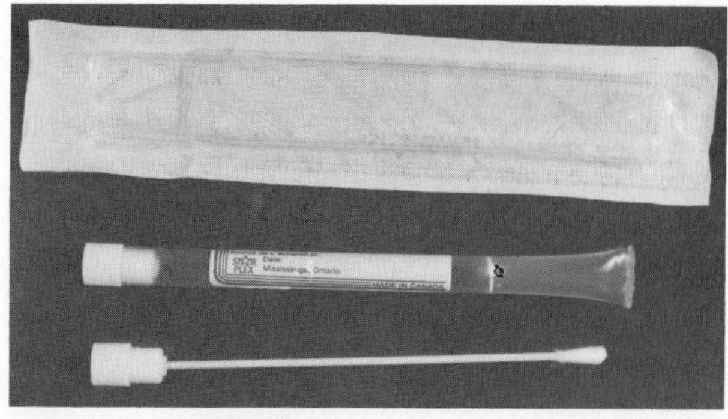

Figure 21–1 A sterilized swab and a tube of transport medium are dispensed in the disposable paper container. After the swab has been employed, it is placed in the tube of transport medium and the tube cap is discarded.

Rationale of Routine Macroscopic and Microscopic Examination of Specimens

A macroscopic examination of a specimen will often determine its suitability for culture. A worker will quickly become adept at recognizing the signs of a poorly taken specimen, e.g., a throat swab that smells of antiseptic, a leaky urine container, or a watery specimen of supposed sputum that is really saliva. These specimens are of little value, and to proceed further, in most cases, simply would be a waste of time. Such specimens should be discarded and replacements requested.

Macroscopic and microscopic examinations should complement one another. The microscopic examination of stained films or wet preparations prior to culture achieves the following objectives:

1. Demonstration of the *general nature* of the specimen, and in particular, the proportions of the different organism types present. On occasion bacteria will be reported in a direct film, yet the aerobic and anaerobic cultures are sterile following overnight incubation. This may be owing to the fact that the organisms were already dead, or perhaps that the incubation period was too brief. Bacteria are seen if the concentration in the original specimen was between 10^4 to 10^5 per mL. The relative proportions of epithelial cells and leukocytes in specimens labeled "sputum" are helpful in differentiating real sputum from saliva and may thus save unnecessary culturing (see below). On occasion, the direct microscopy of a specimen is almost diagnostic. For example, the presence of gram-negative intracellular diplococci in cerebrospinal fluid (CSF) leukocytes is very strong evidence of meningococcal meningitis. Conversely, the presence of large numbers of gram-positive bacilli in urine with only a few leukocytes indicates contamination in a specimen that has been kept at less than optimal conditions for a long period before submission to the laboratory.

2. Microscopic evidence may stimulate a departure from the normal routine. For example, a CSF exudate may be found to be predominantly lymphocytic with no bacteria demonstrable with Gram's stain, indicating that in addition to the employment of routine culture methods, cultures for tubercule bacilli and viruses also should be considered.

In addition to using specific gaseous and cultural environments, e.g., selective and differential media in the isolation of certain pathogens, one can also employ antimicrobial discs on primary cultures to assist in the rapid selection and identification of particular pathogens and the possible employment of anaerobic methods.

EXAMINATION OF MATERIAL FROM SITES NORMALLY STERILE

BLOOD CULTURE

The following organisms may be found in blood cultures:

Streptococcus viridans
Str. pyogenes
Staphylococcus aureus and *albus*
Str. pneumoniae
Neisseria meningitidis
Brucella spp.
Proteus-Providencia-Morganella
Pseudomonas aeruginosa
Enterococci
Anaerobic streptococci
Salmonella spp.
Francisella tularensis
Leptospira spp.
Streptobacillus moniliformis
Escherichia
Citrobacter
Klebsiella
Haemophilus influenzae
Bacteroides spp.
Clostridia
Listeria monocytogenes
Str. agalactiae

The organisms found are naturally related to the clinical status of the patient. Thus, *H. influenzae* may be found in children with meningitis or epiglottitis, and *Str. pneumoniae* septicemia may be confirmatory of lobar pneumonia. Gram-negative bacteremia such as with *E. coli* may be related to urinary tract infection and catheterization or other instrumentation, whereas *Ps. aeruginosa* bacteremia is not uncommon in patients with advanced malignant disease. About 15% of positive cultures yield more than one species of bacteria.

Taking the Specimen

If the bacteremia is continuous, as it often is in endocarditis, the timing of the taking of specimens is of little importance. In intermittent bacteremia, the resultant fever may occur up to 1 hour after the bacteremic episode. In such cases, specimens of blood should be obtained at the first sign of fever, and up to three specimens may be collected within 24 hours. Experience has shown that more than 90% of cases of bacteremia will be disclosed within the first three specimens.

The skin of the proposed venipuncture site should be cleansed with 70% alcohol followed by a solution of 2% tincture of iodine. In patients with known or suspected sensitivity to iodine, the skin is cleaned using only alcohol. If the blood is taken by syringe, then not only must precautions be taken to ensure sterility of the skin before puncture but the stopper of the bottle must be given similar care before the blood is transferred to the culture medium within.

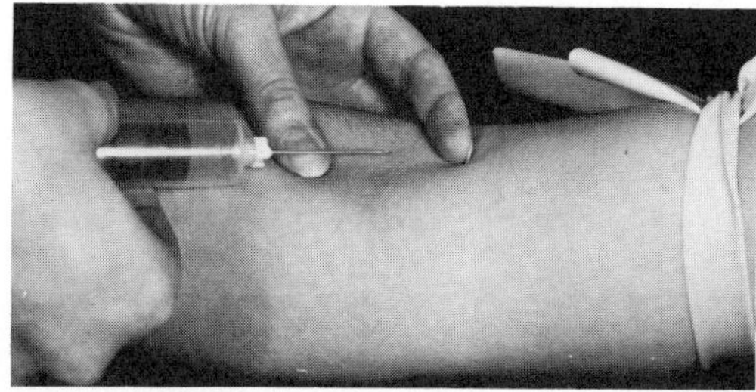

Figure 21–2 Vacutainer blood culture. The assembled apparatus is used to take the blood specimen from the patient, and in the laboratory, a venting unit is placed over the top of the syringe (now the blood culture tube).

The Culture Medium

Trypticase soy broth is a well-recommended medium, but other broths are also satisfactory. An atmosphere of 10% CO_2 within the culture tube or bottle is also advised. Penicillinase may also be added if desired, as may *p*-aminobenzoic acid to neutralize sulfa drugs. Most important, anticoagulants are included; of these, sodium polyanetholsufonate (SPS) has anticomplementary activity and inactivates the phagocytic properties of leukocytes as well as some aminoglycoside and polymyxin antimicrobials. However, SPS has been shown to have some antibacterial activity against anaerobic cocci and meningococci. Therefore, SAS (sodium amylosulfate) has been suggested as a substitute, but it shows some activity against gram-negative bacilli, and at this time SPS is widely employed in a concentration of 0.025-0.05% with 1.2% gelatin, which allows the growth of gram-positive anaerobic cocci.

An antibiotic removal device* is essentially a resin suspended in saline that removes numerous antimicrobials in large amounts (up to 100 μg/mL) from whole blood. Among the antimicrobials removed are amikacin, ampicillin, carbenicillin, cephalothin, cefazolin, chloramphenicol, gentamicin, nafcillin, tetracycline, tobramycin, and vancomycin. Cefoxitin and ticarcillin are removed to low concentrations.

In one method of usage, 5 to 10 mL of blood is added to a 50-mL bottle that holds the resin with 0.025% SPS in saline. The mixture is rotated for more adequate commingling before being added to the blood culture broth. It has been claimed that this method may as much as double the yield of positive blood cultures.

Volume of Blood

The amount of blood to be taken should not exceed 10% of the final mixture with the culture medium. Such dilution decreases the possible effects of immune antibodies and of any chemotherapeutic substances. Ten milliliters of blood from adults and 2 mL of blood from infants have been suggested as reasonable amounts to be taken. In these amounts there is generally an adequate number of bacteria to give a positive culture.

Incubation and Subculture

Incubation should be at 35°C, and a Gram film and subculture should be made on the same day as the blood was drawn (i.e., within a few hours), after 48 hours, and after 7 days. The sample may then be discarded. The practice of taking blood at specified intervals without obvious indication from the appearance in the broth is known as "blind subculture." Often turbidity, hemolysis, or some other evidence of bacterial growth may be seen within the container, although some organisms may grow without any obvious visible effects.

*Marion Laboratories, Kansas City, Mo. 64114.

Acridine Orange Stain* provides a rapid method of screening blood cultures. It is a fluorescent dye and is more sensitive than Gram's stain. Blood cultures are examined at a few hours and at 24 hours of incubation.

Procedure

1. **Make a smear of a drop of blood culture; air dry and fix with 50% methanol for 2 minutes.**
2. **Drain and stain with acridine orange for 2 minutes.**
3. **Rinse in water; drain and allow to dry. Do not blot.**
4. **Examine under fluorescent microscope.**

Result. Bacteria, gram-positive or -negative, and yeasts will appear red-orange (owing to staining of nucleoprotein) against a background of pale green or black.

Subculture is made to appropriate media, which should include blood agar and chocolate agar, and both aerobic and anaerobic incubation follows. On the blood agar, a staphylococcal streak (p. 390) is made to support the growth of haemophili and some types of streptococci. Other media, such as MacConkey, may be used in suspected enteric infections.

If flasks or bottles are used for the blood culture medium, then the broth culture is taken with all possible sterile precautions by a sterile syringe through the sterilized stopper; it is then transferred to the culture plate or to the slide for smear examination.

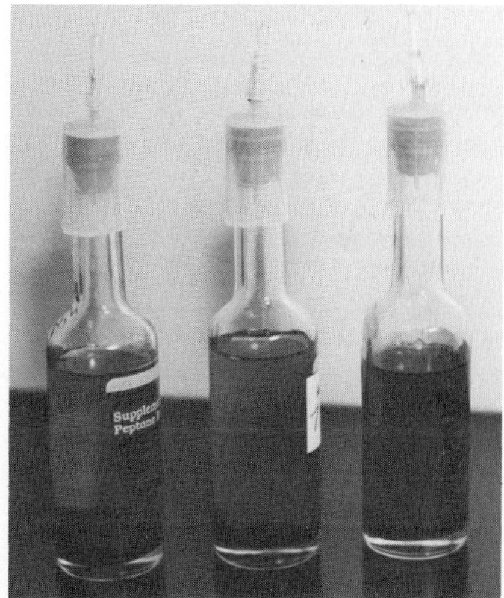

Figure 21–3 Vacutainer blood culture (Becton, Dickinson and Co., Rutherford, N.J. 07070). The Vacutainer system can be purchased with a number of prepared culture media. In the illustration, three blood cultures are shown after 24 hours' incubation. The bottle on the right is opaque as compared with the others, in which the blood has settled, leaving a clear supernatant. The right-hand bottle was from a patient with staphylococcal septicemia.

Blood Culture for Fastidious and Unusual Organisms

For *Brucella*, a Castaneda bottle with a biphasic medium (p. 334) is used in an atmosphere of 10% CO_2. Cultures are kept for four weeks at least.

An improved yield of fungi has been obtained by using a biphasic Castaneda-type medium with brain-heart broth and agar incubated at 30°C for four weeks.

Leptospira organisms are found generally only in the first week of the illness. One to three drops of freshly drawn blood is added to tubes with 5 mL of Fletcher's medium and incubated at 30°C for four weeks. Aliquots of the culture are examined weekly by dark-ground or fluorescence microscopy.

Francisella tularensis requires a liquid medium to which cystine and dextrose have been added.

Interpretation of Positive Results

Because of the widespread distribution of organisms such as *S. epidermis* on the skin, these organisms, along with diphtheroids and *P. acnes* or even *Cl. perfringens*, may be introduced inadvertently into blood culture media, in which they flourish. A contamination rate of 2 to 3% is said not to be unusual. However, although *S. epidermis*, diphtheroids, and *P. acnes* are common contaminants, they may cause bacterial endocarditis, and *Cl. perfringens* may enter the bloodstream from malignant tumors of the GI tract.

If such organisms are obtained from several culture bottles, they become more significant clinically than if they appear in only a single sample. Identical antibiograms or biotypes on organisms obtained from a few samples will also increase the importance of the organisms. Conversely, differing antibiograms or biotypes will diminish their importance. The laboratory must in no circumstance ignore them and must report them to the responsible clinician, informing him of the probability of their significance as the laboratory evidence indicates. The final decision as to the implication of the results is the clinician's.

Commercially prepared blood culture systems are available. Becton-Dickinson makes a series of Vacutainer sets with differing media. Supplemented peptone broth with SPS has worked well in the author's laboratory. Forty-five milliliters of the broth, which includes penicillinase and *p*-aminobenzoic acid, is present in a tube in an atmosphere of CO_2, and it draws 10 mL of blood. A venting tube is provided, and within the virtually closed system both aerobes and anaerobes are grown successfully, although the blood: medium ratio exceeds the suggested 1:10. Since the tubes contain the medium to which blood is directly added, the possibility of contamination during initial specimen taking is reduced. Likewise, risk of contamination is reduced in subculture, which is done through the venting needle and avoids multiple entry into the broth culture.

EXAMINATION OF CEREBROSPINAL FLUID (CSF)

Examination of the CSF yields much information regarding diseases of the central nervous system, since in meningitis (inflammation of the meninges) and other diseases of the central nervous system changes take place in the constituents of the fluid. Meningitis frequently is caused by pyogenic bacteria that apparently have invaded the meningeal sac either via the blood or by the perineural sheaths of the olfactory nerves into the subarachnoid space.

*Vacutainer Acridine Orange Stain, Becton, Dickinson and Co. Rutherford, N.J. 07070, and Mississauga, Ont. L5J 2M8.

The more common organisms that cause meningitis are as follows:

Haemophilus influenzae
Neisseria meningitidis
Flavobacterium meningosepticum
Streptococcus pneumoniae
Mycobacterium tuberculosis
Staphylococcus pyogenes
Group B streptococci
Streptococcus pyogenes
Cryptococcus neoformans
E. coli
Ps. aeruginosa
Other Enterobacteriaceae
Bacteroides spp.
Listeria monocytogenes
Acinetobacter calcoaceticus
Fungi
Acanthamoeba
Naegleria

Treponema pallidum also causes meningitis, but the diagnosis is made serologically. The same may be said for *Leptospira*. Table 21–1 shows the variations of CSF constituents in disease.

As in the case of blood cultures, some types of meningitis have clinical connotations. Infants are more liable to have *E. coli* and Group B streptococcal infections. In childhood, *H. influenzae, Str. pneumoniae,* and *N. meningitidis* are more common, and the same organisms are frequently seen in adults. Anaerobic organisms may spread from brain abscess. *Listeria monocytogenes* occurs as a cause of meningitis in patients with compromised immunoresponses, as does *Acanthamoeba*, whereas the other ameba species, *Naegleria*, causes disease in healthy individuals who have recently swum in man-made lakes or heated swimming pools.

Procedure

Note. The specimen should be cultured as soon as possible after its arrival in the laboratory.

1. Examine and record appearance, and volume of fluid. Usually it is a colorless and watery fluid. However CSF may become blood-stained as a result of either trauma occurring during its collection *or* of pathological hemorrhage within the nervous system or in the subarachnoid space. Following centrifugation the latter fluid will appear yellow or xanthochromic. There are other causes of xanthochromia; for example, a yellow acellular fluid with a very high protein content occurs in Froin's loculation syndrome, in which the noncirculating CSF beneath the blockage becomes altered. Xanthochromia becomes apparent only after a few hours posthemorrhage; consequently, in a fluid aspirated from a patient only freshly suffering from hemorrhage, xanthochromia will not be encountered.

Some physicians obtain CSF as it emerges from the lumbar puncture needle in three separate containers, taken consecutively. If hemorrhage has occurred during passage of the needle, the first container would be the most bloody; the second and third would each be less so. Preexistent hemorrhage would yield three similarly bloody fluid samples.

2. If the fluid is bloody, run dilute or undiluted CSF into a Fuchs-Rosenthal chamber. An excellent diluting fluid is 0.1% toluidine blue, which will stain WBCs blue and leave RBCs unstained. If dilution is performed, it is best to dilute with equal parts of the dye (only a few drops are necessary). *Naegleria* trophozoites have been seen actively motile in freshly obtained unstained CSF by the informed and perspicacious technologist. Red and white cells can be estimated separately. ("White cell" hematological fluid also may be used as diluent, but this destroys red cells.) Normally up to five lymphocytes per μL are present.

3. Centrifuge the CSF and retain the supernate for such biochemical examinations as glucose and protein (pp. 126, 216).

4. If there is pleocytosis, make a smear and examine with Gram's stain. Look carefully for bacteria and make a differential count of cells. Rarely, bacterial meningitis has been said to occur without a raised CSF white count.

5. Plate a loopful of deposit on blood agar and inoculate in a fluid medium such as brain-heart infusion or CTA. If it seems necessary after microscopic examination, incubate in 10% CO_2 atmosphere. If the presence of *Cryptococcus* is suspected, inoculate on Sabouraud's medium and incubate at 37°C and at room temperature. On blood agar, it is good practice to streak a known *Staphylococcus* across the plate after inoculation with CSF. The streak provides V factor and encourages the growth of *Haemophilus* spp. in its vicinity. Routine anaerobic culture is advised by many.

6. If requested, or if suspicion is aroused by other findings, stain by the ZN technique. For example, if a pellicle or "web clot" is seen in the spinal fluid, this may be indicative of *M. tuberculosis*. Remove the pellicle to make smears and apply acid-fast stain. Alternatively, place a drop of centrifuged CSF on a slide and fix it by heat, place another drop over the first, and repeat the process several times, thus building up a "button" of material. This is a fairly effective method of concentration. After staining, examine it very thoroughly. Culture on Löwenstein-Jensen medium.

7. Some special procedures:

(a) *Quellung reaction:* If *Streptococcus pneumoniae* or *Haemophilus influenzae* is suspected, the quellung test can be performed directly on the spinal fluid deposit for an immediate identification of the organism. Often, however, the organisms are not present in sufficient numbers to permit reliable observation of the reaction. Specific antisera are available for these organisms.

(b) *India ink preparation:* This is performed when *Cryptococcus neoformans* is suspected, or if yeasts are seen in the direct smear. One drop of sediment and one drop of India ink are placed on a slide and mixed, and a coverslip is placed over the preparation. Examine microscopically for yeast cells with large clear areas around them (i.e., capsule). If found, a tentative report should be issued stating "encapsulated yeasts present."

(c) *CSF LDH (lactate dehydrogenase)*: LDH in CSF may be helpful in differentiating between bacterial meningitis ($\geq$ 70 u/mL) and viral meningitis ($\leq$ 30 u/mL). Other meningitides caused by tumor, leukemia, and vascular accidents may also raise the level of LDH above 70 u/mL.

(d) *Estimation of immunoglobulin G (IgG) levels:* Refinement of the measurement of CSF protein has made the estimation of IgG levels in the fluid relatively easy. These immunoproteins may be raised either because of local production in the central nervous system or leakage across the vascular/CSF interface. CSF albumin is not made to any significant extent in the CSF,

TABLE 21–1 CSF CONSTITUENTS IN DISEASE

Disease	Macroscopy	No. cells/μL	Protein mg%	Glucose mg%	Other
Normal	Clear	5–10	15–40	50–80	
Acute and amebic pyogenic meningitis	May be turbid	↑ 10000 P	100–500	↓ 0	
Tuberculous meningitis	Clear, possibly fine clot	↑ 1000 L	50–400	↓	
Aseptic meningitis	Variable, usually clear	↑ 400 L > P	20–200	N	Glucose may be down in AM owing to malignancy
Viral meningitis	Clear	↑ 1000 L (P)	50–100	N	
Cryptococcal meningitis	Clear	↑ 1000	50–500	↓	Organism may be seen with India ink, etc.
Subarachnoid hemorrhage	Bloody and xanthochromic	Blood	↑	N or ↑	
Cerebral tumor	Usually clear	5–10	15–100	N	
Spinal block	Xanthochromic	0–10	↑ 2000	N	
Guillain-Barré syndrome	Clear	5–10	50–100	N	
Multiple sclerosis	Clear	5–100	15–50	N	Paretic or negative Lange's test; syphilis serology negative
Syphilis (depends on the stage)	Clear	10–500	25–150	N	Luetic, paretic, or negative Lange's test; syphilis serology positive

P = polymorphs, L = lymphocytic cells, (P) = polymorphs may be present early in the disease, N = normal, ↑ = raised (to), ↓ = lowered (to).

Other laboratory measurements may be helpful in the differentiation of some of these conditions. They are explained in the text, since their interpretation is not always clear-cut without clinical data.

and thus the ratio $\frac{\text{CSF IgG}}{\text{CSF albumin}}$ provides a reference of possible manufacture or permeability. The normal value is 17.5 ± 5%. However this result may be compromised if the patient has hypogammaglobulinemia or hypergammaglobulinemia. A method of obviating this difficulty is to calculate the following ratio, which will cancel the effects of the levels of serum proteins: $\frac{\text{CSF IgG/serum IgG}}{\text{CSF albumin/serum albumin}}$. The normal value is below 0.7, and the range is 0.34 to 0.66. Locally produced IgG may be featured in syphilis and polyneuropathy as well as in multiple sclerosis. Indeed, in a clinical setting, its measurement may be of great assistance in the diagnosis of the latter disease. Likewise, increased permeability of the blood/CSF interface occurs in tumors and infarction.

(e) *Counterimmune electrophoresis*: This is becoming a valuable instrument in rapid bacteriological diagnosis (see p. 552).

(f) *Culture methods for suspected ameba*: These are described in larger works.

8. If requested, freeze material for viral studies.

EXAMINATION OF PUS FROM ABSCESSES

The investigating procedure is the same as that used for wound swabs except that here the possibility of anaerobic infection is always suspected. The specimen is best obtained in a glass syringe without air or in prereduced transport medium (see p. 337). The organisms found in abscesses are similar to those found in infected wounds. However, in addition, *M. tuberculosis* and fungi may be found.

Procedure

1. Make a gross examination of the pus; describe the approximate volume, color, and consistency, and examine for "sulfur granules" (*Actinomyces* and *Nocardia*).
2. Prepare a Gram film. Examine it for pus cells and note the bacterial forms present. A ZN film should be made and examined, and a drop of pus should be mixed with 10% potassium hydroxide to examine for deep fungi.
3. Proceed with aerobic and anaerobic culture as described in the section entitled "Examination of Swabs from Wounds."

If requested, or if suspicion is aroused in preliminary examination, culture specifically for *Actinomyces, Nocardia*, or other deep fungi or for *M. tuberculosis* as described on p. 425.

Examination of Serous Effusions

Frequently microorganisms are implicated in the inflammatory diseases of serous membranes that can progress to the formation of fibrous adhesions. Under normal physiological conditions such fluids are present in specific quantities and possess specific constituents. For instance, joint fluid is present in only sparse quantities and is a pale viscid fluid. By contrast, the volume of CSF in a normal adult is approximately 130 mL, and CSF is a clear, colorless, nonviscid fluid. For purposes of clarity, CSF examination is discussed elsewhere (see above).

General Procedure of Examination

1. Describe the approximate volume, color, and appearance of the fluid. Look for "sulfur granules." If they are present, treat them as described under *Actinomyces*.

2. The fluid is centrifuged and the deposit is used for further investigation. If cytological examination is required, a smear of the fluid is fixed in Schaudinn's fluid before being stained and mounted.

3. A smear of the deposit is stained by Gram's method and by ZN stain.

4. Two blood agar plates, a MacConkey plate, and a tube of Robertson's meat medium are inoculated. One of the blood agar plates is incubated anaerobically. If requested, or if suspicion is aroused in the preliminary studies, one may use the material to investigate the possibility of tuberculous infection. If the material is otherwise sterile, the specimen will need no concentration technique; but if other organisms are present, concentration will be necessary.

5. The culture plates are examined and the procedure followed is that used for wound swabs.

Procedure for Differentiation of Joint Fluids

Normal synovial fluid has the following characteristics. It is a clear yellow fluid that does not clot spontaneously. There are up to 200 WBC per μL, of which less than 25% are polymorphonuclear leukocytes. There are no crystals, and the total protein is 1.8 g per dL.

Examination

1. Fluid from a normal knee joint is generally less than 3.5 mL in volume. The fluid cell count can be made in the same way as a blood white count, using 0.1% methylene blue in saline as a diluent. A film stained with Wright's stain can be employed for the differential count.

2. Because there is no fibrinogen in normal synovial fluid, it does not clot. Thus the appearance of a clot is pathological per se. There is a normal amount of hyaluronic acid present and it is present in a polymerized form. The degree of polymerization may be judged by a simple mucin test. One mL of joint fluid is added to 4 mL of 2% acetic acid, and the mixture is stirred with a glass rod. Normally a tight, ropy mass results, but softer masses or shredded soft flakes may result and arbitrarily be judged "good" (i.e., hard ropy) or "friable."

3. Protein may be estimated by the usual techniques employed for estimation of serum protein (p. 141). Inflammation causes a rise in protein. Immunoglobulins may be measured by the standard radial immunodiffusion methods; they are elevated in rheumatoid arthritis and SLE. Rheumatoid factor and antinuclear antibodies also may be sought in the elucidation of rheumatoid arthritis and SLE, respectively. Complement may be measured by immunodiffusion, and reduction is seen in some cases of rheumatoid arthritis.

4. Crystals: Direct and polarizing microscopy are used to examine a drop of fresh unpreserved joint fluid. Doubly refractile monosodium urate crystals 8 to 10 μm long are seen in gout and may be intracellular. Calcium pyrophosphate dihydrate crystals are seen in chondrocalcinosis and in pseudogout. They may be broader than uric acid crystals and up to 25 μm long, and they may have a "line" running through them; they are best seen under polarized light. In pseudogout, the serum uric acid level is normal. Cholesterol crystals may be found in any chronic effusion and in familial hypercholesterolemia. Corticosteroid crystals are generally needle shaped and may be intracellular and birefringent. Such crystals are the result of therapeutic injection, and their appearance may be very misleading if no history of injection has been obtained.

The differentiation between these crystals is extremely important to diagnosis and treatment. Cholesterol crystals are fairly easily recognized as parallelograms with a notch in one corner. The differentiation of pyrophosphate and uric acid crystals is more difficult. Their needle shape is not very different (although the former may be more "platelike"), and both are refractile. A compensating polarizing microscope that retards red light can differentiate between them but is expensive and not generally available. The first-order red filter required for the compensator can be replaced by two layers of cellophane tape on a clean slide (Owen, 1971). The slide is placed over the polarizer (i.e., the lower polarizing filter) and rotated until the background is red when viewed through the analyzer (i.e., the ocular polarizing filter). Crystals of uric acid seen through this system will appear bright yellow (strong negative birefrigence), and pyrophosphate crystals are faintly blue (weak positive birefringence).

With the use of relatively few criteria, the arthritides can be arranged into five etiological groups, which may help to narrow down the clinical diagnosis. A specific

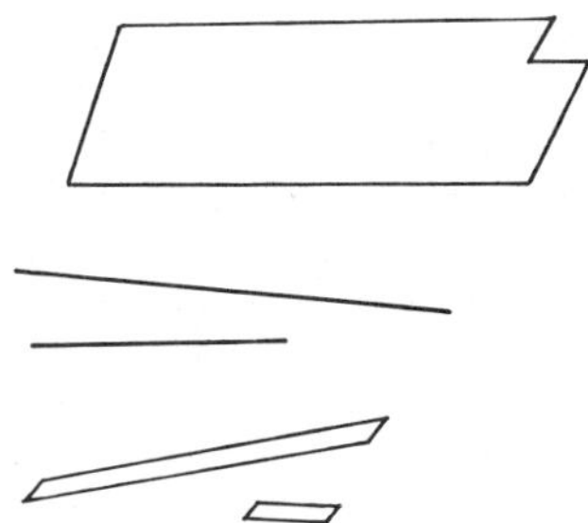

Figure 21–4 Joint crystals. The upper crystal represents cholesterol. Those in the middle are needle shaped, and the lower ones are platelike. Needle shaped crystals may be urates or corticosteroid. Calcium pyrophosphate crystals may be needleshaped or platelike.

diagnosis is possible in the case of crystal-induced arthritis, and with a positive culture in the infectious group. The results of synovial fluid examination in the groups and a list of the diseases in each group are given in Table 21–2.

Among the causes of infectious arthritis are:

N. gonorrhoeae
N. meningitidis
Staph. aureus
Streptococci
Enterobacteriaceae, including *Salmonella* spp.
H. influenzae
Streptobacillus moniliformis
M. tuberculosis
M. kansasii
Fungi

Examination of Tissue

Occasionally, surgical biopsies are submitted for bacteriological examination. The mode of investigation depends largely on the clinical suspicions of the surgeon submitting the material.

Procedure

1. Record size and nature of tissue specimen.

2. If specimen is large enough, cut off a small piece and make impression smears for Gram stain and ZN.

3. If tissue is large, mince it with sterile scissors before transferring it to a sterile Griffith tube for maceration. Addition of a small quantity of peptone water will make the material more manageable.

4. The resultant emulsion may be smeared, stained, and cultured, as desired.

5. For routine cultures incubate at 35°C and examine at 24 and 48 hours. If no growth occurs, continue incubation for 7 days before issuing a "no growth" report. In some cases (tuberculosis or deep fungal infections) a small amount of the material may be planted directly on the appropriate medium.

Examination of Urine

The presence of pus cells in the urine (pyuria) used to be considered a classic sign of urinary infection, but screening studies of large numbers of patients have shown that in some groups, half the patients with significant bacteriuria do not have pyuria or that the presence of pus cells is intermittent. Thus, other methods have had to be devised to assess bacteriuria.

The process of catheterization, once considered essential to obtain a suitable sample for bacteriological work, especially in the female, has been shown to carry with it an inherent risk of infection of 4 to 6% each time the catheter is passed. Thus the trend has been toward obtaining urine specimens without catheterization, in men by "midstream" specimens and in women by the "clean catch" method. The male patient is instructed to wash his hands thoroughly with soap and water and then to rinse and dry them. He then retracts the foreskin and cleans the glans penis with gauze sponges soaked in 5% tincture of green soap in water. The glans is then rinsed with swabs soaked in warm sterile water. He then micturates, passing the first few milliliters of urine into the toilet bowl but the next portion (midstream) into an awaiting sterile specimen container. The female patient also is instructed to thoroughly wash her hands and then to spread the labia and keep them apart until the specimen is taken. She washes the vulva from front to back with a soap sponge and repeats this three times. She then rinses away the soap with swabs soaked in warm sterile water. She passes the first few milliliters of urine into the toilet bowl and, without stopping the act of micturation, then catches a midstream specimen in a sterile container (clean catch). She must avoid contact of the specimen with her thighs or vulva or with any clothing. In young children and infants, aseptic application of an adhesive plastic bag over the genitalia may suffice, but this is tedious, and suprapubic aspiration of the bladder with a syringe is more satisfactory, especially in boys (girls may be catheterized easily).

It is now generally agreed that a count of more than 100,000 bacteria per milliliter of urine is a significant level and indicates a urinary tract infection. A count of less than 10,000 bacteria per milliliter is likewise considered to be the result of contamination. Counts between these levels are of debatable significance and may be caused by slow delivery to the laboratory or severe contamination. In any case, such results require a second specimen to elucidate the first.

Methods of Urinary Bacterial Counts

During the last decade or more, several techniques (both chemical and cultural) have been devised to assess significant bacteriuria. The chemical tests, often devised for screening purposes, have been variations of the nitrate reduction test and the tetrazolium reduction test. The problem with the chemical tests is that they lack specificity. On microscopic examination a Gram film of a drop of unspun urine that has been allowed to dry without spreading and that shows one or more bacteria per oil immersion field usually has a count of $> 10^5$ bacteria per milliliter of urine. The cultural methods are seen to have developed from the classic pour-plate method, through the surface drop method; the standard loop method; filter-paper method; and the dip-inoculum method.

All standard methods require prompt delivery of urine to the laboratory. Specimens may be stored at 4°C for limited periods for some methods.

Procedures

1. The use of pour plates is the classic method of performing bacterial counts. A known amount of urine is diluted in a medium, poured into Petri dishes, allowed to solidify, and incubated. Then the colonies in or on the medium are counted.

2. Standard loop methods are commonly used. Loops may be made (or purchased) to deliver 0.01 mL or 0.001 mL of urine. Inoculate a loopful of uncentrifuged urine onto a plate of blood agar and another onto a plate of MacConkey's agar. Incubate overnight and count the colonies. Multiply the number by 100 or 1000, depending on the loop used, to give the number of organisms per milliliter of urine. If fresh urine cannot be plated promptly, samples may be refrigerated at 4°C for up to 48 hours without significant alteration in bacterial counts.

TABLE 21–2 LABORATORY GROUPING OF ARTHRITIDES

Group I *Noninflammatory*	**Group II** *Inflammatory*	**Group III** *Infection*	**Group IV** *Crystal-induced*	**Group V** *Hemorrhagic*
Osteoarthritis	Rheumatoid arthritis	Bacterial	Gout	Hemophilia and other bleeding diatheses
Traumatic arthritis	Reiter's syndrome	Fungal and mycobacterial infections	Pseudogout	Trauma
Osteoarthritis dissecans	Ankylosing spondylitis			Neuropathic osteopathy
Osteochondromatosis	Rheumatic fever			Pigmented villonodular synovitis
	SLE			
Neuropathic osteoarthropathy	Scleroderma			Tumors
Pigmented villonodular synovitis	Ulcerative colitis			
	Regional ileitis			
	Psoriatic arthritis			

	Normal	**Group I** *Non-inflammatory*	**Group II** *Inflammatory*	**Group III** *Infections*	**Group IV** *Crystal-induced*	**Group V** *Hemorrhagic*
Appearance	Clear, almost colorless	Clear, yellow, slightly turbid	Cloudy, turbid	Turbid opaque	Turbid	Bloody
Mucin clot	Good	Good–friable	Friable	Friable	Friable	Friable
WBC/μL	< 200	200–1000	2000–100,000	10,000–100,000	1000–100,000	75,000
% Neutrophils	< 25%	< 25%	> 50%	> 75%	> 70%	> 25%
Protein (g/dL)	1.8	Raised	Raised	Raised	Raised	Raised
Glucose (mg/dL) compared with blood glucose	Slightly lower	Slightly lower	> 25% lower	> 40% lower	Slightly lower	Slightly lower
Crystals	–	–	–	–	+	–
Culture	–	–	–	+	–	–

Table adapted from Rippey, JH. Synovial fluid analysis. Lab Med 1979, *10*:140; and Rodnam, GP, et al. Primer on the rheumatic diseases. JAMA 1973, 224:661.

3. The Dip Slide method has a plastic slide with raised edges to give an even thickness of medium and a molded grid to simplify the task of enumerating colonies. The slide is enclosed in a clear plastic container, of which the screw cap is an integral part of the slide assembly. One side of the plastic slide is covered with MacConkey agar; the other is covered by Cysteine-Lactose-Electrolyte Deficient medium. Details of MacConkey's agar are given elsewhere (see p. 335). CLED medium will support the growth of usual urinary tract pathogens, and its salt deficiency ensures prohibition of swarming by *Proteus* spp. Yellow colonies are given by lactose-fermenters, and nonlactose fermenters have blue colonies. Different organisms will give different appearances and colors so that it is possible to recognize contaminated specimens quickly. It is generally agreed that a yield of three or more varieties of colony, i.e., types of organism, indicates contamination of the specimen. A contaminated urine specimen is not examined further.

The laboratory may accept the Dip Slide already inoculated with urine under the direction of the physician or a member of the nursing staff. If urine is sent to the laboratory for culture, then it must be exposed to the Dip Slide while it is fresh or within 2 hours of passage at room temperature. If the specimen is refrigerated immediately after it is voided, it may be used for colony counting up to 24 hours. Obviously if these limits are exceeded, normal bacterial proliferation in such an excellent medium will negate any accuracy in the colony count and thus in the decision as to whether the patient has a true urinary tract infection. A time clock in the laboratory reception area can be helpful in checking on the timing of collection and examination of specimens.

The presence of pus cells in the urine may indicate bacterial infection, but some cases of urinary tract infection do not continually exhibit pyuria. In addition, some cases of infection display pyuria subsequent to antibacterial therapy, although cultures are sterile. Pyuria caused by tuberculosis or by mycoplasmal infections also must be considered. It is our practice to make a Gram film on uncentrifuged urine and to record the number of pus cells per high-power field and the presence of bacteria. It is difficult to lay down hard and fast rules for the interpretation of appearances, but the following indicates some of the possibilities:

Pus Cells/HPF	Bacteria	Likely Conclusion
> 3	Gram-positive cocci or gram-negative rods	Genuine urinary tract infection
< 3	Gram-negative rods or mixed appearance	Contaminated specimen; specimen not fresh
< 3	Gram-negative rods or gram-positive cocci, but not mixed	Bacteriuria without pyuria
> 3	None	Urinary tract infection by usual pathogens unlikely; post-antibacterial therapy; ?tuberculosis; ?mycoplasma

Samples obviously contaminated or kept too long before culture can be disposed of, and a fresh specimen requested. Other specimens are subject to the Dip Slide, and the results are recorded and acted upon. In cases of doubt or when the specimen has been obtained by cystoscopy or some other surgical maneuver, it is best to deal with the specimen and leave the decision about the acceptability of the result to the surgeon. The report issued should contain all the pertinent information.

To use the Dip Slide, the cap is removed and the attached slide is immersed in the fresh urine specimen. Excess fluid is allowed to drain. The slide is then returned to the bottle and the assembly is incubated overnight at 35°C. The kit supplies a regression slope that permits estimation of bacterial numbers by inter-

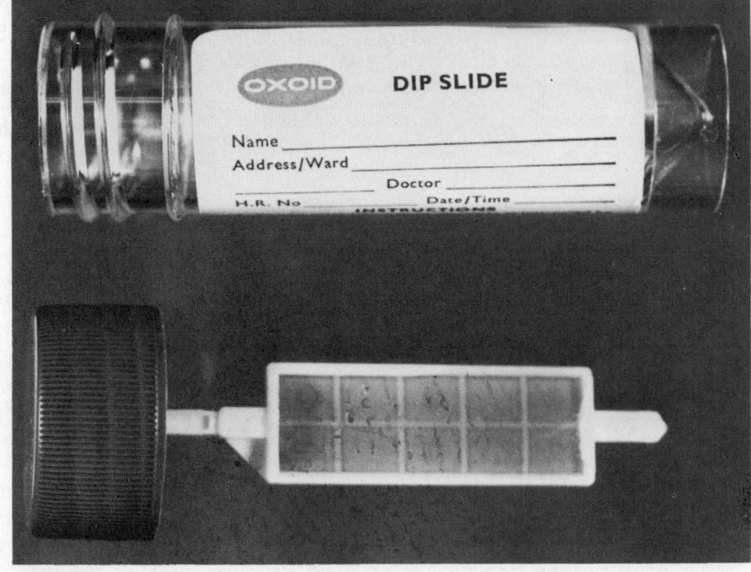

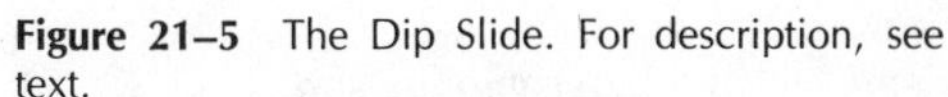

Figure 21–5 The Dip Slide. For description, see text.

polating counts of numbers of colonies on a single face of the slide. Typical results are:

Less than 20 colonies—equivalent to 10,000 organisms per milliliter.

Between 20 and 200 colonies—equivalent to 10,000 to 100,000 organisms per milliliter.

More than 200 colonies—equivalent to more than 100,000 organisms per milliliter.

Organisms Found in Infected Urine

E. coli	*Morganella*
Proteus spp.	*Citrobacter*
Ps. aeruginosa	*Serratia*
Enterococci	*Acinetobacter calcoaceticus*
Staphylococci	*Alc. faecalis*
Salmonella	*Candida albicans*
Mycobacteriaceae	*Klebsiella*
Providencia spp.	*Enterobacter*

Examination of Urine for Tuberculosis of Renal Tract

There seems to be no particular advantage to collecting a 24-hour specimen of urine for this purpose. An early morning specimen appears to be just as informative, is easier to arrange and handle, and is less likely to become contaminated. Concentration on the deposit is performed as described elsewhere (p. 425).

EXAMINATION OF SWABS FROM WOUNDS

Wound infections can occur: (i) when an organism from a normal commensal site is introduced into a new area, as a result either of intentional or accidental trauma, and (ii) when a causal agent is spread from person to person by aerosol formation and other modes of transmission.

The following organisms may be found:

Staph. aureus	*Ps. aeruginosa*
Str. pyogenes	Clostridia spp.
Proteus	Anaerobic Streptococci
Providencia	*Peptococcus*
Morganella	*Staph. epidermidis*
Escherichia	Diphtheroids
Enterococci	*Serratia*
Citrobacter	*Bacteroides* spp.
Klebsiella	

Obtaining the Specimen

If the wound is completely superficial, then it is clinically very unlikely that anaerobic organisms will have any significant part in the etiology of the wound infection. Swabs received from such wounds are plated on blood agar plates and on MacConkey's medium and are incubated at 35°C aerobically for 24 hours. On the blood plate is placed a disk of nitrofurantoin (100 mcg/mL). This allows the growth of *Pseudomonas* and *Candida* to be better appreciated, since most other genera are inhibited. A Gram film is also made, and the presence of pus cells and different bacterial forms is noted.

In cases in which there is a possibility of anaerobic infection, a liquid specimen taken in a glass syringe and kept anaerobic by expelling air and capping the needle with a rubber stopper is preferable to a swab. If swabs have to be used, they should be transported in prereduced anaerobic Carey Blair medium, which is commercially available. A swab for a Gram film should be submitted separately. Speed in plating is most important, and plating at the bedside is advocated by some. Fortunately anaerobic pathogens associated with human infections tolerate exposure to air much better than has been suggested, so that failure to grow suspected anaerobes is generally the result of faulty laboratory techniques rather than the exquisite sensitivity of such organisms to atmospheric oxygen. Nevertheless, efforts should be directed to obtaining specimens under optimal conditions. Gram films assume great importance in the diagnosis of anaerobic infections, since cultures take at least 48 hours, and, from the appearance of films, it may be possible to forewarn the clinician of the possibility of clostridial infections especially. If no swab is specifically available for a Gram film, material should be expressed from the specimen in the syringe or aspirated from the transport medium with another syringe.

Cultures are put up aerobically as above and on modified Schaedler's medium (p. 335) and are incubated at 35°C for 48 hours anaerobically. The plate, after inoculation, has a disk of metronidazole (5 μg/mL) placed on it. This substance is active in vitro against obligate anaerobes but not other organisms (with the exception of *Campylobacter* and *Gardnerella vaginalis*). Among the obligate anaerobes it is most active against *Bacteroides, Fusobacterium,* and *Clostridium* but less so against nonsporing gram-positive organisms such as *Actinomyces, Propionibacterium, Peptostreptococcus,* and *Peptococcus*. In practice, organisms growing close to the disk are unlikely to be true obligate anaerobes. The latter are generally seen beyond a zone of growth inhibition (Fig. 21–6). A chopped meat broth is also inoculated and incubated. In case of questionable results from cultures, the broth serves as a reference for both aerobes and anaerobes.

EXAMINATION OF MATERIAL FROM SITES POSSESSING NORMAL FLORA

INTESTINAL TRACT

Examination of Feces and Isolation of Pathogenic Bacteria

Pathogenic microorganisms found in stool cultures are:

Salmonella spp.	*Aeromonas* spp.
Shigella spp.	*Bacillus cereus*
Arizona	*Campylobacter jejuni*
Escherichia coli	*S. aureus*
Y. enterocolitica	*Cl. perfringens*
V. cholerae	*Cl. difficile*
V. parahaemolyticus	

Common intestinal parasites are:
Entamoeba histolytica
Giardia lamblia

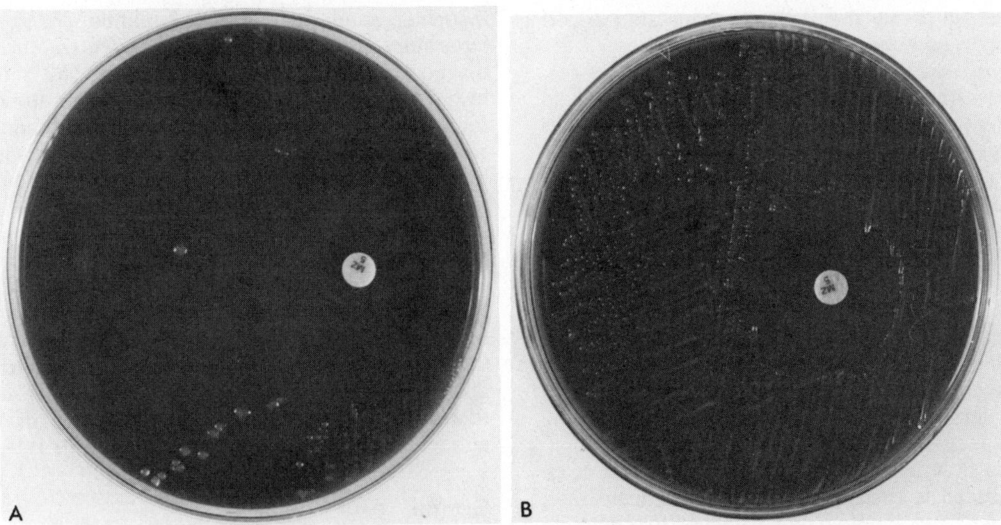

Figure 21–6 The action of metronidazole against *B. fragilis* (**A**) and *C. perfringens* (**B**) is seen in the zone of inhibition around the discs on these anaerobic cultures.

In addition it must be remembered that, especially in children, viral agents such as rotaviruses and the Norwalk agent are common causes of nonbacterial gastroenteritis.

Procedure

Macroscopic and Microscopic Examination. Make a gross examination of the stool, noting color, consistency, and the presence of blood or excess mucus. Bacillary dysentery typically gives a stool that is largely mucus, pus, and blood, with little fecal material. Suspicion of melena or obstructive jaundice may be aroused by color changes.

Microscopic examination should be done by making a light emulsion in saline to search for blood, pus, and ova and cysts (for methods employed in parasite studies, see p. 485). Gram stains are of limited value. However, in rare cases of staphylococcal enterocolitis clusters of gram-positive cocci may be seen to predominate in the film. With polychromic methylene blue, an invasive bacterial disease may be suspected if many pus cells are present. Such diseases include shigellosis and salmonellosis. In typhoid, mononuclear cells will predominate, but in cholera, which is noninvasive, there is no inflammatory exudate.

Obtaining the Specimen. One to two grams of feces is sufficient for culture and should be delivered to the laboratory as soon as possible. Shigellae may not survive the acidification of feces, which happens with cooling. Generally, feces are delivered to the laboratory in transport medium. Because of the newly appreciated importance of *Campylobacter jejuni,* Cary Blair medium is suggested to preserve a more alkaline milieu than glycerol-saline transport medium.

Routine Cultures and Identification Procedure. The following is an example of a routine that may be followed and that will allow salmonellae, shigellae, *Yersinia,* and *Aeromonas* to be isolated and identified. A sample of feces is inoculated onto several types of solid media and also into a fluid enrichment medium, which permits the multiplication of enteric pathogens while inhibiting the growth of intestinal commensal flora for a period of time. As mentioned in Chapter 14, several methods for rapid screening of the Enterobacteriaceae have been developed, of which the API system is considered to be superior. On the third day, suspicious colonies can be inoculated alternatively into this system for rapid presumptive diagnosis and confirmed when applicable by serology.

First day: (a) Plate on bile-lactose media (MacConkey, Hektoen) and also on blood agar and Yersinia selective medium (p. 335). Unlike other plates, this is incubated at 32°C. for 48 hours.

(b) Inoculate a small piece (about pea size) into selenite F broth or GN broth.

Second day: (c) After overnight incubation at 35°C, examine the blood agar plate for staphylococci, *Candida,* evidence of spreading colonies, and so forth. Transfer nonlactose-fermenting colonies from the bile-lactose media to the API system. Leave the plates at room temperature for a further 24 hours. Colonies of *Yersinia* may appear or become more apparent. Since the colonies are small, examination of the plate under a dissecting microscope may be advantageous.

(d) Subculture selenite F broth or GN broth to bile-lactose medium.

Third day: (e) Note the pattern of reaction in the API set. Many organisms may be identified at this stage. If the reactions are suggestive of *Salmonella* or *Shigella,* perform a slide test agglutination using polyvalent antisera. Positive reactions should be reported by telephone so that isolation techniques may be instituted. Commence culture for antigen identification.

(f) Inoculate nonlactose fermenters from step (d) into an API set.

(g) Examine the Yersinia selective plate. Typical colonies are dark red and like "bull's eyes" with a transparent surround. Confirmation is made by the API system.

Fourth day: (g) Read the API set from step (f). If indicated, proceed as in (e).

API System (see p. 343). This system can be employed at stages (e) and (g). The following is merely to indicate simplicity of technique; for more complete details consult the manufacturer's instruction sheet.

1. A single colony is emulsified in 5 mL of sterile saline. This suspension can be used for inoculating the API system and a nutrient agar slant for serology, etc.
2. Inoculate each compartment with the bacterial suspension.
3. After inoculation, those compartments containing reagents for arginine dihydrolase, lysine decarboxylase, ornithine decarboxylase, H_2S, and urease are covered with a layer of sterile mineral oil.
4. A plastic lid is placed over the compartments, and the total system is incubated at 37°C.
5. Following 18 hours' incubation, the reactions are read. Reagents are added to cupules for tryptophane deaminase, Voges-Proskauer, and indole compartments to complete these tests. If necessary add reagent to perform oxidase and nitrite tests.
6. After use, the system is disposed of by incineration.

More Specialized Techniques

Campylobacter jejuni. This is a common cause of infectious diarrhea. The diarrhea is watery and stools may be bloody. Culture is made on Skirrow's medium and grown in a microaerophilic atmosphere with increased CO_2. This can be most conveniently obtained in a GasPak jar using a hydrogen- and CO_2-generating envelope (CampyPak II*). The plates are incubated for 24 to 48 hours at 42°C. Colonies are recognized as small, gray, and oxidase and catalase positive. Microscopically a gram-negative, curved, small organism is seen. These features are diagnostic.

E. coli Diarrhea. Some of the mystery of infantile diarrhea has now been cleared up. *E. coli* can cause disease either by producing a toxin or by invading the bowel wall. In the present status of knowledge it would appear that the enteropathogenic *E. coli* serotypes do not cause scattered isolated cases of diarrhea, and thus there is no reason to study *E. coli* recovered in such cases for their serotype. If there is an outbreak of diarrheal disease in a nursery or if travelers return to North America or Europe with diarrhea, it is worth sending representative *E. coli* from stools of such patients to reference laboratories for tests of toxigenicity, invasiveness, and serotyping.

V. cholerae. Enrichment growth can be encouraged by alkaline peptone water (1.5% peptone in 0.5% NaCl at pH 9) in which a portion of stool is inoculated, then incubated at 35°C for 6 to 12 hours, and then subcultured to TCBS agar (see p. 386) for further incubation. Cary Blair transport medium can be used if necessary for conveying specimens to the laboratory.

V. parahaemolyticus has essentially the same requirements as *V. cholerae*.

S. aureus, B. cereus, C. perfringens. These organisms commonly produce gastric and/or enteric symptoms because of an enterotoxin that is ingested with the offending food. In cases of outbreaks of food poisoning, the supposedly responsible food is cultured. In the case of *S. aureus,* if such is found, the material should be sent to a reference laboratory for identification of the toxin. In *B. cereus,* diagnosis is confirmed by the isolation of 10^5 organisms/g in the offending food. With *C. perfringens,* the organism is found in anaerobic culture of the food and a similar serotype in the stool. Since *C. perfringens* is a normal bowel inhabitant, serological identification of the organism in both food and stool is necessary.

Pseudomembranous enterocolitis. This disease, which may follow antimicrobial therapy, appears to be due to the production of a cytotoxin by *Cl. difficile*. The latter organism is presumably enabled to flourish when the flora of the bowel is disturbed by the antimicrobial. At this time, the demonstration of the organism and its toxin is best done by a reference laboratory. Previously, *S. aureus* was thought to be the cause of this disease, but this was before culture of *C. difficile* and recognition of its role.

Genital Tract

It seems logical from both the clinical and the laboratory aspects to consider genital tract infection in women under two headings: puerperal sepsis and septic abortion, or cervicitis and vaginitis. Every effort should be made to obtain sufficient clinical data from medical and nursing staff to indicate the type of disease suspected.

Puerperal Sepsis and Septic Abortion

The pathogens recognized in these conditions include:

Str. pyogenes (Group A)	*Cl. perfringens*
Group B streptococci	*Staph. aureus*
Enterococci	*Peptostreptococcus*
E. coli	*Peptococcus*

Bacterial diagnosis may be complicated by the presence of normal flora, viz., staphylococci, diphtheroids, nonhemolytic streptococci, and so forth. A high vaginal swab is taken, trying to avoid contamination from the introitus and the lower vaginal wall. Possibly, the cervical canal can be sampled with a soft plastic catheter, obtaining the specimen by aspirating with a syringe. A Gram film is done, and the specimen is cultured on blood agar and a MacConkey plate aerobically and a modified Schaedler plate and Columbia starch agar anaerobically.

Cervicitis and Vaginitis

Although there are nonmicrobiological causes of leukorrhea, the major organisms that cause such disease are:

Neisseria gonorrhoeae
Trichomonas vaginalis
Candida albicans
Gardnerella vaginalis

Because of their posible importance in pregnancy, the presence of Group B streptococci should be noted.

The details of the diagnosis of gonorrhea will be discussed below.

If possible, obtain a saline-soaked swab and make a hanging drop examination for *Trichomonas vaginalis*. The swab is also used to inoculate Trichomonas medium

*Baltimore Biological Laboratories, Inc., Cockeysville, Md. 21030.

(Oxoid*), which is incubated at 35°C for 3 to 5 days. A loopful of the liquid culture is examined daily, subsequent to incubation for motile flagellates. It is claimed that such culture yields a considerable increase (> 20%) in the detection of *Trichomonas*. A Gram film is made, and it may yield diagnostic information, particularly in the case of *Candida* infection and occasionally in gonorrhea.

Swabs are also routinely inoculated on Thayer-Martin medium (for gonorrhea), on Columbia starch agar (for Group B streptococci) incubated anaerobically, and on Colistin nalidixic acid agar for the identification of *G. vaginalis*. A modified Columbia CNA agar with Tween 80 and Difco Proteose Peptone No. 3 as well as 5% human blood has worked very well (Totten et al, 1981). The plates are incubated for 48 hours at 35°C in 5 % CO_2 atmosphere. A MacConkey plate is also incubated.

Diagnosis of Gonorrhea

In women, in whom the disease may often be symptomless, endocervical, urethral, and rectal swabs are advised. In males, urethral swabs are taken. In the presence or on the suspicion of pharyngitis a tonsillar and pharyngeal swab is taken. In other disease, such as conjunctivitis, bacteremia, synovitis, and bartholinitis, cultures are taken from the appropriate area. In taking urethral swabs, 1 hour should have passed since the last micturition.

Gram films may show the typical gram-negative intracellular diplococci. Cultures are made on Thayer-Martin medium in a CO_2-rich atmosphere, conveniently provided by the Jembec plate. Incubation is for 48 hours at 35°C.

Male Urethritis

Although a large proportion of male urethritis is due to gonorrhea, another large proportion is due to organisms other than *N. gonorrhoeae*. These latter organisms are difficult to grow and require cell culture substances or complicated media and protocols. They include *Chlamydia trachomatis* and *Mycoplasma* species. The diagnosis of nongonococcal urethritis (NGU) is generally made presumptively by use of Gram stain. The presence of a large number of pus cells in the absence of gram-negative diplococci is accepted as indicative of a diagnosis of NGU.

External Surfaces

Conjunctival Cultures

These are best taken with a sterile bacteriological loop and then plated directly onto chocolate agar, Thayer-Martin medium, and blood agar plates incubated in 10% CO_2. In cases of spring catarrh, staining by the Romanowsky dyes will reveal large numbers of eosinophils. Viral inclusions are also shown by Giemsa staining in cases of inclusion conjuctivitis (see Fig. 24–1). Plates should be incubated at 37°C for 24 to 48 hours.

Pathogens most frequently isolated from eyes are:

Staphylococcus aureus
Haemophilus spp.
Streptococcus pneumoniae
Neisseria gonorrhoeae
Streptococci
Moraxella lacunata
Acinetobacter spp.
Pseudomonas spp.
"Coliform" bacilli
Viruses and fungi

Respiratory Tract

Upper Respiratory Tract

The upper respiratory tract frequently is involved in either generalized or localized infections. Those sites involved are the middle ear, mouth, oropharynx, nose, nasopharynx, larynx, and trachea. The normal flora of the upper respiratory tract comprise a number of organisms, particularly those of the Neisseriaceae, Corynebacteriaceae, Lactobacteriaceae, and Micrococcaceae families. It is possible that viruses also may inhabit the tract in the capacity of commensals. When the patient is healthy it is almost impossible to recover organisms from levels of the respiratory tract below the middle of the larynx.

Primary infection in the upper respiratory tract is generally viral in origin, and secondary bacterial infection is often caused by "opportunists" that are potentially pathogenic, e.g., *Streptococcus pneumoniae*. Diagnosis of upper respiratory tract infections thus rests on the correlation of clinical findings with the findings of films prepared from exudates and so forth, and from cultures. The area involved is usually obvious, and as such, examination is directed toward these sites.

Ear Culture

Ear swabs in cases of otitis media generally are taken by an ordinary cotton-wool swab. The smears are examined after staining with Gram's stain. The swabs are smeared on blood agar and MacConkey's medium and incubated in thioglycollate broth. The more common organisms encountered in otitis media are:

Ps. aeruginosa	*Escherichia*
Proteus-Providencia	*Klebsiella*
Str. pneumoniae	Anaerobic streptococci
Staph. aureus	*B. catarrhalis*
Haemophilus spp.	*Str. pyogenes*

The aerobic organisms will grow on blood agar, chocolate agar, or MacConkey's medium; growth of anaerobic organisms will be allowed and enhanced in thioglycollate broth. Anaerobic organisms may subsequently be subcultured and treated as described under anaerobic techniques.

Otomycosis is a form of otitis externa and is not uncommonly caused by *Aspergillus* spp. Specimens may be taken and examined as described under mycological techniques (p. 459).

*Oxoid, Columbia, Md. 21045, and Nepean, Ont. K2E 7K3.

Nasal and Throat Cultures

Nasal and throat swabs generally are taken with ordinary cotton-wool swabs, although in cases of suspect whooping cough, a long curved wire swab is used to reach the nasopharynx.

One disadvantage to the use of ordinary swabbing technique in collection of these specimens is that the areas are not very moist and the swab tends to dry out quickly unless it is placed in a transport medium. To overcome this problem it is suggested that the swab be made up with the cotton-wool tip immersed in a small tube containing approximately 0.5 mL of trypticase soy broth. The swab and the small tube are kept together in the carriage tube. For use, the broth-moistened swab is applied to the area and then replaced in the small tube. On receipt in the laboratory, the swab is squeezed against the side of the small tube to discharge its material into the broth. The broth is then used in the bacteriological studies.

Acute Pharyngotonsillitis. It is now generally accepted that the principal bacterial cause of "sore throat" is Group A streptococci and that normal inhabitants of the pharynx, such as *Str. pneumoniae, Staph. aureus, H. parainfluenzae,* and *H. influenzae,* are not significant. There is some limited evidence that streptococci of Groups B, C, and G may cause sore throat. Another, and now a mercifully rare, bacterial cause of sore throat is *C. diphtheriae*.. Most causes of acute pharyngotonsillitis are viral, including of course those viruses of the common cold as well as the Epstein-Barr virus of infectious mononucleosis and that of herpangina.

Subsequent to the making of a Gram film, which may be helpful in the identification of *C. albicans,* in cases of suspected diphtheria, and in Vincent's angina, the swabs are inoculated to blood agar plates, to a MacConkey plate for aerobic culture, and to another blood agar plate and an enriched blood agar plate for anaerobic culture. The latter includes 7.5 mg nalidixic acid and 5 mg colistin sulfate/500 mL blood agar (Oxoid*), which encourages the growth of streptococci. The additional anaerobic culture of throat swabs increases the yield of positive cultures for streptococci that are recognized by hemolysis, since streptolysin O is the only hemolysin produced by some strains. This hemolysin will not survive in oxygen but will endure under anaerobiosis. Streptococci of Groups C, F, and G will also be more easily recognized under anaerobiosis.

In cases of suspected diphtheria or in a screening program, swabs are inoculated on a tellurite medium and a Loeffler's slope (see Fig. 19–4).

Although cases of gonococcal pharyngitis are well documented, they are usually symptomless, and culture on Thayer-Martin or similar medium with the purpose of growing *N. gonorrhoea* is not attempted unless specifically requested by the attending physician.

Vincent's angina is an ulcerative condition of the gums and throat caused by the anaerobes *B. vincentii* and accompanying fusiform bacilli. The appearance of these organisms with pus in direct films is diagnostic, and culture is not undertaken.

*Oxoid, Columbia, Md. 21045, and Nepean, Ont. K2E 7K3.

Epiglottitis. This acute and potentially fatal infection is caused almost exclusively by *H. influenzae* type b. Culture is made on blood agar plates using a disk of bacitracin with X and V factors,* which will inhibit many organisms but allow *Haemophilus* spp. to flourish.

Sinusitis. The more common bacterial pathogens in the paranasal sinuses are:

Str. pneumoniae	Enterobacteriaceae
H. influenzae	*Neisseria* spp.
Str. pyogenes	*B. catarrhalis*
S. aureus	Anaerobic organisms

Swabs or, better, material from needle aspirations are examined by direct Gram films and cultured on a blood agar plate with a BXV disk and on a MacConkey plate. Anaerobic cultures are made on BA (blood agar) and on a Schaedler's plate.

Diagnosis of Whooping Cough. As indicated elsewhere (p. 393), *B. pertussis, B. parapertussis,* and *B. bronchiseptica* all may produce a similar picture of clinical whooping cough. Nasopharyngeal swabs mounted on a wire applicator may be passed through the nasal passage to the posterior pharyngeal wall. There the swab may be left during several coughs, while the head is carefully supported. Immediately on withdrawal of the swab, it is inoculated onto Bordet-Gengou medium or a medium of Oxoid charcoal agar with 40 μg cephalexin/mL and 10% defibrinated horse blood. If this method is considered impractical, the patient is allowed to cough directly into an opened Bordet-Gengou plate. Experience has shown, however, that the former method has a higher success rate of "positive" cultures than the latter, and thus is the method of choice.

The plate should be cultured for up to 6 days at 37°C before being discarded as negative. The colonies of all three bacterial species are smooth, raised, entire, and pearly. Swabs may be smeared and directly examined for *B. pertussis* by an immunofluorescent technique so that results are available quickly (p. 548), or suspected colonies may be screened by this technique.

Lower Respiratory Tract

As mentioned earlier, in the healthy patient the mucous membrane of this portion of the tract is sterile. For a variety of reasons, certain microorganisms and viruses of pathogenic status, or mere "opportunists" from the upper respiratory tract, are able to invade the lower tract and precipitate inflammation.

Examination of sputum from patients with acute bronchitis, bronchiolitis, and pneumonia will be complicated by a number of factors: (i) the sputum will consist of a mixture of exudate from the affected mucous membranes and material (i.e., saliva, etc.) containing commensals from the upper respiratory regions and (ii) in most cases the expectorated specimen very often is thick and tenacious, representing a formidable barrier to sampling. In the latter case, the specimen can be homogenized by a mucolytic agent prior to sampling for culture.

The first problem facing the laboratory is to differen-

*Difco Laboratories, Detroit, Mich. 48232.

tiate sputum from saliva or from sputum grossly contaminated during oropharyngeal passage. By taking a purulent or bloody flecked portion of the submitted specimen and subjecting it to a direct Gram film, one can resolve this problem. Under × 100 magnification, the specimen is examined for epithelial cells and leukocytes and can be classified as follows:

Group	Epithelial Cells	Leukocytes
1	>25	<10
2	>25	10–25
3	>25	>25
4	10–25	>25
5	<10	>25

There has been established a good correlation between transtracheal aspirations (real sputum) and Group 5 specimens of sputum. Thus only Group 5 specimens are accepted and dealt with. Others are rejected, and the physician is informed so that a better specimen can be obtained.

Common pathogens in the sputum include:

Str. pneumoniae
H. influenzae
S. aureus
Enterobacteriaceae
Ps. aeruginosa

Some specimens of sputum are viscid, and it is difficult to obtain a good representative plating without liquefying the specimen. This may be performed as follows:

1. To 45 mL of Thiol broth* add 5 mL of Sputolysin.†

2. Add 5 volumes of diluted Sputolysin to 1 volume of sputum and rotate.

3. Incubate at 35°C for about 30 to 45 minutes, until the mixture is homogeneous.

4. Inoculate on BA with a BXV disc and on a MacConkey agar plate.

(Sputolysin is a sterile solution of dithiothreitol.)

After 18 to 24 hours' incubation, predominant growths of potentially pathogenic organisms are reported. Particularly important here is the definition of *predominant growth.* For example Enterobacteriaceae are not unusually present in the upper respiratory tract. This is especially true in hospitalized patients, where their growth may be encouraged by antibiotic therapy. However, in large numbers, they may be significant and the etiological agent of pneumonia. Such situations, even with organisms like *Str. pneumoniae* are not uncommon, and good screening of specimens of sputa and close clinical-laboratory liaison will help in making the efforts of the laboratory meaningful.

Other Pulmonary Pathogens in Sputum. Viral and fungal agents that produce lower respiratory tract disease are further discussed in the appropriate section.

Methods of Diagnosis in Tuberculosis

Tubercle bacilli may be present in such specimens as sputum, urine, gastric washings, cerebrospinal fluid, pleural fluid, feces, pus, and tissue. Many of these specimens normally contain a large number of organisms (feces, sputum, and gastric washings); others usually are contaminated (urine), and usually tuberculous pus is secondarily infected. Cerebrospinal and pleural fluids, however, are normally sterile, and if they contain tubercle bacilli, there is unlikely to be any other organism present. Concentration methods are used for those specimens that contain organisms other than mycobacteria, since they destroy the contaminant bacteria, leaving the mycobacteria viable. Nevertheless, concentration methods may destroy some mycobacteria; therefore for specimens such as CSF and pleural fluids, concentration is not employed, although centrifugation is used. In addition to destroying contaminant organisms, concentration methods reduce the bulk of specimens, making them more manageable. For urine, the best specimen is an early morning sample. Gastric washings also are optimally taken at this time. A 24-hour "pool" of sputum is the best respiratory tract specimen, and a first morning specimen, although not as good, is better than random samples. Tissues are initially minced with scissors and then ground in a Griffith tube with saline. Further treatment is as with other specimens.

Precautions

In dealing with tuberculous material, the airborne particle is the particular danger. All precautions taken against the production or dissemination of such particles are worthwhile.

Technologists working primarily with tuberculous material should, if possible, be Mantoux-positive (i.e., have some immunity to the disease) and should be warned of the dangers of eating or smoking when manipulating tuberculous material. Routine annual chest x-rays of such persons are desirable. If possible, the laboratory area in which work with tuberculous material is done should be enclosed and used for no other purpose. It should be air-conditioned and have benches, walls, and floors that can easily be washed. Safety cabinets with exhaust ventilation providing small enclosed areas for manipulation are available. Ultraviolet irradiation of the air (above eye level) has been used. Centrifugation presents definite hazards from aerosol formation and also breakages. Ideally, centrifuges should be enclosed in safety cabinets. Failing that, scrupulous care and cleanliness should be observed. Discarded material should receive preliminary disinfection in hypochlorite solution and then be autoclaved.

Besides taking precautions against laboratory infections, one must beware of introducing saprophytic mycobacteria into specimens and thus possibly confusing diagnosis. New slides should be used; material should not be blotted with absorbent paper; rubber bungs and tap water are to be avoided. The smegma bacillus (in Runyon group IV), a harmless commensal in urine, is acid-fast but not alcohol-fast.

N-Acetyl-L-Cysteine (NALC) Method of Concentration

Preparation of Digestant

4% w/v sodium hydroxide 25 mL

*Difco Laboratories, Detroit, Mich. 48232.
†Calbiochem-Behring Corp, La Jolla, Calif. 92037.

2.94% (M/10) trisodium citrate	25 mL
N-acetyl-L-cysteine (NALC)	0.25 g

The NALC should be added to the mixture just prior to use, but the solution will remain stable for 2 days if refrigerated and tightly stoppered. The solution is also self-sterilizing.

Procedure for Sputum, Bronchial Secretions, etc.

1. Using approximately 10-mL quantities, equal volumes of sample and digestant are mixed.
2. Transfer to 50 mL plastic graduated centrifuge tube with cap. Allow to stand at room temperature for 15 to 30 minutes, mixing periodically by gentle rotation to ensure complete liquefaction.
3. Fill tubes with sterile M/15 phosphate buffer at pH 6.8
4. Centrifuge at 3000 rpm (1800-2400 g) for 15 minutes.
5. Discard supernatant into disinfectant.
6. Smear the sediment onto new glass slides for microscopic study.
7. Add 1 mL of sterile 0.2% bovine albumin fraction V (pH 6.8) to the remainder of sediment. The albumin is made as follows: 2 g of bovine albumin in 100 mL of saline adjusted to pH 6.8 with 10% sodium hydroxide and sterilized by Seitz filter. Dilute 1:10 in M/15 phosphate buffer.
8. Examine smears and inoculate medium from albuminized sediment. A dilution of the sediment 1:10 in sterile water also may be inoculated. This dilution reduces the toxic properties of the digest and aids in production of discrete colonies.

Procedure for Urine, Gastric Washings, etc.

The centrifuged deposit of urine is treated like sputum. Pus is similarly treated. For gastric washings, a pinch (50 to 100 mg) of NALC powder is added directly to the specimen, mixed, and then centrifuged. After centrifugation, the sediment in a small amount of distilled water is treated like sputum. Whether it is worth examining feces for mycobacteria (which have probably been swallowed) is questionable. In rare cases where a need is shown, Petroff's method is used (see 3rd edition).

Inoculation and Culture

Two media are widely used for culture of *M. tuberculosis.* These are the coagulated egg-based medium of Lowenstein and Jensen (L-J) and the agar-based medium of Middlebrook and Cohn (7H-10). They each have advantages and disadvantages. The latter medium is clear, so small and early colonies may be seen, thus hastening diagnosis. L-J medium is more apt to become contaminated, but it supports the growth of a wide diversity of mycobacteria and is more easily stored than the agar-based medium. Ideally, both media are used in parallel. They are cultured at 35°C in an atmosphere of 10% CO_2. Some mycobacteria, as will be seen, grow at lower temperatures and can produce pigment either in darkness or in the light. Tubes are examined at least weekly for 10 weeks before being discarded as negative. A dissecting microscope can be used with the agar-based and transparent medium to see tiny early colonies.

Microscopic Examination

1. Ziehl-Neelsen and Kinyoun methods are described under staining techniques. Smears of sputum often are examined directly without concentration, although concentration will increase the number of "positive" smears. CSF is examined by the technique described in that section; a similar technique may be applied to centrifuged pleural fluid. With other specimens, the concentrate is always examined.
2. The method of fluorescent microscopy is described under staining techniques (p. 349). Specialized equipment gives the best results and is safer for the observer to use.

Investigation of Fever of Unknown Origin

In addition to addressing a common clinical problem, the principles employed in investigations of fever of unknown origin serve as a summary of this chapter.

Patients who have a significant and persistent fever, greater than 37.8°C (100°F), the cause of which cannot be readily diagnosed by clinical examination, are referred to as having "fever (or pyrexia) of unknown origin" (FUO).

Such cases are seen to fall into three categories: those caused by (i) noninfections, (ii) systemic infections, and (iii) localized infections.

Some probable causes of the first category of fever are:

- Neoplasms, including the leukemias and lymphomas
- Fear and hysteria
- Myocardial infarction
- Infarction of fibroid of uterus
- Drug hypersensitivity
- Cirrhosis
- Ulcerative colitis and regional ileitis
- Familial Mediterranean fever
- Collagen-vascular disease
- Moschcowitz's syndrome (TTP)
- Blood in serous cavity: peritoneum, pleura, pericardium, joints, etc.
- Sarcoidosis
- Factitious fever
- Pulmonary emboli
- Whipple's disease

The diagnosis of infections in FUO cases will depend upon the employment of both direct and indirect methods, implying that the recovery of a causative agent may not always be possible. Hence, dependence often is placed on the demonstration of the presence of specific antibodies circulating in the patient's serum. Thus, investigations of an FUO usually proceed along the following lines:

Examination of Blood

This should involve:

(a) Determination of general blood picture, i.e., full blood count. The demonstration of a leukocytosis or leukopenia, and so forth, may be *indicative* of a systemic infection.

(b) Direct blood films should be prepared and examined to exclude the presence of circulating parasites such as the malaria plasmodia, *Borrelia,* and *Trypanosoma.*

Blood Culture

Serial blood cultures should be performed. Definitive diagnosis may be made by this method in such conditions as subacute bacterial endocarditis (SBE), salmonellosis and typhoid, brucellosis, gonococcemia, chronic meningococcemia, tularemia, and forms of rat-bite fever.

Serological Examination of the Blood

An effort should be made to perform serological studies at different stages in the disease process to see if any rise in antibody titer occurs (p. 536). Such examination is particularly valuable in the elucidation of disease caused by *Salmonella* and *Brucella*. The Weil-Felix (p. 538) reaction is helpful in the diagnosis of rickettsial disease. Antibodies to *Toxoplasma,* the deep fungi, and heterophil antibodies in the diagnosis of mononucleosis and serum sickness may be valuable. Antistreptolysin antibodies are useful in the diagnosis of rheumatic fever and the presence of circulating rheumatoid factor in rheumatoid arthritis. Other tests of value in autoimmune and collagen disease are listed elsewhere. Serological studies are particularly valuable in the diagnosis of viral disease.

Swabs from the Upper Respiratory Tract

Generally, clinical symptoms are overt in upper respiratory tract infections, but throat swabs and sputa should be examined in case of an overlooked throat infection or the possibility of tuberculosis.

Examination of the Urine

This should be performed to exclude urinary infection. Repeated examination may be necessary. Genitourinary tuberculosis and leptospirosis also should be considered.

Examination of Feces

Culture methods are designed to reveal the presence of organisms of the *Shigella, Salmonella, Yersinia,* and *Campylobacter* groups. The presence of protozoa and of helminths may be significant.

Examination of Tissue and of Body Fluids

Surgically removed lymph nodes and portions of lung or other viscera may be macerated or otherwise treated before culture to reveal the growth of such organisms as the deep fungi, tuberculosis, and so forth. The bone marrow may be cultured in cases of suspected histoplasmosis or miliary tuberculosis. In all these situations, careful histological examination and the use of specific staining methods may be diagnostic. However, after the tissue has been placed in fixative fluid it is too late for cultural studies; therefore surgeons should be encouraged to bisect lymph nodes and viscera and to submit half of the specimen in saline.

In cases of FUO resulting from localized infections such as subphrenic abscesses or pelvic, perinephric abscesses, or in diverticulitis and prostatic abscess, cholangitis, and liver abscesses, the laboratory can give only very general indications of infection. The elucidation of the condition requires much clinical acumen and the expertise of other departments of the hospital outside the laboratory.

Collection of Specimens for Diagnosis of Viral Disease

Although many laboratories in community hospitals do not have facilities for culture of viruses and do not keep a range of viral antigens or antibodies with which to do viral serological studies, it is most important that all laboratory workers have a reference laboratory where such material may be sent and that they be able to obtain satisfactory specimens for examination.

The type of specimen to be submitted will depend on the specific disease and for culture purposes may include nasal washings, nasal or throat swabs, throat washings, vesicular fluids, stools or rectal swabs, spinal fluid, and surgical or autopsy material. All specimens should be deep frozen immediately and shipped with dry ice.

Nasal washings are obtained with sterile saline. Throat swabs are placed in buffered tryptose phosphate broth with gelatin or in Hanks balanced salt solution with 1/2% gelatin (Lennette et al., 1980). Eye swabs and vesicular fluid are treated similarly; vesicular fluid may also be collected in small capillary tubes and the ends sealed with paraffin wax. Stool samples can be sent without a transport fluid, as may spinal fluid. Urine for cytomegalovirus or throat washings for a similar purpose are best sent in an equal amount of 70% sorbitol (w/v) in water. Blood used for viral isolation is anticoagulated with citrate, oxalate, or heparin and is sent to the laboratory by some rapid means *without freezing.* For serological study, blood is obtained without anticoagulating and the clot is separated. The serum is sent frozen. Autopsy or surgical material, unfixed and frozen, is required.

In varicella-zoster, rabies, and herpes, viral particles in cells may be diagnosed by immunofluorescent techniques. Direct electron microscopy of stool is the diagnostic method in diarrhea caused by rotavirus and in some other viral causes of diarrhea.

Serological tests are very numerous. Neutralization tests add the serum to a cell culture with living virus. Without antibodies, a cytopathic effect on the cells would occur; its prevention by serum indicates immune antibodies. Complement-fixing antibodies are demonstrated by tests that employ the classic method (see Fig. 26–6) and known viral antigens. Some viruses (including that of rubella) will agglutinate red cells, and this hemagglutination will be prevented by specific antibodies. There are several tests, including radioimmunoassay, for the diagnosis of hepatitis B, and the heterophil agglutination test has been used widely in the diagnosis of mononucleosis for many years. In viral disease, paired sera are very often important. The first sample is taken at the onset of illness and the second 2 to 3 weeks later. A fourfold or higher increase in titer is considered significant.

Cytological and Histological Diagnosis

Although many hospital laboratories do not, as noted, perform serological or cultural studies in viral disease,

TABLE 21–3 HISTOLOGICAL AND CYTOLOGICAL EXAMINATION IN CHLAMYDIAL AND VIRAL DIAGNOSIS*

Virus	Smear	Section	Material	Result	Method†
Rabies	+	+	Brain	Negri bodies (cytoplasmic), especially in Ammon's horn	Seller's for smears or sections, or Giemsa for sections
Yellow fever		+	Liver	Eosinophilic (intranuclear) inclusions in liver cells. Councilman bodies	Hematoxylin-eosin
Ornithosis	+	+	Avian spleen or air sac; human lung	Red elementary bodies in cytoplasm	Macchiavello, Giménez, Giemsa
Lymphogranuloma venereum	+	+	From buboes	As ornithosis	As ornithosis
Vaccinia-variola	+	+	Scrapings from lesions	Guarnieri inclusion bodies. Paschen elementary bodies in cytoplasm	Guttstein's
Herpes simplex	+	+	Scrapings from lesions	Lipshutz (intranuclear) inclusions. Multinucleate cells in base of lesion. Margination of nuclear cytoplasm.	Hematoxylin-eosin, Giemsa, Papanicolaou
Varicella-zoster	+	+	Scrapings from lesions	Intranuclear, and later cytoplasmic inclusions. Multinucleate cells in base of lesion. Margination of nuclear chromatin in tissues early in disease.	Hematoxylin-eosin, Giemsa
Trachoma-inclusion conjunctivitis	+		Conjunctival scrapings or follicular expression	Cytoplasmic inclusions	Giemsa, Wright, iodine
Molluscum contagiosum	+	+	Exudate or biopsy	Cytoplasmic inclusions or histological pattern	Cresyl blue, iodine, hematoxylin-eosin
Verruca vulgaris		+	Biopsy	Intranuclear inclusions. Vacuolation of cell. Histological pattern.	Hematoxylin-eosin
Measles	+	+	Exudate from nose. Appendix, tonsils.	Intranuclear and cytoplasmic inclusions in exudate. Giant cells in tissues and exudates.	Hematoxylin-eosin
Adenovirus		+	Lung	Scanty nuclear inclusions. Associated necrosis.	Hematoxylin-eosin
Cytomegalic inclusion disease	+	+	Urinary epithelial cells. Biopsy	Cytomegalic inclusions.	Hematoxylin-eosin, cresyl blue

*After Lennette, EH: *In* Diagnostic Procedures for Virus and Rickettsial Diseases, 2nd ed. New York: American Public Health Association, 1956.

†Many specific fluorescent antibody techniques are also available and are often preferable.

there are numbers of cytological or histological examinations that can be done without any special techniques. These essentially attempt to show the presence of inclusion bodies (the viral aggregates) within affected cells. Some specialized stains are used and are briefly listed in Table 21–3.

CHAPTER 21—REVIEW QUESTIONS

1. (a) Ninety per cent of bacteremias will be revealed by taking:
   Three specimens in 24 hours.
   Four specimens in 18 hours.
   Six specimens in 48 hours.
   (b) What are the useful properties of SPS (sodium polyanetholsulfonate) in blood culture media?
   (c) The amount of blood added to fluid blood culture medium should not exceed:
   1%, 10%, or 0.1%.
   (d) Is the finding of *S. epidermidis, Cl. perfringens,* or *P. acnes* ever significant in blood cultures? When?
2. Explain the terms *midstream* and *clean catch.*
3. Outline a method of examining feces for *Salmonella* or *Shigella*.
4. Describe the culture media used for throat swab culture.
   (a) Why is one plate incubated anaerobically?
   (b) Why does it contain nalidixic acid and colistin.
   (c) Is Thayer-Martin medium ever used? When?
   (d) Why is a disc with bactracin and X and V factor used on BA plates from throat swabs?

22 ANTIMICROBIAL SUSCEPTIBILITY AND EPIDEMIOLOGY IN HOSPITALS

ANTIMICROBIAL AGENTS

Although Semmelweis (1818-1865) recognized the importance of infection and the need for antisepsis to prevent puerperal sepsis, he had no clear notion of the bacterial nature of the disease. Lister (1827–1912) appreciated the bacterial nature of wound infection and advocated the use of the carbolic spray in surgery. However, both these famous figures—one showered with honors and the other dying disappointed and demented—aspired only to *antisepsis.* This term means the carrying out of procedure to *avoid* infection. Paul Ehrlich (1854–1915) was the first to explore *chemotherapy*, the introduction of chemicals into the organism to combat infection already present. It is quite different from immunization and vaccine therapy. Ehrlich's ambition was to find the *therapia magna sterilisans,* the chemical that would be bactericidal to the pathogen without killing the cells of the organism. Disinfectants may kill the pathogenic organism but are too toxic for the host cells to allow therapeutic use. Antimicrobials, on the other hand, show selective toxicity, singling out the offending microbiological agent and attaching itself to some receptor in the agent, all without significantly affecting the cells of the host. In 1906 Ehrlich discovered salvarsan, or "606," an organic compound of arsenic that is very effective against the *Treponema pallidum.* Domagk and others in 1935 described sulfamidochrysoidine (Prontosil rubrum), which was the first therapeutic sulfonamide drug; many others followed. For many years it had been known that microorganisms are occasionally antagonistic to each other; it had been reported as early as 1874 and by Pasteur in 1877. In 1929 Fleming noted the inhibition of staphylococci by *Penicillium* (an airborne fungus). He subcultured this fungus, and in 1939-1940 Chain and Florey were able to isolate more adequately the actual inhibitor produced by *Penicillium.* Large pharmaceutical companies learned how to produce the substance in quantities sufficient for more widespread use. This was the dawn of the era of antimicrobials, an extension of chemotherapy. In 1944, Waksman isolated streptomycin from a soil fungus.

On these foundations a vast new industry was founded that today produces an immense quantity of antimicrobials. Initially some distinction could be drawn between chemical substances such as the sulfa drugs, which were considered chemotherapeutic, and substances like penicillin, produced by microbiological agents and considered as antibiotics. With the artificial synthesis of antibiotics and their chemical manipulation, the term *antimicrobial* appears preferable at this time.

DEFINITIONS

Some antimicrobials are *bacteriostatic*, e.g., sulfonamides, chloramphenicol, and erythromycin. They inhibit replication of the organisms but do not prevent them from reproducing once more when the drug is withheld. Such bacteriostatic agents are effective because they give natural defense processes great advantage while the bacterial agent is unable to continue the disease process. Other antimicrobials are *bactericidal*, e.g., streptomycin and penicillins. These produce death of the challenged organism, with obvious beneficial effects. Some drugs, e.g., tetracyclines, are bacteriostatic at usual therapeutic blood levels but bactericidal at higher concentrations.

It is generally sufficient to produce bacteriostasis in any given situation in order to achieve sufficient advantage with antimicrobials. To obtain such bacteriostasis, the drug must be given in a therapeutic dose that is adequate to raise the concentration of the drug in the vicinity of the offending bacterium to a level of *minimal inhibitory concentration* (MIC). This may be defined as that concentration of the antimicrobial which results in virtually complete inhibition of growth of an organism under specific test conditions. Proceeding from this, a susceptible or sensitive organism is one that is inhibited by a concentration of a drug that is equal to or less than that usually obtained in the blood of patients treated with usual therapeutic doses of the drug. Conversely, a resistant organism is not inhibited by a similar concentration but requires blood levels much higher than those usually obtained. Strains of organisms inhibited by levels slightly higher than usual blood levels are considered of intermediate sensitivity.

The situation is not as clear-cut as described above, since the concentration of the antimicrobial blood level will vary with the same dose of drug in different individuals, the drug level in tissues will generally be lower than that in the circulation, and so forth. Likewise, MIC measurment in vitro must be performed under standard conditions of inoculum size, medium pH, presence of protein, and drug stability. Nevertheless the concept of MIC is extremely valuable and is used as a slightly imperfect yardstick in discussing sensitivity and resistance.

In concentrations slightly higher than MIC, a lethal effect on test bacteria often occurs. This level is considered the minimal bactericidal concentration, or minimal lethal concentration (MBC or MLC). Although this may be important in cases of impaired immunological response, such a level is not often necessarily required, and its measurement is less standardized than that of the important MIC.

REVIEW OF ANTIMICROBIALS

Sulfonamides

There are a number of sulfonamide drugs used in clinical medicine. They owe their efficacy to their clinical and morphological resemblance to para-aminobenzoic acid, which is an essential metabolite to the bacterial cell, as a precursor of folic acid, but is not needed by mammalian cells. When the organism takes the sulfa drug instead of para-aminobenzoic acid the process is known as competitive inhibition.

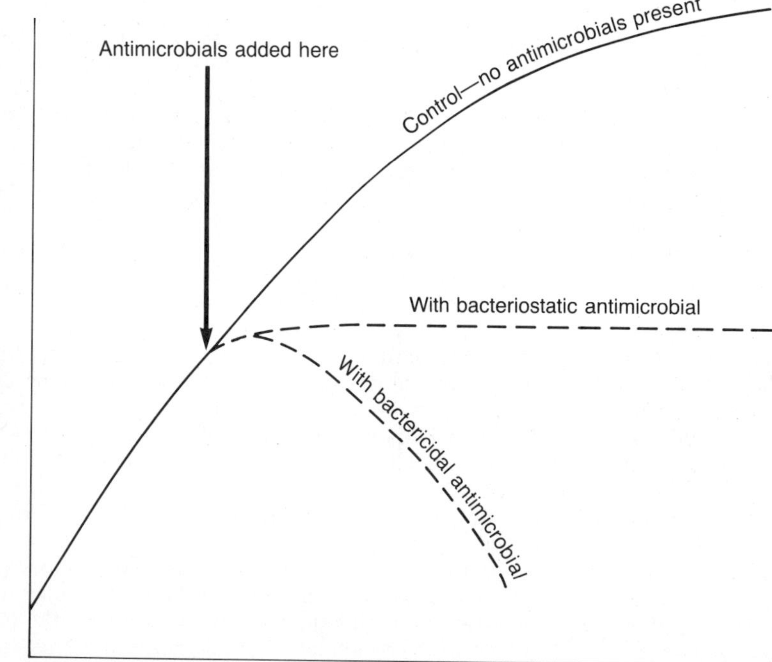

Figure 22–1 A proliferating broth culture is divided into three parts. One part is the control. To a second part a bacteriostatic agent is added, and a bactericidal agent to a third part. At intervals, small aliquots of each part are taken, diluted, and inoculated on solid medium. The number of colonies resulting is a measure of the number of viable organisms in each culture at specified time intervals.

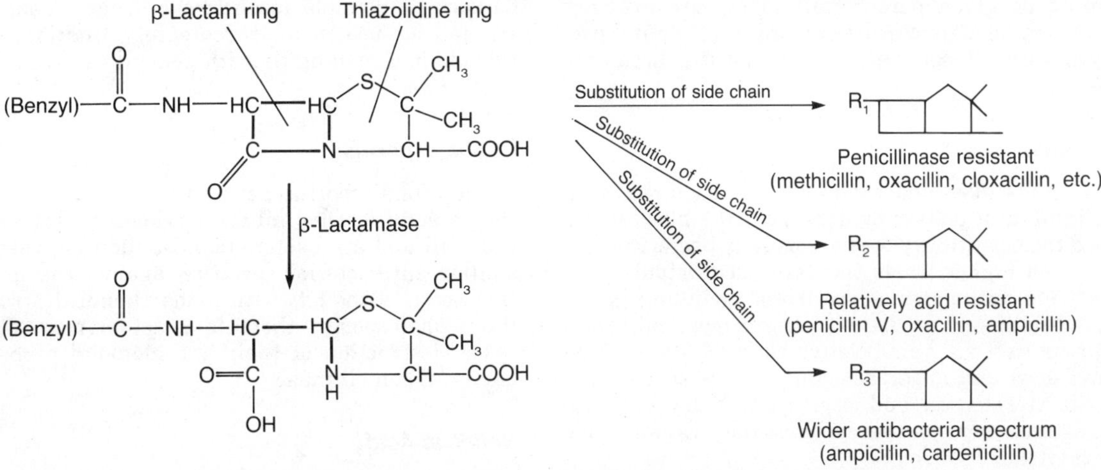

Figure 22–2 Action of penicillinase (β-lactamase) and relationships of penicillins.

When the sulfa is taken up by the bacterial cell instead of its metabolite, *p*-aminobenzoic acid, the production of essential folic acid is arrested. There is inhibition of bacterial growth, i.e., bacteriostasis. With the advent of newer antimicrobials the use of sulfa drugs has diminished. They are effective against the gram-positive cocci, *H. influenzae*, some *Shigella* organisms, *Nocardia*, some *Chlamydia* organisms, and most types of *E. coli*.

Cotrimoxazole

This drug includes a sulfa compound together with trimethoprim. The latter acts in another phase of folic acid synthesis. The combination of these two agents results in a complete block in the folate cycle and thus has a bactericidal action. The dual action (synergism) also reduces the MIC of each drug. The drug is effective against many gram-positive cocci, *H. influenzae, N. gonorrhoeae,* and many gram-negative bacilli, including members of the *Salmonella* genus.

The Penicillins

Penicillin G (benzyl penicillin) is produced in almost pure form by the fungus *Penicillium notatum*. This preparation is used parenterally and like the other penicillin derivations is bactericidal. By inhibiting the formation of the chemical cross-linkages of the bacterial cell wall it prevents wall formation. The cell membrane is left unprotected. The cell is unable to withstand the osmotic tensions to which it is subject and undergoes lysis. All the penicillin derivatives have a similar action on susceptible organisms. The latter, in the case of penicillin G, include the gram-positive cocci, the gram-negative diplococci, *Cl. perfringens, B. anthracis, T. pallidum, A. israelii,* leptospires, *C. diphtheriae,* and *L. monocytogenes.*

By chemical manipulation, the side chain attached to the essential thiazolidine and β-lactam ring can be altered, producing penicillins that may have a broader bacterial spectrum (ampicillin, etc.), or that are resistant to penicillinase (methicillin, oxacillin, cloxacillin), or that are relatively acid-resistant and so may be given by mouth (penicillin V, oxacillin, etc.).

Advantages of these preparations, apart from pharmacological benefits, include the wider antibacterial spectrum of ampicillin, extending to *H. influenzae, Proteus mirabilis, E. coli, Salmonella,* and *Shigella* species. Carbenicillin is usually effective against *Ps. aeruginosa* and indole-positive *Proteus* species.

Penicillinase or β-lactamase is produced by a number of medically important bacteria, including a large majority of *S. aureus* and an apparently increasing percentage of strains of *H. influenzae* and *N. gonorrhoeae.*

β-lactamase is released by the producing cell and inactivates susceptible penicillin by splitting the β-lactam ring. Synthetic penicillins such as methicillin and so forth are resistant to penicillinase and so may be used in infections when the offending organism is suspected as a penicillinase producer. Indeed methicillin is the drug of choice in severe *S. aureus* infections.

The chemical relationships of these types of penicillins and the action of penicillinase is shown in Figure 22–2. It should be remembered that some penicillins may belong in more than one category of penicillin, e.g., oxacillin may be given by mouth (relatively acid resistant) and is also penicillinase resistant. Ampicillin has a wide antibacterial spectrum and can also be given orally.

The Aminoglycosides

This designation usually includes streptomycin, neomycin, kanamycin, gentamicin, tobramycin, and amikacin. Their antimicrobial action, which is bactericidal, is due to their interfering with genetic transcription by binding themselves to bacterial ribosomes. Since they bind themselves only to bacterial and not to mammalian ribosomes, they have selective toxicity.

They are of particular value against gram-negative rods, including *E. coli, K. pneumoniae, Serratia, Proteus* species, and *Ps. aeruginosa.* Streptomycin has also been used in *M. tuberculosis* infections and is effective in plague (*P. pestis*) and tularemia (*F. tularensis*). The drugs are not absorbed from the bowel, so generally they must be given parenterally. They are also not easily transferable across the cerebrospinal fluid. Spectinomycin also belongs to this group, but it is used only in gonorrhea.

Tetracyclines

These drugs also bind themselves to bacterial ribosomes, inhibiting protein synthesis. At the blood levels achieved therapeutically they are usually bacteriostatic, but at much higher levels they are bactericidal. They have a wide antimicrobial spectrum, including gram-negative bacilli such as *Brucella, H. ducreyi,* and *Vibrio cholerae* as well as gram-positive cocci (*S. aureus* and *Str. pyogenes*) and anaerobes (*Bacteroides* species and anaerobic streptococci and peptococci). They are also active against *Mycoplasma pneumoniae,* Chlamydiae, and Rickettsiae.

Polymyxins

These drugs work by altering the physicochemical bonds of the cell membrane, causing ultimate disruption of the membrane. The action is bactericidal against gram-negative bacilli (except *Proteus* and *Serratia*). Although polymyxins are relatively toxic, their action against *Ps. aeruginosa* is particularly valuable at times.

Macrolides

Erythromycin is the only important member of this chemical group. It works by inhibiting protein synthesis when it binds to bacterial ribosomes, and it is bacteriostatic. It is effective against gram-positive cocci and is often used as a clinical alternative to penicillin against *Staph. aureus* and the pneumococcus. It also is effective against *M. pneumoniae* and Chlamydiae and is the drug of choice against *Campylobacter jejuni*.

Clindamycin

Clindamycin achieves antibacterial action in the same way as erythromycin and is also bacteriostatic. It is a clinical alternative to other drugs in the treatment of gram-positive coccal infections. Clindamycin is also effective against the anaerobic cocci and streptococci and *Bacteroides fragilis*.

Chloramphenicol

This substance also inhibits bacterial protein synthesis by attaching itself to the bacterial ribosome and again is bacteriostatic. It has a very wide antibacterial spectrum (against gram-positive cocci and many gram-negative bacilli as well as species of *Bacteroides* and anaerobic cocci). However it may cause fatal aplastic anemia in some patients who have this idiosyncratic response to the drug. This type of reaction is not related to drug dosage and may occur days or months after cessation of chloramphenicol therapy. Toxic bone marrow depression, another adverse effect that occurs during therapy, is related to the dose of chloramphenicol and is accompanied by anemia, perhaps leukopenia, and thrombocytopenia, which are reversible when the drug is discontinued. Because of these ill effects with the dangers of possible fatality, the drug is generally restricted for use in life-threatening situations, such as typhoid and meningitis with penicillinase-producing *H. influenzae.*

Cephalosporins

The cephalosporins have an action similar to that of the penicillins: they inhibit production of the bacterial cell wall and are bactericidal. In addition, they have a similar antibacterial spectrum against the gram-positive cocci. Although within the chemical structure of the cephalosporins there is β-lactam ring, the drugs resist destruction of their antimicrobial properties by bacterial penicillinase.

Nalidixic Acid

This substance's mechanism of antimicrobial activity has not been elucidated. It is effective against gram-negative bacilli and clinically is used particularly in gram-negative bacillary urinary infections.

Nitrofurantoin

Again the method of antibacterial action is unknown. It is useful against the gram-positive cocci, including the enterococci, as well as in infections with *E. coli* and *Citrobacter*. It is of no value against *Pseudomonas*. It is given orally and achieves blood levels that are low but urine levels that are useful therapeutically.

INDICATIONS FOR PERFORMING SENSITIVITY TESTS

1. If the organism isolated as a pathogen has an unpredictable antimicrobial susceptibility spectrum, e.g., staphylococci.
2. If the patient has immunodeficiency and has an impaired defense against microorganisms, even those of usually low pathogenicity, e.g., as in chronic granulomatous disease. In such conditions, bactericidal drugs are desirable.
3. If streptomycin or erythromycin is being used. Resistance to these antimicrobials may develop rapidly, and thus the susceptibility should be monitored.
4. When the infection is life threatening. For example in meningitis with *N. meningitidis*, in which the organism has a predictable sensitivity, there is always the outside chance that a resistant strain may occur, and this may cost the patient his life.

OCCASIONS WHEN ANTIMICROBIAL SENSITIVITY TESTS NEED NOT BE PERFORMED

1. If the cultures yield a mixed growth of organisms of questionable pathogenicity, an antibiogram is positively misleading in that it will create a false sense of security in the mind of the clinician.
2. If the organism is predictably susceptible to a range of antimicrobials, as below:

Str. pyogenes: penicillin(s), cephalothin, and erythromycin.

Cl. perfringens: penicillin(s), cephalothin, and tetracycline.

N. meningitidis: penicillin G and ampicillin.

Ps. aeruginosa: polymyxin, colistin, and gentamycin.

Use of such a list not only may save time in emergency situations, but probably will save time and materials in more usual circumstances.

In cases of non–life-threatening *Salmonella* infections, antimicrobial therapy is at least unhelpful. However, sensitivity tests may be done and recorded but reported only as "available if desired" so that the use of antimicrobials in these conditions will be discouraged.

THE CHOICE OF ANTIMICROBIALS FOR IN VITRO TESTING

The choice of antimicrobials to which an organism should be exposed in testing for sensitivity is partly a matter of individual choice, but based on the experience of many, the following list is suggested. Modifications may be made in conformity with clinical practice.

Gram-positive

Penicillin G
Methicillin
Ampicillin
Erythromycin
Clindamycin
Tetracycline
Cephalothin
(Streptomycin, sulfa, and novobiocin may be used)

Gram-negative

Ampicillin
Cephalothin
Streptomycin
Kanamycin
Gentamycin
Tetracycline
Polymyxin B *or* colistin
(Carbenicillin for *Ps. aeruginosa;* nitrofurantoin and nalidixic acid for urinary tract infections only)
Trimethoprim-sulfamethoxazole
Tobramycin
Amikacin

METHODS OF ANTIMICROBIAL SUSCEPTIBILITY TESTING

There are essentially two methods: (1) antimicrobial dilution tests and (2) the agar diffusion method.

Resistance

Some organisms become resistant to antimicrobials after a particular drug has been used for some time. For example, many of the staphylococci are resistant to penicillin, although when this drug was first used there were virtually no resistant strains. Resistance may be the result of several different mechanisms:

1. The organism produces a substance such as penicillinase, which destroys the antimicrobial (penicillin).
2. The bacteria become adapted to living without the particular enzyme system that the antimicrobial attacks.
3. The cell wall becomes impermeable to the antimicrobial.
4. Phage transfers resistance to antimicrobials by the process of transduction (see p. 359).
5. The killing off of susceptible strains by the antimicrobial uncovers an apparently increased number of resistant strains that survive because of the process of natural selection.
6. Mutant strains emerge (p. 358).
7. Nonchromosomal transfer of drug resistance from other bacteria takes place (see p. 360).

Antimicrobial Dilution Tests

These methods will not be described in detail but only in principle. The antimicrobial is incorporated into broth or agar in varied concentrations. The test organism is then inoculated and the culture appropriately incubated. At the minimal concentration of the antimicrobial in which growth fails to appear, the organism has found its MIC (minimal inhibitory concentration). A useful way to conduct such tests is with the Steer's replicator, which will inoculate 36 different strains of bacteria onto a single plate in a known pattern. This inoculation may be repeated on several plates, each containing a different concentration of antimicrobial agent, and after incubation the MIC of each of the 36 organisms can be read off (Fig. 22–3).

Agar Diffusion Method

This method employs an agar plate inoculated with the test organism. Discs of filter paper containing known amounts of antimicrobial are placed on the plate. As the organism begins to grow, the antimicrobial diffuses from the disc. When the antimicrobial reaches inhibitory or greater concentrations in the agar, there will be no growth of the organism, and zones of inhibition will be found around the antimicrobial disc.

For many years there was considerable confusion over this remarkably simple method. Finally a standarized method (Kirby-Bauer) was designed, by Bauer et al., that recognized the importance of various factors that contributed to the size of inhibition zones around the discs. It furthermore employed concentrations of antimicrobial within the discs that gave levels of antimicrobial expected therapeutically. Results of the Kirby-Bauer technique thus were directly related to the expected results of antimicrobial therapy in the patient.

In standardizing the test, the following factors have to be considered:

The Medium. The pH will influence some antimicrobials; e.g., streptomycin is more efficient at an alkaline pH. Plates incubated under increased tension of CO_2 also show changes in the size of inhibiting zones, probably owing to the change in pH. Thus CO_2-rich atmospheres for sensitivity tests are to be avoided. Electrolyte concentration, dextrose, the purity of the agar, and the

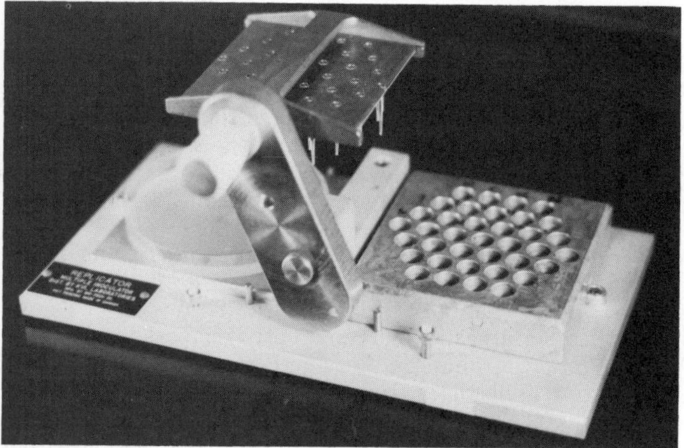

Figure 22–3 Steer's replicating device. The small wells on the right are charged with liquid cultures of as many as 36 organisms. The corresponding metal tips are then placed in these wells and, by a single movement of the handle, are moved over to the left and made to inoculate bacterial plates, always in the same relative positions. A series of plates is used with antimicrobial dilutions or biochemical substrates, and each plate is later examined in each of the 36 separately inoculated areas.

presence of serum protein also will cause changes in the size of inhibitory zones around the antimicrobial discs. However, the addition of 5% defibrinated or chocolatized blood has little effect, except in the case of novobiocin, which is bound strongly to protein. A low concentration of agar yields larger inhibitory zones than a higher concentration.

The Depth of the Medium. This obviously will alter the concentration of diffusing antimicrobials, since in thicker agar an equal amount of antimicrobial will be held beneath a smaller surface area and thus the inhibitory zone will be relatively smaller than in a thinly poured plate.

The Antimicrobial. A more rapidly diffusible antimicrobial obviously will give a wider zone of inhibition than one that is less diffusible. Thus in reading results, the width of a significant (i.e., *clinically* significant) inhibitory zone will differ from one antimicrobial to another. A further feature to consider in standardizing the test is that some antimicrobials lose part of their activity on incubation, e.g., chloramphenicol, and this must be considered in the design of the test in order to correlate the inhibitory zone size with the expected therapeutic level. Likewise, a long period of incubation will allow less susceptible strains of the organism to emerge as the antimicrobial deteriorates.

The Organism. The method described here is exclusively for organisms that grow rapidly. It will be appreciated that in some respects the test is a competition between the diffusing antimicrobial and the growing organism. Standardized methods for slow-growers and fastidious organisms have not yet been developed. Heavy inocula yield small inhibitory zones, whereas light inocula give larger zones. A single colony of the isolated organism should not be used, since it may represent an atypical or resistant clone.

The Disc. Discs should be purchased from reputable suppliers. (In the United States, they are certified by the Food and Drug Administration.) They should be stored at −20°C in a jar containing desiccant, and they should be protected against humidity at all times. The potency of the discs should follow the standards shown in the zone interpretive chart (Table 22–1). Discs should be discarded by the expiry date given by the manufacturer.

Timing of the Application of the Disc. After the plates are inoculated and the discs applied, the cultures are placed within the incubator within a defined period. This is to prevent any possibility of solution of the antimicrobial from the disc onto the surface of the culture, which would confuse the test result by putting the organism at a disadvantage.

The Kirby-Bauer Single Disc Agar Diffusion Test

1. The medium used is Mueller-Hinton agar (Diagnostic Sensitivity Test agar [Oxoid*] is also satisfactory) which is prepared in accordance with the manufacturer's instructions. The pH at room temperature should be 7.2 to 7.4. Sixty milliliters of the medium is poured into 150 mm diameter Petri dishes (glass or plastic) so that the depth of the medium should be 4 mm. Plates may be stored in a refrigerator (2 to 8°C) in plastic bags to reduce evaporation. Just before use, they are placed in an incubator at 35°C for 30 minutes to remove excessive moisture. 5% defibrinated blood may be added to the medium for fastidious organisms (*Haemophilus* and so forth).

2. Five colonies of the organism are touched with a loop, seeded into 4 mL of trypticase soy broth containing 1% yeast extract, and incubated for 2 to 5 hours. To this suspension is then added sterile water or saline to make the density comparable with a barium sulfate standard. (The standard consists of 0.5 mL of 0.048 M $BaCl_2$ (1.175% $BaCl_2.2H_2O$) in 99.5 mL of 1% H_2SO_4 v/v [0.36 N]. The standard needs to be replaced monthly and stored in the dark. It corresponds to approximately 10^8 Enterobacteriaceae per mL).

3. Within 15 minutes of diluting the broth culture, the organisms are streaked evenly on the medium in three directions, using a wooden-stick cotton swab. Excess suspension is removed from the swab by rotating it firmly against the side of the tube before seeding the plate. When the inoculum has dried (3 to 5 minutes), the discs are placed on the plate. The large Petri dishes can accommodate nine discs in an outer ring and three or four in the center. The discs can be applied with a dispenser and then gently pressed down to make a good contact with the agar with a flamed pair of forceps. Vancomycin, polymyxin B (or colistin), and kanamycin have small inhibition zones and so may be placed conveniently in the central area of the plate. The plates are incubated within 15 minutes of these procedures, aerobically and without added CO_2.

*Oxoid, Columbia, Md. 21045 and Nepean, Ont. K2E 7K3

TABLE 22–1 CONTROL LIMITS FOR MONITORING PRECISION AND ACCURACY OF INHIBITORY ZONE DIAMETERS (MM) OBTAINED IN GROUPS OF FIVE SEPARATE OBSERVATIONS AND AS INDIVIDUAL DETERMINATIONS

Antimicrobial Agent	Disc Content	Individual Daily Test Control Zone Diameter (mm)	Accuracy Control Zone Diameter (mm) Mean of 5 Values	Precision Control Range[a] of 5 Values: Maximum	Precision Control Range[a] of 5 Values: Average[b] (mm)
E. coli (ATCC 25922)					
Amikacin	30 μg	19-26	20.2-24.8	8	4.1
Ampicillin[c]	10 μg	16-22	17.0-21.0	7	3.5
Carbenicillin[c]	100 μg	23-29	24.0-28.0	7	3.5
Cefamandole[c]	30 μg	24-30	25.0-29.0	7	3.5
Cefotaxime[c]	30 μg	29-35	30.0-34.0	7	3.5
Cefoxitin[c]	30 μg	23-29	24.0-28.0	7	3.5
Cephalothin[c]	30 μg	17-21	17.7-20.3	4	2.3
Chloramphenicol	30 μg	21-27	22.0-26.0	7	3.5
Colistin	10 μg	11-15	11.7-14.3	4	2.3
Erythromycin	15 μg	8-14	9.0-13.0	7	3.5
Gentamicin	10 μg	19-26	20.2-24.8	8	4.1
Kanamycin	30 μg	17-25	18.3-23.7	9	4.7
Nalidixic acid[d]	30 μg	23-28	23.8-27.2	6	2.9
Neomycin	30 μg	17-23	18.0-22.0	7	3.5
Nitrofurantoin[d]	300 μg	21-26	21.8-25.2	6	2.9
Polymyxin B	300 units	12-16	12.7-15.3	4	2.3
Streptomycin	10 μg	12-20	13.3-18.7	9	4.7
Sulfisoxazole	250 μg or 300 μg	18-26	19.3-24.7	9	4.7
Tetracycline	30 μg	18-25	19.2-23.8	8	4.1
Tobramycin	10 μg	18-26	19.3-24.7	9	4.7
Trimethoprim[d]	5 μg	21-28	22.2-26.8	8	4.1
Trimethoprim-sulfamethoxazole	1.25 μg-23.75 μg	24-32	25.3-30.7	9	4.7
S. aureus (ATCC 25923)					
Amikacin	30 μg	20-26	21.0-25.0	7	3.5
Ampicillin[c]	10 μg	27-35	28.3-33.7	9	4.7
Cefamandole[c]	30 μg	26-34	27.3-32.7	9	4.7
Cefotaxime[c]	30 μg	25-31	26.0-30.0	7	3.5
Cefoxitin[c]	30 μg	23-29	24.0-28.0	7	3.5
Cephalothin[c]	30 μg	29-37	30.3-35.7	9	4.7
Chloramphenicol	30 μg	19-26	20.2-24.8	8	4.1
Clindamycin[d]	2 μg	23-29	24.0-28.0	7	3.5
Erythromycin	15 μg	22-30	23.3-28.7	9	4.7
Gentamicin	10 μg	19-27	20.3-25.7	9	4.7
Kanamycin	30 μg	19-26	20.2-24.8	8	4.1
Methicillin[d]	5 μg	17-22	17.8-21.2	6	2.9
Nafcillin[c]	1 μg	18-24	19.0-23.0	7	3.5
Neomycin	30 μg	18-26	19.3-24.7	9	4.7
Nitrofurantoin	300 μg	20-24	20.7-23.3	4	2.3
Oxacillin[c]	1 μg	21-26	21.8-25.2	6	2.9
Penicillin G	10 units	26-37	27.8-35.2	13	6.4
Polymyxin B	300 units	7-13	8.0-12.0	7	3.5
Streptomycin	10 μg	14-22	15.3-20.7	9	4.7
Sulfisoxazole	250 μg	24-34	25.6-32.4	12	5.8
Tetracycline[d]	30 μg	19-28	20.5-26.5	11	5.2
Tobramycin	10 μg	19-29	20.6-27.4	12	5.8
Vancomycin	30 μg	15-19	15.7-18.3	4	2.3
Trimethoprim[d]	5 μg	21-28	22.2-26.8	8	4.1
Trimethoprim-sulfamethoxazole	1.25 μg-23.75 μg	24-32	25.3-30.7	9	4.7
P. aeruginosa (ATCC 27853)					
Amikacin	30 μg	18-26	19.3-24.7	9	4.7
Carbenicillin[c]	100 μg	18-24	19.0-23.0	7	3.5
Cefotaxime[c]	30 μg	18-22	18.7-21.3	4	2.3
Gentamicin	10 μg	16-21	16.8-20.2	6	2.9
Ticarcillin[c]	75 μg	21-27	22.0-26.0	7	3.5
Tobramycin	10 μg	19-25	20.0-24.0	7	3.5

a. Maximum value minus minimum value obtained in a series of five consecutive tests should not exceed the listed maximum limits, and the mean should fall within the range under "accuracy control."

b. In a continuing series of ranges from consecutive groups of five tests each, the average range should approximate the listed value.

c. To be considered tentative for twelve months from publication of this Supplement.

d. Many laboratories have reported difficulties with these quality control parameters, therefore, the parameters are currently being re-evaluated and revised figures will be published in the future supplements if needed.

Reproduced by permission of the National Committee for Clinical Laboratory Standards, 771 E. Lancaster Ave., Villanova, Pa. 19085, from their publication *Performance Standards for Antimicrobic Disc Susceptibility Tests* May 1981 (M2-A2S1). This material is under constant review, and current revisions may be obtained from the NCCLS.

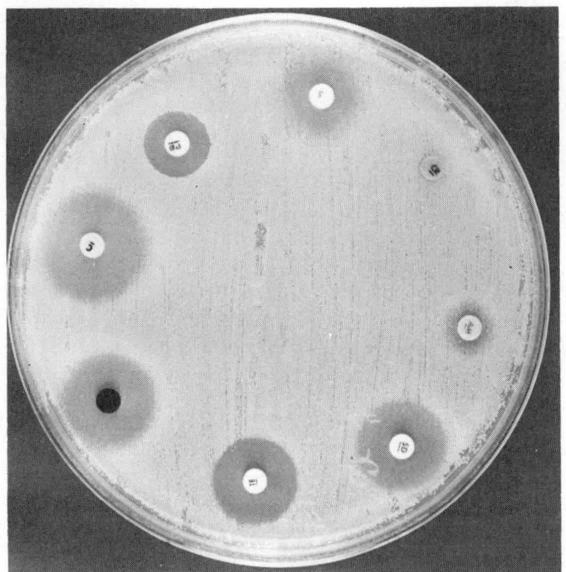

Figure 22–4 The Kirby-Bauer agar diffusion test. The inoculated plate after overnight incubation. The zones of inhibition of growth around the discs impregnated with antibiotic are well illustrated.

4. After 16 to 18 hours' incubation, inhibition zone diameters are measured (including the 6 mm of disc) with calipers at the agar surface or with a ruler, calipers, or other measuring device at the back of the plate (Fig. 22–5). The end point is taken as the complete inhibition of growth as it appears to the unaided eye. In the case of the sulfonamides, however, a slight growth (80 per cent or more inhibition) is disregarded because the organisms grow through several generations before inhibition takes effect. The margin of heavy growth is regarded as the end point in this instance. Penicillinase producers show a sharp, heaped, clearly defined edge of the zone. Although the zone size is generally within the resistant belt, regardless of the size of the zone, such organisms should be reported as resistant. The patient, if given penicillin, should receive one of the penicillinase-resistant forms.

Swarming of *Proteus mirabilis* and *vulgaris* is not inhibited by all antimicrobials, and a film of swarming is ignored. It is not uncommon to find a ring of inner colonies at the periphery of the zone, and the inhibition zone reading should be made within this ring. Often with *Serratia* and polymyxin, several colonies are scattered through the inhibition zone, and this is significant; the strain is regarded as resistant. With other organisms and antimicrobials, the same phenomenon is regarded with suspicion, and the strain should be checked first for purity. If subsequent plates show the same result, the strain is considered resistant.

The zone diameters are recorded and interpreted according to Table 22–2. Organisms are reported as either resistant, intermediate, or sensitive to each antimicrobial tested.

Although the method is designed to challenge an organism with a level of antimicrobial that it may meet in a therapeutic setting in the tissues, it cannot completely re-enact the in vivo situation. The method will not be valid, for example, in the case in which an undrained abscess is present or in the case of organisms present across the blood-brain barrier, which may not be spanned by the antimicrobial. Other causes of therapeutic failure are well described in textbooks of medicine. One, of especial interest to the laboratory worker, is in the usual case of salmonellosis. Here, the antimicrobial is more effective against normal flora than it is against the pathogen. The former normally exert an antimicrobial effect against the invader so that, paradoxically, the invaders proliferate when antimicrobials are given and the carrier state is prolonged.

Control Procedures

Because of the great importance of sensitivity testing, the method must be kept under tight control so that no transmission of inaccurate information to the attending physician can occur.

Stock control organisms are readily available from various suppliers, most conveniently in a lyophilized form on paper discs. The following are needed:

S. aureus (Seattle strain), A.T.C.C. (American Type Culture Collection) No. 25923

E. coli, A.T.C.C. No. 25922

Ps. aeruginosa (Boston strain), A.T.C.C. No. 27853

Cultures—which are treated like clinical specimens—are subjected to the Kirby-Bauer method daily, and careful records are maintained. The inhibition zones for

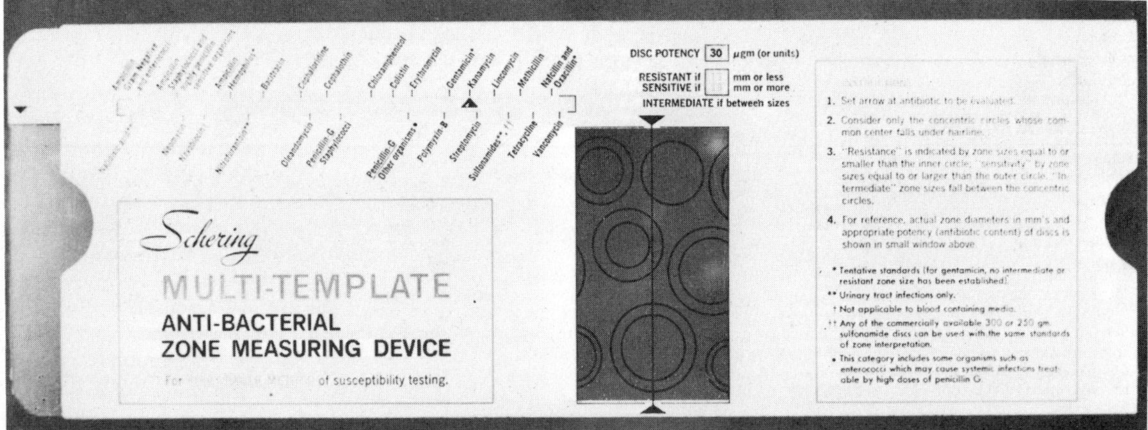

Figure 22–5 Zone measuring device for use with the Kirby-Bauer technique. A template indicating significant or insignificant inhibition is presented in the central window to correspond with the arrow indicating the antibiotic under test. The device may be used by applying it directly to the underside of the plate.

each organism and each antimicrobial are recorded in batches of five serial observations from Monday through Friday. For example, using ampicillin and *E. coli* A.T.C.C. No 25922, the mean of the five values collected should be within 17.0 and 21.0 mm. If the mean value or the range exceeds permissable values, then some technical error is occurring. The errors may include:

1. Factors in preparation, pouring, storage, or length of storage of plates.
2. Storage of discs.
3. Inaccuracies in turbidity standard, size of bacterial inocula, or both.
4. Excess fluid on inoculating swab.
5. Delay in preparing inocula and plating, or delay in applying discs.
6. Incorrect incubating temperature, or use of CO_2 atmosphere.
7. Inaccurate mensuration of inhibition zones.

Special Situations

The standard Kirby-Bauer technique was designed for antimicrobial sensitivity testing for moderately rapidly growing nonfastidious aerobic organisms. However, a number of common pathogens do not fall within this category and must be dealt with by some other technique.

N. gonorrhoeae. This organism grows best in the presence of serum and in an atmosphere of 5 to 10% CO_2. If sensitivity tests are required it is best to do agar dilution methods. It is permissible to test isolates for a preliminary test for β-lactamase production (see below), and this is often done by laboratories in community hospitals. In such a way resistance to penicillin may be suspected correctly before the organism is sent to a more specialized center for agar dilution antimicrobial studies.

N. meningitidis. Although the Kirby-Bauer method is not ideal in the antimicrobial investigation of isolates of this organism, it may be modified by fortifying the Mueller-Hinton medium with 1% Iso-vitalex and 1% hemoglobin (or 5% horse blood). 5% CO_2 may be used if necessary for growth.

H. influenzae. This fastidious organism is first grown on an enriched medium, and then a suspension from such a medium is made up on broth to conform to the turbidity standard. It is inoculated to a modified Mueller-Hinton medium similar to that used for *N. meningitidis*. With a 10 μg ampicillin disc, a zone of 20 mm or more is considered susceptible and a lesser zone resistant. Other zone sizes are similar to those of other organisms.

Str. pneumoniae. Until 1967 all strains of *Str. pneumoniae* were thought uniformly sensitive to penicillin, but then resistant strains were reported, and in 1974 such strains occurred in Canada and the United States. These strains cannot be detected routinely with the standard Kirby-Bauer technique. It must be modified, with a 1 μg oxacillin disc replacing the 10 unit penicillin G disc. With the oxacillin disc the zone of inhibition of a resistant organism is absent or very narrow around the disc, but a sensitive strain has a zone of more than 28 mm. A recent stardardization ruling is that zones ≥ 20 mm are to be considered susceptible and those ≤ 12 mm resistant.

Methicillin-resistant Staph. aureus. Strains of *S. aureus* that are resistant to the β-lactamase–resistant penicillins (methicillin, oxacillin, or nafcillin) or to cephalosporin can be overlooked if incubated at 37°C. They are more easily discovered at a temperature of 30°C, but 35°C is adequate if it is well controlled and a 1 μg oxacillin disc is used. A 5 μg methicillin disc may also be used, but preferably at 30°C.

The Presence of Bacterial β-Lactamase. Many organisms produce β-lactamase. In some gram-negative organisms, the enzyme is bound in the bacterial cell wall and the cell must be disrupted to demonstrate the enzyme. It is fortunate that in the case of *H. influenzae* and *N. gonorrhoeae*, the enzyme diffuses from the cell and may easily be detected.

There are several possible methods of demonstrating β-lactamase. The principle of one of these (acidometric) is to allow the suspected organism or its enzyme to react with a solution of penicillin G at a pH of 8.5. At this pH, the solution of penicillin will be violet when phenol red or bromcresol purple is used as an indicator. β-lactamase will react with the penicillin G to produce penicilloic acid. The indicator will then change from violet to yellow. The reaction is most easily performed with commercially available paper discs or strips that incorporate penicillin and indicator.* A young culture growing on medium without fermenting carbohydrates is best used, and several colonies are smeared on a strip moistened with distilled water. A positive reaction will occur within 10 minutes. Known β-lactamase–producing and β-lactamase–nonproducing organisms are used simultaneously as controls. β-lactamase will also act as a cephalosporinase and will convert the chromogenic cephalosporon Nitrocefin, which is yellow, to a red substance. A commercial paper test† is available, and the result should be given up to 1 hour to develop. It is the only commercial preparation that will identify β-lactamase from the *B. fragilis* group.

Because of the importance of *H. influenzae* as a cause of severe illness, this test should be applied to all isolates of this organism from meningitis, septicemia, or epiglottitis and reported urgently even before other tests for antimicrobials are available. Likewise, although antimicrobial studies on *N. gonorrhoea* are best done in specialized centers, preliminary screening for β-lactamase producers may be done at a primary level so that inadequate penicillin therapy is not commenced or continued.

Anaerobic Organisms. **Since the Kirby-Bauer method was designed for use with rapidly growing aerobes, it cannot be used without considerable modification with anaerobic isolates. A modified disc broth method has worked well in practice and needs no unusual equipment. Brain-heart infusion broth is prepared according to the manufacturers' specifications and supplemented with menadione (2 μg/mL), 0.5% yeast extract, and hemin (5 μg/mL). Five-milliliter aliquots are prepared in tubes. To obtain initial anaerobiosis, the broth is boiled and then cooled immediately before usage, when the supplements are added to the cooled broth. To a series of such tubes, regular**

---

*Beta-Lactamase Detection Papers, Oxoid, Columbia, Md. 21045, and Nepean, Ont. K2E 7K3.

†Cephinase discs, Baltimore Biological Laboratories, Cockeysville, Md. 21030.

TABLE 22–2 Zone Diameter Interpretive Standards and Approximate Minimum Inhibitory Concentration (MIC) Correlates

Antimicrobial Agent	Disc Content	Zone Diameter, nearest whole mm Resistant	Intermediate[q]	Susceptible	Approximate MIC Correlates[a] Resistant	Susceptible
Amikacin[b]	30 μg	≤ 14	15–16	≥ 17	≥ 32 μg/mL	≤ 16 μg/mL
Ampicillin[c] when testing gram-negative enteric organisms and enterococci	10 μg	≤ 11	12–13	≥ 14	≥ 32 μg/mL	≤ 8 μg/mL
Ampicillin[c] when testing staphylococci[d] and penicillin G-susceptible microorganisms	10 μg	≤ 20	21–28	≥ 29	β-lactamase[d]	**≤ 0.25 μg/mL**
Ampicillin[c] when testing *Haemophilus* species[e]	10 μg	≤ 19	—	≥ 20	**≥ 4 μg/mL**	≤ 2 μg/mL
Bacitracin	10 units	≤ 8	9–12	≥ 13	—	—
Carbenicillin when testing the ***Enterobacteriaceae***	100 μg	≤ 17	18–22	≥ 23	≥ 32 μg/mL	≤ 16 μg/mL
Carbenicillin when testing *Pseudomonas aeruginosa*	100 μg	≤ 13	14–16	≥ 17	**≥ 256 μg/mL**	**≤ 128 μg/mL**
Cefamandole[f]	30 μg	≤ 14	15–17	≥ 18	≥ 32 μg/mL	**≤ 8 μg/mL**
Cefotaxime[f]	**30 μg**	**≤ 14**	**15–22[q]**	**≥ 23**	**≥ 64 μg/mL**	**≤ 8 μg/mL**
Cefoxitin[f]	30 μg	≤ 14	15–17	≥ 18	≥ 32 μg/mL	**≤ 8 μg/mL**
Cephalothin[g]	30 μg	≤ 14	15–17	≥ 18	≥ 32 μg/mL	**≤ 8 μg/mL**
Chloramphenicol	30 μg	≤ 12	13–17	≥ 18	≥ 25 μg/mL	≤ 12.5 μg/mL
Clindamycin[h]	2 μg	≤ 14	15–16	≥ 17	≥ 2 μg/mL	≤ 1 μg/mL
Colistin[j]	10 μg	≤ 8	9–10	≥ 11	≥ 4 μg/mL	j
Erythromycin	15 μg	≤ 13	14–17	≥ 18	≥ 8 μg/mL	≤ 2 μg/mL
Gentamicin[b]	10 μg	≤ 12	13–14	≥ 15	≥ 8 μg/mL	≤ 4 μg/mL
Kanamycin	30 μg	≤ 13	14–17	≥ 18	≥ 25 μg/mL	≤ 6 μg/mL
Methicillin[k]	5 μg	≤ 9	10–13	≥ 14	**≥ 16 μg/mL**	**≤ 4 μg/mL**
Nafcillin[k]	**1 μg**	**≤ 10**	**11–12**	**≥ 13**	**≥ 8 μg/mL**	**≤ 2 μg/mL**
Nalidixic Acid[l]	30 μg	≤ 13	14–18	≥ 19	≥ 32 μg/mL	≤ 12 μg/mL
Neomycin	30 μg	≤ 12	13–16	≥ 17	—	—
Nitrofurantoin[l]	300 μg	≤ 14	15–16	≥ 17	≥ 100 μg/mL	≤ 25 μg/mL
Oxacillin[k]	**1 μg**	**≤ 10**	**11–12**	**≥ 13**	**≥ 8 μg/mL**	**≤ 2 μg/mL**
Penicillin G when testing ***staphylococci[m]***	10 units	≤ 20	21–28	≥ 29	β-lactamase[d]	≤ 0.1 μg/mL
Penicillin G when testing other microorganisms[n]	10 units	≤ 11	12–21	≥ 22	≥ 32 μg/mL	≤ 1.5 μg/mL
Polymyxin B[j]	300 units	≤ 8	9–11	≥ 12	≥ 50 units/mL	j
Streptomycin	10 μg	≤ 11	12–14	≥ 15	—	—
Sulfonamides[l,o]	250 or 300 μg	≤ 12	13–16	≥ 17	≥ 350 μg/mL	≤ 100 μg/mL
Tetracycline[p]	30 μg	≤ 14	15–18	≥ 19	≥ 12 μg/mL	≤ 4 μg/mL
Ticarcillin when testing *P. aeruginosa*	**75 μg**	**≤ 11**	**12–14**	**≥ 15**	**≥ 128 μg/mL**	**≤ 64 μg/mL**
Trimethoprim[l,o]	**5 μg**	**≤ 10**	**11–15**	**≥ 16**	**≥ 16 μg/mL**	**≤ 4 μg/mL**
Trimethoprim-sulfamethoxazole[o]	1.25 μg, 23.75 μg	≤ 10	11–15	≥ 16	≥ 8/152 μg/mL	≤ 2/38 μg/mL
Tobramycin[a]	10 μg	≤ 12	13–14	≥ 15	≥ 8 μg/mL	≤ 4 μg/mL
Vancomycin	30 μg	≤ 9	10–11	≥ 12	—	≤ 5 μg/mL

a. **These correlates are not meant for use as breakpoints for susceptibility categorization with dilution MIC tests as described in NCCLS M7-P.**

b. **The zone sizes obtained with aminoglycosides, particularly when testing *Pseudomonas aeruginosa*, are very medium dependent because of variations in divalent cation content. The zone diameter interpretive standards for amikacin, gentamicin, and tobramycin are shown in Table 2. These interpretive standards are to be used only with Mueller-Hinton medium that has yielded zone diameters within the correct range shown in Table 3 when performance tests were done with *P. aeruginosa* ATCC 27853. In addition, the amikacin disc must be 30 μg rather than the 10 μg disc used previously. Organisms in the intermediate category may be either susceptible or resistant when tested by dilution methods and should therefore more properly be classified as "indeterminate" in their susceptibility to aminoglycosides.**

c. **Class disc for ampicillin (amoxicillin), cyclacillin, and hetacillin.**

d. **Resistant strains of *S. aureus* produce β-lactamase and the testing of the 10 unit penicillin disc is preferred.**

e. For testing *Haemophilus* use Mueller-Hinton agar supplemented with 1% hemoglobin and 1% IsoVitaleX (BBL), Supplement VX (Difco) or an equivalent synthetic supplement. Adjust pH to 7.2. Prepare the inoculum by suspending growth from a 24-hour chocolate agar plate in Mueller-Hinton broth to the density of a turbidity standard. The vast majority of ampicillin-resistant strains of *Haemophilus* produce detectable β-lactamase.

f. **Cefamandole, cefoxitin and cefotaxime are recently released cephalosporins having a wider spectrum of activity against gram-negative bacilli than do other previously approved cephalosporins. Therefore, the cephalothin disc cannot be used as the class disc for these three drugs.**

g. **The cephalothin disc is used for testing susceptibility to cephalothin, cefaclor, cefadroxil, cefazolin, cephalexin, cephaloridine, cephapirin, and cephradine. Cefamandole, cefoxitin and cefotaxime must be tested separately. *Staphylococcus aureus* exhibiting resistance to methicillin, nafcillin or oxacillin discs should be reported as resistant to cephalosporin-type antimicrobics, regardless of zone diameter, because in most cases infections caused by these organisms are clinically resistant to cephalosporins. Methicillin-resistant *S. epidermidis* infections also may not respond to cephalosporins.**

h. The clindamycin disc is used for testing susceptibility to both clindamycin and lincomycin.

j. Colistin and polymyxin B diffuse poorly in agar, and the diffusion method is thus less accurate than with other antimicrobics. Resistance is always significant, but when treatment of systemic infections caused by susceptible strains is being considered, results of a diffusion test should be confirmed with those of a dilution method. MIC correlates cannot be calculated reliably from regression analysis.

k. **Of the antistaphylococcal β-lactamase resistant penicillins, either oxacillin, nafcillin, or methicillin may be tested, and results can be applied to the other two of these drugs and to cloxacillin and dicloxacillin. Oxacillin and nafcillin are more resistant to degradation in storage. Cloxacillin discs should not be used because they may not detect methicillin-resistant *S. aureus*. When an intermediate result is obtained with *S. aureus*, the strains should be further investigated to determine if they are heteroresistant.**

l. **Susceptibility data for nalidixic acid, nitrofurantoin, sulfonamides and trimethoprim apply only to organisms isolated from urinary-tract infections.**

m. **Penicillin G should be used to test the susceptibility of all penicillinase-sensitive penicillins, such as ampicillin, amoxicillin, hetacillin, carbenicillin and ticarcillin. Results may also be applied to phenoxymethyl penicillin or phenethicillin. The intermediate category usually contains penicillinase producing isolates and should be considered resistant to therapy.**

n. Intermediate category includes some microorganisms, such as enterococci, and certain gram-negative bacilli that may cause systemic infections treatable with high parenteral dosages of benzyl penicillin but not of orally administered phenoxymethyl penicillin or phenethicillin. For pneumococci and gonococci refer to special interpretations applied in section 4.4.

o. The 250 or 300 μg sulfisoxazole discs can be used for any of the commercially available sulfonamides. Blood-containing media, except media containing lysed horse blood, are not satisfactory for testing sulfonamides. The Mueller-Hinton agar should be as thymidine-free as possible for sulfonamide and/or trimethoprim testing. (See Sec. 3.1.1)

p. Tetracycline is the class disc for all tetracyclines, and the results can be applied to chlortetracycline, demeclocycline, doxycycline, methacycline, minocycline, and oxytetracycline. However, some *in-vitro* data show that certain organisms may be more susceptible to doxycycline and minocycline than to tetracycline. (See Table 1)

q. **The category "Intermediate" should be reported. Infections with bacteria of "intermediate" susceptibility may be considered moderately susceptible and may respond to antimicrobial agents with a wide safe dosage range.**

Reproduced by permission of the National Committee for Clinical Laboratory Standards, 771 E. Lancaster Ave., Villanova, Pa. 19085, from their publication *Performance Standards for Antimicrobic Disc Susceptibility Tests* May 1981 (M2-A2S1). This material is under constant review, and current revisions may be obtained from the NCCLS.

antimicrobial discs are added as shown in Table 22–3 to achieve a calculated concentration in each tube as indicated. A drop of culture from cooked meat broth is added to each tube, and one tube is left inoculated but without antimicrobial as a control. The tubes are incubated anaerobically overnight or longer at 35 to 37°C. Then, the growth turbidity in each tube is compared with the control. The organism is recorded as resistant if the turbidity is 50% or more than that of the control. In practice, most tests appear as "growth" or "no growth."

An even less complicated method employs thioglycolate broth with the discs as before. The broth and discs are left for 2 hours at room temperature to allow the antimicrobial to diffuse into the sloppy agar of the thioglycolate broth. The bacterial inoculum is made, and the tubes may be incubated aerobically without any anaerobic device, since the broth maintains its own anaerobic milieu. Subsequently, results are read as above.

Microdilution methods that lend themselves to some automation have also been devised, using a disc-broth basis and replacing turbidity estimation with an oxidation-reduction indicator.

Modifications of the Standard Kirby-Bauer Technique

One modification of the classic Kirby-Bauer method uses 25 mL of Mueller-Hinton medium in plates of 9 cm diameter in order to give a depth of 4 mm. The plates should be used within 7 days of preparation unless stored at 2 to 8°C in plastic bags. Methods of making suspensions of organisms and standardization are identical, as is the method of plating, although an alternative method of pouring inoculated agar is given. Antimicrobial discs should be no closer than 15 mm from the edge of the plate, and no discs should be closer, one to the other, than 24 mm from center to center. Reading of results is done as before, and tables of significant inhibition zones have been drawn up.

An agar overlay method (Barry et al, 1970) has been designed and standardized. A broth culture of the organism is seeded into agar and subsequently poured into a plate with Mueller-Hinton agar, following which the antimicrobial discs are applied.

Serum Bactericidal Levels (Schlicter Test)

Since this measurement is rarely required, as, for example, in some cases of bacterial endocarditis, only the principle of the method will be discussed here. Dilutions of the patient's serum are tested against the infecting organisms, and in this way, the adequacy of the level of antimicrobial in the patient's serum may be judged.

The isolated infecting organism is grown in Mueller-Hinton broth, and a young (5 to 6 hour) culture is used in the study. Serum samples from the patient are collected, and if possible, a sample of serum taken before the start of antimicrobial therapy is obtained. The serum taken after therapy commenced is then serially diluted using inactivated pooled serum or a suitable broth (Mueller-Hinton, brain-heart, etc.) as a diluent. The pretreatment serum (if available) is used as a control to exclude the effects of immune mechanisms. The serum dilutions and controls are inoculated with the young culture of the infecting organism, and viable cell counts are made using a standard inoculum loop technique and blood agar plates. The serums and controls are then incubated. After incubation, each tube that shows no macroscopic evidence of bacterial growth is subjected to a viability count as before. The greatest dilution of serum that kills 99.9% of the original organism is the minimal lethal concentration. Generally a satisfactory level of antimicrobial has been obtained if the patient's serum diluted 1:8 shows this level of bactericidal activity.

Use of Antimicrobials in Diagnostic Bacteriology

The student will recall that many diagnostic media are selective, i.e., there are components in the medium that are inhibitory to unwanted species and thus select and allow growth of the required species. For example, MacConkey agar has bile salts and crystal violet included to inhibit the growth of gram-positive organisms. Many other media have similar components. Antimicrobials have been used in this way and may be incorporated in the medium, or antimicrobial discs or an enriched medium may be employed to produce an inhibitory zone.

As examples of antimicrobials incorporated in media, cyclohexamide and chloramphenicol are present within commercially available agar for the growth of fungi (Mycosel*, which has components supporting dermatophyte growth, and the antimicrobials inhibit contaminant bacteria and fungi. Schaedler's medium, used in anaerobic work, is often made with included antimicrobials such as nalidixic acid, which inhibits facultative anaerobic gram-negative rods but allows obligate anaerobes to grow. A kanomycin-vancomycin combination is used in a similar fashion and inhibits facultative gram-negative bacilli as well as streptococci and staphylococci. Cycloserine and cefoxitin are added to brain-heart infusion agar to inhibit gram-negative and gram-positive bacteria but allow the growth of *C. difficile.*

*Baltimore Biological Laboratories, Cockeysville, Md. 21030.

TABLE 22–3 ANTIMICROBIAL DISCS TO BE ADDED TO ANAEROBIC CULTURE TUBES IN ANAEROBIC TUBE DILUTION SENSITIVITY TESTS

Antimicrobial	Disc Content	Number of Discs/Tube	Antimicrobial/mL of Broth
Penicillin G	10 u	1	2 u
Ampicillin	10 μg	2	4 μg
Cephalothin	30 μg	1	6 μg
Tetracycline	30 μg	1	6 μg
Clindamycin	2 μg	8	3.2 μg
Chloramphenicol	30 μg	2	12 μg
Erythromycin	15 μg	1	3 μg

Discs with bacitracin (10 units and X and V factors) are used on blood agar after inoculation of upper respiratory tract specimens. The antimicrobial will inhibit most streptococci, staphylococci and neisseriae but will allow the growth of gram-negative rods, haemophili, and yeast species. A furadantin disc (300 μg/disc) in wound swab and genital swab inocula will allow the growth of *Pseudomonas* and yeast species but will inhibit most gram-negative bacilli and gram-positive organisms. Optochin, which was originally developed as an antimicrobial, has a specific inhibitory effect on pneumococci but will not inhibit similar-appearing colonies of α-hemolytic streptococci.

A neomycin (30 μg/disc) disc in inocula that are expected to yield mixed growths will inhibit most gram-negative bacilli (except *Pseudomonas*) but will allow gram-positive cocci such as streptococci and pneumococci to flourish. A penicillin disc (10 units/disc) may also be used to select gram-negative bacilli and species of *Candida* as well as *B. pertussis* on nasopharyngeal cultures.

A disc of 5 μg metronidazole is used in anaerobic bacteriology. It is placed, after bacterial inoculation, on a Schaedler's plate (with incorporated nalidixic acid or kanomycin/vancomycin). Within its zone it inhibits virtually all obligate anaerobes and is therefore most useful in identifying such colonies growing beyond its inhibitory diffusion.

In a similar fashion, discs are used to identify specific organisms or groups. One such example is the employment of bacitracin discs (0.04 units/disc) to identify, presumptively, Group A β-hemolytic streptococci. Any zone of inhibition around the disc is considered positive for the Group A streptococcus. Other groups of streptococci are not inhibited by the small amount of bacitracin. *Citrobacter diversus* is susceptible to discs of 8μg/mL of cephalosporin and resistant to discs of 8μg/mL carbenicillin, but the reverse is true of *C. freundii*. Among the Group D streptococci, the enterococci are resistant to penicillin, but *S. bovis* and *S. equinus*, which are nonenterococcal members of this group, are sensitive. *Ps. cepacia* is insensitive to polymyxins, but most pseudomonads are sensitive.

THE LABORATORY'S ROLE IN INFECTION CONTROL

In most community hospitals there is an infection control committee composed of members drawn from the medical, nursing, and other staffs, as well as from the laboratory. In addition, there is a full- or part-time nurse whose function is that of an executive to the deliberations of the committee. The nurse epidemiologist obviously also maintains a close relationship with the laboratory. The function of the committee will not be detailed here, but obviously much of its investigative and monitoring functions depends to some extent on laboratory surveillance. Some aspects of this laboratory function will be described here.

Laboratory Reports

In urgent situations, e.g., the isolation of a probable *Salmonella* sp., there should be immediate notification of the clinician and the infectious disease control nurse before the more detailed identification of the organism and its antibiotic sensitivity is carried out. However, the detailed identification of the organism must be made with an awareness of the possibilities of any epidemic consequences of that organism in the hospital and the community. Care should be taken in identifying organisms that are considered pathogenic, so that their epidemiological significance can be appreciated. Conversely, it is wasteful and inefficient to identify obvious contaminants and to investigate their antimicrobial sensitivity. Such practices promote initiation of unnecessary antimicrobial therapy.

In cases of suspected epidemics, phage typing of staphylococci and serotyping of other organisms are often important.

Types of Infection Encountered in Hospitals

Patients who come to the hospital with infections that they have contracted outside are considered to have *community acquired* diseases. They may include a number of diseases that, by law, must be reported to health authorities so that they may investigate and prevent epidemics in the community. Such diseases include salmonellosis, tuberculosis, gonorrhea, and others. Within the hospital, policies are in place to determine the type of isolation to be applied to such patients in order to prevent the spread of the infection to other patients and the hospital staff.

More recently it has become very apparent that many infections are manifested by the patient after hospital entry. These are considered *nosocomial*, or hospital acquired. The most important of these are:

1. Postoperative wound infection (25% of nosocomial infections).
2. Urinary tract infections (33 to 50%).
3. Respiratory tract infections (20%).
4. Bacteremia (5 to 10%).
5. Others (salmonellosis, hepatitis, etc.).

Although most of the categories above are fairly self-explanatory, the bacteremias demand some further explanation. About 50% of these arise from contaminated intravenous instrumentation or from respiratory or urinary tract or wound infections. Another 50% of these are considered as *primary*, since the source of bacteremia is unknown. The extent and cost of nosocomial disease is not generally appreciated. It has been estimated that in the United States, one patient in every twenty admitted to the hospital will develop an infection that was not present at admission. The cost of this currently has been estimated at more than one billion dollars per annum.

General Measures Against Nosocomial Disease

Generally these follow sound hygienic practices and good nursing care and techniques. The infection control committee will have policies regarding various types of isolation measures that will be employed for different infectious diseases. These policies will be focused on the type of disease; e.g., in pulmonary tuberculosis particular effort will be made to prevent the spread of disease by droplets or aerosols, but in dysentery, measures against the spread of disease by the fecal-oral route will be emphasized.

Hand washing, good wound dressing technique, instrument care and handling, care of thermometers, proper disposal of urine and feces, proper food handling, and similar skills should be taught to nurses, aides, and orderlies. In addition, specific measures against the major types of nosocomial infections should be taken. These include the following:

1. Good operating room practice in the prevention of skin and wound infections.
2. Avoidance of unnecessary catheterization, and meticulous care if catheters are used to avoid urinary tract infections.
3. The use of sterile or disinfected respiratory equipment to prevent nosocomial respiratory disease.

Preventive Measures Involving Employees

It is obvious that hospital workers as well as patients may bring infections into the hospital, but it is possible for the infection control committee to exert more supervision over the former than the latter. No extensive discussion of the measures will be made here, and naturally details of policy will vary from place to place.

Before beginning employment, all prospective employees should have a physical examination, and persons who are possible carriers of hepatitis or who have tuberculosis should be excluded. After an employee is hired, infections such as diarrhea, skin lesions, febrile exanthems, sore throats, and so forth should be reported promptly and dealt with by the delegate of the infection control committee. Advice regarding immunization against rubella, poliomyelitis, and other infectious disease should be freely available.

Environmental Cultures

Until relatively recently, routine cultures of samples of operating room air, floors, walls, ice machines, and other equipment were made. Unfortunately it became apparent that, despite sincere efforts, the results in the face of experience were of little value. However, in specific situations, environmental cultures may be of some significance, and an example of such a situation is the periodic bacteriological examination of respiratory equipment, humidifiers, or nebulizers. Control of operating room sterilization has already been discussed (p. 26), and this subject retains its importance.

CHAPTER 22—REVIEW QUESTIONS

1. Define (a) *bacteriostasis,* (b) *bactericidal,* and (c) *minimal inhibitory concentration.* Give the principle involved in the performance of the Schlicter test for serum bactericidal levels.
2. Give examples of antimicrobials that act (a) by competitive inhibition, (b) by disturbing cell wall formation, and (c) by interference with bacterial ribosomes.
3. (a) Give the names of three penicillin derivatives that are resistant to β-lactamase.
   (b) Give the principle involved in the detection of β-lactamase.
4. Briefly describe the variables that have to be controlled in the performance of an acceptable disc agar diffusion method.
5. Briefly describe the principles of an acceptable method for determining antimicrobial sensitivity of anaerobes.

23 MYCOLOGY

INTRODUCTION

Before discussing the pathogenic fungi and diagnosis of fungal disease, we should consider the place of the fungi in the classification of living organisms.

Organisms may be divided into five kingdoms, viz., Monera (this includes the bacteria as well as *Actinomyces, Nocardia,* and *Streptomyces*), whose organisms are prokaryotic, and the Protista (protozoans, etc.), Fungi, Plantae (plants, moss, and so forth), and Animalia, all of which are eukaryotic.

Briefly, fungi differ from plants in that they do not have leaves, stems, roots, or chlorophyll, and from bacteria in that they are eukaryotic and have cell walls of polymers of hexose or hexosamine or of chitin.

There are between 100,000 and 200,000 species of fungi. Fortunately, only a few of these are pathogenic to humans; of these, only the most common and the medically important will be considered here.

The medically important fungi are found in four of the several classes of the fungal kingdom. The Zygomycetes include *Rhizopus, Mucor,* and *Absidia,* which occasionally cause disease, especially in patients with defective immune mechanisms. These fungi have nonseptate hyphae. Ascomycetes and Basidiomycetes have septate hyphae and include a few possible pathogens. Most disease-causing fungi are found in the Deuteromycetes or Fungi Imperfecti. In these organisms, no sexual phase was originally observed, and hence the designation "imperfect." The perfect state in some of them has now been identified, but the class name has been retained. The history of discovery of some of the species in this class may be seen in the changes in nomenclature. For example, a fungus that causes maduromycosis was thought imperfect and was named *Monosporium apiospermum*. Later, the perfect stage was called *Allescheria boydii*. Finally, it was shown that the organisms were essentially identical but were found in two states: it was then renamed *Pseudoallescheria boydii*.

Taxonomy plays a lesser part in fungal identification than it does in bacterial recognition. Much fungal diagnosis is made by recognition of structures displayed in the asexual phase as well as by knowledge of the clinical condition of the patient and the possibilities it presents.

FUNGAL ANATOMY

Many of the fungi have long tubelike filamentous structures known as *hyphae*. The hyphae are often divided by septa, and if so are known as *septate hyphae*. The mass of hyphae is called the *mycelium*. Vegetative mycelium is buried in the nutrient medium, and aerial mycelium grows above. Reproductive spores on the hyphae may be of several types. One variety of spore is the *conidium*. Conidia may be present in groups, supported at the end of a specialized branch of mycelium known as a *conidiophore*. Conidia may be borne on specialized parts of the conidiophore known as *sterigmata*. Small unicellular conidia are often called *microconidia* or *microaleuriospores*; multicellular large conidia are often referred to as *macroconidia, fuseaux,* or *macroaleuriospores*. Microconidia may be arranged in bunches *(en grappe)* or singly at the sides of hyphae *(thyrses)*. Pear-shaped conidia are called *pyriform*; club-shaped conidia are *clavate*. In some spores, the hyphae fragment and the resultant conidia are called *arthrospores* or *arthroconidia*. Some fungi produce resting spores, especially in an adverse environment, with peculiarly thick walls; such spores are called *chlamydospores*. The yeastlike fungi differ from the true yeasts in that they do not produce sexual spores in an ascus. In addition, the yeastlike fungi produce a tubelike extension of their protoplasm that differs from hyphae in that there is no separation apparent from the parent cell. These tubelike structures are known as *pseudohyphae*. Yeasts and yeastlike fungi reproduce by budding; the bud is known as a *blastoconidium*.

All fungi are gram-positive, and some species of *Nocardia* are also acid-fast. The fungi give a positive PAS staining. The *Cryptococcus* gives a positive mucicarmine staining reaction.

SYSTEMATIC MYCOLOGY

As stated previously, only the more common or important fungi are dealt with in this section. If the technologist has mastered the techniques of preparation and culture of specimens, many of the pathogenic fungi may be identified from the descriptions to be given. However, it is not within the scope of this work to provide a comprehensive description; for this, reference must be made to larger works.

In medical diagnosis, the fungi fall into three main groups: (1) superficial mycoses and dermatophytes, (2) deep fungi, and (3) contaminant fungi that rarely cause disease.

SUPERFICIAL MYCOSES AND DERMATOPHYTES

In this group there are several fungi that are not biologically related but that cause skin or hair lesions. The dermatophytes share certain features and cause disease of the skin, hair, and nails but do not involve other tissues.

Malassezia furfur. *Malassezia furfur* is responsible for the disease pityriasis versicolor, characterized by a patchy brown desquamating rash involving mainly the trunk. The disease is worldwide in distribution. Diagnosis is made by direct examination of skin scrapings from the lesions, which show small, thick, branching hyphae and round or oval conidia (3 to 8 μm) together. The presence of the hyphae and spores together is diagnostic. Artificial culture is difficult, except with medium with added fatty acid, and it is considered unnecessary for clinical diagnosis.

Nocardia minutissima. *Nocardia minutissima* was thought to produce erythrasma, a discolored desquamating lesion in the axilla or groin, but this disease is now more generally believed to be caused by *Corynebacterium minutissimum*. The disease distribution is worldwide. Diagnosis is made by examination of skin scrapings, which show very slender (less than 1 μm in diameter) interlacing threads, often with small bacillary forms. The organism is not generally cultured artifically.

Nocardia tenuis. *Nocardia tenuis* was thought to cause trichomycosis axillaris, in which condition there are small hard nodules along the course of the axillary (and, more rarely, pubic) hairs. The nodules may be red, yellow, or black. When the nodules are crushed and examined directly, slender (1 μm or less) rods may be seen in them. Culture has yielded *Corynebacterium tenuis,* and it is now generally thought that the disease is not fungal in origin.

Trichosporon beigelii. *Trichosporon beigelii* causes white piedra, an infection of the beard, mustache, or more rarely the scalp or genital hair. The disease has a worldwide distribution. The affected hairs have white nodules along the shaft composed of hyphae and arthroconidia. Culture yields cream-colored yeastlike colonies that become gray and wrinkled. Microscopically there are septate hyphae with arthroconidia and some blastoconidia.

Piedraia hortae. This organism is the agent that causes black piedra, occurring mainly in the tropics of the Americas and Asia and in Africa. The hairs of the head, beard, or mustache have hard black nodules superficially resembling the nits of lice but microscopically demonstrating hyphae and asci. Black, smooth, raised colonies are formed on Sabouraud's agar and show septate hyphae and chlamydospores. Asci are rare in culture.

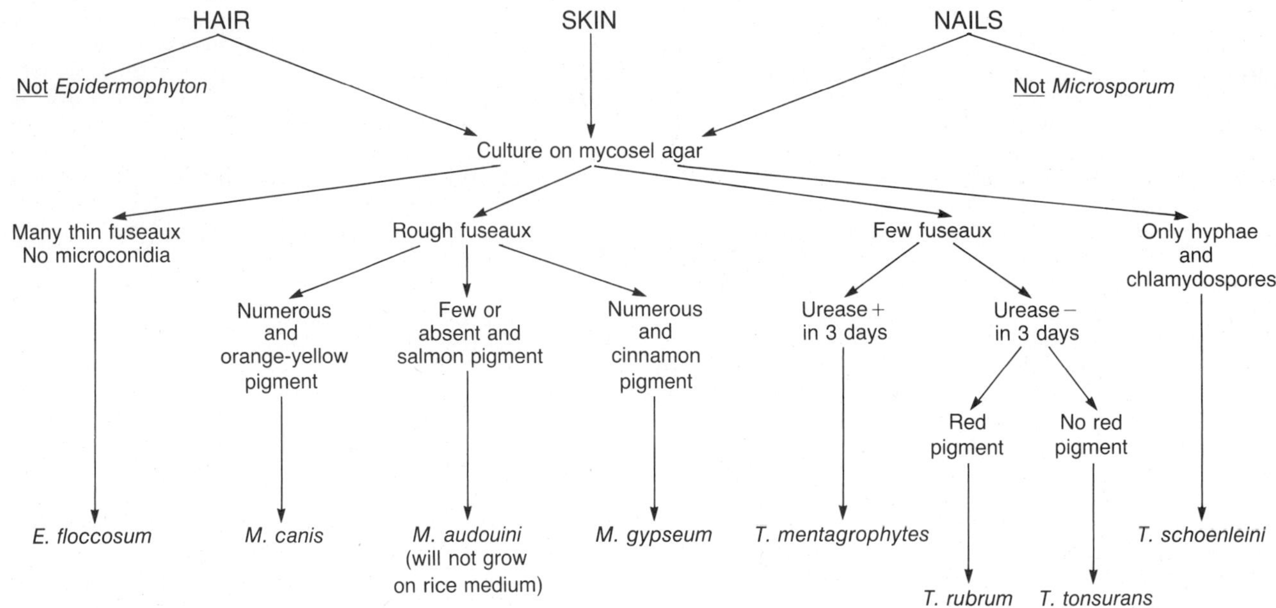

Figure 23–1 Diagnosis of common dermatophytes.

THE DERMATOPHYTES

This group of organisms has certain features in common but is divisible into three main genera: *Trichophyton, Microsporum,* and *Epidermophyton*. They cause diseases of the keratinized structures—skin, hair, and nails—but not of deeper structures. It should be remembered, however, that *Microsporum* does not infect nails and that *Epidermophyton* does not cause disease of the hair. Some species of *Microsporum* and *Trichophyton* cause hair to fluoresce under ultraviolet light. On culture, macroconidia, microconidia, and chlamydospores are seen, but their appearance and relative number differ from one group to the other. In addition, they may show *racquet* mycelium, in which there is terminal expansion of one end of a segment of hypha; *spirals,* in which the mycelium is coiled; and *favic chandeliers,* which are multibranchings at the distal ends of hyphae. All of these features vary in prominence in different groups. Many varieties produce pigment that is often typical enough for diagnosis. Some differential features of the commoner dermatophytes are given in Figure 23–1. The dermatophytes are cultured on Sabouraud's medium at room temperature. Cultures should be maintained for 4 to 6 weeks before discarding. Until recently, it was considered that all the dermatophytes were Fungi Imperfecti; i.e., the sexual stage had not been observed. But ascigerous forms have been described in the genera *Trichophyton* and *Microsporum (Arthroderma* and *Nannizzia,* respectively), which suggests that the dermatophytes ultimately will be classified as Ascomycetes.

Trichophyton

Trichophyton, characterized by multinucleate, clavate macroconidia that are thin-walled (not exceeding 2 μm), smooth, and have 1 to 7 septa, is divisible into numerous groups and species. *T. mentagrophytes* and *T. rubrum* have a worldwide distribution, but some other members are confined to certain geographic regions. All members of the group have certain features in common, but particular properties separate one from the other. Species cause various types of ringworm and athlete's foot. Direct examination of material from skin, hair, or nails will show chains of arthroconidia. Hairs may be covered by the spores, in which case there is said to be *ectothrix* infection; or invaded by them, *endothrix* infection; or characteristically, in infections caused by *T. schoenleinii* and less often by other species, the hairs contain mycelium, some of which has degenerated to leave empty spaces. The hair is not brittle as in the other infections, and thus may be relatively long. This type of infection is known as "favic." The appearance is similar to that seen in other dermatophyte infections, and no diagnosis other than fungal infections can be made on the basis of the direct examination. Cultural features of the group are illustrated in Table 23–1. *T. tonsurans* may be spread by combs or clothing. *T. schoenleinii* may be transmitted directly from one person to another, whereas *T. verrucosum* is often spread from cattle.

T. rubrum. Growth is fairly rapid on Sabouraud's agar, with a cottony white appearance subsequently becoming powdery, and with radial grooves. A deep red-purple pigment produced by the growth diffuses into the medium and is visible on the back of the plate.

T. mentagrophytes. Growth is rapid on Sabouraud's agar, yielding a powdery or cottony white colony, occasionally pink on the reverse side, with a few irregular grooves. The organism produces urease within 3 days, unlike *T. rubrum,* which generally takes about 5 days to become positive. These two species are the ones most commonly found in the United States.

Hair Perforation Test. This may be used to differentiate *T. rubrum* from *T. mentagrophytes.*

Method. **In a sterile Petri dish several sterile hairs from a normal child are added to a culture medium (10 g yeast extract in 90 mL of distilled water). The medium and hairs are then inoculated with the fungal culture in question and**

Figure 23–2

Figure 23–3

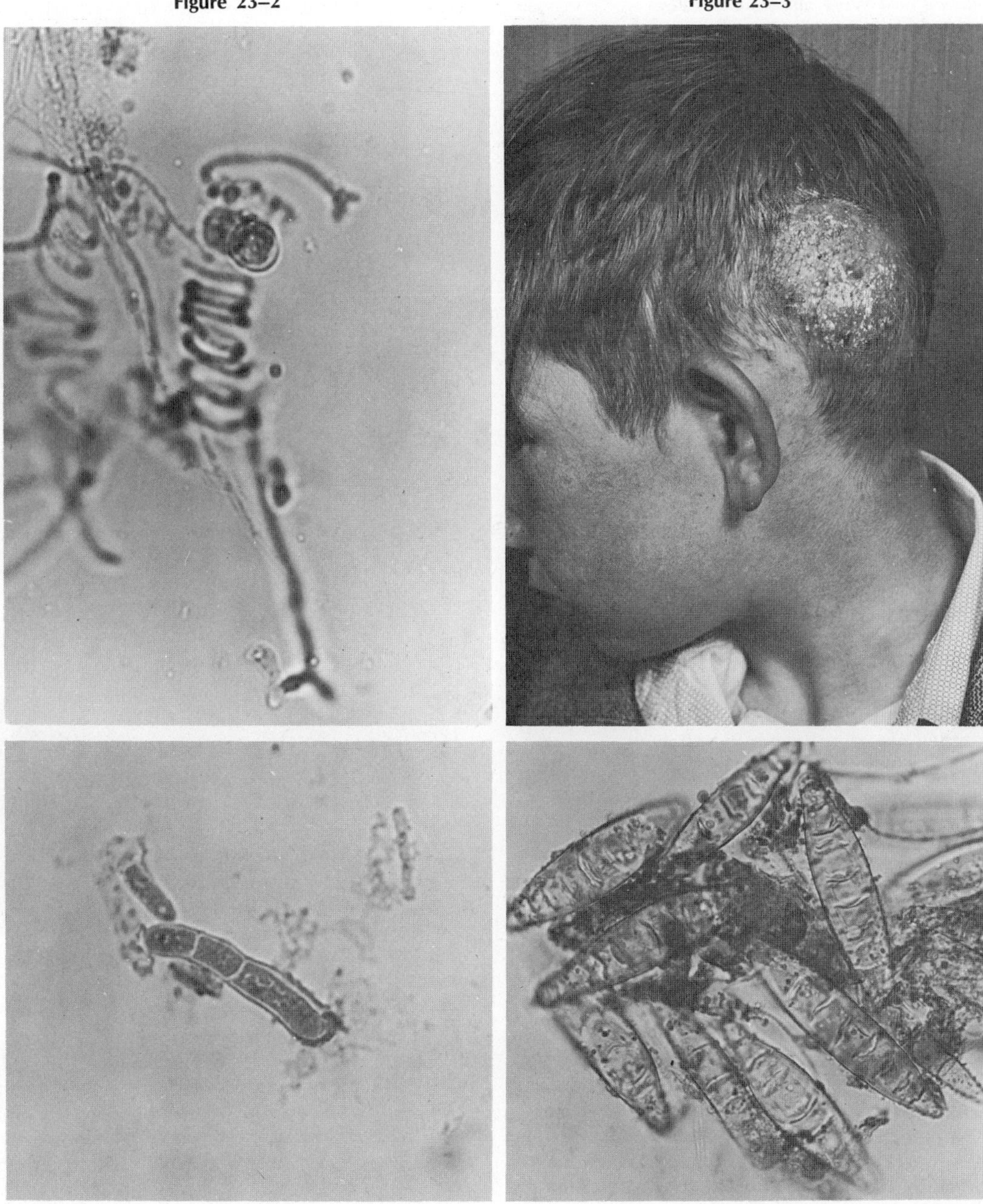

Figure 23–4

Figure 23–5

Figure 23–2 *Trichophyton mentagrophytes* culture showing spirals and chlamydospores. Wet mount; lactophenol cotton blue × 1050.

Figure 23–3 Kerion, caused by *Trichophyton verrucosum*.

Figure 23–4 Macroconidium of *Trichophyton* spp. Wet mount; lactophenol cotton blue × 1050.

Figure 23–5 Fuseaux of *Microsporum canis*. Wet mount; lactophenol cotton blue × 630.

TABLE 23–1 KEY TO DERMATOPHYTES

	Microconidia	Fuseaux	Position of Microconidia	Shape of Fuseaux	Infection of Hair, Nails, Skin
Trichophyton	Very numerous	Few	En grappe or thyrses	Pencil thin; 4–6 μm × 20–50 μm	H, N, S
Microsporum	Few to moderate	Few to many	Thyrses	Spindle-shaped, rough, thick-walled; 3–8 μm × 5–100 μm	H, S
Epidermophyton	Absent	Many	Absent	Ovoid, thin-walled, smooth; may be in clusters; 20–35 μm × 4–6 μm	N, S

incubated at 25° C for up to 4 weeks. The hairs are periodically examined with a drop of lactophenol cotton blue. *T. mentagrophytes* perforates the hair, usually in 4 to 14 days, forming funnel-like channels, but *T. rubrum* does not.

T. verrucosum. *T. verrucosum* affects cattle primarily, but human disease by contact, especially in children, is not uncommon. Growth on Sabouraud's medium is slow, with formation of a waxy or velvety white to yellow colony; microscopic mounts from Sabouraud's medium show only chlamydospores, but enriched media will yield fuseaux and microconidia. *T. verrucosum* is the only dermatophyte that grows better at 37°C than at room temperature. If the organism infects the hair it causes an area of partial alopecia complicated by a boggy infection of the scalp *(kerion)*.

T. tonsurans. Infection with *T. tonsurans* occurs with some frequency in all areas of the United States and in Mexico. Colonies are slow-growing, yellow to tan, and velvety, with a central crateriform depression and radial grooving.

T. schoenleinii. *T. schoenleinii* grows slowly to form a grey corrugated colony, often with a waxlike surface. Culture shows many chlamydospores with few fuseaux and absent microconidia. The organism often causes favus (tinea favosa) in which there is a dense mass of mycelium in the mouth of the hair follicle that, when removed, leaves a red weeping area.

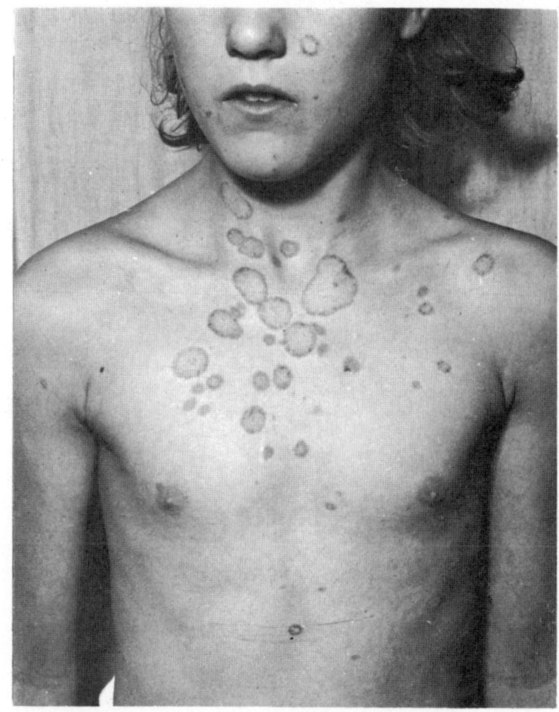

Figure 23–6 Ringworm caused by *Microsporum canis*. The patient contracted the infection from a pet kitten.

Microsporum

This group has fusiform, thick-walled macroconidia with 4 to 15 septa that may bear some prickles or spines. The walls of the macroconidia are thick (up to 4 μm). There are three major species in the group: *M. audouinii, M. canis,* and *M. gypseum*. The organisms have a worldwide distribution, although some species predominate in certain geographic regions. *M. audouinii* is spread from person to person (anthropophilic) and has caused epidemics in children. *M. canis* may be contracted from dogs or cats (zoophilic) or from another human. *M. gypseum* is a dermatophyte of animals but also has been found in the soil and may be contracted from another person. They all cause ringworm.

Direct examination of infected hairs shows ectothrix-type infection; skin scrapings are similar to those seen in other dermatophyte infections.

M. audouinii. *M. audouinii* grows slowly on Sabouraud's medium, with white or tan colonies that develop central elevation but little or no grooving. A red-brown or salmon-colored pigment is produced in the medium. Fuseaux are rare and occasionally poorly formed.

M. canis. *M. canis* grows quickly on Sabouraud's medium, with cottony or powdery colonies with a pale brown center. An intense canary yellow pigment diffuses into the medium.

M. gypseum. *M. gypseum* is rapid-growing and cottony, becoming powdery and turning cinnamon brown. The reverse side of the colony is pigmented red-brown to orange, but there is little diffusion.

Epidermophyton

These are characterized by wide macroconidia with smooth walls and 0 to 4 septa. There is only one species in this group that is pathogenic for humans, *Epidermophyton floccosum*. Colonies are slow-growing on Sabouraud's medium, with a slightly green granular colony developing radial grooves.

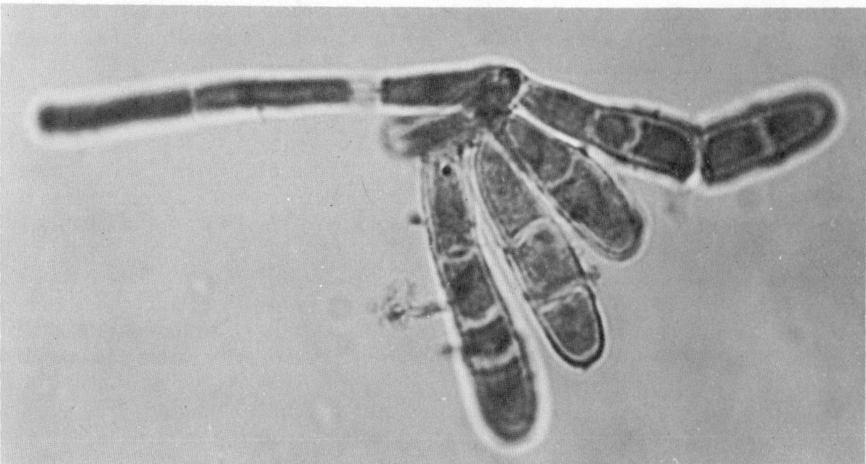

Figure 23–7 Fuseaux of *Epidermophyton floccosum.* Wet mount; lactophenol cotton blue × 1050.

Ultraviolet Light

As mentioned before, certain species of *Microsporum* cause infected hairs to fluoresce, and this aids the dermatologist or laboratory investigator in obtaining infected material.

Species	Fluorescence in Hair with UV Light
T. rubrum	–
T. mentagrophytes	–
T. verrucosum	–
T. tonsurans	–
M. audouinii	+
M. canis	+
M. gypseum	+ or –
E. floccosum	Does not infect hair

Pleomorphism

This is a very common spontaneous mutation occurring in colonies of the dermatophytes. Initially the fuseaux, then the microconidia, and then other structures fail to develop, leaving a mass of featureless fluffy white mycelium. Once the culture has changed, there is no way to reverse the change. The phenomenon makes the maintenance of stock cultures difficult but transfer every 6 weeks or storage below −20°C, preferably the latter, is generally successful in prevention of pleomorphism. Some species *(M. audouinii)* do not become pleomorphic, and this feature may be useful in diagnosis. Longer periods (up to 6 months between subcultures) are successful in some hands in preventing pleomorphism. Storage at 4°C will maintain cultures for 3 to 4 months between subculture, and agar slant cultures covered with mineral oil or sterile distilled water can preserve the growth for 12 months. A method described by the Centers for Disease Control is to place a number of harvested spores from a young culture into sterile water in a screw-capped vessel. The organism is grown on Sabouraud's or potato-dextrose agar slants until a fructifying growth is obtained. Then, 5 mL of sterile distilled water is added to the slant and the surface is aseptically scraped with a loop to harvest spores into the water. This suspension is then poured into a sterile screw-capped vial and kept at room temperature. Yeast-like fungi may be dealt with in a similar fashion. Under such conditions, at room temperature, the spores will remain viable for months or years and can be subcultured to produce typical colonies. Sabouraud's conservation agar (p. 460) may also be useful.

Candida and Some Other Medically Important Yeasts

Candida may reasonably be considered here, since it is often associated with skin and nail disease (intertrigo, cutaneous candidiasis, onychia, and paronychia), although there is some debate as to whether *Candida* is the pathogen or a secondary invader. *Candida albicans,* which is most often cited as a pathogen is also a normal inhabitant of the bowel and is found on the skin and in the sputum of healthy subjects. It used to be thought that *C. albicans* was the only member of the group that was pathogenic, but its common presence without disease as well as the appearances of other species in overt diseases, such as endocarditis due to *C. tropicalis, C. parapsilosis,* and others has shown that species other than *C. albicans* may be disease producing. Apart from skin and nail disease, *Candida* causes thrush, vulvovaginitis, endocarditis, meningitis, and pulmonary candidiasis. The organism is an egg-shaped budding cell that may show small pseudohyphae. Culture is easily made on a variety of media. On Sabouraud's medium at 35°C or at room temperature, there is rapid growth of a creamy white, smooth, shiny colony with a characteristic wine odor. Similar colonies occur on blood agar.

The first problem that the technologist faces after recognizing the growth of *Candida* is deciding whether the isolate has clinical significance. If isolated from the blood or cerebrospinal fluid (CSF), the growth must be considered important. However, a few colonies in a throat swab, or in sputum, or from the skin or vagina may safely be ignored. Recognition of a few colonies from a tracheostomy wound or a fair number of colonies in a stool culture may be a more difficult decision. In those cases, it is better to err on the side of caution. In urine, 10^4 colonies/mL is accepted as a number indicating infection, and specimens with this number of organisms or more are reported and investigated. In patients receiving antimicrobial therapy, or in those with lowered immune responses, the finding of *Candida* becomes more important, and in such cases the appearance of even a few colonies, which in another patient may have been regarded with equanimity, are here regarded with suspicion.

Once it has been decided that the yeast is meaningful, and especially if it has been found in the CSF, *Cryptococcus* is excluded by the absence of a capsule (p. 450). The next step in identification is the germ tube test.

The Germ Tube Test. A small portion of several colonies of the yeast is inoculated into 0.5 to 1 mL of serum and incubated at 37°C for 2 to 4 hours. A drop of the serum is then examined microscopically for the presence of germ tubes (Fig. 23–8). *C. albicans* and *C. stellatoidea* are positive, and other species do not produce them. Some authorities consider *C. stellatoidea* to be a variant of *C. albicans*. Testing may stop at this stage, and a report may be issued.

Chlamydospores. Cornmeal Tween 80 Agar (available commercially) is inoculated with the yeast by making cuts in the agar with the charged inoculating loop. The impregnated area is covered with a flamed coverslip, and the medium is incubated at room temperature for 2 to 4 days. The plate is then examined for chlamydospores, which are produced by *C. albicans, C. stellatoidea,* and some strains of *C. tropicalis.* 2% oxgall agar (20 g oxgall and 18 g agar in 1 liter of water) has been used to demonstrate both germ tubes and chlamydospores. Cultures are streaked onto the oxgall agar and covered by a coverslip. They are incubated at 37°C for 3 or, if necessary, 4 hours and examined microscopically for germ tubes. They are then kept at room temperature for a further 24 or 48 hours and examined for chlamydospores. The advantages of this method, which with practice is reliable, are that it uses only one medium and that it saves time (Yong et al., 1978).

Cornmeal Tween 80 has a much more basic use in that it will support the growth of hyphae or pseudohyphae in many of the yeastlike organisms. The technique for this demonstration, which is pivotal in the differentiation of these fungi, is the same as that used for the demonstration of chlamydospores. After 72 hours at 30°C or at room temperature, *Candida, Geotrichum,* and *Trichosporon* species will produce hyphae or pseudohyphae, but *Cryptococcus, Rhodotorula, Torulopsis,* and *Saccharomyces* (and other true yeasts) will not.

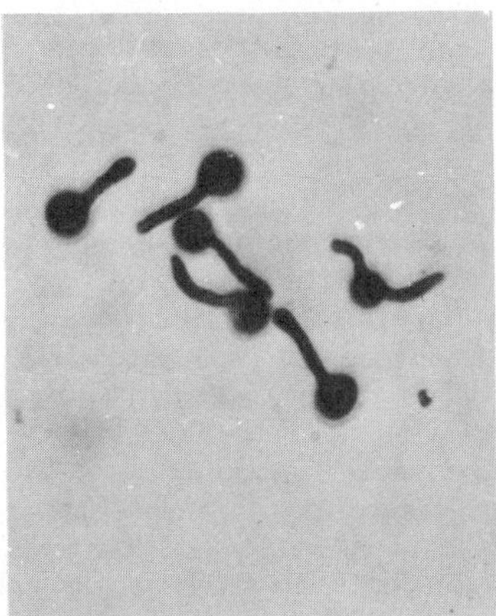

Figure 23–8 Germ tubes of *Candida albicans* after incubation in human serum for about 3 hours. All the yeast cells show one (or more) tubes. Gram stain × 1500.

Fermentation and assimilation tests (aerobic utilization of differing substrates) may also be used to differentiate other species. Several commercial kits for this purpose are now available. With these, one can perform assimilation and fermentation tests rapidly and with a considerable degree of accuracy. The Uni-Yeast-Tek system* is possibly the best. It performs seven carbohydrate assimilation tests as well as testing for chlamydospores in Cornmeal Tween 80 medium, and it tests for urease, nitrate assimilation, and germ tube formation. The API 20C† (Fig. 23–13) is another kit (not unlike the API 20E for the Enterobacteriaceae) that is manufactured to test for carbohydrate assimilation on 19 substrates.

Torulopsis

Torulopsis glabrata is now considered to be a species of *Candida*. It is an occasional pathogen in the urinary tract and has caused fungemia. The round or oval cells show budding that may be multilateral, and colonies look like those of *Candida*. It differs from the *Candida* species in that it does not form hyphae or pseudohyphae on Cornmeal Tween 80 agar and it is inhibited by cyclohexamide (contained in Mycosel agar).

Rhodotorula

This genus is made up of nonpathogenic yeasts that multiply by terminal budding and that have granules within their cytoplasm. They grow well on the usual media and produce a yellow to red pigment. Its importance is in its possible confusion with *Cryptococcus,* since both have a capsule and produce urease. However, the pigmentation and the failure to assimilate inositol are major differentiators.

Trichosporon

T. beigelii has been described above. On culture it produces a growth with many arthroconidia.

Geotrichum

This is a fungus that may initially produce a yeastlike colony but that will also produce hyphae and arthroconidia. It is generally a saprophyte but rarely will occur as an opportunistic pathogen. Differentiation from the yeastlike fungi is made by finding the presence of arthroconidia.

---

*Flow Laboratories Inc., Roslyn, N.Y. 11576.

†Analytab Products, Inc., Plainview, N.Y. 11803 and St. Laurent, Que. H4S 1M5.

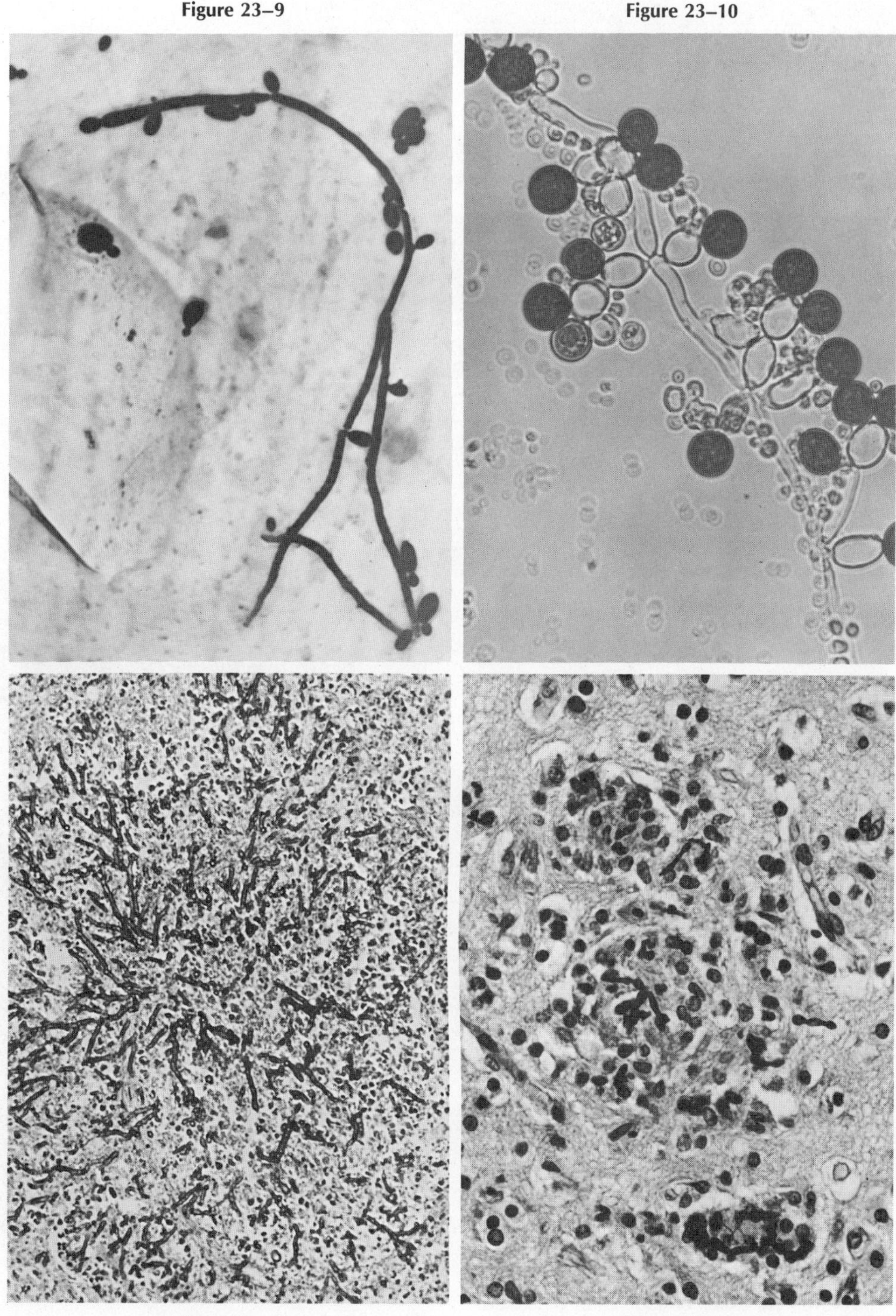
Figure 23–9 Figure 23–10 Figure 23–11 Figure 23–12

Figure 23–9 Candidiasis. Smear from lesion showing budding yeasts and pseudohyphae. Gram stain × 1350.

Figure 23–10 *Candida albicans*. Chlamydospore production on chlamydospore agar (Difco). Chlamydospores are stained by the trypan blue in the medium. Wet mount × 1260.

Figure 23–11 Pulmonary candidiasis. Section of lung. Hematoxylin-eosin × 300.

Figure 23–12 Generalized candidiasis. Section of brain from a child who presented with a skin rash but had no known predisposing condition. PAS and hematoxylin × 500.

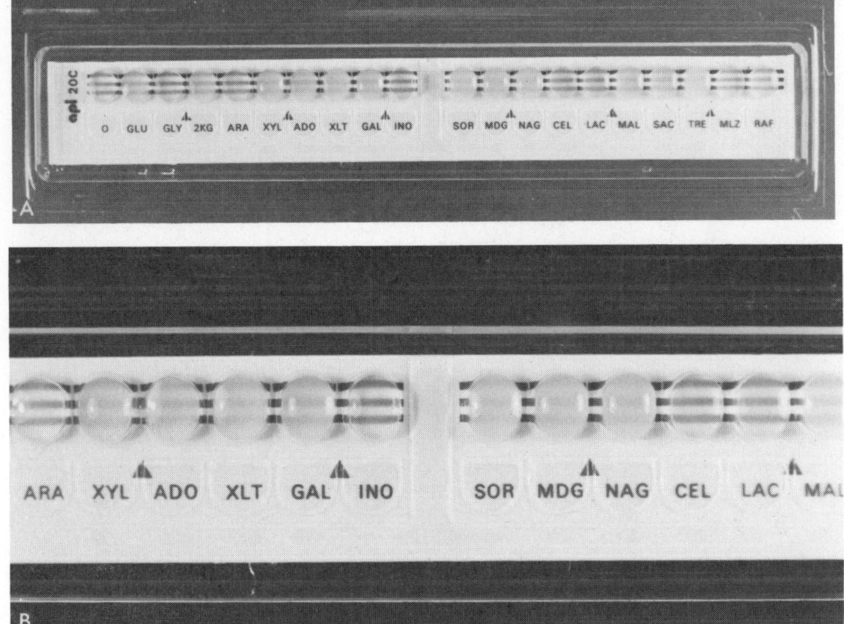

Figure 23–13 API 20C (Analytab Products, Plainview, N.Y. 11803). The apparatus is a plastic strip containing 20 cupules: a control and 19 dehydrated substrates designed to detect assimilation. Yeast suspension is made in API basal medium, which supplies nitrogen growth factors. The suspension is standardized and added to each cupule. Subsequently the tray is incubated at 30°C for 72 hours. Cupules showing more turbidity than the control ("0" on left in **A**) are considered positive. Results are read off from a differential chart. In the illustration, *C. albicans* is shown.

DEEP SYSTEMIC FUNGI

This group includes several species that are largely unrelated but that are all capable of producing disease in the tissues of the body deep beneath the skin. Although taxonomy has placed *Actinomyces* and *Nocardia* with the bacteria, they are by tradition and usage considered within the province of the mycologist. *Cryptococcus* will be considered first, however, since it is one of the yeastlike organisms. Some of the deep fungi display dimorphic growth; i.e., they have a yeast and a mycelial phase. The mycelial form is seen in growth at room temperature in the laboratory, whereas the yeast phase occurs in the tissues and *in vitro* when growth is at 37°C, with, in some cases, additional nutrients in the supporting medium.

Cryptococcus neoformans

C. neoformans is a yeastlike fungus that causes cryptococcosis. The disease is of worldwide distribution and most commonly involves the meninges and brain, although lung, skin, and bone disease are also well recognized. The organism has been isolated from soil and from pigeon droppings. The pigeons do not suffer from the disease, but they carry the organism on their beaks and feet and it survives in their bowel. It is believed that in humans the organism usually gains entry through the respiratory tract, causing disease there or being carried to some other system, probably by the blood. Man-to-man infection does not occur. Infection may be seen as a terminal episode in lymphoma, especially in Hodgkin's disease.

The organisms can be seen by direct examination of sputum, exudate from cutaneous lesions, aspirates from subcutaneous masses, or CSF. They are yeastlike bodies (5 to 20 μm in diameter) demonstrating single budding (rarely, multiple budding) and surrounded by a wide capsule of gelatinous material. In CSF, they must be differentiated from red blood cells and lymphocytes; they are not refractile like red blood cells, and the presence of buds distinguishes them from lymphocytes. The capsule is not easily seen in unprepared CSF, but if the fluid is centrifuged, other cells and debris may delineate the capsular circumference. If a drop of India ink or nigrosin is added to the CSF, capsules become obvious.

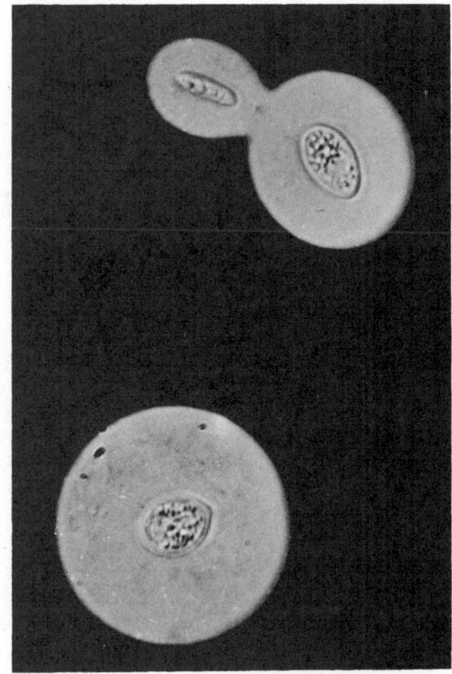

Figure 23–14 *Cryptococcus neoformans.* Wet mount; nigrosin preparation × 750.

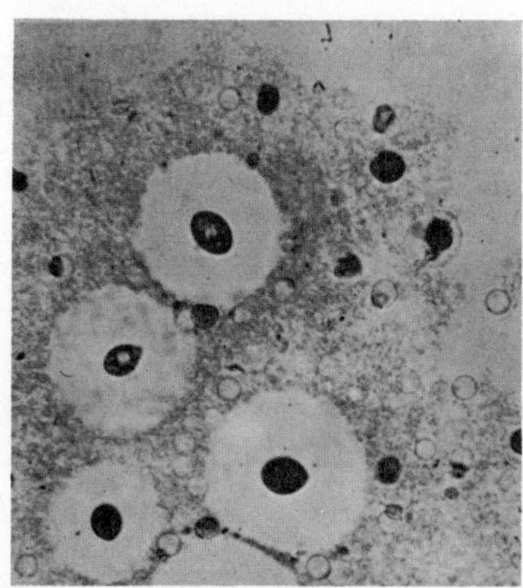

Figure 23–15 *Cryptococcus neoformans*. Centrifuged CSF. Note the ovoid organisms surrounded by a clear capsule thrown into contrast by cellular debris. Lymphocytes and red blood cells are clearly distinguishable. Wet mount; toluidine blue × 500.

Suspicion of the presence of the organisms is often aroused by their slightly ovoid shape or by budding. Toluidine blue 0.1%, which is occasionally used as a stain for counting cells in CSF, colors the organism pink (metachromasia of polysaccharides), whereas lymphocytes become blue and red cells remain unstained. In tissues, Mayer's mucicarmine stain will color the cryptococcal body (*not* capsule) bright red, and when strong this reaction is virtually diagnostic of *Cryptococcus*. The CSF will also show low glucose levels, lymphocytosis, and a raised protein.

In cases in which the clinical suspicion of cryptococcosis is strong, diagnosis has been made on the basis of serological evidence (see further on).

Culture can easily be made on Sabouraud's medium at 37°C or room temperature, and growth is rapid (within 2 to 3 days), but cultures should be kept for 2 to 3 weeks before they are discarded. The colony is initially a white or creamy, glistening, mucoid growth that becomes honey brown and tends to drip down the slope. Mounts of the colony show encapsulated, yeastlike organisms similar to those described, although capsular width appears to become reduced on artificial culture. Urease is produced by all cryptococci but is not produced by *Candida* species. Media containing cycloheximide (Actidione) inhibit cryptococci but have no effect on the growth of *Candida albicans*. On Cornmeal Tween 80 agar, no pseudohyphae will be produced (unlike *Candida*), and it does not produce pigment like *Rhodotorula*,

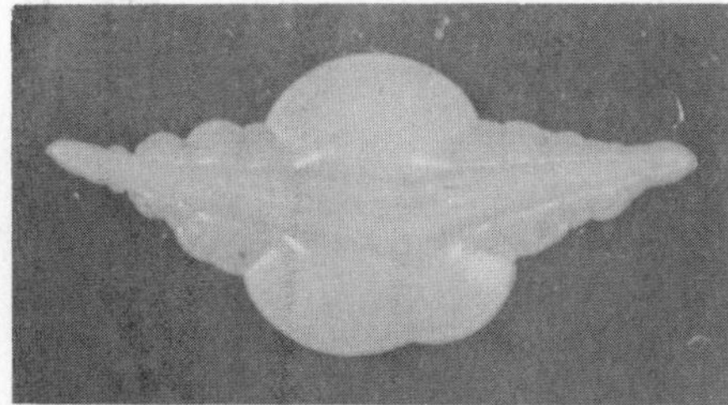

Figure 23–16 *Cryptococcus neoformans*. Culture on Sabouraud's agar. (Courtesy of Dr. Jan Schwarz.)

although like the latter it is urease positive. It was thought that *C. neoformans* was the only species in the genus that would grow at 37°C, but this is not so. To differentiate *C. neoformans* from nonpathogenic cryptococci, growth on Staib's medium (birdseed agar) is employed. The medium is commercially available, and on it, colonies of *C. neoformans* will become tan to brown within 48 hours when incubated at 37°C. Other biochemical tests are available and may best be elucidated by using one of the commercial kits described above.

Cryptococcal antigen may be sought in the CSF or in serum by a fairly simple latex test. The latex particles are coated with anticryptococcal antibody and will agglutinate in the presence of antigen. The test is sensitive, and with the caveat that rheumatoid factor may cause a false positive test, such a result indicates active cryptococcal disease. The sexual stage of the fungus has now been described (*Filobasidiella neoformans* and *bacillispora**).

The relationship between the various yeastlike fungi may be appreciated from Figure 23–17.

Blastomyces dermatitidis

B. dermatitidis is the cause of North American blastomycosis. The disease is characterized by a chronic granulomatous inflammation that may involve the skin, lungs, or other organs. In the skin, lesions tend to be raised and boggy with multiple miliary abscesses and often become pseudoepitheliomatous. In the lung, the spectrum of disease ranges all the way from the subclinical to that resembling tuberculous bronchopneumonia. Hematogenous or disseminated disease may occur in the prostate, kidney, larynx, brain, and so forth, but the gastrointestinal tract is spared. The path of infection is believed to be via the respiratory tract except for rare cases, but the natural habitat of the organism is not known; the organism has been isolated from soil rarely. The explanation for the difficulty in recovering *B. dermatitidis* from the soil is the apparent lysis of this form of the fungus in unsterilized (but not sterilized) soil. The organism probably survives in the sexual (ascigerous) form, which is called *Ajellomyces dermatitidis*. The disease occurs mainly in North America and hence the name; authentic cases have been reported from Africa. Man-to-man infection does not occur.

Direct examination of sputum, pus from the margins of skin lesions or from sinuses, or tissue scrapings taken from skin lesions after they have been cleared with potassium hydroxide may show the single-budding, yeastlike organism (8 to 15 μm in diameter) with its characteristic thick, double-contoured wall. Microforms of the organism (2 to 5 μm) are also known. Culture studies illustrate the phenomenon of dimorphic growth. Cultures should be made for incubation at 37°C and at room temperature. The yeast-phase cultures are best made on blood agar inoculated heavily, and the Petri dish should be sealed with cellulose tape. Cottonseed

*There is some evidence that two of the four separable serotypes of *C. neoformans* are a different species named *C. bacillispora*, of which the perfect form is *F. bacillispora*. The organisms are close to *C. neoformans* biochemically and pathologically.

TABLE 23–2 IDENTIFICATION OF *C. neoformans*

	Capsule	Hyphae On Cornmeal	Sensitivity to Actidione	Pigment of Colony on Sabouraud	Pigment of Colony on Birdseed	Urease	Assimilation of Inositol
C. neoformans	+	–	+	None	Brown	+	+
Torulopsis	–	–	+	None	None*	–	–
Candida	–	+	–	None	None*	–	–
Rhodotorula	+	–		Red	None*	+	–

*Occasionally light brown-yellow.

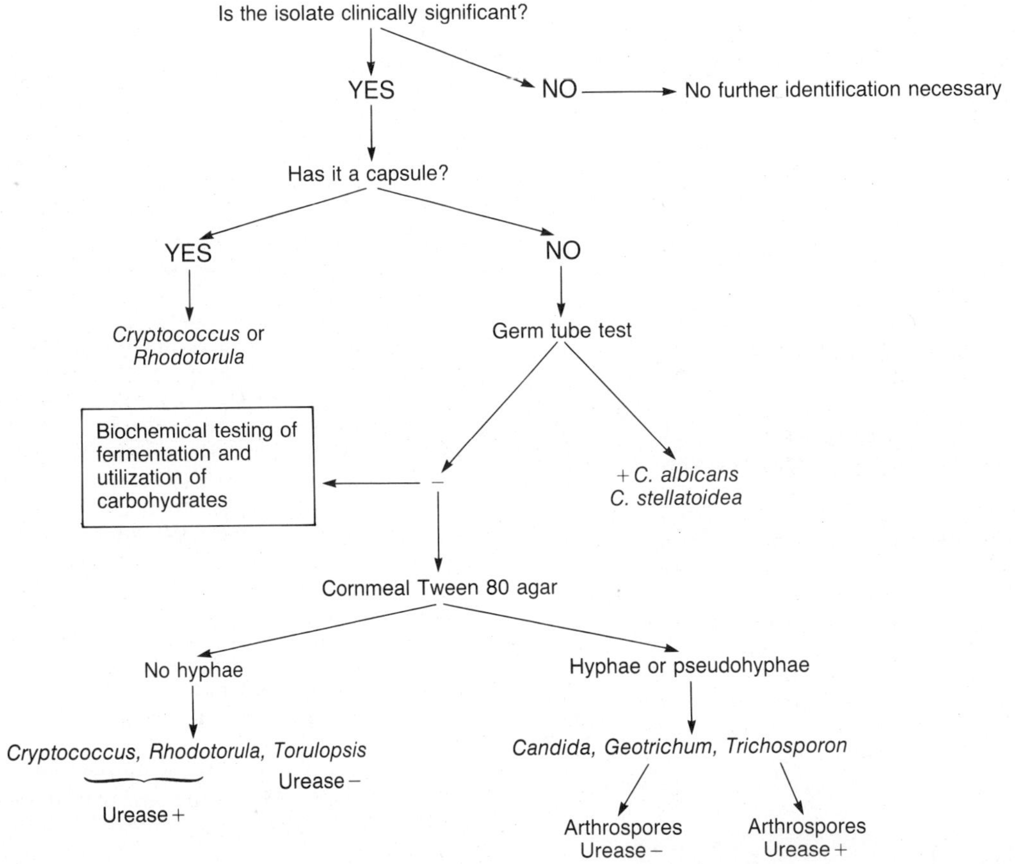

Figure 23–17 Primary differentiation of yeastlike fungi.

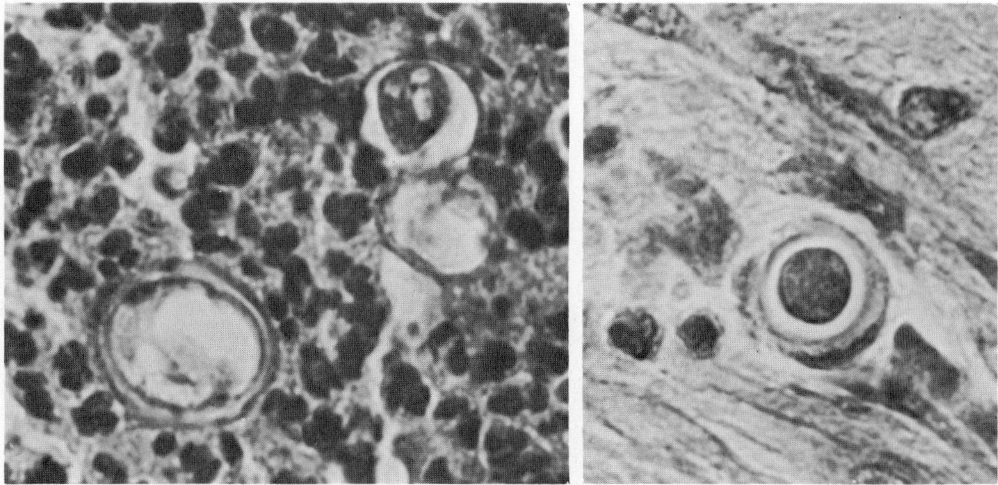

Figure 23–18 Figure 23–19

Figure 23–18 Blastomycosis. *Blastomyces dermatitidis* in pus. × 630.

Figure 23–19 *Blastomyces dermatitidis* in skin. Section of skin. Hematoxylin-eosin × 1050.

agar is best for the conversion of *B. dermatitidis* to the yeast phase. It is made as follows:

Pharmamedia*	20 g
Glucose	20 g
Agar	15 g
Distilled water	1 liter

The reagents are mixed, boiled, and then brought to pH 6 before autoclaving. Yeast-phase colonies are small and shiny, and a mount from such a culture shows numerous budding yeastlike cells with perhaps occasional short, abortive mycelial threads. Mycelial-phase cultures on Sabouraud's medium, grown at room temperature, appear in 2 to 6 weeks, at first are waxlike, and subsequently develop a white cottony aerial growth. A mount from the mycelial phase will show a mycelium of septate hyphae, with round and ovoid conidia (3 to 5 μm in diameter) attached laterally near the septa.

Paracoccidioides brasiliensis

P. brasiliensis is the cause of South American blastomycosis, which differs clinically from its North American counterpart and occurs almost exclusively in Latin America. The disease involves the gastrointestinal tract, its draining lymph nodes, and the skin as well as the viscera (lung, liver, spleen). The organism is dimorphic; the mycelial phase is not unlike *B. dermatitidis* but the yeast form, which is also present in material directly from lesions, differs in that the thick-walled, yeastlike organism shows multiple budding, which is never seen in *B. dermatitidis*. In addition, there is great variation in yeast size. Single-budding organisms are similar in both species, but the multiple budding is diagnostic of *P. brasiliensis*.

*Trader's Oil Mill Co., Trader's Protein Division, Fort Worth, Texas 76101.

Histoplasma capsulatum

H. capsulatum, a dimorphic fungus, is the cause of histoplasmosis, which is endemic in the eastern and central United States, although a few cases have been reported elsewhere. The organism has been isolated from the soil, especially that associated with old, decayed droppings of chickens, other birds, or bats, and appears to enter the body via the respiratory tract. Spontaneous disease occurs in many animals (dogs, rodents, cattle, and others). The sexual phase of the organism has now been identified and is called *Ajellomyces capsulatus.* Local outbreaks of histoplasmosis have been caused by mechanical earth movers disturbing soil. Man-to-man infection does not seem to occur. As with tuberculosis, many persons are infected but the lesion in the lungs heals, although evidence of previous infection is shown by the histoplasmin skin test. A small proportion of those infected by the fungus develop progressive disseminated disease, which is fatal if untreated. The organism lives intracellularly in cells of the reticuloendothelial system and may be seen in the macrophages of the peripheral blood, in cells of the bone marrow, intracellularly in sputum, or in the cells present in effusions. The fungus appears as intracellular tiny oval bodies (from 2 to 4 μm in diameter), with a recognizable clear halo surrounding a small central or eccentric stained "nucleus." The material must be stained in order to visualize the fungi; Romanowsky, Giemsa, hematoxylin, and the PAS reaction are all useful. Culture may be made from peripheral blood, marrow aspirate, gastric washings, and sputum. Liquid media such as brain-heart infusion may be used for primary culture from peripheral blood or from bone marrow fragments. Penicillin, 20 units, and streptomycin, 40 μg, for each milliliter of medium are useful if contamination is suspected. A more chronic variety of pulmonary disease, probably a reinfection, is not unlike pulmonary tuberculosis. It has been shown that the yeast phase is sensitive to chloramphenicol at 37°C. Therefore, *primary* isolation should be made at room temperature if anti-

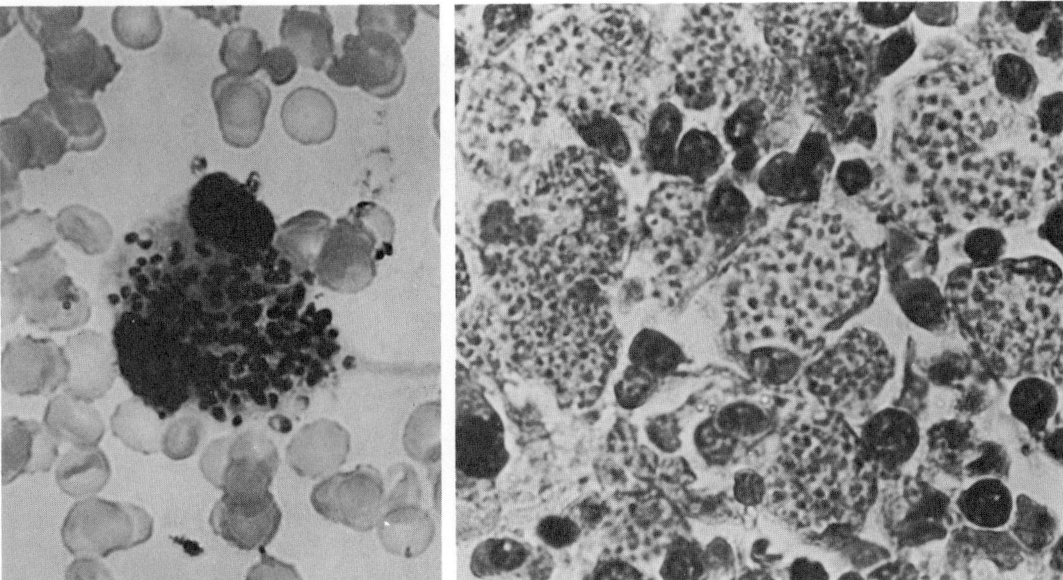

Figure 23–20 Figure 23–21

Figure 23–20 Histoplasmosis. Peripheral blood film. The large phagocytic cell in the center has numerous tiny intracellular organisms and the space around these may be seen in places. Wright's stain × 1350. (From a preparation of Dr. Jan Schwarz, Dept. of Mycology, University of Cincinnati, Ohio.)

Figure 23–21 Histoplasmosis. Bone marrow obtained at autopsy from the same patient as in Figure 23–20; note the large numbers of intracellular organisms. Hematoxylin-eosin × 1260. (Courtesy of Dr. Jan Schwarz.)

biotics such as chloramphenicol are to be employed in the medium. The cultures show dimorphic growth. On blood agar plates incubated at 37°C and tightly sealed, the yeast phase yields small, smooth, cream-colored colonies, and mounts from these show tiny, oval, single-budding, yeastlike bodies (2 to 4 μm) with occasional small abortive mycelia. On Sabouraud's medium at room temperature, the mycelial phase yields a white cottony growth that subsequently becomes brown. Mounts from this later phase show septate hyphae with small spores, perhaps on tiny branches, and the appearance is not unlike that of *B. dermatitidis*. The spores are usually smooth, but some may be irregular. However, older cultures show the diagnostic tuberculate spores. These appear in about 2 to 4 weeks and are 8 μm × 15 to 20 μm in size and have many tiny spiked protrusions (Fig. 23–22).

Figure 23–22 Tuberculate spore of *Histoplasma capsulatum*. Wet mount; lactophenol cotton blue × 1050. (Courtesy of Dr. Jan Schwarz.)

Coccidioides immitis

C. immitis is the cause of coccidioidomycosis, which is endemic in the San Joaquin Valley of California, parts of Arizona, western Texas (although cases have occurred in Mexico), and the Chaco area of South America. The organism lives in the soil and enters the body via the respiratory tract. As with *H. capsulatum,* numerous persons contract the disease in endemic areas, but, apart from a fleeting or subclinical course, there is no further development and the lesion heals. However, in a small proportion of those infected progressive disease develops. This appears to affect the dark-pigmented races such as Negroes, Filipinos, Indians, and Mexicans more often than Caucasians. Progressive disease may present as a granulomatous infiltration or ulceration of skin or lung or as a disseminated systemic infection. In other and more frequently occurring cases, a chronic pulmonary cavitating disease presents.

In tissues, the fungus is typified by the presence of thick-walled spherules (10 to 80 μm in diameter) that are filled with endospores (2 to 5 μm in diameter) (Fig. 23–23). Direct examination of sputum, gastric washings, and pus from skin and subcutaneous lesions may be made by clearing with potassium hydroxide and examining for these spherules. A recommended method is to treat gastric contents or sputum with cupric sulfate to make a 0.5% concentration. After standing for 4 hours,

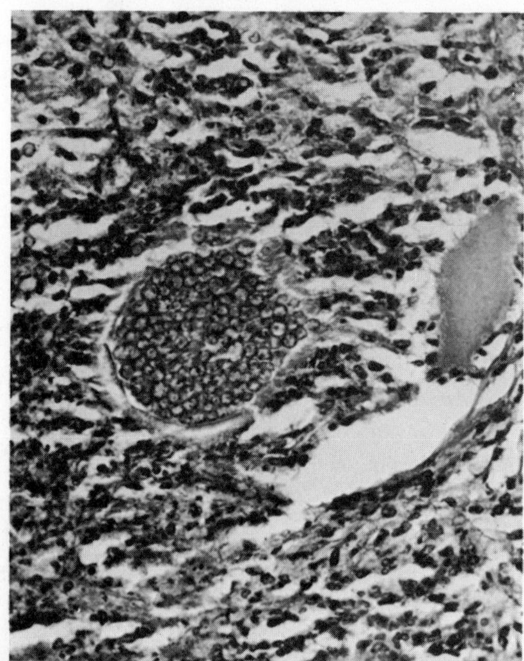

Figure 23–23 *Coccidioides immitis:* Section of mouse spleen with a characteristic spherule filled with small spores and surrounded by inflammatory cells. PAS × 460.

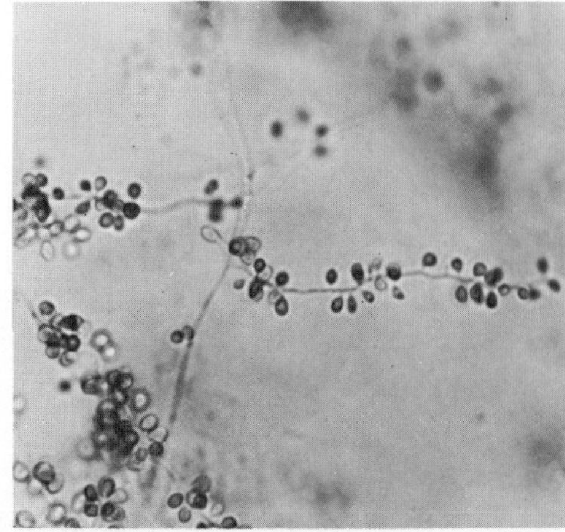

Figure 23–24 *Sporothrix schenkii.* Wet mount; lactophenol cotton blue × 1050. (Courtesy of Dr. Jan Schwarz.)

the treated material is centrifuged and the deposit examined microscopically.

Culture of suspect material should be made on Sabouraud's medium (with added antimicrobials) and incubated at room temperature. The colony develops quickly as a white cottony growth becoming brown. Mounts from such colonies show septate hyphae that are branching. The hyphae form rectangular or barrel-shaped arthroconidia (2 by 4 μm). The arthroconidia are extremely infectious and the greatest care should be employed in examining suspect cultures. A safe method is microscopic examination after autoclaving the culture. The size and shape of the arthroconidia remain unchanged.

Intraperitoneal injection of arthroconidia in suspension or of pus into the testis of guinea pigs will produce characteristic spherules in the animal tissues within 3 to 4 days. Animal tests are important in the diagnosis here, since conversion to the tissue phase *in vitro* is extremely difficult and not easily performed in most laboratories.

Sporothrix schenckii

Sporothrix schenckii is the causative organism of sporotrichosis, which commonly presents clinically as an ulcerative lesion, usually on the hand, with nodules developing along the lymphatic vessels draining the area.

The nodules often break down and form ulcers in the skin. Direct examination from lesions of the disease is almost always negative, and histological examination of biopsy specimens is very difficult, because the demonstrable fungi are few. However, culture from pus or biopsy fragments on Sabouraud's medium at room temperature will give a mycelial phase of growth; culture on blood agar at 37°C under increased CO_2 tension, with the usual technique, yields a yeastlike phase. The latter shows small soft colonies, which on microscopic examination consist of rather ovoid, pleomorphic, multiple- or single-budding, yeastlike bodies (up to 10 μm in diameter). The mycelial-phase colonies appear as tiny, moist, white colonies that later become larger and wrinkled and darken from cream to black. There is no development of aerial mycelium. Mounts of the mycelial phase show slender septate hyphae that bear bunches of pyriform or exceptionally triangular conidia at the tips of lateral branches.

Intraperitoneal injections of infected material into mice or rats usually cause peritonitis and, in contradistinction to human lesions, smears from animal lesions show cigar-shaped and pleomorphic yeast forms occasionally in an intracellular position.

The disease occurs in all parts of the world but is not spread from man to man. The fungus is found naturally growing in timber and on barberry or rose thorns, and it has been found in metal particles, like steel wool, and on sphagnum moss, which is used by florists. It becomes implanted in tissues in the course of minor traumatic incidents. Rare visceral cases of the disease are reported.

Fungi Causing Mycetomas

Numerous fungi and aerobic Actinomycetales (including *Nocardia* and *Streptomyces*) may cause chronic infections of the skin and subcutaneous tissues, including bone. The infections usually involve the feet but may be seen in the hands and more rarely in other parts of the body. The causal organisms are naturally found in the soil and enter the skin through traumatic incidents such as minor wounding by thorns or wood splinters.

Clinically, if the disease involves the foot, it is swollen, possibly discolored, and has numerous draining sinuses. Pus, draining from the sinuses, will contain granules that may be white, yellow, brown, black, or red depending on the etiological agent. The granules may be examined directly with 10% KOH and cultured on Sabouraud's agar. Since the number of fungi causing mycetomas is fairly large, it is advisable that material

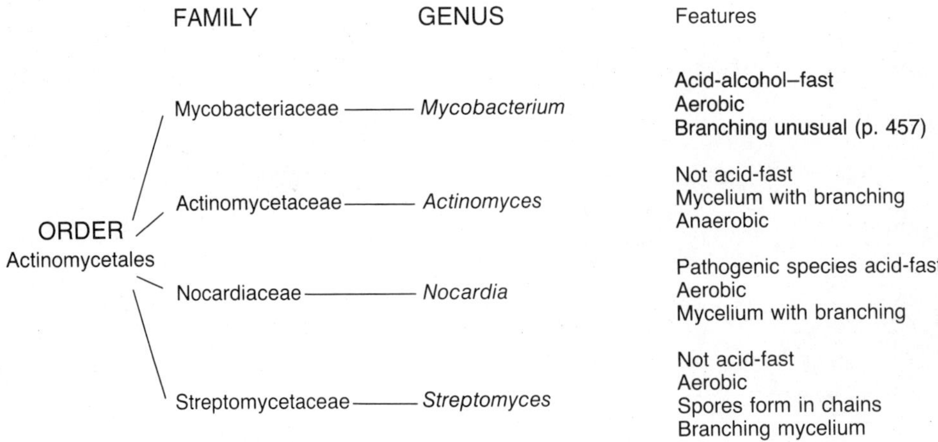

Figure 23–25 Relationships of the Actinomycetales.

from such lesions be forwarded to mycology reference centers. In North America, *Pseudoallescheria boydii* is most commonly isolated from mycetomas.

Dematiacious Fungi

The fungi are related in that they have a brown to black pigment in their cells, conidia, or both. They cause a number of skin diseases, including chromoblastomycosis, which is characterized by a verrucous ulcerated crusted lesion most often seen on the leg. *Phialophora verrucosa, Fonsecaea pedrosoi,* and others are among the most common etiological agents, and, as in mycetoma, they enter the skin through traumatic incidents. Direct examination with 10% KOH may be helpful when the pigmented nature of the fungus is seen and the diagnosis suspected. Culture is made on Sabouraud's agar at room temperature and is best sent to a reference center.

Actinomycetales

The order Actinomycetales, as noted above, truly belongs to the bacteria. However, within the order are several related familes that are medically important. Their relationship may best be seen in Figure 23–25.

Actinomyces (A. israelii and A. bovis)

This organism causes actinomycosis, which is characterized in man by chronic suppurating sinuses on the skin surface leading down to abscess cavities in the underlying tissues. The sinuses are most frequent around the neck (cervicofacial) and in the thorax and the abdomen. The underlying abscess, involving a lung, the bowel, or other organs, besides discharging through the skin, also spreads by extension. It has been shown conclusively that *Actinomyces* lives normally as a saprophyte in the mouth and throat and that some stimulus, as yet unknown, causes the organism to become pathogenic. Saprophytic *Actinomyces* are frequently seen in the crypts of the tonsils. The disease is only rarely transmitted from man to man by inoculation such as human bites. Fairly recently, pelvic inflammatory disease from which *A. israelii* has been isolated has been associated with the usage of intrauterine contraceptive devices.

Direct examination of the pus from sinuses or sputum is most important. A search should be made for small yellow granules; this may be achieved sometimes by examining a gauze dressing that has been left over the sinus for several hours. The granules should be crushed between two slides. Microscopic examination will then show an irregular lobular body with thin interlacing strands (about 1 μm in diameter) at the center and peripherally club-shaped expansions at the end of the filaments. A crushed granule when stained by Gram's

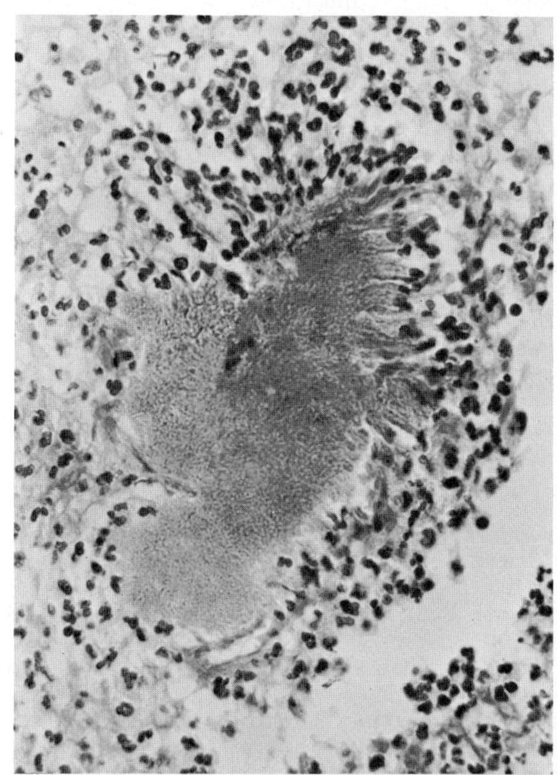

Figure 23–26 Actinomycotic granule. Hematoxylin-eosin × 630.

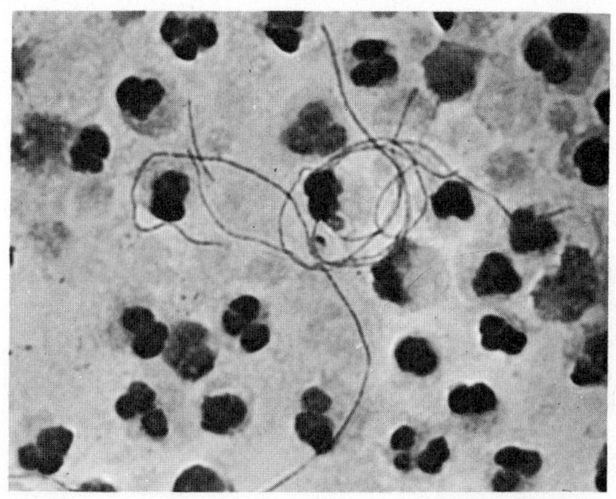

Figure 23–27 Actinomycosis. Portion of mycelium in pus from empyema. Gram stain × 1350.

technique is gram positive, and the finding of true branching of filaments is virtually diagnostic (but see *Nocardia,* following).

Culture of the organism must be made anaerobically, since *A. israelii* is an obligate anaerobe. Culture is further complicated by the fact that the specimen may be contaminated by other organisms; and, since *A. israelii* is sensitive to penicillin, streptomycin, tetracyclines, and chloramphenicol, these antimicrobials cannot be used to obtain a pure culture. Culture is usually attempted in deep tubes of brain-heart infusion agar, glucose agar shake tubes, and thioglycollate broth at 37°C. *A. israelii* appears as small, easily broken, fluffy balls in a layer about 10 mm below the surface in 4 to 6 days. On blood agar incubated anaerobically, colonies appear in 5 to 7 days as white rough colonies that adhere to the medium and are difficult to emulsify. Microscopically, the culture shows small, thin, gram-positive hyphae that demonstrate branching; bacillary rods are also seen. Subculture is difficult. The diagnosis may also be made histologically from biopsy material.

A. bovis, which is a very similar organism, has probably been isolated only from bovine sources, in which it causes "lumpy jaw."

Nocardia and Streptomyces

There are several species in this group and they are very similar biologically to *A. bovis* except that they are aerobic. In addition, *Nocardia* are found in the soil and do not appear to be saprophytic in man. *Nocardia* cause diseases similar to actinomycosis and may also mimic pulmonary tuberculosis. Clinical disease may present as mycetoma, as pulmonary nocardiosis, clinically similar to pulmonary tuberculosis, or as thoracic or cervicofacial "actinomycosis." Cerebral abscesses owing to *Nocardia* are well recognized and are secondary to pulmonary disease. The streptomyces do not cause generalized disease but only mycetomas.

The pathogenic species in the group are *N. asteroides, brasiliensis,* and *caviae* and *Streptomyces madurae, pelletieri,* and *somaliensis.*

Direct examination of pus may show granules similar to those of *A. bovis* but different in color. However, granules are often absent and the diagnosis is then suggested by the presence of slender branching gram-positive rods or hyphae. *N. asteroides, brasiliensis,* and *caviae* are weakly acid-fast, unlike other members of the group, and differentiation may be helped by this staining procedure; however, decoloration should be brief when using the technique, and 0.5% aqueous sulfuric acid is recommended as the decolorizing agent instead of acid-alcohol. Care should be taken not to confuse the acid-fast filaments with *Mycobacterium tuberculosis;* the latter do not show branching except very rarely. Since clinical disease and appearance on direct examination of specimens are so similar in actinomycosis and nocardiosis, cultures of suspect material should be made both aerobically and anaerobically in all cases.

The *Nocardia* and *Streptomyces* are easily grown on Sabouraud's agar either at 37°C or at room temperature. Antimicrobials in the medium may inhibit the growth of *Nocardia.* The colonies are slow-growing and may be moist or powdery, chalky white, or pigmented. Growth is inhibited by chloramphenicol, penicillin, and streptomycin. The appearance of some colonies is not unlike that of some mycobacteria.

Microscopic examination of the colonies may reveal either bacillary forms or long slender hyphae, depending on the species. The bacillary form is considered as evidence of fragmentation of the colony. Species differentiation is best made by a reference laboratory.

OPPORTUNISTIC FUNGI THAT CAN CAUSE DISEASE

This group includes fungi such as *Aspergillus, Penicillium,* and *Phycomycetes.* Spores of these fungi are present in the atmosphere and may contaminate specimens or cultures, or the organisms may be present in material from patients but secondary to primary pathogens. Simple demonstration of the presence of such organisms in specimens is not considered proof of their pathogenicity, but occasionally authentic cases of disease caused by these fungi are reported, especially as opportunistic infections in debilitated or immunodeficient patients. Repeated isolation of the fungus in the absence of other etiological agents, recovery from closed sites, and recognition in biopsy material as evoking specific histological responses are all factors to be considered in judging the pathogenicity of these fungi.

Aspergillus

Aspergillosis of the external ear, nasal sinuses, and lungs is well authenticated. In the lung, the fungus may cause "fungus ball" (aspergilloma), in which the fungus with mucus and debris fills an ectatic bronchus or other cavity, and there is no invasion of the lung substance. Direct examination of material from such sites may show fragments of hyphae accompanied by small rounded spores. In tissue biopsy, hematoxylin-eosin may fail to show the fungus, which will be better shown by the Gridley stain. Culture on Sabouraud's medium at room temperature quickly yields a white cottony growth that subsequently becomes green, dark green or even black. A mount from such a culture shows the typically swollen conidiophore (vesicle) supporting flask-shaped processes known as sterigmata, which bear spores pro-

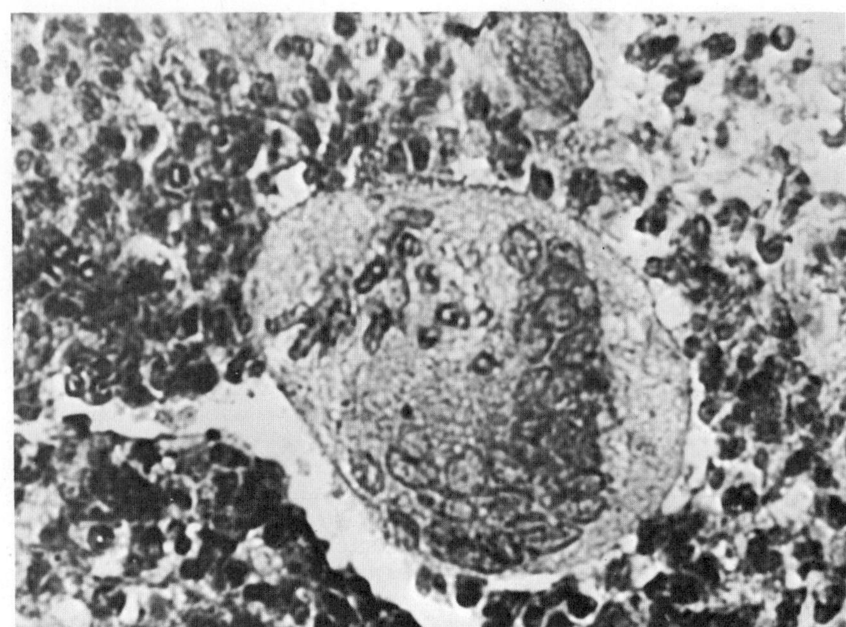

Figure 23–28 Aspergillosis. Hyphal fragments are present in a giant cell. Section of granulation tissue from the chest wall of a patient with proved primary pulmonary aspergillosis. PAS × 1050.

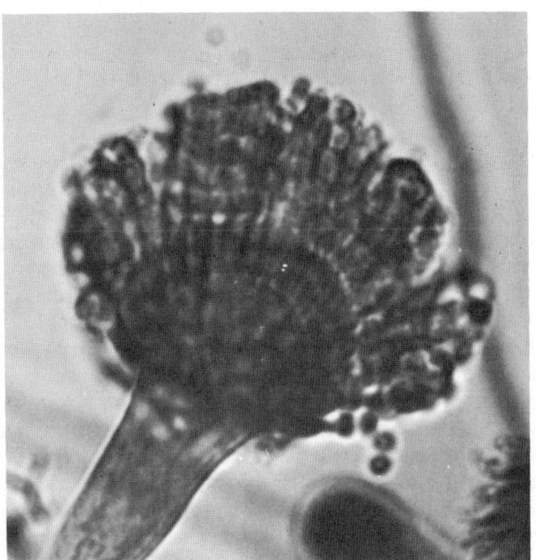

Figure 23–29 *Aspergillus fumigatus*. Slide culture of an organism obtained from the patient shown in Figure 23–28. Note the typically swollen conidiophore. Lactophenol cotton blue × 1050.

duced in short chains. The structure is best observed on slide cultures. Cyclohexamide will inhibit the growth of *Aspergillus*. There are numerous species of aspergilli, and speciation is best made by reference laboratories. The species most often seen in pathological processes is *A. fumigatus*.

Penicillium

Species of *Penicillium* may rarely cause disease of the lungs and of the external ear. Direct examination of submitted sputum or epithelial material from the ear may show an appearance similar to that described under *Aspergillus*. On Sabouraud's agar at room temperature, growth is rapid, producing most often green velvety or cottony colonies, although other pigments are produced. Culture mounts or slide cultures of *Penicillium* show a characteristic penicillus or brush, with an unexpanded conidiophore that branches. The branches may have secondary branches, at the distal end of which are sterigmata bearing chains of spores.

Phycomycetes (Mucormycosis)

The large nonseptate fungi belonging to this class (species of *Mucor, Rhizopus, Absidia,* and possibly others) are common household and laboratory saprophytes. They produce disease (mucormycosis) in humans only rarely and then generally are not cultured but are recognized histologically. The most characteristic form of the disease occurs in poorly controlled diabetics with acidosis, who develop phycomycotic sinusitis in the re-

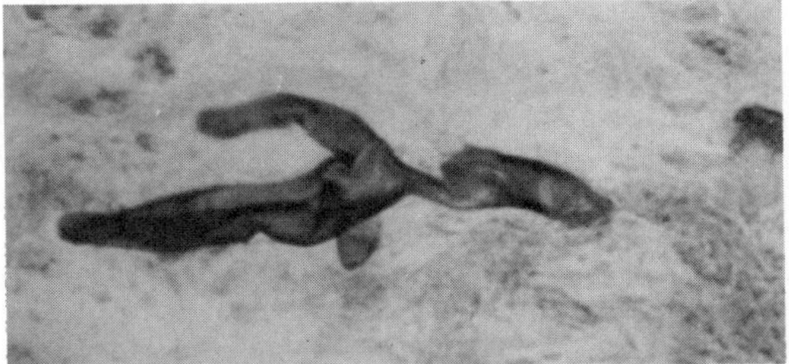

Figure 23–30 Phycomycetes. Section of necrotic tissue from the sinus of a poorly controlled diabetic patient with acidosis, ulceration of the palate, and multiple cranial nerve palsies. The fungus, which failed to grow in vitro, is characteristically nonseptate, thick, branching, and twisting. It also showed invasion of walls of blood vessels. Iron hematoxylin-eosin × 1115.

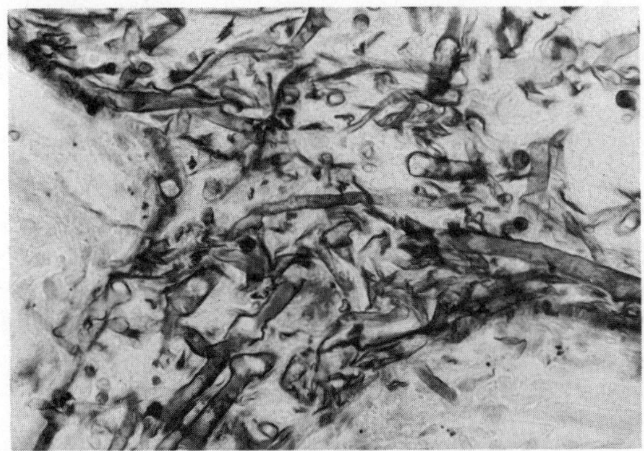

Figure 23–31 Phycomycetes. Heavy infiltration of a pulmonary vein by the characteristic hyphae. From a patient with acute leukemia. × 575.

tro-orbital tissues, and at the base of the skull with involvement of cranial nerves. Other varieties, disseminated, pulmonary, gastrointestinal, and subcutaneous, are documented.

Histologically, the fungi are recognized in biopsy (or necropsy) tissues in hematoxylin-eosin preparations; they show more clearly if iron hematoxylin is used. The large (5 to 50 μm in diameter), nonseptate, branching, twisting hyphae are characteristic and have a propensity to grow into the walls of blood vessels, initiating thrombosis and subsequent necrosis. If culture is attempted, Sabouraud's medium is satisfactory provided no cycloheximide is included.

Nonpathogenic Fungi

There are numerous fungi that contaminate plates and that either originate in the atmosphere or are present on clinical specimens. The student is advised to study these when they present themselves. A guide to the contaminant fungi is to be found in many larger texts on mycology.

MYCOLOGICAL METHODS

Direct Examination of Specimens

Skin scraping examinations are often requested. Occasionally, the technologist may be requested to obtain the specimen. The technique is very simple and requires only two clean slides or one slide and a scalpel blade. The active periphery of the lesion should be swabbed gently with 70% alcohol and then scraped gently with the side of one of the slides or the scalpel blade to dislodge flakes of desquamating epidermis or keratin onto the other slide, which is held below. At the same time some scrapings may be collected in a sterile dry Petri dish for culture studies. Scrapings on the slide are covered by 10 to 20% potassium or sodium hydroxide and a coverslip is gently lowered onto the preparation. The preparation should be left for 20 to 30 minutes, during which time the epidermal cells will become clear and flattened out. Alternatively, the slide may be passed several times through a small flame: the heat will hasten the clearing process. The slide is then examined microscopically under low illumination. Mycelia have to be differentiated from cellular walls, but whereas the latter show some pattern, the branching mycelia are quite irregular and are thicker than the cell walls, and in addition, their septa may be recognized.

A mixture of one part of Parker superchrome blue-black ink and one part of 20% NaOH may be used as a simple stain and clearing agent. The preparation is covered by a few drops of this mixture, which clears the material and selectively stains the mycelia.

Mayer's albumin may be placed on the margin of the lesion to be scraped. The scrapings are then obtained in the usual manner but adhere to the knife so that there is no loss of material. The mixture of scrapings and albumin is then smeared on a slide and may be examined with 10 to 20% KOH or by the PAS method. The PAS method is relatively simple and is especially useful if permanent preparations are required. The slide is cleared with KOH in the usual manner, and the preparation is frozen with a piece of dry ice or on the stage of a frozen-section microtome. The coverslip is removed with the point of a knife, and the preparation is allowed to dry at room temperature. It is fixed for a few minutes in methyl alcohol, drained dry for 5 minutes, and washed for 30 minutes in running tap water. Subsequently it is treated as follows:

1% periodic acid	10 min
Wash in running water	10 min
Flood with Schiff's reagent	10 min
Wash in running water	10 min

Dehydrate in alcohol, clear, and mount as tissue section. By this method fungi are stained bright red; background material is colorless or pale pink.

Affected hairs individually pulled out with forceps are examined with KOH in the same way as skin scrapings. Hair clippings are not acceptable.

Nail scrapings are made with a scalpel, and the material obtained is examined, as are skin scrapings.

Pus may be examined in several ways; the procedure for skin scrapings may be followed or Gram's stain may be used in cases of candidiasis, nocardiosis, or actinomycosis; acid-fast stains may also be used in cases of nocardiosis.

Sputum may be examined in the same way as pus. Giemsa or hematoxylin and eosin stains may be made if *H. capsulatum* is suspected.

Smears of peripheral blood or bone marrow for *H. capsulatum* are satisfactory if stained by the Romanowsky stains.

Examination of CSF for *C. neoformans* is described under discussion of that organism.

Cultural Methods

Mycological studies require relatively few media.

Sabouraud's Glucose Agar (Emmons' Modification)

This is the most useful medium and is used in investigation of numerous fungal infections. The medium may be purchased commercially in dehydrated form.

If desired, 20 units of penicillin and 40 μg of streptomycin or 0.05 mg of chloramphenicol may be added, when the mixture is cool but not solid, for each milliliter of medium. The antimicrobials prevent the possible growth of bacterial contaminants. Cycloheximide (Acti-

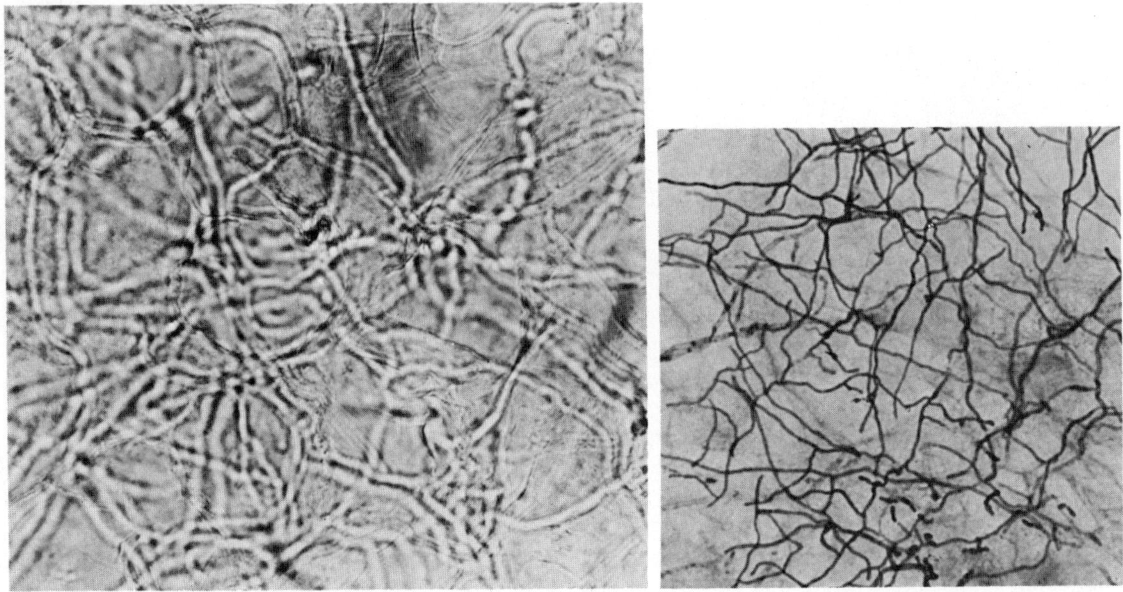

Figure 23–32 Figure 23–33

Figure 23–32 Dermatophyte. Appearance of skin scraping. Wet preparation; KOH × 1350.

Figure 23–33 Dermatophyte. Appearance of skin scraping. PAS method × 300.

dione) and chloramphenicol (Chloromycetin) are added to commercially available antibiotic-Sabouraud's media (Mycosel and Mycobiotic agar), but it should be remembered that this substance inhibits the growth of *Cryptococcus* and some other fungi. Generally two types of media are used to obviate the possibility of antibiotic inhibition. The glucose in the medium is responsible for pleomorphism (p. 447), so that Sabouraud's conservation medium, which is glucose-free, may be used for maintaining stock cultures.

Dermatophyte Test Medium*

This is a dextrose agar with peptone and the indicator phenol red. It also contains cycloheximide, gentamycin, and chlorotetracycline. The skin, hair, or nail sample is inoculated directly on the medium and is kept at room temperature for two weeks. Most saprophytes are inhibited, whereas the dermatophytes will produce a growth that will alkalinize the medium, turning the indicator red. An occasional saprophyte may cause a false positive result, so any growth should be checked microscopically. This technique is valuable in office practice or in a small laboratory in which the specimen turnover is small.

Cornmeal Tween 80 Agar

This medium is described above and is especially useful in the differential diagnosis of yeastlike organisms and the induction of sporulation in most fungi.

Staib's Medium (Birdseed Agar)

This is particularly useful in the recognition of *Cryptococcus neoformans*.

*Charles Pfizer and Co., Diagnosis Division, New York, N.Y. 10017.

Cottonseed Agar

As noted, this medium is used for the conversion of *B. dermatitidis* to the yeast phase.

Urea Agar

Urea agar is useful in the differentiation of the yeastlike fungi. Christensen's urea agar, which is commercially available, is employed and is incubated at 30°C for 5 days. Cryptococci, *Rhodotorula, Nocardia* species described above, and some *Trichosporum* species are positive. *Candida* are generally negative, as are *Geotrichum* and *Torulopsis*.

Other Media

In culture of *A. israelii* anaerobic media (p. 335) are used. Brain-heart infusion blood agar is an excellent substrate for the yeast phase of the dimorphic fungi.

Methodology

A specimen of hair, skin, or nail is obtained after preparation of the area with 70% alcohol. The specimen is directly plated onto Sabouraud's agar, both with and without cycloheximide and chloramphenicol. Incubation is at room temperature or at 30°C. Cultures are kept at least four and preferably six weeks before discarding.

"Contaminated" specimens, such as sputum, urine, and bronchial washings, are plated onto Sabouraud's agar with and without cycloheximide and chloramphenicol and onto blood agar similarly treated or untreated. Incubation should be at both 37°C and at room temperature. Cerebrospinal fluid, tissues, bone marrow, and other such "clean" tissues can be inoculated onto blood agar and onto Sabouraud's medium without antifungal or antimicrobial agents and incubated at 37°C and at room temperature. Feces are unsuitable for mycological studies.

Slide Cultures

Slide cultures are useful if one wishes to preserve the intact fructifying fungus for study. A small square piece of Sabouraud's medium is cut from a plate and placed on a sterile slide. The vertical sides of the square piece are inoculated from a culture of the fungus, and then the medium is covered by a coverslip. In effect, one then has a sandwich with a slide on one side, a coverslip on the other and a piece of Sabouraud's medium between. The whole is then placed in a Petri dish, which is kept moist by a piece of filter paper soaked in 50% glycerol. Growth of the fungus from the vertical sides of the square piece of medium can be observed microscopically through the coverslip, using low illumination. Often some of the fungi stick to the coverslip and, if desired, the coverslip may be lowered onto a drop of lactophenol cotton blue on another slide. By this technique stained fungi, their architecture preserved intact, can be studied.

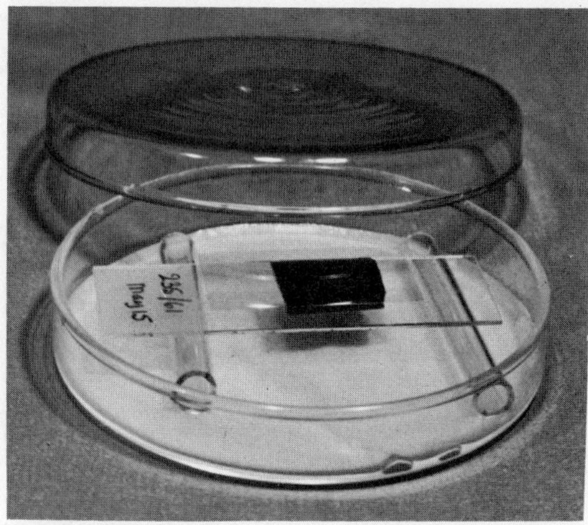

Figure 23–34 Slide culture technique.

Microscopic Examination of Cultures

The most useful stain for examining mounts of cultures is lactophenol cotton blue, which is made as follows:

Lactic acid	20 mL
Phenol	20 g
Glycerol	40 mL
Distilled water	20 mL

This mixture is heated gently in hot water to dissolve the solid components and then 0.05 g cotton blue is added. A small portion of the fungal colony is picked off the medium with a sterile mounted needle and placed in a drop of the stain previously placed on a slide. The drop is then covered by a coverslip. Fungal elements are stained deep blue and the background is pale blue. To make the mounts permanent the edges of the coverslip are sealed with cosmetic nail varnish.

CHAPTER 23—REVIEW QUESTIONS

1. Define *hyphae, mycelium, conidiophore, blastoconidium, favic chandeliers, zoophilic, pleomorphism, dimorphic growth.*
2. Give the three main genera of the dermatophytes. escribe how you would collect samples of skin for direct examination and culture for dermatophytes. What medium would you use and what temperature is optimal? How long would you keep the culture before discarding it as nondiagnostic? Describe the macroscopic and microscopic appearances of *M. canis.*
3. Give criteria for considering a growth of *C. albicans* significant. Describe the cultural appearance and the importance of the germ tube test in diagnosis.
4. What is *Ajellomyces capsulatus?* How does one prepare a culture to demonstrate diagnostic tuberculate spores of *H. capsulatum?* How long do they take to appear?
5. Describe the microscopic appearances of a sulfur granule in a case of actinomycosis. How would you culture it? What would the colonial appearance be in the medium you have selected, and what would be the microscopic appearance of the growth?

24

AN INTRODUCTION TO MYCOPLASMAL, CHLAMYDIAL, RICKETTSIAL, AND VIRAL DISEASE

In a book of this type, no more than a general introduction to this subject can be made. The outlines of the subject will be given and stress will be laid on those aspects that are important to the general hospital laboratory and to the technologists working in such institutions. We will assume that because of the basic differences in working with *Rickettsia, Mycoplasma, Chlamydia,* and viruses, most moderately sized general hospitals do not attempt culture but are concerned with the collection of specimens for culture by more specialized laboratories and with those diagnostic tests that have close similarity with methods employed in other branches of microbiology. The relationships and differences between these genera themselves and the viruses are shown in the accompanying table (Table 24–1).

MYCOPLASMAS

These organisms are the smallest free-living organisms known, and unlike other bacteria, they have no cell wall but are bounded merely by a cell membrane. They have a pleomorphic morphology and may be spheres (0.3 to 0.5 μm) or filaments. The cells do not stain with Gram's method but are poorly shown by Giemsa stain. There are at least 11 recognized species, some of which appear to be commensals. However, mycoplasmal (primary atypical) pneumonia is due to *M. pneumoniae,* whereas *M. hominis* and *Ureaplasma urealyticum* may cause nongonococcal urethritis as well as pelvic inflammatory disease in women. The latter organisms may behave as commensals and not as pathogens in the genital tract, and *M. pneumonia* may be found in the absence of pneumonia.

Diagnosis of Mycoplasma Infection

Many hospitals do not attempt culture of these organisms but send suitably collected samples to reference laboratories. Specimens on swabs are sent expeditiously and without any chance to dry, in a transport medium of 2 mL of trypticase soy broth with 0.5% bovine albumin and penicillin to prevent bacterial overgrowth. Sputum and blood may be submitted "as is." *M. pneumoniae*

TABLE 24–1 Relationships and Differences between *Mycoplasma*, Schizomycetes, *Chlamydia*, *Rickettsia*, and Viruses

	Mycoplasma	Schizomycetes ("Bacteria")	*Chlamydia*	*Rickettsia*	Viruses
Grow on cell-free medium	+	+*	−	−*	−
Generate metabolic energy	+	+	−	+	−
Cell wall present	−	+	+	+	−
Synthesize own protein	+	+	+	+	−
Both RNA and DNA present	+	+	+	+	−
Host cell DNA mechanism responsible for reproduction	−	−	−	−	+
Filtrable through 450 nm pore size filter	+	−*	+	+	+
DNA and RNA present	+	+	+	+	Either DNA *or* RNA: not both
Require sterols for growth	+*	−	−	−	−

*Some exceptions.

Adapted from Charnock, R.M., and Tully, J.G.: Mycoplasmas. *In* Davis, B.D., et al., eds.: Microbiology, 3rd ed. Hagerstown, Md., Harper & Row, 1980.

survives at 4°C for several days, but *M. hominis* may not survive.

Culture is made on complex media, which include agar and broth and diphasic medium (E. media). These incorporate such substances as yeast dialysate and horse serum as well as penicillin and thallium to inhibit bacteria. Colonies are very small (10 to 100 μm) and may take up to a month to appear after incubation at 37°C aerobically. The colonies are not only small but grow imbedded in the agar, presenting a typical "fried egg" appearance. *M. pneumoniae* causes hemolysis in overlaid guinea pig red cells (80% in saline agar) when the colonies are reincubated with the overlaid blood cells for 48 hours.

In mycoplasmal pneumonia, the diagnosis is generally made by the presence of cold agglutinins to human red cells. A titer greater than 40 is suggestive but not diagnostic of atypical pneumonia (p. 539). Occasionally this antibody is sufficient to cause hemolytic anemia in the patient. A complement fixation test is available and is more specific.

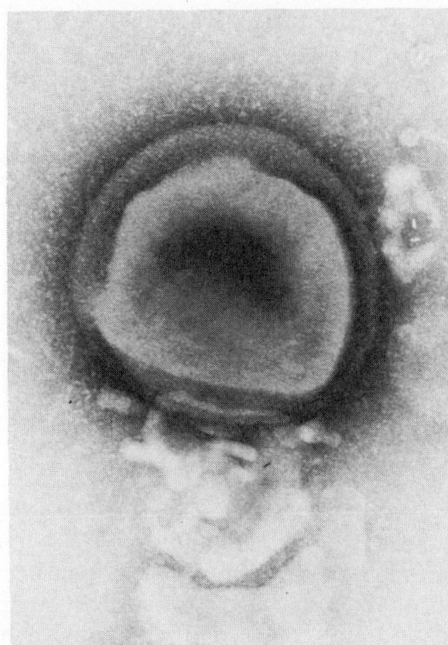

Figure 24–2 Chlamydia. Organism: *C. psittaci*. PTA stain × 100,000. (Courtesy of Dr. P. Blaskovic, Virus Laboratory, Public Health Laboratory, Province of Ontario.)

CHLAMYDIAE

These organisms are much like most bacteria but can only grow within host cells (obligate intracellular organisms). They depend on host cells for the production of their metabolic energy. There are two species. *C. trachomatis* causes the severe disease trachoma as well as benign inclusion conjunctivitis. In addition it is also causative of nongonococcal urethritis and lymphogranuloma inguinale. More recently it has been found responsible for pelvic inflammatory disease in women and for a type of pneumonia in the newborn. *C. psittaci* causes disease in birds that is transmissible to man and here is responsible for ornithosis or psittacosis. The organisms are small (0.25 to 0.35 nm) and can be stained, but not very well, by Gram's method; Giemsa stain is preferable.

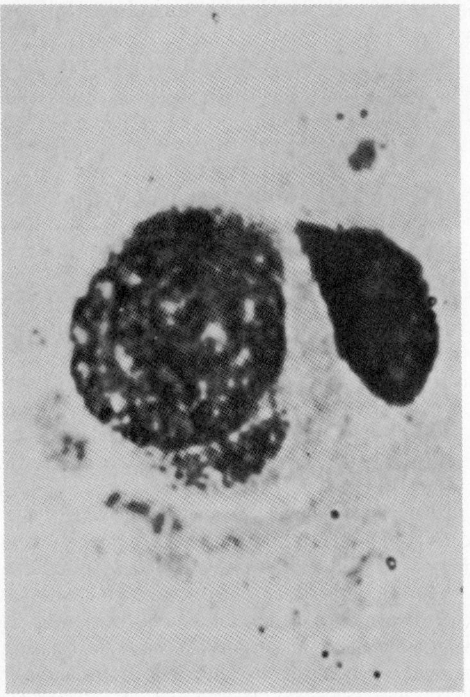

Figure 24–1 Inclusion conjunctivitis. Two typical crescents of granular bluish violet bodies are present close to the nucleus. Giemsa × 2250.

Specimens of pus, blood, sputum, and tissues can be kept at −20°C and referred to more specialized centers for culture. However, if the period of storage needs to be prolonged, −70°C should be employed. A transport medium of 0.2 M sucrose in a 0.02 M phosphate buffer at pH 7 and 5% fetal calf serum is said to keep the organism viable until it reaches cell culture. Material from psittacosis, it should be remembered, is very infectious, and all precautions must be taken. In trachoma–inclusion conjunctivitis infections, scrapings of conjunctival or other epithelium can be stained by a variety of methods, including Giemsa, and the inclusion particles can be seen as a crescentic mass in the cell cytoplasm.

RICKETTSIAE

These are also obligate intracellular organisms but in other respects are not unlike bacteria. There are a number of species, and with one exception (*Coxiella burnetii*), they are carried by lice, ticks, and mites. They are coccobacillary and are about 0.5 μm in greatest diameter. They are stained poorly by Gram's method and better with Giemsa. In North America, *R. rickettsii* causes Rocky Mountain spotted fever, which is spread to humans from rodents, dogs, or foxes by ticks. Elsewhere in the world, other rickettsiae are spread by arthropods from other mammalian hosts to man. Typhus (*R. prowazekii*) is worldwide and is spread from man to man by the body louse.

Diagnosis is often made serologically by the Weil-Felix test (see p. 538). Tissue and blood for culture should be kept frozen in dry ice (−70°C) and shipped expeditiously to the reference laboratory.

VIROLOGY

Definition of a Virus

A virus may be defined as an intracellular parasite that is unable to reproduce itself outside a living host cell, but these properties it shares with the rickettsiae and chlamydiae. In addition, viruses contain one type of nucleic acid (RNA or DNA) and at least one antigenically active protein. They are small but vary in size from about 10 or 20 nm to about 300 nm. Some other general features will become apparent in the description of the varieties.

Structure of Virus

The mature virus particle (virion) has a central core of DNA (deoxyribonucleic acid) or RNA (ribonucleic acid) surrounded by a protein coat (capsid) composed of a varied number of identical protein units (capsomeres). The capsid and the enclosed nucleic acid comprise the nucleocapsid. The virus has a determinable shape. Some are icosahedral, a pattern presenting 20 equal surfaces, each an equilateral triangle, with the capsomeres forming the surfaces; others have the capsomeres wound around the core; and some are tadpole shaped. Some icosahedral viruses contain an inner protein core in addition to the capsid. The helical viruses have their nucleocapsid arranged in a spiral, and some of the viruses in this group, as well as some icosahedral viruses, have an envelope of lipid. The envelope is obtained when the nucleocapsid is released from an infected cell. The capsule is not merely an acquired eukaryotic cell membrane, since the protein of the membrane is virus coded. These protein molecules of the envelope are known as peplomers (peplos = envelope).

Viruses appear to be the sole group of living things in which RNA may be the lone carrier of genetic information. The nucleic acid may be either single- or double-stranded.

Reproduction

The virus is able to multiply only within the cells of the host, and some viruses naturally require specific cell hosts in order to procreate. Thus, some prefer human cells, e.g., measles; others, animal cells, e.g., distemper. Others are less specific, e.g., the arboviruses, which may infect insects and man. Within the host, the virus may be discriminative; e.g., poliomyelitis enters the cells of the anterior horn of the spinal cord; mumps virus enters the cells of the salivary glands, pancreas, and nervous system; and bacteriophages are specific as to the strain of bacteria (often within a species) that they will infest. The selectivity, certainly in some cases, appears to be owing to the presence of receptor sites on the membrane of the cell and recognition attachment sites on the virion surface. When the virus is attached to the cell, it becomes engulfed or phagocytosed. Once within the cell, it loses its protein coat, possibly by lysosomal action. The naked DNA or RNA is then free to replicate, but the process in each instance is, of course, essentially different.

The genetic material seizes control of the host cell and replicates itself as well as organizing the manufacture of protein capsids that are then assembled to form new viral particles.

The inhibition of normal cellular DNA-RNA interactions by viral DNA is a highly specific action, since viral DNA-RNA interchanges continue apace. Whatever the messenger substances are in this inhibition, they are able to differentiate between viral and cellular chemicophysical activities. New units of virus appear and may be seen in the nucleus or cytoplasm of the cell as elementary bodies or as inclusion bodies. The latter presumably are aggregated elementary bodies. Finally, the virus breaks out and infects other cells, leaving the original host a gutted remnant.

METHODS OF CULTURE AND RECOGNITION

Since growth of virus can take place only in living cells, artificial culture demands either living animals or tissue culture.

Although many viruses are naturally cell specific, they may be grown artificially in other types of cell; e.g., polio virus may be grown in monkey kidney tissue. A tissue culture technique giving a monolayer of cells has been developed and has aided observation.

To prepare material for cell culture, the tissue is minced and subsequently the fragments are dispersed with trypsin. The cells are then resuspended in a growth medium generally consisting of a balanced mixture of salts, glucose with serum, albumin, or some more chemically defined nutrient (amino acids and vitamins) with sodium bicarbonate and antimicrobials. The cells are incubated at 37°C, and when they have formed an adequate monolayer, subcultures are made to a maintenance medium. This medium is designed to keep the cells alive and healthy but not to encourage growth.

The type of cells used will depend partially on availability and partially on the nature of the virus expected to be isolated. Monkey kidney, human amnion cells, and human thyroid are used but will die out. Continuous cell lines that are malignant or transformed cells are potentially immortal, and thus are always readily available. Such cells include HeLa cells from carcinoma of the cervix and KB cells from nasopharyngeal cancer. They grow quickly but are less susceptible to viral infection than diploid cells. Among the latter, human fetal cells can be preserved after primary growth at −70°C almost indefinitely, and although they will die out eventually in subculture, they live longer than other diploid forms and retain greater susceptibility to viral infection. Specimens received by the virology laboratory are processed in a number of ways before inoculation, and subsequently evidence of viral infection in monolayered culture may be recognized by any of four effects: the cytopathic effect, plaque formation, hemagglutination and hemadsorption, and interference.

The Cytopathic Effect (CPE). These may appear in a day or two, or may take up to several weeks. Essentially, they are morphological changes in the cells owing to viral proliferation. Some of the effects are shown in Figure 24–3. Some changes are specific enough for an experienced virologist to diagnose the type of viral infection. For example, the fusion of cells to form syncytia is highly suggestive of the paramyxoviruses and the herpes virus groups. Staining of the cultured cells

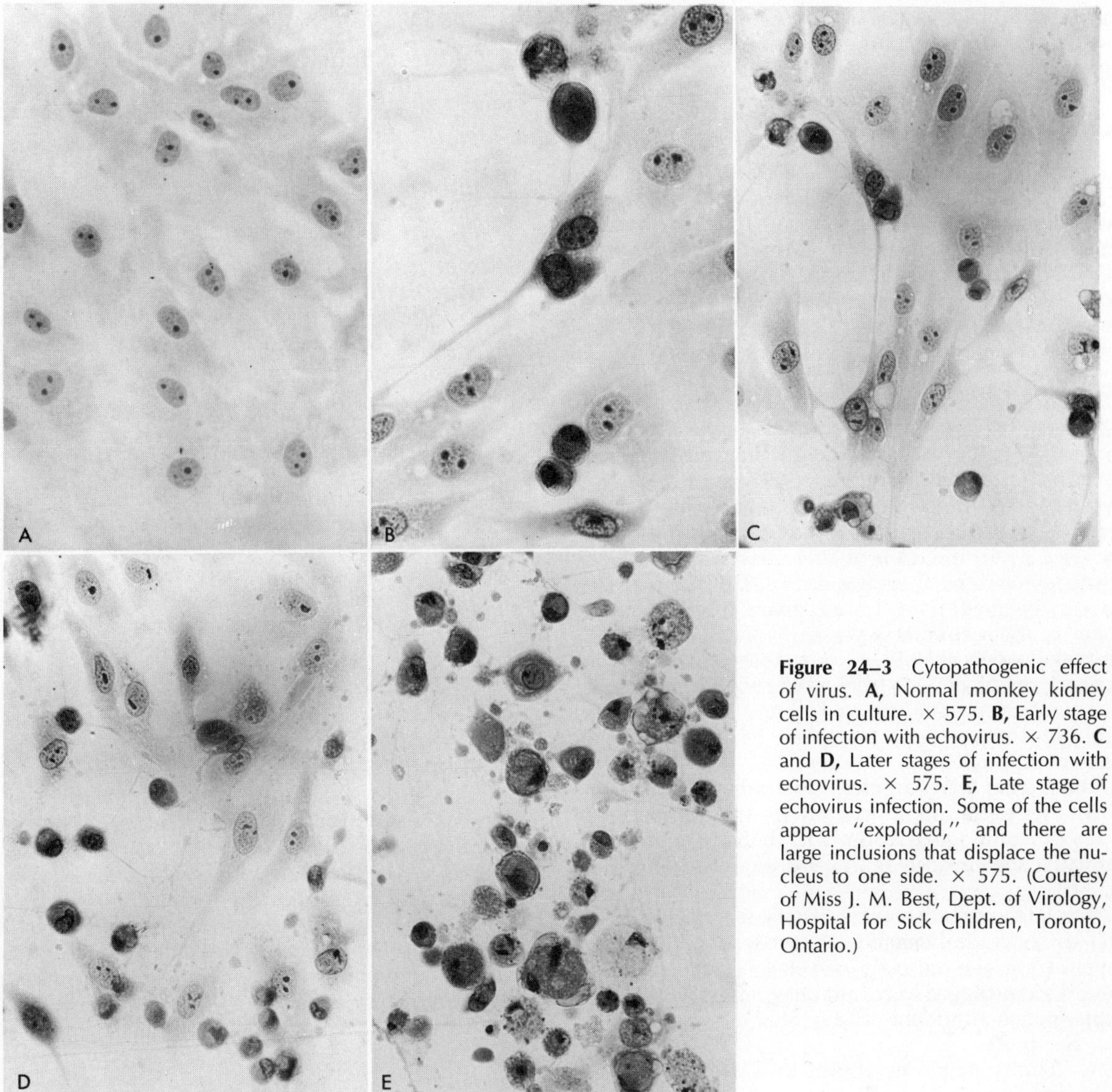

Figure 24–3 Cytopathogenic effect of virus. **A,** Normal monkey kidney cells in culture. × 575. **B,** Early stage of infection with echovirus. × 736. **C** and **D,** Later stages of infection with echovirus. × 575. **E,** Late stage of echovirus infection. Some of the cells appear "exploded," and there are large inclusions that displace the nucleus to one side. × 575. (Courtesy of Miss J. M. Best, Dept. of Virology, Hospital for Sick Children, Toronto, Ontario.)

may show diagnostic inclusion bodies, and fluorescent staining methods may yield an even more specific diagnostic pattern.

Plaque Formation. If a small amount of agar is incorporated in the maintenance medium, viral spread is somewhat reduced and infection more restricted to localized zones of the monolayer. This "plaque" effect may be well illustrated when present by staining with a vital dye such as neutral red. The monolayer then appears as a pink sheet with areas of clearness owing to the cytopathic viral effect preventing uptake of the dye.

Hemagglutination and Hemadsorption. Orthomyxoviruses (including influenza) and the paramyxovirus group have a glycoprotein in the outer part of the virion that will attach to a red cell bearing the required reception areas. The attachment of the virus to the red cells causes the latter to agglutinate. This phenomenon forms the basis of several tests for infection by this group of organisms, which parenthetically do not give a CPE in cell culture. However, cells of the infected culture will agglutinate introduced sensitive red cells around the cell membrane.

Interference. This method was used for viruses that showed no CPE. The principle is that superinfection by viruses does not generally occur. Thus a cell culture showing no CPE following inoculation, then resisting infection by a known CPE producing organism, was presumed to be infected by the first inoculum. The method is not used much now, since cell types demonstrating CPE with such viruses are much more readily available.

Fertilized chick eggs culture is much less used today than previously, but methods are available for the growth of viruses in one of several layers, e.g., the yolk sac, amniotic cavity, or chorioallantoic membrane. Some viruses growing on these structures produce grossly recognizable features or lesions resembling bacterial colonies.

Animal inoculation is also used to a lesser extent than previously, but suckling and adult mice as well as guinea pigs occasionally are used diagnostically.

Serological Methods in Diagnosis

The serological methods are essentially similar to those employed in other areas of microbiology, adapted to the phenomenon of virus infection. It is worthwhile emphasizing the importance of "paired" sera in virus disease diagnosis. Using this method, serum is taken in the acute and then in the convalescent stage of the disease (7 to 21 days apart). The rise in titer in the interval is considered highly significant if it is fourfold or higher.

The major serological methods are as follows:

Complement Fixation. The method employs known inactivated or even live virus as antigen and the other elements as described elsewhere (p. 527 and Fig. 26–6).

Neutralization. Immune serum can inactivate the potential infectivity of viruses. Thus prevention of CPE can be used as an indicator of such inactivation and of the antibody content of such a serum. Dilutions of the serum can be made and a titer given to express the efficiency of the serum in neutralizing CPE.

Hemagglutination Inhibition. For those viruses that agglutinate red blood cells (including rubella, influenza, California virus encephalitis, and others) immune serum will inhibit the response and thus be a test of the presence of antibodies.

Agglutination of Inert Particles. Red cells with antigen attached are used. Agglutination in the presence of antibody in challenging serum will indicate degrees of immunity. A system such as this is used in the detection of anti-HBs.

Indirect Immunofluorescence. Cells infected with a specific virus are challenged with test serum. Then, the presence of antigen-antibody complex is demonstrated by a fluorescein-tagged anti-immunoglobulin.

Counterimmunodiffusion. See p. 552.

RIA. See p. 91.

ELISA. The principle is similar to EMIT (p. 93) but is not a competitive system.

Electron Microscopy

This is now increasingly being used to differentiate, for example, pox viruses from herpes and to show rotavirus and other viruses in infantile or epidemic diarrhea.

Resistance of Virus

1. Viruses are resistant to antibacterial antimicrobials. The chlamydiae, which are sensitive to several such antimicrobials, are not viruses.
2. They are generally more resistant to antiseptics than bacteria but sodium hypochlorite, formaldehyde, and dilute hydrochloric acid are efficient.
3. Viruses can survive long periods at −70°C when freeze-dried. They are killed easily with moist heat but are somewhat more resistant to dry heat. Some are able to survive relatively long periods in dust.
4. Ultraviolet and X-irradiation inactivates viruses.
5. Chloroform and ether will inactivate viruses that have a lipid envelope.

Transmissions of Viral Disease

1. Droplet infection as in the common cold and influenza, or carried from skin lesions in smallpox.
2. Ingestion: poliomyelitis and probably infectious hepatitis.
3. Direct contact: verrucae.
4. Insect-borne: arboviruses.
5. Direct inoculation: serum hepatitis and rabies.
6. Latent: herpes virus may remain latent after initial infection, giving rise to no symptoms but becoming reactivated by some nonspecific stimulus such as fever.
7. Transplacental: the classic examples of viral infections passing from mother to child by this route are rubella, cytomegalovirus infection, and serum hepatitis.

CLASSIFICATION OF VIRUS DISEASE

Classification is difficult because the more usual methods (such as biochemical reactions, physical properties, and enzyme activity) are not available. To complicate matters, similar diseases may be caused by one of several types of virus, and conversely, similar viruses may produce many varieties of disease. However, classification may be based on the following factors: (1) size and morphology, (2) serological relationship, and (3) presence of a DNA or an RNA nucleus.

PICORNAVIRUS

Picornaviruses (pico = small, rna = RNA) include the enterovirus group; poliomyelitis, Coxsackie, and members of the echo group; the rhinovirus types; and the virus that causes foot and mouth disease in cattle. They are small nonenveloped icosahedrons 20 to 30 nm across and probably have 32 capsomeres. The *enterovirus group* is found primarily in the intestine but also in the upper respiratory tract.

Poliomyelitis

There are three types of poliomyelitis virus (1, 2, and 3) that may cause the disease. Entry is by mouth, and multiplication of the virus occurs in the alimentary tract and lymphoid tissue. Invasion of the central nervous system may be subsequent to later viremia or by retrograde direct spread along peripheral nerves from the sites of viral proliferation. The anterior horn cells of the spinal cord are most commonly affected, but the motor nuclei of the pons and the medulla are involved also in some cases.

Only about 1% of infections are clinically apparent. Other patients may merely exhibit slight fever, sore throat, or other minor disability recognized only when the virus is fortuitously recovered or the antibody identified. This is the abortive form. Some cases present as aseptic meningitis without paralysis, in which recovery is complete, and only the small minority have evidence of damage to the anterior horn cells with consequent flaccid paralysis.

It is believed that sewage contamination of drinking water or bathing water or dissemination by flies of contaminated sewage is most important in the spread of the disease, and this fits in well with the time of

TABLE 24–2 CLASSIFICATION OF VIRUSES

Nucleic Acid of Genome	Shape	Type	Human Disease and Viral Species
DNA	Icosahedral	Adenovirus	Upper respiratory tract diseases, follicular conjunctivitis, infantile diarrhea.
		Papovavirus	Papillomas, progressive multifocal leukoencephalopathy.
		Herpes virus	"Cold sores," herpes genitalis, varicella-zoster, cytomegalic inclusion disease, infectious mononucleosis, Burkitt's lymphoma, kerato-conjunctivitis, herpetic whitlow, Hass's disease of the newborn.
	Brick shaped, ovoid, complex	Pox virus	Smallpox, vaccinia, molluscum contagiosum.
RNA	Icosahedral	Picornavirus	Enteroviruses (including those of poliomyelitis), echovirus. Coxsackie—responsible for encephalomyelitis, myocarditis, meningitis. Rhinovirus—common cold.
		Reovirus	Rotavirus—gastroenteritis in children.
		Togavirus	Arbovirus causing encephalitis, dengue, hemorrhagic fevers, yellow fevers. Rubella.
	Helical	Coronavirus	Upper respiratory tract disease, infantile diarrhea.
		Bunyavirus	California encephalitis
		Orthomyxovirus	Influenza
		Paramyxovirus	Mumps, measles, respiratory syncytial disease.
	Bullet shaped	Rhabdovirus	Rabies
DNA or RNA	Bacteriophages		
	Hepatitis	Hepatitis A (RNA)	
		Hepatitis B (DNA)	
		Hepatitis non-A, non-B (?)	

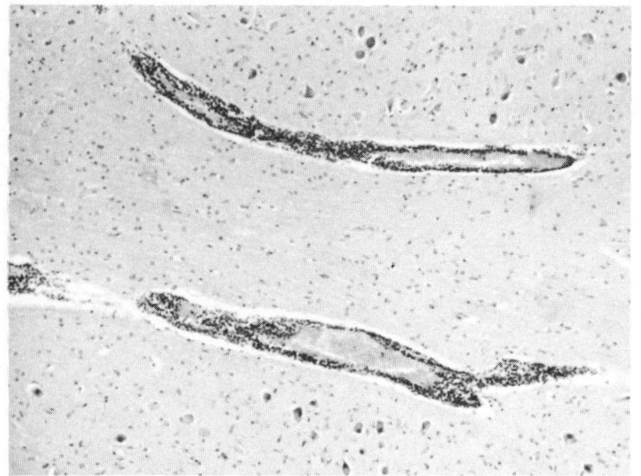

Figure 24–4 Poliomyelitis. Section of medulla showing perivascular cellular infiltration. × 115.

epidemics in the summer and fall. Virus has been recovered from house flies *(Musca domestica)* and other flies.

Epidemics of poliomyelitis are events of the past, however, since the introduction of Salk vaccine in the mid-1950's. This vaccine is of killed (formalinized) virus cultured on monkey kidney cells. Living but attenuated virus of all three types has virtually replaced the Salk inactivated vaccine.

In suspected cases, the virus may be recovered from throat washings and later from the feces. It is not recoverable from the CSF but is recoverable from the spinal cord of deceased patients. A fourfold increase in titer between acute-phase and convalescent sera is diagnostic.

Coxsackie Virus

The Coxsackie virus group includes numerous varieties responsible for a wide range of human disease. They have been divided into two groups, A and B; there are approximately 30 types in group A and six in group B. Group A virus types have been found responsible for herpangina, a disease of children that produces sore throat, vomiting, abdominal pain, and vesicular lesions in the throat or on the tongue. Type A 16 mainly has been found etiological in the hand-foot-and-mouth syndrome, which occurs in children and presents with stomatitis and a vesicular rash of the dorsal and palmar surfaces of the feet and hands, respectively.

Pleurodynia (Bornholm disease) is caused by types of B virus and is typified by chest and pleural pain with fever. Aseptic meningitis, myocarditis, acute pericarditis going on to constrictive pericarditis, and skin rashes are also produced by Coxsackie B viruses. Some meningitic patients may have paralysis, and some "colds" have been found caused by Coxsackie virus types.

Like other enteroviruses, Coxsackie may be isolated from pharyngeal washings early in the disease, and from the stool at later stages. It may also be found in the CSF. Rapid diagnosis is possible by immunofluorescent techniques, which have shown the presence of Coxsackie virus in circulating leukocytes. Paired serological samples are also useful in retrospective diagnosis. Dissemination of this group is probably associated with sewage and with flies.

Echoviruses

Echoviruses (*e*nteric *c*ytopathogenic *h*uman *o*rphan) were so named for their cytopathic effect on tissue culture cells; they were called "orphan" because when they were originally described, they had no "parent" disease. The word *enteric* refers to the primary site of proliferation. There are more than 30 types, and several have been proved pathogenic. Aseptic meningitis, occasionally with a rash, encephalitis, various exanthems with fever, isolated myocarditis, pericarditis, gastroenteritis, and vaginitis have been reported to be caused by echovirus types, as well as "colds" and other upper respiratory tract infections, but some still remain "orphans." The epidemiology is similar to that of other members of the enterovirus group and the virus is recovered from the stool, or from CSF in cases of aseptic meningitis.

The Rhinovirus Group

There are many varieties in this group, and many of them are responsible for "colds." In tissue culture, they require a lower temperature and pH than most viruses. Symptoms of the common cold need no description. Immunity appears independent of serum antibody and is probably more closely related to IgA secretion of the nasal mucosa. Type specific immunity lasts for several years. Immunity to other serotypes, initially complete, decreases over 3 to 4 months.

Nasal and pharyngeal washings are suggested methods for obtaining the virus.

REOVIRUSES

*R*espiratory *E*nteric *O*rphan virus is a double-stranded RNA virus (unlike other RNA viruses, which have a single strand) about 75 to 80 nm in diameter, which is icosahedral and has a double-layered capsid. Many of the genera in this group are not important in human disease, but one variety is causative of a common variety of infantile gastroenteritis.

Rotavirus

The organism so far has not been cultured, but diagnosis is made by electron microscopy, in which the characteristic appearance of the virus particles is diagnostic. About half of the severe cases of infantile gastroenteritis are due to this infection, which is particularly common in winter and fall. Other viruses that have also been associated with infantile diarrhea are adenovirus, calicivirus, astrovirus, and some coronavirus, all of which may be seen by electron microscopy. Epidemic diarrhea occurs in school-age children and adults in outbreaks, and one cause appears to be a type of parvovirus that has been called Norwalk agent. Again, it is seen under electron microscopy but has not been cultured.

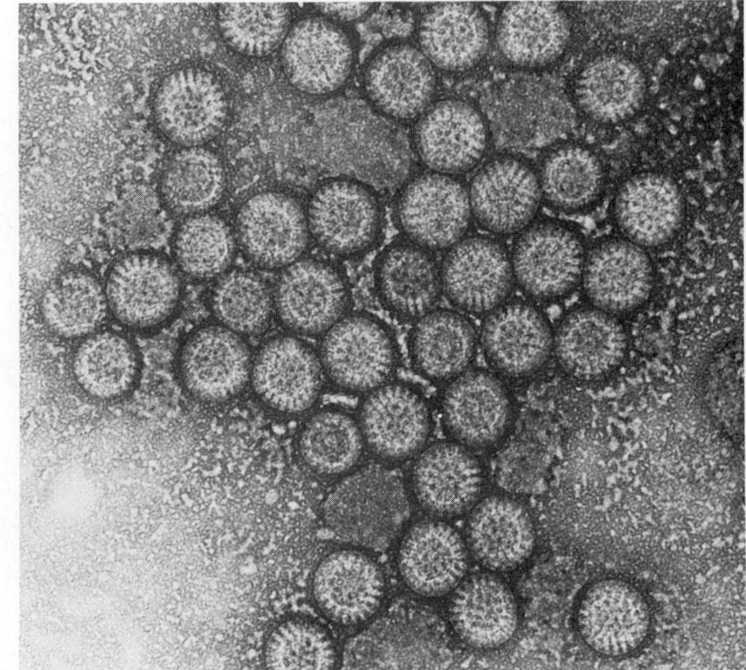

Figure 24–5 Rotavirus. Both smooth and rough forms are shown. The smooth (larger) particles resemble a wheel with short spokes. Uranyl formate stain × 200,000. (Courtesy of Dr. P. Blaskovic, Virus Laboratory, Public Health Laboratory, Province of Ontario.)

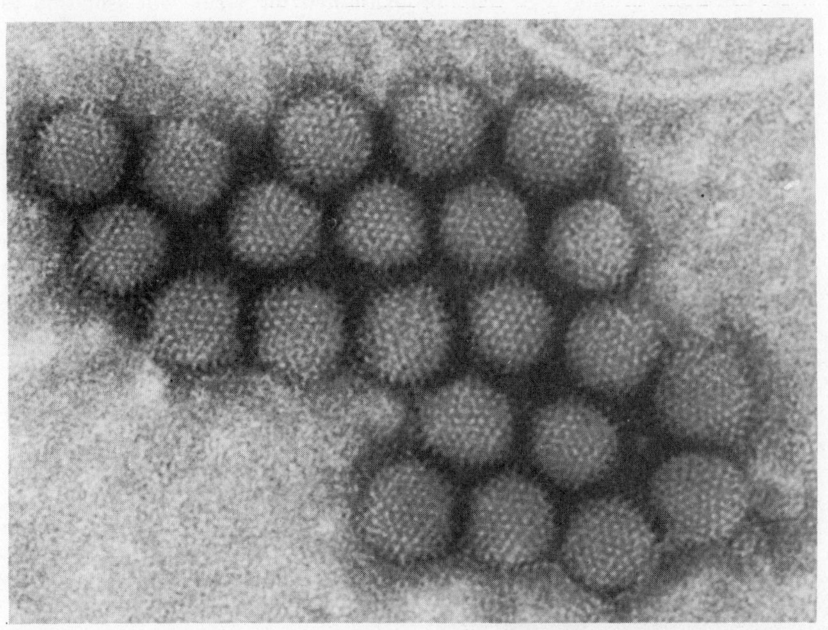

Figure 24–6 Adenovirus. Hexagonal particles with typical arrangement of surface capsomeres. PTA stain × 200,000. (Courtesy of Dr. P. Blaskovic, Virus Laboratory, Public Health Laboratory, Province of Ontario.)

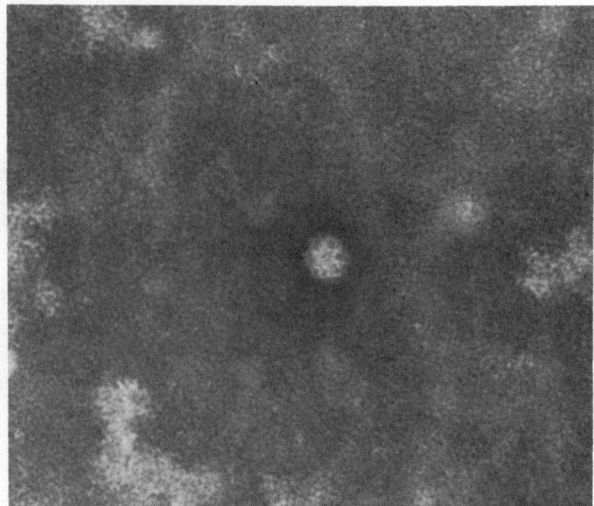

Figure 24–7 Calcivirus. The surface has rounded hollows arranged to give a Star of David pattern; the edges of the hollows form the arms of the star. PTA stain × 200,000. (Courtesy of Dr. P. Blaskovic, Virus Laboratory, Public Health Laboratory, Province of Ontario.)

ARBOVIRUSES (TOGAVIRUSES, BUNYAVIRUSES, AND OTHERS)

There are about 260 types of arboviruses (*ar*thropod *bo*rne = carried by insects), of which about 50 to 60 have caused disease in man. Morphologically, they are spheres of 40 to 60 nm in diameter, with a central icosahedral nucleocapsid around which there is a lipoprotein membrane. The single-stranded RNA of the nucleocapsid has a molecular weight of 3 to 4 million. Hemagglutination is shown by some of the arboviruses under certain conditions. Because of the desire to make viral nomenclature relate more to chemical and physical data, many in this group now are referred to as togaviruses, whereas some members have been reclassified as bunyaviruses and so forth. However, we shall retain the term *arbovirus*. The arbovirus is carried by a vector (mosquito, mite, or tick) from one host to another. Often humans are infected accidentally, since they are not part of the natural cycle (e.g., Murray Valley encephalitis normally is a disease of birds carried by mosquitoes). In other arbovirus diseases, humans may be the natural vertebrate reservoir (as in dengue). Many such diseases are found only in tightly localized geographic endemic areas, for example, the Murray Valley and Japan. Others are more widespread, such as the viruses causing sandfly fever, dengue, or yellow fever.

The Encephalitides

The infections are primarily of mammals and birds, and humans are involved as accidental hosts, as a result of a chance bite by a mosquito, tick, or mite.

The virus is maintained by the animal host in a particular geographic location and may be maintained in winter (when arthropods are absent) by migratory birds, in hibernating creatures, or by transovarial transmission by the arthropods.

The mosquito-borne varieties of the disease are believed spread by the natural host, the horse, and include Western and Eastern equine, Japanese, St. Louis, and Murray Valley encephalitides. The tick-borne conditions include Russian spring encephalitis, carried by ticks infected transovarially and from animals and also disseminated in goat's milk, and louping ill, which occurs in England and is carried from sheep. Powassan virus is maintained by groundhogs in Ontario and by squirrels in other parts of North America and is conveyed to man by ticks. California encephalitis is carried by mosquitoes, probably from rabbits, squirrels, and field mice.

Following the bite of the infected vector, the brain, especially the cerebral cortex, basal ganglia, cerebellum, and pons, is affected. Infiltration of perivascular spaces and meninges by mononuclear cells is seen, with the nonspecific changes of ganglion cell degeneration. Blood and CSF can be examined for virus, but isolation is difficult. Serological tests are available.

RUBELLA

On the basis of its physical and chemical properties, rubella is considered a togavirus, but it is not an arbovirus. It has an internal structure of RNA and protein and a lipoprotein envelope that is about 60 nm in diameter. The envelope possesses a hemagglutinin. The

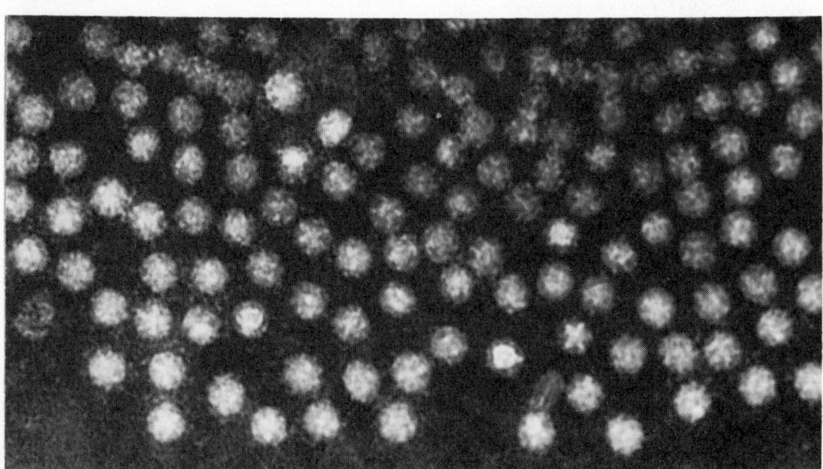

Figure 24–8 Astrovirus. The surface of the particles exhibits a starlike appearance. PTA stain × 200,000. (Courtesy of Dr. P. Blaskovic, Virus Laboratory, Public Health Laboratory, Province of Ontario.)

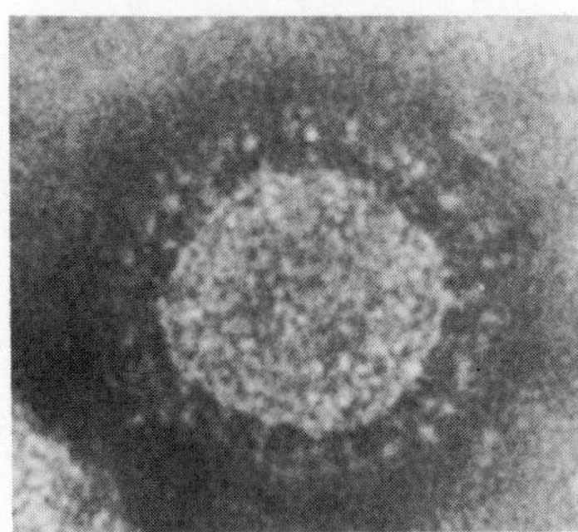

Figure 24–9 Coronavirus-like particles. The peripheral knobs give an appearance that resembles a crown. PTA stain × 200,000. (Courtesy of Dr. P. Blaskovic, Virus Laboratory, Public Health Laboratory, Province of Ontario.)

disease is benign in children, spread by droplet infection and entering the body through the respiratory tract. Subsequently there is viremia, and a rash appears about 3 weeks after the contact infection. Just after the rash appears, antibody is demonstrable in the circulating blood. There is generally little fever, and the rash is not as conspicuous as in measles; indeed, it may never appear. Lymph nodes are enlarged, especially those of the posterior occipital group.

The real importance of the infection is its effect on the fetus, especially if the mother suffers the disease during the first trimester of pregnancy. Infants affected by congenital rubella may show a remarkable spectrum of pathology that includes cataract, deafness, and microcephaly, and there is an increased incidence of spontaneous abortion and stillbirth. The infected fetus shows no immune tolerance to the virus and is born with circulating IgM that cannot be of maternal origin. A surviving child often excretes virus up to a year after birth. Other infectious diseases capable of producing congenital disease are the TORCH group (*T*oxoplasmosis, *O*ther agents such as syphilis, *R*ubella, *C*ytomegalovirus, *H*erpes simplex). Several manufacturers supply commercial kits to detect antibodies to *T. gondii*, rubella, CMV, and herpes simplex virus by ELISA or indirect fluorescent immunoassay.

Live attenuated vaccines are protective but do not appear to give as durable an immunity as the natural disease.

Virus may be obtained from throat washings early in the disease, but in congenital rubella, virus may be obtained from CSF, urine, amniotic fluid, and many other sites. A major effort is being made to identify teenage girls and prospective brides who have not yet had rubella, and also those women in the first trimester who are at risk of contracting the disease. The method of choice for detection is the serum hemagglutination inhibition (HI) test, and other tests are also available.

Other methods employ cells previously infected with rubella virus. Antibodies in serum will attach to such cells and can be demonstrated by fluorescent methods. In additional refinements, the attached antibody is revealed by an anti-immunoglobulin tagged with an enzyme. The latter, in turn, can be displayed by its reaction with its specific substrate. The amount of substrate that is altered is directly proportional to the amount of antibody. Such tests are available commercially and are also available extensively in reference centers.

CORONAVIRUSES

These are spherical single-stranded RNA viruses, 80 to 120 nm in diameter, in which the surface is covered by small pedunculated protrusions (peplomers) with club-shaped ends. These give the appearance of a crown and hence the name *coronavirus*. They are causative of many types of "cold" and upper respiratory tract infections as well as, possibly, some cases of diarrhea. Isolation is very difficult, and as a rule, serological testing is used in diagnostic efforts.

ORTHOMYXOVIRUSES

Myxoviruses are single-stranded RNA viruses (MW about 3 million) that are spherical or filamentous, about 80 to 120 nm in diameter, and that have a lipoprotein envelope. The latter has peplomers that exhibit hemagglutination properties.

The group is represented by the influenza virus.

Influenza

There are three types of the virus, A, B, and C. Type C is the only one that remains antigenically stable. Types A and B are clinically important; each includes numerous strains, and there is continual "antigenic drift." The latter results in the continual appearance of new strains that are related to changes in the envelope antigens. It is also possible that some new strains are from animal sources and are novel human pathogens. The sudden appearance of such different varieties ex-

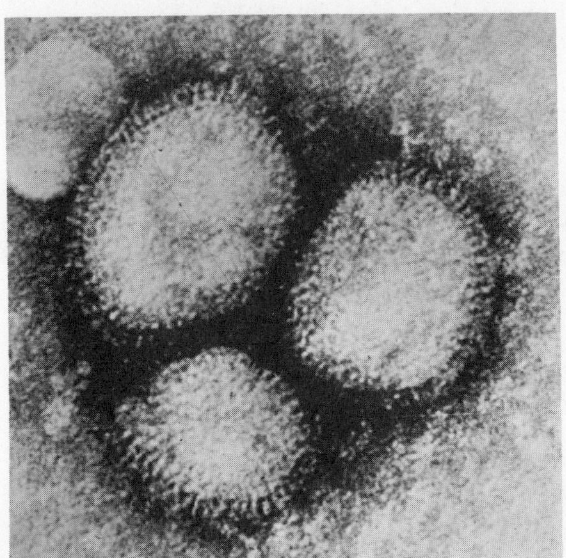

Figure 24–10 Influenza virus. Original magnification × 35,000. A group of viruses showing the characteristic projections on the lipoprotein envelope. These projections carry the hemagglutinins and the neuraminidase. (From the collection of the late Dr. M. J. Lynch.)

plains the pandemics of 1918, 1957, and 1968. The disease is spread by droplet infection and is manifested by fever, respiratory passage infection, and muscle aches. Epidemics or pandemics may occur. The viral infection is often complicated by secondary bacterial inflammation, especially by *Haemophilus influenzae,* and occasionally there is severe and even fatal pneumonia.

Diagnosis is by culture of throat washings on hens' eggs or on primate cell culture. Despite lack of CPE on the infected cell, hemadsorption is well illustrated. Serological studies employing the hemagglutinating properties of the organism are also employed. Rapid diagnosis may be made by using fluorescent-labeled antibody on cells from nasal swabs or throat washings. Immunity of the natural acquired type to any particular strain lasts for about a year and is more closely related to IgA in the respiratory secretions than to circulating IgG.

PARAMYXOVIRUSES

These are single-stranded RNA viruses (molecular weight about 7 million) in which the nucleocapsid is helically arranged with an irregularly shaped envelope of 100 to 300 nm that has tiny spiked protrusions. The envelope has a hemagglutinin, and some varieties have a neuraminidase whereas others have a hemolysin. The group includes parainfluenza, mumps, measles, and the respiratory syncytial virus.

Parainfluenza

There are four types, 1, 2, 3, and 4, and like influenza they will produce hemadsorption that can be inhibited by specific antisera. All produce acute respiratory tract infections, especially in children. Diagnosis is generally made by serological methods. Because of the lability of the virus, throat washings, if taken, should be inoculated into cell culture as soon as possible and not frozen.

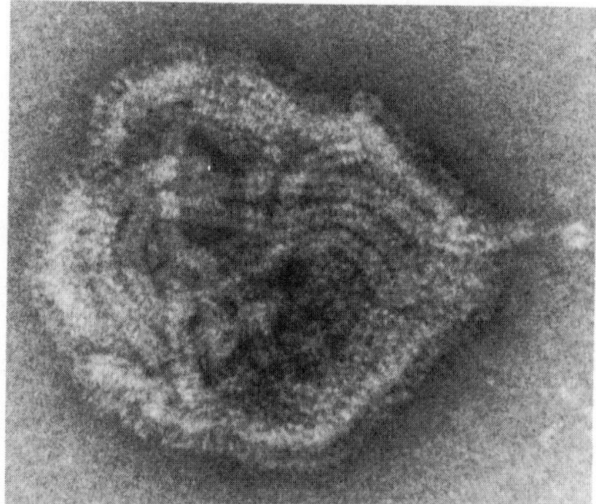

Figure 24–11 Paramyxovirus: mumps. The internal RNA strands and outer fringes of protrusions are visible. PTA stain × 200,000. (Courtesy of Dr. P. Blaskovic, Virus Laboratory, Public Health Laboratory, Province of Ontario.)

Mumps

This disease is carried by airborne particles or fomites, or it may be transferred by direct contact. The features of infection are well known. Generally both, or more rarely one parotid is enlarged and painful with pyrexia. Submaxillary glands are often involved and epididymo-orchitis occurs not infrequently in postpubertal cases. Pancreatitis, inflammation of the ovaries, and meningoencephalitis are well-known complications. The last-mentioned is sufficiently frequent to make mumps a comparatively common cause of aseptic meningitis. Infection originates in the respiratory tract, subsequently followed by viremia, which distributes the infective agent to the various loci described earlier. The virus may be obtained from throat washings, salivary gland ducts, and urine early in the disease and from the CSF in cases of mumps encephalitis. It is useful to know that in mumps, serum amylase is raised even though there may be no pancreatitis. Serological tests are also available. Complement fixation tests are of two types. Antibody to a soluble antigen (nucleoprotein) appears and disappears earlier than that to a V antigen (the viral surface), which persists for years. Hemagglutination inhibition (HI) may also be used, as well as a plaque reduction test in which the inhibitory effect of serum on the formation of viral plaques in culture medium can be measured.

Measles (Rubeola)

Infection is by droplet spread from other children in the catarrhal phase of the disease who remain infectious until a few days after the exanthem appears. The virus multiplies in the respiratory tract and is subsequently distributed elsewhere by macrophages and lymphocytes. Koplik's spots, part of the exanthem, appear as tiny red patches with white centers on the buccal mucosa and are present a day or two before the skin rash appears. The rash is probably allergic in origin, resulting from reaction of antigen in the skin and sensitized cells. Circulating antigen commences to appear in the blood about 2 weeks after the initial viral infection of the lung.

Because of the potential dangers of superimposed bacterial infections, vaccine to measles is now widely used, and a satisfactory attenuated virus vaccine is now available.

Apart from the complications of secondary bacterial infection in the natural disease, there is the possibility of encephalitis, but this is relatively rare (0.1% of cases). The encephalitis has a high mortality, with a death rate of about 15%. If encephalitis occurs, it commences about 2 weeks after the rash and histologically it appears to resemble an allergic encephalomyelitis rather than a primary viral infection. Another cerebral complication is subacute sclerosing panencephalitis, a chronic, slow progressive encephalitis now found to be caused by measles. The virus, possibly carried by lymphocytes, is tolerated by the host in an immunologically sequestered area where it can proliferate and cause anatomic damage. Infants with defects of their cellular immune mechanisms who acquire measles have no rash, and the disease is generally fatal. In the lungs there is a characteristic histological picture of Hecht's giant cell pneu-

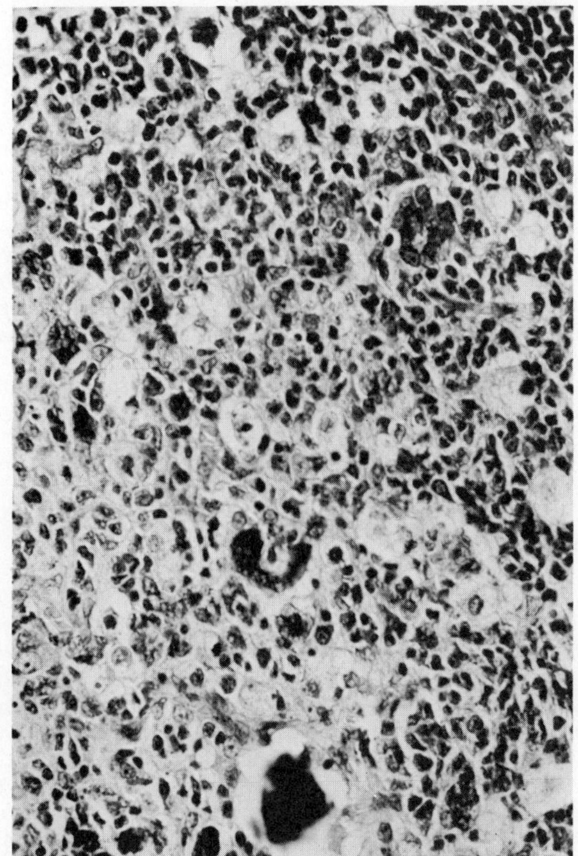

Figure 24–12 Measles. Giant cells (Warthin-Finkeldey) in lymphoid tissue of appendix. × 460.

monia. Some of these cases have occurred in leukemic patients either because of the immunosuppressive nature of the disease or because of the effect of therapeutic agents. In these patients, there is a remarkable persistence of measles virus in the upper respiratory tract. It should be noted that measles virus involves the leukocyte, especially the lymphocyte, and this has been cited as the basis for the loss of tuberculous hypersensitivity in patients with measles.

Laboratory diagnosis is made if required from nose or throat washings or from the blood before the appearance of the rash. After the rash appears, viral isolation may be made from the urine. Characteristic giant cells (Warthin-Finkeldey) with viral cytoplasmic and nuclear inclusions can be found in smears from nasal mucus. They are also seen in lymphoid tissue, particularly in the appendix, removed in the prodromal period. The virus cannot be isolated from cases of encephalitis for the reasons already cited. Virus has, however, been obtained with difficulty from the brain in subacute sclerosing panencephalitis. Rapid diagnosis of measles may be made by fluorescent techniques on the cells of the urinary sediment. Serological methods are also available; commonly hemagglutination inhibition is used.

Respiratory Syncytial Virus

Measles, mumps, parainfluenza 2, and respiratory syncytial virus produce syncytial cells in tissue culture, and the respiratory syncytial virus appears to be a common cause of respiratory disease in small infants (Adam's epidemic pneumonitis of infants). In adults, reinfection may be responsible for some "colds." In the lungs of deceased infants, giant cells are seen that have cytoplasmic inclusions (but not cytoplasmic and nuclear inclusions, as are present in measles).

The virus is somewhat different from other paramyxoviruses. It does not have a hemolysin or a neuraminidase, and will not survive more than a few hours at 4°C. Infants are not protected by maternal antibodies, since the essential IgA does not cross the placenta. Laboratory diagnosis can be made by culturing the virus from throat or nasal washings, but the time between collection and culture should be minimal (up to 3 to 5 hours at 4°C).

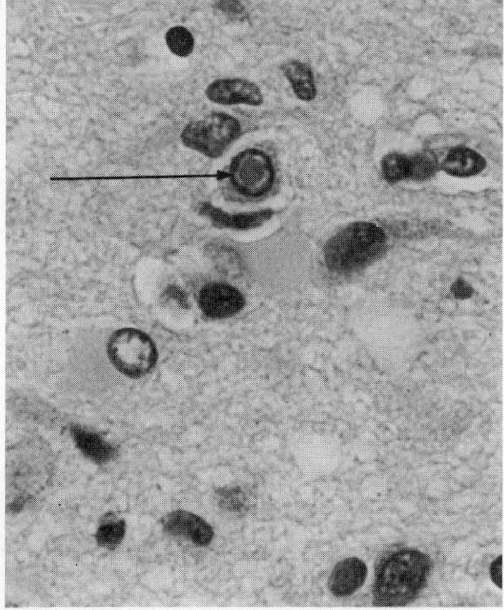

Figure 24–13 Subacute sclerosing panencephalitis due to measles virus. The eosinophilic intranuclear inclusion is indicated by the arrow. Note also the margination of the cytoplasm around the nucleus. Hematoxylin-eosin × 730.

RHABDOVIRUSES

The viruses in this group have a single-stranded RNA in a helical capsomere and a molecular weight of about

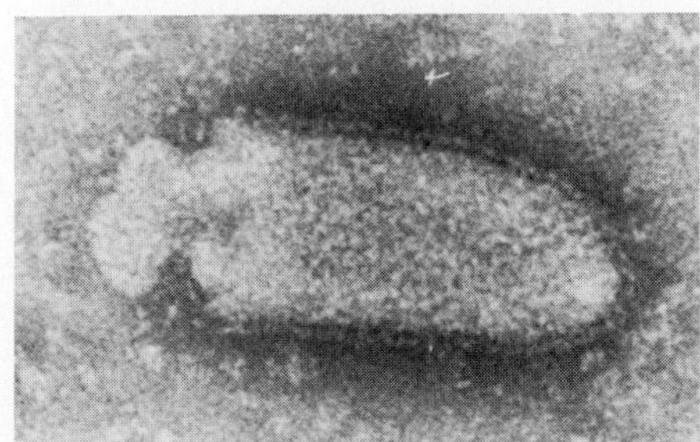

Figure 24–14 Rhabdovirus: rabies. A bullet-shaped particle covered by a fringe of tiny projections. PTA stain × 200,000. (Courtesy of Dr. P. Blaskovic, Virus Laboratory, Public Health Laboratory, Province of Ontario.)

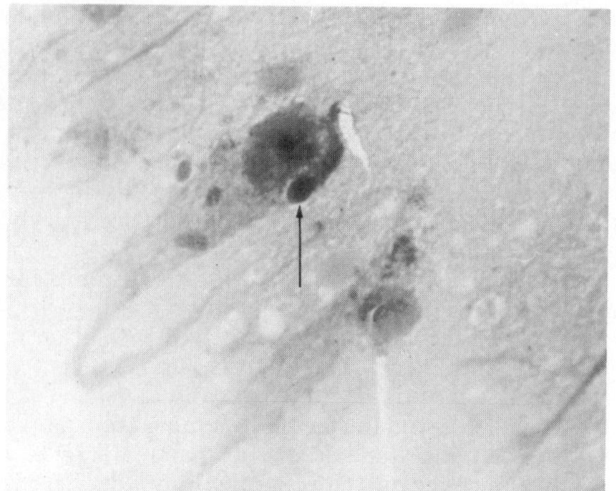

Figure 24–15 Rabies. Touch preparations of hippocampus showing Negri body indicated by arrow in the cytoplasm of the nerve cell. From a boy who died after being bitten by a rabid skunk. Mann's stain × 730. (Courtesy of Dr. W. L. Donohue, Hospital for Sick Children, Toronto, Ontario.)

5 million. There is a lipoprotein capsule, and the virion is bullet-shaped (180 × 75 nm). The important medical member of the group is rabies. Marburg disease, which is a natural disease of monkeys, has occasionally been fatal in humans.

Rabies

In nature, rabies causes disease in carnivores or omnivores who transmit the disease by bites. The vampire bat can transmit the disease without being infected. Infection has occurred subsequent to corneal transplantation in which the transplant was taken from a patient dying of rabies undiagnosed at the time of death. The incubation period is from less than 2 weeks to several months. About 10% of those bitten by rabid animals contract the disease, which when established, with rare exceptions, has been fatal. Diagnosis is confirmed by postmortem examination of the rabid animal, in which typical Negri bodies are seen in the cells of Ammon's horn and the Purkinje cells of the cerebellum. However, since 10 to 20% of infected animals do not have demonstrable Negri bodies, suspension of the brain tissue is inoculated intracerebrally into young mice. The latter will develop clinical symptoms and show Negri bodies and circulating antibodies. Negri bodies may be shown more readily by immunofluorescent techniques than by the conventional histopathological methods. In the infected patient, virus may be recovered after animal passage from the saliva or the CSF.

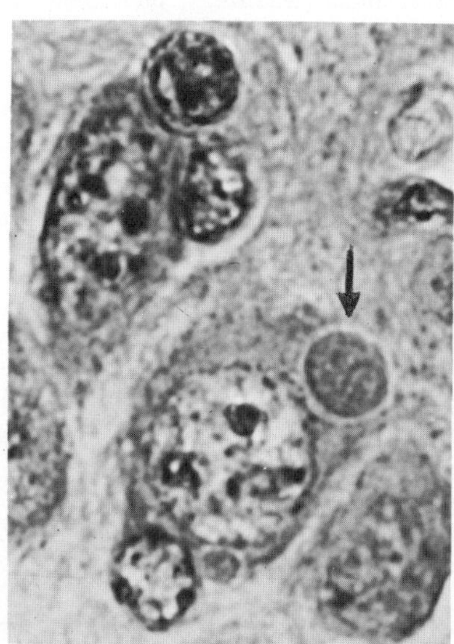

Figure 24–16 Negri body (arrow) in nerve cell of cerebellum from a rabid dog. Mann's stain × 2250.

Protection may be given passively by antirabies human immunoglobulin. Active immunization is by killed vaccine from duck embryo culture (DEV) or from a vaccine grown on human embryo lung cell culture.

ADENOVIRUSES

These were so called since they were first isolated from surgically removed tonsils and adenoids. There are about 30 human types; they have a DNA double-stranded core with a molecular weight of 20 to 25 million, an inner protein core, and an outer icosahedral capsid 70 to 80 nm in diameter. There are 252 capsomeres, and from 12 of these, there are "antennae" with a terminal "knob." There is no envelope. They cause a wide range of diseases, mainly respiratory, including one type of "atypical pneumonia," and also follicular conjunctivitis or pharyngoconjunctival fever, epidemic keratoconjunctivitis, and some cases of infantile diarrhea. The organisms may be found in cases of aseptic meningitis and febrile myalgic conditions. The virus may be recovered from the appropriate site, or diagnosis may be made by serological means.

Generally, the diseases caused by adenoviruses run a relatively benign course, and even the corneal opacities caused by keratoconjunctivitis resolve.

A few fatal cases have occurred in infants (Goodpasture's disease), when there is predisposition by debilitating conditions. In normal children the tonsils and adenoids often carry apparently saprophytic adenovirus, which appears to survive there in a few cells multiplying at a slow rate.

Laboratory diagnosis may be made by recovering the virus from throat washings or from the conjunctiva. Complement fixation tests are also available.

PAPOVAVIRUSES

The name is taken from the descriptive words, *pa*pilloma, *po*lyoma, and *va*cuolating, which summarize the oncogenic activities of this group. They are double-stranded DNA viruses with a molecular weight of 3 to 5 million and have 72 capsomeres. The virion is about 45 to 55 nm in diameter. There is no envelope. They cause warts and condylomas in humans. They are the only definite viral cause of tumors in humans known at this time. However, it is widely accepted that Epstein-Barr virus (of the herpes group) has a role in the etiology of Burkitt's lymphoma. Type 2 herpes simplex virus is suspected of having some part in the causation of cancer of the cervix, but the evidence here is weaker. Polyoma virus, simian virus 40, adenovirus, and Marek's disease virus are DNA viruses that cause cancer in animals. Rous sarcoma virus, avian leukosis virus, and others are RNA viruses that are also oncogenic in animals.

In some cases of advanced malignant disease, progressive multifocal leukoencephalopathy occurs. This is a diffuse degenerative disease of brain neurones with gliosis. Virus particles resembling papovavirus have been found in this condition (Fig. 24–17).

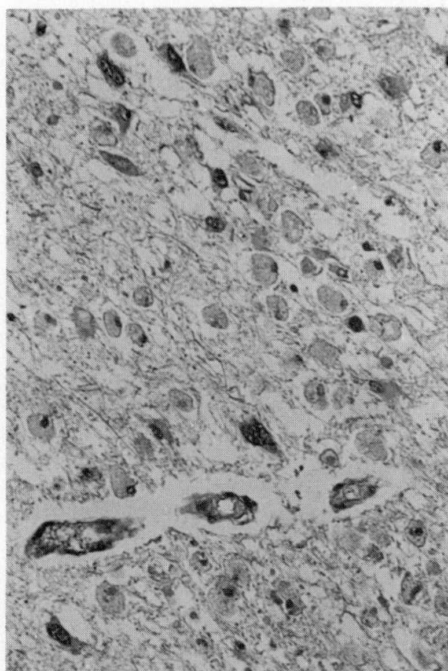

Figure 24–17 Progressive multifocal leukoencephalopathy. From the brain of a patient with Hodgkin's disease. Enlarged nuclei and inclusions are found in the supporting cells of the cerebral substance. SV40, a papovavirus, has been isolated from the brain in some cases. Possibly disturbance of immune mechanisms with the neoplastic process plays some part in such infections. Hematoxylin-eosin × 80.

HERPES VIRUS GROUP

These include the viruses that cause herpes simplex, varicella, and zoster, and also the Epstein Barr virus and cytomegalovirus. The viruses are icosahedral and about 150 to 200 nm in diameter with a double-stranded DNA core (MW 70 to 100 million) and 162 capsomeres. There is a lipoprotein capsule obtained which the newly assembled virion takes from the nucleomembrane when it leaves the nucleus of the cell in which it is formed.

Herpes Simplex

The virus may produce a wide range of clinical infections. Acute gingivostomatitis (one form of aphthous stomatitis) is an acute disease occurring in early childhood with vesicular lesions of the mouth and fever. The condition must be differentiated from herpangina (see under *Coxsackie Virus*), in which the lesions are generally on the fauces. After the primary infection, the virus may lie dormant and be stimulated into activity by fever, producing herpes labialis or other herpes, generally at a mucocutaneous border. Such herpes is recurrent but in the intervals between eruptions there is no evidence of the symbiotic virus. It appears that the virus remains dormant in the sensory ganglion of the trigeminal nerve. Fever or some other stimulus causes the virus to become reactivated and to spread down the sensory fibers to the nerve endings and the skin. There it proliferates and produces the characteristic "cold sore."

Eczema herpeticum is herpes infection complicating infantile eczema. Keratoconjunctivitis may be owing to primary or recurrent herpetic infection. Herpes virus may cause benign aseptic meningitis or encephalitis with a mortality as high as 70%. Herpetic whitlow, which follows minor trauma to the finger, is an unusual occupational hazard of doctors, dentists, and nurses involved in the care of patients with herpetic lesions. Hass's disease, or disseminated herpes of the newborn, is transferred from genital lesions in the mother either in the birth canal or possibly transplacentally. The child

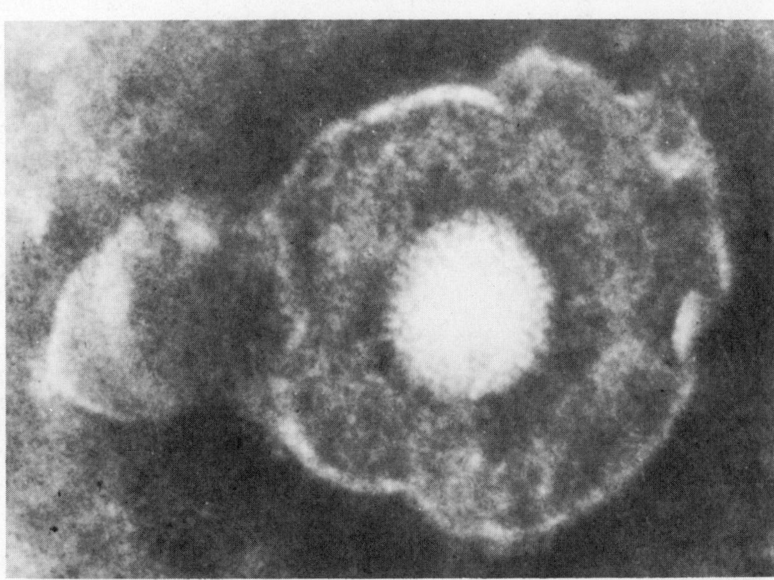

Figure 24–18 Herpes simplex. Original magnification × 40,000. The icosahedral capsid is seen within a lipoprotein envelope. (From the collection of the late Dr. M. J. Lynch.)

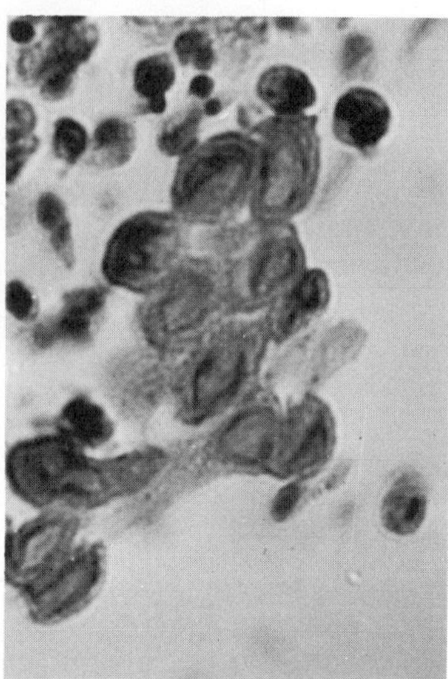

Figure 24–19 Herpes simplex: Section from a lesion of the scalp. A group of typical epithelial cells with large hyalinized nuclei is well illustrated. Hematoxylin-eosin × 133.

becomes ill a few days after birth and is dead in a few more days. At autopsy, necrosis is seen in the liver and adrenal glands especially, and cells at the margins of such lesions often show typical intranuclear inclusions. Vulvovaginitis occurs both in children and in adult women. Type 2 herpes simplex virus is the cause of genital herpes. It is recurrent, like labial herpes, which is described above and is generally caused by herpes simplex type 1. The herpes type 2 virus may remain dormant in the ganglia of the sacral plexus. With the routine Papanicolaou technique in female patients, typical multinucleate cells are seen and the viral inclusions may be recognized. The presence of such cells is diagnostic of genital herpes. The virus may be isolated from vesicles, ulcers, saliva, or CSF. The immunofluorescent techniques are used on smeared preparations or histological material. Since the genital lesion, when it is active, is infectious by contact, genital herpes is a venereal disease that in recent years, with greater promiscuity, has become widespread. Numerous serological tests are also valuable. A rising titer on serial specimens is, of course, significant. Acute and convalescent sera from those with recurrent herpes have a continually high antibody titer that is not altered with the clinical status of the disease. Scrapings from the lesion stained by simple techniques (H and E, Papanicolaou or Giemsa) will show the characteristic giant cells and the typical nuclear changes.

Varicella-Zoster

The viruses that cause varicella (chickenpox) in children and zoster (shingles) in adults appear to be identical. Adults with zoster may infect children, who develop varicella. Both diseases are too well known to require any description. Varicella pneumonia is not uncommon but is usually benign. However, in children with impaired immunological defenses, fatalities occur. Children with leukemia are prone to disseminated varicella, because of either the disease or the antileukemic measures. Zoster occurs in those who have had varicella in the past. The virus remains latent in the posterior root ganglia until reactivated by some stimulus. In some cases, the stimulus may be a condition such as leukemia or Hodgkin's disease, but in the vast majority of cases the nature of the stimulus is obscure and benign.

The virus may be recovered from skin vesicles, spinal fluid, or autopsy material. Biopsy or smeared preparations may be examined for inclusion bodies, and serological tests are available. The latter include complement fixation tests and indirect fluorescence.

Cytomegalovirus

The manifestations of infection by the virus are extremely varied. In infants, the disease is acquired early, and these cases are subclinical. Disseminated or fulminating disease is also seen in infants and is contracted *in utero*. Less acute disseminated disease is a second clinical form, and an opportunistic type occurs with leukemia and malignant disease. Cytomegalovirus has been incriminated in posttransfusion mononucleosis or the "post-pump" syndrome following open heart surgery. Intact leukocytes can carry the virus. In this condition examination of the peripheral blood shows features of infectious mononucleosis, but the serological tests for this condition are persistently negative. However, antibody titers against CMV will show a diagnostic quadrupling during the course of the disease, and the cytomegalovirus may be isolated from the throat. Other varieties of "seronegative infectious mononucleosis" include Q fever and toxoplasmosis. An occasional case of CMV mononucleosis without a history of blood transfusion has been encountered. Liver disease, the result of a chronic, slow-developing CMV infection, has been described occurring in children between 6 months and 8 years old.

The affected cell typically shows both nuclear and cytoplasmic inclusions. In hematoxylin-eosin preparations the nucleus is shown to be enlarged by red-violet inclusions and is surrounded by a halo and then by thickened nuclear membrane. The cytoplasm of such a cell is more basophilic and granular than usual. Freshly collected urine from cases of suspected disseminated disease should be diluted with equal quantities of 70 to 90% alcohol to preserve the diagnostic cells. Cell excretion is not continuous, and several specimens should be obtained. Concentration by a Millipore technique may be advantageous. Congenitally infected infants, as indicated, may show differing clinical syndromes, but among the more common symptoms in clinical cases are low birth weight, splenomegaly and hepatomegaly, microcephaly, mental retardation, petechiae and hemorrhagic pneumonitis owing to thrombocytopenia, inclusion pneumonitis, jaundice caused by hemolytic anemia, chorioretinitis, and cerebral calcification. A postnatal infection in children may result in hepatitis.

The virus may be isolated from urine, leukocytes, saliva, and biopsy material. It is not stable at low temperatures, and the specimen should be dealt with as soon as possible. Specimens should be kept at 4°C rather than in dry ice. Urine can be mixed with an equal volume of 70% sorbitol in distilled water. Swabs, throat washings, tissues, and other specimens are also kept in

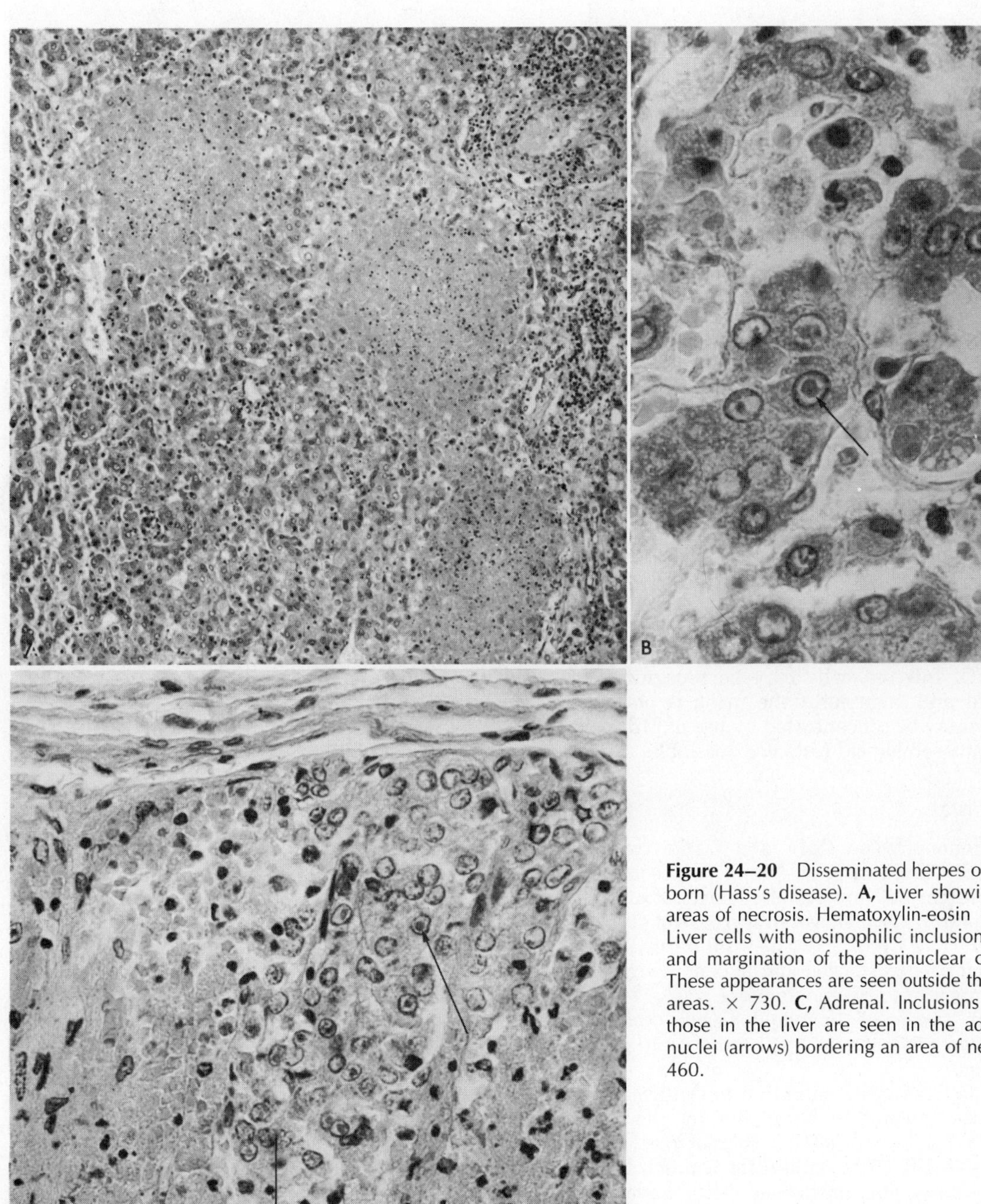

Figure 24–20 Disseminated herpes of the newborn (Hass's disease). **A,** Liver showing typical areas of necrosis. Hematoxylin-eosin × 115. **B,** Liver cells with eosinophilic inclusions (arrows) and margination of the perinuclear cytoplasm. These appearances are seen outside the necrotic areas. × 730. **C,** Adrenal. Inclusions similar to those in the liver are seen in the adrenal cell nuclei (arrows) bordering an area of necrosis. × 460.

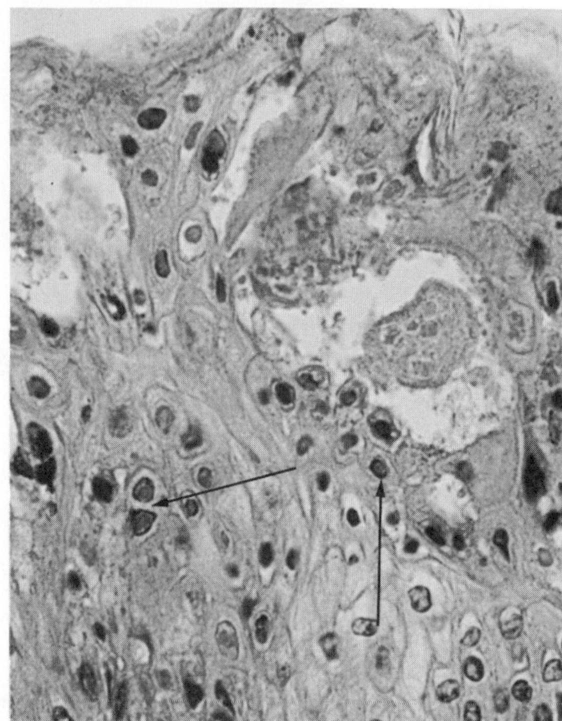

Figure 24–21 Varicella. Early vesicle of chickenpox showing eosinophilic intranuclear inclusions (arrows). Hematoxylin-eosin. × 460.

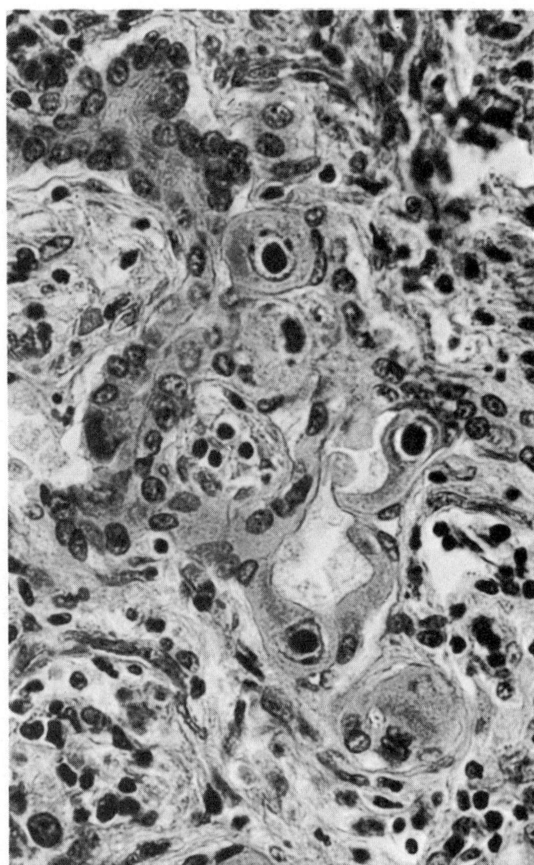

Figure 24–22 Cytomegalovirus. Liver in generalized cytomegalic inclusion disease. Note the dense amphophilic intranuclear inclusions in the epithelial cells of an interlobular bile duct. There is also the typical clear area around the inclusions, and paucity of inflammatory response.

sorbitol diluent (50% aqueous sorbitol and an equal volume of tissue culture medium) if it is desired to keep them at −70°C. Infected cells may be recognized in biopsy material and in urine if the urine is obtained fresh, and they may be concentrated by use of Millipore filters. Numerous serological tests are available.

Epstein-Barr Virus

Infectious mononucleosis (IM) is a fairly common disease, generally presenting in young people as malaise, fever, sore throat, and lymphadenitis. Examination of the peripheral blood shows an increase of atypical lymphocytic cells (see Chap. 29). The viral nature of the disease has long been suspected and it is now virtually proven. Most infections are symptomless.

A malignant tumor of lymphoid tissue occurring mainly in African children (Burkitt's lymphoma) is also due to this virus.

The current laboratory examination to confirm IM is by review of the peripheral blood and by the Paul-Bunnell test or some modification thereof (see Chap. 26). Antibodies to EB virus remain for a much longer period than do heterophil antibodies. They have been found as late as 37 years after the acute disease, whereas the heterophil antibodies are demonstrable in abnormal titer for only a few months. It is likely in the future that the presence of antibody to EB virus will be the parameter of measurement in the diagnosis of IM.

POX VIRUSES

Pox viruses are oval or brick shaped and up to 300 nm in diameter. They have a core of double-stranded DNA with a molecular weight of 160 to 200 million. There is a complicated envelope of lipoprotein, of which the lipid is uniquely virus specified. Within the group are the viruses that cause vaccinia and variola (smallpox), numerous animal and bird pox viruses, the virus of molluscum contagiosum, and that of rabbit myxomatosis.

Variola and Vaccinia

The last natural case of smallpox occurred in Somalia in 1977. The defeat of this historic affliction of humans was a great victory for preventive medicine. The smallpox virus (variola) is now kept alive in a few research centers only. In one of these centers, in England, the virus escaped in 1978, and two cases of smallpox resulted. Nevertheless, for all intents and purposes, the disease is no longer extant. Vaccinia was originally cowpox virus maintained through animal inocculation and was the virus used to immunize against smallpox. This followed the classic observations of Jenner in 1798 that cowpox—a benign disease in humans—protects against the severe and often fatal smallpox. Over the course of time, the original cowpox underwent antigenic change and may have been mistakenly replaced by attenuated smallpox virus.

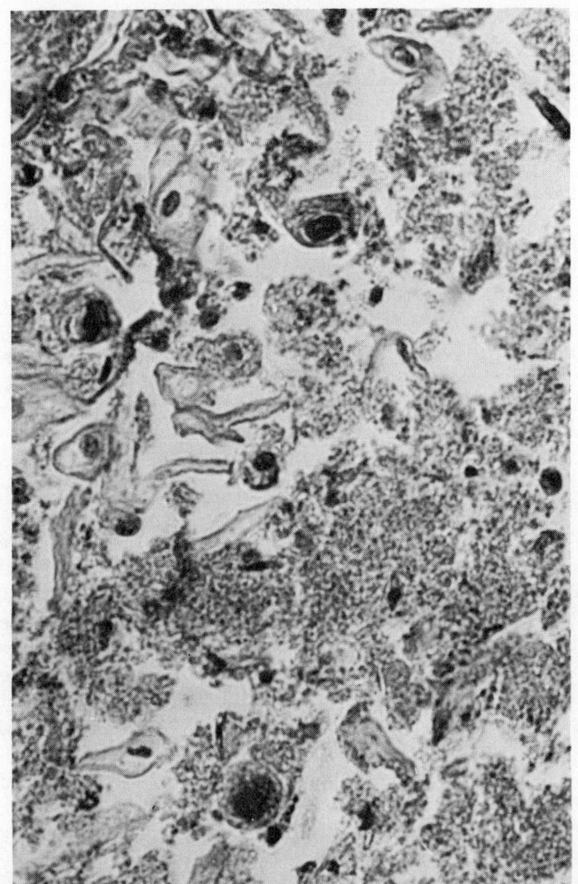

Figure 24–23 Cytomegalovirus. Cell block of urinary sediment. Note the several epithelial cells with the large dense nuclei. The infant had hepatosplenomegaly, thrombocytopenia, and jaundice. He survived the infantile illness but was left mentally retarded. Hematoxylin-eosin × 83.

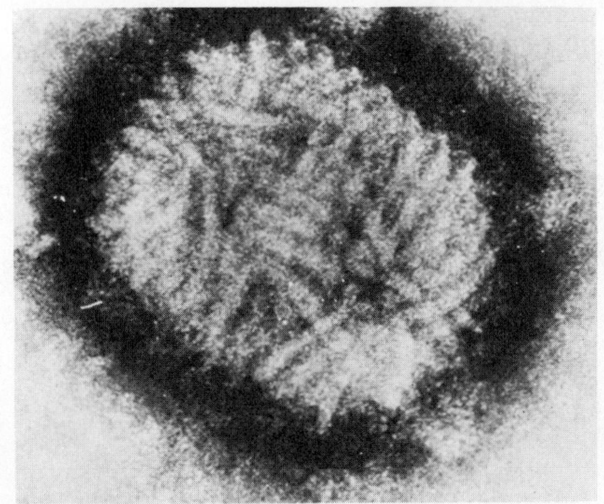

Figure 24–24 Pox virus (molluscum contagiosum). Original magnification × 40,000. The complicated tubular lipoprotein membrane covering of the squat brick-shaped virion is illustrated. (From the collection of the late Dr. M. J. Lynch.)

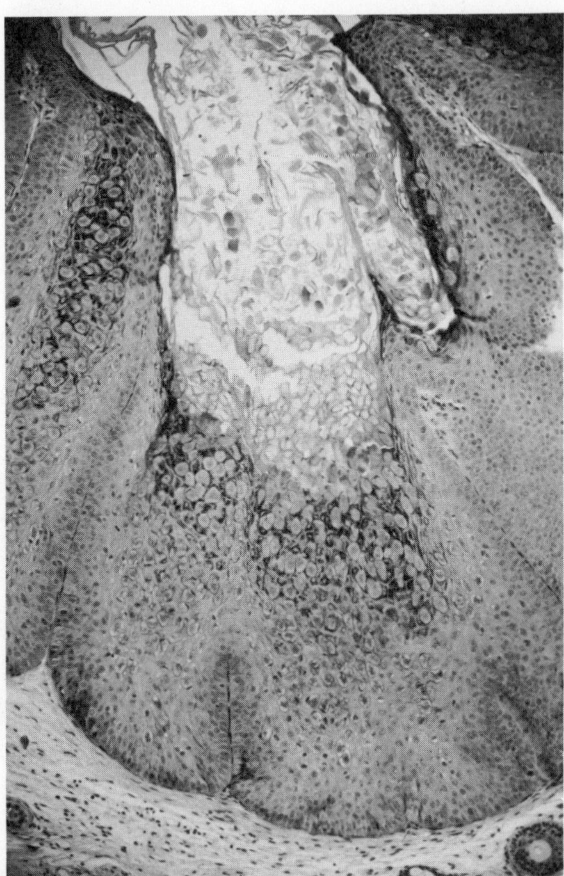

Figure 24–25 Molluscum contagiosum. Section of skin showing the typical molluscum bodies maturing as they approach the surface. Hematoxylin-eosin × 115.

Molluscum Contagiosum

The virus causes small pearly or waxy umbilicated lesions on the face, conjunctiva, limbs, and trunk which can be made to discharge a small amount of yellow material from which virus can be grown. Biopsy of such lesions shows a characteristic histological pattern. The virus of molluscum contagiosum is the largest virus causing human disease.

ASEPTIC MENINGITIS

Numerous unrelated organisms may cause meningitis characterized collectively by similar clinical signs and symptoms and a CSF in which there is lymphocytic increase, an elevated level of protein, and a normal or elevated glucose level, and which is sterile on routine bacteriological culture. Lymphocytic choriomeningitis accounts for 10% of cases, mumps virus, 10%, and herpes simplex virus, 5%; other cases are caused by the arbo group, the Coxsackie and echo groups, and poliomyelitis, varicella-zoster, measles, and the herpes group, including the Epstein-Barr virus of mononucleosis. In cases of "sterile" meningitis one should also consider the possibility of leptospirosis, syphilis, and parasitic infestation (e.g., cysticercosis cellulosae), leukemic or neoplastic infiltration of the meninges, "space-occupying" cerebral lesions, and the Guillain-Barré syndrome.

UNCLASSIFIED VIRUSES

The Hepatitis Viruses

The viral causes of hepatitis are being elucidated slowly. In addition to those viruses that specifically cause hepatitis, it will be recalled that Epstein-Barr virus (in infectious mononucleosis), herpes virus, and cytomegalic virus may also produce hepatitis as well as varicella-zoster. Of the specific hepatitis viruses, they were first clinically recognized as infectious hepatitis and serum hepatitis. They differed as follows:

	Infectious Hepatitis	Serum Hepatitis
Usual method of transmission	Fecal-oral	Parenteral
Incidence	Fall and winter especially	All year
Incubation	15–40 days	60–160 days
Onset	Abrupt	Slow
Mortality	< 0.1%	< 1%
Value of γ-globulin prophylaxis	Protects	Only some pools of γ-globulin (if it has antibody to HBsAg)

The first virus recognized was that of serum hepatitis, which was originally called Australia antigen. Subsequently, the virus of infectious hepatitis was identified. More recently, another variety of hepatitis has been revealed that appears to be caused by other agents.

Serum Hepatitis (Hepatitis B Virus, HBV)

Serum from patients with hepatitis B commonly contains three particles. These are spherical particles of 22 nm diameter that are of surface antigen (HBsAg) and tubular forms of 50 to 230 × 22 nm diameter that have a similar antigen. These particles are not infectious. A third form is the Dane particle, which is less numerous but has a more usual viral structure. It is a 42 nm sphere with a 28 nm core. The spherical portion is of surface antigen (HBsAg), and the core antigen is labeled HBcAg. The latter may be released by treatment of the Dane particle with detergent; it contains a partially double-stranded DNA genome. HBeAg is another portion of the core particle closely associated with the DNA. There are further subdivisions of the antigens,but they will not be discussed here.

Antibody to the surface antigen is given the notation anti-HBs; to the core antigen, anti-HBc; and to HBeAg, the antibody is anti-HBe.

Since the infection is spread parenterally and there are many carriers of the infection, it will be appreciated that laboratory workers, physicians, nurses, dentists, and so forth must take especial care in their work. Those who work in dialysis units are at particular risk. Persons who have had hepatitis must be excluded from donating blood for transfusion, and blood for transfusion must also be screened for HBV. Disposable syringes and needles are obviously advantageous. Many cases of hepatitis occur in illicit parenteral drug users because of contamination of their intravenous devices and needles. Hepatitis B during pregnancy is usually followed by disease in the baby, who becomes a carrier and may develop persistent hepatitis. Sexual contacts of patients with hepatitis B often acquire the disease.

Laboratory Diagnosis. The virus has not been artificially cultured. Diagnosis can be made by liver biopsy and chemical liver function tests as well as by serological tests. Among the latter for antigen are included methods

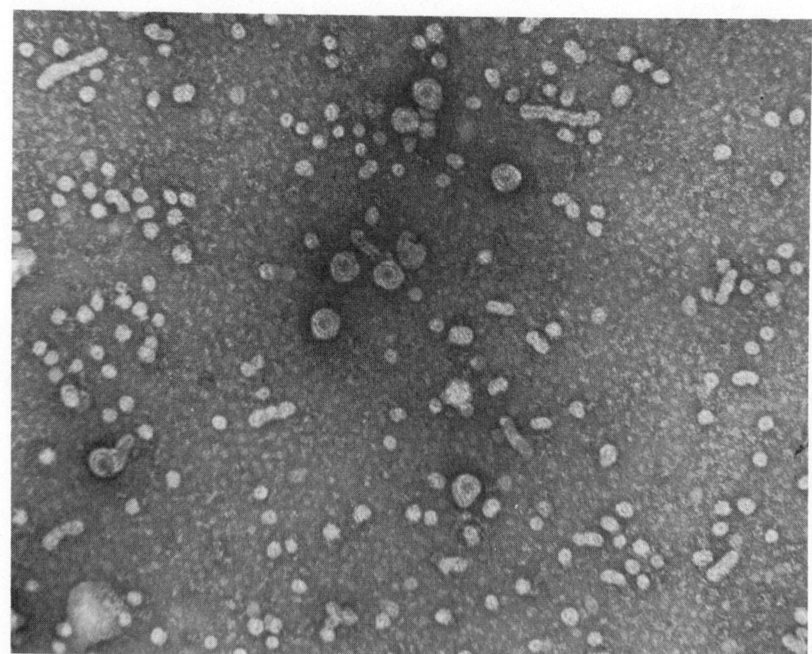

Figure 24–26 Hepatitis B. Serum preparation in which the three typical morphological forms—viz., spherical, rod, and Dane particles—are visible. PTA stain × 200,000. (Courtesy of Dr. P. Blaskovic, Virus Laboratory, Public Health Laboratory, Province of Ontario.)

Figure 24–27 HBV in liver. The virus aggregates are seen as dark areas within the cells, often surrounding the nuclei. The section is from a patient with cirrhosis and liver cancer. Aldehyde-fuchsin × 60.

based on counterimmunoelectrophoresis, tests using red blood cells or latex coated with anti-HBs RIA tests, and enzyme immunoassays. Most of these tests are for HBsAg, but materials for the recognition of HBcAg and HBeAg are becoming available. Likewise HBsAg is marketed and can be used to assay anti-HBs. Patients with viral hepatitis B will have HBsAg in their serum for about 12 weeks after the onset of the disease and will also demonstrate anti-HBc and anti-HBs. Those who became carriers or in whom chronic hepatitis develops will have persistent HBsAg and anti-HBc but not anti-HBs. The presence of HBeAg is associated with the continued infectivity of the blood. There are other markers whose significance as yet is not elucidated. The interpretation of the presence of the commoner antigens and antibodies is given in the following table:

Marker	Significance
HBsAg	Active hepatitis or persistent carrier
HBeAg	Active hepatitis or chronic hepatitis with infectivity of blood
Anti-HBs (in absence of HBsAg)	Evidence of previous infection, and protection against re-infection
Anti-HBc (in absence of anti-HBs)	Evidence of acute or chronic active hepatitis

Surveys have been done and have revealed the widespread presence of anti-HBs, which indicates exposure to HBV. It differs widely from population to population, but in the United States, it occurs in 10.8% of the general population.

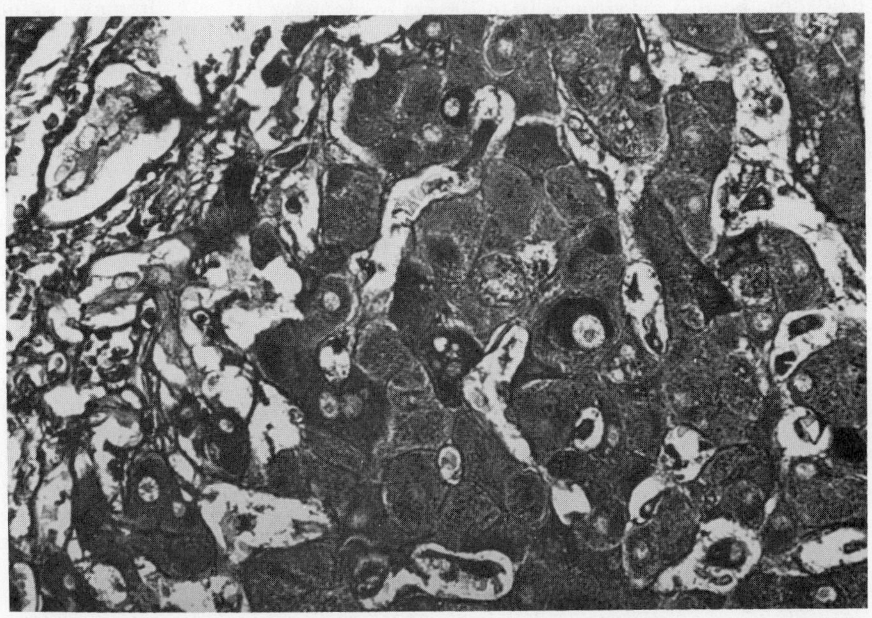

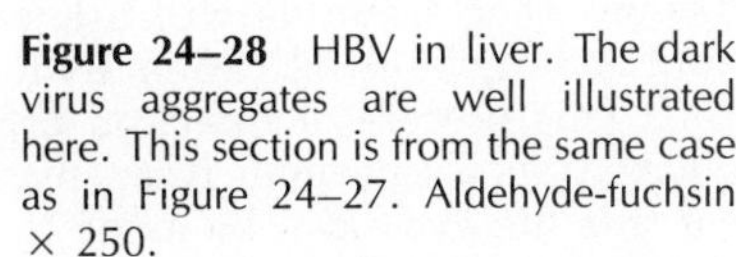

Figure 24–28 HBV in liver. The dark virus aggregates are well illustrated here. This section is from the same case as in Figure 24–27. Aldehyde-fuchsin × 250.

A vaccine made from the plasma of HBsAg carriers, using the HBsAg spherical particles treated with formalin to kill any residual infective virus, has been used in a clinical trial with considerable success to protect individuals at high risk to HBV. A vaccine made on these principles is now commercially available.*

Infectious Hepatitis (Hepatitis A Virus, HAV)

This virus is found in the stools of patients with active disease. It is a 27 nm icosahedral structure reminiscent of the picornaviruses. It has a single strand of RNA. At this time it has not been cultured artificially.

Laboratory Diagnosis. Serologic methods, especially techniques of RIA, have been used to detect the HAV antigen in the stool and blood, and kits for this purpose are commercially available. Anti-HAV appears in the blood in about the third week of the disease and may be measured by RIA or ELISA (*e*nzyme-*l*inked *i*mmuno*s*orbent *a*ssay).

Prevention of the disease among contacts may be achieved with γ-globulin, which is about 80% efficient if given within two weeks of exposure.

Non-A, Non B-Hepatitis (NANB)

Once the diagnosis of hepatitis A and B could be made with some certainty it became apparent that some cases of hepatitis belonged to neither category. It appears that these cases are due to several agents, and now that HBV can be screened out before it is given in blood transfusion, these unknown organisms cause 90% of the cases of post-transfusion hepatitis. In addition it is believed that they cause 15 to 25% of non–transfusion-associated hepatitis. Currently, much work is being done to elucidate NANB hepatitis.

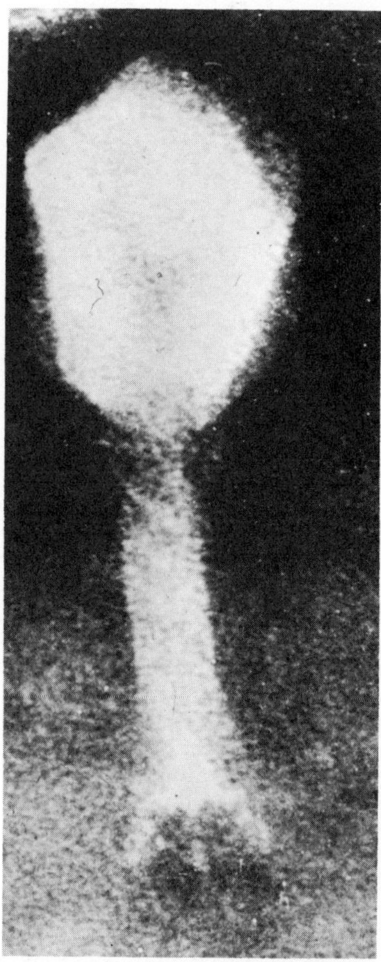

Figure 24–29 *E. coli* phage T4. Original magnification × 90,000. Note the characteristic tadpole shape. (From the collection of the late Dr. M. J. Lynch.)

BACTERIOPHAGE

These are tadpole-shaped organisms that infest bacteria and show a high degree of species and type specificity. The head of the virus is 10 to 100 nm in diameter, and the tail is a hollow tube of protein. In some varieties, the tail is surrounded by a retractile sheath. Within the head there is DNA, but there are some varieties of phage that contain RNA. The phage becomes adherent to the bacterial wall by its tail, and this process is highly specific, depending on chemical receptor areas in the bacterial wall. Phage typing of bacteria is dependent on this exquisite sensitivity. After adherence to the bacterial wall, phage nucleoprotein is passed through the hollow tail, rather like an injectible material through a syringe, into the bacterial substance. Unlike invasion by animal viruses, in most cases the protein coat of the phage remains outside the invaded cell. After entry, the subsequent history of the phage nucleoprotein may vary. In the case of RNA phage, the viral phage acts as mRNA and organizes its own replication.

Events with viral DNA may follow one of several courses:

1. It may synthesize new phage particles until the cell is lyzed (by phage lysozyme), releasing new infective virions. The lysis of bacterial colonies occurs by such a mechanism.

2. Phage may enter the cell and become a "prophage" or quiescent virus, integrating usually with the chromosome of the bacterium and replicating with it. One phage type does not combine with the host chromosome but replicates separately but synchronously. Induction by ultraviolet light or some other stimulus will allow the prophage to merge and undergo multiplication, with resultant lysis of the cell. This process of infection by prophage and induction with lysis is known as lysogeny. Some parallel of parts of this life cycle can be made to transformation of cells by viruses in cell culture.

3. Phage that can become prophage is called temperate phage. It may be released from the cell carrying some of its former host's DNA. This DNA may then become incorporated in a new host when it becomes infected by the phage. This transfer of genetic material from one bacterium to another by phage is known as transduction.

*Heptavax-B, Merck, Sharp, and Dohme, West Point, Pa., 19486.

DIAGNOSIS OF VIRAL DISEASE

General guidelines for the collection of specimens for viral diagnosis are given on p. 427.

MICROSCOPIC EXAMINATION

Some viruses are visible in cells as elementary bodies or as inclusion bodies. These may be studied without specialized equipment, although some special stains are advantageous and of course the specimen must be collected properly. Fixation is important in demonstration of inclusion bodies. In alkaline or neutral fixatives (neutral formalin or osmium tetroxide) the bodies stain poorly, but when fixatives with acetic acid are employed (e.g., Zenker's, Carnoy's, Bouin's), the inclusion body shrinks and is better seen in the stained preparation. Urine for cytomegalovirus must be delivered fresh or properly preserved (p. 476) to the laboratory for microscopy of the cellular sediment.

Immunofluorescent techniques with a high degree of specificity using tagged antisera are being used with increased frequency to identify inclusion bodies.

The results of regular microscopic examination may be seen in Table 24–4. Many of the staining methods are given elsewhere in this volume. Others are to be found in its third edition or in manuals of stain technology.

OTHER MISCELLANEOUS METHODS IN DIAGNOSIS

1. In viral meningitis there is generally pleocytosis with lymphocytes, although early in the disease there may be some polymorphs present. Protein is elevated but, unlike bacterial or fungal meningitides, sugar levels are normal or even raised.

TABLE 24–3 SOURCE OF DIAGNOSTIC SPECIMENS IN RICKETTSIAL, CHLAMYDIAL, MYCOPLASMAL AND VIRAL DISEASE*†

Organism	Specimen: Clinical	Specimen: Autopsy	Other Diagnostic Features
Mycoplasmas	Sp, B, P		Cold agglutinins
Rickettsiae	B		Weil-Felix agglutinations
Psittacosis	Sp, B	Lung	
LGV	P		Frei test
TRIC	C, Sp, S		
Cat scratch			Cat scratch skin antigen
Enterovirus			
Polio	T, F	Spinal cord, medulla, feces	
Coxsackie, Echovirus	T, CSF, F	Brain, etc.	
Rhinovirus	N, T		
Arbovirus	B, CSF	Brain, etc.	
Influenza	T	Lung	
Paramyxovirus			
Parainfluenza	T, N	Lung	
Mumps	Sa, CSF, U	Brain, salivary glands	Serum amylase
Measles	B, T	Brain, lung	
RSV	T, N	Lung, blood	
Rubella	T, U, B	All organs in rubella syndrome	Rubella HI; IgM titer
Rabies	Sa	Brain	
Adenovirus	T, F, Sp		
Coronavirus	Ph		
Papovavirus		Brain	
Herpes viruses			
Simplex	V, CSF, T	Brain, etc.	
Varicella-zoster	V, Sp	Lung	
CMV	U, Sp, T	All organs	
EB	L		Paul-Bunnell or some modification; peripheral blood picture
Reovirus			
Rotavirus	F		
Hepatitis			
HAV			Antigen in blood or stool
HBV			Antigen or antibodies in blood

*Key: B = blood cell culture or animal inoculation; Sp = sputum; P = pus; C = conjunctival swabs or scrapings; S = scrapings of urogenital epithelium; T = throat washings; F = feces; CSF = cerebrospinal fluid; N = nose washings; Sa = saliva; Ph = pharyngeal washings; V = vesicle or skin lesions; L = leukocytes; U = urine.

†Adapted from Behbehani, A. M.: Viral and rickettsial disease. *In* Graber, C. D., ed.: Rapid Diagnostic Methods in Medical Microbiology. Baltimore, Md., Williams & Wilkins Co., 1970; and Jawetz, E., Melnick, J. L., and Adelberg, E. A.: Review of Medical Microbiology, 14th ed. Los Altos, Calif., Lange Medical Publications, 1980.

TABLE 24–4 HISTOLOGICAL AND CYTOLOGICAL EXAMINATION IN VIRUS DIAGNOSIS*

Disease	Smear	Section	Material	Result	Method
Ornithosis	+	+	Avian spleen or air sac; human lung	Red elementary bodies in cytoplasm	Macchiavello, Noble, Giemsa
Lymphogranuloma venereum	+	+	From buboes	As ornithosis	As ornithosis
Trachoma-inclusion conjunctivitis	+		Conjunctival scrapings or follicular expression	Cytoplasmic inclusions	Giemsa, Wright, iodine
Measles	+	+	Exudate from nose. Appendix, tonsils	Intranuclear and cytoplasmic inclusions in exudate. Giant cells in tissues and exudates.	Hematoxylin-eosin
Rabies	+	+	Brain	Negri bodies (cytoplasmic), especially in Ammon's horn	Seller's for smears or sections, or Giemsa for sections
Adenovirus		+	Lung	Scanty nuclear inclusions. Associated necrosis.	Hematoxylin-eosin
Verruca vulgaris		+	Biopsy	Intranuclear inclusions. Vacuolation of cell. Histological pattern.	Hematoxylin-eosin
Herpes simples	+	+	Scrapings from lesions	Lipshutz (intranuclear) inclusions. Multinucleate cells in base of lesion. Margination of nuclear cytoplasm.	Hematoxylin-eosin, Giemsa, Papanicolaou
Varicella-zoster	+	+	Scrapings from lesions	Intranuclear, and later cytoplasmic inclusions. Multinucleate cells in base of lesion. Margination of nuclear chromatin in tissues early in disease.	Hematoxylin-eosin, Giemsa
Cytomegalic inclusion disease	+	+	Urinary epithelial cells. Biopsy	Cytomegalic inclusions.	Hematoxylin-eosin, cresyl blue
Molluscum contagiosum	+	+	Exudate or biopsy	Cytoplasmic inclusions or histological pattern	Cresyl blue, iodine, hematoxylin-eosin
Hepatitis B	−	+	Liver	Cytoplasmic inclusions	Shikata's orcein, aldehyde-fuchsin

*After Lennette, E. H.: *In* Diagnostic Procedures for Virus and Rickettsial Diseases, 2nd ed. New York, American Public Health Association, 1956.

2. Mumps, even when it does not produce clinical pancreatitis, generally gives raised serum amylase levels. This simple chemical test will often help differentiate mumps parotitis from other causes of neck swelling.

3. The Frei test is an intradermal test using yolk sac culture of lymphogranuloma venereum inactivated by heat, formalin, or phenol. The test is read like the tuberculin test and becomes positive within 2 to 3 weeks of the appearance of the primary lesion.

4. Cat-scratch disease: An antigen derived from nodes infected by the agent of cat-scratch disease may be used in a manner similar to the Frei antigen.

5. Infectious mononucleosis: Details of hematological and serological tests are given elsewhere (Chaps. 26 and 29). About 50% to 80% of patients with IM develop a morbilliform rash if given ampicillin, although only about 3% to 8% of the general population so react.

CHAPTER 24—REVIEW QUESTIONS

1. Give a short account of the five serological methods used in viral diagnosis and the principles that govern them.
2. Explain the terms *cytopathic effect, plaque formation, hemagglutination inhibition, neutralization,* and *Dane particle.*
3. (a) Describe the disease caused by the rotavirus. How is the condition diagnosed? What other organisms may cause similar disease?
   (b) What diseases are possibly due to the EB virus?
   (c) Name three viruses that commonly produce aseptic meningitis.
4. Give the methods employed in the laboratory diagnosis of rubella. What is the importance of the diagnosis, especially in women? How can the severe consequences of rubella be prevented? What other infectious agents may cause similar disease?

25 PARASITOLOGY

All species of animals or plants that parasitize man, including the bacteria, fungi, viruses, and parasitic worms and insects could be considered under this heading, but the term is usually reserved for what might more reasonably considered protozoology, helminthology, and entomology as related to medicine.

Previously, reference has been made to the divisions of the plant kingdom, and in this section we shall consider animal parasites. The organisms with which we are concerned in this chapter are Protozoa, single-celled animals; Platyhelminthes, invertebrates compressed dorsoventrally and without a body cavity; and Nematoda, invertebrate, unsegmented roundworms possessing a mouth, anus, and body cavity.

HOST/PARASITE RELATIONSHIP

Symbiosis is the relationship that exists between two dissimilar organisms living together. When this relationship is beneficial to one at the expense of the other, the relationship is said to be parasitic. Those parasitic organisms causing systemic or localized damage to a host's tissues are regarded as pathogens, whereas those parasites living in apparent harmony with a host are considered to be commensals.

Although this text will be largely limited to a consideration of pathogenic parasites, some of the nonpathogenic commensals will be briefly mentioned in order to provide the reader with sufficient information to be able to distinguish between these organisms and the pathogenic species.

Parasitization occurs when the infective stage of a parasite is transmitted to a susceptible host. There are several ways transmission can occur; for example, (1) unwitting ingestion by the host of infective stages of the parasite (pinworm), (2) inoculation by an insect vector (malaria), (3) active skin penetration (schistosomes), (4) transplacental transmission (Toxoplasma), and (5) accidental transmission—passive inoculation during procedures like blood transfusions.

Following transmission, a parasite's ability to survive successfully and to reproduce in a host's tissues will depend on such variables as (1) the number of organisms, (2) the organism's virulence, (3) its location in the host's body, and (4) the immunogenetic status of the host. Likewise, a host's response to a parasite is, in addition to the above, influenced by such factors as age, sex, immunity, nutritional status, and general health.

During their evolution, many of the parasites have developed complex life cycles, sometimes involving several intermediate hosts. A case in point is *Diphyllobothrium latum*, which has two such hosts: the copepod *Cyclops* and a species of freshwater fish (see p. 496). In each of these, the parasite undergoes a particular stage of its development before returning to the definitive host, where it matures to the adult form. Generally, this maturation of the parasite takes place in a specific location; for example, *D. latum* completes its life cycle in the small intestine. In most of the cases described in this chapter, the definitive host is human.

LABORATORY INVESTIGATION OF PARASITIC DISEASE

Intestinal Parasites

The usual specimen required for the investigation in intestinal parasitism is feces, which should be collected in containers that will prevent contamination with urine or water (which may cause lysis). Previous administration of antimicrobial agents may depress the growth of protozoa, and the presence of barium, laxative mineral oil, and so forth makes the recognition of parasites difficult. The stool may be brought to the laboratory within 30 minutes, or, if there is to be delay or the specimen is to be mailed to a reference center, a portion of stool may be preserved by mixing with a fixative preparation (see below). An unpreserved specimen or one in 10% formalin is also obtained for concentration. This is the so-called "2-vial method." It is usual to submit several daily samples, since the number of parasites excreted may have considerable daily variation.

Simple Wet Mounts

A small amount of feces, collected within 30 minutes of examination, is emulsified in a drop of saline or 10% formalin on a slide. It should be of sufficient transparency to allow one to see newspaper print through it. Trophozoites of amebae, flagellates, and ova may be identified by using a × 10 × 40 and an oil-immersion lens. By using saline, one can appreciate the motility of amebae. If 10% formalin is used, motility is lost but nuclei of trophozoites are more easily visible. Lugol's iodine (iodine 5 g, KI 10 g, water 100 mL) in varied dilutions (often 1:5 in water) may be used as an emulsifying agent that will stain nuclei and other structures, making them more easily visible. The iodine solution

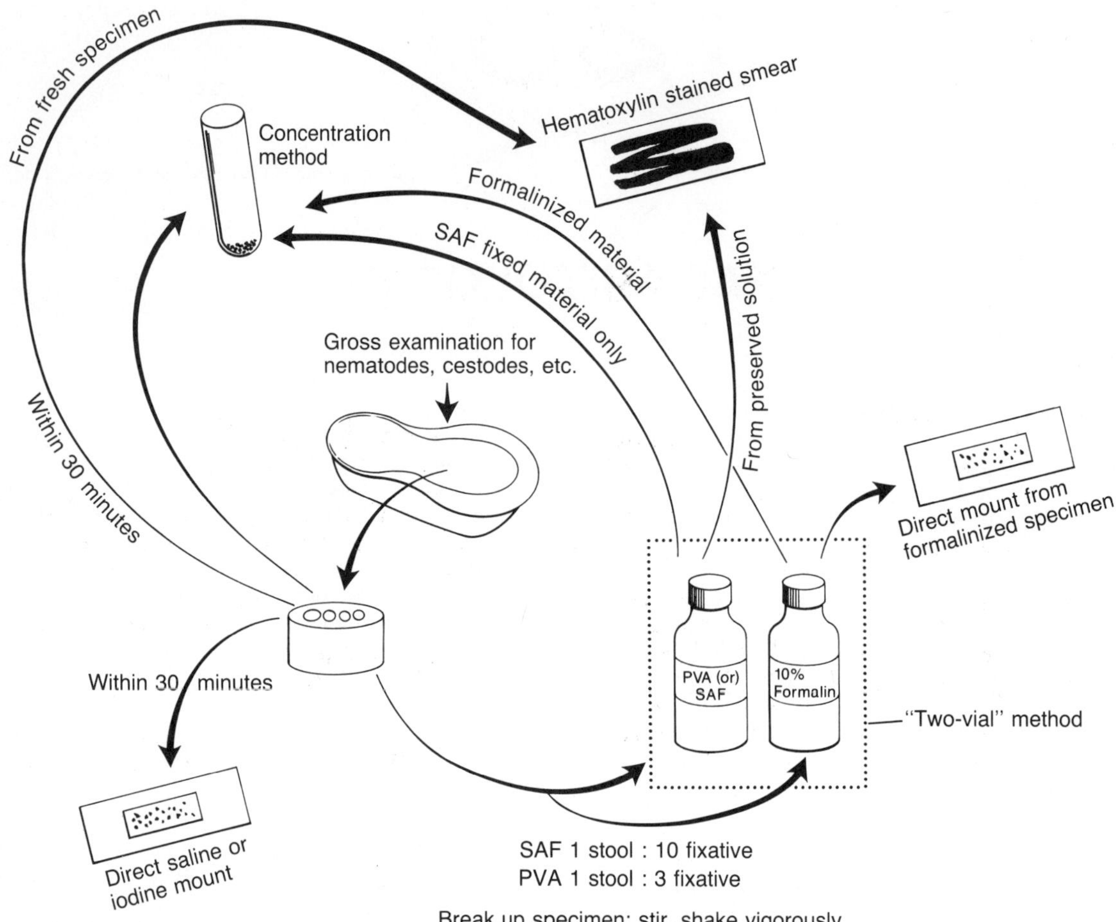

Figure 25–1 Methods of examination for parasites in stools.

should be used within 21 days of preparation. Although heavy infestations are identified by these simple methods, a concentration method must be employed to elucidate lesser degrees of infestation.

Concentration

As the name implies, the method concentrates cysts and ova (but not trophozoites). Some samples with *Giardia lamblia, Endolimax nana* cysts, and ova of *Ascaris lumbricoides* and *Hymenolepis nana* will not concentrate well with this formalin-ether method, but it is relatively easy to perform and commonly used. It produces little morphological distortion and is effective with formalinized specimens.

1. Mix 1 g of fresh feces with 15 mL of saline, and filter the suspension through a double gauze layer into a centrifuge tube. This procedure removes gross fecal material, mucus, and so forth.

2. Centrifuge one minute at 2000 rpm (450 to 500 G).

3. Decant the supernatant, and wash the sediment in saline, repeating the centrifugation until the supernatant is reasonably clear. The final sediment suspension should be about 1 mL.

4. Add to the sediment 10 mL of 10% formalin, and allow to stand for 5 to 10 minutes.

5. Add 3 to 5 mL of ether, stopper the tube, and shake energetically for 30 seconds.

6. Remove the stopper with care and centrifuge at 2000 rpm for 1 minute.

7. Loosen the plug or ring of debris (below the ether layer) with an applicator stick and decant everything except the sediment.

8. Resuspend the sediment in the small amount of remaining formalin and examine as a simple wet mount.

If the specimen has been formalinized (by processing in 10% formalin) as in one of the 2-vial specimens (see above) the concentration method is modified as follows:

1. Strain the suspension through gauze into a centrifuge tube.

2. Add sufficient tap water so as to almost fill the tube, and centrifuge at 2000 to 2500 rpm for 1 minute (500 to 650 G).

3. Decant the supernatant and wash again with tap water, leaving about 0.5 to 0.75 mL of suspension.

4. Add 10 mL of 10% formalin and proceed as in step 5 above (with 3 to 5 mL of ether), completing through step 8.

Preserved Specimens

Formalinized preparations for concentration are described above, but for delicate trophozoite preservation a more subtle method is desirable. Several fixatives for this purpose are available, and two will be described.

SAF Fixative. This fixative is made as follows:

Sodium acetate	1.5 g
Glacial acetic acid	2.0 mL
Formaldehyde	4.0 mL
Water	92.5 mL

About 1 g of fresh feces is emulsified in about 10 mL of the fixative.

PVA Fixative Solution. The preparation of this fixative solution is as follows:

1. Saturated aqueous mercuric choride

Mercuric chloride crystals	130–140 g
Distilled water	1000 mL

Dissolve by heating, and then allow to cool (this is when the excess of mercuric chloride will crystallize out). However if there is no crystallization, add more mercuric chloride and reheat and cool the solution until it is saturated.

2. Modified Schaudinn's fixative:

2 parts of solution number 1 (above) 1 part of 95% ethyl alcohol	93.5 mL
Glacial acetic acid	5.0 mL
Glycerol	1.5 mL

3. Slowly add 5 g PVA (polyvinyl alcohol) powder* to 100 mL of solution number 2 (above) at room temperature with constant stirring. Heat to 75°C or even higher, but do not boil, until the powder dissolves. Stirring will help. Cool to room temperature. The solution should be clear and without lumps, but a slight degree of abnormality will not hinder satisfactory performance. Three parts of fixative are used to one of feces, which is emulsified.

Advantages and Disavantages of Fixation Methods. Both methods will preserve the fine details of diagnostic morphology, including those of trophozoites. SAF fixed material may be used for both concentration and staining procedures; thus only one vial of material need be taken, whereas with PVA fixed material, an additional vial of formalinized stool must be preserved for concentration. SAF fixative is less toxic and corrosive than PVA fixative, but it will preserve less fecal material than an equal amount of PVA fixative (1 in 10 parts of SAF, compared with 1 in 3 parts of PVA). The quality of fixation is better with PVA fixation.

Stained Preparations

Such preparations may show details of trophozoites or other stages that are not apparent in simple wet mounts.

Hematoxylin Staining from SAF Fixed Specimens

1. Add 15 mL of saline to 2 to 3 mL of the suspended fixed fecal specimen.
2. Centrifuge at 2000 rpm for 1 minute.
3. Discard the supernatant and wash twice again with saline.
4. To a slide albuminized with Mayer's albumen, transfer 1 to 2 drops of the fecal sediment and spread with an applicator stick, making "dabbing" rather than "streaking" movements so as to avoid making too thick or too thin a film.
5. Dry at room temperature for 10 minutes.
6. Add 70% ethyl alcohol and leave for 10 minutes.
7. Add tap water and leave for 10 minutes.
8. Stain 10 minutes with iron hematoxylin that has previously been prepared by adding equal parts of the following solutions:

Solution 1	Hematoxylin	1 g
	95% ethyl alcohol	100 mL
	Sodium iodate ($NaIO_3 \cdot H_2O$)	0.1 g
Solution 2	Ferrous ammonium sulfate	1 g
	Ferric ammonium sulfate	1 g
	Concentrated hydrochloric acid	1 mL
	Distilled water	100 mL

9. Wash with distilled water for 30 seconds.
10. Flood with 50% saturated picric acid* for 8 minutes. (This removes excess hematoxylin and is critical.)
11. Wash in alkaline tap water for 10 minutes.
12. "Blue" with ammonaical alcohol (0.5 to 1% ammonia in 80% ethyl alcohol) for 10 minutes.
13. Dehydrate thoroughly with 95% and absolute ethyl alcohol.
14. Clear in xylol.
15. Mount in permount.

Hematoxylin Staining from PVA Fixative. The specimen is treated in a manner similar to the SAF treated material through Step 5 above. Then proceed as follows:

6. Cover the slide with alcohol iodine (to remove the mercury in the fixative) for 10 to 20 minutes. Alcoholic iodine is made as follows:

Solution 1	Add sufficient crystalline iodine to 95% ethyl alcohol to saturation.
Solution 2	Alcoholic iodine: Add 3 mL of the saturated iodine solution to 100 mL of 70% ethyl alcohol.

7. Replace the alcoholic iodine with 95% ethyl alcohol and leave for 10 minutes.
8. Replace with 70% alcohol for another 5 minutes.
9. Proceed to completion through steps 7 to 15 above.

Hematoxylin Staining of Fresh Unpreserved Feces. Such a procedure must be done within 30 to 60 minutes after the stool is passed. Delay results in autolysis of trophozoites, and the stained preparation is of little value.

1. Smear the fresh fecal specimen on a slide, and fix immediately in Schaudinn's fixative at least 1 hour or overnight (working solution for the latter is made as follows:

Solution 1	*Stock solution*	
	Mercuric chloride	45 g
	Ethyl alcohol	310 mL
	Distilled water	625 mL
Solution 2	*Working solution*: Add 5 mL of glacial acetic acid to 100 mL of stock solution.	

Proceed as in steps 6 to 9 under *Hematoxylin Staining from PVA Fixative*.

Ideally, stained organisms are blue-gray with black nuclear structures. Nonstaining organisms may be due to poor fixation. Smears are examined under the oil-immersion objective.

*Elvanol, E. I. DuPont de Nemours and Co., Inc., Wilmington, Del. 19898; DelKote, Inc., Penns Grove, N.J. 08069.

*Solid picric acid is explosive and must be stored under water.

Examination of Urine

T. vaginalis is relatively often seen in the urine sediment and may be seen in male infections as well as those in women.

Schistosoma haematobium may be sought in direct films from urinary sediment.

Examination of Sputum

Ova of *Paragonimus westermani*, the scolices of *E. granulosus*, and the trophozoites of *Entamoeba histolytica* may be found in sputum. The latter two are found in instances of rupture of a pulmonary hydatid or amebic abscess, respectively. Sputolysin (p. 425) or 3% NaOH may be used as a liquefying agent if the specimen is tenacious.

INTESTINAL PROTOZOA

The following species are found in the human intestinal tract:

Retortamonas intestinalis
Enteromonas hominis
Chilomastix mesnili
Giardia lamblia
Dientamoeba fragilis
Entamoeba gingivalis
Entamoeba coli
Entamoeba histolytica
Entamoeba hartmanni
Entamoeba polecki
Endolimax nana
Iodamoeba butschlii.

Although *E. histolytica* is generally recognized as a pathogen and the cause of amebic dysentery and *Giardia lamblia* and *Dientamoeba fragilis* are also accepted as pathogens, none of the organisms is considered as normal fauna. Their presence indicates that the patient has ingested fecally contaminated material at some time. Thus the presence of these other protozoa may alert the technologist to the possibility of parasitic disease, and their identification provides a diagnostic exercise and an index of the level of sanitation in the community.

In this book, no effort will be made to discuss the extensive detailed differentiation of these organisms, but Table 25–1 shows the differentiating features of the commoner intestinal ameba and there is discussion of the commoner and more important organisms.

Entamoeba histolytica

Entamoeba histolytica is the cause of amebic dysentery, which is a type of dysentery usually much less acute than the bacillary form. The organism is capable of producing severe ulceration of the large intestine, penetrating the submucosal layers, and finally reaching the muscle. Such activity may stimulate excessive pro-

TABLE 25–1 DIFFERENTIATION OF INTESTINAL AMEBAE

	Entamoeba histolytica	*Entamoeba coli*	*Entamoeba hartmanni*	*Endolimax nana*	*Iodamoeba bütschlii*	*Dientamoeba fragilis*
Amebae (trophozoites)						
Size (length)	12–20 μm	20–25 μm	5–12 μm	6–15 μm	8–20 μm	5–12 μm
Inclusions	Red blood cells, no bacteria in fresh specimens	Bacteria	Bacteria	Bacteria	Bacteria	Bacteria
Karyosome	Tiny and central	Large and eccentric	Small central	Large and central or eccentric	Large, granular, central or eccentric	4–8 chromatin granules, often binucleate
Motility	Very active, progressional	Sluggish, no progression	Nonprogressive, sluggish	Sluggish but progressive	Sluggish but progressive	Active and progressive
Cysts						
Size (length)	10–20 μm	11–35 μm	6–8 μm	5–14 μm	7–13 μm	No cysts
Shape	Round	Round	Round	Round, ovoid, or ellipsoidal	Irregular	No cysts
Glycogen mass	Present	Present	Present	Present	Present; large, compact, prominent	No cysts
Nuclei	1–4	1–8	1–4	1–4, perinuclear "halos"	1 usually, nuclear membrane indistinct	No cysts
Chromatoidal bodies	Bars, 2 × 4 μm with rounded edges	Rare; if present threadlike with square or pointed ends	1 or more, but may be absent in mature cysts	Absent	Absent	No cysts
Karyosome	Central	Eccentric	Central	Eccentric, may be divided	Central or eccentric, surrounded by large granules	No cysts

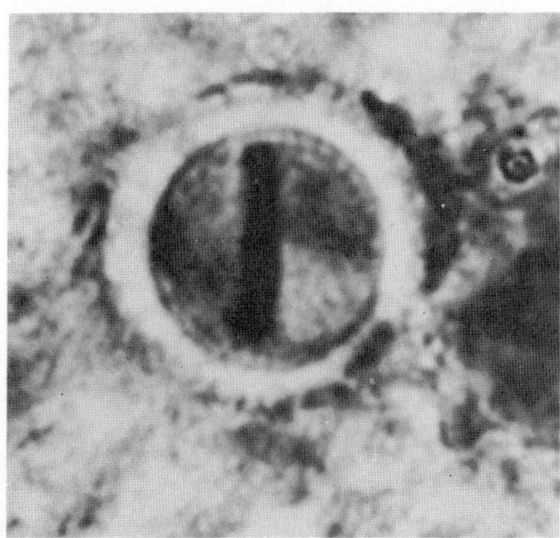

Figure 25–2 *Entamoeba histolytica.* Cyst in stool showing chromatoidal bar. Iron hematoxylin × 2250.

liferation of histiocytes and connective tissues, resulting in the formation of a granuloma found particularly in the walls of the cecum and sigmoid colon and known as ameboma. These tumors have been known to obstruct the lumen of the gut. Furthermore, amebic infection and abscesses of the liver may occur and other organs may be infected as a result of the erosion of the intestinal mucosae by the parasites, subsequent invasion of the bloodstream, and so forth.

The disease may be extremely chronic, and subclinical infections are common; according to some authorities, 10% of the inhabitants of the United States harbor the parasites. Other factors, especially intestinal pathogens, appear to aid *E. histolytica* in gaining a foothold and causing disease. The distribution of *E. histolytica* is worldwide, and infection is contracted by ingestion of food or water contaminated by cysts of the organism. There is no intermediate host, but flies may act as carriers.

Life Cycle and Morphology. The cysts of *E. histolytica* are swallowed and pass through the gastrointestinal tract, protected against the various enzymes by the cyst wall. At the ileocecal valve, the trophozoite is liberated and this form colonizes the large bowel mucosa. Cysts from different strains of the organism vary in size from small to large, between 10 and 20 μm. They may have a delicate wall or a thick wall with a double outline. There are one to four nuclear structures, each containing a central karyosome. Within the cyst are one or two chromatoidal bodies measuring about 2 by 4 μm. An irregular mass of glycogen may also be demonstrated.

The trophozoite ameba is between 12 and 20 μm with pseudopodia. When stained with iron hematoxylin a nuclear membrane is seen, encircling a small central dot of chromatin, the karyosome. Within the protoplasm, even in the unstained state, red blood cells may be seen.

Free-living amebae of the genera *Hartmannella, Acanthamoeba,* and *Naegleria* have been isolated from the human nasopharyngeal cavity and central nervous system; in the latter they cause a fatal infection.

The Flagellates

Man is host to several nonpathogenic, cosmopolitan flagellate species; *Chilomastix mesnili, Retortamonas intestinalis, Enteromonas hominis,* and *Trichomonas hominis. Giardia lamblia* is the only intestinal flagellate that is considered pathogenic. A pathogenic trichomonad, *Trichomonas vaginalis,* occurs in the urogenital tract.

Giardia lamblia

Giardia lamblia causes a relatively mild type of diarrhea with bulky yellow stools, abdominal pain, and loss of appetite. The trophozoite is found in the duodenum and the upper gastrointestinal tract; the cysts are present in the lower part of the small intestine and in the

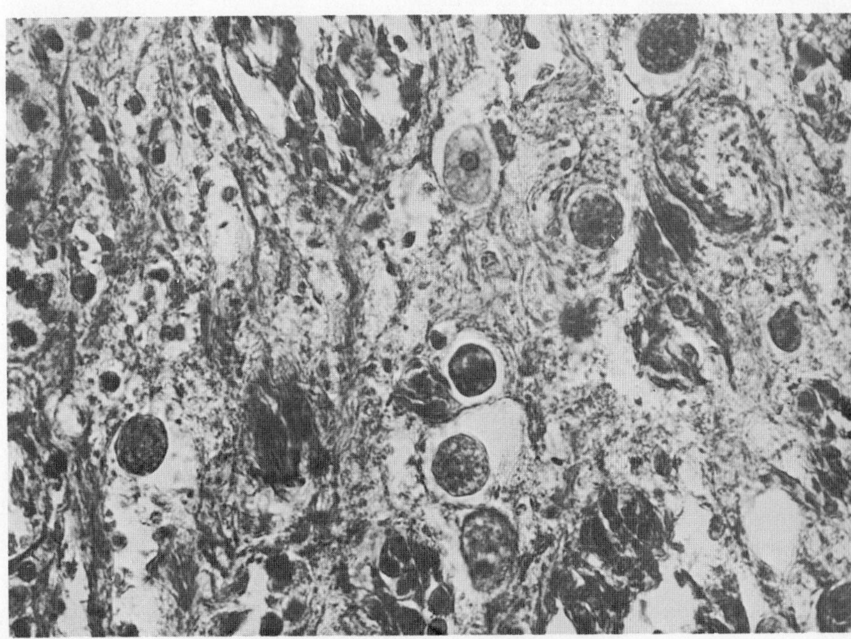

Figure 25–3 *Entamoeba histolytica.* Trophozoites in tissue. Section; iron hematoxylin × 630. A periodic acid Schiff stain is very useful in identifying these organisms, since they are strongly positive. (Courtesy of Dr. L. S. Mautner, St. Joseph's Hospital, Toronto, Canada.)

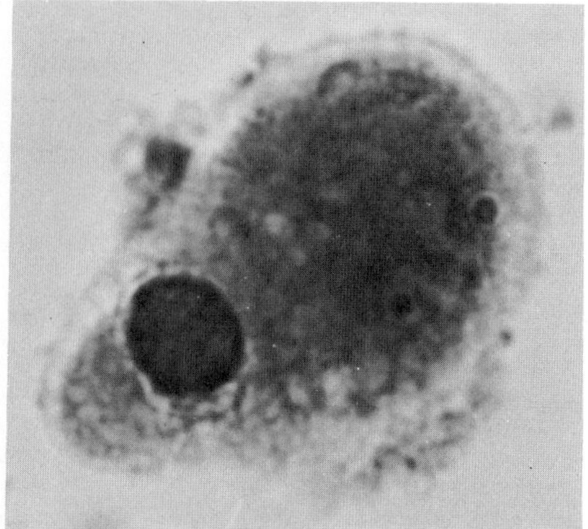

Figure 25–4 *Entamoeba coli.* Vegetative (trophozoite) form. Iron hematoxylin × 2250.

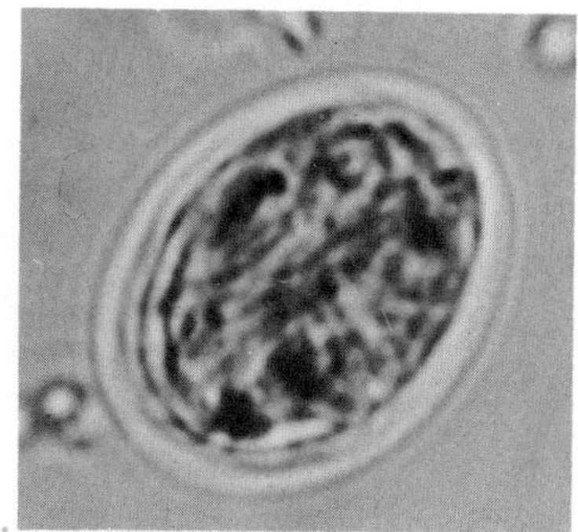

Figure 25–5 *Giardia lamblia.* Cyst in stool. Unstained × 2500.

colon. The organism is not uncommonly found in stools of patients, especially children, who have no symptoms. However, in some cases there is evidence of malabsorption. Infection is contracted by ingestion of water or food contaminated by cysts. The organism has a worldwide distribution.

Although generally infestation may be asymptomatic or possibly endemic, epidemics of diarrhea owing to *G. lamblia* have been reported in tourists returning from the USSR or the Mediterranean area. One should be aware of this possibility as a cause of "traveler's diarrhea."

Life Cycle and Morphology. The life cycle is similar to that of *E. histolytica.* Cysts are visible in stool when unstained and appear as ovoid bodies measuring approximately 10 by 7.5 μm with a relatively thick wall. Stained preparations show two to four nuclei, and there is often a spiral structure running across the long diameter of the cyst and dividing it in two.

The trophozoite is less likely to be present in the stool unless at the time of examination there is active diarrhea. The flagellate is pear-shaped and measures approximately 10 to 20 μm, and, in a fresh warm stool, there is characteristic jerky progressive movement; however, unless the organism is stained, no details of structure can be made out. A stained preparation will show two anterior nuclei, and, running the length of the parasite, there are two linear structures known as axonemes; in addition, eight long, thin flagella are apparent. Cysts are more often found in stools and flagellates in duodenal aspirates. Enterotest* is a gelatin capsule on a length of nylon thread. The patient swallows the capsule, which is withdrawn after 4 hours. Adherent mucus is microscopically examined for flagellates. Table 22–4 may be of some assistance in the differentiation of flagellates in stool specimens.

Diagnosis. The diagnosis is made by recognition of the trophozoites or cysts in the stool.

Cells and Materials in Stools that May be Confused with Protozoa

Polymorphonuclear leukocytes and macrophages may be confused with amebae, but definition of the leukocytic, coarser, more elongated nuclei should differentiate them. Epithelial cells are larger and less likely to be mistakenly identified: the cytoplasm has no inclusions. Yeasts are not unusual. They are often oval and measure 4 to 6 μm in length, and they may be seen budding. *Blastocystis hominis* is a larger yeastlike plant cell structure that often assumes a green tint. It has no visible nucleus and peripherally includes some refractile granules.

*Health Development Corp., Palo Alto, Calif. 94303.

TABLE 25–2 Differentiation of Intestinal Flagellates

	Giardia lamblia	Chilomastix mesnili	Retortamonas intestinalis	Enteromonas hominis	Trichomonas hominis
Trophozoite					
Size (length)	10–20 μm	6–20 μm	4–9 μm	4–10 μm	8–20 μm
No. of nuclei	2	1	1	1	1
No. of flagella	8	4	2	4	4
Shape or specific feature	Pear-shaped axonemes	Pear-shaped spiral groove in body	Pear-shaped	Ovoid, flattened one side	Pear-shaped undulating membrane may contain RBS
Cysts					
Size (length)	8–13 μm	8 μm long	5 × 4 μm	8 × 4 μm	No cysts
Shape	Ovoid	Ovoid or pear-shaped with small anterior knob	Pear-shaped	Ovoid, or round	No cysts
Nuclei	2–4	1	1	1–4	No cysts

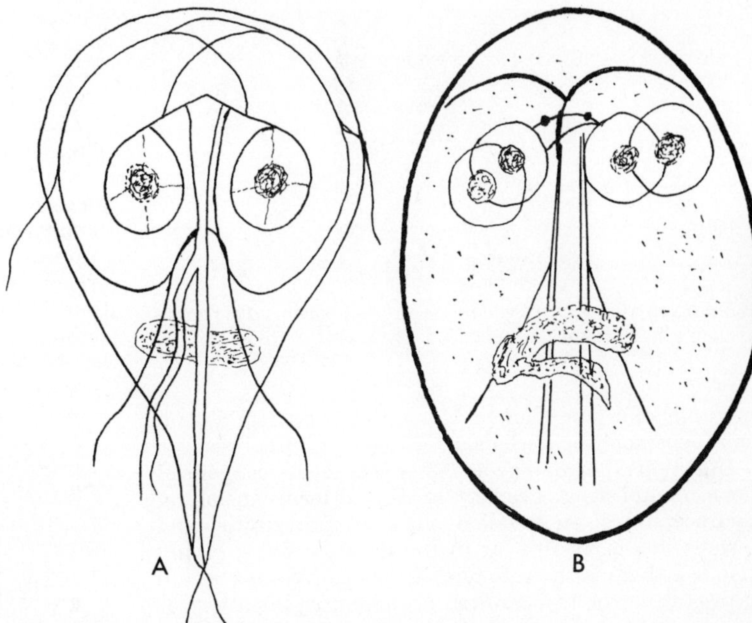

Figure 25–6 Detailed sketch of *Giardia lamblia*. **A,** Trophozoite; **B,** cyst.

Errors are often made because the organisms or suspected organisms are not measured. Size is most important, for example, for separating *E. histolytica* from *E. hartmanni* and for identification of helminth eggs. A properly calibrated occular micrometer is a most important diagnostic instrument.

Trichomonas vaginalis

T. vaginalis is considered to be the cause of one variety of vaginitis characterized by abundant foul-smelling leukorrhea and pruritus vulvae. Others think the organism is a secondary invader and is not pathogenic *per se*. *T. vaginalis* is also associated with one variety of nonspecific urethritis in men, but it should be remembered that the organism is found in urine of men and women who are symptomless. At one time the organism was thought to be identical with *T. hominis*, but in spite of close morphologic similarity the organisms do not survive if transplanted to each other's natural habitat.

Morphology. The organism is found only as a trophozoite and measures about 12 to 26 μm long and is pear shaped. There are four anterior flagella and an undulating membrane running on one side of the organism for about half the body length. A single nucleus and slender axostyle in a granular cytoplasm complete the anatomy (Fig. 25–7).

Diagnosis. A swab from the vagina should be placed in a tube so that it is partially covered by warm saline. The tube should be delivered immediately to the laboratory and, if it cannot be examined at once, may be left temporarily in the 37°C incubator. A "hanging drop" preparation (see p. 346) is made from the moist swab. *T. vaginalis* is easily recognized as a motile, pear-shaped flagellate. Urethral discharge from a male, or material from prostatic massage, may be examined similarly. The organisms may be seen (often fortuitously) in urinalysis while examining urinary deposit. There is a fair amount of truth in the somewhat cynical remark that *Trichomonas* is recognized because it is "a pus cell that moves."

COCCIDIANS

Toxoplasma gondii

Toxoplasmosis is a disease caused by *Toxoplasma gondii*, an intestinal coccidian of the Felidae. In the human host, *toxoplasma* is seen as a small organism (often crescentic in shape), measuring approximately 2 to 3 by 4 to 6 μm, often found in an intracellular position. Furthermore, they are frequently grouped together in pseudocysts that measure 10 to 50 μm. The organism may be seen in tissues or in exudate smears stained by hematoxylin and eosin, the Romanowsky stains, or Giemsa. They are not unlike *Leishmania*, but do not

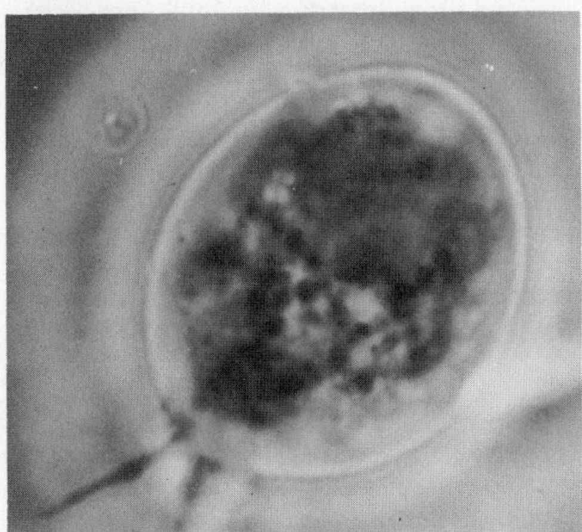

Figure 25–7 *Trichomonas vaginalis*. Trophozoite in vaginal discharge. Phase contrast × 2250.

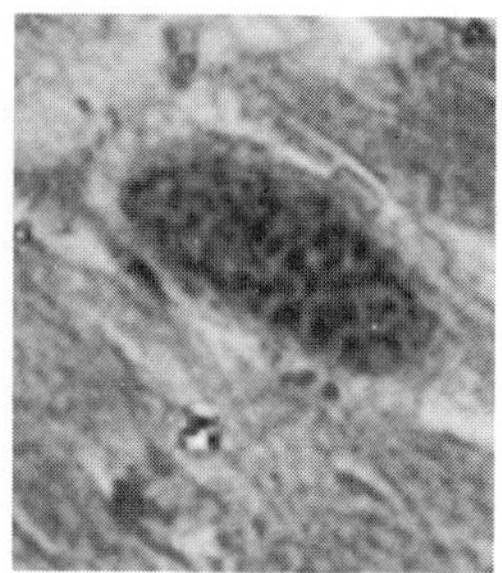

Figure 25–8 *Toxoplasma gondii* pseudocyst in myocardial fiber of a kitten's heart. Hematoxylin-eosin, original print × 135.

have flagella, and show a basophilic cytoplasm with a small eosinophilic nucleus.

Infections in man may be either in a severe congenital form, manifesting a variety of clinical forms including hydrocephalus, encephalomyelitis, chorioretinitis, and lesions in the viscera, or in the acquired form, giving rise to either (a) an acute lymphadenopathy, (b) a severe illness in which myocarditis, pneumonitis, hepatitis, or meningoencephalitis may predominate in the clinical picture, or (c) ocular disease.

Aspects of the Life Cycle. The parasite *Toxoplasma* has a cosmopolitan distribution and is able to develop in a wide variety of vertebrate hosts; the complete life cycle occurs only in the Felidae. It would appear that the organism was originally an intestinal coccidian that subsequently has evolved to multiply in extraintestinal sites, in both the definitive host (the cat) and other susceptible species.

Following ingestion of *Toxoplasma* trophozoites (tachyzoites), schizogony and gametogony occur in the feline gut epithelium, particularly in the ileum, resulting in the formation of oocysts (bradyzoites) typical of Coccidia. Sporozoites are excreted in the cat's feces and thus may infect children who play innocently in soiled areas. The feces may also contaminate vegetation, which, if poorly washed before eating, may infect humans and other animals. *Toxoplasma* tachyzoites in the feline (definitive host) can be found in the mesenteric lymph nodes and other organs. Oocysts (bradyzoites) are ingested subsequently by intermediate hosts, e.g., man, rodents, birds, and so forth, among which infection appears to be disseminated principally by carnivorism. Thus, *Toxoplasma* in the feline host has a coccidian life cycle, yet unlike typical coccidians, it deviates with respect to the multiplication of the organism in other tissues and hosts. Figure 25–9 summarizes the essential features of the *Toxoplasma* life cycle.

Congenital transmission in man, though medically important, is probably of minor epidemiological importance, whereas transmission via the ingestion of cysts or trophozoites in raw and undercooked meats is of prime concern. Organ transplantation has been shown to be another rare cause of transmission of the disease.

Diagnosis

1. Diagnosis is made by recognition of organisms in cytological, hematological, or histological material. Generally, in biopsy material, appearance of identifiable organisms is rare. However, their presence may be suggested very strongly by a particular histological pattern in lymph nodes. The picture is not completely diagnostic without supporting serological evidence. Giemsa staining of smears or sections from putty-like areas of affected brains is recommended.

2. Serological methods are largely used in diagnosis. There are numerous methodologies.

3. Enzyme-linked immunosorbent assay (ELISA) methods are available commercially. Antigens in one commercial test* are bound to beads made of ferrous material. The beads are challenged with the test serum and then are washed to remove unattached serum protein. The washed beads are then exposed to a peroxidase-conjugated antiglobulin that will attach to the antibody bound to the bead. The beads are washed again to remove unattached peroxidase and placed in a substrate solution. The appearance of color indicates the presence of antibody.

4. Indirect fluorescent antibody kits for the diagnosis of toxoplasmosis are also available.‡ The organisms are present on slides and are exposed to the patient's serum. After washing, fluorescent-labeled anti-human globulin is added. Should antibody be attached to the organism, a green fluorescence will be seen under fluorescent microscopy.

THE CESTODES

Basic Characteristics

The cestodes or tapeworms are parasitic flatworms and comprise a class of the phylum Platyhelminthes. The tapeworms have certain features in common. The cestode body consists of an anterior attachment organ or scolex, followed by a series of flat rectangular segments known as proglottids. This chain of proglottids is called the strobila (see Fig. 25–10). Since new segments are produced by the scolex, the distal segments of the worm are the oldest. Each proglottid is hermaphroditic, each segment having a testis, ovary, and uterus. The male and female organs of each proglottid meet at the *genital pore.* The scolex varies from species to species but is provided with sucking discs or hooklets by which it attaches itself to the bowel of the host. Distal proglottids containing mature ova become detached from the main body of the worm and are passed in the feces. Subsequently, they are ingested by an animal known as the *intermediate host* and, in this animal, the worm larvae migrate to muscle where they are found in the cystic stage. Ingestion of the meat of this animal, poorly cooked, by the *definitive host,* which often is man, will liberate the cysts, which become adult worms in the bowel. In the life cycle of *Echinococcus granulosus,* the definitive host is the dog, with man, sheep, and moose acting frequently as intermediate hosts. *Echinococcus multilocularis* has the fox or dog as its definitive, and rodents or man as its intermediate, host. Occasionally in the life cycle of *Taenia solium* man is the intermediate host. *Hymenolepis nana* is the only one in which there is no intermediate host and infection is from man to man. Table 25–3 summarizes the basic characteristics of the cestodes.

---

*Bionetics Laboratory Products, Kensington, Md. 20795.

‡Zeus Scientific, Inc., Raritan, N. J. 08869.

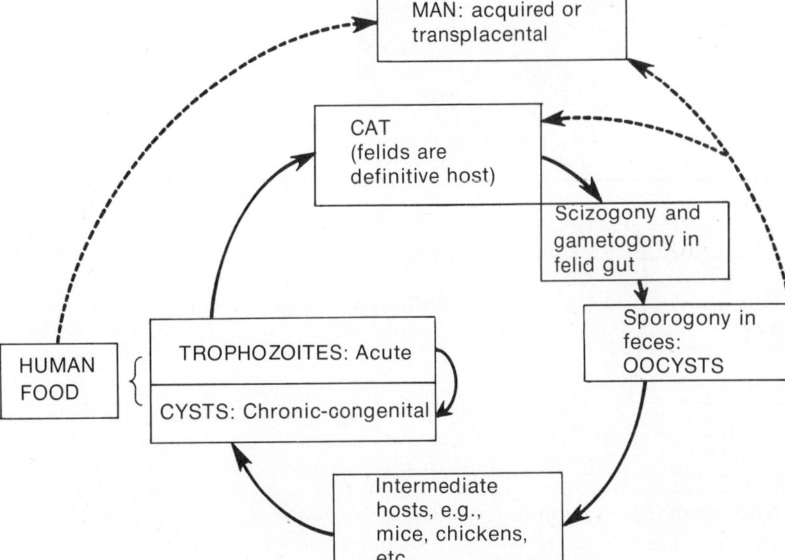

Figure 25–9 Life cycle of *Toxoplasma gondii*.

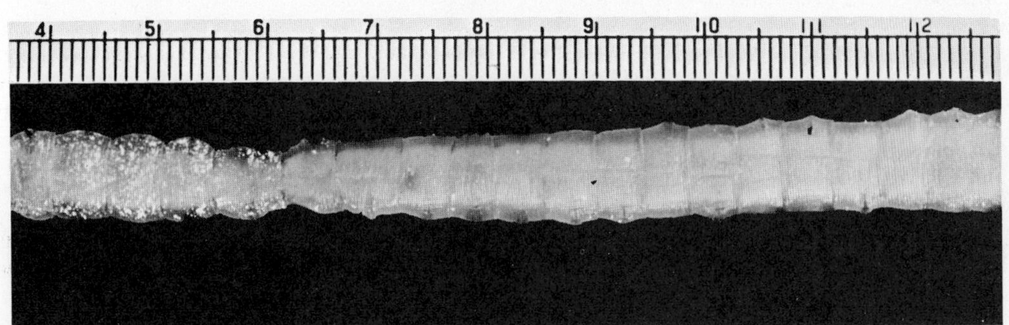

Figure 25–10 Proglottids of the tapeworm (scale in centimeters).

TABLE 25–3 Key to Tapeworms

	Taenia solium	*Taenia saginata*	*Diphyllobothrium latum*	*Hymenolepis nana*	*Echinococcus granulosus*	*Echinococcus multilocularis*
Definitive host	Man	Man	Man	Man	Dog	Foxes, wolves, dogs
Intermediate host(s)	Pig (man)	Cattle	Crustacea Fish	None	Sheep, cattle, man	Mice, voles, man
Length	2–7 m	10–12 m	4–10 m	4 cm	3–6 mm	1.2–3.7 mm
Suckers	4 lateral	4 superolateral	2 lateral grooves	4 lateral	4	
Hooklets	2 rings	Nil	Nil	Single ring	28–50 (usually 30–36)	
Uterus	7–13 lateral branches	15–20 lateral branches	Few convolutions	Sacciform	Lateral pouches often present	No lateral pouches
Genital pore	Regular alternation, lateral	Irregular alternation, lateral	Central	Unilateral	On equator of proglottids	Anterior to equator of proglottids
Ova	40 μm (both *Taenia*): With radial striation of capsule		70 × 45 μm operculated	30 × 50 μm thick capsule	30–40 μm, indistinguishable from *Taenia* or *Multiceps*	

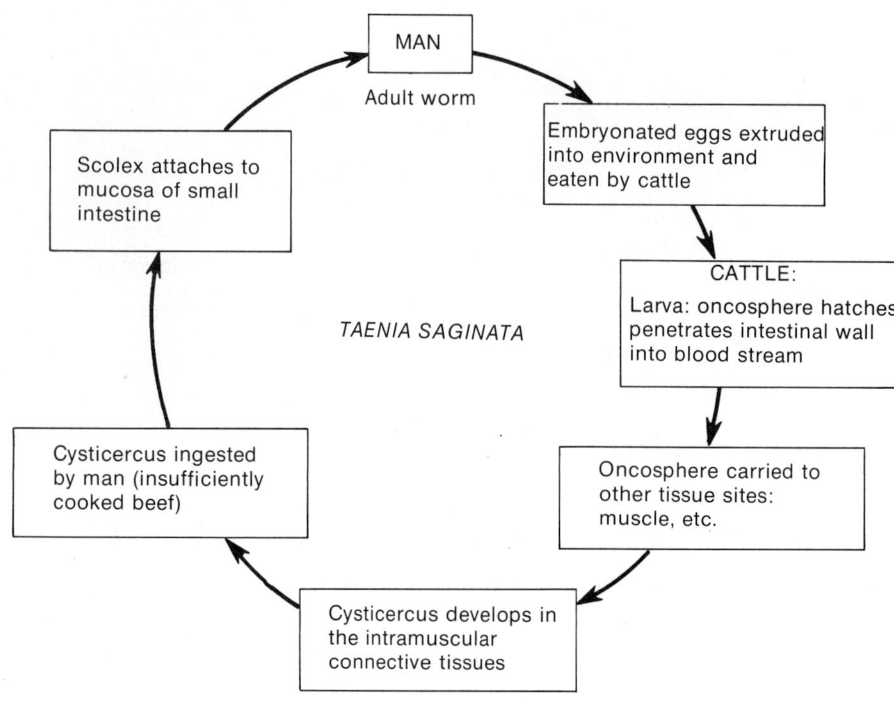

Figure 25–11 Life cycle of *Taenia saginata.* N. B. Cycle is same as that of *T. solium,* except that intermediate stages occur in pigs.

Taenia solium

The adult worm usually produces few symptoms, and the patient generally first notices proglottids in the feces. However, if the patient becomes the intermediate host, cysts are formed in many tissues of the body. Often these cause little trouble while they are alive, but when they die there is a severe tissue reaction (often with calcification) and symptoms appear. Quite often, cysts develop in the brain, producing epilepsy or hydrocephalus. When the cystic stage occurs in man, the disease is known as cysticercosis cellulosae *(vide infra).*

Life Cycle and Morphology. The adult worm measures from 2 to 7 meters long and lives in the small bowel. The scolex measures only about 1 mm in diameter and has four lateral sucking pads and, superiorly, a rounded projection known as a rostellum which supports a double row of small hooklets around the circumference. The proglottids vary in size, with small ones superiorly and larger segments inferiorly. The uterus has 7 to 13 lateral branches and, if several segments are obtained, the genital pore is seen alternating regularly from side to side in adjacent segments. Mature ova may be present in excreted proglottids or may be passed free. They are round and measure about 40 μm in diameter, with a thick shell often appearing radially striated. Within the shell in the ovum, linear markings representing hooklets may be seen.

The life cycle (Fig. 25–11) requires one intermediate host, the pig. Embryonated eggs in the soil may be ingested by this animal. In the pig the cystic stage occurs in muscle. By eating poorly cooked, infected pork, man becomes infected, and the adult worm develops from the ingested larvae. In some instances, as implied earlier, man is infested but becomes not the definitive but the intermediate host, developing cysticercosis cellulosae (see Fig. 25–12). This results from eating food contaminated by ova. The most common sites are striated muscle and the brain. In muscle the cysts frequently calcify without causing too much trouble to the host. However, in the central nervous system calcification is rare; instead, tissue reactions occur, often precipitating motor and sensory impairment. If the cerebrospinal fluid drainage is blocked, internal hydrocephalus may develop.

Diagnosis. In the laboratory, diagnosis is made by the identification of ova or proglottids in feces. Since the eggs of *T. solium* are infectious to man and can cause

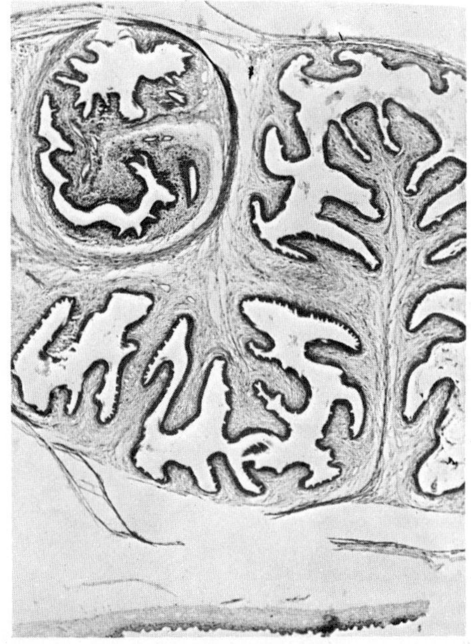

Figure 25–12 *Cysticercus cellulosae.* Section; hematoxylin-eosin × 60.

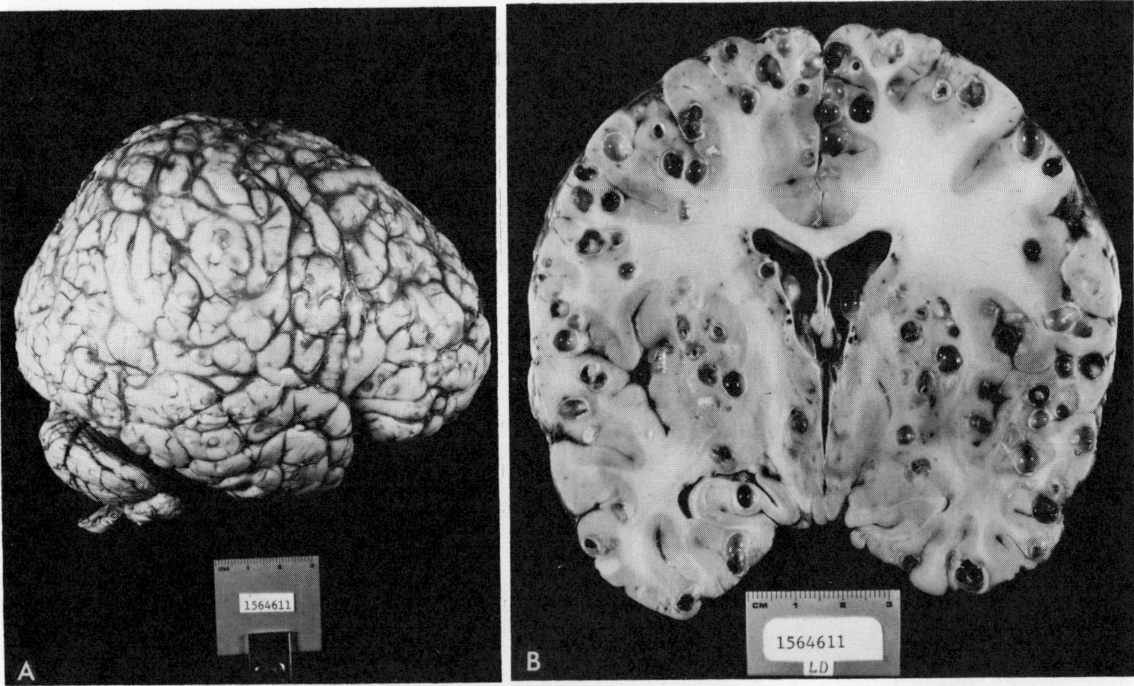

Figuure 25–13 Cerebral cysticercosis. Brain of an Ekari girl aged 13. **A,** Lateral and, **B,** coronal section with multiple cysts, particularly in the gray matter. The estimated total number of cysts in the brain exceeded 20,000. (Courtesy of Dr. D. C. Gajdusek and the Armed Forces Institute of Pathology, Washington, D.C.)

fatal cysticercosis, it is important to commence treatment immediately following diagnosis. The ova are identical in appearance with those of *T. saginata* and so are not completely diagnostic (Fig. 25–14). Proglottids may be identified by the number of branches of the uterus and position of the genital pore (Fig. 25–14). If the proglottids are pressed between two slides, enough detail is often revealed under a hand lens or dissecting microscope for recognition of distinguishing features. Immersion in a solution of carbolxylene (25 g of phenol in 75 mL of xylene) will often clear the specimen sufficiently to see detail more clearly. If desired, the segments or the worm may be fixed in saturated aqueous mercuric chloride, followed by immersion in 50% alcohol containing iodine. The iodine is removed with 70% alcohol and the slide is transferred to a solution of carmalum:

Cochineal or carmine	25 g
Glacial acetic acid	25 mL
Potassium alum	25 g
Distilled water	1000 mL
Salicylic acid	1 g

The specimen is stained for at least 12 hours, differentiated with acid alcohol, dehydrated, and cleared. The worm or proglottid is cleared and the viscera are shown in different shades of red. The diagnosis of cysticercosis cellulosae is usually histological. Since the proglottids are produced by the scolex anteriorly, the head of the worm must be dislodged by therapy in order to effect a cure. Treatment by a vermifuge or vermicide is often followed by a purge and an enema. All material passed is sent to the laboratory and passed through a sieve in order to trap the head. The head is diligently sought among the narrow segments (Fig. 25–14).

Taenia saginata

As with *T. solium*, there are usually few clinical symptoms of infection. Man never becomes the intermediate host in this infestation.

Life Cycle and Morphology. The adult worm lives in the small intestine of man and measures usually 10 to 12 meters. The scolex is expanded terminally (measuring approximately 2 mm in diameter) to support four sucking pads, but there are no hooklets. The proglottids have a uterus with 15 to 20 lateral branches, and the genital pore alternates irregularly. Ova are identical in appearance to those of *T. solium*. The life cycle of *T. saginata* is summarized in Figure 25–11. The eggs are ingested by cattle, the intermediate host, in which the cystic stage occurs. Ingestion of raw or poorly cooked infected beef containing the larvae will cause their liberation, and the maturing worm will infest the small bowel.

Diagnosis. The diagnosis is made by the presence of typical proglottids in the stool (Fig. 25–15). The ova are only diagnostic of either *T. solium* or *T. saginata* infestation. Following therapy, the head of the worm may have to be identified by the method described under *T. solium*.

Diphyllobothrium latum

The fish tapeworm is not uncommon in parts of eastern and northern Europe and also around the shores of the upper Great Lakes in North America. Usually, as with the other tapeworms, there is little clinical symptoma-

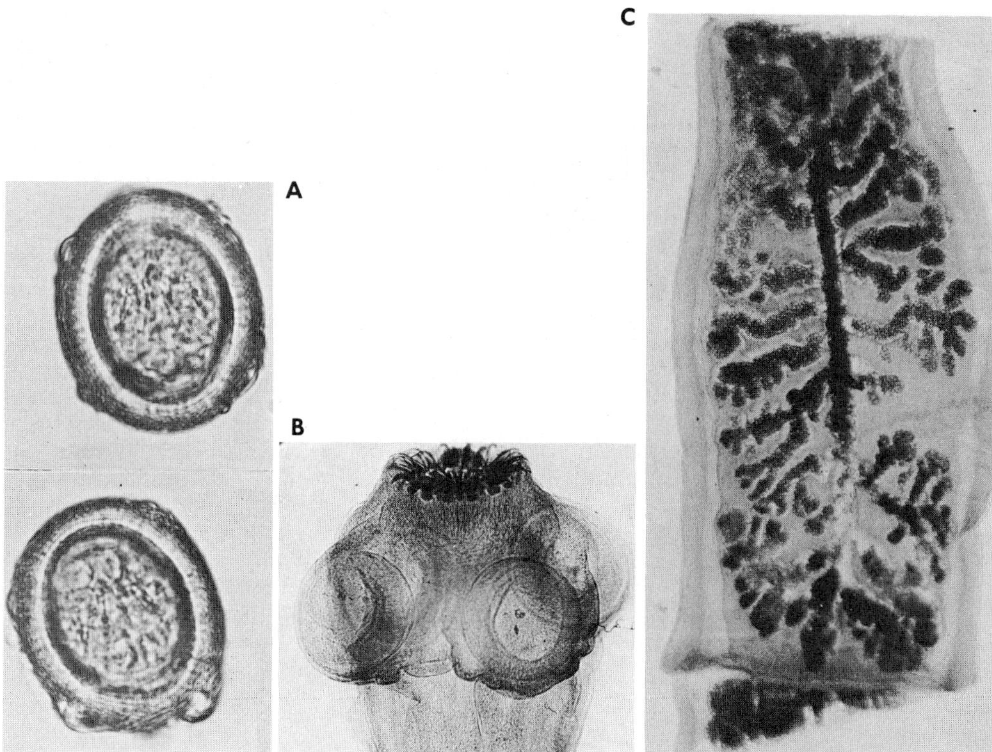

Figure 25–14 *Taenia solium.* **A,** Ova. × 1050. **B,** Scolex. × 48. **C,** Proglottid. Gravid segment showing a branched uterus filled with ova. × 13. (**B** courtesy of Dr. A. M. Fallis, Toronto, Ont. **C** courtesy of the late Col. C. A. Bozman, Wellcome Museum of Medical Science, London, England.)

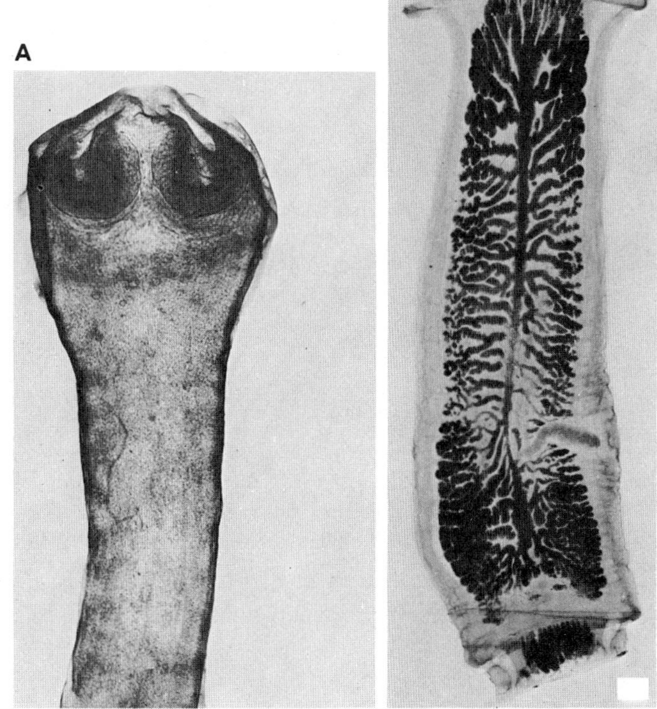

Figure 25–15 *Taenia saginata.* **A,** Scolex. × 60. **B,** Proglottid. Gravid segment. × 5. (**A** courtesy of Dr. A. M. Fallis, Toronto, Ont. **B** courtesy of the late Col. C. A. Bozman, Wellcome Museum of Medical Science, London, England.)

tology. However, in a few cases of the infestation, the patient may present with macrocytic anemia, which is cured if the worm is dislodged and passed. It is believed that the worm competes with the host for vitamin B_{12}. If the worm uses more of this essential metabolite than the host can spare, the latter becomes vitamin B_{12}-deficient and develops macrocytic anemia.

Life Cycle and Morphology. The essential features of the life cycle of *D. latum* are summarized in Figure 25–16. The adult worm is usually about 4 meters long and lives in the small bowel. The scolex measures about 1 mm in diameter in the same axis as the body; there are no hooklets or suckers as such, but there are two relatively long grooves that serve functionally for the same purpose (Fig. 25–17). The proglottids have a uterus that occupies little space as compared with *T. saginata* or *T. solium*, with only few coarse convolutions (Fig. 25–17). The genital pore is centrally situated. The ova are ovoid and yellow-brown in color, measuring approximately 70 by 45 μm, and are provided with a hinged lid known as an operculum at one end of the shell (Fig. 25–17). Within the thin shell, several cells of the developing embryo are usually apparent. The ova mature in water and a free-living ciliated embryo (coracidium) develops. This form is ingested by minute crustaceans, which subsequently are eaten by freshwater fish (mainly species of pike). The organisms break out of the alimentary tract of the fish and infest muscle, not as cysts but as wormlike larvae. The crustacean and the fish are considered first and second intermediate hosts. A man who eats raw or poorly cooked, infested fish will become the next or definitive host.

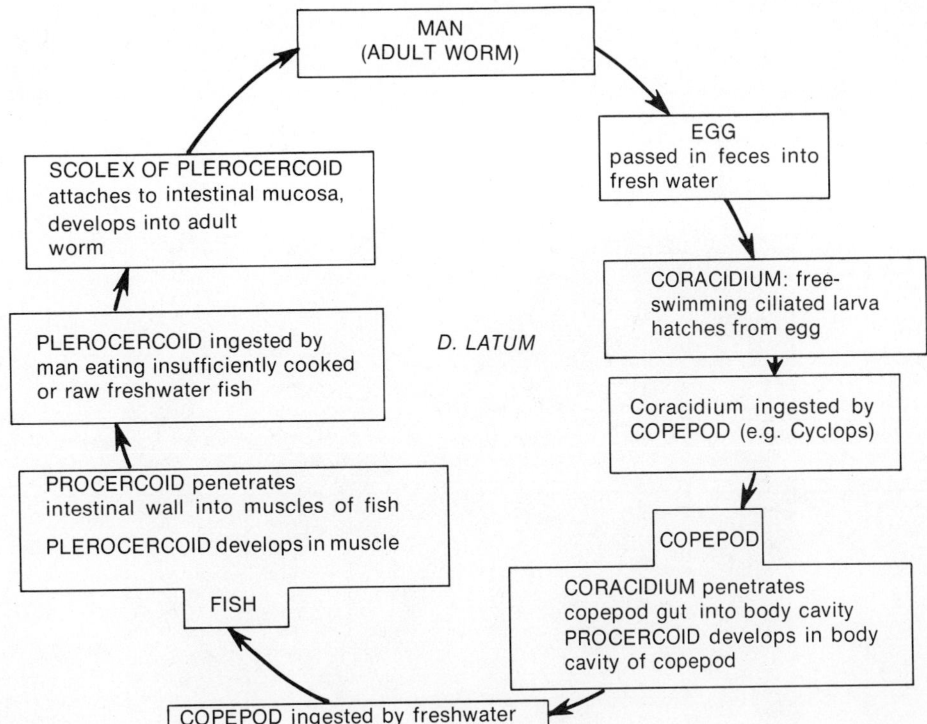

Figure 25–16 Life cycle of *Diphyllobothrium latum.*

Diagnosis. The finding of the proglottids or the operculated ova in the stool is diagnostic. The only other parasites of man that produce ova with opercula are liver flukes.

Hymenolepis nana

The dwarf tapeworm is not uncommon in southern Europe and in the southern part of the United States and in Latin America. In small children multiple infection may cause intestinal symptoms such as pain and diarrhea, as well as convulsions. Unlike the tapeworms, there is only one host and infection is believed to be from man to man.

Life Cycle and Morphology. The adult worm measures up to 4 cm long and has a maximum diameter of 1 mm. The tiny scolex is only 0.3 mm in diameter and has four lateral suckers and a retractable rostellum with a single row of hooklets (Fig. 25–18). The proglottids in the distal part of the worm are rounded rather than flattened and the largest are relatively small as compared to the other species of tapeworms. The maximum size is approximately 1 by 0.3 mm. The uterus is saccular and irregular, and the genital pores in adjacent segments are arranged on the same side. The ova are round or slightly ovoid, measuring about 50 μm in diameter and having a thick gelatinous capsule between two thick walls. Within the gelatinous material at each pole there are some rather indistinct filamentous markings. Within the inner capsule is the mature ovum, which is provided with three distinct pairs of hooklets (Fig. 25–18). The life cycle of *Hymenolepis nana* is summarized in Figure 25–19. This parasite is unique in that the adult worm develops following ingestion of the egg by man, the six-hooked oncosphere burrowing into the villi of the intestinal mucosa, where it develops into a cysticercoid larva. When matured, the larvae "hatch" into the lumen of the small intestine in which they grow into adult worms. It is also possible that *H. nana* may develop into infective cysticercoids in various arthropod intermediate hosts, e.g., fleas, grain beetles, etc.; the latter can be ingested inadvertently with contaminated grain products. Similarly, larval fleas can be ingested, particularly by children.

Hymenolepis diminuta is similar to *H. nana*, and is a cosmopolitan cestode of rats and mice. Children appear to be more prone to infestation by this species. The cestode has a short life and infections are generally light. The absence of polar filaments in the egg readily distinguishes this species from *H. nana*. The life cycle of *H. diminuta* is shown in Figure 25–19.

Diagnosis. Diagnosis is made by identification of the ova in the stool (Fig. 25–18).

Echinococcus granulosus

Man is an intermediate host in this infestation. The usual definitive host is the dog or wolf; sheep and cattle as well as man may be the intermediate hosts. The incidence of human infestation is high in sheep-raising areas and especially in Iceland, Australia, Wales, Italy, and the southern part of South America. The cystic stage in man involves the liver particularly, but hydatid cysts of the lungs, and to a lesser extent of other viscera, are well documented. The cysts give rise to symptoms by mechanical pressures in their different sites; rupture may cause serious allergic reactions.

Life Cycle and Morphology. The adult worm, which lives in the small bowel of the dog, has only three or four segments and measures 3 to 6 mm long. The head

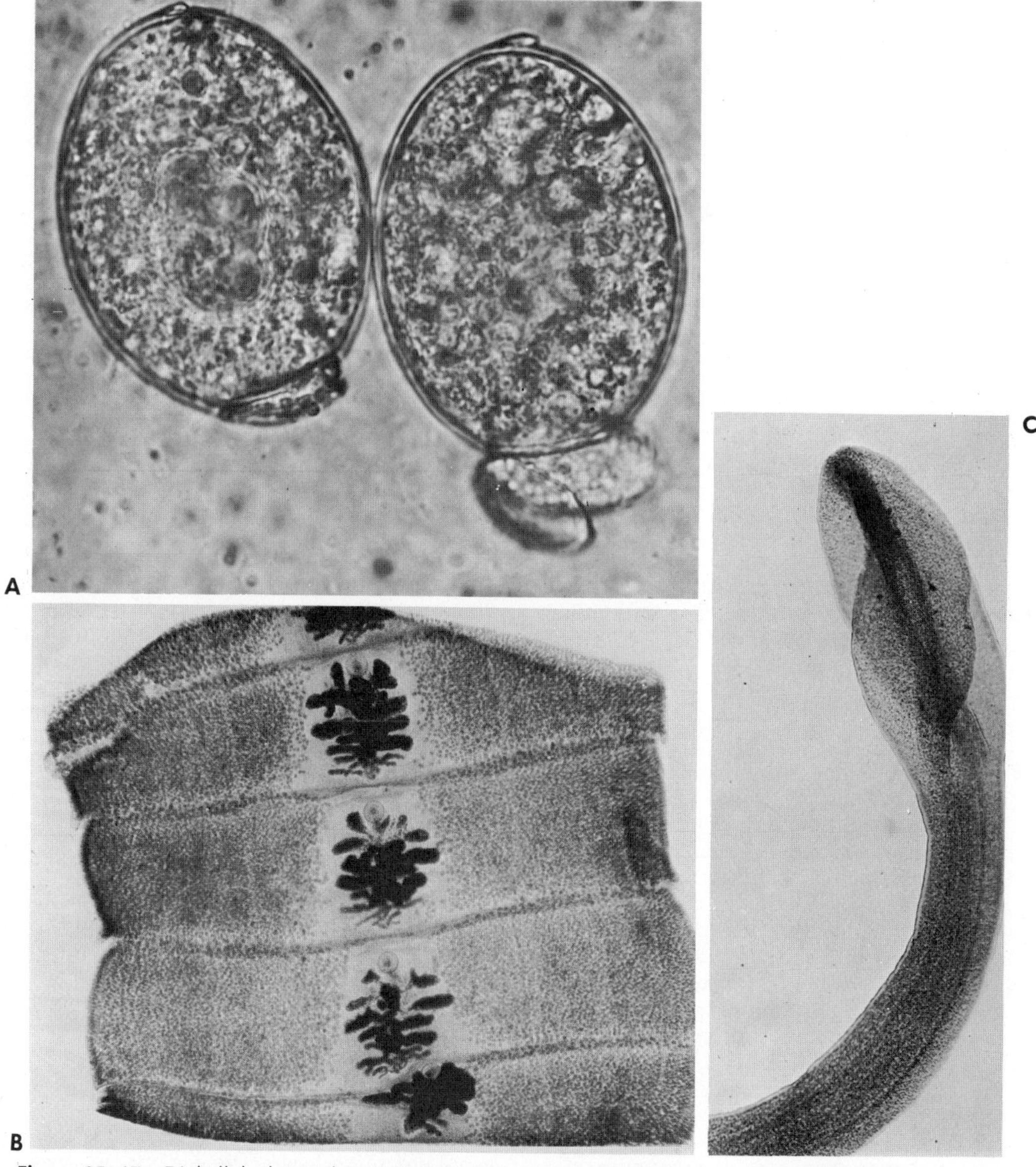

Figure 25–17 *Diphyllobothrium latum.* **A,** Ova. One ovum shows an open operculum and an extruding embryo. × 1050. **B,** Proglottids. Mature segments showing arrangement of genitalia and situation of the genital pore. × 15. **C,** Scolex. × 60. (**B** courtesy of the late Col. C. A. Bozman, Wellcome Museum of Medical Science, London, England. **C** courtesy of Dr. A. M. Fallis, Toronto, Ont.)

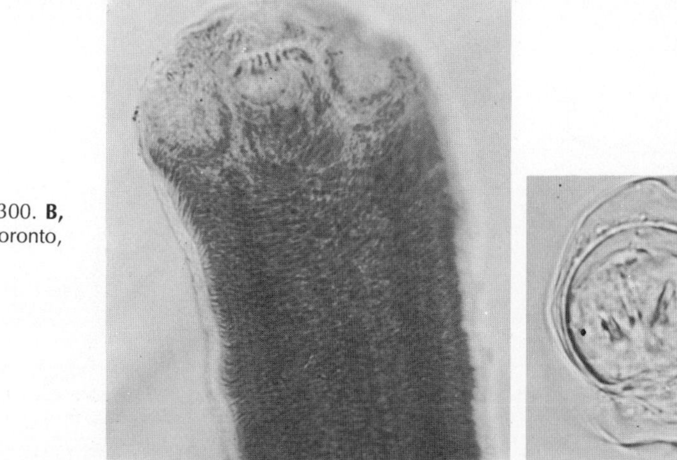

Figure 25–18 *Hymenolepsis nana.* **A,** Scolex. × 300. **B,** Ovum. × 1050. (**A** courtesy of Dr. A. M. Fallis, Toronto, Ont.)

has four suckers and two rings of hooklets. The ova are similar to those of *T. saginata* and are passed in the dog's feces. When ova are ingested by man, the larvae are liberated, enter the venules of the small bowel wall, and are transported in the portal system to the liver; less commonly, they are taken to the lungs or other organs. In the organs, the larvae form cysts that may ultimately reach 25 cm in diameter. The cyst has two layers, and from the inner membrane there develop "daughter cysts," which are ovoid structures containing the invaginated scolex of a mature worm complete with suckers and a rostellum bearing hooklets. The dog becomes infected by eating infected viscera from sheep and cattle, and the cycle is complete (Fig. 25–20).

Diagnosis. Serological examination is often diagnostic. There are numerous methodologies, which include an indirect hemagglutinin test, bentonite and latex flocculation tests, and indirect fluorescence. Generally, serum is sent to reference laboratories for such investigation.

Surgical Exploration. Surgical exploration of the cyst will yield hydatid fluid, and microscopic examination of such material will show the characteristic barbed hooklets or even "daughter cysts." In looking for the hooklets, much help can be obtained, especially in old cysts, by having sections stained with Ziehl-Neelsen. The hooklets are acid-fast.

Echinococcus multilocularis (Alveolar Hydatid)

The usual definitive host is the white or red fox or wolf, and the intermediate hosts are voles, field mice, or

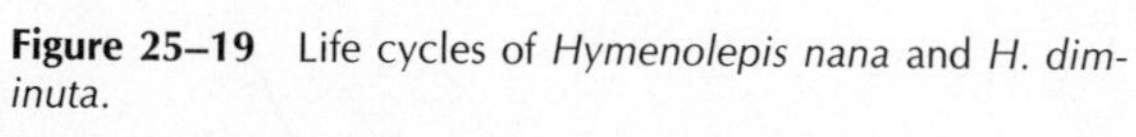

Figure 25–19 Life cycles of *Hymenolepsis nana* and *H. diminuta.*

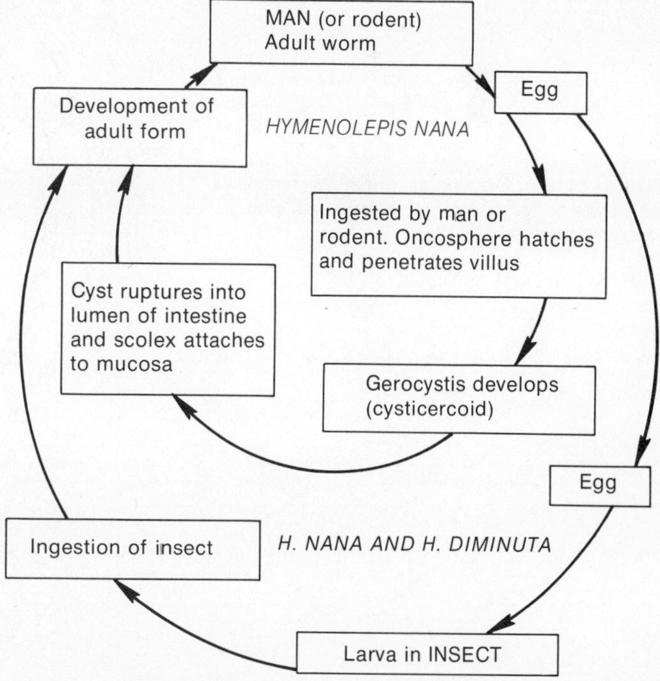

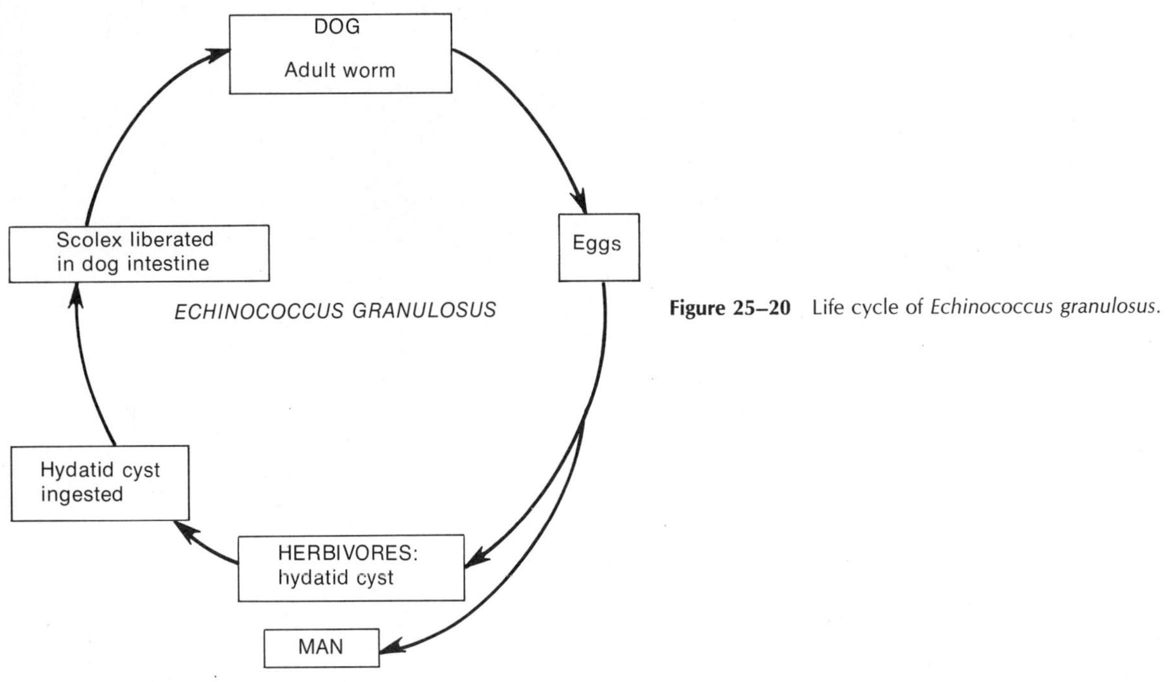

Figure 25–20 Life cycle of *Echinococcus granulosus*.

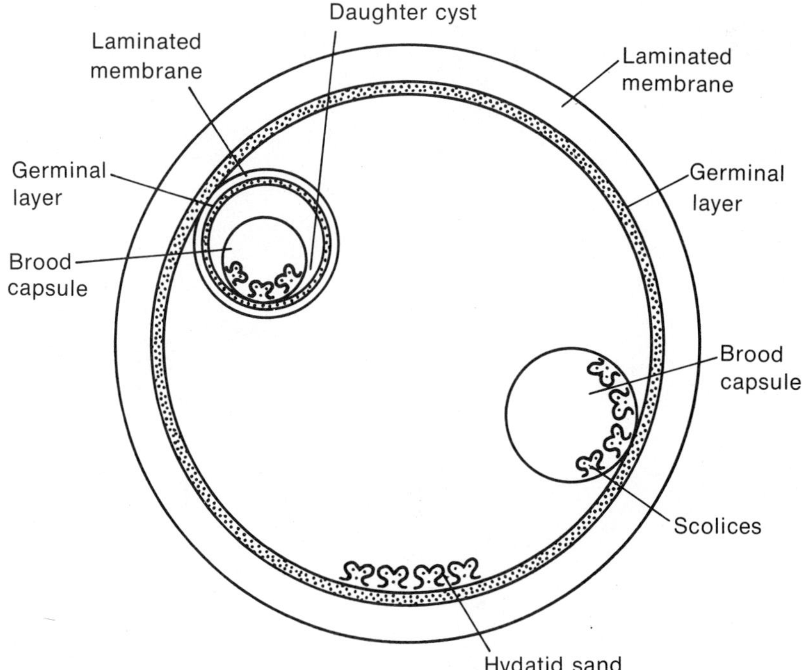

Figure 25–21 Diagrammatic representation of *Echinococcus granulosus*. Hydatid cyst, with daughter cysts (see Fig. 25–23).

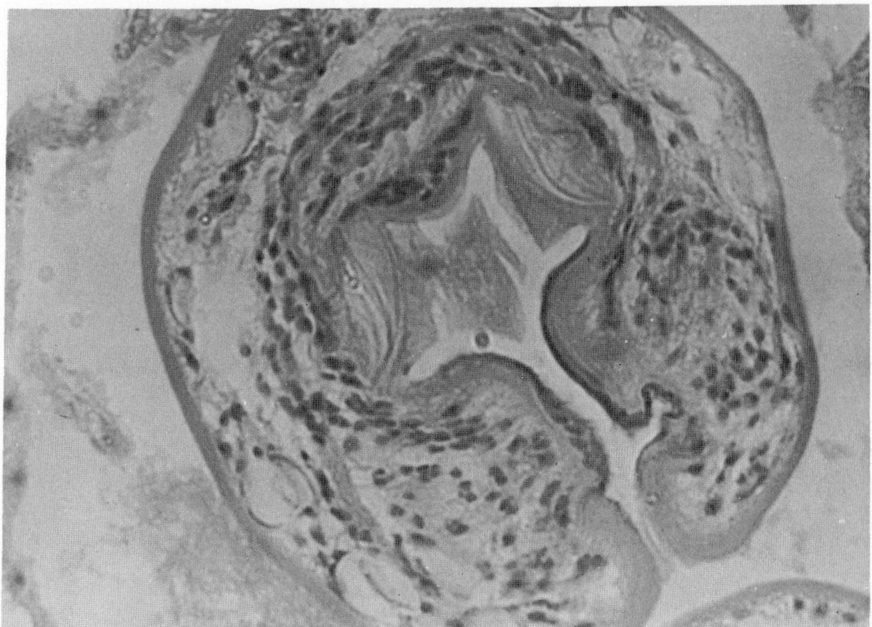

Figure 25–22 *Echinococcus granulosus.* Daughter cyst showing invaginated scolex and hooklets. Hematoxylin-eosin × 1050.

ground squirrels. Even in this sylvatic setting, man may become the occasional intermediate host by ingesting berries contaminated with ova or by manual contamination in trapping or skinning infested wild animals. Domestic dogs and cats may become definitive hosts by eating infected mice, and man in an urban setting may then become the intermediate host by ingesting material contaminated with cat's or dog's feces. The disease has a remarkably wide geographic distribution, causing infestation in Europe, USSR, Japan, South America, and Australasia. In this continent, cases have occurred in the prairie provinces of Canada and in North Dakota, Alaska, and the Arctic. In man the cyst in the liver forms small vesicles without ectocyst (about 0.5 cm in diameter) filled with mucoid material containing few or no scolices. Spread is by budding at the periphery, around which there is inflammatory exudate of the host's cells and in time a fibrotic response. Thrombotic infarction is common. Destruction of the liver and metastases to the lungs and brain occur. The outlook for the disease is very poor unless the proliferating cysts are surgically removed and this is rarely possible. This course of the disease contrasts sharply with the relatively, occasionally completely, benign course of infestation with *E. granulosus*.

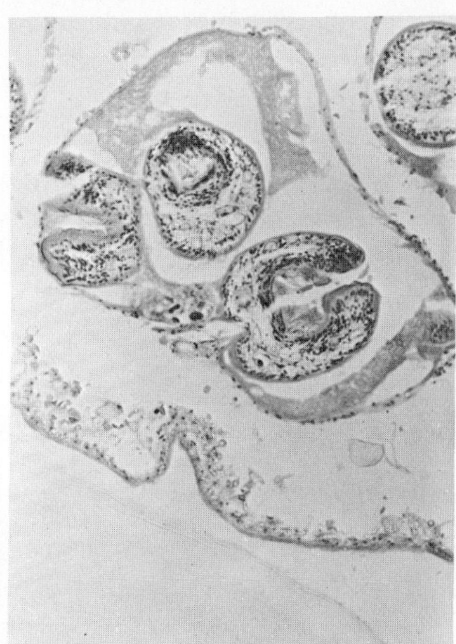

Figure 25–23 *Echinococcus granulosus.* Daughter cysts. Hematoxylin-eosin × 300.

Life Cycle and Morphology. The adult worm in the small bowel of the dog or fox is similar to *E. granulosus* but smaller (1.2 to 3.7 mm). The ova passed in the feces are also similar to those of *E. granulosus*. In the natural cycle of the disease, the dog or fox is infected by eating mice or voles and the canine droppings infect a further group of rodents. When man becomes the intermediate host, the multimicrovesicular disease of the liver may produce no definitive symptoms, but there may be jaundice, hepatomegaly, and possibly slight eosinophilia. Metastatic lesions will produce focal symptoms.

Diagnosis. Serological tests similar to those employed in the diagnosis of *E. granulosus* are used. There is cross-reaction between *E. granulosus* and *multilocularis*.

THE TREMATODES

Basic Characteristics

The Trematoda or flukes are one class of the phylum Platyhelminthes. The majority of the species parasitic in man are digenetic (hermaphroditic) and capable of self-fertilization; the exceptions are the schistosomes, and these will be discussed separately. All flukes have complex life cycles, requiring one or more intermediate hosts. Eggs are laid by the adult within the vertebrate host, which when discharged into the external environment may contain fully developed larvae. The larva or miracidium escapes via a lid in the eggshell, if operculated, or through a longitudinal split if nonoperculated. The miracidium then seeks out its aquatic intermediate host, generally a mollusc (snail or clam). Within the mollusc, the miracidium undergoes metamorphoses into sporocysts, which serve as a brood sac for the development of a generation of daughter sporocysts known as rediae. Ultimately a large number of larvae are produced called cercariae. In some species the cercariae are able to penetrate the definitive host directly, as is the case with *Schistosoma*; or they enter an insect, fish, or some other second intermediate host; in others, they become attached to vegetation to await ingestion by the definitive host. Those cercariae requiring a second intermediate host are referred to as metacercariae. Figure 25–24 summarizes the essential morphologic features of an adult trematode and its life cycle.

Liver Flukes

There are several genera and species that particularly involve the liver and the biliary passages. Among these are *Fasciola hepatica*, which is primarily a disease of sheep but also infests man; *Opisthorchis felineus*, which infests dogs, cats, and foxes, but also may affect man; and *Clonorchis sinensis*, which is endemic in the Orient but may also be found in Oriental immigrants living in North America.

Clonorchis sinensis (Opisthorchis sinensis)

The adult worms infest the biliary passages, and the disease often must be differentiated from liver disease.

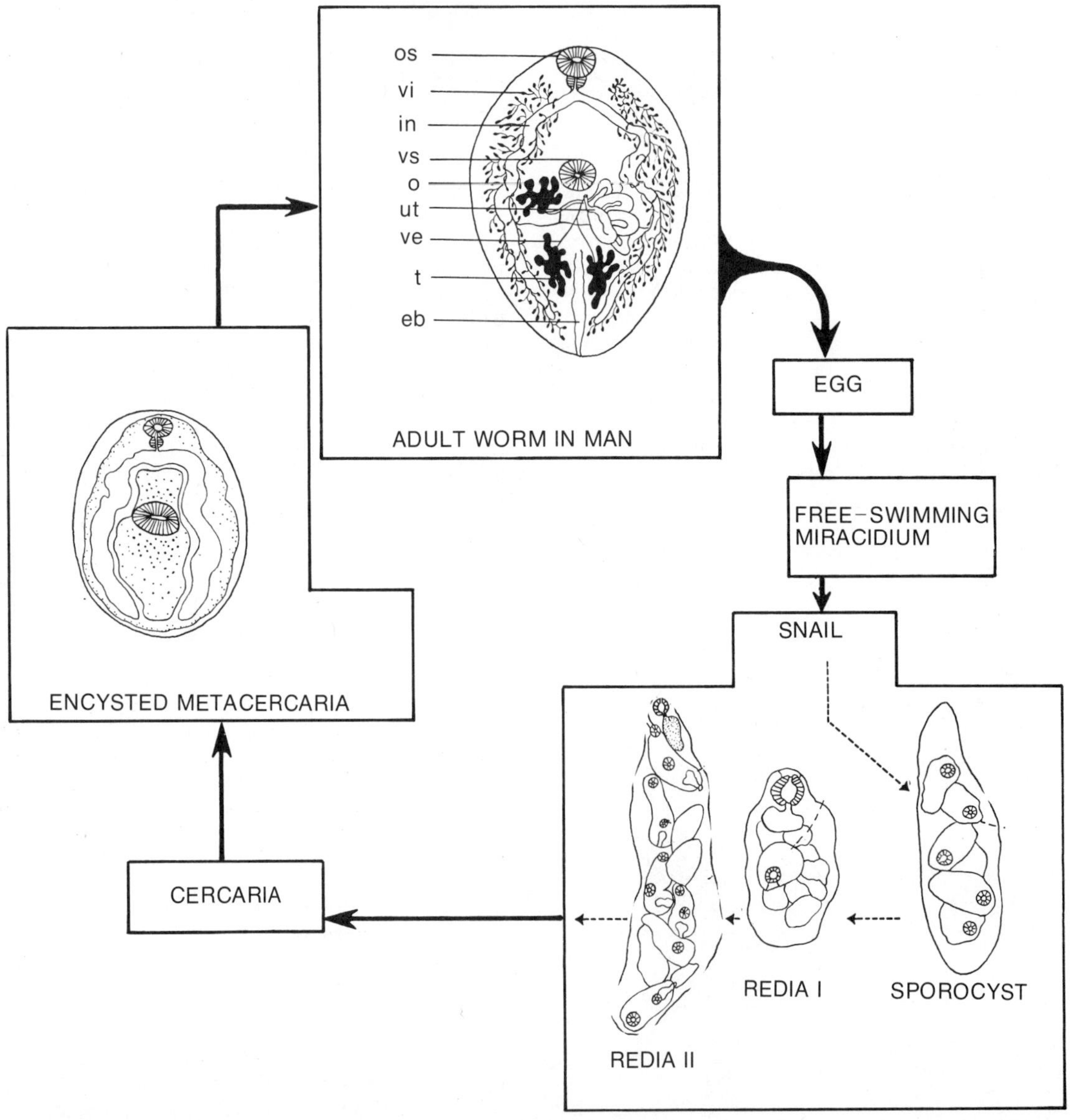

Figure 25–24 Summary of essential morphological features of an adult trematode, and its life cycle. Adult trematode: *eb*, excretory bladder; *in*, intestine; *o*, ovary; *os*, oral sucker; *t*, testis; *ut*, uterus; *ve*, vas efferens; *vi*, vitellaria; *vs*, ventral sucker.

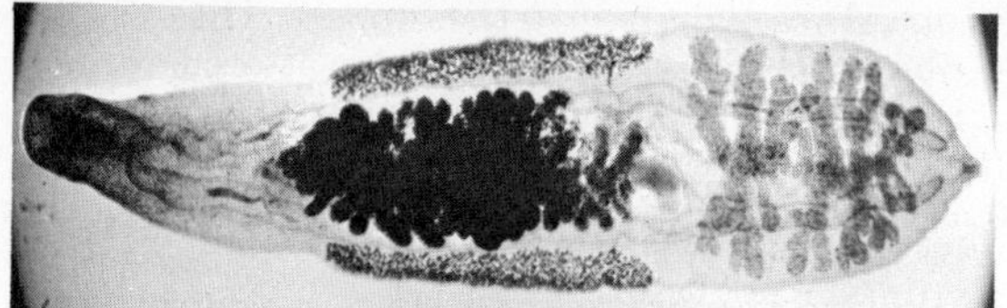

Figure 25–25 *Clonorchis sinensis* adult. × 10.

Symptoms and signs suggestive of hepatitis, cholangiolitis, and cirrhosis may be prominent. The adult worm is a boat-shaped, fleshy mass measuring 10 to 25 by 3 to 5 mm (Fig. 25–25). Ova are approximately 15 to 30 μm and have an operculum at one pole, and at the other pole a small projection from the shell (Fig. 25–26). With fine microscopic focusing, the egg shell has an irregular linear pattern like "cracked dry mud." Ova pass through the bile passages into the bowel and are excreted in the feces. In water the ova produce a free-living form or miracidium, which is ingested by a water snail. In the snail several stages of development are accomplished until free-living cercariae escape and infest fish, invading the latter between the scales and encysting in the superficial flesh. Ingestion of poorly cooked fish will cause infestation in man and, during digestion, the cysts liberate metacercariae, which migrate up the biliary ducts and mature to adult worms. Since this worm is endemic to Vietnam, laboratory workers should be aware of its possible presence in American war veterans. The life cycle is summarized in Figure 25–27. Diagnosis is made by finding characteristic ova in the stool, or by histological examination of liver biopsy.

Opisthorchis felineus

This is a parasite generally found in cats, though man can also become infected. The adult worm inhabits the bile ducts and causes a disease similar to that produced by *O. sinensis*. The life cycles of the two parasites are similar. There are subtle structural differences between the two adult forms. The ova of *O. felineus* are considered to be narrower than those of *O. sinensis*; otherwise they are morphologically indistinguishable.

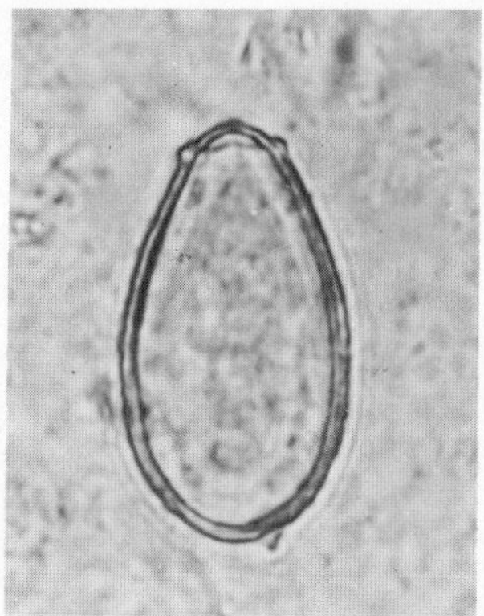

Figure 25–26 *Clonorchis sinensis* ovum. × 1050. (Courtesy of Dr. D. S. Ridley, Hospital for Tropical Diseases, London, England.)

Fasciola hepatica

This is a common parasite of herbivores often referred to as the sheep liver fluke. It has a cosmopolitan distribution. Human infestations are not infrequent and are of considerable public health importance in Latin America. The adult worm of *Fasciola hepatica* is smaller than its relative *Fasciolopsis buski*; in addition to size, it can be readily differentiated from the latter by its characteristic shape, a "cephalic cone" at the anterior end.

Infestation occurs following ingestion of aquatic vegetation (e.g., watercress) upon which *Fasciola* metacer-

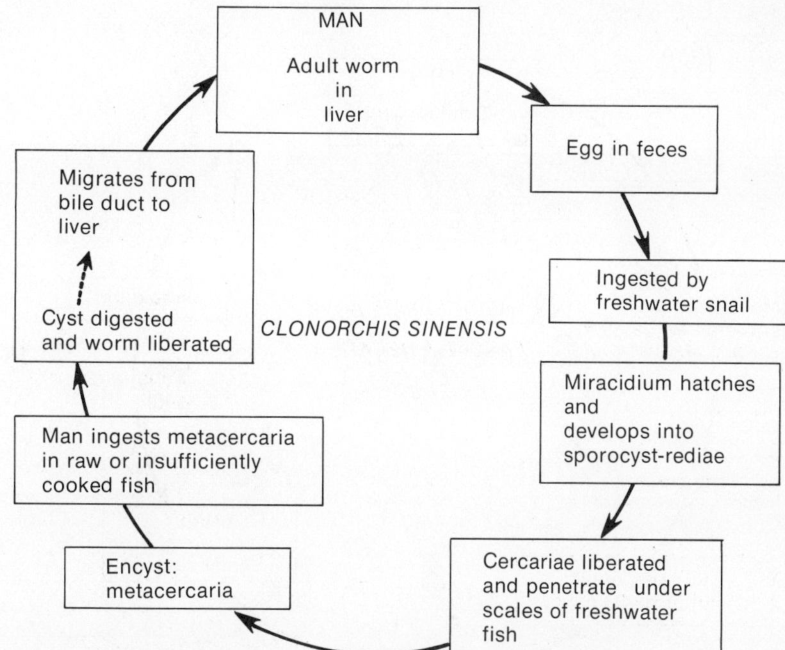

Figure 25–27 Life cycle of *Clonorchis (Opisthorchis) sinensis*.

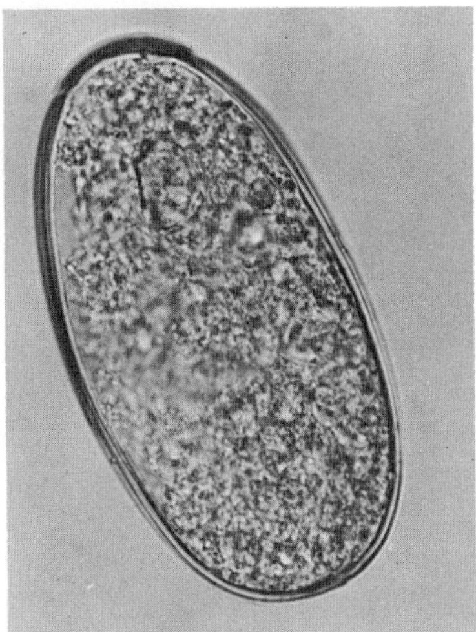

Figure 25–28 *Fasciola hepatica* ovum. Note the operculum with its convex joint surface. × 6030.

cariae have become encysted. These metacercariae burrow into and through the wall of the duodenum and enter the bile ducts, where they mature. In human infections considerable local irritation may result during the migration of immature worms to the liver region. Resulting pathology includes damage to liver tissues, mechanical obstruction, and so forth. Diagnosis depends on finding eggs in the feces (it should be noted that they are not readily distinguished from those of *Fasciolopsis*). They are large operculated eggs measuring 130 to 150 by 60 to 90 μm (see Fig. 25–28). The life cycle is summarized in Figure 25–29.

Lung Flukes

Paragonimus westermani

This fluke and related species are to be found parasitizing human lung tissue, often encapsulated in cystic-like structures adjacent to the bronchi. These flukes are distributed throughout Asia, and scattered throughout the islands of the South and Southwest Pacific.

The adult worms are dark brown in color, measuring from 0.8 to 1.5 cm in length, 0.5 to 0.8 cm in width, and 0.3 to 0.6 cm in thickness (Fig. 25–30). The eggs of this parasite are operculated and large, measuring from 75 to 120 μm in length and by 45 to 60 μm in breadth, and dark brown in color (Fig. 25–30). They are to be found in expectorate or fecal specimens.

Infestation results from the consumption of raw or insufficiently cooked freshwater crustaceans, e.g., crayfish, in which the encysted metacercarial stage occurs. The larval stages occur in an appropriate species of snail (e.g., *Melania*). Following ingestion, the metacercariae are liberated into the lumen of the host's intestine, where they penetrate, and enter the peritoneal cavity. From here they enter the pleural cavity and subsequently gain entry into the lungs, where they mature. Here, the worm provokes a pronounced tissue reaction, resulting in the formation of "pulmonic" cysts (a fibrous capsule surrounding the parasite). *Paragonimus* is known to cause lesions in other sites, e.g., brain, but extrapulmonary paragonimiasis is rare. Extruded eggs infiltrate into the bronchioles, where they find their way to the external environment either via the sputum or feces.

Patients infested with *Paragonimus* frequently experience hemoptysis following a paroxysm of coughing, the expectorate of which will often contain numerous dark brown eggs; the appearance of these in the sputum has been likened to "iron filings."

Diagnosis is dependent on the demonstration of the characteristic operculated eggs in either the sputum or feces.

Blood Flukes

There are three important species in this group that cause chronic and severe disease in man: *Schistosoma*

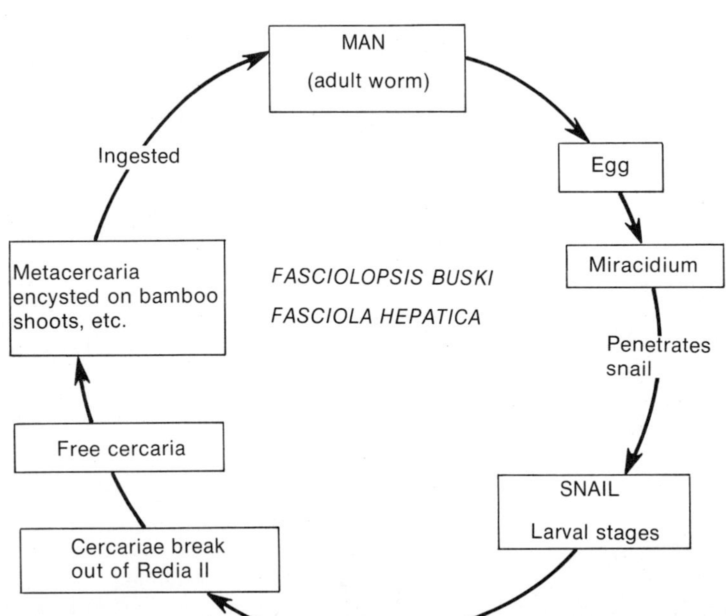

Figure 25–29 Life cycles of *Fasciolopsis buski* and *Fasciola hepatica*.

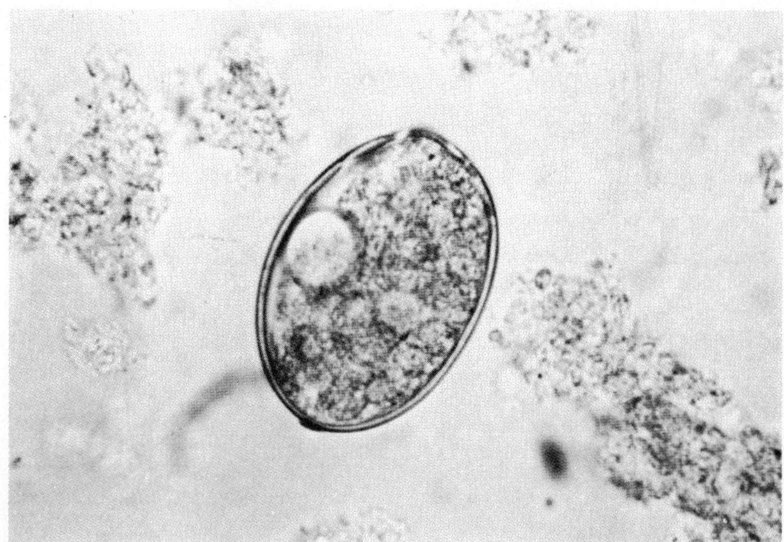

Figure 25–30 *Paragonimus westermani* ovum. (Reprinted by permission. From Blecka, Lawrence J.: *Concise Medical Parasitology*. Copyright 1980. Menlo Park, California: Addison-Wesley Publishing Company.)

haematobium, S. mansoni, and *S. japonicum*. The first is widespread in the Middle East and Central and South Africa; the second occurs in Egypt, Central and East Africa, South America, and some Caribbean areas (in particular Puerto Rico); *Schistosoma japonicum* occurs only in the Orient.

Schistosomes

The schistosomes differ from other trematodes in that (i) they are diecious (i.e., there are 2 sexes and the organisms are either male or female but not hermaphroditic), (ii) they are adapted to an intravascular existence, (iii) ova are not operculated, but hatch via a longitudinal rupture in the eggshell if liberated into fresh water, and (iv) all other trematode parasites of man are acquired through ingestion of metacercariae, but infection with schistosomes takes place by direct penetration of the cercariae through the skin.

Life Cycles of *Schistosoma*. The life cycles of the three species are similar (Fig. 25–31). The mature worms live in the veins of the pelvis or mesenteric veins and are about 6 to 15 mm long, varying from species to species, with the female always larger than the male. Ova are laid in the veins, often over a period of years, and they finally rupture through the vein walls into the tissues and the viscera. *Schistosoma haematobium* ova most often pass from the pelvic veins into the urinary bladder and can be found in the urine; ova from other species more often rupture into the bowel and are passed in the

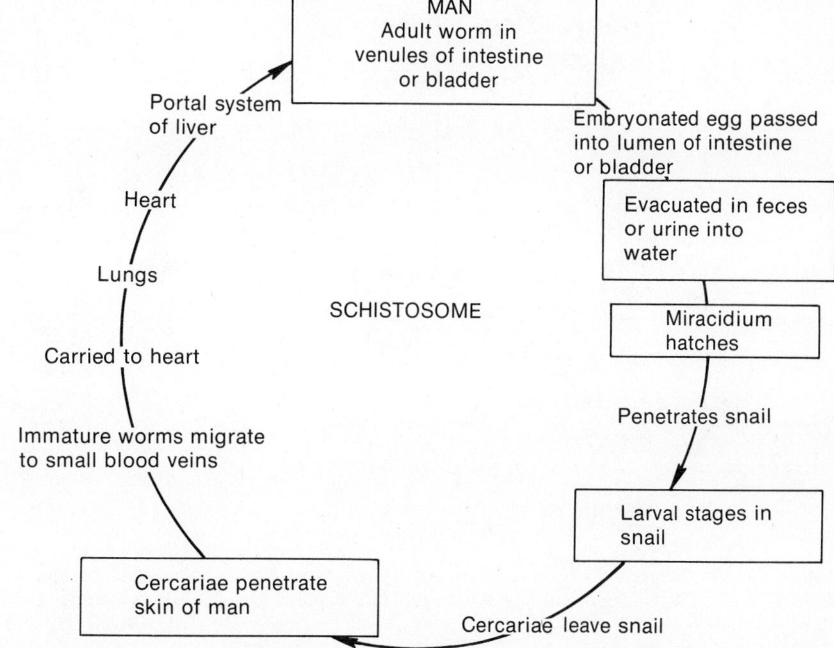

Figure 25–31 Life cycle of the Schistosomes.

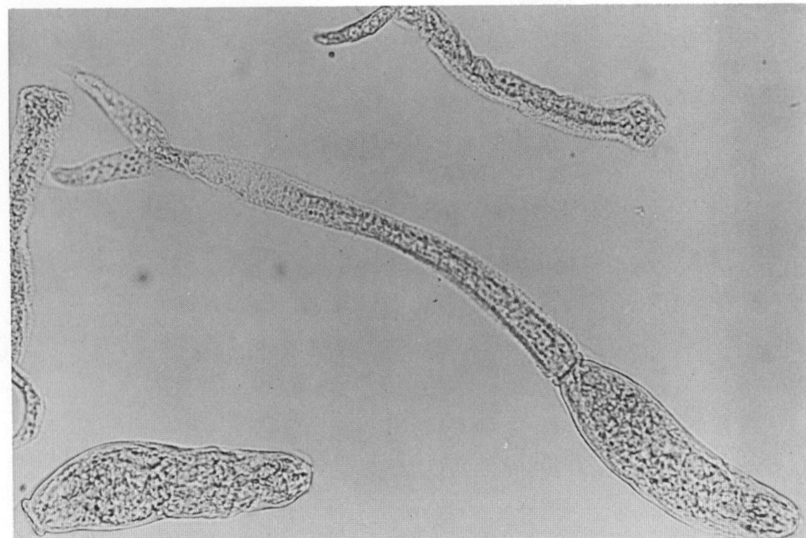

Figure 25–32 *Schistosoma mansoni*. Cercariae. × 300.

feces. In the excreta, the ova reach water where they become free-living miracidia, which infect water snails. In this host, maturation continues until another free-living form, the cercaria, is produced (Fig. 25–32). Cercariae then swim until they come in contact with human skin, which they pierce to invade the small veins. They are carried in the blood to the right ventricle and actively force themselves through the pulmonary circulation into the systemic circulation. Finally, they arrive in the mesenteric artery and the portal veins, where they mature and subsequently infest these and other abdominal vein systems.

Schistosomiasis. In the diseases produced by all three organisms, there is an initial period characterized by irritation at the point of entry of the parasite through the skin, urticaria, fever, abdominal pain, and perhaps diarrhea. A second stage follows which in *Schistosoma haematobium* infestation is shown by urinary symptoms, in *Schistosoma mansoni* infestation by abdominal pain and diarrhea, and in *Schistosoma japonicum* infestation by diarrhea and fever. A third stage in the disease caused by *Schistosoma haematobium* is that of severe chronic urinary disease; in the mansoni type, this stage is typified by colitis, fissures, ischiorectal abscesses, and hepatomegaly and splenomegaly; and in the japonicum type, by hepatomegaly, splenomegaly, colitis, and ascites.

Morphology of Ova of *Schistosoma*. The ova of *Schistosoma haematobium* measure about 150 by 60 μm and are provided with a spine projecting from the shell, characteristically situated at one pole (Figs. 25–33 and 25–34). Ova of *Schistosoma mansoni* are similar in size and are differentiated by the site of the spine, which in this species is lateral to one pole (Fig. 25–35). The ova of *Schistosoma japonicum* are smaller, measuring ap-

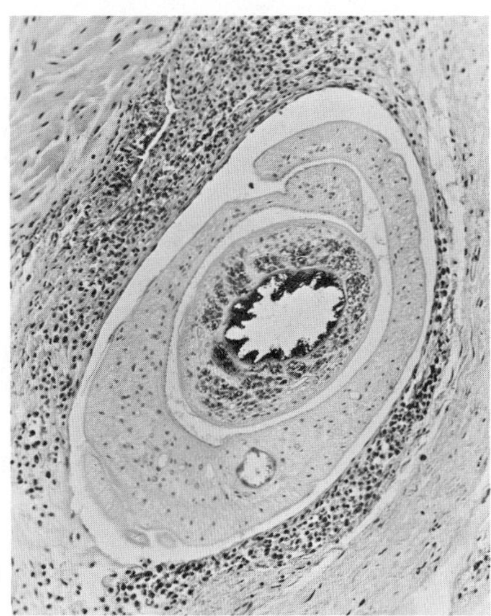

Figure 25–33 *Schistosoma haematobium*. Adults in vessels of the bladder wall; the female is within the gynecophoric canal of the male. Hematoxylin-eosin × 180.

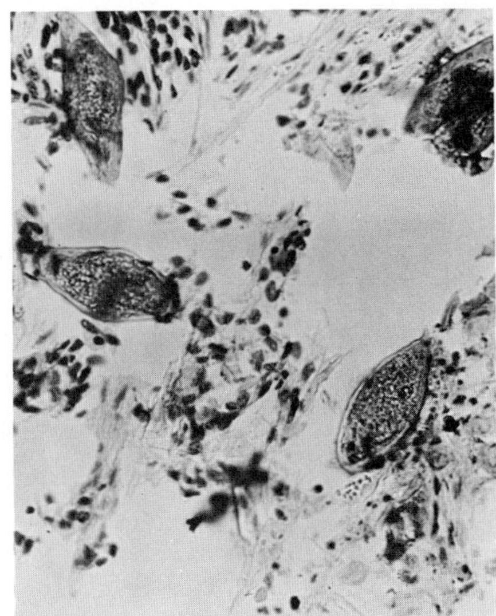

Figure 24–34 *Schistosoma haematobium*. Ova in the bladder wall. Note the position of the spine at one pole. Hematoxylin-eosin × 300. (Courtesy of Prof. Besium Turhan, Dept. of Pathology, Istanbul University Medical School, Turkey.)

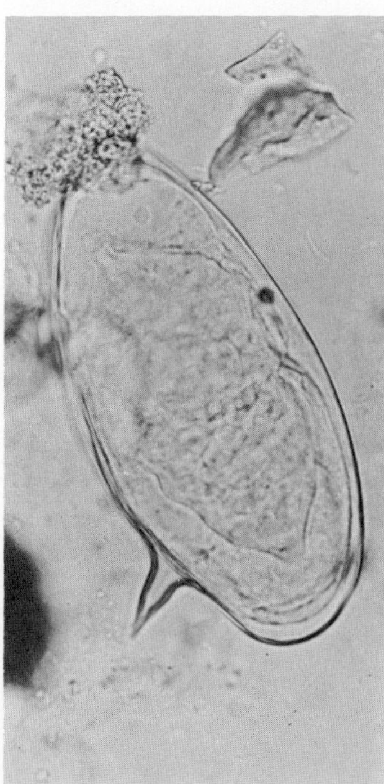

Figure 25–35 *Schistosoma mansoni*. The long spine is laterally situated. Ovum in feces. × 630. (Courtesy of Dr. Jan Schwarz.)

proximately 80 by 60 μm, and on the lateral surface there is a small depression, one side of which is extended to form a small curved hook (Fig. 25–36).

Diagnosis. The diagnosis may be made by finding ova in the urine (*Schistosoma haematobium*) or in the stool (*Schistosoma mansoni* and *japonicum*). Although urine (for *S. haematobium*) may be collected at any time, it is said that the best collection time is between noon and 2 p.m. The urine may be filtered by the Millipore method to achieve concentration. Surgical biopsy from affected areas will often reveal ova surrounded by inflammatory and scar tissue. Intradermal, complement fixation, indirect fluorescence, and flocculation tests are also used.

THE NEMATODES

Basic Characteristics

Compared with the digenetic trematodes and certain cestodes, the majority of the nematodes have relatively simple life cycles. Typically, larvae are required to undergo a free-living stage of development (external to the host) in order to mature to the infective stage. Such larvae are often referred to as rhabditiform, which is a reference to the type of esophagus they possess. Hookworm and *Ascaris* are examples of such species requiring this stage of external development. By contrast, *Enterobius* and *Trichuris* adult worms lay eggs that are infective immediately upon expulsion from the host environment, if fully embryonated. Variations in the life cycles of nematode worms are shown in Figure 25–37.

Morphologically, the nematodes are nonsegmented round worms, covered by a tough protective cuticle. The anterior end of the worm may be equipped with teeth or plates as is the case with the hookworms, whereas in primitive forms the mouth is surrounded by three lips. The nematodes have a complete digestive tract, extending from mouth to anus, an opening on the ventral surface not far from the posterior extremity. The anterior segment of the digestive canal is generally a muscular esophagus. The sexes are separate and generally exhibit considerable sexual dimorphism. Fundamental features of nematode anatomy are depicted in Figure 25–38.

Intestinal Nematodes

Trichuris trichiura (Whipworm)

This nematode parasite has worldwide distribution. The adult worms live in the mucosa of the cecum or the mucosae of nearby bowel, and usually only a relatively small number are present. In the majority of cases, infestation is asymptomatic, but occasionally it produces abdominal pain and vomiting or, in very heavy infestation, there may be bloody diarrhea and anemia. Rarely, mechanical obstruction of the appendix lumen may initiate appendicitis. Rectal prolapse can also occur in heavy infections.

Life Cycle and Morphology. Infection is from man to man by ingestion of food soiled with developed viable ova (see Fig. 25–37). The shell of the ovum is digested in the small intestine and the larval form of the worm attaches itself to the bowel mucosa, later moving to the site of choice in the cecum. The adult worm measures 3 to 4.5 cm (male) or 3.5 to 5 cm (female). Both forms are

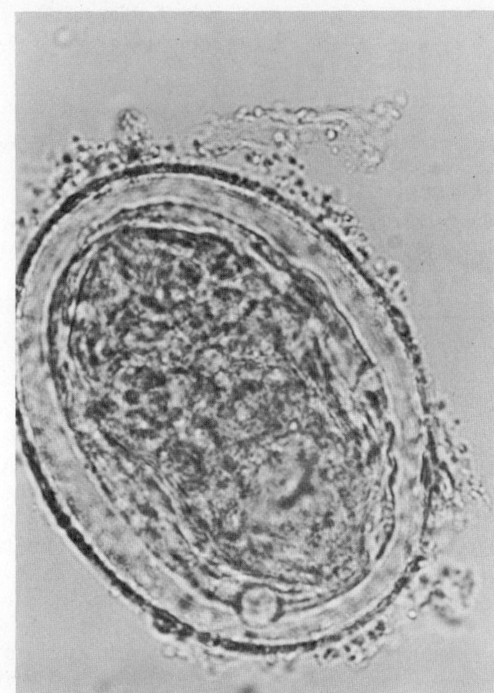

Figure 25–36 *Schistosoma japonicum*. The small lateral spine can be seen, with a small corresponding depression in the wall of the ovum. Ovum in feces. × 1050. (Courtesy of F. R. N. Pester, Dept. of Helminthology, London School of Hygiene and Tropical Medicine, England.)

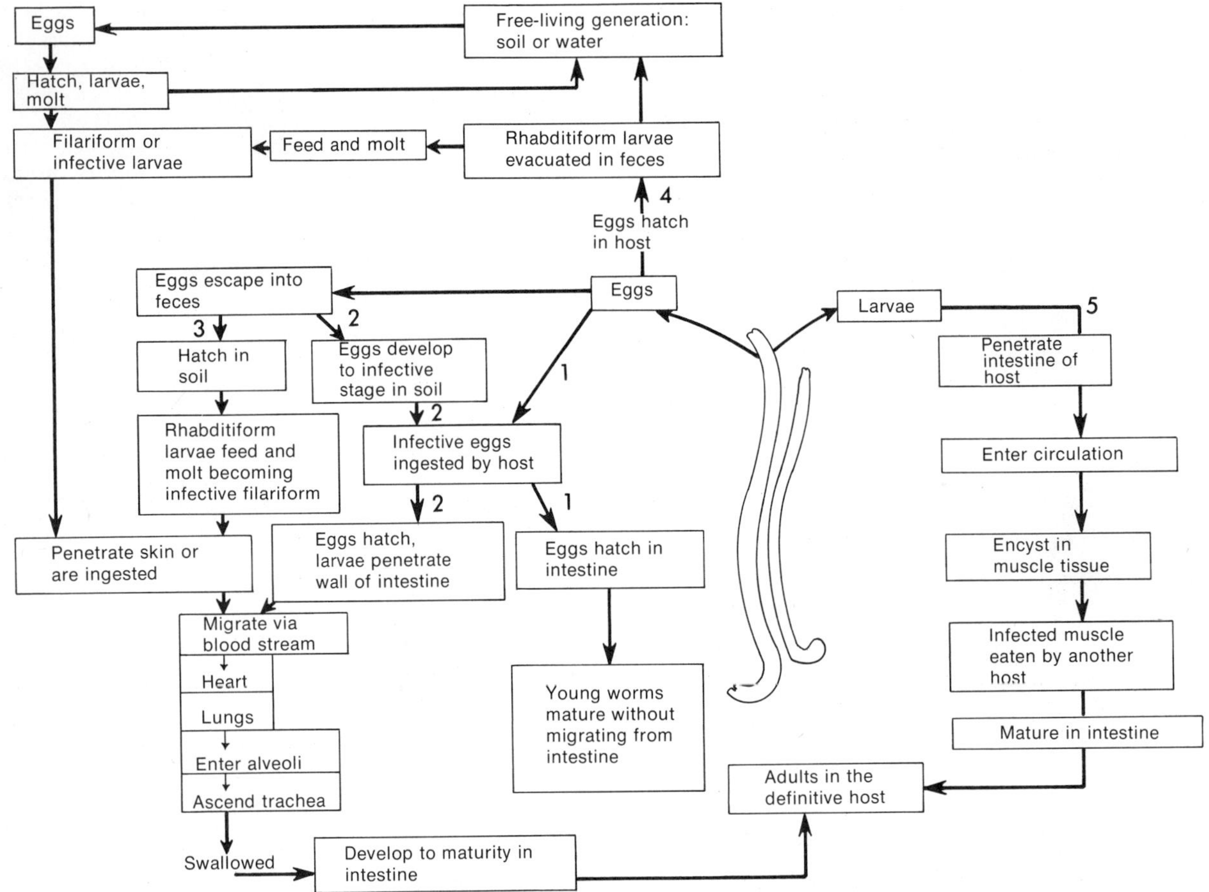

Figure 25–37 Variations in the life cycle of nematode worms. 1. *Enterobius vermicularis* and *Trichuris trichiura;* 2. *Ascaris lumbricoides;* 3. *Necator americanus* and *Ancylostoma duodenale;* 4. Strongyloides stercoralis; 5. *Trichinella spiralis.*

thin in their anterior parts but wider posteriorly; the male has a coiled caudal end. The adult worms are rarely seen in the feces, but the ova are easily recognized. They measure approximately 50 by 22 μm and have caps at either end, giving them a "Chinese lantern" appearance.

Diagnosis. Diagnosis is made by recognition of the ova in stool (Fig. 25–39).

Enterobius vermicularis (Pinworm, Threadworm)

The pinworm is of worldwide distribution, although its incidence varies from place to place. In North America and western Europe, children are more often infested than adults. The adult worms live in the cecum, appendix, and adjacent colon and ileum, but the female migrates to the anus to deposit her ova. The infestation does not, as a rule, produce any severe disease, although if the worms invade the appendix they may be factors in causation of appendicitis. Also, pruritus ani and vulvae caused by pinworms may be quite distressing.

Life Cycle and Morphology (Fig. 25–37). The adult worms are small and resemble fragments of cotton thread. The male measures 2 to 5 mm long and is about 0.2 mm thick at its greatest diameter; the caudal end is curved. The female is up to 13 mm long and 0.5 mm thick. At each side of the head, there is a slight expansion which is striated. When gravid, the female's body appears filled with ova (Fig. 25–40). At this stage, the female migrates down to the anus and beyond, laying her eggs on the perianal skin. The ova measure approximately 50 by 20 μm and are oval, with one characteristically flattened side; there is a thick chitinous capsule, and within, a coiled, occasionally motile, embryo is apparent (Fig. 25–41). The ova are carried by the fingers of the patient either to reinfect himself or to infect others who swallow them.

Diagnosis

1. The adult worms or ova may be recovered in the feces of the patient, but this method is not as efficient as others.

2. *Cellophane Tape Method*: **This method involves the collection of ova deposited on the perianal skin during the night on "sticky" tape that can be examined by direct microscopy. The procedure for preparing and collecting this specimen is summarized in Figure 25–42. As shown, the sampling "swab" consists of a length of cellophane tape attached to a microscope slide that in turn is fixed to a wooden spatula with a rubber band. The tape is carefully reversed over the end of the spatula and then pressed firmly to the perianal skin early in the morning before defecation.**

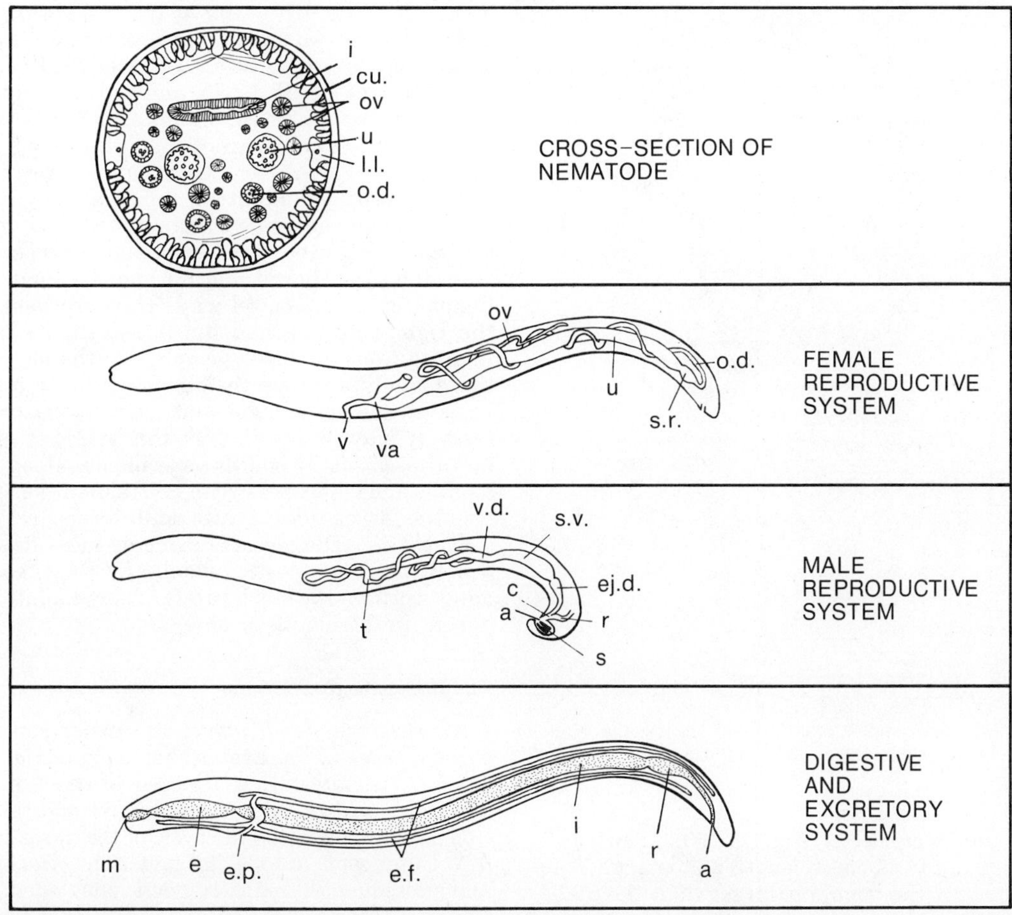

Figure 25–38 Basic anatomy of nematoid (ascarid): *a*, anus; *c, cloaca; cu*, cuticle; *e*, esophagus; *e.p.*, excretory pore; *e.t.*, excretory tubules; *ej.d.*, ejaculatory duct; *h*, hypodermis; *i*, intestine; *l. l.*, lateral line; *m*, mouth; *m.c.*, muscle cells; *n*, nucleus; *ov*, ovary; *o.d.*, oviduct; *r, rectum; s*, spicules; *sa*, sarcoplasm; *s.r.*, seminal receptacle; *s.v.*, seminal vesicle; *t*, testis; *u*, uterus; *v*, vulva; *va*, vagina; *v.d.*, vas deferens.

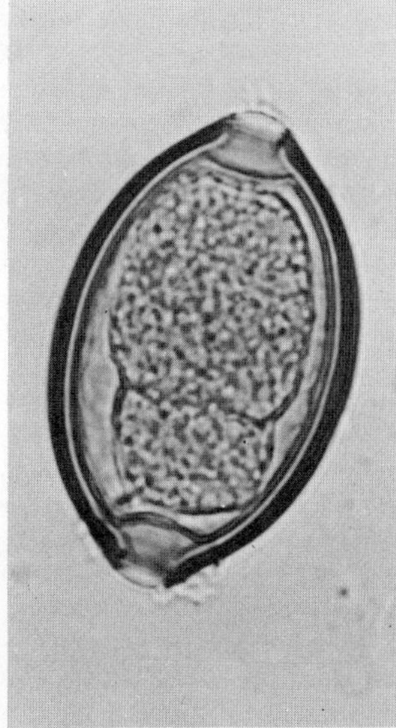

Figure 25–39 *Trichuris trichiura* ovum. × 1050. (Courtesy of Dr. A. M. Fallis, Toronto, Ont.)

Afterward, having detached the slide from the spatula, the tape is returned to the original position and smoothed down with a cotton ball. Direct microscope examination is then possible through the transparent tape. If desired, a drop of toluene may be placed on the slide before smoothing down the tape. The toluene clears epithelial cells, debris, and air bubbles. Specimens should be collected as soon as the patient arises, before bathing and defecation. Furthermore, unless positive, the test should be repeated on at least two other occasions.

Ascaris lumbricoides (Roundworm)

The roundworm has worldwide distribution and is the most common helminth infestation. Adult worms live in the small intestine and often produce no recognizable physical symptoms. However, they do cause abdominal pain and may produce symptoms by mechanical blockage of the bowel, the appendix, or the bile ducts. In the stage of migration of larvae there may be pneumonitis with fever, and systemic effects such as urticaria and asthma are not uncommon. Such systemic effects may also be seen in laboratory workers who become allergic to antigens of the worms encountered in handling them.

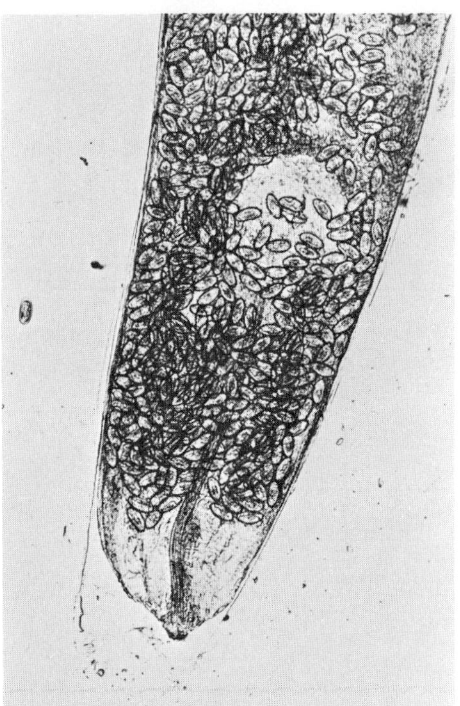

Figure 25–40 *Enterobius vermicularis.* Gravid female; the body cavity appears completely filled with ova. × 300.

Life Cycle and Morphology (Fig. 25–37). The adult worm measures up to 35 cm in length and is about 2 to 4 mm in diameter; the female is larger than the male, and diagnosis from the appearance of this large nematode and its superficial resemblance to the earthworm is not difficult (Fig. 25–43). Both ends are pointed, and at the anterior end, three lips can be identified under a hand lens. The distal end of the male worm is curled and there are two small sharp protrusions here known as the copulatory spicules. The fertilized ova measure 35 to 50 μm by 45 to 75 μm and are clothed in an irregular, mammillated, albuminous coat within which there is a thick transparent shell containing a granular protoplasm (Fig. 25–44). Ova may be brown or yellow in microscopic examination. Infection is by ingestion of ova from the soil or in contaminated food or drink. In the small intestine, the ova produce larvae that penetrate the small bowel mucosa and the small veins and lymphatics of the bowel wall. They are then carried to the right ventricle and the lungs. In the lungs, they migrate from the blood vessels into the air spaces, and there is migration up the air passages, across the epiglottis into the esophagus and down the gastrointestinal tract. It may be possible, at this stage, to observe the larval ascarids in sputum specimens, along with eosinophils and Charcot-Leyden crystals. In the small intestine the larvae develop into adult forms.

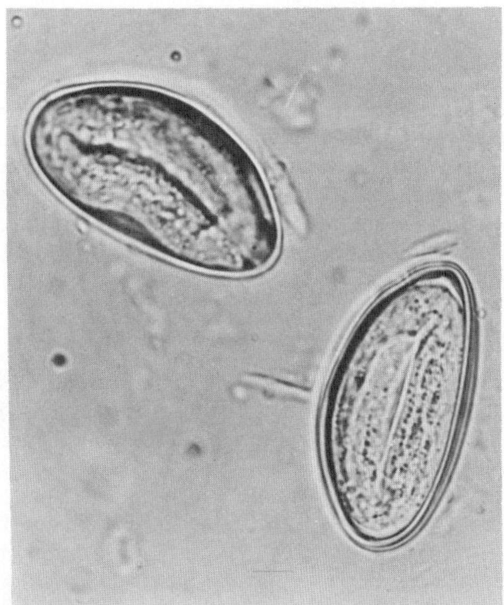

Figure 24–41 *Enterobius vermicularis* ova. Scotch-tape preparation cleared with immersion oil × 810.

Diagnosis. Diagnosis is made by identification of the ova in stool or, less commonly, by the presence of an adult worm in the stool; rarely, a small adult worm may appear in the mouth or nose.

Ancylostoma duodenale

Ancylostoma duodenale is the major cause of hookworm disease in the Eastern hemisphere, but occasional cases of the infestation are seen in the Americas. The disease may present in several ways and the presentation depends upon the life cycle of the parasite (Fig. 25–37). Cutaneous lesions (ground itch), transient fever, and subsequent chronic iron-deficiency anemia occur in stages of the disease.

Life Cycle and Morphology. The adult worms measure approximately 1 cm by 0.5 mm and live attached to the mucosa of the upper jejunum. The worms are provided with a buccal capsule, reinforced by chitin and including two fused teeth. The tail of the female terminates in a simple pointed extremity, but that of the male is complicated, with several specialized endings forming a definitive pattern. The worms feed on blood and lymph sucked from the host's intestinal mucous membranes. The female passes her fertilized ova directly into the lumen of the host's intestine, and they appear in the feces. The ova are ovoid and measure 60 by 40 μm; within the capsule there are usually two to eight cells that represent the developing embryo; occasionally, a small motile embryo may be seen. If feces are passed into soil, the ova mature in several days and a free-living form is hatched. These larvae may then come in contact with human skin, which they breach to invade small veins. This part of the life cycle is responsible for ground itch. Through the veins the larvae are carried to the heart and lungs. From the vessels of the lungs they pass into the pulmonary air spaces, up the air passages into the oropharynx, and down the esophagus toward the jejunum.

Diagnosis. The diagnosis of infection is usually made by the demonstration of typical ova in the stool; worms are rarely seen. In endemic areas, specialized techniques are employed to evaluate the intensity of infestation by making ova counts of the stool.

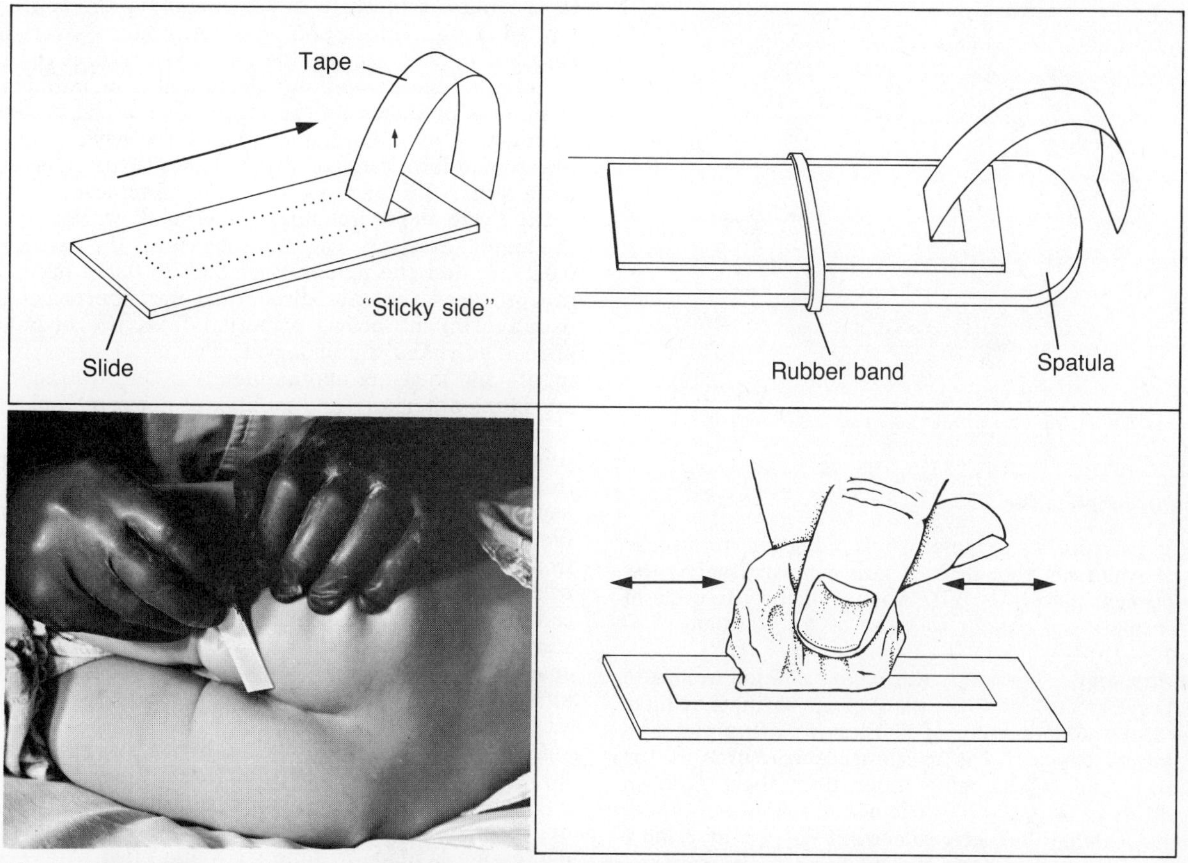

Figure 25–42 Technique of the cellophane-tape method of obtaining ova of *Enterobius vermicularis* from the perianal skin.

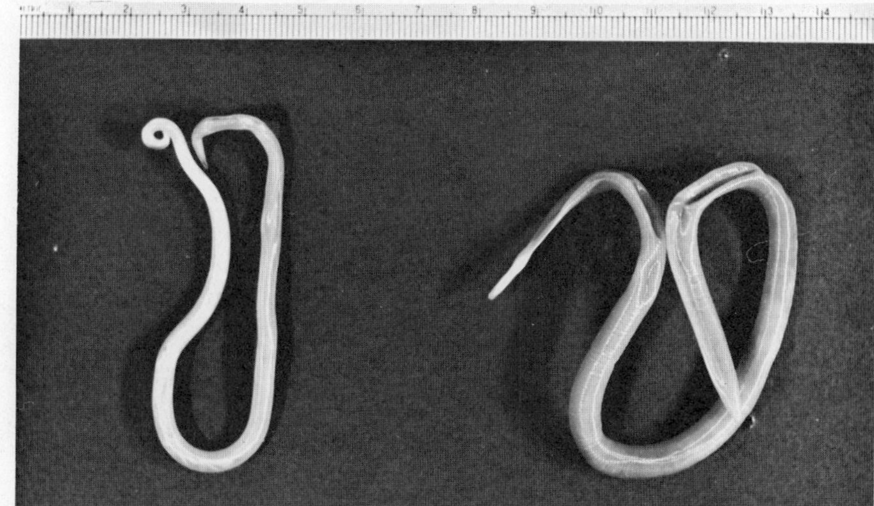

Figure 25–43 *Ascaris lumbricoides.* Adult male and female.

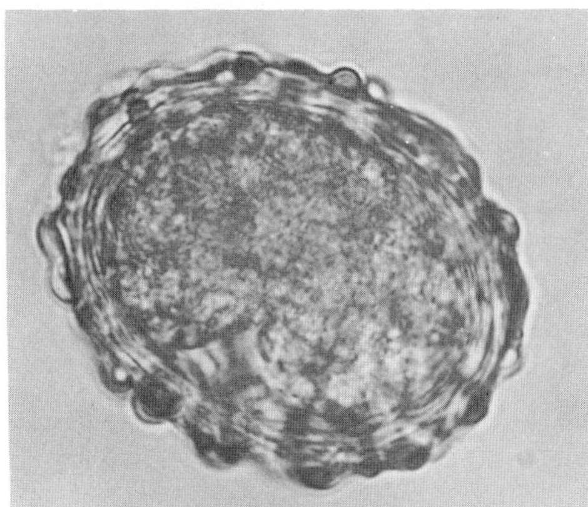

Figure 25–44 *Ascaris lumbricoides* ovum. × 1050.

Necator americanus

This parasite is the major cause of hookworm disease in the Americas though it is now comparatively rare. The clinical picture of infestation and the life cycle of the parasite are similar to those of *Ancylostoma duodenale*.

Morphology. The adult worms are similar in size to the *Ancylostoma* but in the place of the teeth, they have a ventral and dorsal pair of semilunar cutting plates in the buccal capsule. The specialized structures at the posterior end of the male differ from those seen in *Ancylostoma* (Fig. 25–45). The ova are similar to those of *Ancylostoma* but are somewhat longer and more narrow, measuring 30 to 40 μm by 64 to 76 μm (Fig. 25–46).

Strongyloides stercoralis

This worm causes strongyloidiasis, mainly in tropical America and southeastern Asia, but it has also occurred in the more temperate areas, including the southern United States. Infestation does not produce severe disease but may be responsible for a skin rash at the site of inoculation, as well as abdominal and pulmonary symptoms produced by the migrations of the parasite. About 50% of individuals infested are asymptomatic. Severe and fatal cases of strongyloides (hyperinfections) have occurred in patients who were immunosuppressed.

Life Cycle and Morphology. The adult worms live in the small intestine. The male measures 0.7 by 0.04 to 0.05 mm and the female 2 by 0.03 to 0.075 mm. Ova are produced that are discharged into the bowel and usually "hatch" before excretion from the body and appear as rhabditiform larvae. The latter are actively motile and measure approximately 300 by 20 μm; they are blunt anteriorly and pointed posteriorly, and have a small ovoid body in the center of the trunk. Rhabditiform larvae may, under favorable conditions, become free-living forms in the soil, reproducing themselves usually as rhabditiform varieties that molt to become filariform larvae. The latter forms also develop directly from the rhabditiform variety without an intermediate free stage. Filariform larvae invade human skin on contact and enter small veins through which they are transported to the lungs, where they break into the air spaces and migrate up the trachea and down the esophagus to continue the life cycle. Variations in this parasite's life cycle are summarized in Figure 25–37.

Diagnosis. Diagnosis is made by identification of the larvae in stool. If the stool is left in a stoppered container at about 30°C, the larvae will migrate from the feces and be found crawling up the glass. Alternatively, a depression is made in solid feces and filled with water. The preparation is kept warm for several hours; larvae will be found in large numbers on microscopic examination of the water. If strongyloidiasis is suspected and fecal examination is negative, duodenal fluid should be sampled and examined. The Enterotest is useful for this purpose (see p. 490 for details).

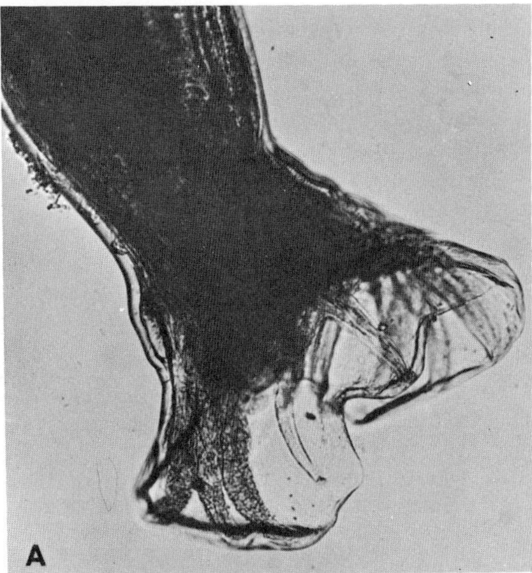

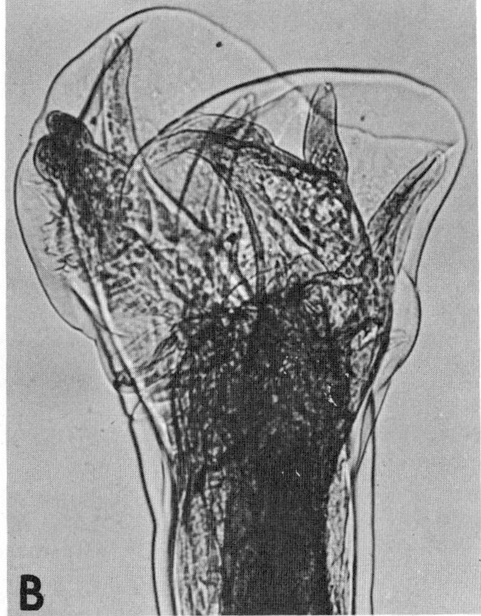

Figure 25–45 **A,** Posterior end of male *Anycylostoma duodenale*. × 100. **B,** Posterior end of male *Necator americanus*. × 100. The caudal bursa of *Ancylostoma duodenale* is open; that of *Necator americanus* is closed.

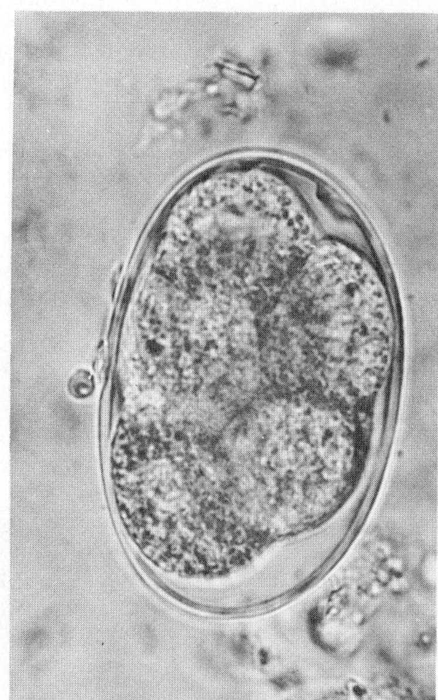

Figure 25–46 *Necator americanus* ovum. × 1050.

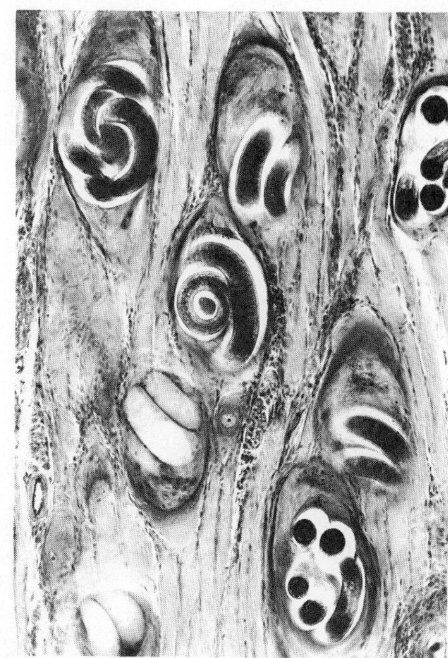

Figure 25–47 Trichinosis. Muscle biopsy. Hematoxylin-eosin × 180.

Tissue Nematodes

Trichinella spiralis

Infestation by *Trichinella spiralis* has a worldwide distribution and is quite common in North America. Trichinosis is caused by eating poorly prepared trichinous pork. It is important to note that U.S.D.A. inspection does not include inspection of pork for *T. spiralis*. Hence, transmission can be prevented only by thoroughly cooking all pork products before consumption. The disease in man is often characterized by an initial period of gastroenteritis, accompanied *occasionally* by a skin rash. Subsequently, there is severe muscular pain with characteristic edema of the eyelids and scrotum, fever, and intense eosinophilia (up to 75%) in the peripheral blood. Severe systemic symptoms may occur in this stage or subsequently including heart failure and bizarre neurological disorders. About 1 in 20 patients is said to die in this stage; in others, recovery may take a long time. The causes of the different stages are apparent from the life-cycle (Fig. 25–37).

Life Cycle and Morphology. The natural reservoir of the disease appears to be in rats, and they have infected domesticated pigs. Since swine are usually raised on offal and garbage, there is much opportunity for trichinous hog meat to be fed to them, and so a vicious cycle is set up in the pig population. The parasite encysts in the muscles of the pig and survives inadequate cooking. If such meat is swallowed, larvae are released in the duodenum and develop into adult male and female worms. The males measure approximately 1.5 by 0.05 mm and the females are 3 to 4 by 0.075 mm. After copulation the female lays fertilized ova, initially into the bowel lumen, but subsequently they are carried into the lymphatics and small blood vessels and are disseminated throughout the body. One female may discharge more than a thousand such ova over the space of several weeks. After deposition in tissues an elongated ovoid capsule develops around a coiled larva, which measures 0.8 to 1 mm long.

Diagnosis. Laboratory diagnosis is usually made by histological examination of a muscle biopsy (Fig. 25–47). However, other methods are available.

Commercial latex reagents and materials for the Bentonite flocculation test for the diagnosis of trichinosis are available.* During the early stages of the disease, while there is gastroenteritis, adult worms may be identified in feces. Larvae have been rarely seen in the blood or cerebrospinal fluid during the stage of dissemination.

Toxocara canis and *T. cati* (Visceral Larva Migrans)

Visceral larva migrans (VLM) occurs when fertile eggs of certain nematodes, which require the enteroportal-pulmono-esophageal cycle for maturation, are ingested by unnatural and incompatible hosts. In the case of man, the ova involved are usually those of *T. canis* (dog ascarid), and less often those of *T. cati* (cat ascarid). The larvae are liberated in the upper small intestine and pass through the bowel wall to the portal venous and lymphatic systems. The larvae are arrested in small capillaries, especially in the liver but not infrequently also in the lungs, eyes, brain, heart, and kidneys. They excite an active host inflammatory cell reaction, initially of eosinophils mainly, but increasingly also of plasma cells, lymphocytes, and macrophages. Foreign body giant cell reactions are commonly added.

Children between 1 and 6 years of age who have the habit of pica are at risk of acquiring VLM. The children are infested by playing in soil or dirt contaminated by

*Cordis Laboratories Inc., P.O. Box 523580, Miami, Fla. 33152.

dog or cat excreta bearing infective larvae (fertile eggs) of *T. canis* or *T. cati.* Clinically, there may be no symptoms or signs apart from eosinophilia, which may range up to 80% of total white cell counts as high as 100,000. Hepatomegaly is common, and splenomegaly also may occur. Wheezing or asthma may occur in asthmatics or if there is heavy pulmonary infestation. Granulomas (pseudotubercles) in the retina may affect vision. Nervous system involvement may cause convulsions. Urticarial rashes also occur.

Diagnosis. Visceral larva migrans should be suspected in any young child showing persistent eosinophilia and some or all of the signs and symptoms enumerated. Demonstration of diffuse hypergammaglobulinemia, with increased levels of IgM antibodies, (natural agglutinin titers, e.g, antiA and anti B, often exceed 1024), adds support to, but is not definitive in, diagnosis. Until recently serology was not useful because of cross-reactions with human *Ascaris* and *Strongyloides.* Now there is an improved method available on request from the Centers for Disease Control, Atlanta, Georgia. Serial sections of needle or open biopsy of the liver may reveal parasites if the biopsy is performed within 2 weeks of last exposure to infestation. However, one usually sees only the characteristic eosinophilic granulomas, often showing a small central track or necrotic area. Examination of dirt from the child's usual play areas may reveal fertile ascarid ova. When pulmonary symptoms predominate, human ascariasis must also be considered.

BLOOD PARASITES

In this section, malaria and babesiosis will be considered. Disease due to the blood and tissue flagellates *Leishmania* and *Trypanosma* will not be considered here, since they are rarely encountered in North America and are found naturally in other parts of the world.

INTRACELLULAR BLOOD PROTOZOA

MALARIA (Class: Sporozoa; Order: Haemosporidia; Family: Plasmodiidae; Genus: *Plasmodium*)

The word *malaria* is a contraction of the Italian *mala aria,* meaning literally, bad air. It was so named because for centuries the disease was associated with the miasma of swamps and damp places. However, although this association was correct, the causative agent was not the air, but rather the protozoan *Plasmodium,* nurtured in the swamp-bred mosquito.

In 1956 the World Health Organization launched a campaign to eradicate malaria based primarily on the interruption of malaria transmission through the destruction of anopheline vectors by DDT. Unfortunately the campaign's mission has been frustrated by the emergence of malaria-carrying mosquitoes resistant to insecticides as well as strains of parasites resistant to drugs. As a consequence, malaria is still the most common, and economically the most important, disease of man. In the light of the practical failure of insecticides and drugs to control malaria effectively, an effort is underway to develop a malarial vaccine. The use of a vaccine involving blood stages appears to offer the most promise. Similarly, current research on the apparent relationship of the Duffy-group genotype to innate host immunity to malaria may provide valuable insights into the pathogenesis of malaria.

Malaria is caused by obligatory parasites for which man, along with other vertebrates, is the intermediate host. *Anopheles* spp. of mosquito are the definitive hosts. Four species of the genus *Plasmodium* cause disease in man: *P. malariae, P. falciparum, P. vivax,* and *P. ovale.*

Outline of Plasmodium Life History

When an infested female mosquito feeds on the blood of a human host, the malarial parasites (sporozoites) are injected with the salivary juices of the mosquito. Following the bite, the sporozoites circulate in the blood for not longer than 30 minutes, and cannot be found again in the circulating blood until the expiration of the preerythrocytic cycle (this constitutes the incubation period, which varies according to the malarial species). During this time an exoerythrocytic phase of multiplication of the parasite proceeds in the parenchymal cells of the liver. By repeated division, large numbers of merozoites are produced, some of which continue the exoerythrocytic cycle while others initiate the erythrocytic stage of development. In *P. malariae* and *P. vivax* infections, exoerythrocytic schizogony parallels erythrocytic development, and the former stage may persist, leading to long latent periods and subsequent relapses. Exoerythrocytic schizogony does not continue in *P. falciparum* once the erythrocytic cycle has been initiated; hence relapses do not occur once the erythrocytic parasite has been eliminated by chemotherapy.

The erythrocytic phase of the life cycle in man commences with the merozoites' penetration of circulating red blood cells, within which they enlarge and are known as trophozoites. In Romanowsky-stained smears they are seen in the early stages of their maturation as rings of light blue cytoplasm, with a small eccentric or peripheral dot of red chromatin. This gives rise to the characteristic "signet ring" appearance. The early trophozoites of *P. ovale, P. malariae,* and *P. vivax* usually occupy approximately 1/3 of the red cell interior, whereas *P. falciparum* occupies about 1/5 of the cell. Occasionally, *P. falciparum* may be seen with double chromatin dots (earphone forms), and in comparison the "signet ring" is thin. As the trophozoite grows it becomes ameboid in appearance, which coincides with its destruction of hemoglobin.

It is of interest to note here that the malarial parasites are adapted to a normal red cell environment, and any changes in this environment would seem to interfere with their ability to survive and reproduce. Hemoglobin S (heterozygote) seems to have a marked resistance to *P. falciparum.* Many have suggested that this may be attributable to both the peculiar characteristics of hemoglobin S, the sickling of red cells in an anoxic environment, and the characteristic life cycle of *P. falciparum,* namely, its adherence to the walls of the small blood vessels during its maturation (see Fig. 25–50). Conditions here are essentially anoxic, and sickling of the

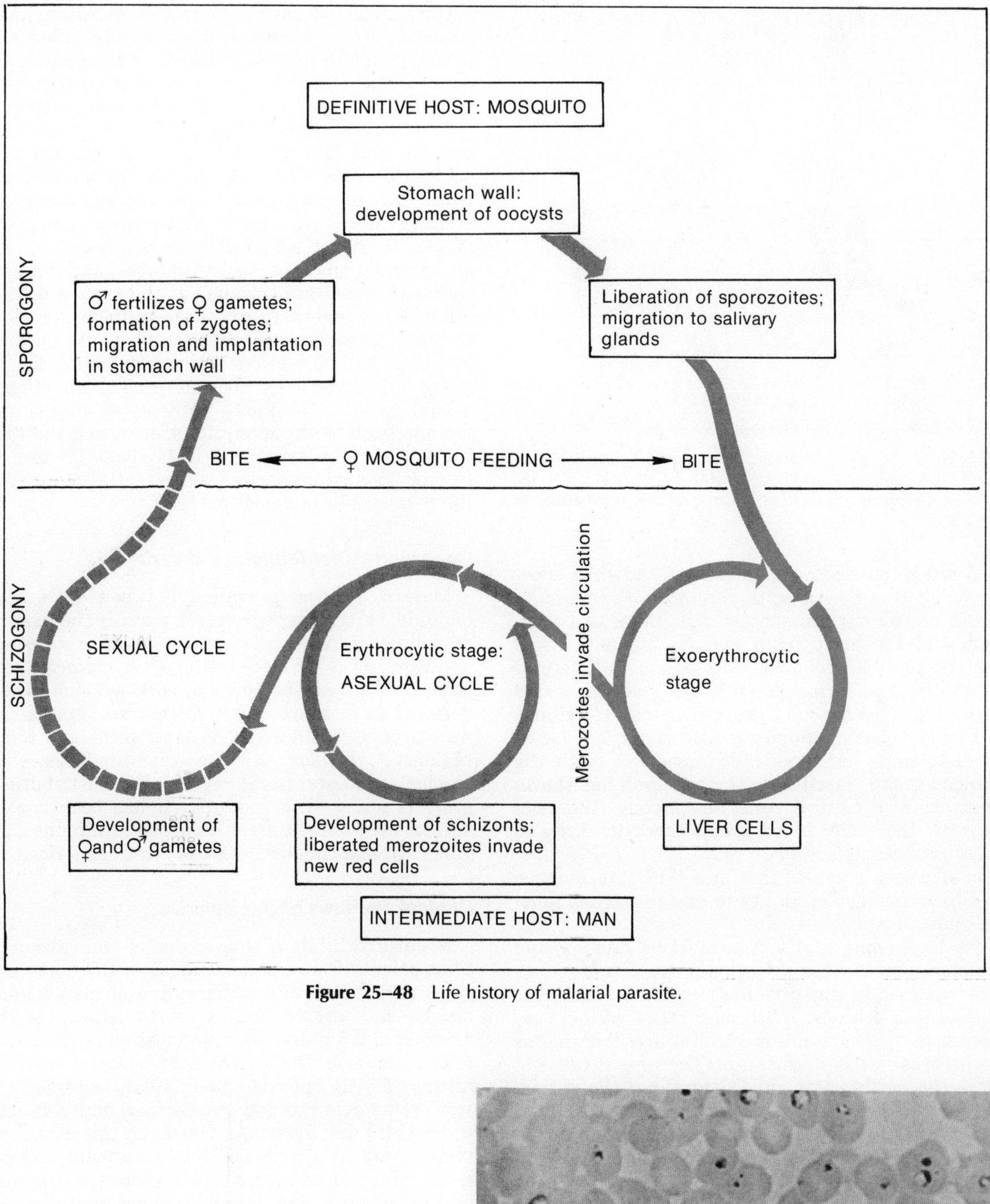

DEFINITIVE HOST: MOSQUITO

Stomach wall: development of oocysts

SPOROGONY

♂ fertilizes ♀ gametes; formation of zygotes; migration and implantation in stomach wall

Liberation of sporozoites; migration to salivary glands

BITE ◄—— ♀ MOSQUITO FEEDING ——► BITE

SCHIZOGONY

SEXUAL CYCLE

Erythrocytic stage: ASEXUAL CYCLE

Merozoites invade circulation

Exoerythrocytic stage

Development of ♀ and ♂ gametes

Development of schizonts; liberated merozoites invade new red cells

LIVER CELLS

INTERMEDIATE HOST: MAN

Figure 25–48 Life history of malarial parasite.

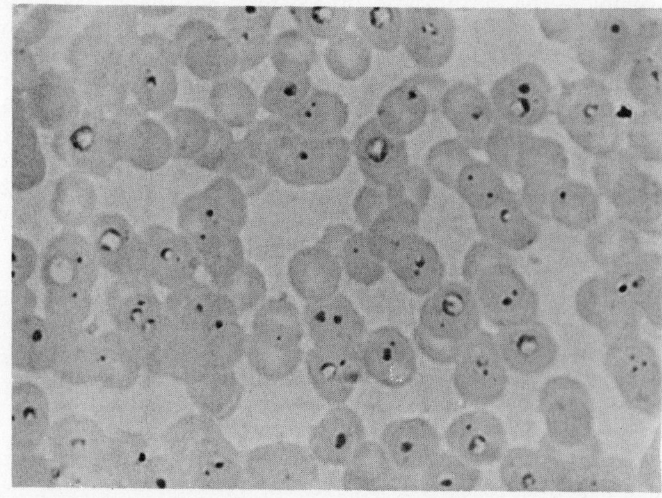

Figure 25–49 *P. falciparum* (malignant tertian malaria). Peripheral blood smear showing the extremely heavy infestation that is rather characteristic of this parasite and that accounts for the incidence of blackwater fever in malignant tertian malaria. × 1350.

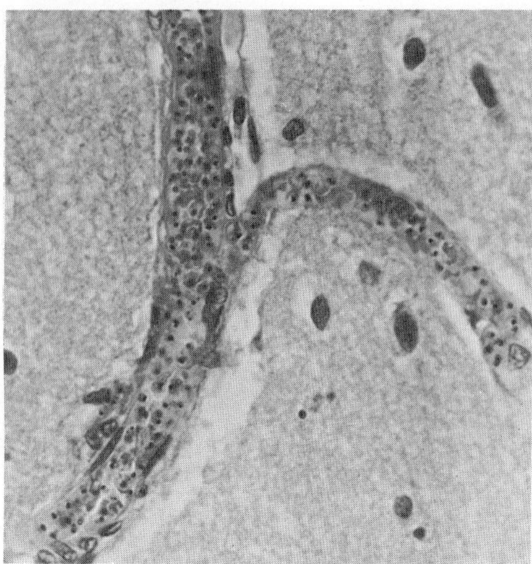

Figure 25–50 *P. falciparum* malaria. Section of brain from a patient who died. The capillaries are clogged with parasitized red cells. Rapid coma and death may occur because of this. Hematoxylin-eosin × 630.

infected red cells would surely have an adverse effect on the survival of the parasite. Similarly, the placenta also is an anoxic environment, so that these two characteristics of the hemoglobin and the parasite could explain the possible higher fertility of female heterozygous sicklers. Also it has recently been demonstrated that infection of the red cell by several species of malaria is apparently dependent upon a specific membrane factor either dictated by or genetically associated with the Duffy blood group. Specifically this research has shown the presence of a natural resistance among American blacks with the Duffy blood group genotype *FyFy* to *Plasmodium vivax* infections.

It has also been proposed that in G-6-PD deficiency, a state of increased susceptibility to oxidant stress, falciparum malaria is suppressed.

As the trophozoite matures its nucleus divides, and these subsequent nuclear divisions produce up to 20 or more merozoites. In this dividing stage, the parasite is referred to as a schizont. With maturation of the schizont, schizogony occurs and merozoites are liberated as free structures in the bloodstream. The time it takes to complete the erythrocytic cycle determines the periodicity of the chills and fever symptomatic of the disease. The liberated merozoites enter fresh red cells and the process is repeated.

After several generations of merozoites have been produced in this way some spontaneously develop into male and female sex cells, called microgametocytes and macrogametocytes, respectively. The mechanism controlling the development of merozoites into either sexual or asexual forms is still unknown. Experiments have shown that some merozoites produced by primary exoerythrocytic schizonts develop directly into sexual forms without an intermediate schizogony in the peripheral blood. These sexual forms grow into large ovoid bluish bodies with a red chromatin mass that is more or less central in position. The microgametocytes tend to be somewhat smaller than their counterparts, and stain a less intense blue. Further development of the gametocytes is dependent on their being ingested by a mosquito.

Once ingested by an *Anopheles* mosquito the male gametocytes, by a process descriptively called exflagellation, give rise to about 5 slender microgametes, which enables the male form to come into contact with the female. Fertilization ensues, and the microgametocyte is known as a zygote. The parasite now migrates to the midgut wall (during this time it is referred to as an ookinette), and settles in the tissues immediately beneath the mucosal cells. Here the zygotes grow and enlarge into round oocysts, within which large numbers of spindle-shaped sporozoites are produced. On reaching an optimum size, the oocyst ruptures, and the liberated sporozoites migrate throughout the tissues of the mosquito. Many find their way to the salivary glands, where they are concentrated in large numbers. As the mosquito bites, its salivary juices are injected into the victim, along with some 3000 sporozoites. The duration of the sexual cycle in the mosquito depends on a number of factors, such as the mosquito species and the temperature, but on the average it lasts about 1½ to 2 weeks. Figure 25–48 summarizes the essential features in the life history of a malarial parasite.

Geographic Distribution of Malaria

Malaria is most prevalent between 45°N and 20°S latitude. Of the four species, *P. vivax* is the most widely distributed and prevails in the temperate zones, extending from 64°N to 32°S latitude. *P. malariae* tends to have a localized distribution, with a much lower incidence than *P. vivax* and *P. falciparum,* and is found in well-circumscribed areas of subtropical and temperate regions. *P. falciparum* is the prevailing species in most tropical and subtropical regions. The distribution of *P. ovale* is not well defined, but it has been reported in Africa, the Middle East, China, the Philippines, Central America, and the west coast of South America.

Clinical Features of the Malarias

Malaria exhibits a wide range of clinical manifestations arising from the destruction of the hosts' erythrocytes and the resultant disruption of metabolism. The disease is characterized by febrile attacks, secondary anemia, and a progression, in most cases, from an acute to chronic state. During the acute stage there are intermittent febrile episodes. In *P. vivax,* the febrile paroxysm occurs every second day (tertian) and in *P. malariae* every third day (quartan). However, this classic picture is now rare as a result of drug treatment and prophylaxis, which often precipitate asynchronous maturation of the parasite and irregular fever patterns. Benign types are usually owing to *P. vivax, P. malariae,* or *P. ovale. Plasmodium falciparum* is generally associated with the malignant form of the disease *(vide infra).*

Differential Features of the Malarial Parasites

Plasmodium vivax (Benign Tertian; see Fig. 25–51)

The asexual cycle takes approximately 48 hours. As maturation proceeds the trophozoite enlarges, loses the classic ring form, and becomes an irregular bluish struc-

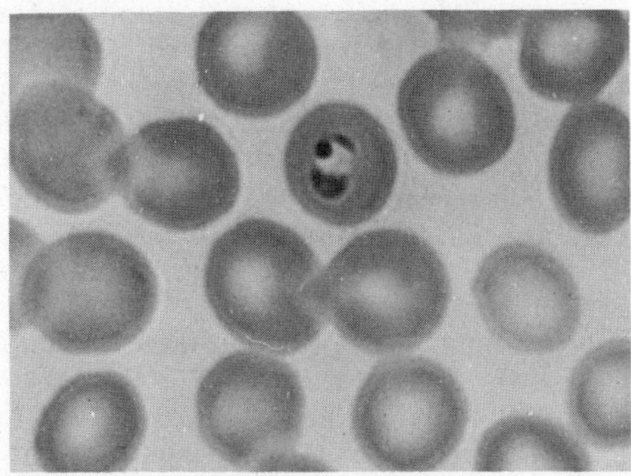

Figure 25–51 *Plasmodium vivax* (benign tertian malaria); young trophozoite (ring form). × 1350.

ture with small red chromatin granules and fibrils and greenish brown granules of "malarial" pigment. This latter is hematin derived from the hemoglobin of the red blood cell. Coincidentally, the parasitized red cell enlarges and becomes noticeably paler because of loss of hemoglobin. Outside the parasite in the red cell, pinkish dots (Schüffner's dots) may become visible and increase in number as the trophozoite matures. The amount of chromatin in the parasite increases and is seen as chunks or many coarse granules of red color. The schizonts are large and "mulberry"-like, consisting of 12 to 25 oval merozoites. The cycle is never entirely scynchronous. Therefore, parasites at more than one stage of development can be seen. After second or third paroxysm gametocytes can be found, which are generally rounded and approximately 1½ times the size of a red blood cell.

Plasmodium malariae (Quartan Malaria)

The asexual cycle takes approximately 72 hours, with fever and chills recurring every fourth day.

Ring forms of *P. malariae* are not readily distinguished from *P. vivax*. It tends to form elongated structures stretching across the red cell, i.e., equatorial band forms. The infected red cell is not enlarged, as with *P. vivax* and *P. ovale*. As the parasite matures it occupies almost the entire red cell. The merozoites of *P. malariae* stain a rather deep blue with Romanowsky stain, and about 6 to 12 of them constitute a schizont. The red cell cytoplasm shows no Schüffner's dots, but many parasitized cells may contain fine pink dots called Ziemann's stippling (seen only in heavily stained preparations). The merozoite arrangement in the schizont has been likened to a rosette. The gametocytes closely resemble those of *P. vivax*. Relapses occur, indicating the persistence of exoerythrocytic schizogony.

Plasmodium ovale

The asexual cycle is approximately 48 hours, producing a paroxysm on every third day. The parasite causes a relatively mild form of malaria, somewhat resembling that of *P. vivax*. In *P. ovale* infections, there is a high rate of spontaneous recovery without treatment. The parasitized red cells have a characteristic oval shape, are slightly enlarged, and generally show abundant Schüffner dots. The red cells may also display ragged, irregular edges. Schizonts usually give rise to an average of eight merozoites. The gametocytes are not characteristic.

Plasmodium falciparum (Malignant Tertian, Estivoautumnal or Tropical Malaria)

This is widely endemic in the tropics and gives rise to the most severe type of disease. Infestation may be so extreme that when schizogony occurs very large amounts of blood are destroyed and hemoglobinuria is very heavy (blackwater fever); it may be so severe as to cause anuria. The tendency for large masses of parasitized red cells to accumulate in the capillary blood vessels of the brain often leads to delirium, coma, and death (Fig. 25–50).

In falciparum infestation certain characteristics may be noted in blood smears (Fig. 25–49). The ring forms frequently show two chromatin dots and two- or three-ring forms in one red cell are common (less common in *P. vivax*). (See Fig. 25–52). Schizonts are not often seen in peripheral smears. (Schizonts of *P. falciparum* develop in capillaries.) Basophilic dots (Maurer's dots) may be seen in the infested erythrocyte; these occur only in the case of *P. falciparum* infestation, in which reddish clefts may also be seen in the red cell. Schizonts may be seen in a heavy infection of moribund patients. A mature schizont may have 8 to 36 merozoites (average 24). The infested erythrocytes do not enlarge but take on a brassy hue. Gametocytes are characteristically crescentic in shape (10 to 12 by 3 μm) and stretch the red cells (Fig. 25–53). Table 25–4 summarizes the microscopic features of the malarial parasites.

Laboratory Diagnosis of Malaria

Malaria produces chronic debility and chronic anemia; the more severe form (malignant tertian) poses a more immediate and grave threat to life. The manifestations of malaria are varied, and the disease should always be

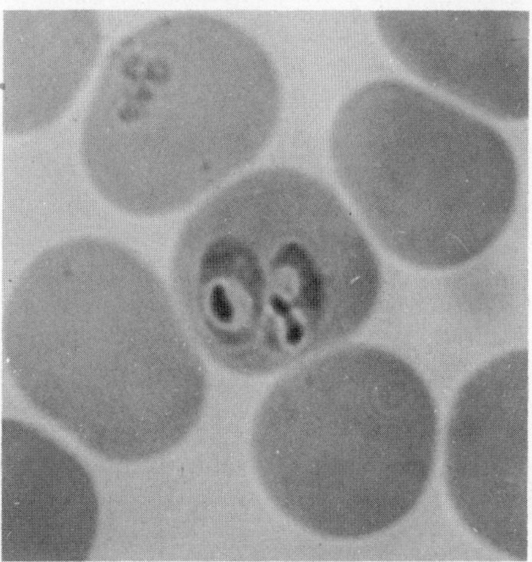

Figure 25–52 *Plasmodium falciparum* (malignant tertian malaria); red blood cell containing two ring forms. Note: although trophozoites of the different malarial parasites cannot be differentiated, double infestation of red cells is much more common in the case of *P. falciparum*, the ring forms of which not infrequently have two chromatin dots. × 2250.

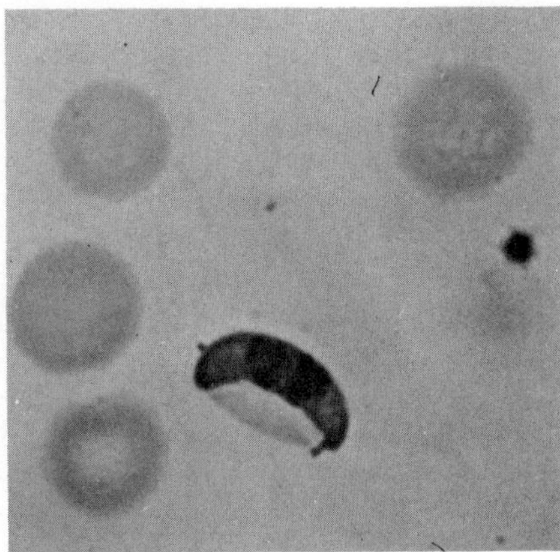

Figure 25–53 Gametocyte of *P. falciparum,* showing the characteristic crescent stretching the parasitized red cell. × 1350.

suspected and looked for in patients in (or from) malarious regions. Usually red cells and hemoglobin are equally reduced. Macrocytosis may be evident because of the increased number of reticulocytes and because of enlargement of parasitized red cells in the case of *P. vivax* and *P. ovale*. Generally, sedimentation rates are increased, whereas prothrombin times are decreased. Other abnormal laboratory data include increased osmotic fragility, reversed albumin to globulin (A/G) ratios, decreased plasma protein levels, and fluctuations in the levels of cholesterol and glucose. Also alkaline phosphatase, SGOT, and SGPT enzyme levels may be slightly elevated. In active phases signs of hemolytic activity are evident (increased indirect-reacting serum bilirubin, methemalbuminemia, and hemosiderinuria). In the chronic forms the leukocyte count is generally reduced, but there is very often an increase in monocytes. Leukocytosis occurs following chills. The organs show abundant malarial pigment. Liver and spleen are enlarged, and material obtained by splenic puncture shows parasites and pigment.

The clinical diagnosis is substantiated by finding the parasites in the peripheral blood. Ordinary Romanowsky-stained smears are quite satisfactory for this, but in endemic areas a more rapid and efficient means of diagnosis is provided by the thick film methods. Some experience is required in the use of this method, which gives higher percentages of positive diagnosis in much less time. Generally, the blood films must be made about 10 times the thickness of normal smears. Ideally, one should be just able to see the hands of an average-sized watch through thick films. These are easily made by placing a good-sized drop of blood on a clean slide and spreading it with the side of a glass rod until it covers an area of approximately 2 cm diameter. It is then allowed to dry (in air or in an incubator at 37°C). Two staining methods will be described.

Field's Rapid Stain Method (Thick Films)

Solution 1:

Methylene blue	0.8 g
Azure B (or azure 1)	0.5 g
Anhydrous potassium dihydrogen phosphate	6.25 g

TABLE 25–4 ESSENTIAL MICROSCOPIC FEATURES OF MALARIAL PARASITES IN BLOOD FILMS

	P. vivax	*P. malariae*	*P. ovale*	*P. falciparum*
Asexual cycle	48 hours	72 hours	48 hours	24–48 hours
Trophozoite appearances	Ameboid Occupies ⅓ diam. erythrocyte Single chromatin dot Appliqué forms at first Double infections	Not unlike *P. vivax* Tends to form equatorial bands Occupies ⅓ diam. erythrocyte	Not typical	Small, occupies approximately 1/5 diam. erythrocyte Often 2 chromatin dots: "ear phones" Multiple infections Appliqué forms
Erythrocytic appearances	Pale, slightly enlarged	Not altered	Ovoid and enlarged; ragged edges Pale	Often unaltered
Predilection of parasite to erythrocytes according to age	Reticulocytes and new erythrocytes	Adult erythrocytes	Reticulocytes and new red cells	Not particular
Cytoplasmic changes	Schüffner's dots	May exhibit Ziemann's stippling	Schüffner's dots	Basophilic stippling Maurer's dots
Schizont characteristics	Large mulberry-like 12–25 oval merozoites	Small, daisy-head like or rosette 6–16 round merozoites	Small 4–12 merozoites	Small 8–32 merozoites
Gametocytes	Rounded 1½ times size of normal erythrocyte	Rounded, same size as normal red cell	Not characteristic	Elongated, crescent or sausage shaped

Distilled water	500 mL
Anydrous disodium hydrogen phosphate	5.0 g
Solution 2:	
Eosin (watery)	1.0 g
Anhydrous disodium hydrogen phosphate	5.0 g
Anhydrous potassium dihydrogen phosphate	6.25 g
Distilled water	500 mL

Note. Dissolve the phosphate salts in the distilled water first and then the dyes. In the case of the azure B it is advantageous to grind it into solution in a mortar with some of the phosphate solution. Let each solution stand overnight and then filter. The solutions may be refiltered if they become "scummy." Staining is effected in Coplin jars; if the jars are covered, the stain will keep for up to 1 to 2 months. When solution 2 becomes greenish it should be discarded.

Procedure

1. Immerse dried, unfixed film for 1 to 3 seconds in solution 1.

2. Remove and rinse immediately for about 5 seconds in clean tap water until no more stain comes from the film.

3. Immerse in solution 2 for 2 seconds.

4. Rinse for 2 or 3 seconds in clean tap water. Let stand to drain and dry.

Leishman Stain (Thin Films)

This method employs a stabilized Leishman solution. The stability of this stain is related to the presence of glycerol, and is an important advantage, particularly in the tropics, where ordinary stains may deteriorate in a few weeks. The stain is used at a pH of 7.2 to give a more intense staining reaction.

Reagents

Leishman dye	3.8 g
Methyl alcohol	250 mL
Glycerol	250 mL

Preparation of Stock Solution of Stain

1. Grind 3.8 g of Leishman stain in a large mortar, and add glycerol to the mortar, a little at a time, grinding and mixing with each addition.

2. Add about half of the methyl alcohol, and continue to grind and mix.

3. Transfer contents of the mortar to glass stoppered bottle.

4. Pour remainder of methyl alcohol into mortar and grind up the residue. Transfer entire contents of mortar to the stock bottle.

5. Label bottle with name of stain, batch number, and date of preparation. Then incubate at 37°C for 24 hours. Intermittent shaking is advocated.

Preparation of Buffer Solution

Potassium dihydrogen phosphate	0.7 g
Disodium hydrogen phosphate (anhyd.)	1.0 g
Distilled water	1000 mL

The pH of the solution, normally 7.2, should be checked and adjusted if necessary before use. Disodium hydrogen phosphate tends to change when exposed to the air; hence an initial checking of the pH is a necessary safeguard. Once adjusted, the pH of the solution should remain stable for several months.

Preparation of Working Solution

FILTER STOCK SOLUTION. Add 3 drops of stain for every milliliter of buffer solution. One slide requires approximately 3 mL of diluted stain.

Method

1. Fix thin films by adding a few drops of methyl alcohol, and leave for a few seconds. For thick films, following drying they should be dehemoglobinized by immersing in water and then treated as for thin films.

2. Pour off alcohol and before films dry, apply diluted stain.

3. Stain for 30 minutes.

4. Differentiate by holding slides under a steady stream of water for approximately 15 seconds. *Do not pour off stain*—always flush—this will prevent desposition of scum on the slide surface.

5. Allow slides to drain and dry before examining.

Serodiagnosis

In cases in which the level of parasitemia is particularly low serodiagnosis may be of value. Here an indirect fluorescent antibody (IFA) test is available.

Differential Diagnosis

The most common error made by inexperienced workers is to mistake platelets lying on red cells for malarial parasites. When parasites are scanty in the peripheral blood, e.g., in chronic forms of *P. vivax* and between attacks of malignant tertian malaria, thick films may be very helpful, and examination of bone marrow smears may be diagnostic in difficult cases. Smears of peripheral blood made ½ to 2 hours after a "provocative" subcutaneous injection of 0.5 to 1 mL of 1:1000 epinephrine may reveal parasites more readily.

BABESIOSIS (Class: Sporozoa; Order: Haemosporidia; Family: Babesiidae; Genus: *Babesia)*

The genus *Babesia* contains 17 species that are distributed widely throughout the world in cattle, goats, equines, dogs, and cats. Occasionally man can become involved in these zoonoses (vide infra).

Unlike most Sporozoa, *Babesia* multiply by binary fission in mammalian erythrocytes and in the organs of hard ticks. The relationship of arthropod to parasite is essentially one of vector, that is, the parasite does not pass through a sexual cycle in the tick. An infected tick passes the parasite to its offspring, which in turn transmits it to a new mammalian host.

Babesia invade red cells in a manner akin to that of *Plasmodium*. Multiple infections of the red cell are characteristic, in which the pear-shaped parasites lie

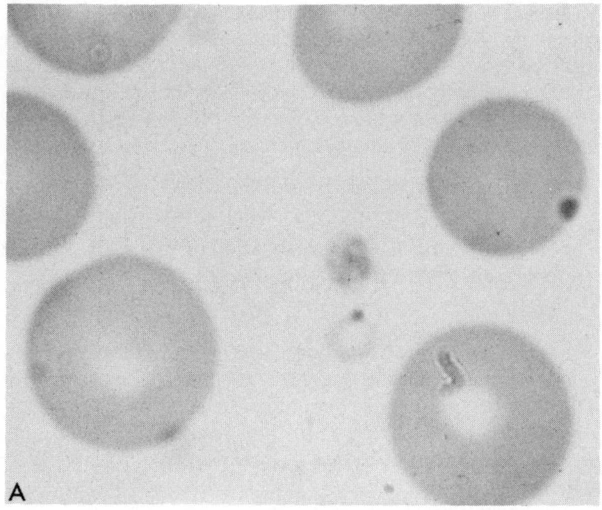

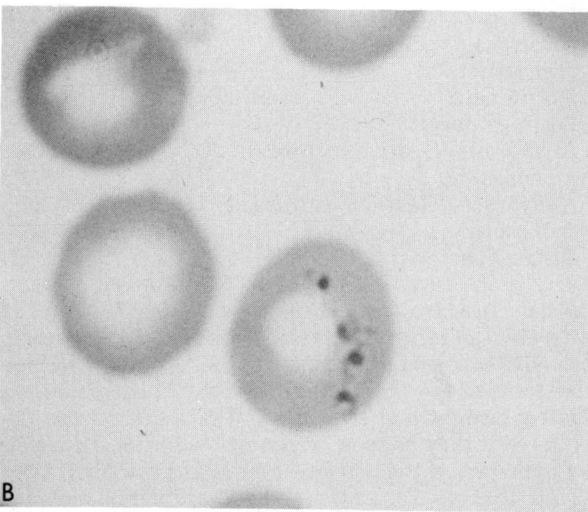

Figure 25–54 *Babesia microti.* **A,** Extracellular ring form (Giemsa stain, × 2000); **B,** intracellular tetrad form (Giemsa stain, × 2000). (Courtesy of William B. Scharfman, Albany Medical College, Albany, New York.)

side by side with their pointed ends in contact, superficially resembling *P. falciparum.* Figure 25–54 indicates typical structures encountered.

Differential features of the blood film between babesiosis and malaria include characteristic tetrads of microzoites in the former. In babesiosis the parasite does not form a haem pigment in the cells; malarial parasites may do so. The number of babesial trophozoites in a red cell may be as many as 12, but malarial trophozoites never exceed 3. Babesial parasites may have 3 chromatin dots, but malarial parasites have only 1 or 2. If the patient's blood is inoculated into hamsters, babesial parasites proliferate in the animal's blood, but in the case of malaria the disease is not so transmissable.

Babesiosis is relatively often seen in patients who have had no functioning splenic tissue, but it has occurred in patients with normal spleens. Because of the problem of transmission by blood transfusion, in 1980, blood was no longer accepted for transfusion from residents of the Cape Cod Islands and the Shelter Island areas, since there is a focus of the disease along the northeastern shore of the United States. Cases, of course, have occurred worldwide.

The illness is characterized by fever, chills, sweating, malaise, myalgia, and possibly by hemolytic anemia. A survey in Nantucket Island, Massachusetts, suggests that *Babesia* spp. can cause asymptomatic and self-limiting infections. Similar asymptomatic disease has been reported from Georgia and Mexico.

Diagnostic procedures should include examination of thick and thin Giemsa-stained blood films and hamster inoculation. An indirect fluorescent antibody test is also available.

CHAPTER 25—REVIEW QUESTIONS

1. Explain the 2-vial method of taking a fecal sample for parasitology. Describe the contents of the vials, how you would prepare the samples, and how they could be examined subsequently.
2. Describe the major differences between the cysts of *E. histolytica* and *E. coli* under the headings of size, position of karyosome, number of nuclei, and presence of chromatodial bodies.
3. Describe the life cycle of *T. saginata* and the characteristics of its ova.
4. Give the differential features of babesiosis and malaria as may be revealed in the laboratory.
5. Describe the life cycle of *E. granulosus.* What methods are available for diagnosis?

26

IMMUNOLOGY AND SEROLOGY

INTRODUCTION

Although since the time of Jenner's introduction of smallpox vaccine in 1798 immunology has been wedded almost exclusively to bacteriology and the study of resistance to disease, other aspects of the subject were apparent by the early part of this century. At that time, while Ehrlich was describing the humoral aspect of immunity, which was to be dominant for so many years, Metchnikoff was introducing the concepts of cellular facets of immune response. Allergy and hypersensitivity (anaphylaxis, hay fever, asthma, and so forth) as adverse effects of the immune response were first appreciated at about the same time. Research into problems of tissue grafting and the new genetic knowledge released a flood of understanding about cellular immunity, which in a sense vindicated the somewhat neglected ideas of Metchnikoff. In the 1940's and 1950's, concepts about the production of antibodies against one's own tissues, thus producing chronic destructive disease, became clarified. These were considered as "autoimmune diseases." Those diseases considered "collagen" diseases (rheumatoid arthritis, lupus erythematosus, and so forth) became related more clearly to immune reactions.

Such knowledge of immune mechanisms helped in the recognition of diseases owing to deficiencies of the immune system (agammaglobulinemia, thymic aplasia, and so forth). More basic research into the chemistry of antibodies yielded information about such conditions as multiple myeloma and Waldenström's macroglobulinemia, in which the immunoglobulin-producing cells are in the grip of uncontrolled malignant proliferation.

Immunology has come a long way since its initial application. In this chapter, aspects of immunology that relate to these varied features will be described. A survey of the subject will be made, but emphasis will be given to those aspects of disease that may be investigated in a general hospital laboratory.

ANTIGEN

It is difficult to define an antigen other than by describing it as a substance that when injected into an animal is recognized as "foreign," and if given access to immunologically competent cells, will provoke an immune reaction. Generally, antigens are large (MW over 10,000) and consequently are usually protein. However, physical size of the molecule is not a controlling factor, since dextran (a carbohydrate) with a molecular weight of 100,000 is not antigenic, but insulin with a molecular weight of 6000 may be. Antigenicity is not necessarily confined to protein substances.

Substances known as *haptens* (Greek = to grasp), which themselves are nonantigenic, may bind themselves to protein, conferring antigenicity on the protein-hapten complex. Examples of such haptens are the carbohydrate capsules of pneumococci and benzylpenicillinic acid. The latter, a breakdown product of penicillin, attaches itself to serum protein, rendering it antigenic and causing the individual to be hypersensitive to further penicillin injections. It may attach itself to red blood cells, thus providing the basis for an immune type of hemolytic anemia following the administration of penicillin. The capsule of the pneumococcus not only confers antigenic specificity on the pneumococcal protoplasm but also contributes to the virulence of the organism.

The shape of the antigen molecule is of importance antigenically, especially the position of chemical groups at the exposed portions of the chains. The chain structure of protein with secondary and tertiary folding of the molecule lends itself to a multiplicity of possibilities of differing spatial presentation and thus antigenic characteristics. Some substances that are usually nonantigenic may be made antigenic by combination with Freund's adjuvant (a chloroform extract of tubercle bacilli in a water-in-oil emulsion). With this substance, the antigen is released over a long period; possibly the histiocytes in the adjuvant stimulated granuloma contribute to antibody production, or possibly the complex lipid-wax-water-antigen molecule configuration is such that it evokes antigenicity. Other adjuvants such as aluminum salts (alum precipitated diphtheria toxoid) and *Bordetella pertussis* are well known and have a practical application in clinical medicine.

Some Important Antigens

Blood group antigens are of great practical importance. They are large molecules of glycolipids with sphingosine and fatty acid, but the determining antigenic substance on the molecule is *N*-acetyl-D-galactosamine (group A) and D-galactose (group B). Similar antigens are found in many plants and bacteria. It is of considerable practical and theoretical interest to consider the production of natural isoagglutinins that do not develop for several months after birth. Germ-free animals do not develop human blood group antibodies, but if *E. coli* O 86 is introduced into the bowel, they will develop anti-B substance in their serum. Presumably this is in response to the B-like antigen present on the *E. coli* O 86 surface. It is believed that in a similar way, infants develop "natural" isoagglutinins in response to colonization of the bowel by bacteria. Antibodies to their own red blood cell group are not produced because such antibodies could only be produced by "forbidden clones" (see p. 533), and because of the phenomenon of immune tolerance (see p. 530).

Bacterial antigens may be extremely complex, since they may be capsular, cell wall, flagellar, exotoxin, or of other bacterial origin.

Heterophil antigens are groups of antigens that occur in apparently unrelated organisms, plants, or animals. They are immunologically identical, reacting with a single antibody. One such example of heterophil antigen is given above in the antigenic relationship between *E. coli* O 86 and human blood group B. Species of *Rickettsia* that cause typhus have antigenic components identical with species of *Proteus*. This relationship is useful in the diagnosis of typhus; hence its use in the Weil-Felix test.

The Forssman antigen is widespread in nature in the cells of many species, such as guinea pig cells and red blood cells of sheep, as well as in some plants and bacteria. Forssman antibody must be differentiated from another heterophil antibody in the differential diagnosis of infectious mononucleosis.

Histocompatibility antigens have become important since the advent of the possibility of tissue transplantation. These antigens are glycopeptides present on the surface of the cells of the body, including the leukocytes. They differ completely from the system of blood group antigens. The system is known as the HL-A (Human Leukocyte-Locus A) system, and it possesses 21 antigens in a series of genetically determined combinations. Each individual will have four of the antigens identifiable on his cells. Although the HL-A system is of major importance in transplantation, the ABO and P blood group systems are also significant.

ANTIBODY

Antibodies are produced by immunocompetent cells in response to antigenic stimuli. Antibodies are serum proteins, and together they generally are considered as immunoglobulins. Electrophoretically, typically they are γ globulins, but they extend into the β and into the α_2 region (Fig. 26–1).

At this time we recognize five groups of immunoglobulins, which are known as IgG, IgA, IgM, IgD, and IgE.

MOLECULAR STRUCTURE

In the center of Figure 26–2 is a diagram of the IgG molecule. Its molecular weight is about 150,000. The sedimentation coefficient is 6 to 7 Svedberg units.

Figure 26–2 shows each half of the molecule as composed of two units. Each of these is a polypeptide chain, probably folded on itself. The larger of the two chains in the half-molecule has a molecular weight of 50,000 and is known as the "H" or "heavy" chain. The smaller chain is known as the "L" or "light" chain, and has a molecular weight of 23,000.

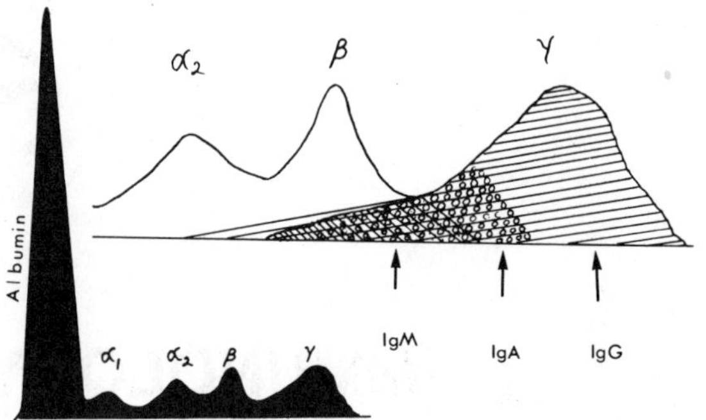

Figure 26–1 Quantitative scan *(solid black)* of serum protein electrophoresis (diagrammatic), and enlargement of a portion of it *(insert)* to show electrophoretic mobility of the three major immunoglobulins. It will be seen that IgG globulins *(oblique hatch)* overlap IgM *(cross hatch)* and IgA *(circles)*.

How the Chains are Held Together. The major bond between the L and H chains, and also between the two halves of the molecule, consists of disulfide linkages between cysteine residues. The entire molecule may contain 15 disulfide bonds, but only three of these hold the chains and half-molecules together (one between each L and H chain, and one between the two H chains holding the halves together); the 12 remaining disulfide bonds are within the chains. However, reduction of these bonds alone is insufficient to break the molecule, and it is assumed that there are other, weaker interchain forces bonding the chains together. An excess of sulphydryl reagent (2-mercaptoethanol) can break the chain, and this reaction has been used in immunology (see section on immunohematology, p. 599).

IMMUNOGLOBULIN CLASSES

The accompanying table shows that all classes share the same two types of light chain, i.e., each immunoglobulin may have either a κ (kappa) or a λ (lambda) light chain. However, each individual molecule has either kappa or lambda light chains, never both. In normal sera about two-thirds of the immunoglobulins have kappa, and one-third lambda-type light chains; they are referred to as type K and L molecules, respectively (see chart below).

Molecular Formulas. From what has just been said, it will be evident that each immunoglobulin may be written as a formula that expresses both its heavy and light chain constitution:

Immunoglobulin	Molecular Formulas
IgGK	$\gamma_2\kappa_2$
IgGL	$\gamma_2\lambda_2$
IgAK	$\alpha_2\kappa_2$
IgAL	$\alpha_2\lambda_2$
IgMK	$(\mu_2\kappa_2)_5$
IgML	$(\mu_2\lambda_2)_5$
IgDK	$\delta_2\kappa_2$
IgDL	$\delta_2\lambda_2$
IgEK	$\epsilon_2\kappa_2$
IgEL	$\epsilon_2\lambda_2$

The light chains, both κ and λ, which are polypeptides, have 214 amino acid residues. Of these, 108 or 109 are

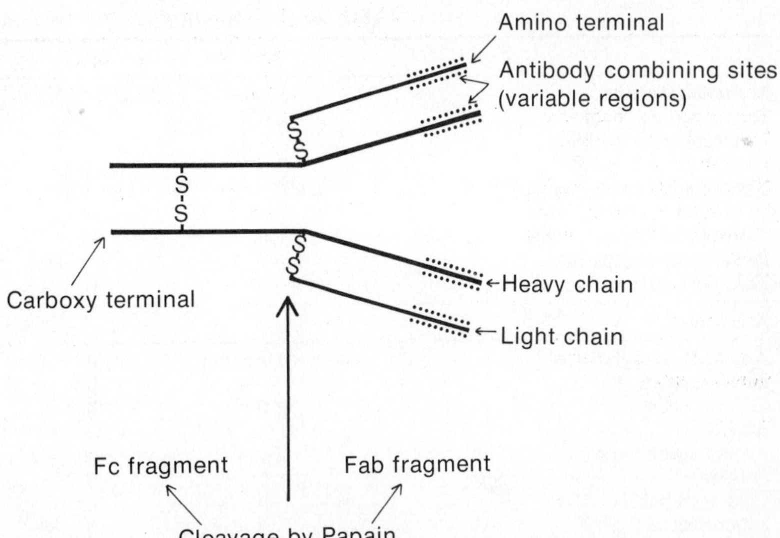

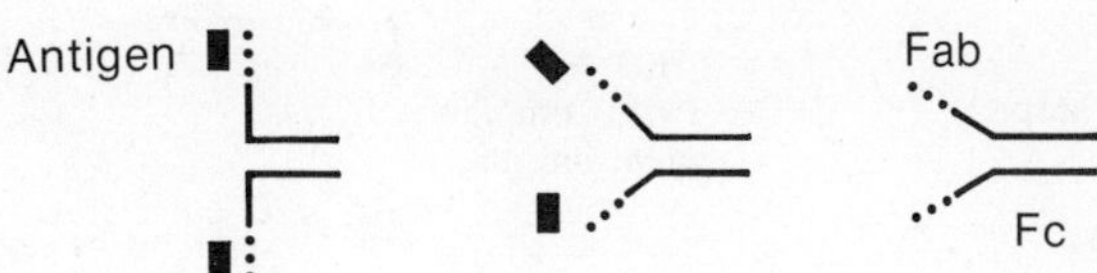

Figure 26–2 Diagram of a simple immunoglobulin on the Porter model. In the lower diagram, the angle between the Fab components widens to accommodate 2 antigenic pieces and at the same time, the Fc contracts.

variable and are sited at the same end of the molecule as the 118 variable amino residues of the heavy chains (Fig. 26–2). The other amino acids in the constant part of the molecule are placed in a regular pattern. The variable part of the immunoglobulin is seen to be at one pole of the molecule, and the antigen binding site resides here.

NORMAL IMMUNOGLOBULINS

IgG

In the normal adult, IgG comprises 70 to 80% of the total immunoglobulins and itself amounts to 1.2 g per dL plasma, on average (range, 0.6 to 1.6 g per dL).

Antibodies Contained in IgG. As may be judged from relative quantities, the IgG class represents a very large number of antibodies. It probably also contains the most sophisticated antibodies from an evolutionary standpoint. Most antitoxins (e.g., antidiphtheria, antitetanus) and most antibacterial (bactericidal, etc.) and antiviral antibodies are present in the IgG immunoglobulin class. Likewise, complement-fixing antibodies (IgM also fixes complement) and antiH (flagellar) antibodies belong here.

In terms of evolution, IgG seems to have evolved later than IgM. In keeping with this, the sequence in the organism's response to antigenic stimulation usually consists of IgM being produced initially, followed later, and ultimately replaced by, IgG. Mature plasma cells produce IgG in their abundant rough-surfaced endoplasmic reticulum. The main, if not the only, stimulus for its manufacture appears to be foreign proteins, i.e., antigens.

IgG may cross the placenta, and thus maternal IgG antibodies may protect the infant during the first few weeks of life; but conversely, in cases of Rhesus incompatibility, this immunoglobulin passage may cause severe and even fatal disease in the unborn or newborn child.

IgA

This immunoglobulin class normally accounts for 10 to 20% of total plasma immunoglobulins in the adult, and itself amounts to 200 ± 50 mg per dL serum (range, 60 to 330 mg per dL). They also are 7S globulins, but differ from IgG globulins in containing four times as much carbohydrate (10%). Molecular weights in the IgA class are from 150,000 to 390,000, and sedimentation coefficients correspond, ranging from 7S to 11S. The 11S variety are dimers of IgA or may possess different alpha chains. The main immunoglobulin present in saliva appears to be IgA. The same is true of tears and nasal, tracheobronchial, and gastrointestinal secretions. The IgA in these secretions and in colostrum is different from that in plasma: its sedimentation coefficient is 11S rather than 7S, and antigenic differences also exist. Plasma IgA is "secreted" into the parotid saliva. In the process, a second protein is added to the IgA molecule. This is called secretory component and it is a glycoprotein. It is manufactured by the breast, salivary, and mucosal glands and is attached to the heavy chains of the IgA immunoglobulins. In addition, a further poly-

TABLE 26–1 PROPERTIES OF THE IMMUNOGLOBULINS

	IgG	IgA	IgM	IgD	IgE
Molecular weights	150,000	150,000–390,000	900,000	185,000	190,000
Sedimentation coefficient	6–7S	7–11S	19S	7–8S	8S
Electrophoretic mobility	$\beta_1 - \gamma_2$	$\alpha_2 - \gamma_2$	$\beta - \gamma$	γ	β
Carbohydrate content	2.5%	10.5%	10%	13%	11
Normal adult levels (mg/dL)	600–1600	60–330	50–200	0.5–40	10–140 ng
% of total immunoglobulin	70–80	15	7	1	0.002
Distribution (% in Plasma)	40	40	80	80	50
Presence in secretions	+	+ + + +	0	?	?
Transport across placenta	+ + + +	0	0	0	0
Antibodies					
AntiA, B isoagglutinins	± (0 usually)	0	+ + + +		
Immune antiA, B	+ +	0	+ +		
saline	0	0	+ + +		
AntiRh					
incomplete	+ + +	0	0 or +		
Forssman	0	0	+ + + +		
Cold agglutinins	0	0	+ + + +		
Heterophil	0	0	+ + + +		
AntiLewis; anti-i	0	0	+ + + +		
Antistreptolysin	+ + + +	0	0		
AntiO, *Salmonella*	0	0	+ + + +		
AntiH, *Salmonella*	+ + + +	0	0		
Antitoxins (diphtheria, tetanus, streptococcal)	+ + + +	0	0		
Antiviral	+	+ + + +	±		
Complement-fixing	+ + + +	0	±	?	–
Reaginic (skin-sensitizing or atopic)	+ (with complement only)	0	0	0	+ + + +
Rheumatoid factor (Rf)	±	0	+ + + +		
Combining with Rf	+ + + +	0	0		
LE factor and antibodies	+ +	0	+ +		
Antipneumococcal (capsular)	+ + + +	0	±*		
Wassermann antibody	0	0	+ + + +		
Antispirochetal antibodies	+ ±	0	+ + +		
Antitrypanosomal	0	0	+ + + +		
Autoantibodies (antithyroid, etc.)	+ +	0	+ +		

Explanation of + Symbols: + + + + means that, in so far as can be ascertained, nearly all the antibody is present in this fraction.

*Species variation in response to certain antigens exists, especially to those containing carbohydrate.

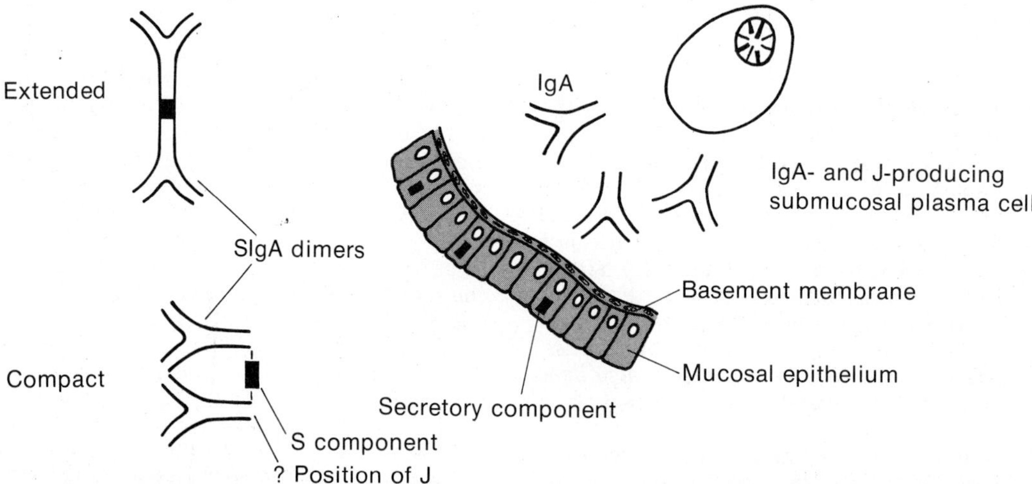

Figure 26–3 IgA and J polypeptide are produced by a submucosal plasma cell. These substances pass the basal membrane and in the mucosal lining cell are joined with secretory component. Subsequently they are expelled into the duct lumen as SIgA dimers, which have been shown by electron microscopy in the configurations illustrated.

TABLE 26–2 SERUM IMMUNOGLOBULIN LEVELS OF NORMAL SUBJECTS OF DIFFERENT AGES*

Age	No. of Subjects	IgG mg/dL (range)	% Adult Level	IgA mg/dL (range)	% Adult Level	IgM mg/dL (range)	% Adult Level	Total Gamma Globulins mg/dL (range)	% Adult Level
Newborn	22	1030 ± 200 (645 – 1245)	89 ± 17	2 ± 3 (0 – 10)	1 ± 2	10 ± 5 (5 – 30)	11 ± 5	1045 ± 200 (660 – 1440)	67 ± 13
1–3 mos	29	430 ± 120 (270 – 760)	37 ± 10	21 ± 13 (5 – 55)	11 ± 7	30 ± 11 (15 – 70)	30 ± 11	480 ± 130 (325 – 700)	31 ± 9
4–6 mos	33	430 ± 185 (205 – 1125)	37 ± 16	28 ± 18 (8 – 95)	14 ± 9	43 ± 17 (10 – 85)	43 ± 17	500 ± 205 (230 – 1230)	32 ± 13
7–12 mos	56	660 ± 220 (280 – 1530)	58 ± 19	37 ± 18 (16 – 98)	19 ± 9	54 ± 23 (22 – 147)	55 ± 23	750 ± 240 (325 – 1685)	48 ± 15
13–24 mos	59	760 ± 210 (260 – 1390)	66 ± 18	50 ± 24 (20 – 120)	25 ± 12	58 ± 23 (15 – 115)	59 ± 23	870 ± 260 (400 – 1585)	56 ± 16
25–36 mos	33	890 ± 185 (420 – 1275)	76 ± 16	71 ± 37 (20 – 235)	36 ± 19	61 ± 19 (30 – 115)	62 ± 19	1025 ± 205 (500 – 1420)	65 ± 14
3–5 yrs	28	930 ± 230 (570 – 1600)	80 ± 20	95 ± 25 (55 – 150)	47 ± 14	56 ± 18 (20 – 100)	57 ± 18	1080 ± 245 (730 – 1770)	69 ± 17
6–8 yrs	18	925 ± 255 (560 – 1490)	80 ± 22	125 ± 45 (55 – 220)	62 ± 23	65 ± 25 (25 – 120)	66 ± 25	1110 ± 295 (640 – 1725)	71 ± 20
9–11 yrs	9	1125 ± 235 (780 ± 1455)	97 ± 20	130 ± 60 (12 – 208)	66 ± 30	80 ± 33 (35 – 130)	80 ± 33	1335 ± 255 (965 – 1640)	85 ± 17
12–16 yrs	9	945 ± 125 (725 – 1085)	82 ± 11	150 ± 60 (70 – 230)	74 ± 32	60 ± 20 (35 – 70)	60 ± 20	1155 ± 170 (835 – 1285)	74 ± 12
Adults	30	1160 ± 305 (570 – 1920)	100 ± 26	200 ± 60 (60 – 330)	100 ± 31	100 ± 25 (50 – 150)	100 ± 27	1460 ± 355 (730 – 2365)	100 ± 24

***Values drawn from Stiehm, E. R., and Fudenberg, H. H.: Serum levels of immune globulins in health and disease: A survey. Pediatrics, *37*:715, 1966. In the case of larger values, figures are presented in this table to the nearest 5. The method used was a modification of the radial agar diffusion plate method, employing sera developed against pure normal protein fractions prepared by the authors cited.**

peptide—"J" (joining)—helps to form the compound IgA or SIgA molecule.

IgA appears to be essential in warding off sinobronchial infections. Occasional, apparently normal persons exhibit isolated absence of this immunoglobulin class. The presence of IgA in colostrum and breast milk is probably of significance in protecting newborn infants at least partially from gastrointestinal infections. It may have an important role in the prevention of viral disease.

IgM

This class normally constitutes about 7% (3 to 10%) of total immunoglobulins in the adult and itself amounts to 100 mg, ± 25 mg per dL (range, 50 to 200). They are the largest of the immunoglobulin molecules, their molecular weights averaging about 900,000. Their sedimentation coefficients range from 17S to 20S (usually stated as 19S).

As indicated by their molecular formulas, $(\mu_2\kappa_2)_5$ or $(\mu_2\lambda_2)_5$, the molecules are pentamers of IgM, each with a molecular weight of 180,000, joined together by disulfide bonds, and probably also by the J-chain, which appears to be associated with polymeric molecules. In theory, therefore, the IgM molecule could contain as many as 10 antigen-combining sites.

As regards antibody functions, it has already been mentioned that the IgM class usually is the first to appear in response to antigenic stimulation. The chief antibody types associated with the IgM class are opso-

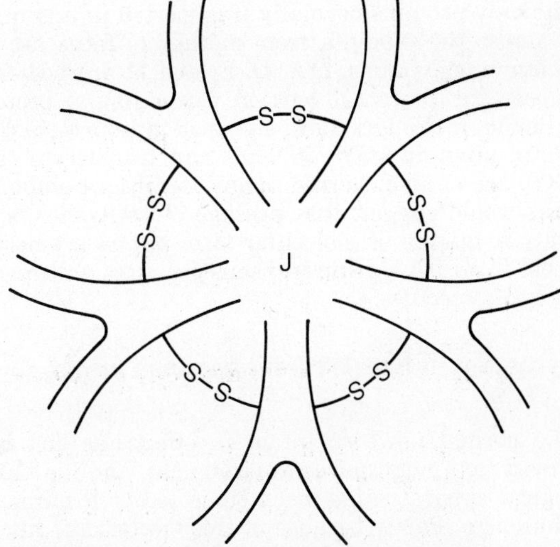

Figure 26–4 A suggested pentameric pattern for IgM.

nins, bacteriolysins, and bactericidins, and isohemagglutinins, cold agglutinins, Forssman antibodies, and heterophil antibodies all belong to the IgM group. AntiLewis and anti-i antibodies and the rheumatoid factor are also IgM globulins, as are antispirochetal antibodies. Peculiarly, the endotoxic or the somatic (O) salmonella antigens evoke 18 to 19S immunoglobulins, whereas the H (flagellar) antigens of the same organisms excite IgG antibody production.

The cell type that manufactures IgM immunoglobulins is probably intermediate in type between large lymphocytes and plasma cells and resembles the lymphocytoid cells of Waldenström's macroglobulinemia.

IgD

This class of immunoglobulins has a molecular structure that conforms to that of the other immunoglobulins; i.e., it has its own specific, delta-type, heavy chains, and either kappa or more commonly lambda light chains.

Its mean concentration in serum is between 0.5 and 40 mg per dL, and its molecular weight is 185,000, which corresponds well to its sedimentation coefficient of 7 to 8S. As yet, it has not been allocated a particular role in the immune reaction, but IgD antibodies against insulin and diphtheria toxoid as well as antinuclear autoantibodies in systemic lupus erythematosus have been found.

IgE

This antibody class is present in only minute amounts in serum (10 to 40 ng per dL). It has a molecular weight of 190,000 and a sedimentation rate of 8S. Unlike other antibodies it is heat labile (at 56°C for 20 minutes) and adheres to tissue mast cells. When exposed to the corresponding antigen or allergen, reactions take place at the surface of the cell, releasing a series of substances. These include histamine, serotonin, kinins, and other substances that are responsible for a spectrum of clinical syndromes, including asthma, urticaria, and anaphylaxis. Patients with asthma have shown raised levels of serum IgE.

Transplacental Immunoglobulin Transport

The only proteins normally transported in any quantity across the placenta from mother to fetus are the IgG immunoglobulins. IgA, D, E, and M antibodies do not pass the placental barrier. Surprisingly, proteins smaller than the IgG class, e.g., acid glycoprotein (MW 35,000), albumin (MW 65,000), and transferrin (MW 90,000) are not transferred in any significant amounts.

This would suggest that passage of antibodies is not merely a matter of molecular size, but is a selective process in which specific transmission sites will readily pass IgG molecules.

Development of Immunity in the Newborn, Infant, and Child

The normal newborn infant in effect has just been removed from a germ-free environment, and his immunological apparatus has been subjected to a minimum of challenge. Partly because of this "isolation," his immune mechanism is immature. However, it is known that after the twentieth week of gestation the normal human fetus is capable of making antibodies. For many decades this has been known in the case of congenital syphilis. Other infections of the TORCH group (*T*oxoplasmosis; *O*ther, including syphilis; *R*ubella; *C*ytomegalovirus disease, and generalized *H*erpes) have also caused a raised IgM level in the fetus.

Nevertheless, under normal circumstances the human fetus does not begin to synthesize antibodies to any significant degree until after birth. IgM is the only type of immunoglobulin normally made by the fetus before and at the time of birth. The neonate then is wholly dependent on transplacental transfer of maternal IgG, a process that is so efficient that cord blood levels of IgG are almost as high as, and sometimes slightly higher than, maternal levels.

In Figure 26–5 the sequence of events in the normal development of immunity (immunoglobulins, to be more correct) from birth to adulthood can be seen. The average full-term infant does not begin to synthesize IgG globulins until between the first and third months of life, i.e., at the time plasma cells begin to appear. By the end of the first month of life the infant's IgG has been reduced by about 50%, because it is all of maternal origin and its half-life is approximately 24 days, although its half-time survival may be somewhat longer in the infant. After the first month the rate of decline in IgG concentration slows considerably, for two reasons: (1) the disappearance of maternal IgG is more or less exponential; (2) about this time the infant's own immune mechanism begins to synthesize IgG globulins.

Figure 26–5 shows that between the third and sixth month the concentration of IgG in the infant's blood reaches its lowest level (about 400 mg per dL, i.e., one-third the adult value). If for any reason the onset of IgG production by the infant is delayed, it is obvious that much lower levels (150 to 250 mg per dL) may be reached by the fifth to sixth months of life.

Normally, however, the rate of IgG synthetic activity, once started, gathers momentum rather steeply, and by the end of the first year average levels of 650 mg per dL are attained. The steep rise continues until the age of about 5 years, after which the rate of increase slows perceptibly and continues in a more gentle slope into adulthood.

Production of IgM, which is the first to be synthesized, follows a gradual rise into the modest adult levels. IgA immunoglobulins, which in all probability begin to be synthesized before IgG proteins, also exhibit a very gentle curve of increment with, however, a slight "spurt" between the ages of 3 and 8 years.

Complement

Complement, which was formerly thought of as a single substance necessary for the completion of certain antigen-antibody reactions in vitro, is now known to consist of at least 14 distinct serum proteins with essential functions in basic biological reactions. The complement proteins react with one another, with antigen, and with receptors on cell membranes. The result of such interplay in vivo is enhanced phagocytosis, chemotaxis of polymorphs, and other reactions of inflammation, including lysis and death of cells. In defense of the body, bacteria are lyzed with obvious beneficial effect.

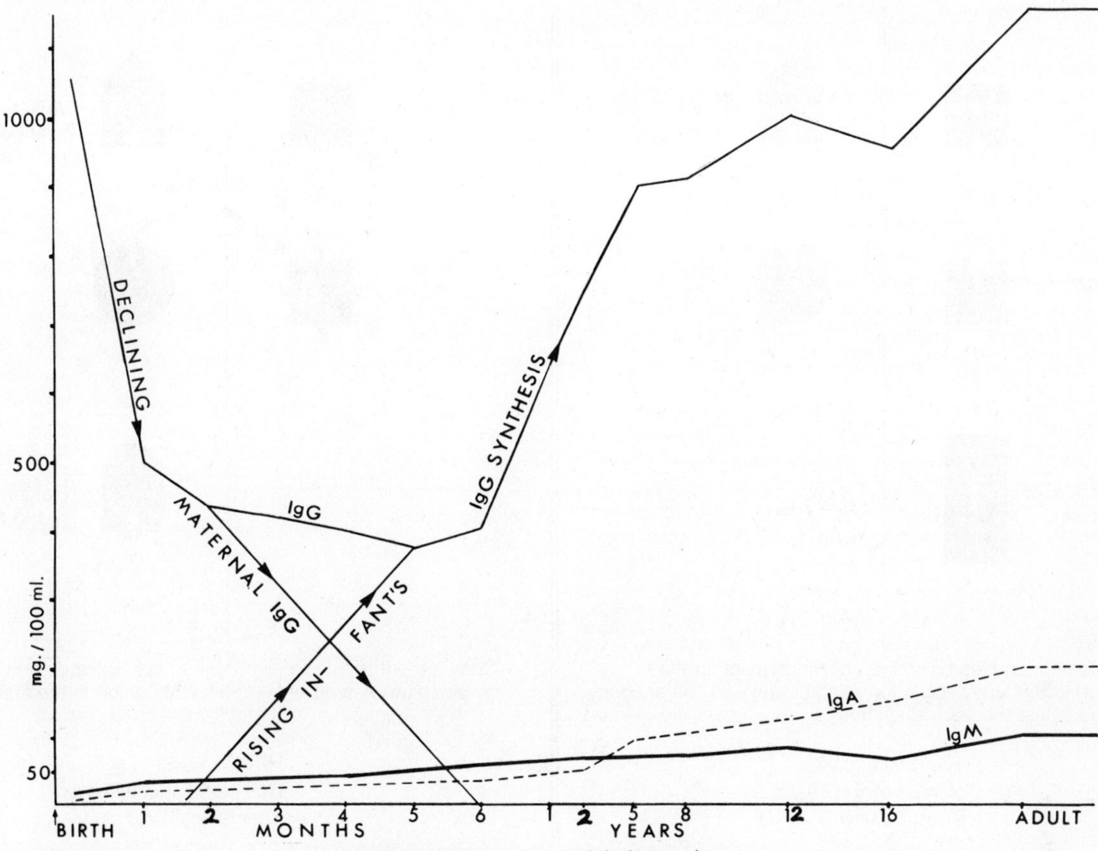

Figure 26–5 Immunoglobulins and age.

Generally in laboratory medicine, knowledge of the complement system is exploited in two ways. First, it is used to determine if a particular antigen-antibody reaction, which shows no physical evidence of union, has occurred. Here a controlled amount of necessary complement is added to the systems. Should it be used up in the test antigen-antibody combination, which is tested first, then it is not available to lyze red cells in a competing test system tried subsequently. Hence nonlysis of red cells in such a system is considered positive for the presence of some specific antibody or antigen (Fig. 26–6).

More recently, circulating complement fractions have been measured to see if complement has been consumed in an extensive antigen-antibody combination, as occurs in diseases such as SLE, acute glomerulonephritis, serum sickness, bacterial endocarditis, and so forth.

The classic complement system has at least nine proteins (C1-C9), which act in sequence when C1 is stimulated. The system is a biological amplifier or cascade. A small chemical change to a few molecules of C1 activates many molecules in the next stage and so on, until thousands of molecules, in the late stages, are implicated. The classic pathway is activated by antigen-antibody reactions or aggregated immunoglobulins.

The alternate pathway may be stimulated by IgA, by complex polysaccharides, and by other, apparently unrelated substances. Several substances are involved in the early phases of the alternate pathway, including properdin, a circulating protein molecule. The fascinating feature of the alternate pathway is that it can be activated in the absence of antibody by polysaccharides in bacterial walls and yet can destroy bacteria and neutralize viruses.

An outline of the classic and alternate complement pathway is shown in Figure 26–7.

In the absence of complement factors that may occur rarely as congenital defects, there are major changes in the susceptibility of the affected individuals to disease. SLE occurs more frequently in those with deficiency of C1q, C1r, C1s, C2, C4, C5, and repeated infections in those with lack of C1r, C2, C3, and C5. C6- and C8-deficient subjects are prone to prolonged systemic gonococcal disease, and in C6 deficiency, recurrent meningococcal meningitis may occur. Absence of a normal inhibitor of C1 is associated with angioneurotic edema.

THE DUAL NATURE OF THE IMMUNE RESPONSE

In the introductory remarks to this chapter, the concepts of humoral and cellular immunity were mentioned. Although these are relatively old concepts, it is only in the last 20 years or so that the two types of immunity have been better defined.

The removal of a lymphoid outpouching of the gut of a fowl (bursa of Fabricius) in early life resulted in the nonproduction of immunoglobulins after potent antigenic stimuli. Subsequently, it was shown that thymectomy in newborn mice resulted in their incapacity to reject skin grafts from other mice; however, these ani-

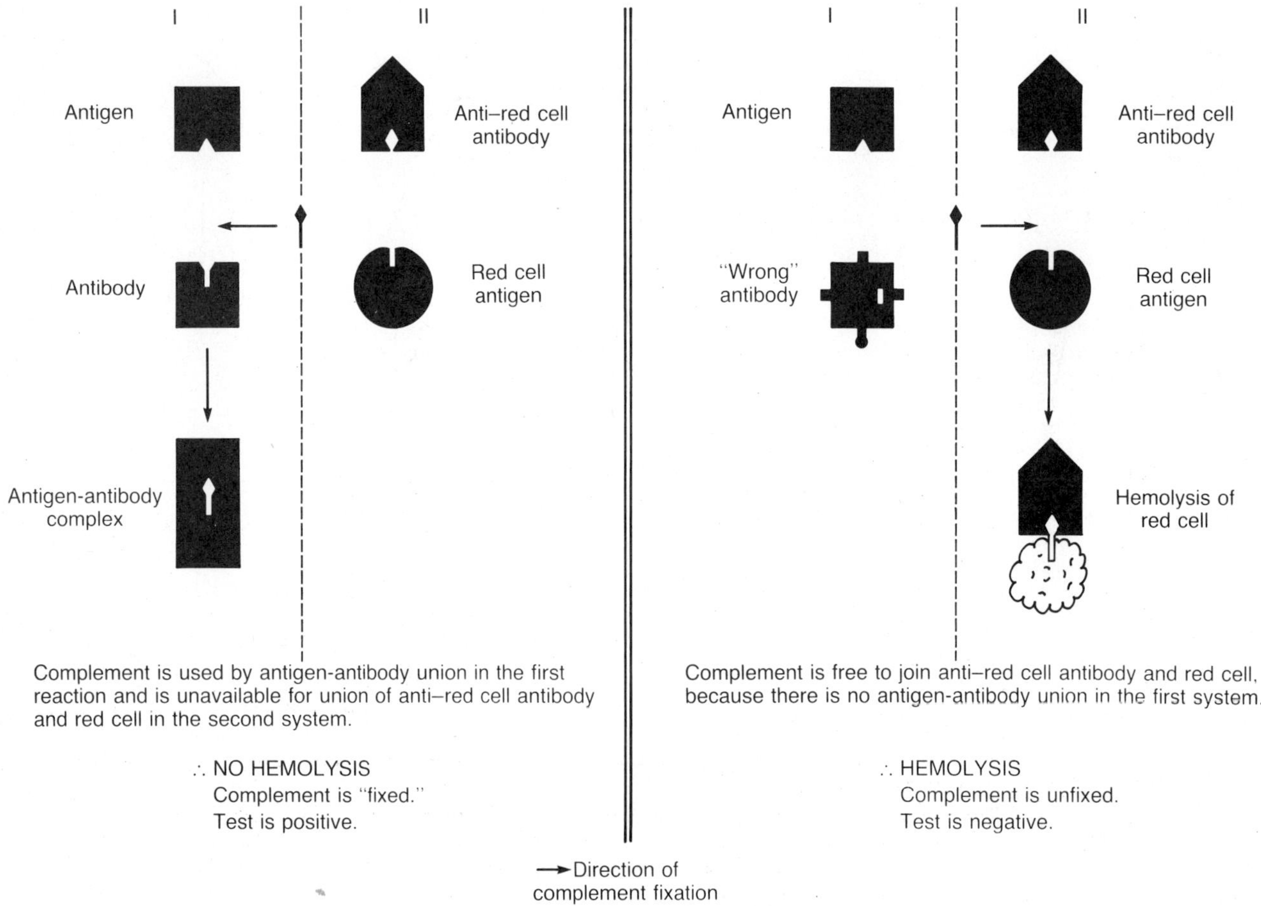

Figure 26–6 Principle of the complement fixation test.

mals could produce circulating immunoglobulins. Removal of the thymus in birds also reduced their capacity to reject grafts. Other combinations of thymectomy and bursectomy were performed, and the stage was set, certainly in the birds, for the dual origin of immune activity: the bursa of Fabricius produces immunocompetent cells that respond to antigen by the production of immunoglobulin; the thymus provides competent cells that have the ability to reject tissue grafts. In humans there is no bursa of Fabricius, but it is believed that Waldeyer's ring (pharyngeal tonsillar ring), with the lymph nodes of the ileocecal region and Peyer's patches, are analogues. The thymus in humans is believed to have the same functions that it has in birds and in the lower animals. This organ develops from the third branchial cleft and has epithelial and lymphocytic components. It would appear that the cells from the marrow enter the thymus, in which they are in some way conditioned or processed to serve cellular immune reactions. They pass from the thymus as so-called T-cells to populate lymph nodes in the paracortical regions and into the spleen in the area immediately adjacent to the central arterioles.

The Bursal Component of Immunity

The cells that are the agents of the bursal component, i.e., Waldeyer's ring and the lymphoid tissue of the small bowel, are lymphocytic, but antigenic stimulation causes proliferation and morphological changes resulting in plasma cells. These originate especially from the germinal follicles of the lymph nodes and from the lymph node medulla (as well as from the spleen). They emigrate to circulate in the blood as lymphocytes. They are known as B-cells. Although they are almost identical to T-cells

TABLE 26–3 Comparison Between Humoral and Cell-Mediated Immune Reactions

	Humoral	Cellular
Passive transfer to another subject	By immune serum	By sensitized leukocytes or transfer factor
Circulating antibody	Present	Absent
Time of maximum response	Within a short time (minutes or hours)	24–48 hours
Effector cell	B-cell; plasma cell	T-cell
Active lymph node area	Germinal follicles, medulla	Paracortical areas

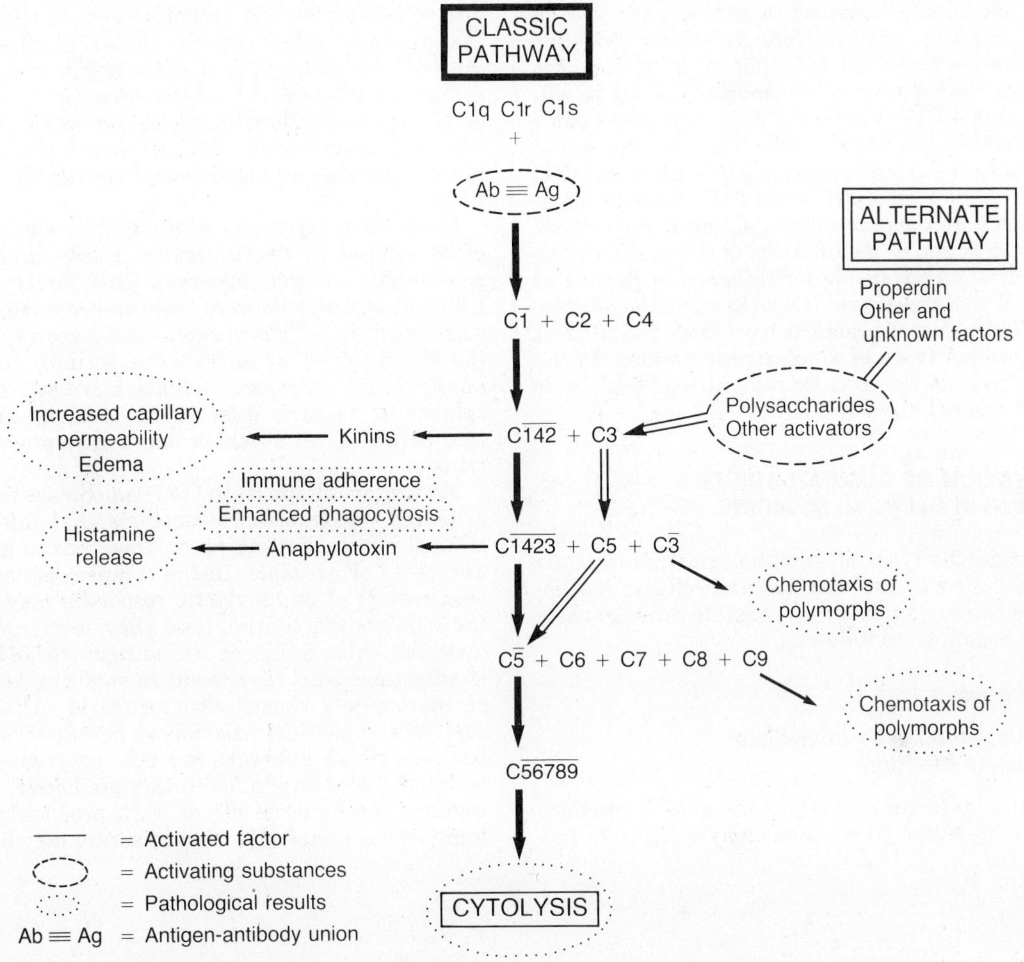

Figure 26–7 Sequence of reaction of complement factors and their pathological results.

under light microscopy, with electron microscopy they are seen to have numerous surface protrusions, unlike T-cells, which have a virtually flat surface. B-cells have many receptor immunoglobulin molecules attached to their cell membrane, but T-cells have relatively few.

B-Cell Response to Antigen

There is evidence for considerable cooperation between T-cells and B-cells. Nevertheless, each has a unique function. It would appear that antigen that stimulates the B-cells is taken up initially by macrophages and partially fixed at the cell surface, where it provides a strong immunogenic stimulus to B-lymphocytes. The macrophages also produce RNA, which is another antigenic stimulus. The antigen at the surface of the macrophage is presented to B-cells and is united with the immunoglobulin on the surface of the B-cell. It is a remarkable and almost unbelievable phenomenon that specific immunoglobulins for each of an almost infinite number of possible antigens are already preformed on the B-cells! At the acceptance of the antigen by the surface immunoglobulins, the cell begins to proliferate to produce a clone of cells with the same immunological specificity as the parent. These become plasma cells and produce humoral and specific antibodies to the offending antigen, which circulates in the bloodstream.

T-Cell Response to Antigen

T-cells are stimulated in the same way as B-cells by the presentation of antigens attaching to their specific surface antibody receptors. Again, a clone of similar cells is stimulated, and again macrophages may play a part in presenting the antigen to the affected cell. The stimulated cells produce substances that attract lymphocytes and macrophages and inhibit migration of lymphocytic cells, which are also cytotoxic for a variety of other cells, including tumor cells, virus-infected cells, and so forth. The phenomenon of delayed type hypersensitivity (see below) is also due to stimulation of a T-cell response.

The Recognition of "Self" and "Nonself"

In this regard the work of Burnet and Medawar was most important, and it subsequently earned them both the Nobel Prize. Initially it was hypothesized by Burnet that if antigen were given to an animal before the lymphoid system was mature, then the animal would consider the antigen as "self." If one attempts to graft skin from one strain of mouse to another, the second mouse will reject the graft as "foreign." If, however, the second mouse is given an injection of cells from the spleen of the first mouse while in utero, then it will accept the skin of the first mouse when it reaches adult life. Thus, having encountered cells from the first mouse while in utero, the second mouse regards them as "self" and preserves the memory into adult life. This phenomenon is known as *immune tolerance,* and it may result from the destruction or modification of the specific clone or clones of cells responsible for recognizing particular antigen(s). It is of great significance in medicine because of its relationship at a practical level with tissue graft and with various types of autoimmune disease. In the latter, the body mechanisms for recognizing "self" in its own tissues are defective.

CLASSIFICATION OF IMMUNOLOGICAL PHENOMENA IN CLINICAL MEDICINE

To illustrate the types of immunological phenomena that are mediated by the humoral and cellular mechanisms described earlier, it is convenient to consider them under four headings, as follows:

Type I Reactions

Anaphylactic Antibodies—Immediate Hypersensitivity Reaction

In humans, only reagins (IgE) are able to produce these reactions, although reactions may occur with IgG and complement. The essential part of the reaction is that antibody is bound to the surface of cells, and in the antibody-antigen reaction some of the cells are able to release substances like histamine (from mast cells), serotonin, kinins, prostaglandins, and slow-reactive substance of anaphylaxis (SRS-A), which contract smooth muscle, as well as heparin and eosinophil chemotactic factors.

In animals, especially in the guinea pig, anaphylaxis often results in death within a few minutes of the challenging antigen injection. This rarely happens in humans, but may do so in instances involving second or subsequent injections of such substances as horse serum (previously used in antitetanus serum). Other severe anaphylactic responses include laryngeal edema, and splanchnic vascular dilatation with shock and generalized urticaria, all of which may follow provoking injections.

Most often, anaphylactic phenomena are fairly benign although uncomfortable reactions that differ in their clinical effects, depending on the mode of entry of the antigen. For example, in the common pollen sensitivities, results of anaphylactic responses may be seen in the eye (conjunctivitis), nose (hay fever), and bronchi (asthma). Absorption of the antigen through the gastrointestinal tract may result in vomiting and diarrhea, or in remotely caused skin urticaria. Although some cases of asthma (intrinsic) have a hereditary and obscure basis in which allergens are not involved, other cases (extrinsic) also have a hereditary predisposition, but the immune mechanisms are at work producing the symptoms, and a raised IgE level in serum may be obtained.

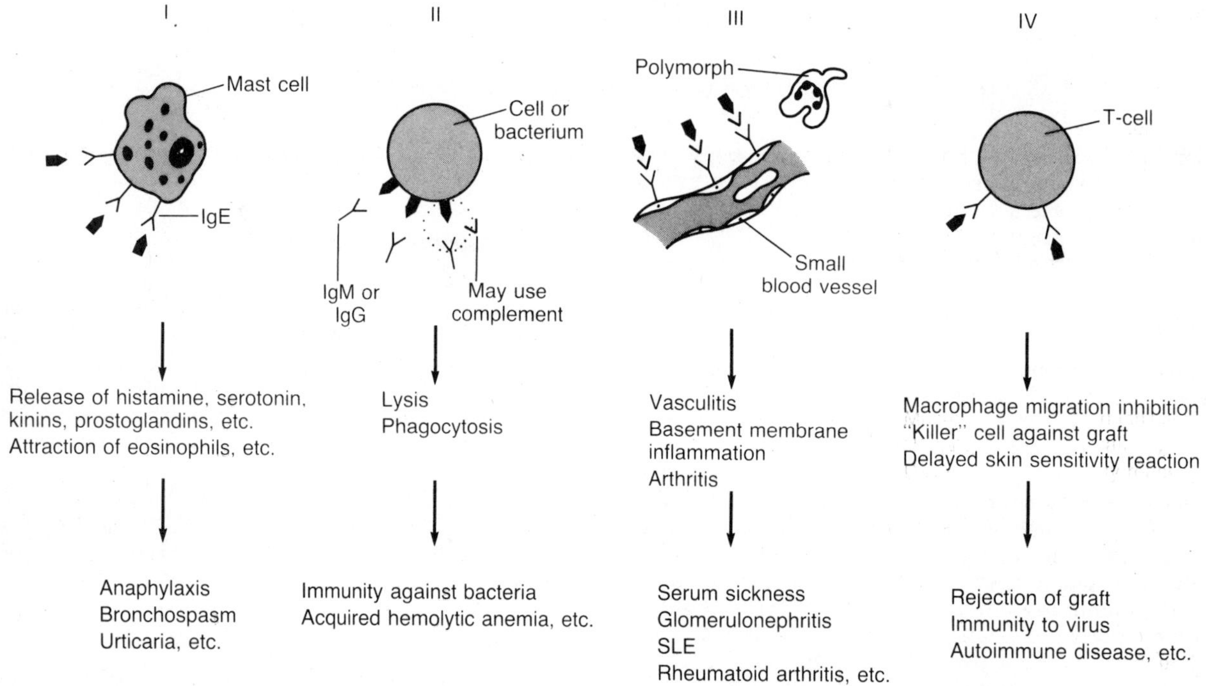

Figure 26–8 Types of immune response (see text).

TABLE 26–4 TYPES OF CLINICAL IMMUNOLOGICAL RESPONSE

Type	Reaction	Antibody	Clinical Examples
I	Anaphylactic	IgE	Asthma, hay fever, helminth infestation
II	Cytotoxic	IgG, IgM	Antibacterial antibodies, autoimmune disease (Hashimoto's thyroiditis, antigastric antibodies in pernicious anemia, hemolytic anemia, etc.), viral disease prevention
III	Antigen-antibody complex	IgG, IgM	Serum sickness, glomerulonephritis, and immune complex disease
IV	Delayed hypersensitivity	Sensitized lymphocytes	Tuberculin skin test (also fungal skin tests, Frei antigen, etc.). rejection of allografts or xenografts, "resistance" to viral disease

Some reactions to drug and other therapy (blood transfusion) may follow the binding of hapten to body protein, resulting in the immediate type of immune response.

TYPE II REACTIONS

Cytotoxic Reaction

These cytotoxic antibodies may need complement to effect the results of cell death or basement membrane damage. Among the diseases so caused are the autoimmune hemolytic anemias (Chap. 29), thyroiditis (p. 288), and idiopathic thrombocytopenic purpura (Chap. 31), and these may be diagnosed by the presence of circulating specific immunoglobulins (either IgG or IgM) in high titer, although in the case of ITP the demonstration of the immune mechanisms in diagnosis has technical problems.

Antipenicillin antibodies may be cytotoxic, causing hemolytic anemia by destroying the red cells that have the hapten, aminopenicillanic acid, attached. Another drug, α-methyldopa, probably binds itself to Rhesus antigen, and this provokes a hemolytic antibody similar to that seen in immune hemolytic anemia. Drugs such as apronalide (Sedormid), quinine, and many others form haptens on the surface of platelets, leading to antibody-mediated thrombocytopenia. On the credit side, such reactions are very important in the immune reaction to bacterial infection.

TYPE III REACTIONS

Immune Complex Disease

Generally, the union of antigen-antibody is disposed of by phagocytosis. However, in some instances, the immune complex becomes deposited and in turn evokes a response that damages tissues. Unlike anaphylactic antibodies, which elicit clinical symptoms within minutes, type III reactions require a build-up of antibody (IgG and IgM) in the circulation and the presence of a continued high concentration of antigen in the tissues.

Serum Sickness

Primary serum sickness occurs in subjects who have had no previous contact with the exciting antigen, and accelerated serum sickness occurs in those who have been sensitized previously. In the primary syndrome, antibody produced in response to the antigen builds up in the circulation over a period of days. If the antigen is still circulating by the time there is a sizable amount of circulating antibody, the stage is set for the formation of immune complexes, and symptoms appear between the 7th to 12th day after antigen administration. The antigen-antibody complex is deposited on a sensitive membrane, such as beneath the glomerular endothelium, where, with complement, it attracts polymorphs and releases inflammatory products causing tissue damage. In accelerated serum sickness, the patient has had previous experience of the antigen, and symptoms will commence between a few hours to a few days after administration, depending on the titer of the circulating antibody. In both instances, there may be production of IgE as well as IgM and G, and in these instances, anaphylactic symptoms may occur. In primary serum sickness, such anaphylactic symptoms will occur in the time limits given, and it should be noted that here, anaphylactic symptoms present *without* provoking previous injections. In the accelerated type of serum sickness, anaphylactic symptoms may occur within a few minutes to a few hours.

The lesion of the immune-complex facet of serum sickness may involve the joints (arthritis), kidney (glomerulonephritis), heart (myocarditis), and skin (vasculitis). The course of the illness is variable and is predicated on the type, extent, and severity of the lesions. Serum sickness provoked by drugs forming haptens with body protein antigen (penicillin, streptomycin, and others) is well known.

Chronic Immune-Complex Damage

A number of naturally occurring diseases are thought to be caused by deposits of immune complex and complement in the tissues. Like serum sickness, these diseases show some or all of the features of arthritis, carditis, glomerulonephritis, and vasculitis. Among the diseases in which this etiology is suspected are systemic lupus erythematosus (SLE), acute diffuse glomerulonephritis, rheumatic fever, rheumatoid arthritis, and periarteritis nodosa.

TYPE IV REACTIONS

Cell-mediated Immune Reactions

These are mediated by cells; circulating antibody and complement are not required. An outline of the mechanisms of stimulation and progression of the cell-mediated response has been given earlier. Although some reactions can be used as pure examples of this type of response, many other reactions to immunological insult may include both cellular and humoral components. Some of the more important examples of Group IV responses will be discussed briefly.

The Tuberculin Skin Reaction

This well-known test has a history that goes back to the end of the 19th century, when Koch introduced tuberculin (a filtrate of a broth culture of *M. tuberculosis)*. Although it was valueless as a therapeutic agent, the purpose for which Koch originally had introduced it, tuberculin was found of value as a diagnostic tool. Koch's "old tuberculin" has now given way to the purified protein derivative of tuberculin (PPD), given intradermally in considerable dilution (1:1000 to 1:10,000), in 0.1-mL amounts. After 48 hours, a positive response is considered to be an area of induration of 5 mm or more in diameter at the site of injection, surrounded by erythema. The reaction is positive in those who have been sensitized by previous or present tuberculosis. It does not indicate the clinical activity of the disease. The exact relationship of the skin sensitivity to the "level" of cellular immunity is not known with certainty, but it is likely that the skin reaction to the protein is a reflection, although perhaps an incomplete one, of cellular immunity to the microbiological agent.

Other skin tests used similarly include histoplasmin, coccidioidin, blastomycin, and the Frei test.

The sensitivity to a particular antigen may be transferred from a sensitive to an insensitive individual by a transfer of lymphocytes but not by transfer of serum. However, it has been found that an extract from these lymphocytes of responsive individuals of a substance known as *transfer factor* can transmit delayed sensitivity to a previously nonreactive individual without cells.

Cell-mediated immune reactions are of great importance in the transplantation of tissues, in immunity to viral disease, in forms of contact sensitivity, and in autoimmune disease.

AUTOIMMUNE DISEASE

Until relatively recently, it was thought that the body would not form antibodies or display an immune response against its own tissues—the so-called horror autotoxicosis of Ehrlich. However, this belief became untenable after the demonstration of antibodies to red blood cells in patients with acquired hemolytic anemia, the lupus erythematosus cells in SLE, and antithyroglobulin antibodies in Hashimoto's thyroiditis.

From the previous discussion on the recognition of "self" and "nonself" by immunocytes, it was concluded that the tolerance of "self" is programmed in utero or in the newborn period. Foreign antigen introduced before that time will be regarded subsequently as "self," and thymectomy will also result in tolerance of the cell-mediated mechanism toward the introduced antigen. It is not known how this occurs at the cellular level except that if a cell produces immunocytes against the body's

TABLE 26–5 OUTLINE OF INVESTIGATION IN AUTOIMMUNE DISEASE

Disease	Antigen	Method of Detection of Antibody
Thyroiditis	Thyroglobulin Epithelial microsomal antigen Second colloid antigen	IFA on unfixed monkey thyroid
	Thyroglobulin	Tanned red cell antibody
	Epithelial microsomal antigen	Tanned red cell antibody
Rheumatoid arthritis Sjögren's syndrome, lupus erythematosus	IgG (altered)	Identification of RF
Scleroderma Rheumatoid arthritis Sjögren's syndrome Lupus erythematosus	Nuclear antigens	IFA on cell nuclei LE cell test
	DNA	IFA or unfixed kintoplast of *Crithidia luciliae*
Primary biliary cirrhosis	Mitochondria	IFA on unfixed rat kidney tubule cells
Chronic active hepatitis	Smooth muscle	IFA on unfixed rat stomach smooth muscle
Autoimmune hemolytic anemia	Red cell	Coomb's test
Autoimmune skin disease	Various skin constituents	IFA or DFA on patients' skin biopsy or on "normal" skin
Pernicious anemia	Parietal cell microsomes	IFA on unfixed rat gastric mucosal cells
Addison's disease	Adrenal cortical cell cytoplasm	IFA on unfixed adrenal cortex cells
Renal disease	Basement membrane: deposit of antigen antibody complex	IFA or DFA on patients' renal biopsy or on "normal" human kidney

IFA, indirect fluorescent antibody; DFA, direct fluorescent antibody; RF, rheumatoid factor; CF, complement fixation; DNA, desoxyribonucleic acid. Most of these tests are available in kit form from commercial suppliers.

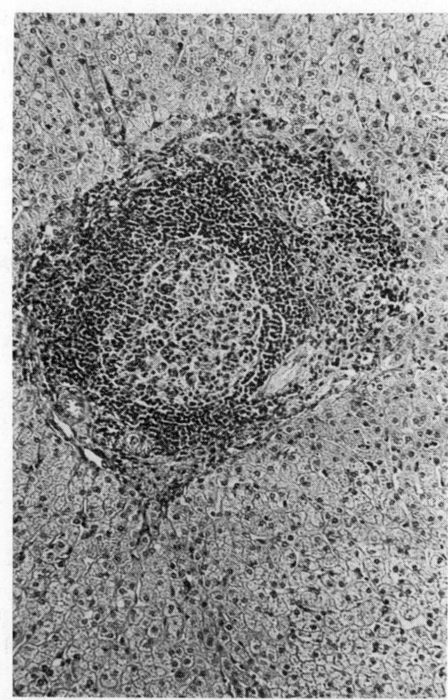

Figure 26–9 Primary biliary cirrhosis. The 48-year-old woman had progressive painless obstructive jaundice. Note the well-defined lymphoid follicle involving the biliary triad. Hematoxylin-eosin × 33.

tissues, there is some censorship mechanism that suppresses their proliferation. In autoimmune disease it is considered that the censorship breaks down, and forbidden clones producing self-destructive immunocytes commence to flourish. Such a mechanism has been proposed for the etiology of rheumatoid arthritis, myasthenia gravis, SLE, and other conditions. There is an increased incidence of autoimmune disease with advancing age. To explain this, it has been suggested that the censorship of "forbidden clones" becomes less strict with age, and as an example of this, the age-related incidence of biologically false positive tests for syphilis is quoted.

The change in body protein that makes it "nonself" to normal immunocytes may occur in several ways. Antibodies against microbiological antigens may cross-react with body tissues; e.g., streptococcal antibodies cross-react with myocardium and thus form a basis for the streptococcal etiology of rheumatic carditis, colon antibodies in ulcerative colitis cross-react with a serotype of *E. coli.* Viral infections may alter the antigenic nature of cells, and this is probably of some significance in mumps and measles encephalomyelitis. Numerous drugs, as we have seen, are capable of inducing autoimmune processes. The adjuvant properties of mycobacterial extracts and other substances have been described previously. In chronic granulomatous disease (leprosy and syphilis) many autoimmune phenomena have been described. Possibly granulomatous disease may play a part, at present only suspected, in autoimmune pathogenesis. Some body protein normally is excluded from the circulation and thus is never recognized as "self." If exposed subsequently, then it is regarded as "nonself," and an immune reaction is mounted. Examples possibly include the uveitis following the escape of eye-lens protein and spermatic granuloma. The protein of sperm is of course not present in the fetus.

These examples do not explain all the so-called autoimmune diseases, but they point a way to understanding their etiology. It should be added that there does appear to be a genetic propensity to autoimmune disease.

A list of the more common diseases considered to be autoimmune in nature is appended. The list is not exhaustive and does not include all the diseases suspected of autoimmune pathogenesis.

Many of the tests used to detect autoimmune diseases are not specific. For example, RF is found not only in rheumatoid arthritis but also in other disease, such as lupus erythematosus. Some tests are more specific, e.g., mitochondrial antibody is positive in about 90% of cases of primary biliary cirrhosis but in only a small percentage of other types of autoimmune disorders. The explanation of the presence of such antibodies as anti–smooth muscle in active chronic hepatitis is unknown, and their common presence in a completely unrelated disorder, such as infectious mononucleosis, only adds to the complexity of the problem at this time.

IMMUNODEFICIENT SYNDROMES

These can be considered most rationally under three headings:

1. The primary immunodeficiencies are those conditions in which, as a primary hereditary condition, either cellular or humoral immune mechanisms are deficient.

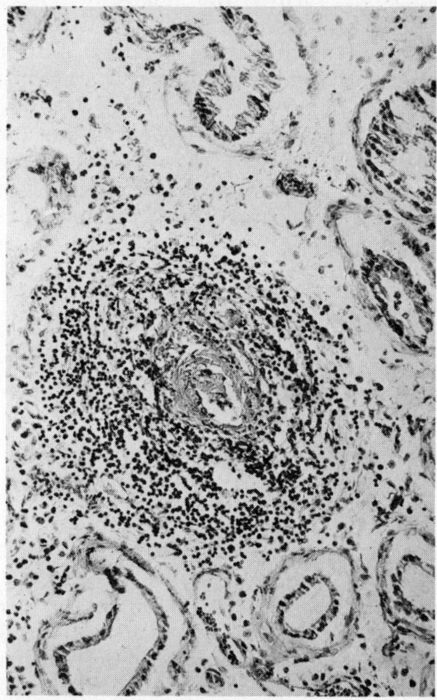

Figure 26–10 Arteritis in rheumatoid arthritis. The patient had suffered progressive active arthritis for many years. At autopsy, arteritis was also demonstrated, and it is seen in a small artery of the testis. The wall of this artery is acellular and hyaline and shows infiltration by inflammatory cells. Hematoxylin-eosin × 33.

2. The secondary immunodeficiencies result from involvement of the immunogenetic system in the course of another disease. This group also includes the phagocytic dysfunction disorders.

3. Acquired immunodeficiency syndrome (AIDS) is discussed on p. 607.

Primary Immunodeficiency Syndromes

These diseases are congenital defects of T- or B-cells and consequently may involve the cellular arm, humoral arm, or both arms of the immune mechanism. Thus, on the one extreme, there may be agammaglobulinemia or dysgammaglobulinemia in which several or individual immunoglobulins are absent because of deficiency of B-cells. On the other end of the disease spectrum, thymic dysplasia will produce deficiency of T-cells with lack of cell-mediated immune mechanisms. Combined deficiencies occur, such as the Wiskott-Aldrich syndrome in which deficiency of immunoglobulin(s) is combined with loss of cell-mediated responses.

For completeness, primary deficiencies also include disorders of phagocyte functions, such as Chédiak-Higashi syndrome, and a group of derangements of the complement system, to which some reference is made above.

Secondary Immunodeficient Syndromes

Such diseases include tumors of the lymphoid system involving B- or T-cells, which therefore do not function adequately, as well as hematological disorders in which phagocytes are quantitatively or qualitatively deficient, e.g., leukemia, aplastic anemia, and so forth. Protein-losing conditions, such as the nephrotic syndrome, deplete the body of immunoglobulins, and there are less well understood mechanisms affecting patients with diabetes mellitus and renal failure who exhibit diminished resistance to infection.

Drugs like cortisone and cytotoxic agents as well as x-irradiation used in cancer therapy affect immunological function. Many drugs are used therapeutically deliberately as immunosuppressives in transplant surgery, immune complex disease (e.g., glomerulonephritis), and so forth.

CONDITIONS ASSOCIATED WITH HYPERIMMUNOGLOBULINEMIA

Polyclonal Reactions

In the normal individual the serum immunoglobulins exhibit some normal variation that, in part at least, is due to the great variation possible in the standard immunoglobulin molecules in the variable regions of that molecule. The pattern, then, is the product of numerous different clones of cells, each producing a specific immunoglobulin in response to specific antigens in its experience.

If the individual is then subjected to some prolonged antigenic stimulus, as occurs with some chronic diseases, he will produce a wide spectrum of antibodies in response to the individual antigens in the stimulus. It will be appreciated, in this regard, that even a relatively simple bacterium has a number of antigenic constituents; thus, the usual response to infection is the production of immunoglobulins (usually IgM followed by IgG) from a number of immunoglobulin-producing clones of lymphocytes. This reaction is considered polyclonal, and in some conditions the level of immunoglobulin is unusually high and may be of diagnostic importance.

Polyclonal gammopathy occurs in liver disease and particularly in chronic active hepatitis but also in cirrhosis. It occurs in many types of chronic infections, such as chronic osteomyelitis, as well as in the parasitic infestations of leishmaniasis, chronic malaria, and congenital toxoplasmosis. Autoimmune diseases such as Sjögren's syndrome, Hashimoto's thyroiditis, and others also exhibit polyclonal gammopathy.

In a physico-chemical sense, polyclonal response will yield differing immunoglobulins, each with distinctive light and heavy chain variable zones.

Monoclonal Reactions

Neoplastic proliferation, unlike physiological or hyperplastic proliferation, is not of varied cells but of a single clone that is proliferating in an uncontrolled fashion independent of the body's demands and needs. In the case of neoplasia of the B-cells, the immunoglobulin is monoclonal; thus one type of immunoglobulin with a constant pattern of heavy and light chains and variable region pattern is produced. The immunoglobulin produced may be IgG, A, M, D, or E. Generally, IgM is produced in a condition known as Waldenström's macroglobulinemia and the others in multiple myeloma. In the latter condition, about three-quarters of the patients excrete monoclonal light chains in the urine, where they are known as Bence Jones protein. They are produced by the malignant cells in some excess over complete immunoglobulin. One type of multiple myeloma produces only light chains, and these are also

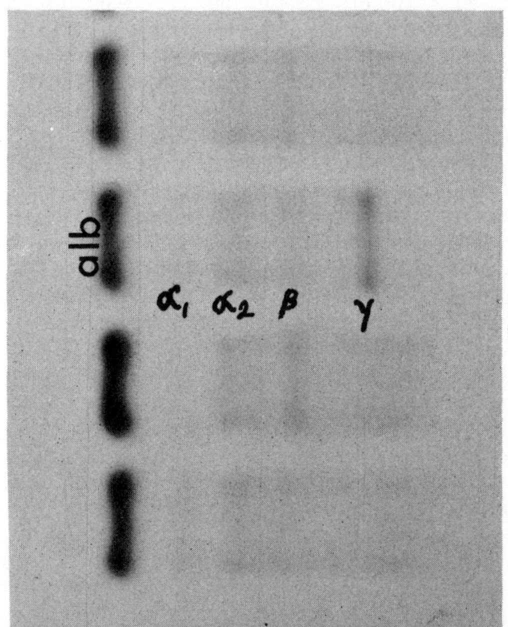

Figure 26–11 Cellulose acetate electrophoresis of serum from a patient with plasma cell myeloma, showing an abnormal protein in the gamma region. Figure 26–12 shows the Bence Jones protein (*A*) of the same patient. The strips immediately above and below are of normal sera for reference.

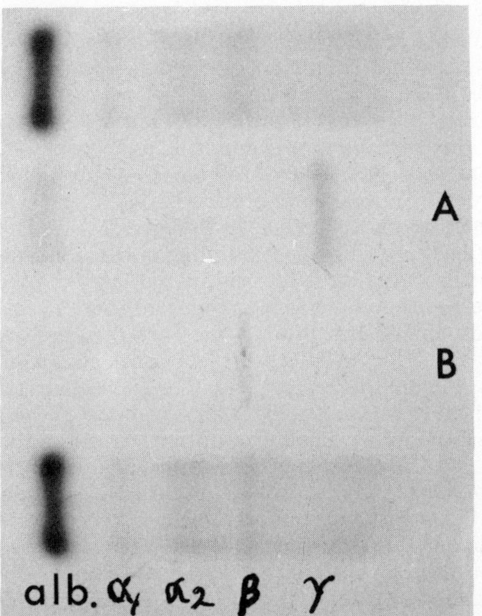

Figure 26–12 Bence Jones proteinuria. Microzone cellulose acetate electrophoresis, showing typical Bence Jones protein (*A*) in urine concentrated fiftyfold by dialysis; *B,* Urine from another myeloma patient, showing a faint "band" in the beta region, which is an application artifact. The patterns immediately above and below are those of normal sera for reference.

excreted, but in the serum there is no abnormal monoclonal immunoglobulin. In another related disease, only heavy chains are produced; γ, μ, and α are found in the blood and may also appear in the urine, but there are no κ or λ chains.

Some lymphomas and leukemias will also produce monoclonal gammopathies. Biclonal gammopathy has two distinct monoclonal immunoglobulins (usually IgM). Generally, the patients have lymphoma or macroglobulinemia.

There are some further conditions in which monoclonal proliferation of immunoblasts occurs but which are not considered necessarily neoplastic. Monoclonal gammopathy has been found with increasing frequency in the older age groups. Some of these will develop myeloma, but the ultimate nature of this condition is not yet apparent.

CRYOGLOBULINEMIA

Cryoglobulins are monoclonal or polyclonal immunoglobulins that precipitate from solution at temperatures of less than 37°C down to 4°C. In such a situation, the skin of course is mainly affected and shows cold urticaria, microthrombosis, Raynaud's phenomenon, and even gangrene. The globulin may be IgG, which at low temperatures becomes crystalline, or it may be cryoprecipitable IgM or IgG, a mixture of these, or, rarely, IgA or even Bence Jones protein. Most cases occur in association with multiple myeloma or Waldenström's macroglobulinemia, but some have been reported in association with rheumatoid arthritis, in cirrhosis, in sarcoidosis, and in some instances without obvious associated disorders.

PYROGLOBULINEMIA

Such proteins are precipitated at 56°C. Bence Jones protein normally has this property, but so do some monoclonal IgG immunoglobulins. The phenomenon is of interest only in vitro, but half of the sera that show this property come from patients with multiple myeloma.

PROTECTIVE MECHANISMS AGAINST INFECTIOUS DISEASE

It will be appreciated that immune mechanisms have been evolved to protect the body from, and if necessary to rid the body of, potentially harmful foreign material. Although much of our work in the laboratory is devoted to demonstration of humoral antibodies and to a lesser extent to the cell-mediated mechanisms, there are other protective means. These will be described briefly under the heading of innate mechanisms.

NATURAL (INNATE) PROTECTIVE MECHANISMS

Innate protective mechanisms against disease are provided by a combination of genetic, nutritional, and environmental factors that may be considered under the headings of species, racial, and individual, as follows:

Species Immunity. Some species are naturally protected against certain infections, and the protection does not depend on circulating antibody. For example, lower animals are not susceptible to gonorrhea, man is immune to distemper, and the turtle is not liable to tetanus.

Racial Immunity. In this group, a race within the species has a relative immunity. For example, types of grain can be bred that are immune to diseases that affect the species generally. Algerian sheep are naturally immune to anthrax, but European sheep are not. Men with sickle cell anemia are relatively resistant to malaria.

Individual Immunity. The unbroken skin is probably impervious to bacteria, although some infections gain some degree of entry into hair follicles and sweat and sebaceous glands. It is claimed that some bacteria penetrate intact skin, but this claim is unproven. Sweat and sebaceous glands produce an oily and acidic secretion that is inhospitable to bacteria. Keratinizing skin cells are shed along with their resident bacteria. The upper respiratory tract is lined by a mucous membrane that secretes mucus. The latter entraps bacteria and is constantly moved upward by mucosal ciliary action into the nose and mouth, from which it is excreted. In tears, there is an enzyme, lysozyme, that digests the walls of gram-positive bacteria, thus protecting the conjunctivae. Lysozyme is also present in skin and in nasal secretions. Gastric acid and enzymes destroy most ingested bacteria, and protection is also given to the gastrointestinal tract by secretion of IgA into the lumen by many glands in its course from the parotid gland to the mucous glands of the intestine. The bacterial population of the large bowel is kept within bounds by peristalsis and excretion. In the urinary tract, the flushing action of urine, together with its osmolarity and acidity, is important. Acidity in the adult vagina also aids in the maintenance of a stable normal flora.

Other defensive mechanisms include the cough reflex and the conjunctival reflex. Age, alcohol, diet, debility, and factors in the environment (air, housing, standards of hygiene, and so forth) all play roles in the individual response to infection.

ACQUIRED IMMUNITY

Active Acquired Immunity. Such immunity may be obtained naturally by the individual after diseases such as chickenpox, measles, or typhoid. The individual may be stimulated to achieve the same type of immunity by exposing himself to innate components of the microbiological agents of the respective diseases, to attenuated (avirulent) but similar organisms, or to the detoxified but antigenic products of the disease-causing organisms. Examples of these types of artificially acquired immunity are typhoid immunization (with dead organisms), polio immunization (with ingestion of attenuated polio vaccine of Sabin), and diphtheria toxoid (made nontoxic by formalin or alum).

Passive Acquired Immunity. This is an immunity acquired by passage of antibodies, either naturally across the placenta or artificially by intramuscular or even intravenous injection of antibodies. Diphtheria and tetanus antitoxin are examples.

"NATURAL ANTIBODIES"

The bacterial origin of natural isoagglutinins has already been related (p. 521). The titer of normal serum against typhoid and other members of the salmonellae is probably owing to the antigens shared by these organisms with the more usual inhabitants of the bowel. The antigens of normal flora will provoke antibody reactions and some of these, by cross-reaction, can be measured in diagnostic tests for the presence of antibody against *S. typhi* and other organisms of the enteric fever group.

THE MEASUREMENT OF IMMUNE RESPONSE

The basic methodologies used are those of precipitation, agglutination, complement fixation and cytolysis, phagocytosis, fluorescent antibody studies, investigation of cell-mediated responses, and some miscellaneous and less easily classifiable methods. This classification will be adhered to except when continuity and clarity of diagnosis require otherwise.

PRECIPITATION

This reaction may be defined as the visible result of an antigen-antibody reaction between a soluble antigen and its antiserum. In addition to these two substances, electrolytes are necessary to bring the process to its desired conclusion, and pH and temperature of the mixture also have an effect. Antigen and antibody molecules are bound together in a lattice of alternate molecules if the reaction is successful. Since both substances in the original mixture are soluble, relatively large lattices of antigen-antibody must be formed to be visible. If there is an excess of either antigen or antibody, the resultant amount of precipitation is less than when optimal proportions are present. The reason becomes apparent by reference to Figure 26–13. In the situation shown on the lefthand side of the figure, there is excess of antibody, so that the combining sites on antigen are "over-filled" and large lattices are not formed. Likewise, on the righthand side of the diagram there is excess of antigen and the combining sites are "under-filled," so that again, large lattices are not formed. In a more usual fashion, the reactions may be expressed as shown in the chart below. Thus, the most sensitive zone of the test for the given amount of antigen is in the range of 1/320 to 1/640 dilution of antiserum.

Note particularly that with low dilutions of antiserum there is no precipitation, and likewise, a relative excess of antigen will yield a negative test. This latter phenomenon is known as the *prozone* phenomenon. The excess of antigen is owing to the fact that there is insufficient antibody to combine with the abundant antigen to form visible precipitates. When there is a relative abundance of antibody, the cause may be that the combining sites of the antigen particles are occupied by antibody and the lattice structure—antigen-antibody-antigen-antibody-antigen-antibody—is not constructed, but only small groupings using more antibody, e.g., antibody-antigen-antibody · antibody-antigen-antibody · antibody-antigen-antibody.

The practical application of this phenomenon is evident. Optimal proportions of antigen and antibody dictated by previous experience are chosen; single dilution tests are avoided if possible.

AGGLUTINATION

This reaction is essentially the same as precipitation. The difference is in the size of the reacting particles of antigen. In precipitation, the results of antigen-antibody union optimally result in the appearance of visible precipitation of antigen-antibody complex in a previously clear solution. In agglutination, the antigen particles are visible before the immune reaction occurs, and the union of antibody is aggregation of the antigen particles into larger aggregates. Prozone phenomena occur here, as in the precipitin reaction, and they result in the nonclumping of antigen particles, cells, or inert antigen carriers such as latex.

TITER

In the various procedures for identifying antibodies that are conducted in diagnostic tests, the strength of the antibody demonstrated is often significant. For example, antibodies to typhoid are found in nearly all

Amount of antigen	constant							
Antiserum titer	20	40	80	160	320	640	1280	2560
Amount of precipitate	−	−	−	+ +	+ + + +	+ + + +	+ +	−

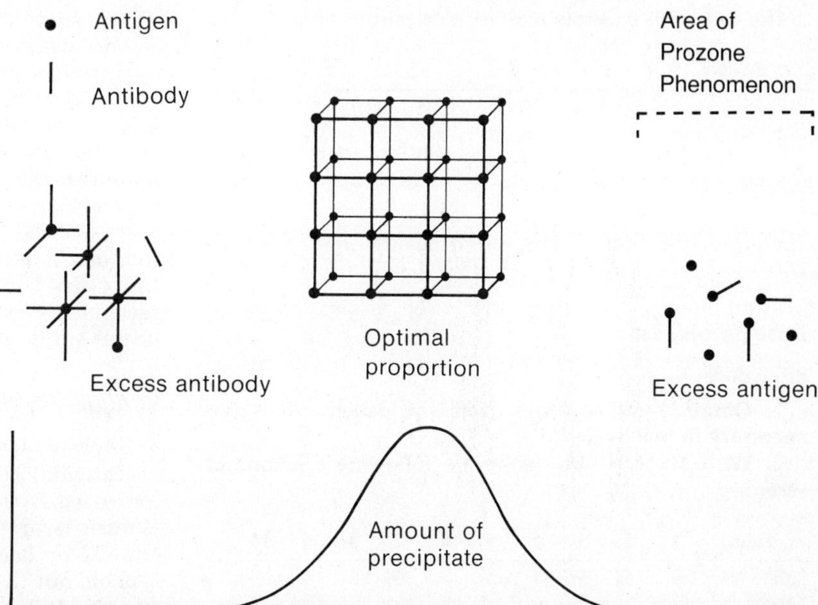

Figure 26–13 Precipitation; to explain the importance of optimal amounts of antigen and antibody (see text).

sera, but this does not mean that everybody has typhoid. Naturally, the presence of antibodies to some antigens, e.g., Rh antigens, is always significant. The strength of the antibody solution in producing antigen-antibody phenomena is an indication of the reaction of the patient to the offending antigen and, if it is above a certain level, may be of diagnostic value. It is not practically possible to weigh out the amount of immune protein present in the serum, but the dilution of a serum producing a visible agglutination or precipitation with an antigen is obviously related to the amount of immune antibody present. The more dilute the serum that is able to produce the anticipated result, the more antibody present. The reciprocal of the highest dilution giving the anticipated result is known as the titer. Thus, if a serum in a dilution of 1 in 250 gives a visible antigen-antibody result, but the same serum in a dilution of 1 in 300 does not, the serum is said to have a titer of 250.

SOME PRACTICAL APPLICATIONS OF PRECIPITATION AND AGGLUTINATION REACTIONS

Typing and Grouping of Bacteria

Using known antisera and extracted soluble antigen from streptococci, Lancefield grouping (p. 369) may be performed.

Blood Banking

Many of the methods employed in blood banking are agglutination reactions using unknown cells with known antisera or vice versa.

Widal Reaction (Febrile Agglutinins) and Slide Agglutination Tests

The Widal reaction is a serological method commonly used in the diagnosis of typhoid, enteric, and undulant fevers. The reaction measures the titer of serum against suspensions of known organisms. The classic method is a tube agglutination technique; a slide method is also available.

Slide Agglutination Method

Salmonella O and H antigens and *Br. abortus* antigen are commercially available for this purpose. The method is rapid. The following apparatus is required:

Large glass slide rule into squares, preferably 5 rows of 6 squares
0.2-mL graduated pipette
Illuminated Diamond Rh typing box

Procedure

1. Deliver 0.08, 0.04, 0.02, 0.01, and 0.005 mL of the serum to the squares in each row.

2. Add to each row 0.03 mL of antigen suspensions and mix with applicator sticks.

3. Rock the slide on the illuminated box for 3 minutes and read the agglutination.

4. The degree of agglutination is read in accordance with the following scale:

Complete agglutination	**4 plus**
75% agglutination	**3 plus**
50% agglutination	**2 plus**
25% agglutination	**1 plus**

5. The serum dilutions on the slide are considered to correspond with the following dilutions in the tube test:

0.08 mL serum	**1/20**
0.04 mL serum	**1/40**
0.02 mL serum	**1/80**
0.01 mL serum	**1/160**
0.005 mL serum	**1/320**

The titer of the serum against the antigen is considered to be shown by that serum giving a 2 plus agglutination.

The following example may be illustrative:

Square	1	2	3	4	5
Serum mL	0.08	0.04	0.02	0.01	0.005
Corresponding titer of serum	1/20	1/40	1/80	1/160	1/320
Agglutination	4 plus	4 plus	3 plus	2 plus	1 plus

Therefore, the titer of this serum against this antigen is 160.

Tube (Widal) Test

Procedure

1. Obtain 1 mL of serum from the patient. (It is not necessary to inactivate it.)

2. With 10 test tubes make the following dilutions of serum:

Tube	1	2	3	4	5	6	7	8	9	10
Saline mL	9	5	5	5	5	5	5	5	5	5
Serum mL	1	5 mL of tube 1	5 mL of tube 2	—	—	etc.	etc.	—	dis-card	5 mL
Dilution	$\frac{1}{10}$	$\frac{1}{20}$	$\frac{1}{40}$	$\frac{1}{80}$	$\frac{1}{160}$	$\frac{1}{320}$	$\frac{1}{640}$	$\frac{1}{1280}$	$\frac{1}{2560}$	$\frac{1}{5120}$

3. To a rack of small round-bottomed tubes in four rows of 10 tubes each, add 0.5 mL of the dilutions and to an eleventh tube in each row add 0.5 mL saline (negative control).

4. Add 1 drop of concentrated O antigen to each tube by using *S. typhi O, S. paratyphi A O, S. paratyphi B O,* and *Br. abortus* in the four rows, respectively.

5. In another rack, four rows of Dreyer's tubes are set up in a similar fashion, each with 0.5 mL of the serum dilutions and the eleventh row with 0.5 mL of saline.

6. To each row of these tubes add 0.5 mL of the dilute H suspensions of *S. typhi, S. paratyphi A, S. paratyphi B,* and nonspecific *Salmonella H.* The serum dilutions in these tubes will be double those in the previous set, i.e., 1/20, 1/40, 1/80, and so on.

7. The O tubes are placed in a water bath at 56°C for 4 hours and then left at room temperature overnight before reading, with the aid of a convex mirror, for agglutination. The H tubes are incubated at 37°C for 2 hours and read immediately and again the next morning. The fluffy type of H agglutination is easily seen with the naked eye in the conical-bottomed Dreyer's tubes.

A significant and suspicious O titer for *S. typhi* is 160, but a rising titer on repetition is considered more important (see below). H titer is nonspecific, especially in persons who have received TAB inoculations, and may rise with any fever. In brucellosis, a titer of 160 is significant. A zone phenomenon in the first few tubes of the *Brucella* series is not uncommon and is due to excess of antibody.

Interpretation of Results

The slide test is a screening test and should be regarded as such, and the Widal test is liable to a number of variables. For example, results will depend on the stage of the disease, and titer rises only in the second week of the disease. The "Normal" level of agglutinins will vary in different populations and circumstances; for example narcotic addicts have higher levels of *S. typhi* O and H antibodies. Early antimicrobial therapy will retard the rise of titer, and previous immunization will increase O and H antibodies, which may also rise in *any* febrile episode. Added to these, there are the technical variables in the performance of the test. The concept of "normal" titer in febrile agglutinins has become somewhat irrelevant, and it is more rational to examine for an increase in titer after an initial study. A fourfold increase is considered suspect.

Vi Agglutination

As previously described, the Vi antigen may mask the O antigen. Thus, in some cases of typhoid, only the increased H titer may be demonstrable, and the result is misinterpreted. When there is strong evidence, either clinical or bacteriological, that the patient may have typhoid but the Widal test is inconclusive, the Vi agglutination test should be done.

Vi antibody is frequently found in typhoid carriers, although O antibody may be of usual titer. The antiVi titer does not become high, and a titer of 10 or above is considered significant. *S. typhi* Vi is commercially available, and the methodology for estimation of antiVi titer is the same as in the Widal test. There is unfortunately a high incidence of false negative and false positive results.

Weil-Felix Reaction

As described elsewhere (p. 522), in the course of rickettsial infections, antibodies of the heterophil type are produced against species of *Proteus* (OX-19, OX-2, OX-K). Antigens of unflagellated organisms are commercially available, as are reagents for a rapid slide test. The latter should be confirmed, if positive, with the tube test. The methodology of the tube test parallels that given for the Widal, using a row of tubes with serum dilutions of 1/10 to 1/5120 for each *Proteus* strain. To each 0.5 mL of serum dilution add 0.5 mL of the respective antigen suspension. Mix well, incubate for 2 hours at 37°C, and then keep overnight at 4°C. Caveats similar to those given above in reading Widal results are worth considering. Titers over 160 are regarded with suspicion, and the serum is reexamined at a later date for an increase in titer. A fourfold increase is definitely suspect.

Identification of the Enterobacteriaceae

In a sense these serological tests are reversed Widal reactions in which unknown organisms are challenged with sera of known antibacterial titer. Both slide and tube tests are performed. Such tests are important in identification and are detailed under *Salmonella* (p. 378) and *Shigella* (p. 381).

STREPTOCOCCUS MG AGGLUTINATION TEST

Patients with viral pneumonia (more specifically, that caused by *Mycoplasma*) develop heterophil antibodies to

Streptococcus MG. Thus the titer of the patient's serum against the organism may be used in the diagnosis of nonbacterial pneumonia. *Streptococcus* MG suspensions are available commercially, as is *Streptococcus* MG antiserum.

Method

1. Set up eight 3 by ½ inch test tubes. In the first, place 0.8 mL saline; place 0.5 mL saline in the other seven. Add 0.2 mL of serum from the patient to the first tube, mix, and transfer 0.5 mL to the second tube. Continue doubling the dilutions to the end of the row and discard 0.5 mL from the seventh tube.

2. Add 0.5 mL of 1:10 saline-diluted *Streptococcus* MG suspension to each tube. Serum titers in each tube are 10, 20, 40, 80, 160, 320, and 640; the eighth tube acts as an antigen or negative control.

3. A set of tubes using a positive serum of known titer should be run in parallel.

4. Tubes are shaken, incubated at 37°C for 2 hours, and placed in the refrigerator overnight. They are then reincubated at 37°C for 2 hours and read for agglutination. The titer is that of the tube in which small clumps appear and there is incomplete supernatant clearing.

5. A titer of 20 is significant, as is a fourfold increase between the acute and convalescent specimens. A negative result is not necessarily clinically significant.

Cold Agglutinins

In atypical pneumonia caused by *Mycoplasma* infection, a nonspecific cold agglutinin appears in the patient's serum. A normal titer of cold agglutinins up to 16 may be found, but titers above 40 should be viewed with suspicion.

Method

1. Obtain a sample of blood from the patient and place immediately in an incubator at 37°C to clot. This will avoid adsorption of agglutinins on the patient's own cells. Centrifuge to obtain clear serum, and remove to a new tube.

2. Prepare a 5% suspension of Group O (or patient's own) cells in saline.

3. Make a series of doubling dilutions of the patient's serum (0.25 mL should remain in each tube).

4. Add an aliquot (0.25 mL) of the 5% suspension of red cells to each tube.

5. Mix and place in a refrigerator at 4°C for 2 hours. Immediately on removal from the refrigerator note agglutinating titer of the serum.

6. Place tubes in a 37°C water bath for 15 to 30 minutes. Any agglutination resulting from cold agglutinins then should be dispersed.

Serology in Syphilis

There are numerous antibodies produced when the body is invaded by *T. pallidum*. These can be considered as of two types.

1. Nonspecific antibodies (reagins) possibly are in response to the lipoidal antigen of *T. pallidum* or to a lipoidal antigen resulting from the invasion of host tissues. It has been suggested that such antibodies formed by the latter mechanisms may be considered as autoantibodies produced against host tissue altered in some way in the course of treponemal infection. This view would help in the understanding of false positive serological tests, which can be regarded as resulting from the production of antibody (or reagin) to cardiolipin-like substances released from cells in the course of disease other than syphilis. The antigens used in tests for reagins are cardiolipin-lecithin substances prepared from normal animal tissues. Initially Wassermann, in 1906, used the liver from a dead syphilitic infant as antigen, since *T. pallidum* that cannot be artificially cultured is present in large numbers in congenital syphilitic livers. Subsequently, organs from nonsyphilitic individuals were found to be just as effective as an antigen, and finally heart muscle of cattle with cholesterol and lecithin was used. Such a nonspecific antigen is used in numerous complement fixing and precipitation tests (nontreponemal).

2. Specific antitreponemal antibodies are formed specifically to treponemes and in these tests, a treponeme itself is used as the antigen.

Nontreponemal Tests

The VDRL (Venereal Disease Research Laboratory) Slide Test

This is probably the most commonly performed test for syphilis, since it is easily standardized and performed, and is inexpensive. It becomes positive 1 to 3 weeks after the appearance of the primary lesion and is present in all cases of secondary syphilis but in only 75% of tertiary cases. It is not as sensitive or as specific as the fluorescent treponemal antibody absorption test (FTA-ABS; see further on). However, the FTA-ABS is much more difficult to perform and may remain positive in old treated syphilis. The VDRL is more responsive to treatment and thus acts as a clinical guide; it also will pick up false positive reactions. These, which were formerly considered as "biological false positives," may be identified by a negative FTA-ABS. Nevertheless, their identification is important.

False Positive Serological Tests

These may be considered as either acute or chronic, separable by the period of reactivity of the serum with antigen. In those cases in which the serum is reactive for a period of less than 6 months the condition is considered as acute, whereas a reactivity for a longer period is regarded as chronic. The causes are listed below.

Acute False Positive	Chronic False Positive
Atypical pneumonia	Systemic lupus erythematosus
Leprosy	Hashimoto's thyroiditis
Narcotic addiction	Cryoglobulinemia
Aging	Some patients with ANA, RF, or elevated gamma globulin, usually without clinical signs

Treponemal disease other than syphilis, such as yaws, bejel, and pinta, will also give reactive VDRL tests, as well as a positive FTA-ABS.

VDRL Slide Qualitative Test

Reagents and Apparatus

1. Antigen. An alcoholic solution containing 0.3% cardiolipin, 0.9 % cholesterol, and lecithin 0.21 ± 0.01% supplied in brown screw-capped bottles or in small sealed glass ampules. The antigen should be stored at room temperature and should contain no precipitate.

2. Buffered saline solution

Sodium chloride	10 g
Neutral, reagent-grade formaldehyde	0.5 mL
Disodium hydrogen phosphate, hydrated ($Na_2HPO_4 \cdot 12H_2O$)	0.093 g
Potassium dihydrogen phosphate, anhydrous (KH_2PO_4)	0.17 g
Distilled water	1000 mL

3. Control sera.

4. Rotating machine to rotate 180 times per minute circumscribing a circle ¾ inch in diameter on a horizontal plane.

5. Glass slides with ceramic rings enclosing areas of 14 mm in diameter.

6. One ounce bottles with screw cap, Vinylite or tinfoil liners, narrow mouth, and a round or flat bottom. (A bottle with a convex bottom is unsatisfactory since the preliminary 0.4 mL of buffered saline will be distributed in the periphery and not cover the bottom.)

7. Syringe, 2 mL.

8. Hypodermic needles, 18-gauge and without bevel point which will deliver 1/60 mL per drop.

9. Water bath with thermostat set at 56°C.

Preparation of Serum. Serum is obtained from clotted centrifuged blood and inactivated for 30 minutes at 56°C in a water bath. If sera are kept for 4 hours or more after inactivation, they should be reinactivated at 56°C for 10 minutes. Those containing particulate debris should be recentrifuged.

Preparation of Slides. New slides are cleaned with Bon Ami and wiped with a soft cloth after drying. Used slides are washed with detergent or soap, rinsed in water, and then cleaned with Bon Ami and wiped with a soft clean cloth after drying. Sera will spread within the circles of a clean slide; if they do not spread, the slide is not clean. Glass slides with concavities and glass rings are not recommended for the test.

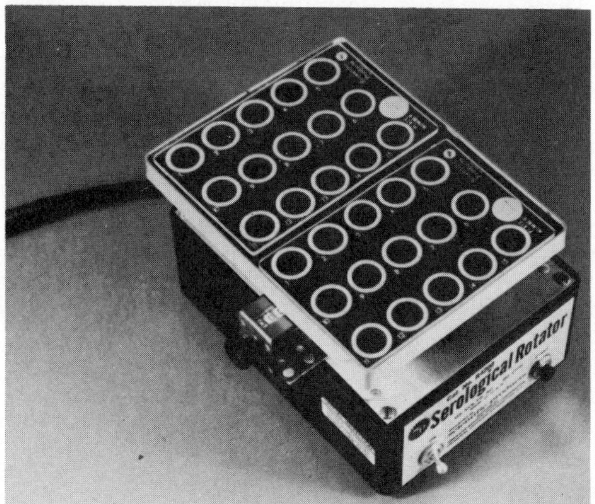

Figure 26–14 Rotating machine for use in the VDRL test. On the rotating platform are two glass slides with ceramic rings. To the left of the platform is a counter that records the number of rotations.

Preparation of the Antigen Emulsion

1. Pipette 0.4 mL of buffered saline into the bottom of a 1-ounce, round, screw-cap, stoppered bottle.

2. Add 0.5 mL of antigen, drop by drop, within 6 seconds (from the lower half of a 1.0-mL pipette graduated to the tip) directly onto the saline solution while continuing to rotate the bottle gently on a flat surface. The temperature of both solutions should be between 23 and 29°C, and the speed of rotation of the bottle is correct when the bottle describes a circle of 2 inches in diameter three times per second.

3. Blow the last drop of antigen from pipette without allowing the pipette to touch the saline solution.

4. Continue to rotate the bottle 10 seconds more.

5. Add 4.1 mL of buffered saline from a 5-mL pipette.

6. Place the top on the bottle and shake vigorously for approximately 10 seconds.

7. The antigen is now ready and may be used for 1 day.

Preparation of Positive and Negative Control Sera. Serum that will give a weakly reactive flocculation in dilution of 1 in 4, a reactive test at a dilution of 1 in 2, and a negative reading at 1 in 8 is commerically available. It is our custom to make the doubling dilutions with buffered saline and to inactivate the dilutions with the batch of sera to be examined in parallel.

Methodology of VDRL Slide Qualitative Test

1. Pipette 0.05-mL aliquots of inactivated sera into each ring of the slide.

2. Add one drop (1/60 mL) of antigen emulsion to each serum.

3. Rotate the slide on the rotating machine for 4 minutes.

4. Read tests immediately after rotation microscopically at ×100 magnification. The antigen appears as short rod forms. Aggregation is interpreted as positive reactivity as follows:

No clumping or slight Roughness	Nonreactive
Small clumps	Weakly reactive
Medium or large clumps	Reactive

Occasionally zonal reactions owing to excess of reactive serum are seen. These are recognized by the presence of large or small clumps of nonuniform size with loosely bound particles. The clumps are intermingled with free antigen particles. The reaction may be reported as weak, but a quantitive procedure will reveal a stronger reaction. Such sera are, of course, examined further.

Because of the possibility of prozone phenomenon, all weakly reactive sera must be diluted and retested. If positive reactions are found, the titer should be estimated. A positive-reacting serum should be confirmed by the FTA-ABS test as described further on.

The RPR (Rapid Plasma Reagin) Test

This is a rapid method that can be adapted to field surveys in the diagnosis of treponemal disease using disposble cards, a small lancet, and a toothpick. It gives results closely parallel to the VDRL. The antigen is similar to the VDRL antigen, modified by the addition

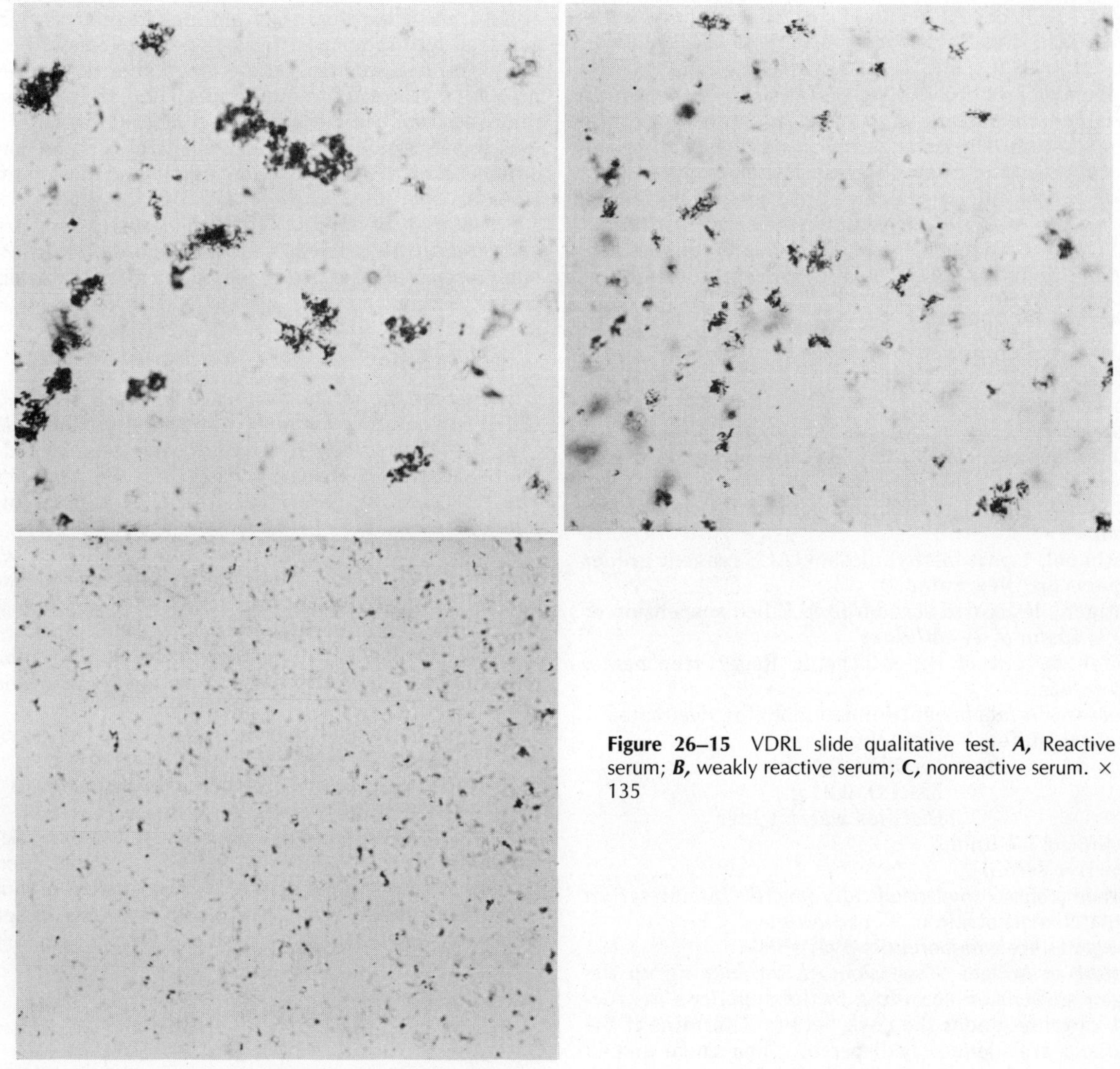

Figure 26–15 VDRL slide qualitative test. ***A,*** Reactive serum; ***B,*** weakly reactive serum; ***C,*** nonreactive serum. × 135

of choline chloride and charcoal and is commercially available.* Under usual laboratory conditions, the RPR test may be performed as follows:

Either 3 drops of unheated plasma or 0.05 mL of serum is added to one drop (through an 18-gauge needle) delivering 45 drops per mL of antigen. The slides on which the mixtures are made are rotated at 180 rpm for 4 minutes and then read at a magnification of 100. Results are read as follows: no clumping—nonreactive; small or slight clumps—weakly reactive; medium and large clumps—reactive.

In the field, plasma can be collected simply without complicated apparatus by the use of a Brewer collection slide,† which is partially coated with an anticoagulant, and with lectin, which will agglutinate red and white cells leaving plasma. With a capillary tube, 0.03 mL of the plasma is placed on the prepared area of the diagnostic card. Then one drop antigen (approximately 1/70 mL) is added. The fluids are mixed with a toothpick to spread the mixture in the entire designated area. The card is tilted to and fro for 4 minutes, allowing time for the mixture to flow into the narrow part of the test area and then into the wider area. Clumping of particles is regarded as reactive, whereas no clumping is regarded as nonreactive.

Treponemal Tests

The FTA-ABS (Fluorescent Treponemal Antibody Absorption) Test

This is the treponemal test used in the confirmation of reactive VDRLs. It is more sensitive and more specific than the VDRL, but is not as easily performed and is

*Hynson, Westcott, and Dunning, Baltimore, Md. 21201.

†Becton, Dickinson and Co., Rutherford, N.J. 07070 and Mississauga, Ont. L5J 2M8.

more expensive. Whether the laboratory will attempt to confirm its own reactive VDRL tests or send them elsewhere will depend on the expected volume of such work and the time and space available to the technical staff.

In principle, a virulent (Nichols) strain of *T. pallidum* maintained in rabbits is allowed to react with the patient's serum. The latter has been previously absorbed with an extract of nonpathogenic Reiter treponeme to remove nonspecific treponemal antibodies. Specific *T. pallidum* antibodies attached to the Nichols *T. pallidum* on a slide are demonstrable with fluorescein-labeled antiglobulin, using a dark-field fluorescent microscope.

Reagents and Apparatus

Dark-field fluorescent microscope
Incubator (35° to 37°C)
Moist chamber
Slide carrier
Bacteriological loop, 2 mm, 26-gauge platinum wire
Dropper bottle
Glass slides and coverslips, cleaned for 1 hour in alcohol
Methanol, 1 part methyl alcohol (ACS reagent grade) to 9 parts distilled water
Antigen, desiccated standardized killed suspension of Nichols strain of *T. pallidum*
Reiter sorbent of nonpathogenic Reiter treponeme, ready to use
Fluorescein-labeled antihuman globulin, desiccated
Phosphate buffer NaCl 7.65 g
Na_2HPO_4 0.724 g
KH_2PO_4 0.21 g
Distilled water 1 liter
Mounting medium
Reactive serum
Sorbent control (nonspecifically reactive human serum against Nichols strain of *T. pallidum*)
Reagents are commercially available.

Testing of Antigen Suspension. After making up the antigen suspension according to the supplier's instructions, examine under the dark field to determine if the organisms are adequately dispersed. Then smear and fix to slides (see further on). Check for fluorescence with control sera.

Testing of Fluorescein-Labeled AHG. Rehydrate the conjugate in accordance with the manufacturer's instructions. Make up serial dilutions with 2% Tween 80 solution in buffer; the dilutions so made should include the titer specified on the manufacturer's vial. Each dilution is tested with reactive serum diluted 1:5 in buffer, and the dilution selected is one that gives maximum fluorescence.

Serum Controls

4+ control: Reactive 4+ serum diluted 1:5 in buffer and in sorbent. Both should give a 4+ fluorescence.

Minimal positive control: A dilution of reactive serum (4+) to give 1+ fluorescence only.

Nonspecific serum: Sorbent control diluted 1:5 with buffer and with sorbent. The buffer dilution will give a 2+ to 4+ response. The sorbent control should be negative.

Nonspecific staining: Using buffered saline in the place of serum and Reiter sorbent in the place of serum. Both should be negative.

Preparation of Antigen Slides. Two circles, each 1 cm in diameter, are made on clean slides with a diamond stylus, and one loopful of the rehydrated antigen is smeared within each of them. They are allowed to dry for 15 minutes at room temperature and then immersed in 10% methanol for 5 minutes. The slides are then removed from the methanol, and blotted dry with bibulous paper. Each test and each control is to be done in duplicate on the same slide employing both antigen smears.

Preparation of Serum. Test and control sera are inactivated at 56°C for 30 minutes before testing. Previously prepared sera are reheated for 10 minutes on the day of testing.

Methodology

1. Prepare 12 × 75 mm tubes for each serum to be tested and one tube for each control, as described earlier.

2. 0.2 mL of sorbent is placed in each test tube and 0.05 mL of serum. Mix at least 8 times with the same pipette. The test must be performed within 30 minutes of this dilution.

3. Cover each antigen smear with 0.03 mL of serum-sorbent dilution. Treat control mixtures similarly. Place in a moist chamber and incubate at 35°–37°C for 30 minutes.

4. Rinse in buffered saline for 5 seconds. Soak in two changes of buffer for 10 minutes. At the 5-minute change, dip and rinse in buffer 10 times. Rinse and dry with bibulous paper.

5. 0.03 mL diluted fluorescein-labeled AHG (in buffer and 2% Tween 80) is added to each smear.

6. Place again in moist chamber in incubator at 35°–37°C for 30 minutes and repeat rinsing as in step 4.

7. Mount slides in mounting medium and examine at a magnification of 400 under ultraviolet light. *Note.* Exposure to light before examination will cause fading of fluorescence, but storage in the dark for up to 4 hours is permissible.

Results

Moderate to strong fluorescence	++ to ++++	reactive
Weak fluorescence (equivalent to 1+ control)	+	reactive
No fluorescence or barely visible	− to ±	nonreactive

AGGLUTINATION TESTS USING INERT PARTICLES

Using inert particles coated with antigen (or antibody), it is possible to perform tests against serum with circulating antibody (or antigen), which when reactive will cause agglutination of the particles. The materials used are polystyrene latex particles (8 μm in diameter), bentonite, which is a colloidal hydrated aluminium silicate, or erythrocytes treated with tannic acid. These inert particles, when agglutinated, will present a much more apparent reaction than the essential precipitation that has taken place.

The RA Test (for Rheumatoid Factor)

Rheumatoid factor (RF) is found circulating in the blood of patients with rheumatoid arthritis. It is not by any means specific for this disease and is found in other diseases both related and nonrelated to rheumatoid arthritis. Among these diseases are SLE, polyarteritis, tuberculosis, leprosy, syphilis, bacterial endocarditis, and Waldenström's macroglobulinemia, as well as some cases of ankylosing spondylitis, juvenile rheumatoid arthritis, psoriatic arthritis, sarcoidosis, cirrhosis, and mononucleosis. It is believed that during some infection of a joint, IgG antibody is produced. Subsequent to its production, the antibody becomes altered for some reason, and against this altered antibody a second antibody is formed. Usually this second antibody is IgM, but it may be IgG or even IgA. To demonstrate this antibody, which is RF, the serum is challenged with IgG latex-coated particles. Agglutination indicates the presence of RF.

Reagents (commercially available)

Latex-Globulin. With added blue dye to facilitate reading.

Positive Control Serum. Already diluted 1/20.

Negative Control Serum. Normal serum diluted 1:20 in buffer diluent.

Glycine-Saline Buffer Diluent.

Divided Slide.

Method

1. Add 1 drop of heat-inactivated (56°C for 30 minutes) test serum (0.05 mL to 1 mL of buffer diluent (approximately 1/20 dilution).

2. Place 1 drop of this diluted serum in a space on the divided slide.

3. Place 1 drop of positive control serum (without further dilution) in another space of the slide.

4. Add 1 drop of diluted normal serum to a third space.

5. Add 1 drop of latex antigen to each specimen, mix with the applicator stick, tilt the slide, and read after 1 minute. Visible flocculation from fine to large aggregates and complete clumping are grades of positive reactivity.

The test is not entirely specific, as noted above. False negatives are rare. Serum in which there is a high titer of RF may give false positive results with a latex test for cryptococcosis. Incomplete heat inactivation, some hyperlipidemic conditions, and cryoglobulins may also occasion false positive results.

Many other similar tests using carrying inert particles such as latex are commercially available. These include pregnancy tests that detect chorionic gonadotrophin in urine and tests to detect fibrin-fibrinogen degradation products, cryptococcus antigen, trichinella antigen, DNA, and others.

STAPHYLOCOCCAL COAGGLUTINATION (COA)

The staphylococcus has a covalently bound protein (A) in its wall. This protein binds IgG antibody by its Fc portion, leaving the antigen-binding portion (Fab) free. There are an estimated 80,000 binding sites of protein A in each *Staphylococcus,* so the antibody-tagged bacterial body has considerable ability to combine with bacterial cells or their antigens. The combined cells form a lattice of antigen and antibody, giving a heavy coagglutination on a slide that is visible within a minute.

Currently, the determination of streptococcal Lancefield groups can be performed with this technique, as can the serological confirmation of *N. gonorrhoeae, Str. pneumoniae,* and *H. influenzae.* The test is available commerically.* The pneumococcus and *H. influenzae* can be detected as bacterial antigens in CSF even before Gram films or culture results are available. In cases in which the CSF is sterile because of antimicrobial therapy, the correct diagnosis may be made retrospectively by the presence of inanimate bacterial antigen material in the fluid.

QUELLUNG TESTS

These tests have been referred to in the serological identification of pneumococci and can be used similarly in the serotyping of klebsiellae and *H. influenzae.* Although the word *quellung* literally means swelling, it is now believed that the capsules of the organisms do not swell when challenged with the specific antiserum, but rather that a precipitin reaction takes place on the surface of the bacterial capsule. This reaction makes the capsule highly refractile and thus more easily visible in most unstained preparations.

C-REACTIVE PROTEIN

In the acute phase of inflammation, as well as fever and leukocytosis, changes also occur in the plasma proteins. These proteins are considered acute-phase proteins that rise in early inflammatory response. They are a disparate group that includes haptoglobins, ceruloplasmin, α_1-glycoprotein, and others. One of them is

*Pharmacia Diagnostics, Piscataway, N.J. 08854, and Dorval, Que. H9P1H6.

IgG
Staphylococcal cell
Fab
Fc
Protein A
Antigen

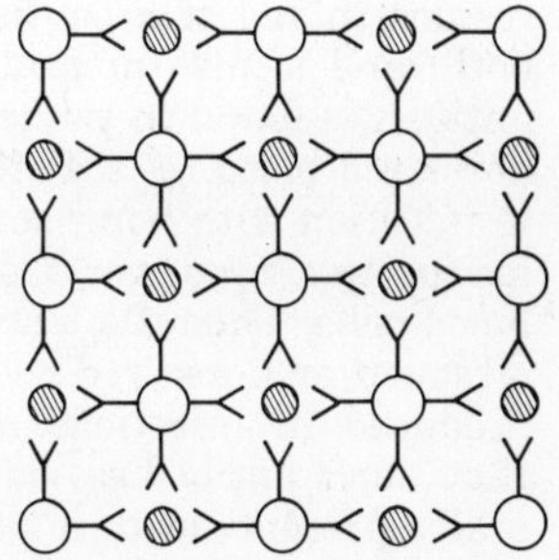

Figure 26–16 Principle of the staphylococcal agglutination technique. On the left is a diagram of the positioning of IgG and its components, the antigen, and the staphylococcus. On the right, the lattice formed by staphylococcal cells and the antigen-antibody combination is shown.

fibrinogen, which is one of the factors in blood clotting but also is related to erythrocyte sedimentation rate (ESR). C-reactive protein was originally so named, since it precipitated with the C-polysaccharide of the pneumococcus, but its appearance was later shown to be a nonspecific response to almost any inflammatory process.

Normally the level of C-RP is very small (below 0.5 mg/dL) and is not detected by capillary precipitate or latex agglutination. Latex agglutination is simple to perform. One drop of the patient's serum is mixed with one drop of latex C-RP (commercially available) and mixed thoroughly on a slide. Control positive and negative sera are similarly treated. Agglutination in the test serum occurring after 3 to 5 minutes is considered positive. Since prozones may occur, it is advisable in case of negative reactions to repeat the test with serum diluted 1 to 10 with normal saline. Although the appearance of a positive reaction can be regarded as significant and reported to the physician in a short time, all tests should also be performed using the radial immundiffusion technique (see below). The latter is less capricious than the latex test and is quantitative. Serial levels of C-RP may be obtained during the course of the disease, aiding the physician in its management.

Although the ESR and C-RP both reflect an inflammatory process, the C-RP is not disturbed by such phenomena as anemia, hyperglobulinemia, age, abnormality of red cell size and shape, and so forth. On the other hand, in tuberculosis in which the process of inflammation is chronic, the ESR is more reliable.

Serology in Infectious Mononucleosis (IM)

IM is a common disease, detailed elsewhere (pp. 478 and 657), and due to infection by Epstein-Barr virus. The disease most often is definitively diagnosed by serological means. During the course of the disease, antibodies to a number of antigens are produced, including several to the E-B virus and to antigen i of red blood cells. Not infrequently, reagins to syphilis (giving false positive serological tests for syphilis) and rheumatoid factor are also produced, as well as others. The latter include antibodies to the red cells of sheep and horses.

Antibodies stimulated by one antigen that react with an entirely unrelated antigen from another species are known as *heterophil antibodies*. The antibody to E-B virus that agglutinates the red blood cells of sheep or horses is such an antibody. There are other heterophil systems, such as the antibody in typhus that agglutinates bacteria of the *Proteus* genus and the antibody against *Mycoplasma* that agglutinates human red cells.

Forssman antigen is a widespread antigenic substance present in many species (horse, cat, mouse, etc.). It resides in red cells or tissue cells, but usually not in both, and is also present in some bacteria. Forssman antigen is found in tissues and is present in sheep and horse red blood cells. Patients with serum sickness due to injection with horse serum will also develop antibodies (up to a titer over 224) against sheep and horse red blood cells. Thus if a test were set up for agglutination of sheep or horse red cells by the heterophil antibody produced in infectious mononucleosis, the possibility that such antibodies were Forssman antibodies (normally present up to a titer of 320) or serum sickness antibodies would have to be excluded.

Forssman antigen may be adsorbed from serum by pretreatment with guinea pig kidney, and serum sickness antibody by pretreatment with ox red cell and partially with guinea pig kidney. Relationships are best seen in the table below.

Antibody	Absorbed by Guinea Pig Kidney	Absorbed by Ox Red Cell
Forssman	Yes	No
Infectious mononucleosis	No	Yes
Serum sickness	Yes (partially)	Yes (completely)

Screening tests based on these principles are commercially available, and one is detailed below:

Citrated Horse Cells Test*

Reagents

1. 10% suspension of guinea pig kidney antigen (reagent I).
2. 10% suspension of beef stromata antigen (reagent II).
3. 20% suspension of horse erythrocytes in 3.8% sodium citrate. Glass slide divided into two squares, marked I and II.

Procedure

1. **Place one drop of reagent I in square I and one drop of reagent II in square II.**
2. **Place one drop of patient's serum in each square, avoiding reagents I and II.**
3. **Place 10 μL of horse red blood cell suspension in each square, avoiding other reagents.**
4. **Mix patient's serum in square I with reagent I and patient's serum in square II with reagent II, and then blend in horse red blood cells.**
5. **Agglutination should occur within one minute.**

If the agglutination in square I is stronger than that in square II, the test is positive. Positive and negative controls should be included with each test.

The Paul-Bunnell Davidsohn Differential Test for Heterophil Antibody

Because of the specificity and sensitivity of the Monospot or other similar test and its simplicity, the full differential tube test is not done unless some particular problem arises. The reagents, which include guinea pig emulsion, ox red cell suspension, and sheep red blood cells, can be purchased.

Method

1. **Inactivate 1 to 2 mL of the patient's serum at 56°C for 30 minutes.**
2. **Set up three tubes, A, B, and C, as follows:**

	A	B	C
Inactivated serum	0.25 mL	0.25 mL	0.25 mL
Normal saline	1 mL	—	—
Guinea pig kidney	—	1 mL	—
Ox cell suspension	—	—	1 mL

*Monospot, Ortho Diagnostics, Raritan, N.J. 08869 and Don Mills, Ont. M3C 1L9.

Antibody Type	Titer of Unabsorbed Serum	Titer of Serum Absorbed by Guinea Pig Kidney	Titer of Serum Absorbed by Ox Cells
Normal Forssman	40	0	40
Infectious mononucleosis	1280	1280	160 or less
Serum sickness	160	0	0–40*

*Owing to Forssman

3. Mix contents of each tube well and leave at room temperature for 15 minutes; the exact time will depend on the reagents used. Shake and centrifuge at 2000 G for 5 to 10 minutes. Remove and retain the supernatants. They each represent a 1 to 5 dilution of patient's serum.

4. For each of the supernatants A, B, and C set up a row of nine tubes. To the first two tubes add 0.2 mL of the appropriate supernatant. To each of tubes 2 through 9 place 0.2 mL of normal saline. Mix the contents of tube 2 well, and make doubling dilutions in the succeeding tubes. Set up a tenth tube in each row as a control with 0.2 mL of saline.

5. To each tube add 0.2 mL of 1% sheep red cell suspension; mix and leave at room temperature for 2 hours. For quicker results, centrifuge at 1000 G for 1 minute.

6. Flick each tube to resuspend sheep cells, and look for a granular or clumped agglutination with the aid of a concave mirror. Read the titer of the last tube in each row showing agglutination. Typical readings for each of the antibody types are as listed at top of page.

Interpretation. There is a 96 to 97% correlation of the Monospot tests with the longer Paul-Bunnell Davidsohn test. It is worth remembering that a positive heterophil agglutination generally appears in the second or third week of the illness but may be delayed until the fifth week and also that the test may remain positive for a year subsequent to infection.

CYTOLYSIS AND COMPLEMENT FIXATION

Lysins. Some antigen-antibody reactions are demonstrable by disintegration of the antigenic cell. This phenomenon is seen in blood bank technology when certain immune sera cause hemolysis of red blood cells containing specific antigens. If the serum containing lysing antibody is heated for 30 minutes at 56°C, lysis of the antigenic cell does not occur. However, if fresh guinea pig serum (containing no antibody) is added to the heated serum and cellular antigen, lysis will occur. Thus it is apparent that unheated serum contains a substance, also present in guinea pig serum, that is necessary for the demonstration of lysis. This substance is known as *complement* (see p. 526). Although hemolysis is a fairly commonly observed result of lysins, lysis of bacteria is uncommon. However, the bactericidal activities of certain immune sera also need complement, and this type of antigen-antibody reaction is considered to be caused by lysins. Lysis, therefore, is an antigen-antibody reaction that requires a third substance, complement, for demonstration. During the reaction, the complement is bound in a complex with the other two substances. Complement is present in the serum protein of all animals, but the guinea pig seems to provide a particularly rich source. The complementary power of serum may be destroyed by heating to 56°C for 30 minutes, a process known as inactivation. Likewise, if sera are left at room temperature, complement is destroyed in a few hours; conversely, it is preserved by freezing. Many chemical substances, including soaps, alcohol, chloroform, acids, alkalis, and proteolytic enzymes, may destroy complement. Physical agents other than heat also may inactivate complement by altering the colloidal or particulate status of the solution. Examples of such agents include bacteria, yeasts, and tissue cells, as well as adsorbent particles such as charcoal. Such contamination is responsible for the anticomplementary nature of some sera and may be responsible for false positive results in a test performed without adequate controls. Violent shaking for long periods (30 minutes) may also inactivate complement. A brief discussion of the role of complement in immune processes is given on p. 526.

The principles of complement fixation are given in Fig. 26–6. Such tests are used in the diagnosis of various infectious diseases and were particularly widely employed in the classic Wassermann test for syphilis. Nowadays, their major application is in the diagnosis of viral and rickettsial infections and to some extent in parasitology and mycology.

MEASUREMENT OF COMPLEMENT

Complement levels are most conveniently measured by radial immunodiffusion methods (see p. 550). Plates to measure C3 and C4 levels are commercially available, and others can be prepared if desired. Levels of C3 and C4 are depressed in immune complex disease, glomerulonephritis, SLE, subacute bacterial endocarditis, and so forth.

Another method employs sensitized erythrocytes (i.e., cells coated with antibody) suspended in buffered saline. Dilutions of the patient's serum are added to provide the necessary complement, and the tubes are incubated at 37°C for 30 minutes. The titer of complement is the reciprocal of the highest dilution of serum allowing 50% hemolysis of the sensitized erythrocytes (CH_{50}). Normal values will vary with the method employed. This method measures total complement.

Antistreptolysin O Titer. This test, commonly referred to as the ASO, is used as an aid in the diagnosis and management of rheumatic fever, acute glomerulonephritis, and other group A streptococcal infections. In such conditions the ASO titer frequently is raised. In the test a series of mixtures is set up in which different quantities of serum are incubated with standard amounts of streptolysin. The mixtures are then challenged by a red blood cell suspension. The tube that has the least serum

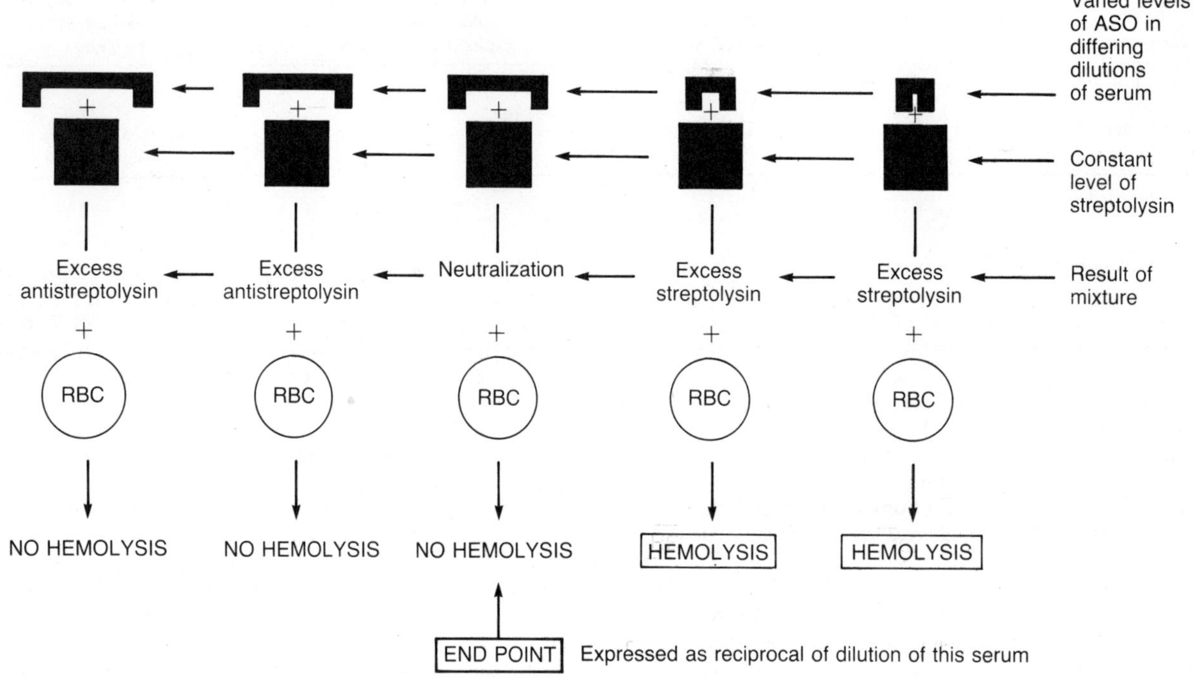

Figure 26–17 Principle of the ASO titer test.

but no hemolysis has the amount of immune antistreptolysin that exactly neutralizes the standard amount of streptolysin. Results are expressed in Todd units.

Latex-ASL

This test may be used as a screening test if desired, and positive sera may be confirmed by the standard ASO technique. The reagents are commercially available. In the test, a solution of streptolysin O containing 200 IU per milliliter is added to serum, and subsequently this mixture is added to the latex reagent on a slide. The latex is coated with streptolysin O. Thus if agglutination of the latex occurs, the patient's serum has an antistreptolysin titer of at least 200 IU per milliliter, and this is considered a value of significance. A modification of this test has been introduced to yield a quantitative titer. The results are said to compare well with those of the standard test and can be made available within 20 minutes.

Microtitration techniques are preferred over tube tests. The former need less serum and fewer reagents and cost less per test. In addition, more tests may be performed by the technologist in the same period of time. The materials for the microtitration tests are available commercially, and the details of the test provided by the manufacturer should be rigidly followed.

In essence, as in the tube test, dilutions of inactivated serum are mixed and incubated with a standard amount of streptolysin O and then sheep or rabbit erythrocytes. Controls of the red cells, serum, and the ASO are run, as well as a standard serum control. In the test, the highest serum dilution showing no hemolysis (i.e., in which the streptolysin is neutralized by ASO) is the end point. The controls should show no lysis in the serum or erythrocyte test, and with standard serum, hemolysis should occur up to the predetermined titer. The end point is expressed as a titer that is reported in Todd units.

Interpretation

The ASO titer is raised in about 80% of patients with rheumatic fever. It reaches its zenith 3 to 5 weeks after infection and falls to normal levels within 6 to 12 months. An ASO titer of $>$ 120 Todd units in a preschool-age subject or adult, or of $>$240 in a school-age patient, is suspicious of a recent streptococcal group A infection. A rise in titer of two or more dilutions from acute to convalescent tests is certainly significant. In fact, the rise in titer is correlated with the development of rheumatic fever but not the level of the initial titer.

Although acute glomerulonephritis very often follows streptococcal disease, the ASO titer may not be raised if the infection was that of the skin, and other tests, such as the antihyaluronidase or anti-DNase tests, must be performed.

It should be remembered that a rise in ASO titer will occur in uncomplicated group A streptococcal disease, and the test is used as a diagnostic indicator in suspected rheumatic fever and glomerulonephritis.

ANTIHYALURONIDASE TITER

Like the antistreptolysin titer, this examination reveals the presence of antibody to an exotoxin of group A streptococci and thus indirectly, of group A streptococcal infection. About 80% of these infections are revealed by the ASO, and it is estimated that an additional 10% can be exposed by the AHT used in parallel. A third antistreptococcal exotoxin titer measurement, such as anti-DNase B, will yield still another 5% unrevealed by using only two. The test consists of setting up a series of dilutions of serum with a standard amount of hyaluronidase, then adding a substrate (hyaluronate), allowing the mixture to incubate and then testing for the survival of the substrate by attempting precipitation with acetic acid. The antihyaluronidase titer is the reciprocal of the serum dilution in which clot can be demonstrated. Normally, this does not exceed 1/250; a rising titer over a period of 3 to 5 weeks is significant.

Reagents and Method

1. Set up a row of clean 13 by 75 mm tubes, numbered 1 through 7, for each serum to be tested. Behind this row, set up another row of tubes numbered 8 through 14.

2. The patient's serum should be sterile if possible and stored in refrigerator until use. Contaminated, chylous, or hemolyzed samples should not be used. Either fresh or inactivated serum is suitable.

Serum dilutions are made as follows: Add 0.25 mL distilled water to tubes 2 through 7 and 9 through 13. Add 0.5 mL distilled water to tube 14. Prepare a 1/32 dilution of serum by adding 0.1 mL serum to 3.1 mL distilled water and mixing. Add 0.25 mL of the 1/32 dilution to tubes 1 and 2. Mix the contents of tube 2, transfer 0.25 mL to tube 3, and continue doubling the dilutions to tube 7, from which 0.25 mL is discarded.

3. AHT standard is made by rehydrating one vial of the reagent (commercially available) with 1 mL of distilled water and dissolving by gentle end-over-end rotation. Add 0.25 mL of this solution to tubes 8 and 9. Then transfer 0.25 mL from tube 9 to 10 and continue doubling the dilution to tube 12, from which 0.25 mL is discarded.

4. AHT enzyme is rehydrated just before use. To one vial add 4 mL distilled water and dissolve in the same manner as the standard. Add 0.25 mL to tubes 1 through 13.

5. Mix by shaking the tubes and incubate at 37°C in a water bath for 15 minutes.

6. Cool in the refrigerator at 6 to 10°C for 10 minutes.

7. AHT substrate is made by rehydrating one vial with 8 mL of distilled water, shaking vigorously to dissolve thoroughly. Store in the refrigerator until use. Add 0.5 mL to all tubes and shake well.

8. Incubate at 37°C for 20 minutes.

9. Cool at 6 to 10°C for 30 minutes.

10. Add 0.1 mL of 2 N acetic acid to all tubes and shake vigorously.

11. Examine all tubes for presence of clot. Tube 13, the enzyme control, should have no clot; the substrate control, tube 14, should have a definite clot.

PHAGOCYTOSIS AND OPSONIC ACTIVITY

Apart from the neutropenias in which there is a quantitative reduction of phagocytes in the peripheral blood owing to drugs, myeloproliferative disease, neoplastic replacement of the marrow, hypersplenism, and so forth, qualitative defects are also identifiable.

Tests for such defects are generally sophisticated and include the nitroblue tetrazolium dye reduction test and the Holmes test (both of which are described in the third edition of this work). The former examines the oxidative mechanisms within leukocytes that destroy ingested bacteria; the latter tests the ability of polymorphs to kill phagocytosed organisms.

TABLE 26–6 THE ANTIHYALURONIDASE TEST

	Step 1		Step 2				Step 3			
	Tube No.	Serum Dilution	Ml Diluted Serum	Ml AHT Enzyme	Ml Distilled Water		Ml AHT Substrate		Ml 2 N Acetic Acid	
Patient's serum	1	1/32	0.25	0.25	—		0.5		0.1	
	2	1/64	0.25	0.25	—		0.5		0.1	
	3	1/128	0.25	0.25	—		0.5		0.1	
	4	1/256	0.25	0.25	—		0.5		0.1	
	5	1/512	0.25	0.25	—		0.5		0.1	
	6	1/1024	0.25	0.25	—		0.5		0.1	
	7	1/2048	0.25	0.25	—	Shake thoroughly and incubate at 37°C for 15 minutes. Cool in the refrigerator at 6–10°C for 10 minutes.	0.5	Shake thoroughly and incubate at 37°C for 20 minutes. Cool in the refrigerator at 6–10°C for 30 minutes.	0.1	Shake vigorously and record presence or absence of clot.
AHT standard	8	1/32	0.25	0.25	—		0.5		0.1	
	9	1/64	0.25	0.25	—		0.5		0.1	
	10	1/128	0.25	0.25	—		0.5		0.1	
	11	1/256	0.25	0.25	—		0.5		0.1	
	12	1/512	0.25	0.25	—		0.5		0.1	
AHT enzyme control	13	—	—	0.25	0.25		0.5		0.1	
AHT substrate control	14	—	—	—	0.5		0.5		0.1	

First steps in the killing of organisms by phagocytes are motility and chemotaxis of the cells and then their recognition and opsonization. Opsonins are substances that enhance the capacity of the phagocyte to consume the bacteria, and among the most important opsonins are antibodies and complement.

A measurement of opsonophagocytic function of cells may be made by incubating washed leukocytes with, say, staphylococci for 30 minutes at 37°C in both the presence and absence of immune serum and complement, then comparing the results with cells from a presumably normal individual. The cells are examined microscopically after staining for ingested bacteria.

In comparing sera, washed leukocytes are incubated with saline and staphylococci, with normal serum and staphylococci, and with test serum and staphylococci.

The average number of bacteria/leukocytes in each mixture is called the *phagocytic* index, and the ratio of ingested bacteria to cells in the third mixture as compared with the second is the *opsonic* index.

So many variables are encountered in this test that it has found no important place in the clinical laboratory.

FLUORESCENT ANTIBODY STUDIES

Besides substances that are naturally fluorescent, there are dyes that will absorb light of a certain wavelength and emit light of a different wavelength. The exciting light is of short wavelength, blue or ultraviolet, and the emitted light is of longer wavelength, green, orange, or yellow. For example, acridine orange absorbs light at 365 nm and emits it at 542 nm. The science of fluorescent microscopy depends on the physical law that if an excited molecule cannot pass on energy to adjacent molecules, it will emit the energy; in this case it does so in the form of light at a longer wavelength.

Numerous kinds of apparatus are available for use in this field, but all employ certain basic components: an illuminating source, selective exciter filters, and secondary eyepiece filters, all adapted to the microscope. The illuminant is generally a high-pressure mercury vapor burner chosen for its maximal emission of light, which is in the 300 to 400 nm range, and for its high light intensity. The maximum absorption of the dye used to stain the specimen governs the choice of the primary filter, which is placed between the light and the specimen. In the eyepiece is a secondary filter, which has two functions: first, it absorbs the wavelength of the stimulating light so that stained bodies appear bright on dark backgrounds; second, the filter absorbs ultraviolet radiation, which is dangerous to the eyes of the observer.

Figure 26–18 *Bordetella pertussis*: smear from a culture identified by FITC-conjugated antibody. The small coccobacilli are seen as relatively bright structures on a dark background. × 2300.

The mounting material and the immersion oil must, of course, be nonfluorescent. Mineral oil and glycerol are suitable substitutes for immersion oil.

Fluorescence is a property of certain substances, e.g., some minerals and lipochrome fragments. It may be induced by staining, as in the auramines staining of acid-fast bacilli (p. 349) and in procedures in histochemistry. A very wide application, however, is in immunology. Dyes such as fluorescein and rhodamine may be attached to antibodies without interfering with their immunological characteristics. Thus, antigen in bacteria or in tissues may be identified when coupled with its specific antibody marked with a fluorescent dye. There are three main methods of immunofluorescent marking.

1. *The direct test:* The antibody is attached to the fluorescent dye and then applied directly to the tissue or to the suspect organism. Such a method may be used in the rapid diagnosis of *N. gonorrhoeae, B. pertussis*, and so forth.

2. *The indirect test:* Here, the unlabeled antibody attaches to the antigen of the tissue or bacterium, and then fluorescein-tagged anti-immunoglobulin is applied. If the latter remains attached, then by implication antigen-antibody union has occurred and antigen is thus present. An advantage of this method is that several fluorescent anti-immunoglobulin molecules attach to each immunoglobulin molecule, and thus fluorescence is brighter. This method is used in the FTA-ABS and in many tests in the elucidation of autoimmune disease.

3. *The "sandwich" technique:* By this method, antibody produced and present on the surface of cells is identified. First antigen is added and then fluorescent-tagged antibody. The antigen is sandwiched between the antibody on the surface of the cell and the marker fluorescent-tagged antibody.

MISCELLANEOUS SEROLOGICAL TESTS

Tularemia

Serological tests are performed in a fashion similar to the Widal test, using a heat-killed suspension of *F. tularensis*. Agglutinins appear 8 to 10 days after infection, and their level rises for 8 weeks. Agglutinating titers of 40 to 80 and rising titers are considered diagnostic of infection. It should be noted that cross-reactions with *Br. abortus* and *Y. enterocolitica* or *pseudotuberculosis* may occur. Rapid diagnosis of an exudate or culture may be made by direct immunofluorescence.

Leptospirosis

The most commonly performed test is a slide agglutination against a pooled killed suspension of different serotypes of leptospires. The pooled antigens can be purchased. Agglutinating titers appear in the second week of the illness and rise until about the fourth week.

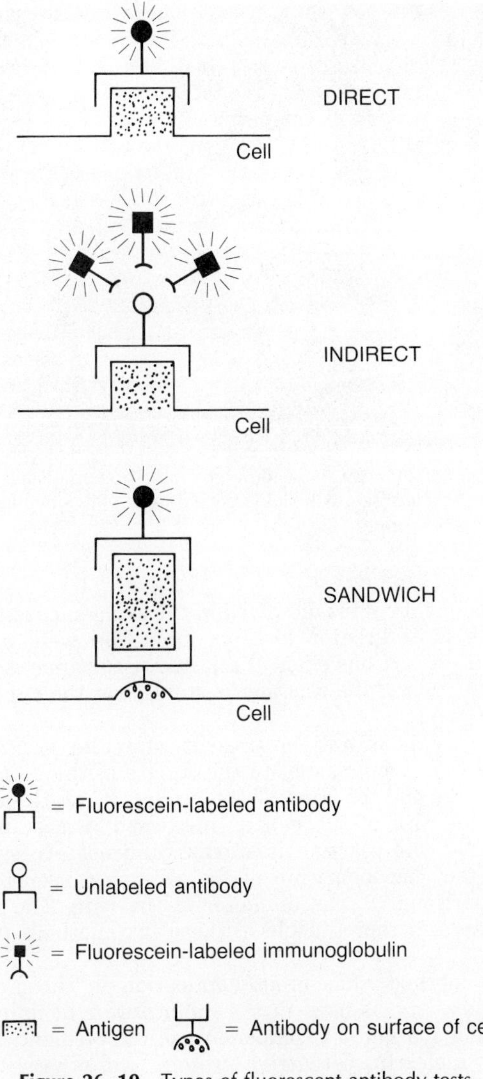

Figure 26–19 Types of fluorescent antibody tests.

Toxoplasmosis

The commonest serological method used is the indirect immunofluorescent test using the patient's serum, a preparation of *Toxoplasma gondii* on a slide (commercially available), and fluorescein-labeled anti–human IgG.

Echinococcus

There are numerous techniques applicable to serological diagnosis of this infestation, including complement-fixation tests, tests based on immunofluorescence, and tests using tanned red cells coated with echinococcal antigen. However, since the tests are infrequently required in community hospitals and antigens are not commercially available, generally serological examination for this disease is performed in reference laboratories. There is cross-reaction between *E. granulosus* and *E. multilocularis*.

Trichinosis

The bentonite flocculation test is generally performed. As will be recalled, bentonite is an inert particulate substance that may be coated with antigen and that will agglutinate on challenge with specific antisera. A similar latex test is commercially available. The test becomes positive relatively late in the disease (by the third week 90% are positive but in the first week only 25%).

IMMUNODIFFUSION

When antigen and antibody are allowed to react in gels, they will diffuse toward one another, and at the point at which they meet in optimal proportions, they will form a visible precipitate.

Double Diffusion in Two Dimensions (Ouchterlony)

Here, basically, an agar plate is used in which holes (wells) are cut and filled with antiserum and antigen. The plates are kept moist, and within days, or longer, lines of precipitate appear between the wells containing reactive substances. Each antigen and antibody diffuses at different rates through the medium, so that each separate line of precipitation between wells indicates a distinct antigen-antibody reaction. If lines are continuous, then antigens and antibodies are identical, and if discontinuous, then they are nonidentical. The concept may be appreciated more easily in Figure 26–20.

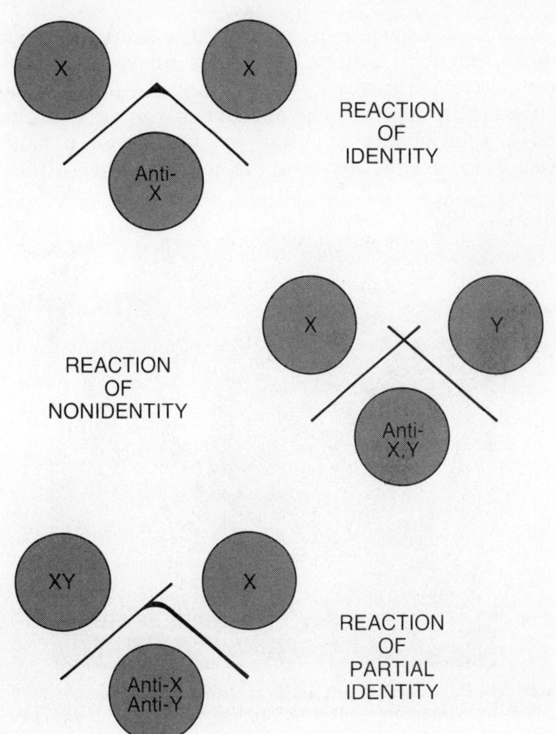

Figure 26–20 Patterns of antigen-antibody reaction in double-diffusion precipitin tests.

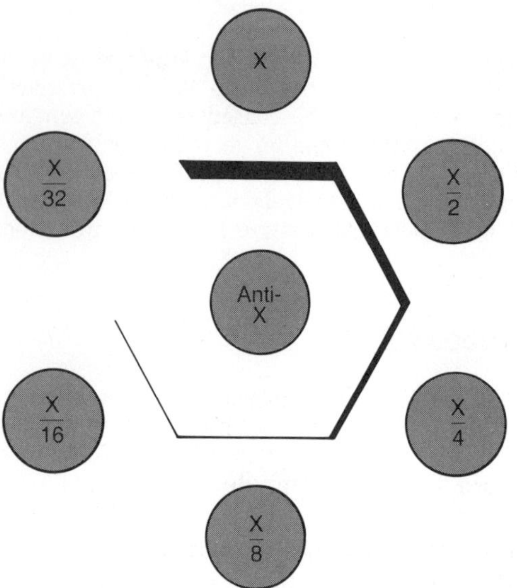

Figure 26–21 Quantitation of antigen by the double-diffusion precipitin test. X = Antigen; $\frac{X}{2}, \frac{X}{4}, \frac{X}{8}$, etc. = Dilutions of antigen. Note that the thickness of the precipitin lines is roughly proportional to the amount of antigen present.

Double immunodiffusion can also be used to quantitate roughly the amount of antigen or antibody present in reactions. The thickness of the precipitin lines is semiquantitatively proportional to the amount of antigen-antibody complex (Fig. 26–21).

Single Radial Immunodiffusion (Mancini)

As a more accurate extension of the semiquantitative measurement of antigen described above, antibody is here present diffusely in the gel, and the antigen alone is present in the well. The antigen only (singly) diffuses, and a relationship is found in the size of a ring of precipitation that appears. As more antigen diffuses,

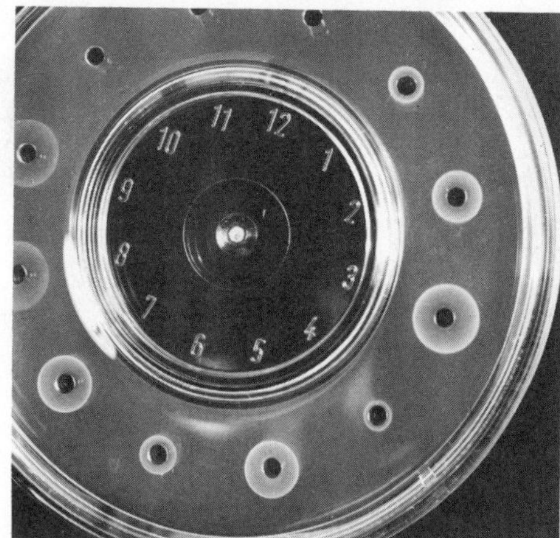

Figure 26–22 Tri-Partigen plate. Zones of precipitation between the serum containing immunoglobulins within the wells and the specific antibody in the agar (antiIgA, M, or G) are illustrated. The first three wells are used for control sera. The size of the precipitin ring is proportional to the concentration of antigen (IgA, M, or G).

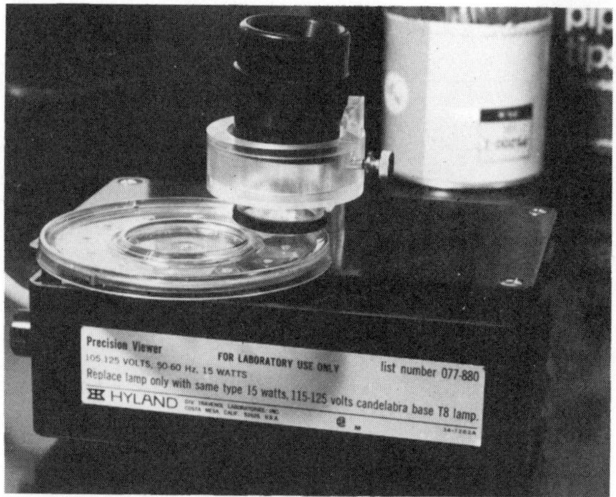

Figure 26–23 Viewer for reading precipitin zone diameter. Their relation to control sera will yield concentration of the immunoglobulin in the test serum.

the precipitin ring is dissolved in the antigen excess and appears at a greater distance from the well, where optimal proportions exist. If allowed to continue, a time will come when the reaction is stable and the ring will stop growing.

The amount of antigen present, after the reaction is complete, is proportional to the square of the diameter of the ring (or the area of the circle). If, on the other hand, the size of the ring is measured in a standard time after the reaction is started, and not necessarily completed, the logarithm of the antigen concentration is proportional to the diameter of the ring. The more accurate and reproducible of these two methods is the first.

This method finds great application in the clinical laboratory and is used in the quantitation of immunoglobulins, C3 and C4 components of complement, albumin, transferrin, C-reactive protein, and others. Commercially prepared plates are generally made to go to completion in 18 hours at 20 to 25°C in a humidity chamber and are provided with control sera. After incubation, the ring sizes are measured in an illuminated and magnifying measuring device. The ring diameters squared of the standard sera are plotted against the known concentrations of the particular protein. The diameter squared of the test sera on the same plate can be plotted on the standard curve, and the concentration is read off from the curve.

Immunoelectrophoresis

The technique is a further refinement of the precipitin reaction in gels. Here, a serum sample is initially electrophoresed through an agarose matrix that, as explained elsewhere (p. 88), will separate the various protein components of the serum according to electrophoretic mobility. The most mobile are prealbumin and albumin, and the least mobile is gamma-globulin. When this is achieved, antisera containing specific antibodies are applied parallel to the direction of migration and allowed to diffuse toward the separated protein antigens (Fig. 26–24).

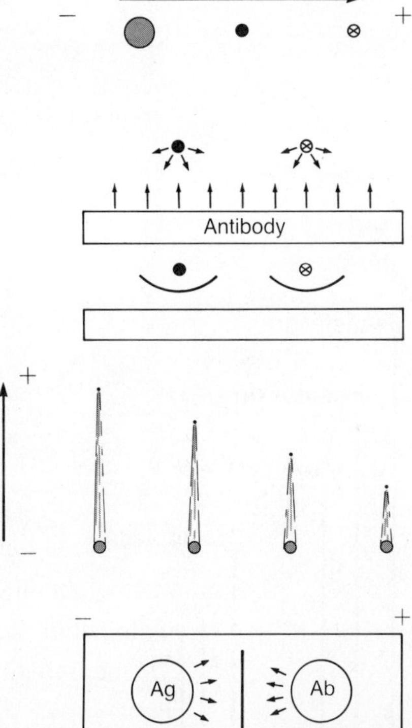

① Specimen in well is subjected to electrophoresis. Proteins migrate.

IMMUNOELECTROPHORESIS

② Antibody now placed in trough migrates, and there is also diffusion from electrophoretically separated protein fractions.

③ Precipitin arcs occur at sites of antigen-antibody combination.

"ROCKET" IMMUNOELECTROPHORESIS

Antigen migrates into an antibody-containing gel electrophoretically. "Rocket" areas of precipitation occur as antigen meets antibody. The height of the rocket is proportional to the amount of antigen in the well.

COUNTERIMMUNOELECTROPHORESIS

Antigen and antibody migrate rapidly toward one another under electrophoresis. A line of precipitation between the wells indicates antigen-antibody reaction.

Figure 26–24 Techniques of immunoelectrophoresis.

Many manufacturers now provide complete kits for this estimation, and as a rule the electrophoretic agarose plates have a number of alternating wells in which to place the patient's serum and a normal serum control. Between the wells of normal serum and test serum is a prepared, precut, but not evacuated trough (see Fig. 26–25). In outline, the wells are filled with their respective sera and the correct voltage is applied through a barbital buffer in an electrophoretic chamber. The migration of albumin through a dye marker can be observed so that satisfactory separation of the protein components of the sera can be achieved.

After electrophoresis, which generally takes 30 to 60 minutes depending on the plate and the amperage, the plate is removed and the agarose in the troughs is removed. Then, appropriate antiserum is placed in each trough, and the plates are closed with a lid and put into a humidity chamber at room temperature for 24 hours. Finally, precipitin arcs are viewed on an illuminated box through a magnifier, or they may be stained with Amido black or some similar protein stain.

The precipitin lines are curved, since during electrophoresis the protein with the serum is distributed in foci from the cathode to the anode and subsequently diffuses radially; the antiserum in the troughs diffuses in a linear fashion.

Commercial kits usually allow one to detect alterations in IgG, IgA, and IgM, kappa and lambda chains. The technique is widely used in the investigation of immunoglobulin disorders.

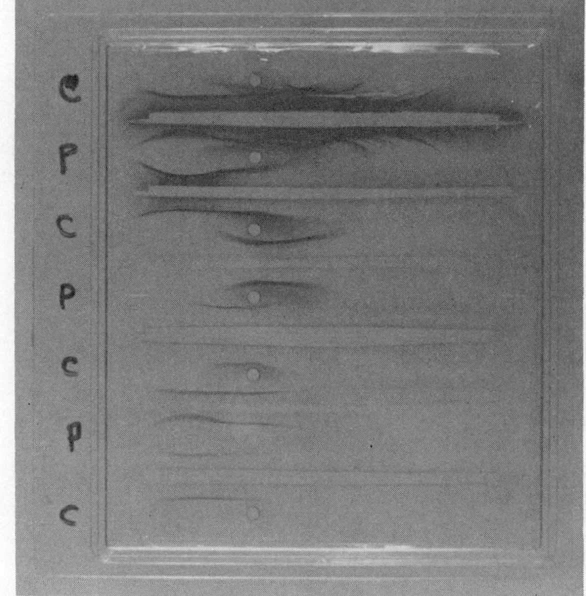

Figure 26–25 Immunoelectrophoresis (ICL Scientific, Fountain Valley, Calif. 92708). In the illustration, *C* indicates control serum and *P* the patient's serum. Briefly, 4 μL of serum is placed in each well, and the plate is subjected to electrophoresis on an ICL Power Supply I. Subsequently, the precut troughs of agar between the wells are removed, and 80 to 90 μL of appropriate serum is pipetted into each trough. The antisera used are (from above down): (1) anti-human polyvalent, (2) anti-IgG, (3) anti-IgA, (4) anti-IgM, (5) anti-kappa (free and bound), and (6) anti-lambda (free and bound). The sera are allowed to diffuse into the agar at room temperature in a moist atmosphere for 24 to 48 hours. After diffusion, white precipitate arcs may be examined against a dark background, or the plates may be washed and stained. This plate was stained with amido-black and was from a patient with an abnormal peak in IgG and in kappa, indicating an abnormal clonal production of a protein with the molecular formula $\gamma_2\kappa_2$.

Rocket Immunoelectrophoresis (Laurell)

This is another development in which a gel medium incorporating antibody is used. Wells are cut into the medium, and serum (containing antigens such as immunoglobulins) is placed. The plate is then subjected to electrophoresis, and the protein antigen in the well

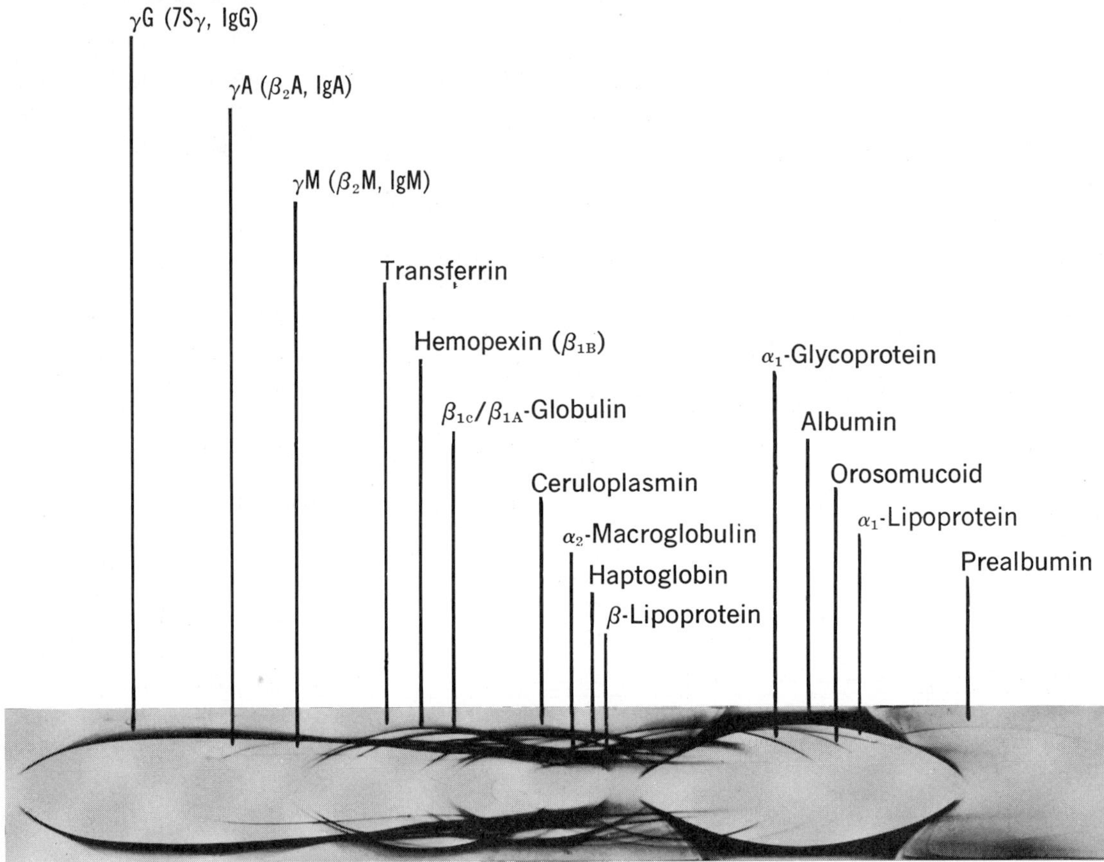

Figure 26–26 Immunoelectrophoretic pattern of pooled human serum *(center well)*, electrophoresed and then reacted against goat antihuman serum *(bottom trough)* and horse antihuman serum *(top)*. (Courtesy of Hyland Laboratories, Costa Mesa, Calif. 92626.)

moves from the cathode to the anode. The resultant pattern of precipitation of antigen-antibody occurs in a spike or rocket form (Fig. 26–24). The distance of migration of the protein, or the length of the rocket, is directly proportional to the amount of antigen in the well. Commercial kits are available, and the procedure is a rapid method of quantitating immunoglobulins, but it requires considerable technical time.

Counterimmunoelectrophoresis

A further and growing application is based on the fact that soluble antigen migrates toward the anode, whereas antibody mobility is less than that of water moving toward the cathode. Thus antibody is carried toward the cathode (endosmosis). When antigen and antibody are placed in wells in a gel and current applied, the migration and diffusion of the one toward the other can be accelerated (i.e., the negative electrode is placed on the antigen side and the positive electrode on the antibody side). Within 30 minutes under suitable conditions, a precipitin line is seen if the antigen and antibody are reactive (Fig. 26–24). The procedure is being used increasingly to identify bacterial antigens in body fluids and to a lesser extent in the identification of antibodies. In the first application, the advantages are that the method is more rapid than culture and that it is not affected by antimicrobial therapy in which culture of the fluid may prove sterile. Staphylococcal coagglutination (p. 543) techniques have been used similarly.

CHAPTER 26—REVIEW QUESTIONS

1. Define *antigen, hapten, antibody, immunoglobulin,* and *B-cells.*
2. a. Which immunoglobulin can cross the placenta? Give two possible effects on the newborn of such passage.
   b. What intrauterine infections occur that may cause the fetus to produce its own immunoglobulin? Which class is the latter?
3. a. Explain the difference between polyclonal and monoclonal gammopathy. What is the significance of the monoclonal type?
   b. What method is usually used in serology to measure the amount of immunoglobulins present?
   c. Explain the theoretical basis of the test.
4. What are reagins? What is the antigen used in tests for reagins? How does one confirm a positive result?
5. Explain with a diagram the basis of immunoelectrophoresis, direct immunofluorescence, and coagglutination.

REFERENCES FOR MICROBIOLOGY SECTION

American Society for Microbiology. Cumulative Techniques and Procedures in Clinical Microbiology (Cumutech Series). Washington, DC, American Society for Microbiology, 1974–1983 (continuing series).

Barry AL. The Antimicrobic Susceptibility Test: Principles and Practices. Philadelphia, Lea & Febiger, 1976.

Barry AL, Garcia F, and Thrupp LD. An improved single disk method for testing the antibiotic susceptibility of rapidly growing pathogens. Am J Clin Pathol 1970, *53*:149–158.

Blacklow NR, and Cukor G. Viral gastroenteritis. N Engl J Med 1981, *304*:397–406.

Blazevic DJ, and Ederer GM. Principles of Biochemical Tests in Diagnostic Microbiology. New York, John Wiley & Sons, 1975.

Carroll JA, Gados M, and Chen HP. Counterimmune electrophoresis: a method for the determination of bacterial polysaccharide antigens. Lab Med 1980, *11*:541–544.

Cowan ST. Cowan & Steel's Manual for the Identification of Medical Bacteria, 2nd ed. New York, Cambridge University Press, 1974.

Davis BD, Dulbecco R, Eisen HN, and Ginsberg HS. Microbiology Including Immunology & Molecular Genetics, 3rd ed. Hagerstown Md., Harper & Row, 1980.

Dolan CT. A practical approach to identification of yeast-like organisms. Amer J Clin Pathol 1971, *55*:580–590.

Dowell VR Jr, Lombard GL, Thompson FS, and Armfield AY. Media for the Characterization and Identification of Obligately Anaerobic Bacteria. Atlanta, U.S. Dept. of Health, Education, and Welfare, Public Health Service, Center for Disease Control, 1980.

Flynn J, and Wattkins SA. A serum free medium for testing fermentation reactions in *Neisseria gonorrhoeae*. J Clin Pathol 1972, *25*:525–527.

Goldberg RL, and Washington J. Comparison of isolation of *H. vaginalis* from peptone starch dextrose agar and Columbia Colistin–Nalidixic acid agar. J Clin Microbiol 1976, *4*:245–247.

Granato PA. Evaluation of a dip-slide device for enumeration of bacteria in urine. Lab Med 1980, *11*:246–250.

Gubash SM. Synergistic haemolysis test for presumptive identification and differentiation of *Clostridium perfringens. C. bifermentans, C. sordellii*, and *C. paraperfringens*. J Clin Pathol 1980, *33*:395–399.

Islams, AKMS. Rapid recognition of Group B streptococci. Lancet 1977, *1*:256–257.

Koneman EW, Allen SD, Dowel VR Jr, and Sommers HM. Color Atlas and Textbook of Diagnostic Microbiology. Philadelphia, JB Lippincott Co., 1979.

Koneman EW, Roberts GD, and Wright SF. Practical Laboratory Mycology, 2nd ed. Baltimore, The Williams & Wilkins Co., 1978.

Kubica GP, and Dye WE. Laboratory Methods for Clinical and Public Health—Mycobacteriology. Atlanta, U.S. Dept. of Health, Education, and Welfare, Public Health Service, National Communicable Disease Center, 1967.

Land GA, Fleming WH III, Beadles TA, and Foxworth JH. Rapid identification of medically important yeasts. Lab Med 1979, *10*:533–541.

Leigh DA, and Simmons K. Identification of non-sporing anaerobic bacteria. J Clin Pathol 1977, *30*:991–992.

Lennette EH, Balows A, Hausler WJ, and Truant JP, eds. Manual of Clinical Microbiology, 3rd ed. Washington, DC, American Society for Microbiology, 1980.

MacFaddin JF. Biochemical tests for the identification of medical bacteria, 2nd ed. Baltimore, The Williams & Wilkins Co., 1980.

McGinnis MR. Laboratory Handbook of Medical Mycology. New York, Academic Press, Inc., 1980.

Martin WJ. Practical method for isolation of anaerobic bacteria in the clinical laboratory. Appl Microbiol 1971, *22*:1168–1171.

Murphy DB, and Hawkins JE. Use of urease disks in the identification of mycobacteria. J Clin Microbiol 1975, *1*:465–468.

Nakamura RM, and Deodhar S. Laboratory Tests in the Diagnosis of Autoimmune Disorders. Chicago. American Society of Clinical Pathologists, Educational Products Division, 1976 (reprinted 1979).

Owen DS. A cheap and useful compensated polarized microscope. N Engl J Med 1971, *285*:1152.

Park CH, Fauber M, and Cook CB. Identification of *Haemophilus vaginalis*. Am J Clin Pathol 1968, *49*:590–593.

Phelps P, Steel AD, and McCarty DJ Jr. Compensated polarized light microscopy: identification of crystals in synovial fluid from gout and pseudogout. J.A.M.A. 1968, *203*:508–512.

Rose NR, and Friedman H, eds. Manual of Clinical Immunology, 2nd ed. Washington, DC., American Society for Microbiology, 1980.

Rytel, MW. Counterimmunoelectrophoresis: a diagnostic adjunt in clinical microbiology. Lab Med 1980, *11*:655–658.

Schieven BC. *Haemophilus vaginalis* vaginitis: a laboratory approach. Ontario Medical Technologist 1980, *1*:15–16.

Shikata, T, Uzawa T, Yoshiwara N, Akatsuka T, and Yamazaki S. Staining methods of Australia antigen in paraffin section: detection of cytoplasmic inclusion bodies. Jap J Exp Med 1974, *44*:25–36.

Sutter VL, Citron DM, and Finegold SM. Wadsworth anaerobic bacteriology manual, 3rd ed. St. Louis, CV Mosby Co., 1980.

Yong DCT, Smitka C, Prytula A, and Kane J. The comparison of two agar media for germ tube and chlamydospore production by *Candida albicans*. Health Lab Science 1978, *15*:197–200.

Youmans GP, Paterson PY, and Sommers HM. The Biologic and Clinical Basis of Infectious Disease, 2nd ed. Philadelphia, WB Saunders Co., 1980.

Section III

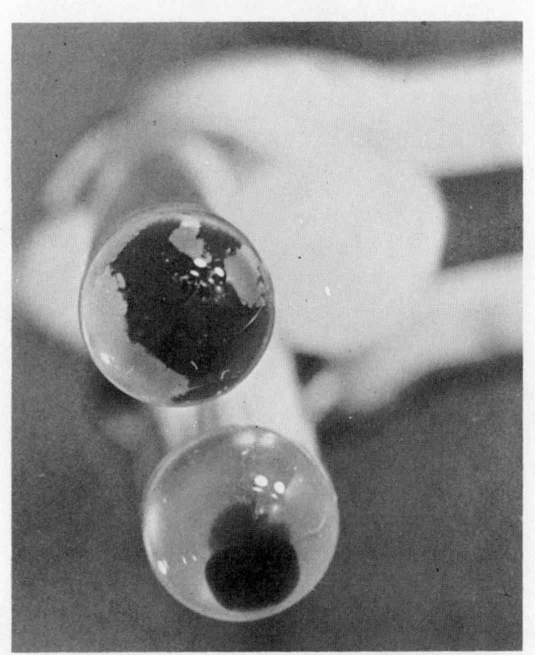

IMMUNOHEMATOLOGY

PRINCIPLES OF IMMUNOHEMATOLOGY

INTRODUCTION

Immunohematology is one of the oldest disciplines of applied immunology, representing a distinct subspecialty that incorporates principles of other disciplines, such as genetics, biochemistry, and, particularly, hematology and immunology.

The purpose of this and the next chapter will be to introduce the newcomer to the principles and practice of the science of immunohematology according to the syllabus requirements of the Canadian Society of Laboratory Technologists (CSLT) and the American Society of Clinical Pathologists (ASCP). Students requiring more detailed information are referred to the list of general references following Chapter 28. The explanation of many of the genetic terms used will be found in Chapter 1.

ANTIGENS AND ANTIBODIES

By broad definition, an antigen is a substance (usually protein in nature) that, when introduced parenterally into an individual whose tissues do not possess that particular substance, is capable of instituting the production of antibody specific to itself. In order to act as an antigen, a substance must be of sufficiently high molecular weight, the lowest limit for a substance to be a good antigen being in the 40,000 to 50,000 MW range. Substances below 5,000 MW generally fail to act as antigens and, if so, are known as *haptens*. In addition to this, the substance must be foreign to the host and it must be "antigenic" (i.e., potent), which depends to some extent on the *form* of the antigen and the route of administration.

On the surface (membrane) of the red blood cell are minute glycoproteins and glycolipids that are under genetic control. These substances are of sufficiently high molecular weight to act as antigens and are known as *blood group antigens*. It is these antigens that are of primary interest to the immunohematologist.

The specificity of the blood group antigens studied so far has been shown to be determined by the sequential addition of sugar residues to a common precursor substance as a result of indirect gene action. The precursor substance, which is located on or within the red cell membrane, is composed of four molecules of three different sugars, D-galactose (two molecules), *N*-acetylgalactosamine (one molecule) and *N*-acetyl-glucosamine (one molecule). There are two types of precursor substance, known as Type 1 and Type 2, which differ in terminal *linkage*. The action of the genes causes the production of an enzyme that, in turn, causes the addition of another sugar to the basic precursor substance, which determines the specificity of the antigen. (For further discussion, see *The ABO Blood Group System.*)

The number of antigen sites on the red cell varies according to the specificity involved. Thus there are approximately 1 million ABO sites and 250,000 D antigen sites on the red cell membrane of individuals possessing these antigens. Red cell antigens not only are present on the red cells but have also been detected on leukocytes and platelets and in saliva, milk, seminal fluid, plasma, and most tissues of the body, although many specificities do appear to be confined wholly to the red cell membrane. In addition, blood group substances, particularly ABO substances, have been found in certain plants and bacteria.

The antigens on the red cells are not always constant throughout life. Some specificities are poorly developed at birth (e.g., I, Lewis) and some can be altered in certain disease states (e.g., A,B). Changes in blood group antigens have also been noted during pregnancy (e.g., Lewis).

The introduction of a blood group antigen into a "foreign" circulation may stimulate the production of a blood group (or red cell) antibody. This may occur as the result of transfusion therapy or as a result of fetomaternal transfusion in pregnancy. Certain antibodies occur without known antigenic stimulus, and these are known as non–red cell immune, non–red cell, or naturally occurring antibodies. Antibodies are not generally produced by individuals whose red cells possess the corresponding antigen (Landsteiner's law) although there are exceptions to this, as will be discussed below.

Blood group antibodies belong to a family of proteins known as *immunoglobulins,* all of which have the same basic structure (i.e., two heavy chains and two light chains, held together by disulfide bonds) and function. There are five classes of immunoglobulin, known as IgG, IgM, IgA, IgD, and IgE. Blood group antibodies are IgG, IgM, or IgA. IgG and IgA molecules in serum are composed of a single structural unit (respectively, two gamma and alpha heavy chains and two light chains, which are either kappa or lambda, but not both). The IgM molecule, on the other hand, consists of five basic structural units arranged in a circular fashion and is known as a cyclic pentamer. The heavy chains are mu, and the light chains, again, are kappa or lambda, but not both (see Fig. 26–4).

A portion of the immunoglobulin molecule has a variable amino acid sequence and is thought to determine antibody specificity. The remainder of the molecule has a constant amino acid sequence, which is similar for each type and subtype. The hinge region of the molecule allows for flexibility. The antigen binding site is believed to be at the end of the heavy and light chains in the variable portion of the molecule. The immunoglobulin molecule can be split into fragments by certain enzymes—these fragments are called Fab (*F*ragment capable of *A*ntigen *B*inding) and Fc (*F*ragment *C*rystalline). The action of the enzyme papain splits the molecule into 2 Fab and 1 Fc fragments. Other enzymes (e.g., pepsin, trypsin) produce slightly different fragments. The Fc fragment of the molecule directs the biological activity of the antibody, whereas the Fab fragment is involved in antigen binding (see Fig. 26–2).

Immunoglobulin molecules combine with antigens on cellular surfaces, resulting in the destruction of the cells *extravascularly* (outside of the blood vessels) or *intravascularly* (within the blood vessels through the action of complement—see below).

In addition to this, immunoglobulin molecules are responsible for the neutralization of toxins and the facilitation of phagocytosis.

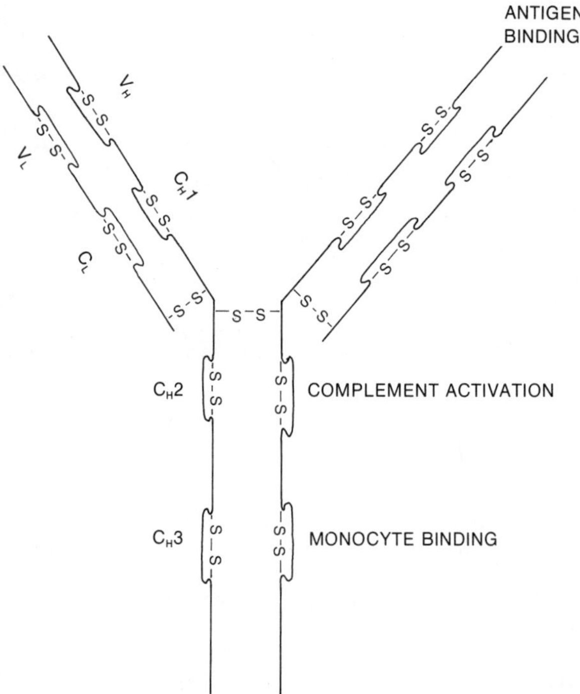

Figure 27–1 Immunoglobulin domains. (From Bryant, N. J.: Laboratory Immunology and Serology, rev. ed. Philadelphia, W. B. Saunders Co., 1979.)

Immunoglobulin Domains

Each immunoglobulin molecule has internal disulfide links, forming loops in the peptide chains that are known as *domains* (Fig. 27–1). Each of these domains has a distinct function: the *variable-region domains* (V_L and V_H) form a specific antigen-binding site, and the *constant-region domains* (C_H2 and C_H3, respectively) initiate the complement sequence and cause the adherence of the molecule to the monocyte surface.

Types of Immunoglobulin

As mentioned, there are three main classes of immunoglobulin: IgG, IgM, and IgA. The immunoglobulin classes IgD and IgE do not apply to the study of immunohematology. These three main classes differ in structure and in properties, as summarized in Table 27–1.

The Immune Response

There are three main types of immunity: so-called natural immunity, humoral immunity, and cell-mediated immunity. (See Chapter 26 for an explanation of these terms.)

The so-called primary response occurs after first encounter with a foreign antigen. Antibody production is usually slow and is, to some extent, dependent on the dose of the challenging antigen and on the route of administration. It is not clear if IgM antibody is formed initially in the primary response.

The so-called secondary response occurs after second or subsequent encounter with the same foreign antigen. Small doses of challenging antigen, in this case, may produce large amounts of antibody, which is usually IgG. The secondary response occurs as a result of immunological memory, the information about the challenging antigen being carried by the small lymphocytes (B-cells).

When an individual fails to produce an antibody to foreign stimulus, this is referred to as *tolerance* or *immunological tolerance*. Dizygotic twins (human and animal), who share the same placental circulation, are tolerant of each other's antigens and possess a dual population of red cells. Such twins are known as *chimeras*. Temporary chimerism occurs in multitransfused patients or in patients who have received a graft of bone marrow. Individuals receiving large doses of antigen become temporarily tolerant to these antigens. This is known as *high-dose tolerance* or *immunological paralysis*. Antibody response can also be suppressed by the administration of passive antibody.

Antibody Activity In Vivo

Antibodies do not directly damage red cells carrying the corresponding antigens but are instrumental in their destruction. Red cells may be destroyed in either of two ways:

1. *Extravascular*—The attachment of antibody to antigenic receptors on the red cells causes them to lose their elasticity and become spherical. These "changed" red cells are unable to pass through the sinusoidal tissue in the spleen and are therefore removed from the circulation.

2. *Intravascular*—Destruction of the red cells takes place within the blood vessels through the action of complement.

Complement. The term *complement* refers to a complex set of several distinct proteins that react sequen-

TABLE 27–1 Properties of the Main Immunoglobulins in Serum

Characteristic	IgG	IgM	IgA
Heavy chains	γ	μ	α
Light chains	κ or λ	κ or λ	κ or λ
Molecular formula	$\gamma_2\kappa_2$ or $\gamma_2\lambda_2$	$(\mu_2\kappa_2)_5J$ or $(\mu_2\lambda_2)_5J$	$\alpha_2\kappa_2(\alpha_2\kappa_2)_2$* $\alpha_2\lambda_2(\alpha_2\lambda_2)_2$*
Molecular weight	150,000	900,000	160,000 330,000*
Sedimentation coefficient	7S	19S	7S,105S*
Percentage carbohydrate (serum)	3	11.8	7.5
Normal serum concentration (mg/100 mL)	1275(±280)	125(±45)	225(±55)
g/L adult range	7.3–23.7	0.47–1.47	0.61–3.3
g/L newborn	Slightly higher than adult	±0.1	Undetectable
Catabolic rate (T½(d))	23	5	6
Percentage intravascular	44	80	40
Fractional catabolic rate (%/d)	7	18	33
Crosses placenta	Yes	No	No
Usual serologic behavior	"Incomplete" antibody	Agglutinin ("complete" ab)	Agglutinin ("complete" ab)
Serologic behavior after heating to 56° C for 3 hours	Unaffected	Reduced	Unaffected
Effect of alkylating agents on serologic behavior	May develop agglutinating activity	No longer agglutinates	Partially inactivated
Turnover rate (synthesis, mg/kg/d)	28	5–8	8–10
Complement fixation	Yes	Yes	No
Presence in colostrum	Yes	No	Yes
Usual temperature of reaction	37° C	20° C	37° C
Usual antigenic stimulus of red cell antibodies	Transfusion or pregnancy	Often "naturally occurring"	
Isoelectric points	6.2–8.5	5.5–7.4	4.8–6.5
Electrophoretic migration	Slow gamma	Slow gamma	Slow beta
Water solubility	Soluble	Insoluble	Soluble
Gm specificity (on gamma chains)	Yes	No	No
Km specificity (on kappa chains)	Yes	Yes	Yes
Antibody activity	Yes	Yes	Yes
External secretions	No	No	Yes
Effect of 2-ME and DTT	Not affected	Inactivated	Partial inactivation

*In serum, 10 per cent of IgA is in the form of dimers.
(From Bryant, N. J.: An Introduction to Immunohematology, 2nd ed. Philadelphia, W. B. Saunders Co., 1982, p. 39.)

tially and cause such biological effects as immune adherence, phagocytosis, and cell lysis. Both IgM and IgG antibodies can initiate the complement system (with the exception of the IgG4 subclass of IgG). The complement sequence is described in Chapter 26 and Figure 26–6.

Complement can be destroyed in vitro by anticoagulants (which chelate calcium), by heating to 56°C for 30 minutes, by normal serum inhibitor, and as a result of storage.

Antibody Activity In Vitro

The fundamental reaction between antigen on red cells and its corresponding antibody is simply one of *combination,* which may or may not be followed by *agglutination* (i.e., clumping) of the cells concerned.

Sensitization—The simple combination of antigen and antibody, either in vivo or in vitro, with or without subsequent agglutination, is known as sensitization.

An antigen and its specific antibody possess complementary corresponding structures that enable the antigenic determinants to come into very close apposition with the binding site on the antibody molecule, where the two are held together by weak intermolecular bonds. This antigen-antibody reaction is reversible, and therefore, in accordance with the law of mass action, can be written thus:

Antigen (Ag) + Antibody (Ab) $\rightleftharpoons$ AgAb (antigen-antibody complex)

The strength of the antigen-antibody bond depends on how well the antibody complexes with its corresponding antigen. Antibodies, even of the same specificity, contain molecules with a variety of binding strengths, which is reflected in the avidity and strength of the final agglutination reaction. The degree of complexing reflects the *equilibrium constant* of the antibody, which is the average binding strength of the antibody sample. The equilibrium constant can be altered by increasing either the number of antigen sites available or the number of antibody molecules present. Altering the physical environment of the antigens and antibodies, by altering pH or ionic charges, also affects the equilibrium constant.

The most common method of affecting the equilibrium constant is to increase the number of antibody molecules relative to the number of antigen sites available. This has the effect of increasing the likelihood of antigen-antibody complexes forming. This is done by using large volumes of serum (antibody) and weak suspensions of cells (antigens).

Obviously, if the identity of an antibody is known, it will establish the identity of the antigen with which it reacts. Similarly, if the identity of the antigen is known, any antibodies with which it reacts can be identified. In order to do this, it must be possible to establish that an antigen-antibody reaction has, in fact, occurred. In immunohematology, this is done by demonstrating agglutination, hemolysis, sensitization, inhibition (neutralization), precipitation, and complement fixation.

Agglutination. The fundamental and most commonly used reaction in the immunohematology laboratory to demonstrate the interaction of antigen and antibody is the phenomenon of agglutination. By broad definition, agglutination is simply the clumping of cells into aggregates, often as a result of the combination of an antibody's binding sites with antigen sites of adjacent red cells. Certain red cell antibodies will agglutinate cells suspended in saline (i.e., simply by bringing the two components—antigen and antibody—together in a test tube and allowing a period of time for the reaction to take place at room temperature, or by hastening the reaction by immediate centrifugation). These antibodies are known as *saline-active* (complete) antibodies. Other red cell antibodies do not agglutinate in a saline medium but require the presence of a potentiating medium (e.g., bovine albumin, proteolytic enzymes) in order for clumping to occur subsequent to sensitization. These antibodies are sometimes called *saline nonreactive* (incomplete) antibodies, although because saline reactive antibodies are most often IgM and saline nonreactive antibodies are most often IgG or IgA (with some exceptions), it is perhaps best to refer to the antibody by its immunoglobulin class. The reason for this difference in reactivity is believed to be related to the size of the antibody molecule: IgG molecules, consisting of a single structural unit, can bind antigen sites that are up to 14 nm apart, whereas IgM molecules, which consist of five structural units, can bind sites that are up to 35 nm apart.

With respect to red cell antibodies that are IgG (or IgA) and therefore unable to bring about agglutination when antigen sites are more than 14 nm apart, the addition of potentiating medium (albumin or enzymes) is believed to reduce the net negative charge exerted by the red cells, thereby decreasing the degree of repulsion between them and allowing them to approach one another more closely. This explanation is not entirely satisfactory, since it fails to explain why certain IgG antibodies (e.g., IgG anti-A and anti-B) do bring about agglutination in a saline medium. It has been suggested that the attachment of IgM molecules to red cells will alter the degree of repulsion between the red cells (or the net negative charge exerted by the cells, known as the *zeta potential*) and that if enough IgG molecules can be attracted to the red cells, a similar effect is obtained. It has also been shown that some antigen sites may be fairly inaccessible, deep in the red cell membrane, whereas others protrude from the cell surface. It is therefore also possible that, in some instances, IgG molecules may be capable of causing the agglutination of red cells if the corresponding antigen protrudes from the cell but not when the corresponding antigen is buried within the cell membrane.

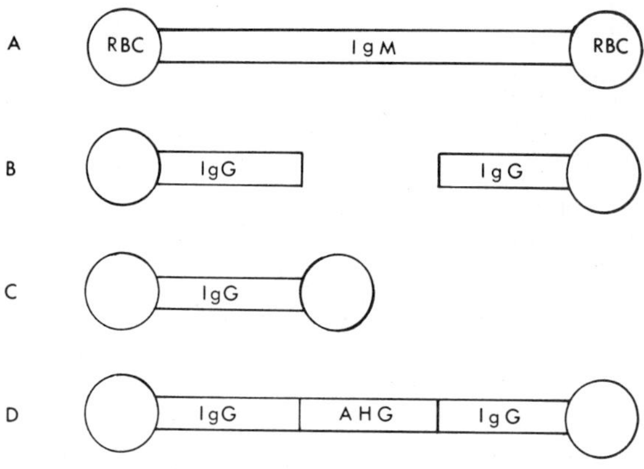

Figure 27–2 The demonstration of red cell agglutination.

Perhaps the most common method of causing agglutination of IgG antibodies, however, is through the use of antiglobulin serum. This is an antibody produced in an animal (usually a rabbit) in response to injection of human globulin, which then interacts with human globulin (antibody) in in vitro tests. The antiglobulin test is more fully described in Chapter 28 (see also Fig. 27–2).

Hemolysis. When certain antigen-antibody reactions have taken place, complement is activated, causing the destruction of the red cells and resulting in the loss (release) of hemoglobin from the cells. Antibodies that have this capacity are called *hemolysins.* In the test system, hemolysis of the cells is recognized by the hemoglobin-tinged supernatant obtained after centrifugation of the test mixture.

Inhibition (Neutralization). Soluble forms of blood group antigens have the effect of neutralizing (or inhibiting) the reaction of the corresponding blood group antibody. In the neutralization test, soluble antigen is added to serum containing antibody; if the strength of the antibody decreases (or if it disappears completely), an antigen-antibody reaction can be assumed. This test is most often used in the determination of secretor status.

Precipitation. Precipitation is the interaction of antigen and antibody in optimal proportions, resulting in the formation of a visible precipitate. The precipitation test is rarely used in the immunohematology laboratory.

Complement Fixation. Complement fixation involves the binding of complement by antigen-antibody aggregation and the lysis of the sensitized red cells. Like the precipitation reaction, complement fixation is rarely used in the immunohematology laboratory.

Reagents. The reagents used in the performance of these tests are discussed in Chapter 28.

Factors Influencing Antigen-Antibody Reactions

Temperature

Certain blood group antibodies react best with their corresponding antigen at warm temperatures (so-called warm agglutinins) whereas others favor a colder temperature for optimal reaction (so-called cold agglutinins). Temperature changes in the surrounding media affect the equilibrium constant, the rate (speed) of the reaction, or both.

Two terms are commonly used in this respect, namely, the thermal *range* and the thermal *optimum.* At the thermal optimum, the antibody molecules will react most quickly with the antigen. As the temperature deviates from the thermal optimum, the speed of the reaction will lessen, until, outside of the thermal range, no reaction will occur.

Several explanations have been offered to elucidate the reasons for the effect of temperature on antigen-antibody reactions, yet none has, so far, proven entirely satisfactory.

pH

Most blood group antibodies demonstrate optimal activity between pH 6.5 and 7.5. Outside of this pH range, antigen-antibody reactions are depressed and have been known to fail altogether. It should be noted, however, that there are exceptions to this generalization.

Time

Incubation time can affect the association of antigen and antibody in saline. If incubation time is too short, reactions will generally be weaker; if incubation time is prolonged, antigen-antibody complexes may disperse (dissociate), and this dissociation rate may overtake the rate of association.

Electrical Repulsion

Red cells carry negative electric charges on their surfaces when suspended in saline and therefore repel one another and attract positively charged sodium ions (cations), resulting in an ionic cloud around each cell.

Some of these cations travel in a constant configuration around each red cell and become a part of the kinetic unit of the cell. The cloud of positively charged cations around the cell causes a reduction in the net negative charge of the cell. When a potentiating medium (e.g., bovine albumin or proteolytic enzyme) is added to the cells, the net negative charge is further reduced so that the cells repel one another less strongly and are mutually able to approach more closely.

The edge of the cloud of cations is known as the *slipping plane* or the *plane (boundary) of shear;* this theoretical boundary separates those cations that move with the cell from those that do not. Zeta potential is a measurement (in mV) of the net charge exerted by the cell at the plane of shear (which differs according to the type of media in which the cells are suspended).

The zeta potential is therefore directly related to the electrostatic repulsion between the cells.

The Effects of the Nature of the Antigen

Apart from the *position* of the antigen on the red cell (i.e., whether it is on, below, or protruding from the membrane) the *amount* of antigen on the membrane is an important influence on antigen-antibody reactions. Different red cell antigens have varying numbers of antigen sites, and even within a specific blood group system an individual may be homozygous or heterozygous for the gene of the particular antigens involved. An individual who is homozygous for a particular gene will have considerably more antigen sites on his red cells than an individual who is heterozygous for the same gene, and antibodies may show different patterns of reactions between the two. If an antibody reacts strongly with red cells from an individual who is homozygous for the causative gene but weakly or not at all with red cells from an individual who is heterozygous for the same gene, the antibody is said to be dose dependent, and the phenomenon is known as *dosage effect.* Examples of this are to be found particularly in the MNSs and Rh/Hr blood group systems.

The Effects of the Nature of the Antibody

The immunoglobulin class and the "strength" of an antibody are important influences on antigen-antibody reactions. The most sensitive technique in practical immunohematology is the antiglobulin test, yet even this test has limits. A very weak antibody may not be detected in the antiglobulin test, because there are two few antibody molecules on the cell. Nevertheless, since the cell is sensitized, it is liable to rapid destruction in the reticuloendothelial system.

Conversely, a very strong antibody may so sensitize the red cell antigen sites that no antigen sites remain vacant. Therefore, the antibody attached to one red cell antigen is unable to unite with an unsensitized antigen site on an adjacent red cell, and agglutination is blocked. To effect agglutination in these cases, the ratio of antigen to antibody must be altered. This is usually done by diluting the antibody to reduce the number of antibody molecules present (see *Prozone Phenomenon,* p. 605).

THE BLOOD GROUP SYSTEMS

Approximately 500 blood group antigens have been described, many of which fall within the 20 to 30 so-called blood group systems. The following discussion will confine itself to those blood group systems that are considered to be of prime importance. Students requiring more comprehensive coverage of this subject are referred to the list of general references following Chapter 28.

The ABO Blood Group System

History

Blood groups and the inherited differences in human blood from one individual to another were first discovered by a German scientist, Karl Landsteiner (1900), who took samples of blood from six of his colleagues, separated the serum, and prepared saline suspensions of the red cells. When each serum sample was mixed with each red cell suspension, he noticed that agglutination of the cells had occurred in some mixtures and not in others.

Landsteiner came to the realization that the agglutination had occurred because the red cells possessed an antigen and that the corresponding specific antibody was present in the serum. When no agglutination had occurred, either the antigen or the antibody was missing from the mixture.

This discovery led Landsteiner to postulate the presence of three distinct blood groups. A fourth group was discovered by his pupils, von Decastello and Sturli, in 1902. We now known these four classifications as the ABO blood group system.

Only two antigens, now known as A and B, were needed to explain the four blood groups; an individual could possess one, the other, both (group AB), or neither (group O). It was further discovered that individuals who lacked either the A,B, or both antigens possessed in their serums the antibodies to these missing antigens. Individuals who possessed the A antigen on their red cells, therefore, also possessed anti-B in their serum; individuals who possessed the B antigen had anti-A in their serum; individuals who possessed neither A nor B antigens (group O) had both anti-A and anti-B in their serum; and individuals who had both A and B antigens (group AB) had neither anti-A nor anti-B in their serum. This information is shown in the following table:

Group	ABO Antigen on RBC	Antibodies in Serum
O	None	Anti-A and Anti-B
A	A	Anti-B
B	B	Anti-A
AB	A and B	None

Later it was discovered that there are "subgroups" (i.e., weaker forms) of the A antigen. The first of these to be recognized was called A_2 (further discussed below), and it allowed for the classification of six main groups:

$$A_1, A_2, B, A_1B, A_2B, \text{and } O.$$

Other subgroups of A have been described, such as A_3, A_x, and A_m. Subgroups of B have also been described, but these are very rare.

The Inheritance of the Groups of the ABO System

That the ABO groups are inherited characters was suggested in 1908 and proved in 1910. At first, three allelic genes—*A, B,* and *O*—were postulated, of which each individual inherits two, one being from each parent. The *O* gene does not produce a product, and is therefore believed to be amorphic.

In 1930, Thompson postulated four allelic genes—A_1, A_2, *B,* and *O*—and this postulation is now accepted as being correct. The four ABO alleles give rise to six phenotypes and ten genotypes, as follows:

Phenotypes	Genotypes
A_1	A_1A_1
	A_1A_2
	A_1O
A_2	A_2A_2
	A_2O
B	BB
	BO
A_1B	A_1B
A_2B	A_2B
O	OO

With the use of anti-A, anti-B, and anti-A_1 sera, all six phenotypes can be distinguished, but only three genotypes (A_1B, A_2B, and *OO*).

The expression of the *A* and *B* genes appears to be dependent on the gene *H*. Most individuals are homozygous for the *H* gene (i.e., *HH*); the *h* gene is amorphic.

The interaction of *H, A,* and *B* genes occurs as follows:

1. The basic precursor substance is converted by the *H* gene to H substance by the addition of the sugar L-fucose to the terminal D-galactose of the precursor substance.
2. The H substance is partly converted by the *A* and/or *B* genes to A and/or B substance by the attachment of *N*-acetyl-galactosamine and/or D-galactose, respectively, to the substrate formed by the *H* gene. Some H substance remains unconverted. The *O* gene, being amorphic, effects no conversion of H substance; therefore, group O individuals have the most H substance.

The amount of H substance (antigen) on the red cell therefore varies with the ABO group (depending on the amount of H substance converted into A and/or B substance). The order of reactivity usually follows the pattern O—A_2—A_2B—B—A_1—A_1B.

The Subgroups A_1 and A_2

Among U.S. whites, 78.48% of group A individuals belong to subgroup A_1 and almost all of the rest are of subgroup A_2. The distinction between these two groups is made with the use of specific anti-A_1, derived from plant (e.g., *Dolichos biflorus* seed extracts) and/or human sources. The difference between A_1 and A_2 may be both qualitative and quantitative (i.e., based on the quality of the antigen itself and on the number of antigen sites), although whether this is actually so is still a matter of controversy.

The Bombay Phenotype

The Bombay phenotype refers to individuals who lack the *H* gene (i.e., they are of genotype *hh*). Since the *H* gene is required for the conversion of precursor substance to H substance, and since the *A* and *B* genes cause the attachment of sugar residues to the substrate formed by the action of the *H* gene, individuals of the Bombay phenotype test as group O even when normal *A* and *B* genes have been inherited.

The sera of Bombay individuals contain anti-A, anti-B, and anti-H. The strong anti-H causes the serum to agglutinate the red cells of normal group O individuals.

Individuals who possess the Bombay phenotype do not secrete A, B, or H substances, even when the *Se (secretor)* gene has been inherited (see *Secretors and Nonsecretors* on p. 563).

Secretors and Nonsecretors

Approximately 75% of individuals secrete substances in their saliva that have the same specificity as the antigens (ABO) on their red cells. The term *secretor* refers to individuals who secrete A, B, and/or H substances. H substance is secreted by all secretors; A and B substances are secreted (in addition to H substance) by individuals of groups A and B, respectively. Group AB secretors secrete A, B, and H substances.

Secretion of ABH substances is controlled by the gene *Se*. Its allele, *se*, is an amorphic gene. Individuals who are homozygous or heterozygous for the *Se* gene are secretors.

It should be noted that the *Se* gene does not control the secretion of Lewis substances, which are also found in saliva (see *The Lewis Blood Group System* below).

Secretor status is determined by the inhibition (neutralization) test, as follows:

Technique 1: Saliva Tests for the Determination of Secretor Status

Method

1. Collect about 0.5 mL of saliva in a clean, dry beaker. This can be accomplished in an infant by using a very small cotton wool swab held in hemostat forceps, which absorbs the saliva and is then squeezed, expressing the drops into a small tube. Alternatively, a plastic pipette can be used by holding the infant's mouth open and recovering saliva from under the tongue. In adults who have difficulty, a wad of wax in the mouth will help to increase salivation.

2. Centrifuge the saliva at approximately 3200 rpm (1000 G) for ten minutes, then pour the supernatant into a hard-glass test tube.

3. Place the supernatant saliva in a boiling water bath for ten minutes; this is most important, since it will destroy the enzymes that would otherwise inactivate the group-specific substances and will also destroy anti-A and anti-B, which are often present in secretions.

4. The saliva, at this point, may be stored, and it will keep well at −20°C. If the saliva is frozen, a clearer supernatant will result.

5. When testing for secretor status, it is normally sufficient to test for H substance alone by preparing a dilution of the extract of *Ulex europaeus* (available commercially) and testing this against group O red cells. If no conclusion can be reached and the subject is group A, B, or AB, an additional test, using dilutions of serum containing the appropriate antibody, can be performed for the presence of A or B substance, using A_2-cells with anti-A and B-cells with anti-B.

6. It is important to run controls in parallel with the test, using the saliva of several secretors and several nonsecretors.

Interpretation. If the test for H substance is negative (i.e., no agglutination of the indicator red cells because of the antibody's activity being completely neutralized by the group specific substance), the individual is a secretor of H substance. Partial or no inhibition (i.e., a positive test) reveals a nonsecretor. (*Note:* In all neutralization tests, no agglutination or hemolysis is a positive result.)

The amount of blood group substance can be estimated by making serial dilutions of the saliva in saline (i.e., by performing a titration).

Note that, despite the difference in the reactivity of A_1 and A_2 red cells with anti-A, saliva from A_1 and A_2 secretors shows virtually no difference in reactivity.

Immune anti-A and anti-B are not neutralized by blood group–specific substances A and B. If potent substances are used, however, partial neutralization may occur.

The Antibodies of the ABO Blood Group System

There are two extreme views concerning the reasons for the development of anti-A and anti-B in all individuals except those of blood group AB:

1. Antibodies are the result of contact with A and B substances in the environment subsequent to birth.

2. Antibodies are wholly genetically determined.

Both of these theories have been supported by scientific observations, and it therefore appears likely that both genetic and environmental influences are involved.

Anti-A and Anti-B. As mentioned, anti-A and anti-B are present in the serum of all individuals whose red cells lack the corresponding antigen. These antibodies may be wholly IgM, partly IgM and IgG, partly IgM and IgA, or a mixture of all three immunoglobulins. IgG anti-A and anti-B may be "naturally occurring" (in group O individuals) or "immune" (i.e. stimulated by transfusion or pregnancy). Immune anti-A and anti-B are recognized by a rise in titer, increased avidity, increased difficulty to neutralize with A or B substance, the appearance of hemolysin, and serological activity that is stronger at 37°C than at 4°C. Both IgG and IgM anti-A and anti-B are capable of binding complement, and most are readily hemolytic. IgA anti-A and anti-B fail to bind complement.

The strength of anti-A and anti-B varies considerably in different individuals, and these antibodies are often present in very low concentrations in patients with hypogammaglobulinemia. The antibodies are usually absent in neonatal sera. They increase in strength between 3 and 6 months of age, reaching a maximum at 5 to 10 years of age, after which they gradually decrease in strength. The agglutinins are found in human milk and in ascitic fluid and saliva.

Anti-A and anti-B sometimes occur as autoantibodies, though in these cases they usually show cross-reactive specificity with the Ii blood groups.

Anti-A. Two separate populations of anti-A molecules occur in group O and group B individuals: anti-A (reactive with A_1 and A_2 red cells) and anti-A_1 (reactive with A_1 red cells only).

Anti-A_1 from group B individuals is usually IgM; anti-A_1 from group O individuals is often IgG. Anti-A_1 occurs as a separate antibody in 1 to 2% of A_2 bloods and 25% of A_2B bloods. This anti-A_1, when reactive below 25°C (most examples), is clinically insignificant. Anti-A_1 reactive above 25°C may bring about the destruction of A_1 red cells in vivo.

Anti-A_1 has been found in a number of seed extracts, the most useful being *Dolichos biflorus*. Lectins (seed extracts) specific for anti-B and anti-A+B have also been described, but these are not generally used. It should also be noted at this time that the snail *Helix hortensis* is a source of powerful anti-A, which agglutinates A_1 and A_2 red cells at about the same strength. The receptor is known as A_{hel}.

Anti-H. Pure anti-H is found in Bombay (O_h) individuals as a hemolysin and as an agglutinin that is almost as active at 37°C as at 0°C. Reagents with anti-H specificity can be prepared from the seeds of the plant *Ulex europaeus,* the extract of which is commonly used in laboratories. Other plant sources of anti-H are less satisfactory.

Anti-A,B. Anti-A,B is derived from the serum of group O individuals. When combined with unknown red cells, anti-A,B will show agglutination with A_1, A_1B (and some A subgroups), and B, yet will show no agglutination with red cells of group O. The main reason for the use of this serum is to allow distinction between red cells of group O and red cells that belong to a subgroup of A and that might otherwise be indistinguishable.

The Clinical Significance of ABO Antibodies

ABO antibodies must be considered of extreme clinical significance, since they are capable of causing rapid red cell destruction in vivo and in many cases may result in the death of the recipient. In addition, ABO antibodies are a common cause of hemolytic disease of the newborn (see discussion below).

ABO Grouping Techniques

Establishing the ABO group of an individual usually involves so-called forward and reverse grouping. The sera for forward grouping is of human origin, usually collected from individuals whose "natural" antibodies have been stimulated to high titers. Anti-A (from group B individuals), anti-B (from group A individuals), and anti-A,B (from group O individuals) are normally used in forward grouping. Red cells for reverse grouping are also of human origin, from group A and B individuals. Both A_1 and A_2 red cells may be used, although A_1 cells are usually sufficient in most routine procedures.

Technique 2: ABO Grouping (Slide or Tile Method)

Method

1. Place one drop of anti-A, one drop of anti-B, and one drop of anti-A,B typing reagents on a divided slide or tile. Place two drops of serum from the individual under test on the same divided slide.

2. To the anti-A, anti-B, and anti-A,B add one drop of washed, 10% suspension of red cells from the individual under test.

3. To the two separate drops of serum from the individual under test, add one drop of known A_1 and B red cell reagents, respectively.

4. Mix each separate cell-serum mixture thoroughly with separate applicator sticks, and rock or rotate the tile until clumping (agglutination) is apparent.

5. Read macroscopically for agglutination.

6. Record results.

Interpretation. Results of ABO grouping are interpreted as shown in Table 27–2.

Technique 3: ABO Grouping (Tube Technique)

Method

1. Set up five 10 × 75 mm test tubes in a test tube rack.

2. Label the tubes as follows: anti-A, anti-B, anti-A,B, A_1-cells, and B-cells.

3. Add one drop of anti-A grouping serum to the tube labeled "anti-A."

4. Add one drop of anti-B grouping serum to the tube labeled "anti-B."

5. Add one drop of anti-A,B grouping serum to the tube labeled "anti-A,B."

6. Add one drop of serum from the individual under test to both the tube labeled "A_1-cells" and the tube labeled "B-cells."

7. Add one drop of a washed 5% suspension of red cells (in saline) from the individual under test to the tubes labeled "anti-A," "anti-B," and "anti-A,B."

8. Add one drop of A_1-cells to the tube labeled "A_1-cells."

9. Add one drop of B-cells to the tube labeled "B cells."

10. Mix each tube thoroughly.

11. Incubate at room temperature for 60 to 90 minutes, or centrifuge at 3400 rpm (Serofuge)* for 15 seconds.

12. Read macroscopically for agglutination and hemolysis, using an optical aid.

13. Record results.

Interpretation. Results are interpreted as shown in Table 27–2. (See also Fig. 27–3.)

(It should be noted that this technique, like all techniques given in this section, are suggestions only. In all cases, the directions given by the manufacturer (when using commercial antisera) should be followed carefully and never modified unless appropriate controls are performed to ensure that the chosen antisera will work properly according to the chosen technique of the laboratory.)

Controls. It is generally unnecessary to run controls each time ABO grouping is performed; however, reagent antisera and cells used should be controlled on a daily basis as part of a routine quality control program.

*Clay Adams Corp., Parsippany, N. J. 07054.

TABLE 27–2 INTERPRETATION OF RESULTS OF ABO GROUPING

Anti-A	Anti-B	Anti-A,B	A_1-cells	B-cells	Group
−	−	−	+	+	O
+	−	+	−	+	A
−	+	+	+	−	B
+	+	+	−	−	AB

Positive (+), cells are agglutinated; negative (−), cells are not agglutinated.

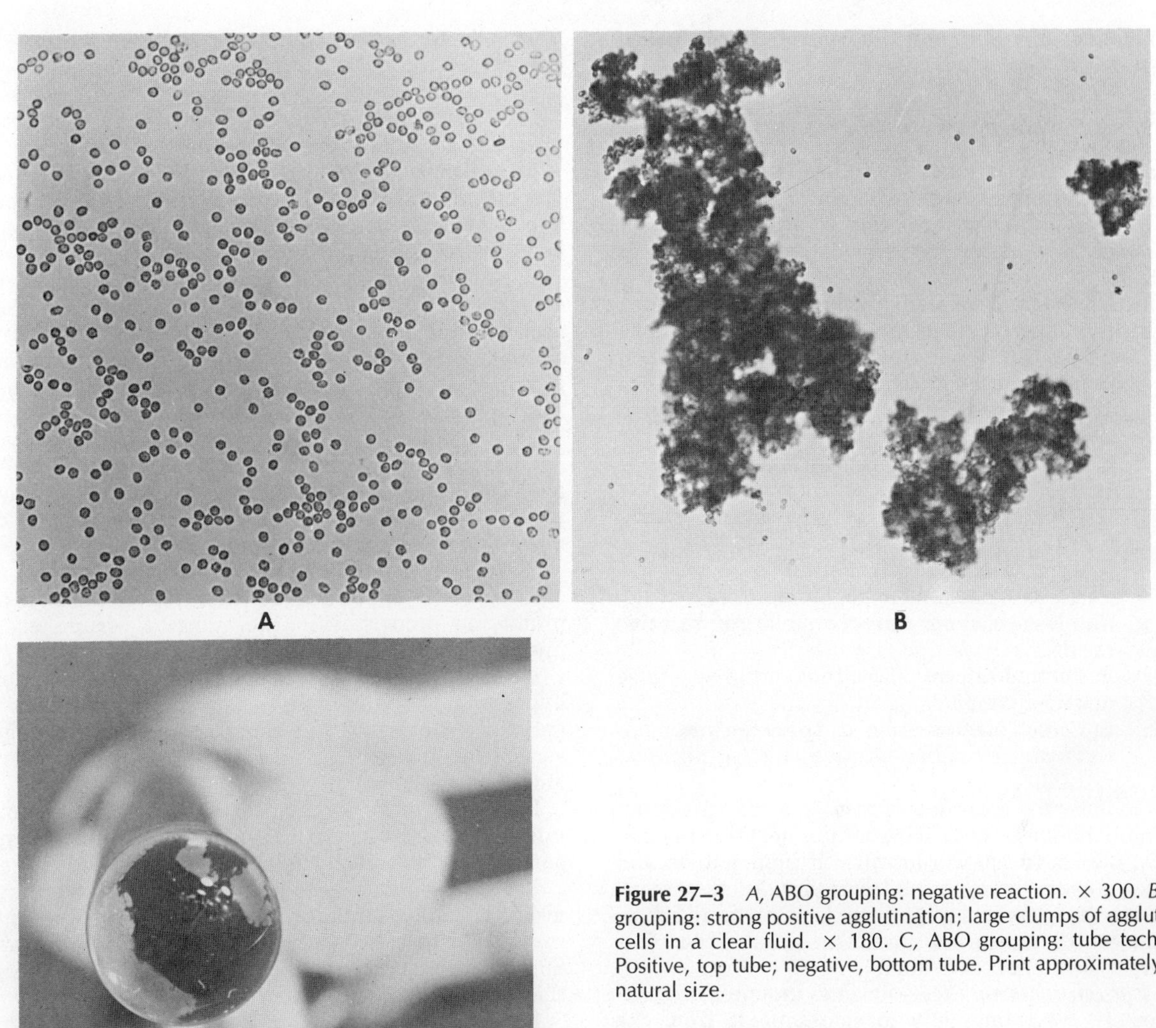

Figure 27–3 *A,* ABO grouping: negative reaction. × 300. *B,* ABO grouping: strong positive agglutination; large clumps of agglutinated cells in a clear fluid. × 180. *C,* ABO grouping: tube technique. Positive, top tube; negative, bottom tube. Print approximately twice natural size.

Technique 4: Subgrouping with Dolichos biflorus Extract (Anti-A_1)

Method

1. Set up three 10 × 75 mm test tubes in a test tube rack, labeled "Test," "Positive control," and "Negative control," respectively.

2. Place one drop of *Dolichos biflorus* extract into all three tubes.

3. Add one drop of a washed 5% suspension of red cells from the individual under test to the tube labeled "Test."

4. Add one drop of known A_1-red cells to the tube labeled "Positive control" and one drop of known A_2-red cells to the tube labeled "Negative control."

5. Incubate at room temperature for 60 minutes, or centrifuge at approximately 3200 rpm (1000 G) (Serofuge) for 15 seconds.

6. Examine macroscopically for agglutination and hemolysis, using an optical aid.

7. Record results.

Interpretation. Agglutination in the tube labeled "Test" indicates that the individual belongs to group A_1. No agglutination in this tube indicates that the individual belongs to a subgroup of A. *Note:* This result should be considered invalid unless the controls have worked as expected.

Anomalous Results in ABO Testing

Anomalous results may be caused in routine ABO testing by a number of factors, including the following:

1. *Technique*—Poor technique is one of the major causes of anomalous results in routine ABO testing. For example:
    a. Dirty glassware can give false positive results.
    b. Improper cell-to-serum concentration can give false positive or false negative results.
    c. Contamination or inactivation of reagents can give false negative or, occasionally, false positive results.
    d. Overcentrifugation can give false positive results.
    e. Undercentrifugation can give false negative results.
    f. Failure to identify hemolysis as a positive result can give a false negative result.
    g. Careless reading can give a false negative result.
    h. Failure to use an optical aid can give a false negative result.
    i. Incorrect identification of specimen or materials can give false positive or false negative results.
    j. Incorrect recording of results or interpretation can give false positive or false negative results.

All of the above can be controlled if rigid policies and procedures are enforced in the laboratory. An anomalous result due to poor technique can lead to fatal consequences for the recipient, and it is always the most difficult type of error to defend.

2. *Serum abnormalities*—Reverse grouping may be affected by Wharton's jelly (a contaminant from the umbilical cord) or serum proteins, causing rouleaux. These factors may be present in the patient's serum and remain in the cell suspension tested.

3. *Sensitization* —Antibody-coated (sensitized) red cells in the patient may agglutinate in a high-protein medium.

4. *Recent transfusion*—A transfusion of blood of another ABO group before testing may provide a sample that is a mixture of cell types, giving a "mixed-field" appearance on testing.

5. *Unusual genotype*—The A or B antigens may be weakly expressed because of an unusual genotype (i.e., subgroups of A and B).

6. *Misgrouping*—A_2B and A_3B samples may react weakly with reagent anti-A. If anti-A_1 is present, the sample may be misgrouped as group B. Sera from samples thought to be of blood group B should therefore be tested against A_2 as well as A_1 red cells to distinguish those with anti-A_1 but no anti-A in their serum.

7. *Disease*—In some subjects with acute leukemia or other nonhemolytic malignant disorders, the red cell antigens in the ABO blood group system may be greatly depressed. Depression of A_1 and H antigens can also occur in refractory anemia.

8. *Polyagglutination*—Red cells may possess genetic or acquired surface abnormalities that render them polyagglutinable.

9. *Chimerism*—A chimera possesses a dual population of red cells, resulting in a classic mixed-field appearance on testing.

10. *Acquired B*—Acquired "B-like" activity can result from the action of gram-negative organisms.

11. *Abnormal proteins*—Abnormal proteins, altered proportions of globulins, and high concentrations of fibrinogen may cause rouleaux formation, which could be mistaken for agglutination.

12. *Blood group–specific substances*—In certain conditions (e.g., patients with ovarian cysts) blood group–specific substances may be of such high concentration that anti-A and anti-B are neutralized when unwashed red cells are used. At least three washes may be necessary before accurate results can be obtained.

13. *Irregular antibodies*—Besides unexpected antibodies reacting with A, B, or H antigens, irregular antibodies in some other blood group system may be present that react with antigens on the A or B cells used in reverse grouping.

14. *Unwashed cells*—The use of unwashed red cells can cause false positive results because of rouleaux-promoting properties in the subject's serum (e.g., in multiple myeloma).

15. *Hypogammaglobulinemia*—The first indication of hypogammaglobulinemia (decreased amounts of gamma-globulin) may be missing or weak reactions in serum (reverse) grouping due to low levels of anti-A and anti-B.

16. *Drugs, etc.*—Drugs, dextran, and intravenously injected contrast materials may cause cellular aggregation that resembles agglutination.

17. *Dyes*—Antibody to coloring dyes (e.g., acriflavine used in some countries as a yellow dye for anti-B reagents) can cause false positive results with anti-B. Such a discrepancy would be recognized, however, by the presence of anti-B in the serum.

18. *False reaction*—When testing with *Dolichos biflorus* extract it should be noted that the lectin will agglutinate strongly positive Sd(a+) red cells irrespective of ABO group, as well as Tn+ cells.

19. *Age*—Anomalous results may occur when testing an infant who has not begun to produce his own antibodies or who possesses antibodies that have been passively acquired from the mother or when testing an elderly person whose antibody levels have declined.

20. *Preservatives*—A patient may possess antibodies to elements of the preservatives, suspending mediums, or reagent solutions used in testing, resulting in errors in ABO group classification.

Steps in the Resolution of ABO Anomalies

Many of the anomalies in ABO testing can be resolved by obtaining a new sample of blood from the individual, carefully washing the cells, and repeating the tests. If problems are still encountered, the antibody screening tests, age, diagnosis, previous medications or transfusions, serum protein findings, antiglobulin test results, and auto-control may all help in establishing the cause. Rouleaux formation can often be diminished by adding additional saline to the cell-serum mixture. If anti-I is the cause, it is usually possible to auto-absorb the antibody, though this should not be attempted if the patient has been transfused with red cells in the preceding four weeks, since the antigens on the transfused cells may absorb a developing allo-antibody of clinical significance.

Weak examples of A or B can be diagnosed in many cases by testing the cells with many different samples of anti-A and anti-B, by incubating them at 18°C or 4°C before testing, by testing the cells for the ability to absorb antibody, by testing the eluate from absorbed cells for agglutinating activity against cells of other usual phenotypes, by testing the saliva, and by studying the blood and saliva from blood relatives to determine a possible hereditary pattern for the abnormality.

If polyagglutinability is suspected, various lectins can be employed to establish the different types.

THE LEWIS BLOOD GROUP SYSTEM

The Inheritance of Lewis Genes and the Expression of Lewis Antigens

In 1946, Mourant reported the discovery of the antibody anti-Le^a. The antithetical antibody, anti-Le^b, was described in 1948 by Andresen.

Lewis is a system of *soluble* antigens present in saliva and plasma; the determinants are not indigenous to the red cells. The red cells, however, *acquire* their Lewis phenotype by adsorption of Lewis substances from the plasma.

In 1955, Ceppellini showed that the presence of Le^a substances in saliva was controlled by a dominant gene, which he called *L*. The allele was originally called *l*, but both genes were later changed by Ceppellini and other workers to *Le* and *le*. The possible Lewis phenotypes in adults are Le(a+b−), Le(a−b+), and Le(a−b−). The Le(a+b+) phenotype is possessed by certain group O and A_2 subjects, although in these cases the reaction with anti-Le^a is usually weak and not consistent with all anti-Le^a sera.

The Lewis phenotype is controlled by the interaction of three sets of independently inherited genes, *Lele, Hh,* and *Sese*. Since Lewis substances (antigens) are formed only in secretions and plasma and not directly on red cells, the interaction of the three sets of genes actually determines which Lewis antigens will be in the serum and will therefore be adsorbed onto the red cells.

Individuals who inherit the *Le* gene can produce Le^a substance, and therefore (provided that they have not inherited either the *H* or *Se* genes) their red cells will have the phenotype Le(a+b−). For Le^b substance to be produced, *Le, H,* and *Se* genes must all be inherited, and the simultaneous presence of these three genes will produce the Le(a−b+) phenotype.

In each of the three systems, the alleles *le, h,* and *se* are amorphic and therefore produce no product. The red cells of *lele* individuals are Le(a−b−), since no Lewis substances can be made. The Le(a+b+) phenotype may be possessed by group O and A_2 individuals who possess the *H, Se,* and *Le* genes. Since the *Sese* genes are inherited independently and control only the secretion of ABO substances, Le(a−b−) indivduals may either inherit the *Se* gene and be secretors of ABH substances or be homozygous for the amorphic *se* gene and be nonsecretors of ABH substances.

In addition to the above, the Lewis phenotype may be modified by the ABO phenotype; e.g., in Le(b+) subjects, the A_1 gene may interfere with the expression of the Le^a antigen.

In summary, therefore

1. The phenotype Le(a+b−) is found in nonsecretors of ABH.
2. The phenotype Le(a−b+) is found in secretors of ABH.
3. The phenotype Le(a−b−) is found in individuals of genotype *lele*. These individuals are usually secretors, since the frequency of the *Se* gene is approximately 80%.
4. Le(a+b−) individuals (nonsecretors of ABH) secrete Le^a substance.
5. Le(a−b+) individuals secrete ABH, Le^a, and Le^b substances.

Characteristics of Lewis Antibodies

Anti-Le^a. Anti-Le^a is a fairly common antibody in human sera when compared with other red cell antibodies. It is found in secretors who are Le(a−b−) (i.e., *lele*). With rare exceptions, all examples of Lewis antibodies have the ability to bind complement and cause hemolysis in vitro. Most anti-Le^a sera also contain some weak anti-Le^b. Both antibodies are usually IgM, and they can be "non–red cell immune" (see p. 557), reacting best at temperatures below 37°C. Some examples are enhanced in the indirect antiglobulin test or through the use of the enzyme papain. Anti-Le^a is occasionally immune in origin and as such has been implicated in hemolytic transfusion reactions. The antibody has been produced in chickens, rabbits, and goats. These antibodies are either the precipitating or the agglutinating type.

Anti-Le^b. Anti-Le^b is usually produced in nonsecretors who are Le(a−b−) (i.e., *lele*). Potent anti-Le^b sera possess properties in common with anti-H, as follows:

1. They react more strongly with O and A_2 red cells.
2. Saliva that inhibits anti-H also inhibits anti-Le^b.
3. Most anti-Le^b antibodies are produced in A_1 or A_1B individuals.

There are two kinds of anti-Le^b sera:

1. Anti-Le^{bH}—This antibody is neutralized by the saliva of all ABH secretors and reacts only with A_2 and O red cells.
2. Anti-Le^{bL}—This antibody is not neutralized by the saliva of ABH secretors but is neutralized by the saliva of Le(a−b+) individuals and reacts with the red cells of all blood groups.

Both anti-Le^{bH} and anti-Le^{bL} are mostly IgM and can bind complement. It is rare for these antibodies to cause hemolytic transfusion reactions, and they have never been implicated in hemolytic disease of the newborn.

Lewis Antibodies and the Routine Blood Bank

Individuals with Lewis antibodies should ideally receive Le(a−b−) blood, when available, especially in the case of potent antibodies that cause in vitro hemolysis. In cases of weaker antibodies, blood of other phenotypes, i.e., Le(a+b−) or Le(a−b+), may be transfused, and these will rarely cause transfusion problems for the following reasons:

1. Lewis substances in plasma, when transfused to a recipient with Lewis antibodies, will wholly or partially neutralize the circulating antibodies.

TABLE 27–3 INTERPRETATION OF SALIVA TESTS FOR THE DETECTION OF LEWIS SUBSTANCES

Dilutions of Saliva				
1/1	**1/80**	**1/320**	**1/1280**	**Interpretation**
2+	2+	2+	2+	Le(a−b−)
—	—	—	1+	Le(a+b−)
—	—	1+	2+	Le(a−b+)

2. Tranfused Le(a+) and Le(b+) red cells lose their Lewis antigens within a few days of transfusion and become Le(a−b−).

In this regard, the injection of plasma in amounts sufficient to neutralize all detectable Lewis antibodies will allow sufficient normal survival of Le(a+b−) or Le(a−b+) blood.

Lewis antibodies are frequently found in pregnant women, but they do not cause hemolytic disease of the newborn, because they are predominantly IgM (and therefore do not cross the placenta) and because most infants type as Le(a−b−). The reason for the increase in the frequency of Lewis antibodies in pregnant women appears to be because Lewis antigens can become weaker through pregnancy to a point at which the woman may type as Le(a−b−).

Technique 5: The Detection of Le^a and Le^b Substances in Secretions (Saliva)

Method

1. Centrifuge saliva at approximately 3200 rpm (1000 G) for ten minutes and recover supernatant into a separate test tube.

2. Immerse the supernatant in a boiling water bath for ten minutes to inactivate the enzymes, which would otherwise inactivate the blood group substances.

3. Dilutions of saliva to be tested are then added to equal volumes of diluted anti-Le^a, mixed with Le(a+) red cells, and subsequently examined macroscopically for agglutination.

***Note:* It can be considered unnecessary to test for Le^b substance, since, when Le^a and H are present, its presence is inferred.**

4. Controls are of major importance. The negative control, saliva from a Le(a−b−) *(lele)* subject, must be carefully selected, since a small proportion of subjects whose red cells group as Le(a−b−) secrete Le^a substance in their saliva. Saliva from a subject of phenotype Le(a+b−) (or Le[a−b+]) may be used as a positive control.

5. Results are interpreted as shown in Table 27–3.

THE RHESUS BLOOD GROUP SYSTEM

The Rhesus system is second in importance to the ABO system.

In 1939, Levine and Stetson found in the serum of a mother of a stillborn fetus an unusual agglutinin that was found to agglutinate 80% of random ABO compatible donors. In 1940, Landsteiner and Wiener injected blood from the monkey *Maccacus rhesus* into rabbits and guinea pigs and found that the resulting antibody agglutinated the red cells of about 85% of human donors.

The two antibodies were considered to be the same. Individuals who possessed the corresponding antigen, therefore, were called Rh-positive, and individuals who lacked the antigen, Rh-negative. It is now known that rabbit anti-rhesus and human anti-Rh are not the same. The rabbit antibody was renamed anti-LW (after Landsteiner and Wiener), and the human antibody retained the title anti-Rh.

Fortuitously, the antibody first discovered (which became the subject of the historic researches just recounted) later proved to be the most common and important among a family of closely related antibodies. Though increased knowledge has in a sense increased the complexity of the whole problem, the fact remains that the antibody first discovered accounts for some 95% of all cases of Rh hemolytic disease of the newborn and Rh incompatibility.

As early as 1941 a new Rh-type antigen and antibody (C,rh′; anti-C, anti-rh′) was discovered by Wiener, Landsteiner, and Levine; in the same year Levine found a serum containing a further antibody (anti-c, anti-hr′) and noted that more than one antibody might occur in the same serum. Within a very short time, the new Rh blood group system was shown to be both independent of known blood group systems and inherited according to mendelian laws. Further alleles were discovered and confirmed independently by many workers, chiefly American and British.

Two theories of inheritance have been proposed for the Rhesus blood groups.

Nomenclatures and Genetic Theories

The Fisher-Race Nomenclature and Genetic Theory. The Fisher-Race genetic theory of Rh inheritance states that there are three closely linked loci, each with a primary set of allelic genes (*D* and *d*, *C* and *c*, *E* and *e*). These loci are so closely linked that crossing over rarely occurs. The Rh gene complex can therefore be assembled in eight different ways (*CDe, cDE, cde, cdE, Cde, CDE, cDe,* and *CdE*). Rh antigens are, therefore, named C, D, E, c, and e. The d antigen has not been discovered and is thought not to exist. The symbol "d" is used to denote the *absence* of D. Other antigens subsequently shown to be part of the Rh system have been classified using the same basic principles.

The Wiener Nomenclature and Genetic Theory. Wiener visualized an infinite number of alleles at a single complex locus, each locus determining its own agglutinogen, which is comprised of multiple factors. The alleles are named R^1, R^2, r, R^o, r', r'', R^z, and r^y. For example, the gene R^1 produces a complex antigen (agglutinogen), R_1, which is made up of at least three factors: rh′ (C), Rh_o (D), and hr′′ (e).

The Rosenfield Nomenclature. Rosenfield proposed a numerical nomenclature that is free of genetic implication. The antigens are numbered in order of discovery (D=Rh1, C=Rh2, E=Rh3, etc.). A comparison of the three nomenclatures is as follows:

Fisher-Race	Wiener	Rosenfield
D	Rh_o	Rh1
C	rh′	Rh2
E	rh″	Rh3
c	hr′	Rh4
e	hr″	Rh5

Owing to the multiplicity of Rhesus groups, the Rosenfield nomenclature, at the time of this writing, has reached Rh42.

Rh Inheritance

Rh inheritance is straightforward. The gene complex (e.g., R^1 or *CDe*) is directly passed on from generation to generation. An individual who is R^1r *(CDe/cde)*, therefore, will pass either R^1 *(CDe)* or *r (cde)* to his or her offspring.

The Rh complex has been assigned to chromosome number 1.

Frequencies

The frequencies of common antigens and genotypes in North American whites are as follows:

Antigen	Frequency
D	85%
C	70%
E	30%
c	80%
e	98%

Genotype	Frequency
R^1r	32.4%
R^1R^1	22.2%
rr	12%
R^1R^2	13%
R^2r	9.4%
R^2R^2	1.8%

The D^u (Rh_o^u) Allele

D^u is a "weak" form of the D antigen, giving some but not all of the reactions of the "normal" D antigen. D^u red cells are agglutinated by some anti-D sera but not by others. In some cases the weak antigen is determined genetically.

There are many grades of D^u. Lower grade D^u's are detectable only by the indirect antiglobulin test, whereas higher grade D^u's react with some but not all anti-D sera. Certain low grade D^u's may be detectable only by absorption and elution of anti-D from the red cells.

D^u may be directly inherited through an allele D^u at the Rh complex locus. Certain examples of D^u are the result of position effect exerted by *Cde* on a normal *D* gene in the opposite gene complex (i.e., in *trans* position). The *C* gene in *cis* position (i.e., on the same gene complex) may also weaken the expression of the D antigen. Alternatively, it has been suggested that the D antigen is not a single entity but a mosaic structure of different component parts, named A, B, C, and D. Individuals possessing all parts are classified as Rh^{ABCD}. Individuals who lack one or more of the component parts may produce an antibody corresponding to the missing part. About 50% of D^u samples lack one or more of the component parts of the D antigen. Tippett and Sanger classify Rh-positive individuals who produce anti-D into six categories.

D^u must be considered clinically significant. It has been implicated in both hemolytic transfusion reactions and in hemolytic disease of the newborn.

In the laboratory, a sample of blood is classified as D^u if it reacts with anti-D in the indirect antiglobulin test *only*. D^u red cells will not react with "genuine" saline anti-D. D^u subjects who are blood donors are classified as Rh_o (D)-positive. D^u subjects who are recipients of blood transfusion are most safely classified as Rh_o (D)-negative.

There is no specific anti-D^u serum.

Characteristics of Common Rh Antibodies

The majority of Rh antibodies are IgG (7S). A few anti-D sera contain IgM antibody (almost always accompanied by IgG antibody), and rare anti-D sera contain a minor IgA component. The IgG antibody molecules are predominantly of the IgG1 and IgG3 subclasses, although some are partly IgG2 or IgG4.

Non–red cell immune ("naturally occurring") anti-D is extremely rare, although several examples of non–red cell immune anti-E and a few examples of non–red cell immune anti-C have been described.

Rh antibodies are commonly stimulated by transfusion or pregnancy. Anti-Rh_o (D) is the most common Rh antibody formed, although Rh-negative blood is routinely used for transfusion to Rh-negative recipients and Rh-immune globulin is used to suppress Rh immunization during pregnancy. After anti-Rh_o (D), anti-G (anti-CD) is probably the most common Rh antibody formed, followed by anti-c and anti-E.

The majority of Rh antibodies do not bind complement, because the antigens are too far apart on the membrane to allow IgG molecules to collaborate with one another.

Rh antibodies are capable of causing severe hemolytic transfusion reactions and are a cause of hemolytic disease of the newborn. Rh-positive blood may be transfused to Rh-negative recipients who do not possess Rh antibodies in extreme emergency cases. This, however, should be avoided when possible, since up to 70% of such recipients will form anti-D following transfusion; it should be specifically avoided in transfusing women of child-bearing age. Large doses of Rh_o (D) immune globulin may be given to Rh-negative recipients of Rh-positive blood to suppress immunization.

Rh_o (D) Typing and Other Techniques

Rh_o (D) typing may be performed on a slide (tile) or in tubes, using saline-reactive or slide-and-rapid-tube reagents. In routine situations, cell typing involves only Rh_o (D), with full phenotyping being performed only in special circumstances. Controls of all tests are essential; with Rh_o (D) typing, a control using immunologically inert reagents must accompany each test. When using saline-reactive antisera, known positive and negative red cells should be included as controls.

Technique 6: Rh_o (D) Typing (Slide Technique)

Method

1. Place one drop of reagent anti-Rh_o (D) on a labeled slide.

2. Place one drop of albumin or other control medium on another labeled slide.

3. To each slide add two drops of well-mixed 40% to 50% suspension of red cells in plasma or serum.

4. Thoroughly mix the cell suspension and reagent, using a clean stick for each slide, and spread the mixture evenly over most of the slide.

5. Place both slides on a viewing surface (lighted); tilt gently and continuously to observe for agglutination. Do not allow cell mixture to come in contact with hands. *Note:* The viewing surface should be kept lighted at all times to preserve a temperature of 45 to 50°C. Reagents placed on a glass slide in contact with the surface should then reach 37°C (the optimum temperature for reaction) within two minutes.

Interpretation. A positive test has agglutination with anti-Rh_o (D) and a smooth suspension of cells in the control. A negative test has a smooth suspension of cells in both the "test" and the "control." If there is agglutination or irregularity in the control, the test results must be considered invalid, and a saline test must be performed.

Causes of False Reaction in Slide Tests

1. *False positives*—False positive reactions may be caused by the following:
   a. Drying on the slide, which may be confused with agglutination.
   b. Small fibrin clots, which may give the appearance of agglutination.
   c. Incompletely anticoagulated blood, which may clot on the heated slide.
2. *False negatives*—False negative reactions may be caused by the following:
   a. Saline-suspended cells, which react poorly or not at all.
   b. A cell suspension that is too weak (as in a severely anemic patient), which may cause cells to agglutinate poorly.
   c. Weakly active cells, which may take the full two minutes to agglutinate and may therefore be misinterpreted if read too soon.
   d. Reagents identified improperly at the time of use, which may result in the wrong reagent's being used in place of anti-Rh_o (D).

Technique 7: Rh_o (D) Typing (Tube Technique)

Method

1. Place one drop of antiserum in a tube labeled "test."

2. Place one drop of albumin or control medium in a tube labeled "control."

3. Add one or two drops (depending on manufacturer's directions) of a recommended cell suspension (usually 2 to 5%) in serum or saline to each tube, or use a clean, separate applicator stick to dislodge sufficient cells from the clot to approximate the cell volume of one drop of 5% suspension in each tube.

4. Mix well and centrifuge according to manufactuer's directions.

5. Gently resuspend the cell button and observe for agglutination. (*Note:* If an applicator stick was used to transfer the cells, the addition of one drop of saline to the tube before resuspending the cell button will provide more fluid and make resuspension and reading easier).

Interpretation. A positive test has agglutination with anti-Rh_o (D) and a smooth suspension of cells in the control. A negative test has a smooth suspension of cells in both the test and the control. If there is agglutination or irregularity in the control, the test results must be considered invalid and a saline test performed.

Causes of False Reaction in Tube Tests

1. *False positives*—False positive reactions may be caused by the following:
   a. The anti-Rh_o (D) used may contain, in addition to anti-Rh_o (D), antibodies of another specificity (e.g., anti-Bg).
   b. If an antibody complex (e.g., anti-G) is used instead of pure anti-Rh_o (D), red cells that lack the Rh_o (D) antigen but possess the C antigen will be agglutinated.
   c. If cells and serum remain together too long before the test is read, the high protein medium may produce rouleaux, which resemble agglutinates.
2. *False negatives*—False negative reactions may be caused by the following:
   a. Inadvertent failure to add the reagent.
   b. Failure to properly identify reagents, resulting in the wrong reagent's being used in place of anti-Rh_o (D).
   c. Cells and serum remaining together too long before the test is read, in which case antibody may elute from weakly reactive cells, and small agglutinates may disperse.

Technique 8: Rh_o (D) Typing (Saline Tube Test)

Method

1. Place one drop of saline-reactive anti-Rh_o (D) in a properly labeled test tube.

2. Add one drop of a 2 to 5% saline suspension of well-washed red cells.

3. Mix gently and incubate at 37°C (time of incubation according to manufacturer's directions).

4. Centrifuge (time and speed according to manufacturer's directions).

5. Gently resuspend the cell button and observe for agglutination. (*Note:* A saline suspension of known Rh_o (D)-positive and Rh_o (D)-negative cells should be run in parallel with the test as a control. Ensure that the concentration of cells in the control is comparable to that of the test cells).

Interpretation. Agglutination in the test indicates that the red cells are Rh_o (D)-positive. D^u cells will not normally be agglutinated. This test is performed only on recipients of transfusion; any seemingly negative recipient should be given Rh-negative blood. *Note:* Saline-reactive anti-Rh_o (D) cannot be used for D^u testing.

Tests for Other Rh Antigens

Both saline-reactive and slide or rapid tube test reagents are commercially available for the Rh antigens rh′ (C), rh″ (E), hr′ (c), and hr″ (e); they should be used according to the manufacturer's directions. Red cells that are known to be positive and negative should be used as controls, and these should be run in parallel with the test unless they are frequently used, in which case, they should be controlled as part of a daily program (see Chapter 28). A high-protein control should be used

TABLE 27–4 REACTIONS OF BLOODS WITH COMMON ANTISERA

Anti C Anti rh′	Anti c Anti hr	Anti D Anti Rh_0	Anti E Anti rh″	Commonest Genotype in Each Reaction Group: *Fisher-Race*	*Shorthand*	Calculated % Frequency of Each Reaction Group in England
+	+	+	−	CDe/cde	R_1r	34.9
+	−	+	−	CDe/CDe	R_1R_1	18.5
−	+	−	−	cde/cde	rr	15.1
−	+	+	+	cDE/cde	R_2r	14.1
+	+	+	+	CDe/cDE	R_1R_2	13.4
−	+	+	−	cDe/cde	R_0r	2.1
−	+	−	+	cdE/cde	r″r	0.9
+	+	−	−	Cde/cde	r′r	0.8
+	−	+	+	CDe/CDE	R_1R_z	0.2
+	+	−	+	cdE/Cde	r″r′	very small
+	−	−	−	Cde/Cde	r′r′	very small
Percentage frequency of positive reactions given by these sera						
68	81	83	29			

with slide or rapid tube test reagents, as for anti-Rh_o (D). It should be noted that these reagents may contain antiglobulin-reactive antibodies other than those specified on the label, and therefore, unless the instructions clearly indicate their suitability, these reagents should not be used in the antiglobulin test. (See Table 27–4.)

Other Causes of False Positive and False Negative Results in Rh Testing

1. *False positives*—False positive reactions in routine Rh typing may also be caused by:
   a. *Contaminating antibody*—A contaminating antibody with specificity other than that indicated by the label could cause false positive results. Although this is not a common problem, it must be kept in mind and tested for when using any reagent.
   b. *Polyagglutination*—Polyagglutinable red cells may be agglutinated by any human protein reagent, because the causative antibodies are present in all human serums. This situation will reveal itself through discrepant ABO cell and serum tests, except in the case of group AB red cells.
   c. *Serum-suspended cells from a patient with abnormal serum proteins*—This situation may cause rouleaux formation, which could be mistaken for agglutination. The situation will reveal itself in a positive albumin or reagent medium control and can be resolved by using well-washed saline-suspended red cells with saline-reactive reagents.
2. *False negatives*—False negative reactions in routine Rh typing can also be caused by:
   a. A reagent antibody that recognizes only a compound antigen and that will not react with red cells that carry the individual specific antigens as separate gene products [e.g., anti-hr (f) or ce] will give negative results with R^1R^2 *(CDe/cDE)* red cells or any other cells on which the hr″ (e) antigen is part of a gene product that does not include the compound antigen. A well-defined quality-control program should obviate the problem.
   b. Red cells with variant antigens (e.g., C^w, ce^s) may fail to react with standard reagents. There is no easy way to detect this problem, which may only reveal itself in family studies or in the investigation of antibody that is directed against the variant.

OTHER BLOOD GROUP SYSTEMS

THE Ii BLOOD GROUP SYSTEM

In 1956, Wiener and co-workers recognized the specificity of a previously known cold agglutinin thought to be nonspecific by showing that a particular example of the antibody was compatible with 5 out of 22,000 donor red cell samples. The antibody was called anti-I and the corresponding antigen, I. Rare individuals who appeared to lack the antigen were classified as belonging to phenotype "i," and subsequent studies led to the discovery of anti-i by Marsh and Jenkins in 1960.

Inheritance

Infants rarely possess the I antigen: most appear to be of phenotype i. During the first eighteen months of life, the red cells gradually come to react strongly with anti-I and weakly with anti-i. The I reactivity then appears to be retained by healthy persons throughout life.

The I antigen has a mosaic structure:

I^F (fetal) is that part of the antigen present in fetal red cells and in the red cells of i-adults.

I^D (developed) is that part of the antigen which is developed after the first eighteen months of life.

Therefore, the genes that control Ii specificity are believed to be involved in assisting with the development of i into I.

Nomenclature

I-adult. The I antigen in random adults shows a great range of strength, yet the I antigen strength of one individual's red cells appears to have a constant level.

The red cells of almost all healthy adults have the I antigen.

I-cord. Very weak reactions can be obtained with powerful anti-I and cord red cells. There are both qualitative and quantitative differences in the I antigen of cord (and adult) red cells.

i-adult and i-cord. Red cells that fail completely to react with anti-I are classed as i_1. Red cells that have a small amount of I antigen are classed as i_2. The phenotype i_1 is found mainly in whites, whereas the phenotype i_2 is found mainly in blacks. The i_1 and i_2 phenotypes can be distinguished by absorption tests: anti-I is not absorbed from an i_1 donor with i_2 red cells.

Characteristics of Antibodies

Anti-I is a common autoantibody in patients suffering from acquired hemolytic anemia of the cold antibody type and is also found as a weak cold agglutinin in the serum of "normal" individuals. Allo–anti-I is rare but is found in the serum of most i subjects. In i_1 individuals, the antibody fails to react with i_1 and i_2 red cells. In i_2 individuals, the antibody does react (though weakly) with i_2 red cells, and these cells can absorb some anti-I from these sera. Allo–anti-I does not reveal the gradation of antigen strength in I people. Virtually all anti-I antibodies are IgM and have the ability to bind complement. Anti-I cold agglutinins commonly show a transient increase in titer following infection by *Mycoplasma pneumonia,* which (in occasional patients) results in an episode of hemolytic anemia.

Anti-i is a cold agglutinin, usually IgM but sometimes IgG. The antibody has not been described as an alloantibody. All examples so far described have been autoantibodies. Transient anti-i has been found in the serum of individuals suffering from infectious mononucleosis. An antibody presumed to be anti-i has also been found to be not uncommon in patients suffering from alcoholic cirrhosis.

Anti-I has never been implicated as a cause of hemolytic disease of the newborn (since it is invariably IgM). Most examples of anti-I do not cause hemolytic transfusion reactions; however, occasional examples that react at 30–37°C in vitro produce variable degrees of destruction of red cells in vivo that are well correlated with their thermal range in vitro.

Anti-i has very rarely been implicated as the cause of hemolytic disease of the newborn, but it has not been known to cause hemolytic transfusion reaction.

The P Blood Group System

The P blood group system was discovered by Landsteiner and Wiener as an unexpected by-product of the experiments in which the MN groups were discovered. Human red cells were injected into rabbits, and the resulting immune rabbit serum, upon subsequent testing, was found to agglutinate some samples of human red cells and not others. The two types of blood were called P+ and P−. The antibody, anti-P, was found in human serum soon afterwards.

In 1951, Levine and co-workers discovered the antigen Tj^a, which was shown, in 1955, to be part of the P system. The antigen P later became the antigen P_1 when it was discovered that individuals who produce anti-Tj^a were P-negative. It was then realized that P-negative individuals share a powerful antigen with P-positive individuals and do not lack an antigen of the P system as was originally thought.

In light of this discovery, the notation of the P system was modified as follows:

The P-positive phenotype became P_1.
The P-negative phenotype became P_2.
Anti-P became anti-P_1.

Inheritance

The P_1 antigen is believed to be inherited as a dominant mendelian character. Individuals of phenotype P_2 are regarded as possessing a silent (amorphic) gene, P_2.

Characteristics of Antigens

The antigen P_1 occurs in a wide variety of strengths. It has been suggested that the differences in strength of the antigen is an inherited phenomenon. The phenotype "p," originally classified as Tj(a−), is extremely rare. All individuals of this phenotype have anti-PP_1P^k (anti-Tj^a) in their serum. The inheritance of this phenotype is unclear, although homozygosity for a third silent allele *(p)* or homozygosity for a regulator gene at some other locus have been suggested as possible explanations.

Characteristics of Antibodies

Anti-P_1 is present in the serum of two thirds of random P_2 individuals, usually as a cold-reacting agglutinin and usually weak. In pregnant women who are P_2, the incidence of anti-P_1 has been found to be almost 90%, even though the antibody is not associated with alloimmunization in pregnancy. Anti-P_1 can occur as a non–red cell immune antibody in human serum, although it is usually stimulated by transfusion. The antibody is usually a cold-reacting IgM agglutinin, although a few examples react at 37°C. These warm agglutinins may fix complement.

Anti-P (Donath-Landsteiner Antibody). In paroxysmal cold hemoglobinuria, the patient's serum contains an antibody that reacts in the cold and classically has anti-P specificity. The antibody, which is known as the Donath-Landsteiner (DL) antibody (after its discoverers), produces hemolysis both in vivo and in vitro when the blood is first cooled and then warmed. The DL antibody has also been found in other disease states (syphilis, following measles and mumps, chickenpox, and so forth), and in these conditions it does not always have anti-P specificity. The DL antibody (i.e., of anti-P specificity) is always IgG.

Clinical Significance

Anti-P_1 can cause severe adverse transfusion reactions, although the destruction of P_1 red cells by anti-P_1 is described as "occasional." Examples of anti-P_1 that sensitize red cells to anti-complement serum should be regarded as clinically significant. Anti-P_1 has not been implicated as a cause of hemolytic disease of the newborn.

THE MNSs BLOOD GROUP SYSTEM

The MNSs blood group system was discovered through the injection of human red cells into rabbits and subsequent absorption of the resulting rabbit serum, which was then tested against other human red cells. As a result of this work (by Landsteiner and Wiener), the M and N (and P) antigens were discovered. During the next thirty years, several rare antigens were discovered, some of which were shown to be alleles of *M* and *N*. The antigen S was discovered in 1947, and the anticipated antithetical antigen, s, was discovered in 1951. In 1954, Greenwalt and colleagues discovered that less than 1% of black blood samples lacked both S and s.

Inheritance

It was originally proposed that two allelic genes, *M* and *N*, determine the presence of the M and N antigens, allowing for three possible genotypes *(MM, MN,* and *NN)* and three phenotypes (M, MN, and N). The recognition of *S* and *s* enlarges the original theory to encompass two sets of allelic genes. The genes *M, N, S,* and *s* are inherited as dominant genes. It has been suggested that N is a precursor of M, although this has not been proved and opposing viewpoints have been expressed.

Characteristics of Antigens

The M and N antigens are glycoproteins and appear to depend on the presence of sialic acid in appropriate linkages, although there is little information on the structures differentiating M and N specificity. It has been concluded, however, the sialic acid is an essential part of the M and N receptors.

The M, N, S, and s antigens are well developed at birth.

Characteristics of Antibodies

Anti-M occurs usually as a cold agglutinin reacting best at 4°C and weakly or not at all at 37°C. The antibody is usually IgG, although examples that are IgM are also frequently found. IgG anti-M may react strongly with albumin or serum-suspended red cells and in some cases may react as well at 37°C as at 4°C. Strong dosage effect occurs with anti-M whereby the antibody may react only with homozygous *(MM)* red cells. Certain examples of anti-M bind complement, though they do not cause in vitro lysis. Anti-M will not react in an enzyme medium because of the effect of enzymes on sialic acid. The antibody may cause the destruction of transfused M-positive red cells, although hemolytic disease of the newborn due to anti-M is rare. Anti-M is also found in the seeds of the plant *Iberis amara*.

Anti-N is found almost exclusively in S-s-individuals. Most examples are non–red cell immune and are typically IgM cold agglutinins that are inactive at temperatures above 20 to 25°C. Immune anti-N is extremely rare. Anti-N will agglutinate M-positive (N-negative) red cells at temperatures of 23°C or lower and will also agglutinate trypsin-treated M-positive (N-negative) red cells. The antibody fails to react with red cells of phenotype MS^u, and the reaction strength between anti-N and M-positive red cells is influenced by the Ss group of the red cells.

Patients on renal dialysis may develop anti-N that is reactive at 4°C and 20°C but never at 37°C. This antibody is believed to be stimulated by small numbers of red cells left in the dialysis equipment that are denatured by formol treatment. This antigen, formed by formaldehyde treatment, is known as "formaldehyde N." Anti-N often shows dosage and may react only with NN red cells. Most examples of the antibody do not bind complement or cause in vitro lysis. The reaction of anti-N is inhibited by enzymes, though trypsin serves to enhance the cross-reaction between anti-N and MM red cells.

Mild hemolytic disease of the newborn has been reported that was due to anti-N, although this is extremely unusual. The antibody has not been implicated as a cause of hemolytic transfusion reactions but must be considered significant when it is reactive at temperatures above 30°C.

Several lectins have anti-N specificity, the most notable of which is the seeds of the plant *Vicia graminea*.

Anti-S is commonly found as an immune antibody in multitransfused patients, although examples that are non–red cell immune have been reported. Most examples of anti-S are IgG. Some examples have the ability to bind complement but do not appear to have the ability to cause in vitro lysis. Anti-S has been implicated in hemolytic transfusion reactions and in hemolytic disease of the newborn.

Anti-s is usually IgG, yet it reacts more strongly at low temperatures than at high temperatures. A few examples appear to bind complement, but most do not. Anti-s has been implicated as a cause of hemolytic transfusion reactions and of hemolytic disease of the newborn.

THE DUFFY BLOOD GROUP SYSTEM

Anti-Fy^a was first described by Cutbush, Mollison, and Parkin in 1950. A year later, anti-Fy^b was described by Ikin and colleagues. The Fy^a antigen was found to occur in 66% of random whites, and the Fy^b antigen was found to occur in 80% of random whites. The majority of blacks are of phenotype Fy(a-b-), a phenotype rarely found in whites.

Inheritance

The genes Fy^a and Fy^b are codominant alleles. The phenotype Fy(a-b-) in blacks is believed to be caused by a third allele, *Fy,* although it has been suggested that this phenotype may be due to the inheritance of an independent modifying gene that inhibits the expression of the Fy^a and Fy^b genes. Whites who appear to be Fy(a-b-) are believed to be homozygous for the gene Fy^x, which makes a small amount of Fy^b antigen. The Fy^x gene is more common in the heterozygous state in whites.

The Duffy locus was assigned to chromosome number 1 in 1963.

Nomenclature

A numerical nomenclature for the Duffy antigens has been devised. Under this system, the Fy^a and Fy^b antigens (names that are still generally used) become Fy1 and Fy2.

Characteristics of Antigens

The antigens Fy^a (Fy1) and Fy^b (Fy2) are the main antithetical antigen pair in the system. Both antigens have low antigenicity. Enzymes markedly reduce or eliminate the activity of the red cell Fy^a and Fy^b receptors.

Duffy antigens do not exist naturally in a soluble form. The Fy^a and Fy^b determinants are thermolabile (they are inactivated by heating red cells to 56°C for 10 minutes), and they are also denatured by treatment with formaldehyde, indicating that they are protein in nature. The Fy^a and Fy^b receptors on the red cell membrane are considered to be associated with susceptibility to malaria.

Characteristics of Antibodies

Most examples of anti-Fy^a are IgG, detectable mainly in the indirect antiglobulin test. About 50% of examples bind complement. Only very rare examples of non–red cell immune anti-Fy^a have been reported.

Anti-Fy^b is most often IgG. Some examples of this antibody show dosage. There has not been a report of a non–red cell immune anti-Fy^b.

The activity of some anti-Fy^a and anti-Fy^b sera is enhanced by reducing the ionic strength of the surrounding medium and by lowering the pH.

Incompatibility involving anti-Fy^a may cause severe hemolytic transfusion reactions, and the antibody has been shown to be a cause of hemolytic disease of the newborn. Anti-Fy^b has also been implicated as the cause of a fatal hemolytic transfusion reaction, but it has not been implicated as the cause of hemolytic disease of the newborn. The antibody has been known to disappear from the sera of immunized patients within a few months of detection, thus producing the conditions for possible delayed hemolytic transfusion reaction.

THE KELL BLOOD GROUP SYSTEM

The Kell blood group system was discovered by Coombs, Mourant, and Race in 1946 through the detection of an antibody (anti-K) in the serum of a mother who had given birth to a child suffering from hemolytic disease of the newborn. The antibody was found to sensitize the blood of her husband and about 7 to 9% of random blood samples. The antibody defining the antithetical antigen, k, was discovered three years later by Levine and co-workers.

Nomenclature

The antigens of the Kell blood group system were originally named after the individuals in whom the antibodies were first found. A numerical nomenclature, patterned after the Rosenfield nomenclature, has been suggested and is now generally used; under it, K becomes K1 and k becomes K2.

Characteristics of Antigens

The antigen K (K1) is found in 7 to 9% of random whites who possess the genotype, *KK* (0.2%) or *Kk* (99.8%). The gene responsible for the K antigen is directly inherited and is codominant with its allele, *k*. K-positive and k-positive individuals, therefore, must have at least one parent who is K-positive or k-positive, respectively. Both the K (K1) and k (K2) antigens are highly antigenic.

Characteristics of Antibodies

Anti-K. Non–red cell immune anti-K (-K1) is rare, though as an immune IgG antibody, it stands secondary in frequency to antibodies of the ABO and Rh systems. The antibody is usually detected by the antiglobulin technique at 37°C, though some examples are detected by enzyme techniques. Many examples of anti-K (anti-K1) will also react in saline if a slide technique is used with red cells suspended in their own serum. Anti-K1 sometimes shows the ability to bind complement, though it is incapable of causing in vitro lysis. The antibody has been implicated as the cause of both hemolytic disease of the newborn and hemolytic transfusion reaction. It usually results from direct stimulation by transfusion or pregnancy. Because the antigen frequency is low, little difficulty is encountered in obtaining K-negative units for transfusion.

Anti-k. When this rare antibody occurs, it is usually IgG and is detectable by the antiglobulin technique. It has been implicated as the cause of both hemolytic disease of the newborn and hemolytic transfusion reactions. It is always stimulated by transfusion or pregnancy.

THE KIDD BLOOD GROUP SYSTEM

The antibody anti-Jk^a was discovered by Allen and associates in 1951 in the serum of a mother whose child suffered from hemolytic disease of the newborn. The corresponding antigen, Jk^a, was found to be present in about 77% of white donors. Anti-Jk^b, which recognized the antithetical antigen, Jk^b, was discovered in 1953 by Plaut and associates.

In 1959, the phenotype Jk (a-b-) was discovered. It was presumed to be due to a third, silent allele, *Jk*. Some Jk(a-b-) individuals possess an antibody giving reactions of anti-Jk^a plus anti-Jk^b; the antibody is known as anti-Jk3.

Inheritance

Jk^a and Jk^b are inherited as mendelian codominants. The most common phenotype in whites is Jk(a+b+), whereas the phenotype Jk(a+b−) is more common in blacks.

Characteristics of Antibodies

Anti-Jk^a. Most examples of anti-Jk^a have been found to be IgG, although occasional examples have been shown to be IgM. The antibody, therefore, is most commonly detected in the antiglobulin and enzyme techniques. The antibody commonly (probably always) binds complement. In fact, it does this so readily that strong examples in fresh serum may actually lyze incompatible red cells during incubation. If the supernatant serum is not examined for hemolysis before the indirect antiglobulin test is performed, there is a risk of overlooking the antibody. Anti-Jk[a] has only rarely been the cause of hemolytic disease of the newborn and of a hemolytic transfusion reaction. It is usually the direct result of stimulation by transfusion or pregnancy.

It should be noted that Kidd antibodies are extremely labile, both in vivo and in vitro. Because of this, they are frequently involved in delayed transfusion reactions (i.e., the antibody may not be detectable in a crossmatch, but may rapidly reappear as a secondary response after transfusion, causing red cell destruction a few days after transfusion).

Anti-Jk[b]. Anti-Jk[b] is usually found in sera that also contain other immune antibodies. It is detectable by the antiglobulin or enzyme techniques and is usually IgG. All examples bind complement. The antibody has been implicated in both hemolytic disease of the newborn and in hemolytic transfusion reaction.

CHAPTER 27—REVIEW QUESTIONS

1. Discuss the genetics of the Lewis blood group system, emphasizing the differences between it and other blood group systems. Include in this discussion the interaction of the genes *Lele, Hh,* and *Sese.*
2. Compare the Fisher-Race and Wiener genetic theories of Rh inheritance, then prepare a table giving the comparative symbols for the five most important antigens in the system (C,D,E,c,e) according to the Fisher-Race, Wiener, and Rosenfield nomenclatures.
3. Write a short paragraph comparing the terms *genotype* and *phenotype.*
4. Describe the sequence of complement activation by the alternative pathway.

PRACTICE OF IMMUNOHEMATOLOGY

BLOOD DONATIONS

The Selection of Blood Donors

The following are the primary criteria for the selection of blood donors:

Age. Prospective blood donors must be within the age limits of 18 to 65.

History of Jaundice. Prospective blood donors should not have a history of viral hepatitis; they should not have received a transfusion of blood or blood products in the last six months; they should not have been in close contact with a case of hepatitis in the last six months. If a donor's blood is suspected of having been responsible for a case of posttransfusion hepatitis, that donor should not be accepted. The prospective donor should not be a known or suspected drug addict (i.e., injected drugs), nor should he or she have been tattooed within the past six months. Ear piercing, especially if performed under questionable conditions, is also reason for deferment. In addition, donors must be rejected if their blood has been found to contain HB_sAg.

Body Weight. Prospective blood donors should weigh at least 110 lbs (50 kg) to be eligible to give a full donation.

History of Malaria. Donors who have had malaria should be deferred for three years after becoming asymptomatic (or after therapy is discontinued). Individuals who have traveled or lived in areas considered endemic for malaria should be deferred for three years after leaving the area.

Present or Recent Illness or Surgery. Although knowledge of specific conditions of recent illness or surgery is not required, prospective donors with long-term illnesses should be excluded. In most other cases of illness, the donor should be rejected until he or she is free of all signs and symptoms and has been so for a period of time (2 to 3 weeks). Donors who have undergone surgery, hospitalization, or illness requiring the care of a physician should be deferred—the period of deferment being dependent on the particular illness involved in each case. Donors who have colds, influenza, or a tooth extraction should be deferred for at least a week. Donors with known drug allergies or with severe allergies to other substances should be rejected. Donors receiving scheduled drugs (particularly antihypertensive agents, antimicrobials, and corticosteroids) should also be rejected.

Recent Immunization. Prospective donors who have recently been immunized (inoculated) should be deferred for at least one week or until any symptoms have subsided. Recipients of inoculations that involve animal agents should be deferred for three months.

Hemoglobin. The hemoglobin of prospective donors should be at least 12.5 g/dL (125 g/L). This should be checked immediately before donation by using the "copper sulfate" test. The copper sulfate solution should have a specific gravity of 1.053, because blood with a hemoglobin concentration of 12.5 g/dL (125 g/L) or greater will sink in this solution.

Frequency of Donation. In general, donors should not donate more than four times a year, although this will depend on the policy of the collecting clinic. It is generally agreed that females should donate less frequently than males because of the loss of blood that occurs during normal menstruation, which may average out to the equivalent of one blood donation per year.

Procedure for the Collection of Blood Donations

1. Place a sphygmomanometer cuff on the donor's arm above the proposed site of venipuncture and raise the pressure to 20 to 40 mm of mercury.

2. Thoroughly cleanse the proposed site of venipuncture, using a disinfectant with rapid bactericidal action. A 0.5% tincture of chlorhexidine diacetate (colored with basic fuschin to demarcate the area of application), a 1% tincture of iodine, or a 1% PVP-iodine tincture is satisfactory.

3. Place the donor pack on an automatic scale, threading the tubing through the notches on the scale lever. The blood pack must be below the level of the donor so that the blood does not have to flow against normal gravity.

4. Raise the pressure in the sphygmomanometer cuff to 60 to 80 mm of mercury and ask the donor to clench his or her fist so as to distend the veins.

5. Insert the needle.

6. As soon as blood enters the tubing, expel the bead that prevents fluid from entering the unit. Reduce the pressure in the sphygmomanometer cuff to 40 mm of mercury and attach the appropriate labels to the blood pack and specimen tube(s).

7. Carefully mix the anticoagulant with the blood as it flows into the pack.

8. When donation is complete, apply forceps to the tubing near the pack, reduce the pressure in the sphygmomanometer cuff to 0 mm of mercury, and remove the needle from the vein.

9. Ask the donor to maintain pressure on the vein with a dry, clean cotton swab for ten minutes, keeping the arm extended during this period. Ensure that the bleeding has ceased before allowing the donor to remove this swab.

10. Collect the necessary specimens for testing, seal the pack, and prepare four or five segments for testing purposes by sealing the tubing that is attached to the pack. The blood, once collected, may be allowed to cool for a short period of time at room temperature before it is refrigerated. This period of time should not exceed one hour.

Testing of Blood Donations

Before being released for transfusion purposes, all blood donations are tested as follows:

Donor's Red Cells

1. ABO grouping (forward, including anti-A, B).
2. Rh$_o$(D) typing (by enzyme methods or slide and rapid tube methods). All Rh$_o$(D) negative units are confirmed, then tested with anti-CD and anti-DE. D^u tests are performed on all r′ and r″ units.

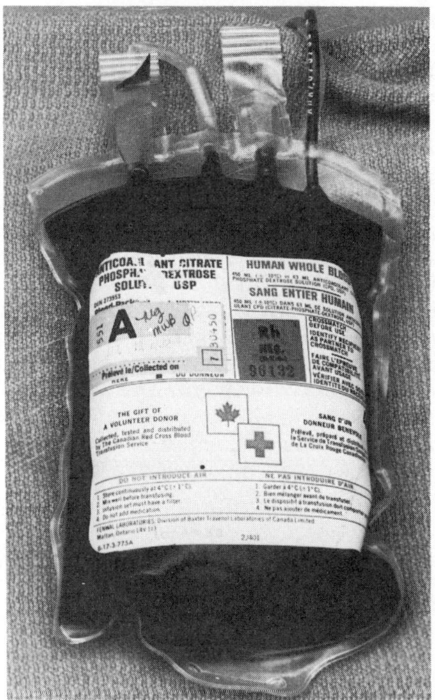

Figure 28–1 CPD blood pack unit.

Donor's Serum

1. Reverse ABO grouping.
2. Antibody screening tests using enzyme and antiglobulin methods.
3. VDRL tests (for syphilis).
4. HB$_s$Ag and HB$_s$Ab tests.

BLOOD COMPONENTS

Whole Blood

Storage Requirements. Proper storage conditions are essential if survival time of stored red cells is to be kept at a maximum. Units should be kept at a constant temperature of 4°C (±1°C), since at this temperature bacterial growth and cell metabolism are reduced. Temperatures of 2°C were claimed to be better by some workers; however, at 2°C, the white cells and platelets become irreversibly clumped. Blood kept below 4°C is also more likely to clog the pores of administration set filters.

At temperatures below 2°C, red cells are swollen by the effects of dextrose, become extremely fragile, and are likely to hemolyze. At temperatures above 10°C, bacterial growth is increased, and cell survival is decreased by as much as 20 per cent.

The Effects of Storage. The effects of storage on whole blood are numerous. Even when blood is stored at a constant temperature of 4°C in CPD (Citrate Phosphate Dextrose anticoagulant) or ACD (Acid Citrate Dextrose anticoagulant), cell deterioration begins within a few days of collection. The cells gradually lose their ability to metabolize glucose; they suffer a loss of potassium to the plasma, the osmotic and mechanical fragility is increased, and there is a loss of membrane lipid. The in vivo survival is diminished: 5 per cent of the red cells are lost after one week's storage, 10 to 15 per cent after two weeks, and 15 to 30 per cent after three weeks. The addition of Adenine (Adenine CPD) will prolong the acceptable shelf life of red cells to 35 days.

There is a decrease in the level of 2,3-diphosphoglycerate (2,3-DPG) and adenosine triphosphate (ATP) on storage. Concentrations of 2,3-DPG are better maintained in CPD stored blood throughout the storage period than in ACD stored blood because of the higher pH. Concentrations of ATP are initially better maintained in ACD (because of the lower pH), though late in storage ATP concentrations are frequently higher in CPD stored blood, probably because of the extra 2 millimoles of phosphate in CPD solutions.

When blood is stored at 4°C, the normal physiological transport of sodium and potassium across the red cell membrane is almost stopped: as storage continues, however, intracellular and extracellular concentrations of sodium and potassium tend toward equilibrium. Within 24 hours after transfusion, red cells stored in CPD correct their sodium imbalance. The potassium content, however, does not become normal for more than six days.

Applications. Whole blood is indicated primarily when a patient has blood loss severe enough to cause symptoms of hypovolemia. Less acute hemorrhage or anemia may be effectively treated with concentrated red cells. There is little justification for the routine use of whole blood. (See Table 28–1.)

TABLE 28–1 Blood Components and Their Use

Blood Component	Use
Fresh whole blood	Acute blood loss requiring massive replacement
Stored whole blood	Acute blood loss
Packed red cells	Correction of anemia
Platelet concentrate	Functional or quantitative platelet defects
Leukocyte poor blood	For individuals with leukocyte antibodies
Washed red cells	To circumvent reactions caused by plasma antigens
Cryoprecipitate	Factor VIII deficiency, von Willebrand's disease
Factor VIII concentrate	Factor VIII deficiency
Fresh frozen plasma	Coagulation factor defects
Serum albumin	Burns, protein depletion, blood volume restorer
II-VII-X-IX Concentrate	Correction of vitamin K dependent factor deficiencies
Factor IX concentrate	Factor IX deficiency
Gamma globulin	Hypogammaglobulinemia, etc.

Plasma (Fresh Frozen and Stored)

Storage Requirements

Fresh Frozen Plasma. Fresh frozen plasma is separated from red cells after centrifugation at 4°C and is frozen as rapidly as possible. The product is stored at −30°C for a maximum of 12 months or at −20°C for a maximum of 3 months.

Stored Plasma. Stored plasma is obtained from whole blood during the first 72 hours of storage at 4°C or is derived from the supernatant plasma after cryoprecipitate production. It may be stored at 4°C for a maximum of 21 days, or may be frozen and stored for up to 24 months.

Effects of Storage

Fresh Frozen Plasma. Deterioration of fresh frozen plasma does occur during storage, although there is no general agreement as to its extent. Storage periods are primarily observed because of the deterioration of labile clotting factors (the principal use of fresh frozen plasma) during storage.

Stored Plasma. Although plasma does not deteriorate greatly on storage, the periods of storage are observed because of the risk of contamination of the unit.

Applications

Fresh Frozen Plasma. Fresh frozen plasma is used for the treatment of deficiencies of labile coagulation factors when concentrated preparations are not available or are not indicated (e.g., mild congenital and acquired deficiencies, transfusion-induced dilution of labile factors) and in combination with concentrated red cells when "fresh whole blood" is required.

Stored Plasma. Stored plasma is effective in the treatment of patients requiring volume or protein replacement: It is also used in cases of burns, hypovolemic shock, coagulation factor deficiencies (other than factor V and VIII), and anticoagulant (vitamin K antagonist) reversal.

Stored plasma is also used as a pump prime for extracorporeal circulation and for the reconstitution of concentrated red cells. (*Note:* Both indications are very rarely clinically necessary.)

Red Blood Cells (Packed Red Cells, Red Cell Concentrates)

Storage Requirements. When red cell concentrates are prepared in a "closed" system with appropriate multiple packs, the sterility of the unit is not affected and the concentrate may be stored for the same period of time as whole blood. If, however, the unit has been entered during preparation, the blood should be administered as soon as possible to avoid multiplication of bacteria that may have gained entry during the collection procedure.

Effects of Storage. Storage of red cell concentrates results in the same deterioration as noted above (see *Storage Requirements, Whole Blood*), provided that the concentrates are prepared in a closed system.

Applications. Red cell concentrates are indicated in all situations in which it is important to increase the hematocrit level with the least disturbance of blood volume (i.e., in cases of anemia as well as many other conditions). Red cell concentrates should be used in preference to whole blood in the vast majority of cases, since they have the following advantages over whole blood:

1. They minimize the possibility of circulatory overload.

TABLE 28–2 CHARACTERISTICS OF WHOLE BLOOD AND RED CELL CONCENTRATES PER UNIT

Characteristic	Whole Blood	Packed Cells
Volume, mL	500 ± 25	300 ± 25
Hematocrit %	40 ± 5	70 ± 5
Red cell volume, mL	200 ± 25	200 ± 25
Plasma volume, mL	300 ± 25	100 ± 25
Albumin content, g	10–12	4–5

(From Herst, R., and Shepherd, F. A. (eds.): Clinical Guide To Transfusion—Products and Practices. Toronto, The Canadian Red Cross Society Blood Transfusion Service, 1979.)

2. They reduce the incidence of transfusion reactions from donor antibodies.

3. They reduce the volume of anticoagulant and electrolytes transfused.

4. They minimize the incidence of transfusion reactions to plasma components.

5. They permit each blood donation to be used as components and fractions in more than one individual.

A comparison of the characteristics of whole blood and red cell concentrates per unit is given in Table 28–2.

Frozen Red Cells

Storage Requirements. Red cells frozen in high concentration glycerol are stored at −65°C or below and preferably −80°C. The duration of storage under these conditions is three years to ten years. Red cells frozen in low concentration glycerol must be stored in the vapor stage of liquid nitrogen at −150°C, and as such may be stored for ten years. Once thawed, the red cells should be stored at 4°C for no longer than 24 hours.

Effects of Storage. Red cells stored in a frozen state do not undergo notable deterioration.

Applications. Frozen-thawed red cells may be used for the following purposes:

1. To minimize severe allergic transfusion reactions.
2. For patients who have IgA–anti-IgA reactions.
3. In cases of paroxysmal nocturnal hemoglobinuria.
4. To minimize sensitization to leukocyte and platelet antigens in prospective transplant patients.
5. For the provision of "rare" blood.
6. For the provision of blood for autologous transfusion.

Human Serum Albumin

Storage Requirements. Human serum albumin (normal serum albumin) is prepared from normal human plasma by cold ethanol plasma fractionation and is available in 5% or 25% concentrations. The 25% concentration should be stored at between 2 and 8°C and should not be frozen. The 5% concentration should be stored at room temperature (which must not exceed, at any time, 37°C) and also should not be frozen. The shelf life for both products is about three years—and the expiry date should be strictly observed.

Effects of Storage. If properly stored, human serum albumin should not undergo any notable deterioration during its shelf life.

Applications. Human serum albumin may be used for the following purposes:

1. In cases of shock due to hemorrhage or surgery.
2. As a fluid replacement during manual or automated therapeutic plasma exchange.
3. To promote a diuresis in edema due to hypoproteinemia.
4. In cases of neonatal hyperbilirubinemia.

It should be noted that unless the pathological conditions responsible for the hypoproteinemia can be corrected, the infusion of human serum albumin will promote only a transient benefit to the patient. The following are some of the complications of the infusion of human serum albumin:

1. Pyrogenic, allergic, or hypotensive reactions (which occur rarely). The symptoms of these reactions usually disappear when the infusion is slowed or stopped.
2. Dilutional anemia (which may occur particularly if the albumin is given for volume replacement after hemorrhage).

It should be noted that human serum albumin is contraindicated for patients in whom a rapid increase in circulating blood volume may be deleterious.

Gamma Globulin (Immune Serum Globulin)

Storage Requirements. Immune serum globulin (gamma globulin) may be stored at 2 to 8°C for two years without notable deterioration.

Applications. Immune serum globulin is given to provide *passive* antibody protection after exposure to certain disease states and also for prophylaxis in congenital antibody and immune deficiency disorders. The product is effective in cases of exposure to the following:

1. Measles (rubeola).
2. Hepatitis A (infectious hepatitis).
3. Hypogammaglobulinemia (*Note:* congenital immune deficiency disorders can be treated by monthly injections of human serum globulin; the effect in acquired hypogammaglobulinemia in less well documented).

Factor VIII Concentrate; Antihemophilic Factor, AHF (Cryoprecipitate)

Storage Requirements. Fractionated factor VIII is obtained by fractionation of pooled fresh frozen plasma. As a lyophilized preparation, it may require refrigeration storage at 2 to 8°C and should not be frozen. It may also be stored at room temperature for limited periods of time. Frozen concentrate (cryoprecipitate) is stored at −18°C or lower for a period of twelve months from the date of blood collection.

Applications. Concentrated factor VIII is used in cases of hemophilia A (congenital factor VIII deficiency) and in cases of acquired factor VIII inhibitors. The lyophilized high-purity fractions do not contain significant concentrations of von Willebrand's factor and are therefore not recommended in von Willebrand's disease. It should be noted that the same preparations contain blood group alloagglutinins (anti-A and anti-B). Therefore, patients of groups A, B, or AB who receive large doses of AHF repeatedly should be monitored for signs of intravascular hemolysis and decreasing hematocrit values. In addition, allergic reactions may occur with the use of AHF, although these are fairly infrequent.

Cryoprecipitated factor VIII is prepared from a single donation of fresh blood by cold precipitation, a process that also concentrates the fibrinogen, although the other plasma proteins are present in cryoprecipitate in the concentrations found in normal plasma. The factor VIII activity in each individual unit cannot be determined at the time of production without contaminating the preparation, but it averages about 80 units of factor VIII, ensured by routine quality control procedures. Cryoprecipitated factor VIII is indicated in cases of hemophilia A (congenital factor VIII deficiency), von Willebrand's disease, and acquired factor VIII deficiency (disseminated intravascular coagulation and transfusional dilution in massive transfusion).

Factor IX Concentrate

Storage Requirements. Factor IX concentrate is obtained from pooled plasma by fractionation. It contains factors II, VII, IX, and X with a minimal amount of total protein. The preparation is lyophilized and stored in the refrigerator at 2 to 8°C.

Applications. Factor IX concentrate (complex) is indicated in cases of congenital factor IX deficiency (hemophilia B), congenital factor VII deficiency, and congenital factor X deficiency for the prevention and control of hemorrhagic episodes. Acquired deficiencies of factor II, VII, IX, and X should not generally be treated with factor IX complex, since these conditions can be treated effectively with plasma with less risk. It should be noted that the risk of transmitting hepatitis virus is present when using factor IX complex (despite testing). Factor IX complex is contraindicated in patients with liver disease and in neonates because of the risk of thrombosis or disseminated intravascular coagulation.

Platelet-Rich Plasma; Platelet Concentrate

Storage Requirements. Platelet concentrates (or platelet-rich plasma) may be stored for up to 72 hours at room temperature with constant agitation (Fig. 28–2). Platelet concentrates so stored should be kept in a volume of approximately 50 mL of plasma.

Effects of Storage. Platelets stored for up to 72 hours as indicated undergo a progressive decrease in their hemostatic effectiveness. After 72 hours of storage, the pH of the preparation may fall below 6.0, a level below which the platelets do not appear to be hemostatically functional. The temperature of storage (22°C) ensures optimal survival and hemostatic function, and the agitation prevents the formation of platelet aggregates.

The use of new types of plastic bags (O_2 diffusible) that are now available allows platelet storage for up to five days.

Applications. Platelets (as concentrates or as platelet-rich plasma) can be used for the prevention and treatment of bleeding due to thrombocytopenia (although they are not generally effective in cases of immune thrombocytopenia). They can also be used for the treatment of bleeding due to proven platelet function disorders, even though the platelet count is not significantly decreased.

Note: Platelet concentrates can also be prepared by pheresis (so-called thrombopheresis) and as such can be obtained from a single donor and HLA matched (if required) using automated cell separation equipment. If so prepared, the platelets should be administered promptly after preparation. If storage cannot be avoided, it should never be for longer than 24 hours, since the cells are prepared in an open system and sterility cannot be assured beyond that time. Again, storage should be at room temperature (22°C) with constant agitation. Platelet concentrates prepared by pheresis are indicated when platelets are required and it is necessary to minimize alloimmunization, as in potential transplant candidates. The preparation is also indicated when an individual requiring platelets has become refractory to standard pooled-platelet preparations. It should be noted that a crossmatch should be performed before the administration of platelets obtained by pheresis, because the product can contain a considerable number of red cells.

Leukocyte-Poor Blood

Storage Requirements. Leukocyte-poor red cells are generally prepared for a specific patient immediately before transfusion and as such are not stored. If storage is essential, it should not be for longer than 24 hours

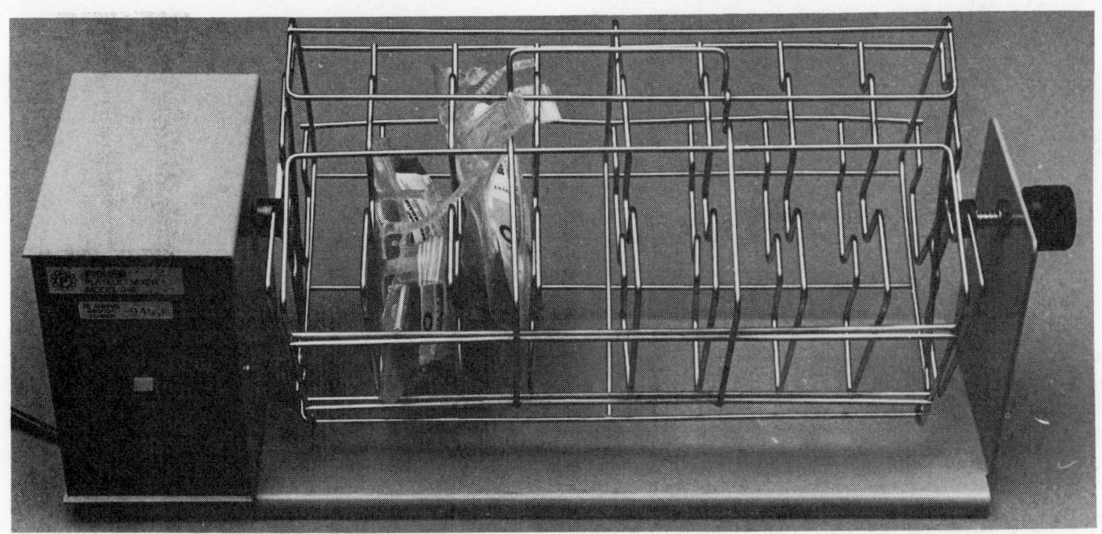

Figure 28–2 Platelet mixer. (Fisher Scientific Co., Pittsburgh, Pa. 15219 and Don Mills, Ont. M3A 1A9.)

after preparation, since (in procedures of preparation that involve entering the bag) there is a risk of contamination. Units prepared in a closed system can be stored for the normal life span of the unit (as whole blood).

Applications. Leukocyte-poor blood is indicated for the following:

1. Patients who have repeated febrile reactions due to leukocyte antibodies.
2. Patients undergoing renal dialysis (to reduce the risk of alloimmunization to leukocyte and platelet antigens).

Note: Frozen-thawed red cells can be used as an alternative to leukocyte-poor blood.

Granulocytes

Storage Requirements. Granulocytes are obtained from a single donor, using automated cell separation equipment, and they cannot be separated from individual routine blood donations. Granulocytes are therefore prepared for a specific patient and are not stored.

Applications. Leukocyte concentrates (granulocytes) may be of value for selected patients with granulocyte counts below 500 × 10^6/L and evidence of continuing infection uncontrolled by antimicrobials. The clinical benefit of prophylactic administration of leukocytes for low granulocyte counts without evidence of infection has not been definitely established.

COMPONENT PREPARATION IMMEDIATELY BEFORE ADMINISTRATION

Fresh Frozen Plasma

Immediately before transfusion, fresh frozen plasma is thawed at 37°C for at least 20 minutes (or until thawing is complete). The product should be administered promptly after thawing, because factors V and VIII deteriorate rapidly. The thawing process can be accelerated by using an agitator, by breaking up the plasma mass, and by using specially designed microwave ovens.

Stored Plasma

Stored plasma is available immediately for clinical use. The unit chosen should be group compatible with the recipient's blood, but not necessarily group specific. The following may be taken as a guide:

Recipient's Blood Group	Donor's Blood Group
O	O, A, B, AB
A	A, AB
B	B, AB
AB	AB

Concentrated Red Cells

Once crossmatching is complete and compatibility has been established, concentrated red cells may be administered without any special preparation procedure. If the unit is stored as whole blood, concentrated red cells can be prepared as follows:

1. Place the sedimented blood on a plasma extractor (Fig. 28–3). *Note:* If the unit has not sedimented on storage for whatever reason, it may be centrifuged at high speed in a refrigerated centrifuge.
2. Aseptically insert the cannula of a transfer container into the outlet site of the bag of blood.
3. Carefully release the spring compressor on the plasma extractor, thus expressing the plasma into the transfer container.
4. Clamp the tubing between the primary pack and the transfer pack in two places, and cut the tubing between the clamps.
5. The packed red cells are now ready for use.

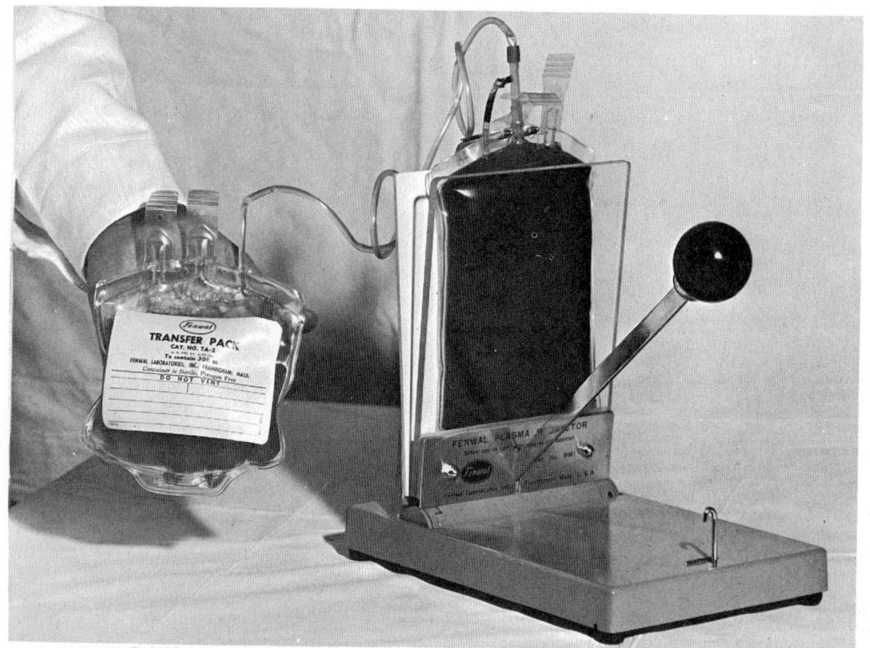

Figure 28–3 Transferring plasma from the plastic pack. (Courtesy of Fenwall Laboratories, Inc., Morton Grove, Ill. 60053.)

Cryoprecipitate

Immediately before use, cryoprecipitate should be completely thawed in a water bath at 37°C. Note that temperatures in excess of 37°C cause loss of factor VIII activity. Complete thawing should be achieved within ten minutes, after which the cryoprecipitate must be administered promptly for maximal in vivo recovery. The product may be administered as individual units or as a pool of several units.

If a diluent is required, small quantities of preservative-free normal saline may be introduced through an outlet site in the cryoprecipitate bag after thawing. Each bag should be gently agitated to ensure complete dissolution of the cryoprecipitate. The dissolved cryoprecipitate requires administration through a filter. It is preferable, though not essential, to administer group-compatible cryoprecipitate.

Factor IX Concentrates

Lyophilized factor IX concentrates should be reconstituted with preservative-free sterile water (usually provided with the preparation) immediately before use. It requires filtration before or during administration.

Leukocyte-Poor Blood

There are several methods of preparing leukocyte-poor blood, each having varying efficiency. It should be noted that those methods that require entering the bag result in potential contamination; therefore, the unit must be infused promptly after processing. Methods of preparing leukocyte-poor blood include the following:

Inverted Centrifugation

1. The unit of blood is centrifuged in an inverted position at high speed.
2. After centrifugation, the red blood cells are transferred to a satellite bag, leaving some residual red cells (15–20%) and the white cell layer in the main bag.
3. The red cells in the satellite bag are then infused.

Augmented Sedimentation

The addition of sedimenting agents such as dextran or hydroxyethyl starch facilitates the separation of white blood cells by centrifugation or gravity.

Manual Wash

By this method, the red cells are washed and centrifuged 4 to 6 times in normal saline. The disadvantages of this technique are that some white blood cells do remain and that there is red cell loss in the processing. In addition, the bag is entered in order to add saline, thus increasing the risk of contamination.

Automated Wash

This method uses special machines designed to wash the cells, a process that can be performed on liquid stored or frozen red cells. There is less red cell loss and white cell removal is more efficient than with the manual method of washing.

Special Filtration

By this method, the red cells are filtered through a micropore (40 microns or less) filter just before administration. Depending on the type of filter used, this may be performed in the laboratory or at the patient's bedside. The efficiency of white cell removal depends on the type of filter used.

REAGENTS

Cell Suspensions (Reagent Red Cells)

Origin. Red cells used as laboratory reagents are of human origin, obtained from individuals of group A and group B for anti-A and anti-B reverse grouping reagent (respectively) or from individuals with useful phenotypes for screening or panel cells. Human red cells are also used in the laboratory as controls for specific antisera.

Storage. Reagent red cells are stored at 2 to 8°C when in general use in the laboratory, or they may be stored in a frozen state (in glycerol or liquid nitrogen) for extended periods of time (see discussion below).

Preparation and Standardization. Most laboratories use reagent red cells that have been produced by commercial houses and as such are ready for immediate use. Cell suspensions are also prepared in the laboratory, however, using the following method:

1. Red cells that have been washed at least twice should be used for all tests, unless the volume of work makes this impractical. If two washes do not result in an absolutely clear supernatant, the cells should not be used.
2. The cells should be washed periodically if a particular sample is being used throughout the day.
3. Accurate suspensions from washed packed red cells must be made whenever possible. Graduated centrifuge tubes are used when large volumes have to be prepared. Alternatively, the color and density of the suspensions can be compared macroscopically in tubes of equal bore to ensure that they are of approximately the same strength. This inspection can be confirmed by examining the color of a drop of blood hanging from a pipette.
4. Ensure that all tubes are labeled with the cell phenotype and the source of the cells (e.g., the unit number or the donor's last name).
5. For best results, use cell suspensions only on the day of preparation.
6. Always use the weakest cell suspension consistent with specific, easily read results. *Note:* The reactivity of the cells must be controlled. This is particularly important if commercially prepared red cell suspensions are used.

Red cell suspensions (reagent red cells) should be standardized in accordance with the requirements of the appropriate licensing authority.

Preservative Solutions. The most common preservative solution used in reagent red cell suspensions is Alsever's solution (a modified ACD solution), which is prepared as follows:

Trisodium citrate (dihydrate)	8.0 g
Dextrose	19.0 g
Sodium chloride	4.2 g
Citric acid (monohydrate)	0.5 g
Distilled water to	1000 mL

One volume of this solution is added to one volume of blood.

Storage in a Frozen State

Glycerol. Red cells may be stored in a glycerol solution using the following method:

1. A buffered citrate-glycerol solution is prepared by adding 19.4 g tripotassium citrate (monohydrate), 3.1 g sodium dihydrogen phosphate (dihydrate), and 2.8 g disodium hydrogen phosphate (anhydrous) to 600 mL of distilled water. Then 400 mL of glycerol is added to 600 mL of buffer citrate. The final pH is 6.9 to 7.0.
2. Pack the anticoagulated blood to be frozen and remove *all* of the supernatant plasma.
3. Note the volume of packed red cells and measure out an equal volume of citrate-glycerol.
4. Add the buffered citrate-glycerol to the red cells in small quantities, mixing constantly. The addition should take at least five minutes, depending on the quantity of red cells to be frozen.
5. Divide the cells into small portions and freeze at −30°C. The proportion of glycerol must be altered for temperatures lower than −30°C.

The Recovery of Glycerolyzed Red Cells By Dialysis

1. Thaw the frozen red cells at room temperature.
2. Pour the thawed red cells into a length of dialysis tubing, and submerge the tubing in a saline bath for 30 to 60 minutes. Constant stirring of the saline with a magnetic stirrer greatly improves the efficiency of this step.
3. Remove the red cells from the saline bath, and pour the cells into conveniently sized test tubes.
4. Wash in saline until the supernatant is free of hemolysis.

Note: The use of citrate-phosphate solution rather than saline has been suggested both for dialysis and for the first wash after dialysis, after which the cells are washed in saline. The method of preparation of the citrate-phosphate solution is provided in Mollison, P.L.: Blood Transfusion in Clinical Medicine, 6th ed., p. 731 (see references).

Liquid Nitrogen. Red cells for storage in liquid nitrogen should be collected in either EDTA, CPD, or ACD. The red cells should not be more than two days old when they are frozen if antigens are to store well. Immediately before freezing, the blood should be mixed with half its volume of 40 per cent sucrose in buffered saline, added slowly and mixed well. The method of freezing is as follows:

1. Two-inch plastic tubing and a transfusion "taking" set needle are fitted on to a siliconed 50-mL syringe.
2. The syringe is suspended over a two-liter beaker (lined with absorbent cotton batten on sides and bottom).
3. The beaker is filled with liquid nitrogen, and the syringe is filled with blood (prepared as above).
4. The blood is dropped from the syringe into the liquid nitrogen. The syringe should be fitted with a clip to ensure uniform drops that do not coalesce on entering the liquid nitrogen.
5. The pellets of frozen blood are transferred with a cooled spoon to cardboard boxes filled with liquid nitrogen, then placed in a liquid nitrogen container.

The Recovery of Red Cells Frozen In Liquid Nitrogen

1. **Remove the pellets of blood from the liquid nitrogen container.**
2. **Place the pellets in 1 per cent NaCl at 45°C.**
3. **Agitate the solution. The pellets will melt quickly.**
4. **Wash the blood in isotonic saline until the supernatant fluid shows no hemolysis.**

Antisera

Origin. Blood grouping antisera used in the laboratory are either of human or of animal origin. Anti-A, anti-B, anti-A_1 (human), and anti-D are all obtained from hyperimmunized human donors who have produced such antibodies as a result of transfusion or pregnancy or whose "natural" antibodies have been stimulated to high titers through the injection of specific substances. Antiglobulin sera (both monospecific and polyspecific) are produced through the injection of human globulins into rabbits, with subsequent recovery of the rabbit "anti-human" antibodies.

Storage. Blood grouping sera generally retain their potency for long periods of time when stored at 4°C. The half-life of antibodies in immunoglobulin solution stored at 4°C has been reported to be not less than 20 years, though IgM antibodies appear to be much more labile than IgG. Of course, blood grouping sera are not stored for that length of time because of the possibility of contamination, and each product is usually assigned an expiry date indicating the "safe" period in which the reagent can be used.

Sera stored at 4°C require some sort of bacteriostatic agent to inhibit growth of contaminants (e.g., 0.1 per cent sodium azide). It should be noted that concentrations greater than 0.1 per cent have been shown to affect the titer of Rh antibodies and the electrophoretic pattern of serum.

Reagent antisera can be stored at −20°C and as such do not require the addition of any bacteriostatic agent. Repeated thawing and freezing of the antisera, however, should be avoided. Antisera containing high concentrations of albumin should be stored at 2 to 8°C and should not be frozen, since these lower temperatures cause crystallization of the albumin, leading to loss of reactivity. Frozen serum that contains antibodies must be completely thawed and the vial inverted several times before use, because the antibodies are usually concentrated in the lower portion of frozen serum.

When donations for antisera are procured, it is always preferable to obtain serum rather than plasma. Blood grouping reagents, however, are now frequently obtained by plasmapheresis, which yields plasma.

Plasma may be clotted by the addition of an excess of calcium chloride ($CaCl_2$) in the ratio of 1 mL of a molar solution to each 100 mL of plasma.

Standard Specifications. All antisera used in the laboratory must meet minimum standards as required by the appropriate licensing authority.

Rh/Hr Control (Suspending Medium Control)

False positive results in Rh_o (D) typing can be caused by the interaction between the red cells and the non-antibody materials in the reaction mixture. Not only the macromolecular nature of the medium, but also specific substances in the reagents may cause cellular aggregation that resembles antibody-mediated agglutination.

Principle of Use. To detect the false positive results mentioned above, the control medium used should contain the materials used in the antisera, lacking only the specific antibody. Many commercial manufacturers offer immunologically inert high-protein mediums that resemble the reagent in all other ways. If this material is available, the test for Rh_o (D) should be controlled with it. In the absence of inert serum diluent, 22 or 30 per cent bovine albumin may be substituted, although this is not as satisfactory.

Rh/Hr control sera should be stored at 2 to 8°C, and the expiry date on the vial should be observed.

Common Lectins

In 1954, Boyd and Shapleigh reopened investigations of the observation that certain seeds contain substances that react specifically with human red cells by studying a vast number of leguminous and nonleguminous plants. The substances in plants that demonstrated specificity with human red cells were called "lectins." A great number of these substances are known. However, in this text, only the most common (and commonly used) will be considered.

Dolichos biflorus. The lectin obtained from the plant *Dolichos biflorus* is virtually specific for A_1 red cells and will react more than 500 times more strongly with A_1 than with A_2 red cells. Its use is the best method of distinguishing between red cells of the two groups. Strong concentrations of the lectin will produce agglutination with A_2 red cells, but this can be corrected by dilution with saline.

It should be noted that the lectin will also react with red cells that are Sd(a+) or Cad-positive—i.e., Sd(a++)—or with red cells that are Tn-activated, regardless of group.

Solutions of *Dolichos biflorus* and other lectins are readily available from commercial companies; however, they can easily be prepared in the laboratory if the seeds are available.

Once prepared, *Dolichos biflorus* solutions retain their avidity for three years when stored at 4°C. (*Note:* Lectin solutions should not be kept at room temperature, nor should they be frozen.)

Ulex europaeus. The plant *Ulex europaeus* is common gorse. The seed extract has anti-H specificity and is used as a standard anti-H reagent by most workers. Its use is valuable in the detection of H substance in saliva, which is demonstrated by testing the ability of the saliva to inhibit (neutralize) the reaction of the lectin with group O red cells.

Anti-H from the seeds of *Ulex europaeus* may be stored at 4°C, its shelf life being at least one year.

Arachis hypogaea. This lectin is prepared from raw peanuts. Once prepared, the solution has anti-T specificity and provides a useful reagent for the detection of polyagglutinable red cells produced by T activation.

Bovine Albumin

Origin. Bovine albumin is one of the plasma proteins obtained from beef blood. Processing includes the biochemical control of protein concentration, pH, and specific conductivity. When properly prepared, it is one of the most successful high-protein media in serological use.

Storage. Bovine albumin is stored at 2 to 8°C for the shelf life recommended by the manufacturer. Bovine albumin should not be stored at room temperature, nor should it be frozen.

Uses. IgG antibodies often agglutinate red cells suspended in bovine albumin, since the use of that substance increases the dielectric constant of the medium and thus reduces the zeta potential (the electric repulsion between the red cells). Although bovine albumin is used in the detection of IgG antibodies, it is doubtful if any "significant" antibody will react *only* in albumin.

In the antiglobulin test, it has been found that sensitivity is greatly increased by the addition of bovine albumin in preference to saline. The reactions are often more rapid, and it has been suggested that incubation time may be cut to 15 minutes. Bovine albumin is usually available in a 22% or 30% solution.

Note: The refractive indices of bacteria and albumin are very similar. Therefore, it is difficult to detect bacterial contamination visually, because no cloudiness appears. For this reason, the solution is maintained at 2 to 8°C when not in actual use, and the manufacturer's instruction as to expiration date is closely observed, although the 4°C shelf life is probably as long as five years.

Saline Solutions

Isotonic Saline. A 0.85% solution of sodium chloride and distilled water is of the same osmotic pressure as the contents of the human red cell (i.e., isotonic). The solution so prepared is known as isotonic saline, and is used in the laboratory as a general cell suspending medium. It is prepared by dissolving 8.5 g of sodium chloride in one liter of distilled water.

The solution should be freshly prepared each day and should not be stored.

Low–Ionic Strength Solution (LISS). Low–ionic strength solution (LISS) contains sodium glycinate, phosphate buffer, and saline. It can be used in the laboratory instead of saline as a suspending medium for red cells in antibody detection tests. The main advantage of the use of LISS is to shorten the incubation time. An incubation time of 10 minutes has been found to be satisfactory for the detection of a wide range of antibodies. A further advantage is to increase the uptake of certain antibodies; this effect has been found to be pronounced with selected Rh antibodies believed to be of low affinity.

Low–ionic strength solution is prepared as follows:

1. Dissolve 18 g of glycine in about 500 mL of distilled water and add 1.0 M NaOH until the pH is 6.7 (about 0.35 mL).
2. Add 800 mL of this solution to 20 mL of 0.15 M phosphate buffer (pH 6.7), and add 180 mL of 0.17 M saline.

Buffered Saline. The pH of isotonic saline is in the vicinity of 5.7, and for this reason, many laboratories add phosphate buffer to bring the pH into the region of 7.2 to 7.4.

Buffered saline can be prepared as follows:

1. Dissolve 90 g sodium chloride crystals in one liter of freshly distilled water.
2. Dilute one in ten with distilled water for use.
3. Add 5 mL/L of phosphate buffer at pH 7.6 (Hendry's buffer or a standard 0.2 M buffer).

4. Store both stock solutions and working solutions at 4°C in polypropylene flasks.
5. Autoclave the working solution at 121°C for 60 minutes.
6. Keep the solutions at 4°C.

Note: The presence of phosphate is believed to offset any impurities in the distilled water.

Proteolytic Enzymes

At present, the proteolytic enzymes in common use in the laboratory are bromelin, trypsin, ficin, and papain. The mode of action of these enzymes varies with antigenic specificity. They react, it is believed, by reducing the net surface-charge density by splitting off negatively charged carboxyl groups of sialic acid and thus reduce the zeta potential. It was shown by Pollack and his associates in 1965 that red cells treated with ficin show the greatest reduction of zeta potential; papain follows closely, and trypsin has the least effect.

In the blood transfusion laboratory, proteolytic enzymes have their main use in their ability to cause saline-suspended red cells to agglutinate with IgG Rh antibodies; in fact, this has been shown to be the most sensitive and effective method of demonstrating these antibodies, though its sensitivity is also valuable for the detection of P_1, Lewis, Kidd, and many other antibodies.

It should be noted that enzyme testing is inadequate as a sole test for compatibility, since certain antibodies of considerable clinical significance (e.g., anti-Fy^a) will not be detected with enzyme-treated red cells.

Papain. The enzyme papain is from the pawpaw (*Carica papaya*) and is in regular use in many blood banks in both one- and two-stage techniques. The enzyme is useful in detecting very low concentrations of certain antibodies, though this sensitivity causes many "cold" autoagglutinins to be detected readily. The two-stage technique has been found to be more sensitive than the one-stage technique, since, if serum is incubated for a long period of time with papain, immunoglobulin molecules will be cleaved.

Papain (stock solution) is usually stored in a frozen state. Cystine-papain is usually stable for four months at −25°C; EDTA-papain is stable for six months at 4°C, though it can be stored for much longer periods of time at −25°C. Stock papain powder deteriorates slowly at room temperature and should always be stored at 4°C. Papain solution, once thawed, should be used immediately and any remaining material discarded. It should never be refrozen. Adequate controls should be included in the test whenever a new vial of the enzyme is used.

Trypsin. The enzyme trypsin is obtained from hog's stomach and has limited uses. One distinct disadvantage of the protease was realized by Heistö and his associates, who, in 1965, found that 94 out of 961 normal donors hemolyzed their own trypsinized red cells. This hemolysin was found to be much more common in women than in men and was shown to be inherited; it is not inhibited by trypsin itself. Moreover, trypsinized red cells mixed with normal serum and incubated for less than 20 minutes will usually be found to be agglutinated, though if incubation is continued for one hour, 99% of the cells will become negative.

A stock solution of trypsin will keep for four months at 4°C.

Bromelin. The enzyme bromelin is an extract from the pineapple (*Ananas sativus*) and appears to be about as effective as ficin (discussed below). It has been used in one-stage and two-stage techniques (the latter proving more sensitive). The enzyme is in fairly general use, yet it appears to have no obvious advantages over the other proteases.

Bromelin is in reasonably common use in autoanalyzers, where it is mixed with polyvinylpyrrolidone (PVP), and it has proved valuable in this application.

The enzyme, like other common proteolytic enzymes, does not detect anti-Fy^a. Antibodies such as anti-M, anti-N, and anti-S are also not detected. It is believed to be the corresponding *antigen* that is affected by enzyme treatment in these cases.

Bromelin (stock solution) can be stored at 4°C, where it remains potent for two months.

Ficin. The enzyme ficin is an extract from the fig (*Ficus carica*). The enzyme is not widely used, though it has been found to be as sensitive as papain, if not more so.

Ficin is usually stored at −20°C, where it retains its potency for several months. At 4°C, ficin is considered potent for only one week.

Anticoagulants

An anticoagulant is a substance that acts to prevent the clotting of red cells. The substance is used in blood donations (in addition to ensuring against the clotting of red cells) to ensure proper maintenance of red cell hemoglobin function and viability and to maintain the delicate biochemical balance of certain elements such as glucose, pH, ATP, and 2,3-DPG.

Anticoagulated specimens are sometimes used in special serological procedures; however, they are never used in crossmatching because of their effect on complement binding.

Citrate Phosphate Dextrose (CPD). This is the anticoagulant most widely used at present in blood donations. Compared with acid citrate dextrose (ACD) (see below) this anticoagulant gives slightly less hemolysis, a slightly smaller "leak" of potassium from the cells, and a prolonged posttransfusion survival of the red cells. All comparisons published so far have supported the indication of better viability of red cells in CPD as opposed to ACD. The favorable effects of this anticoagulant are mainly due to its higher pH.

The citrate ion in CPD solution is present in more than sufficient quantities for anticoagulation. This ion binds plasma calcium in the collected blood, preventing clotting. In addition, CPD contains 2 mM of phosphate, which contributes to the adenosine phosphate pool, important in the glycolytic process and maintenance of cell viability. CPD solutions also contain sufficient quantities of dextrose to allow the stored blood to continue glycolytic metabolism, thereby maintaining adequate concentrations of ATP to ensure sufficient viability for at least three weeks.

CPD solutions generally contain 1.66 g sodium citrate (dihydrate), 0.206 g citric acid (anhydrous), 0.140 g sodium dihydrogen phosphate (monohydrate), and 1.61 g dextrose (monohydrate). Distilled water is added to make 63 mL. This 63 mL of anticoagulant solution is required to prevent the clotting of 450 mL of blood.

The average survival of red cells in CPD is 70 to 75 per cent after 28 days. The addition of adenine to CPD will prolong red cell survival of 70 to 75% to 35 days.

Acid Citrate Dextrose (ACD). This anticoagulant was used until quite recently in blood donations. Various published observations have agreed that red cells stored in ACD for 14 days have a survival of 85% or more; the survival after 24 days is usually 70% or more.

Like CPD, the citrate ion in ACD binds plasma calcium in the collected blood, preventing clotting. The dextrose in ACD is present as a preservative and as a nutrient for the red cells, ensuring sufficient viability for at least three weeks.

ACD solutions generally contain 1.49 g trisodium citrate (dihydrate), 0.54 g citric acid (monohydrate), 1.65 g dextrose (monohydrate), and distilled water to make 67.5 mL—the amount needed to prevent clotting of 500 mL of whole blood.

During exchange transfusion to newborn infants or rapid transfusions to adults with impaired liver function, high levels of citrate may be reached, and serious toxic effects may be observed. These toxic effects are likely to develop when blood is transfused at a rate of 1 liter in ten minutes. The effects can be minimized by administering calcium (10 mL of 10% calcium gluconate for each liter of citrated blood).

Ethylenediaminetetraacetic Acid (EDTA). This anticoagulant is no longer used in blood transfusion work, except in the investigation of autoimmune hemolytic anemia or in certain elution procedures, because it has displayed no distinct advantage over citrate and because it has been shown to damage platelets and greatly inhibit the action of complement. It is, however, commonly used in hematological procedures (e.g., specimens for hemoglobin estimation).

The sodium salts of EDTA are strong chelating agents (as are the potassium salts) that bind calcium and thereby prevent clotting. Thirty milliliters of 1.36% NaH_2EDTA, which provides 1.1 millimoles of EDTA, will prevent the clotting of 500 mL of whole blood.

EQUIPMENT

Unlike other sciences of medical technology, immunohematology involves very little automated equipment. The following is a brief account of the equipment routinely used in the blood transfusion laboratory. This discussion is by no means complete, and it considers only those pieces of equipment that are specified for study by the syllabus of the Canadian Society of Laboratory Technologists (CSLT) and the American Society of Clinical Pathologists (ASCP).

Refrigerated Centrifuge

A refrigerated centrifuge is usually a floor model that is large enough to centrifuge blood packs at a constant speed and temperature. This centrifuge is generally used when preparing packed red cells from units of whole blood, but it is also used in plasmapheresis and in the preparation of platelet concentrates as well as other blood components.

In the blood transfusion laboratory, the refrigerated centrifuge is one of three types of centrifuge required—the other two being the standard bench-type centrifuge for the spinning of blood specimens, which has variable speeds and heads, and a constant-speed centrifuge for the spinning of serum-cell mixtures before reading (Fig. 28–4).

The centrifugal force (G) exerted by a centrifuge can be calculated by using the formula 0.00001118 × r ×

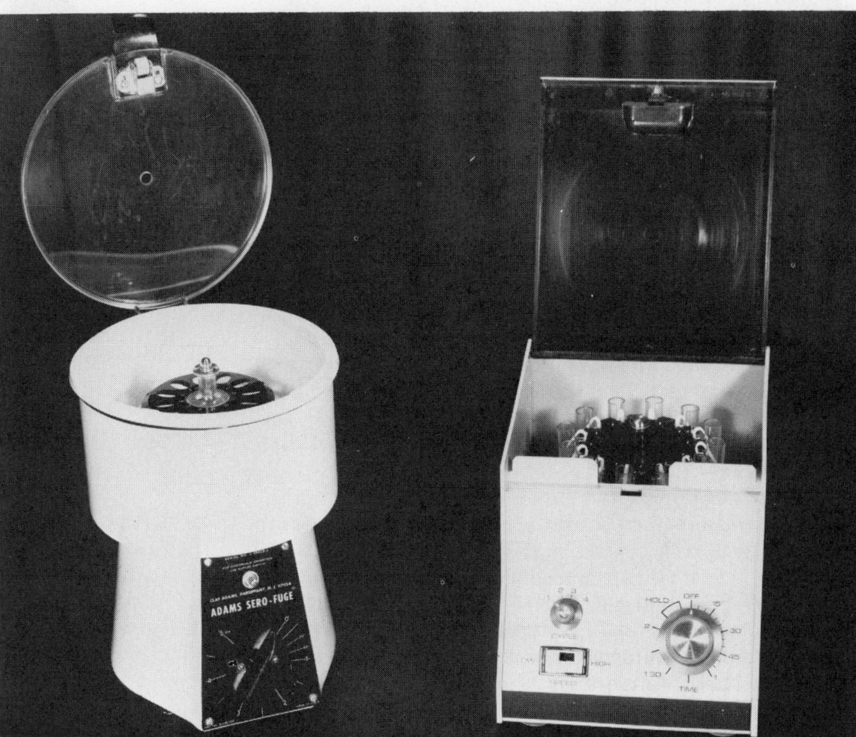

Figure 28–4 Two useful types of blood bank centrifuges. *Left,* Serofuge, Clay Adams, Parsippany, N.J. 07054. *Right,* Immunfuge, Dade, Miami, Fla. 33152.

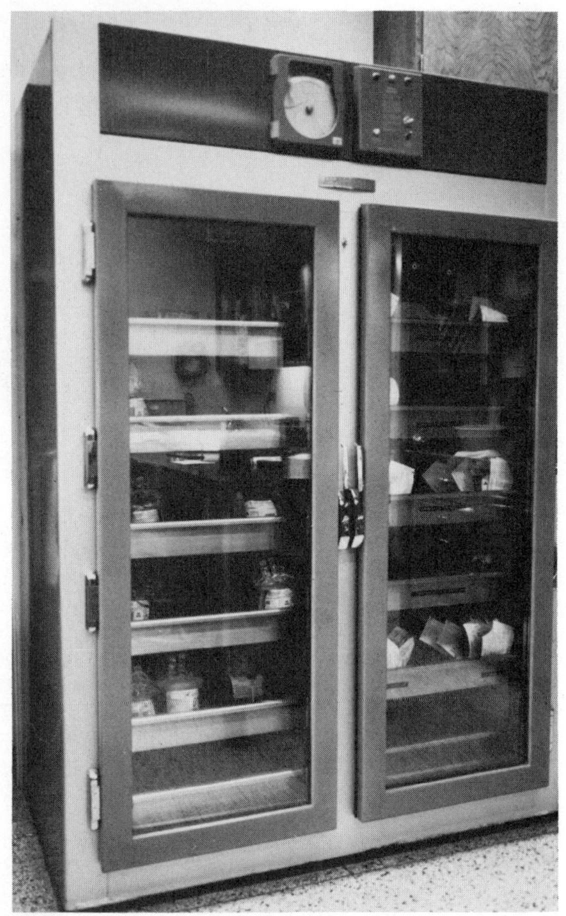

Figure 28–5 Blood bank refrigerator. Note the alarm system, the recording thermometer, and arrangement of the shelves, which pull out on rollers for easy accessibility. (Manufactured by Puffer-Hubbard, Grand Haven, Mich. 49417.)

n^2, where r equals the radius of the centrifuge head in centimeters and n equals revolutions per minute. (See p. 698.)

Blood Bank Refrigerator

Either the cylindrical variety with rotating shelves or the conveniently shaped variety with pull-out shelves is suitable (Fig. 28–5). Blood may be conveniently arranged in this latter type of refrigerator so that all units of the same group are on one shelf. The units should be arranged so that the oldest blood is easily at hand and is used first. Certain shelves should be reserved for blood that is crossmatched, and the bottom of the refrigerator can be used for holding units of plasma and other blood components.

The refrigerator chosen should be of a reliable make, fitted with a safety light and an 8-day continuous temperature recording device. It should also be fitted with an alarm system that sounds when the temperature falls below 2°C or rises above 6°C. This alarm system should be connected with a department of the hospital in which reliable, informed personnel are on duty at all times (e.g., maintenance or engineering), unless the blood transfusion laboratory maintains a 24-hour service (and even then such a safeguard may be desirable). In addition, it is advisable that the blood bank refrigerator and the alarm system be connected to an emergency power system to guard against problems that may be the result of a main power failure. An automatic buzzer that sounds when the refrigerator door is opened is also recommended. Only laboratory staff and certain designated members of the nursing staff should be permitted to open the blood bank refrigerator.

Rh Typing Box

The use of lighted viewing boxes when performing Rh typing on a slide or plate helps to facilitate reading and also to provide sufficient heat so that the temperature of the reaction mixture is approximately 37°C. To this end, the surface of the view box should remain between 40 and 50°C, and this temperature should be checked routinely before use. Slides should be placed in the middle part of the surface to avoid possible cold spots.

Automated Cell Washers

Automated cell washers are primarily designed for use in the washing phase of the antiglobulin test. These machines, which are available from several commercial suppliers in variously modified styles, automatically wash, decant, mix, and rewash red cells from one to four times. Some systems also add the antiglobulin reagent to the tubes.

It should be noted that if any of these systems is used, careful quality control of the instrument is essential to ensure constant and reliable results. (See Fig. 28–6.)

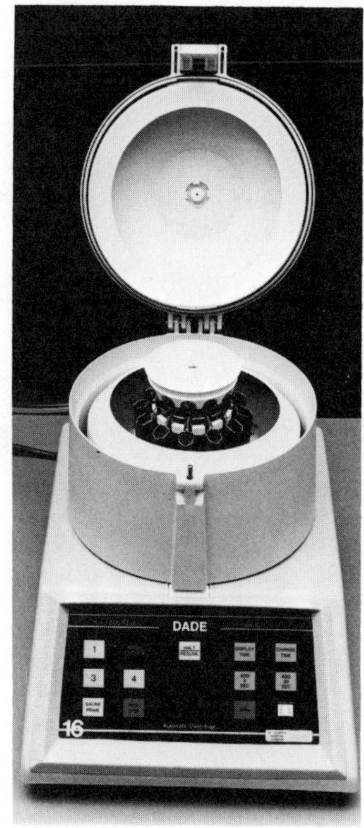

Figure 28–6 Automatic cell washer. (Dade, Inc., Miami, Fla. 33152.)

THE ANTIGLOBULIN TEST

The antiglobulin test is probably the most important and most widely used serological procedure in modern blood banking. It was first described in 1908 by Moreschi and was rediscovered and introduced into clinical medicine by Coombs, Mourant, and Race in 1945. Most antibodies that result in transfusion problems are detectable by the antiglobulin test. The test will detect IgG antibodies that do or do not react in either saline or high-protein media or that react weakly or variably in these media. It will also detect antibodies that bind complement but that may not be capable of binding themselves to red cells in sufficient quantities to give a positive test (e.g., anti-Jk^a).

There are two different forms of the antiglobulin test: the direct test, used to demonstrate the coating (or sensitization) of red cells with antibody, and the indirect test, used to demonstrate the presence of free antibody in the serum. It follows, therefore, that the direct test is performed by using the patient's red cells and the indirect test by using the patient's serum. An important difference between the two tests is that the direct test requires no incubation in vitro, whereas the indirect test does. Both tests are described below.

In compatibility testing (crossmatching), the antiglobulin test is by far the most important single test in current use and comes closest to approaching the "ideal." The main limitation is the large number of factors that may influence or affect the reaction (see later discussion).

The Direct Antiglobulin Test: Theory and Application

The direct antiglobulin test is used to demonstrate that red cells have been coated (sensitized) with antibody in vivo. The test has many applications: in hemolytic disease of the newborn to show whether fetal red cells are sensitized with maternal antibody, in autoimmune hemolytic anemia, and as an indication of incompatible transfusion or delayed hemolytic transfusion reaction.

A positive reaction in the direct antiglobulin test, however, can be confusing, since such a result can be caused by variables other than antigen-antibody sensitization. For example, a positive test can be caused by several disease states (viral pneumonia, infectious hepatitis, infectious mononucleosis, favism, megaloblastic anemia, reticulocytosis, acute intermittant porphyria, and, most important, acquired hemolytic anemia). Many drugs, too, have been shown to be the cause of a positive direct antiglobulin test (e.g., alpha-methyldopa [Aldomet], penicillin, cephalothin, Mesantoin, stibophen, phenylhydrazine, quinine, and others). More causes of a false antiglobulin test result are discussed below.

The Indirect Antiglobulin Test: Theory and Application

The indirect antiglobulin test is used to demonstrate the presence of free antibody in the patient's serum. This is achieved by incubation of the serum with red cells of various antigenic makeup at 37°C, allowing sensitization of the red cells to occur (i.e., sensitization in vitro). The addition of antiglobulin serum (once free antibody has been diluted out by washing the red cells) provides the "bridge" between sensitized red cells by employing an antibody produced in a rabbit, which reacts with antibody or complement attached to the red cells. The rabbit "anti-human" globulin reacts with the sensitized red cells and produces agglutinates. If either antigen or antibody is missing from the mixture, the red cells will fail to aggutinate, and the test is interpreted as negative. (See Fig 28–7.)

The indirect antiglobulin test is the most widely used serological test in modern blood banking. Although its most important application is in the compatibility test, it is also used in antibody identification, in hemolytic disease of the newborn, in cases of autoimmune hemolytic anemia, in the investigation of adverse reactions to transfusion, and in practically all other investigations undertaken by the blood transfusion laboratory.

The Antiglobulin Test: Methods

The Direct Antiglobulin Test

1. Place one drop of a 2 to 5 per cent saline suspension of red cells from the individual under test into a 10 × 75 mm test tube.

2. Wash the red cells four times in large volumes of saline. Care should be taken to ensure adequate removal of the supernatant saline after each wash. (*Note*: Washing accomplishes *dilution* rather than removal of free globulin.)

3. Add one or two drops of antiglobulin reagent (broad spectrum).

4. Mix well.

5. Centrifuge at 3400 rpm (1000 G) (Serofuge*) for 15 seconds.

6. Examine for agglutination by using an optical aid, and record results. Check all negative reactions microscopically. (See *Interpretation of Results,* below.)

7. Add IgG-sensitized red cells as a control, centrifuge, and read. If a negative result is obtained, the test result is

*Clay Adams Corp., Parsippany, N.J. 07054.

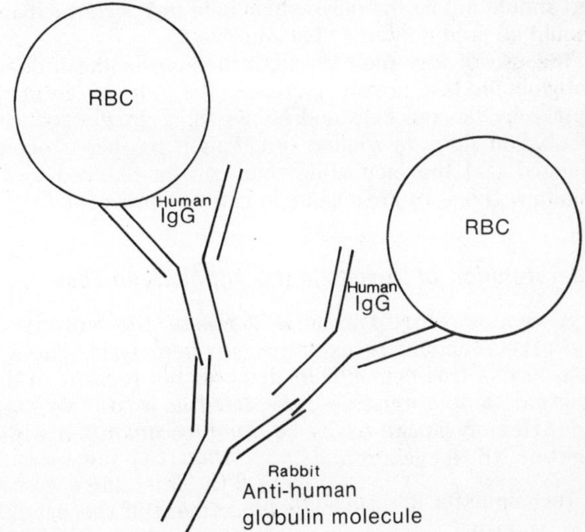

Figure 28–7 Reaction of the anti-human globulin molecule. (From Bryant, N. J.: An Introduction to Immunohematology, 2nd ed. Philadelphia, W. B. Saunders Co., 1982, p. 270).

invalid. If monospecific anticomplement reagents are used, complement-sensitized red cells should be substituted for IgG-sensitized red cells.

The Indirect Antiglobulin Test

1. Place two to six drops of the serum under test (patient's serum) in a 10 × 75 mm test tube.
2. Add one drop of a washed 5% suspension of the test cells (donor's red cells, screening cells, etc.). (*Optional*: Two drops of bovine albumin may be added to the mixture. If this is done, the sensitivity of the test can be increased and it has been suggested that the incubation time may be reduced to 15 minutes. It should be noted that if full incubation is routinely used [30 minutes or longer], the use of bovine albumin is of less importance, since there is no obvious difference in sensitivity with or without the use of albumin after this incubation time.)
3. Mix well.
4. Incubate at 37°C for 15 to 30 minutes (or longer).
5. Immediately upon removal from the incubator, centrifuge for 15 seconds at 3400 rpm (1000 G) (Serofuge): examine for hemolysis and/or agglutination, using an optical aid; record results.
6. Wash the red cells three or four times in large amounts of saline. Decant each wash as completely as possible.
7. Add one to two drops of antiglobulin reagent.
8. Mix well.
9. Centrifuge at 3400 rpm (1000 G) (Serofuge) for 15 seconds.
10. Examine for agglutination, using an optical aid. Check all negative reactions microscopically.
11. Record results.
12. *(Optional)*: Add one drop of known sensitized red cells to all tests giving negative results. Centrifuge at 3400 rpm (1000 G) (Serofuge) for 15 seconds; examine for agglutination. If no agglutination is seen, the test result is invalid and must be repeated.

(*Note*: Enzyme-treated red cells may be used in the antiglobulin test, which will increase the sensitivity of the test with respect to some antibodies. Because of the effect of enzymes on certain blood group antigens, however, this test should not be the only antiglobulin test performed and should be used only as a "back-up" test.

The use of low–ionic strength medium in the indirect antiglobulin test greatly increases the rate of antibody uptake by the red cells and allows for a greatly reduced incubation time. In routine situations it has been recommended that the incubation time can be reduced to 10 minutes. This is of great value in cases of emergency.)

Interpretation of Results in the Antiglobulin Test

A soon as centrifugation is complete, the contents of the tube(s) should be examined for hemolysis. The appearence of free hemoglobin that was not present in the original sample must be interpreted as a positive reaction. Hemolysis can easily be observed against a white light or white background.

Technique for Resuspending the Cell Button

1. Hold the test tube at a sharp angle in such a way that the fluid, moving across the cell button, assists in dislodging the red cells.
2. Shake the tube very gently until all of the red cells have been dislodged from the wall of the tube.
3. Tilt the tube back and forth to obtain an even suspension of cells (or agglutinates).

Precautions

1. Never read more than one tube at a time.
2. Take care not to overshake or undershake. Overshaking can break up fragile agglutinates. Undershaking may give the appearance of a positive reaction.
3. Use a consistent light source with an optical aid.
4. Check all negative reactions microscopically. A microscope can also be useful in distinguishing rouleaux formation from true agglutination.

All reactions should be graded as follows:

4+ One solid aggregate, no free cells, clear supernatant (macroscopic reading).

3+ Several large aggregates, few free cells, clear supernatant (macroscopic reading).

2+ Medium-sized aggregates, some free cells, supernatant clear (macroscopic reading).

1+ Small aggregates, just visible macroscopically; many free cells; turbid reddish supernatant (macroscopic and microscopic reading).

w+ Tiny aggregates, clumps barely visible macroscopically; many free cells; turbid reddish supernatant (microscopic reading).

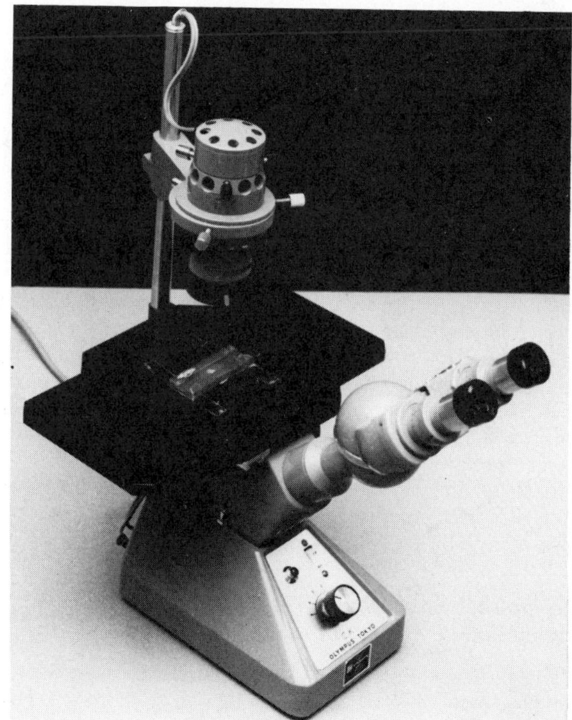

Figure 28–8 Inverted microscope suitable for reading test results directly in test tubes. (Olympus Corp. of America, North Hyde Park, N.Y. 11040.)

MF Mixed field, few isolated aggregates, large areas of free cells, red supernatant.

O Negative, no aggregates, smooth suspension.

Controls for the Direct and Indirect Antiglobulin Tests

Probably the best control for the direct and indirect antiglobulin test is the addition of IgG-sensitized red cells after reading. A positive result indicates the following:

1. The antiglobulin reagent has remained active and has not been neutralized.
2. The red cells have been adequately washed.
3. The final volume of saline did not excessively dilute the antiglobulin reagent.
4. Antiglobulin reagent was added to the test tubes.

A negative result invalidates the result of the test.

Commercially prepared presensitized red cells can be used for this purpose, or they can be prepared in the laboratory by titrating an IgG antibody [anti-Rh_o (D)] and using the dilution that results in a 2+ agglutination. Diluted serum is then prepared and incubated at 37°C with enough Rh_o (D)-positive red cells to provide one drop of sensitized red cells for every negative antiglobulin test in the day's workload.

Sources of Error in the Antiglobulin Test

Causes of False Positive Reactions

1. Traces of species-specific antibodies (heteroagglutinins) due to improper preparation of the antiglobulin serum.
2. Enzyme-treated red cells (because of greater sensitivity) reacting with residual anti-species antibodies.
3. Test cells that have a positive direct antiglobulin test.
4. Anti-T or anti-Tn in the antiglobulin serum reacting with T-activated or Tn-activated red cells. This can be caused by bacterial contamination of the test cells or by septicemia in the patient.
5. Extreme reticulocytosis due to transferrin bound to reticulocytes reacting with antitransferrin in the antiglobulin serum. (*Note*: Most antiglobulin reagents today have little or no antitransferrin activity.)
6. Colloidal silica in saline stored in glass bottles that is leached from the container.
7. Metallic ions in saline stored in metal containers (or used in equipment with metal parts) that may bring about nonspecific protein sensitization of the red cells.
8. Improperly cleaned glassware (or other forms of contamination of cells, serum, or reagents).
9. Overcentrifugation.
10. Autoagglutination before washing, which may persist through the washing phase.
11. Uptake of complement on to the red cells in vitro. After a period of storage, clotted blood samples may react with anticomplement in the antiglobulin serum (anti-C3 and/or anti-C4). A small percentage of samples from segments of plastic tubing (i.e., containing blood stored at 4°C with anticoagulant) will react with anti-C4d. The cause of these false positives has not been definitely established.

Causes of False Negative Reactions

1. Incorrect technique for the particular antibody involved.
2. Inadequate washing of the red cells, causing neutralization of the antiglobulin serum by trace amounts of residual globulin (as little as 2 μg of IgG/mL as a final concentration).
3. Insufficient active complement when the particular antibody is detectable only in the presence of active complement or insufficient anticomplement in the antiglobulin reagent.
4. Improper storage of test cells, test serum, and/or antiglobulin reagent, resulting in loss of reactivity.
5. Delays or interruptions in the test procedure, particularly during the washing phase, which may result in the elution of the antibody from the red cells.
6. Failure to add antiglobulin reagent.
7. Red cell suspensions that are too heavy (which may not permit optimum coating with antibody) or too light (which may make reading difficult).
8. Undercentrifugation or overcentrifugation (the latter because of the excessive force required to resuspend the red cells).
9. Contamination of the antiglobulin reagent with human serum.
10. Incorrect incubation temperature (not allowing for maximum coating of the red cells), or fluctuating incubation temperature.
11. Prozone (See pp. 536 and 605). (*Note*: This should not be a problem with licenced products, provided that the manufacturer's directions are followed.)
12. Insufficient incubation time.
13. Failure to check negative reactions microscopically.

Antiglobulin Reagents: Specificity and Application

The antiglobulin reagent used in routine laboratory work is a pool of serum usually made from two different colonies of rabbits (although goats and sheep can also be used). One colony is immunized with highly purified IgG to produce anti-IgG and the other with human beta globulins to produce anticomplement. The reagent (known as broad-spectrum antiglobulin reagent or "polyspecific" antiglobulin reagent) is then prepared by combining the anti-IgG and anticomplement (anti-C3). As such it contains both components and is able to detect antibodies that do or do not initiate complement sensitization of the red cells.

Anti-IgG. Several so-called monospecific antiglobulin reagents can be prepared by injecting animals with highly purified proteins, such as IgG, IgM, IgA, C3, or C4, or by the absorption of unwanted antibodies from broad-spectrum antiglobulin reagents. These monospecific reagents can be used to determine which protein is responsible for a positive direct antiglobulin test. In the routine laboratory, anti-IgG is most often used, since IgG antibodies are most often clinically important. The specific reagent is also useful in the indirect antiglobulin test in the identification of mixtures of non–complement-binding and complement-binding antibodies.

Anti-C3. The role of anticomplement in the antiglobulin reaction can be summarized as follows:

1. To detect complement-binding, clinically significant antibodies that may be missed by pure anti-IgG in routine testing.

2. To enhance the reactions of complement-binding antibodies.

3. To detect IgM antibodies, which invariably bind complement, yet which may elute off the red cells with increase in temperature.

It is generally agreed that anti-C4 is less important than anti-C3 for the detection of clinically significant complement-binding antibodies. Since red cells stored in CPD have higher than normal levels of C4 and C3d bound to their membrane, antiglobulin serum should have low levels of anti-C4, and anti-C3d levels must be high enough to detect C3d on the red cells that have been sensitized with complement-binding antibodies in vitro but not so high as to cause "false" positive reactions with CPD stored blood.

In the direct antiglobulin test, anti-C3 is important for the following reasons:

1. In cold hemagglutinin disease (cold antibody autoimmune hemolytic anemia), the patient's cold antibody reacts at up to 30 to 32°C. The patient's red cells therefore become sensitized with antibody in the peripheral circulation when the skin temperature drops to this range or below. The antibody, which usually binds complement, may cause hemolysis of the red cells; however, if the red cells escape hemolysis, they will be recirculated and warmed to 37°C when the cold antibody elutes off the red cells into the plasma, leaving only complement components (primarily C3d) attached to the red cells.

2. In as many as one-fifth of patients with warm antibody autoimmune hemolytic anemia, only complement (C3d) is demonstratable on the red cells. It is believed that IgG is present on the red cells, but in amounts below the threshold of the antiglobulin test as routinely performed.

COMPATIBILITY TESTING

The compatibility test (or "crossmatch") is the most important and most frequently performed procedure in the routine blood bank laboratory. There are two kinds of crossmatch: the "major" and the "minor." The major crossmatch is the more important, since its purpose is to prevent a transfusion reaction (adverse) by detecting antibodies in the patient's serum that would reduce the survival of the donor's red cells and to ensure maximum benefit to the recipient. The minor crossmatch detects antibodies in the donor that may be capable of adversely affecting or destroying the recipient's red cells.

Many procedures are available that can, in combination, constitute a satisfactory crossmatch. Since adverse reactions to transfusion can occur if antibodies in the recipient's serum are not recognized or detected in the crossmatch (which may lead to a reduced survival or a rapid destruction of the transfused red cells and even to the death of the patient), it is essential that the crossmatch provide conditions suitable for the optimum reactivity of as many clinically significant antibodies as presently known techniques allow.

Identification

Before a specimen of blood from the intended recipient is accepted for compatibility testing, all clerical details regarding identification must be checked. The patient's full name, hospital number, address, and date of birth must coincide on the specimen tube and on the requisition. Specimens that are unlabeled must be rejected. Under no circumstances should the clerical details be written on the specimen tube after it has been received by the blood transfusion laboratory or after the blood has been taken. Specimens should be also be rejected on the basis of clerical error. In doubtful cases (e.g., when the patient cannot be identified because of unconsciousness when admitted) the laboratory director should be consulted.

It is a sobering thought to realize that the most efficient laboratory using the best equipment and personnel cannot prevent an adverse transfusion reaction caused as a result of inaccurate identification.

Saline Techniques: Applications and Limitations in Crossmatching

Certain blood group antibodies react at body temperature in vivo yet may give optimum reactions in vitro at temperatures below that of the body. Saline techniques are designed to detect IgM antibodies that react optimally at room temperature (22°C) or below. These include anti-M, anti-N, anti-Le^a, anti-Le^b, anti-Lu^a and anti-P_1. The technique also serves to detect major ABO grouping errors, since incompatibility in this phase will result (in potentially serious situations) if red cells of an incorrect ABO group have been mistakenly selected for crossmatching.

As a sole compatibility test, saline techniques are, of course, inadequate, since clinically significant IgG antibodies are not detected in this phase. Note that agglutination in the saline crossmatch may indicate the presence of cold agglutinins (e.g., anti-I) that will often increase in strength with reduction in temperature.

Most laboratories include saline techniques as part of the routine crossmatch. In emergency situations, this test is sometimes eliminated from the procedure, or performed by the "immediate spin" technique. Details of the saline (room temperature and 37°C) technique are included under the heading *Antibody Detection and Identification.*

Albumin Techniques: Applications and Limitations in Crossmatching

The addition of bovine albumin to the crossmatch presents ideal conditions for the detection of Rh/Hr and certain other blood group antibodies. Bovine albumin acts to increase the dielectric constant of the medium (thereby reducing the zeta potential), allowing IgG antibodies to be demonstrated. The majority of IgG antibodies are detectable in this way, although some may only agglutinate very weakly (e.g., anti-Fy^a).

The sensitivity of the antiglobulin test can be increased through the addition of bovine albumin (see further discussion under the heading *The Antiglobulin Test*).

One of the main disadvantages of albumin techniques is the presence of nonspecific aggregates revealed in microscopic reading (especially when 30% albumin is used). Although these aggregates are rarely a problem for the experienced worker, the inexperienced may be confused by them. In appearance, they have smooth edges and leave a trail of unagglutinated red cells. Although a drop of saline will often help to disperse them, it should be noted that this may also disrupt weak agglutination.

A further disadvantage of albumin techniques is the occasional presence in the serum of albumin autoagglutinating factor (AAAF). This is a rare type of autoagglutinin that reacts with red cells only when they are suspended in bovine albumin and not when they are suspended in saline. In fact, the antibody responsible for this phenomenon is not directed against albumin at all but rather against sodium caprylate (used as a stabilizer in some preparations of bovine albumin) or other fatty-acid salts. Details of the albumin 37°C test are included under the heading *Antibody Detection and Identification.*

Enzyme Techniques: Applications and Limitations in Crossmatching

Like albumin techniques, enzyme techniques can provide a satisfactory "back-up" test for the indirect antiglobulin technique in routine crossmatching, since they are capable of detecting many clinically significant IgG and saline-active IgM antibodies. Both one- and two-stage techniques are available. The two-stage technique (i.e., red cells pretreated with enzyme and then tested with the patient's serum) is most widely used. One-stage techniques (i.e., enzyme, patient's serum, and donor's red cells incubated together), though easier to apply in the crossmatch situation and therefore convenient, are less sensitive than two-stage techniques.

The major limitation of enzyme techniques is their inability to detect certain antibodies in the MNSs and Duffy blood group systems. This fact immediately precludes the use of enzyme techniques as a sole test for compatibility. Other limitations include the inactivation of certain enzymes (e.g., papain) if improperly stored and the incidence of "nonspecific" agglutinins as a result of the method's high sensitivity. Moreover, false results can be obtained if the red cells are "overtreated" with certain enzymes (e.g., papain) because of fragmentation of the immunoglobulin molecules by the enzyme.

On the positive side, enzymes occasionally allow for the detection of some antibodies not demonstrable by other techniques—notably some early Rh/r antibodies and certain rare examples of Kidd antibodies.

Enzyme tests may be carried through the antiglobulin technique if required (see under the heading *The Antiglobulin Test*).

Since cold autoagglutinins are enhanced by enzyme technique, a patient auto control should always be run with each test.

The enzymes commonly used in the blood transfusion laboratory are bromelin, trypsin, papain, ficin, and multienzyme preparations, each of which have certain individual characteristics. The use of a specific enzyme in the laboratory is purely a matter of individual preference.

The Antiglobulin Test: Applications and Limitations in Crossmatching

Of all compatibility tests, the antiglobulin test probably comes closest to approaching the "ideal," and its inclusion in the routine crossmatch should be considered essential. The majority of antibodies that could result in transfusion problems are detectable in this test. The technique is capable of detecting many IgG antibodies that do not react in either saline or high-protein media or that react weakly or variably in these media. It also detects antibodies that bind complement but that may not be capable of binding to red cells sufficient IgG to give a positive test. The main limitation of the test is the large number of factors that may influence or affect the reaction (see p. 589).

Selection of Blood for Transfusion: Routine Situations

As a general rule, the blood selected for crossmatch should be of the same ABO and Rh_o (D) type as that of the recipient. In cases in which ABO group-specific blood is unavailable (as in transfusing group A blood to an AB recipient or for ABO and/or Rh hemolytic disease of the newborn), it may be acceptable or even advisable to transfuse packed red cells of a different ABO group, provided that they are compatible.

It is considered unnecessary to be concerned with subgroups of A unless the patient has a clinically significant anti-A_1 or anti-HI (anti-O), in which case the following will apply:

1. Anti-A_1 in the patient's serum. Examples of anti-A_1 that are active in vitro at 30°C or higher have been shown to be capable of causing extensive red cell destruction. These patients should receive blood of subtype A_2. If a powerful anti-A_1 is present that is reactive at room temperature, it is still good practice to give the patient blood of subtype A_2.
2. Anti-HI (Anti-O) in the patient's serum. Examples of anti-HI (anti-O) that are *not* inhibited by H substance are occasionally active at temperatures above 30°C and have been known to cause rapid destruction of transfused (incompatible) red cells. These patients should receive blood of group A_1.

In the case of Rh, matching for the Rh/Hr antigens *other* than Rh_o (D) is considered unnecessary unless, of course, the patient has a known Rh/Hr antibody, in which case blood lacking the corresponding antigen must be selected. Rh_o (D)-negative recipients should receive blood that, in addition to being Rh_o (D)-negative, should also be rh′ (C-negative and rh″ (E)-negative. In cases of shortage or emergency, rh″ (C)-positive (Du-negative) blood may be substituted when transfusing adult Rh_o (D)-negative recipients (although this should be avoided for the transfusion of women of child-bearing age, except in cases of dire emergency). Generally rh″ (E)-positive (D^u-negative) blood is preferable to rh′ (C)-positive (D^u-negative) blood under these circumstances, since the latter, when transfused to an Rh_o (D)-negative recipient, could stimulate the formation of anti-G.

For D^u-positive recipients, the transfusion of Rh_o (D) positive blood appears to involve very little risk of immunization of anti-Rh_o (D).

Selection of Blood for Transfusion: Emergency Situations

In cases in which there is insufficient time to determine the patient's blood group (or in which this is impossible), blood of group O Rh_o (D)-negative (rh′ [C]-negative, rh″ [E]-negative) may be used, *provided that* most of the plasma is removed and that it has been tested and found to be free of hemolytic anti-A and anti-B. Blood of group O Rh_o (D)-positive may be used *only* if Rh_o (D)-negative blood is unavailable.

In the vast majority of circumstances in which blood is required in an emergency situation, there is time to perform a routine ABO and Rh_o (D) typing. If time permits, an emergency crossmatch can be performed, and group- and type-specific blood should be given. It is best to perform all tests in the transfusion facility without relying on previous records. Evidence of the patient's blood group must *not* be taken from cards, dog tags, driver's licences, or other such records.

When an emergency crossmatch is required, the patient's physician must weigh the risk of transfusing uncrossmatched or incompletely crossmatched blood against the consequences of waiting for routine crossmatch tests to be completed. In the laboratory, the following is recommended:

1. Requests for compatibility testing labeled "stat" or "emergency" must take precedence over all other work in the laboratory.
2. The attending physician should indicate the urgent nature of the situation, and, if uncrossmatched or imcompletely crossmatched blood is required, should be made aware of the inherent risks involved.
3. The routine crossmatch should be begun and continued even if the blood is released. The use of low–ionic strength solution as a suspending medium will allow a safe reduction of incubation time.
4. If the incompatibility is detected in any phase of the crossmatch, the patient's physician should be notified immediately, as should the medical director of the laboratory.

Selection of Blood When the Recipient's Specimen is Not Available

In certain rare situations, a specimen from the recipient is not available for crossmatch (e.g., if the patient is being transferred from another hospital and blood is required immediately upon arrival in order to save the patient's life). In cases such as these, group O Rh_o (D)-negative (rh′ [C]-negative, rh″ [E]-negative) blood should be chosen for transfusion. As soon as a specimen from the recipient is available, a routine crossmatch should be performed on the units already transfused and on those that are to be transfused. If incompatibility is noted in any phase of the crossmatch, the patient's physician and the medical director of the laboratory should be notified immediately.

Selection of Blood When Group-specific Blood is Not Available

The transfusion of blood of a group that is not the same as that of the recipient is acceptable when the required group is not available under the following conditions:

1. Blood must be issued as packed red cells whenever possible.
2. If the whole blood is issued, it must be shown to lack hemolysins directed against cells of the recipient's group.

The choices of alternative blood groups that are acceptable are shown in Table 28–3.

In cases in which groups A_1 (or A_2) or B are both acceptable as an alternative first choice for transfusion (see Table 28–3), either group may be chosen, but only one of the two should be used for a given recipient. If the patient has received one of these two and blood of yet another group is needed, it is best to use blood of group O (hemolysin free). Generally in these circumstances, group A blood is chosen preferentially, because it is more readily available than group B blood.

The decision to change back to group-specific blood should be based on the presence or absence of anti-A and/or anti-B in subsequent samples of the recipient's blood. If the crossmatch of a freshly drawn sample from the patient with group-specific blood indicates compatibility (especially in the saline room-temperature phase), then the group-specific blood can be issued. (*Note*: Group-specific transfusions should *not* be given through the same infusion set as was used for the transfusion of red cells of a different ABO group.) The effect of transfused alloantibodies should be evaluated when the emergency is over, since these antibodies may cause hemolysis of the recipient's red cells.

Visual Checking of Donor Units

Before a unit of blood is chosen for crossmatch and before it is issued for transfusion, it is important to check the unit visually. Discoloration of the blood (e.g., purple coloring) indicates hemolysis of the red cells, which may have been caused by improper storage conditions. Clots in the unit (which could be due to inadequate mixing of anticoagulant when the unit was collected), although serologically insignificant, can often cause clogging of the administration set.

Antibodies to High- and Low-incidence Antigens in Crossmatching

Occasionally, a crossmatch will reveal compatibility in the antibody screen with incompatibility involving only one unit selected for crossmatch. This could be due to an antibody to a low-incidence antigen in the recipient's serum reacting with the corresponding antigen on

TABLE 28–3. Choice of Alternative Blood Groups Acceptable for Patients of Particular Blood Groups When Group-Specific Blood Is Unavailable

Patient's Blood Group	Alternative Blood Group *First Choice*	*Second Choice*
A_1	0	None
A_2 with anti-A_1	0	None
A_1 with anti–HI(O)	None	None
B	0	None
A_1B	A or B	0
A_1B with anti-HI(O)	A_1 or B	None
A_2B	A or B	0
A_2B with anti-A_1	A_2 or B	0

the donor cells. If possible, the antibody should be identified and an alternative unit chosen for crossmatch.

The problem is much more difficult in the case of an antibody to a high-incidence antigen. In some cases it is not possible to find compatible units of blood. In cases such as these, the patient's relatives, especially siblings, may be compatible. If not, it may be possible to find compatible donors through a reference laboratory or a rare donor file. If a patient is known to have an antibody to a high-incidence antigen and is likely to require repeated transfusions, the possibility of autotransfusion should be considered.

ANTIBODY DETECTION AND IDENTIFICATION

The detection of incompatibility in antibody detection (screening) tests or crossmatching presents a choice of two courses of action for the technologist:

1. To identify the antibody(ies) and select blood that lacks the corresponding antigen(s) for crossmatching.
2. To perform crossmatching using several other donor units in an attempt to find units that fail to react with the recipient's serum (which are then regarded as compatible and issued for transfusion).

The second choice of action is much less desirable than the first and should be chosen only in cases of extreme emergency in which the provision of blood is the first priority. In following the first course of action—i.e., the identification of the antibody(ies)—a careful, planned methodology will reduce the waste of valuable serum and aid in the final elucidation of the problem.

Selection of Screening Cells

Commercial panels (for antibody identification) are usually accompanied by at least two separate "screening cells" for the *detection* of antibodies. These red cells, which are group O, contain as many common antigens as possible. Pooled reagent screening cells are not recommended for the detection of antibodies in patients (although they are sometimes used when screening the serum of blood donors), since weak antibodies may not be detected because not all of the cells will possess the same antigenic determinants.

Screening cells will, in most cases, not detect antibodies to low-frequency antigens, because these antigens will probably not be present on the cells. Antibodies of this type are therefore detected only when an antibody identification procedure is performed because of the presence of *another* antibody in the serum, or when a crossmatch is found to be incompatible, or if a newborn presents with or develops jaundice after delivery.

Antibody screening tests should be set up in parallel with crossmatching procedures through all phases and with all other laboratory procedures in which it is important to detect the presence of irregular antibodies (e.g., prenatal and postnatal investigations). The screening cells' protocol is provided with the cells and should be closely examined whenever an irregular antibody is detected, since it may, in some cases, serve as an aid in the identification of the antibody.

It should be noted that, if screening cells are prepared by an individual laboratory, the cells chosen should (if possible) provide at least one homozygote for each specificity known to show dosage. This will avoid the problem of an antibody's being missed because it reacts only with homozygous cells and not with heterozygous cells.

A typical screening cell protocol is given in Table 28–4.

Selection of Panel Cells

Antibody identification is performed using a "cell panel." These are commercially prepared, though they can be made up by each individual laboratory. They consist of a number of red cells from different donors (usually eight to ten) of group O that have been carefully selected and tested for the presence or absence of most common antigens. Institutions that prefer to prepare their own panels can fully phenotype individuals on staff and either bleed them regularly or freeze large donations from these individuals in glycerol or liquid nitrogen.

Panels are usually phenotypes for the following red cell antigens: D, C, E, c, e, f, C^w, V, K, k, Kp^a, Kp^b, Js^a, Js^b, Fy^a, Fy^b, Jk^a, Jk^b, Xg^a, Le^a, Le^b, S, s, M, N, P_1, Lu^a, and Lu^b. Additional low-incidence and high-incidence antigens for which the cells have been typed and found to be all negative or all positive, respectively, are usually noted separately on the protocol (or panel sheet). Any "special" typing that has been performed that reveals an "unusual" cell is usually listed in line with the other reactions of the cell. Certain antigens (especially P_1) that show variable antigenic strength are so marked on most panel protocols.

An example of a typical panel sheet (or protocol) is given in Table 28–5.

In general, a useful cell panel will include some red cells that possess and some that lack as many as possible of the common antigenic determinants, chosen in such a way that a distinct pattern of reactions is available for the easy identification of most "single" antibodies and of many "multiple" antibodies.

Red cells that are regarded as special (i.e., those either possessing a low-frequency antigen or lacking a high-frequency antigen) can be stored frozen for future complicated investigations rather than being used in routine situations. In this way, laboratories can develop a "library" of unusual red cell specimens.

Commercial panel cells are usually suspended in modified Alsever's solution to a 3 to 6 per cent suspension

TABLE 28–4 A Typical "Screening Cells" Protocol

Donor No.	Genotype	D	C	E	c	e	f	C^w	K	k	Fy^a	Fy^b	Jk^a	Jk^b	Xg^a	Le^a	Le^b	S	s	M	N	P_1	Lu^a
1	$R_1^wR_1$	+	+	0	0	+	0	+	0	+	+	+	+	+	+	0	+	+	+	+	+	+	0
2	R_2r	+	0	+	+	+	+	0	+	+	0	+	0	+	+	+	0	+	+	+	0	+	0

(From Bryant, N. J.: An Introduction to Immunohematology, 2nd ed. Philadelphia, W. B. Saunders Co., 1982, p. 283.)

TABLE 28–5 A Typical Panel Sheet or Protocol

Donor (Cell)	*Rh/Hr*	*Rh/Hr*							*Kell*		*Duffy*		*Kidd*		*X-linked*	*Lewis*		*MNSs*				*P*	*Lutheran*		*Special Antigen Typing*
No.	Genotype	D	C	E	c	e	f	C^w	K	k	Fy^a	Fy^b	Jk^a	Jk^b	Xg^a	Le^a	Le^b	S	s	M	N	P_1	Lu^a	Lu^b	
1	R_1R_1	+	+	0	0	+	0	0	0	+	0	+	+	0	0	+	0	0	+	+	0	0	0	+	
2	$R_1^wR_1$	+	+	0	0	+	0	+	0	+	0	+	+	0	+	0	+	0	+	+	+	$+^s$	0	+	Bg(a+)
3	R_2R_2	+	0	+	+	0	0	0	0	+	0	+	0	+	+	0	0	+	0	+	0	+	0	+	Kp(a+)
4	R_0r	+	0	0	+	+	+	0	0	+	0	+	+	0	+	0	+	0	0	0	+	$+^s$	0	+	Sd(a+)
5	r′r′	0	+	0	0	+	0	0	+	+	+	0	+	+	+	0	0	+	+	+	+	0	+	+	
6	r″r	0	0	+	+	+	+	0	0	+	+	0	0	+	+	+	0	0	+	+	+	+	0	+	Bg(a+),Wr(a+)
7	rr	0	0	0	+	+	+	0	+	0	+	+	0	+	0	0	+	0	+	+	+	$+^s$	0	+	
8	rr	0	0	0	+	+	+	0	0	+	+	0	+	+	+	0	+	0	+	+	+	+	+	0	Mg+,Co(b+)

(From Bryant, N. J.: An Introduction to Immunohematology, 2nd ed. Philadelphia, W. B. Saunders Co., 1982, p. 282.

and should be stored at 2 to 6°C when not in use. Care should be taken to avoid contamination of the red cells with bacteria or with blood or serum. The "dating period" of the panel (i.e., the date of expiration) should be respected. Note that toward the end of the dating period, the reactivity of some of the more labile antigens may be slightly diminished.

Tests Used in Antibody Detection and Identification

Saline (Room Temperature)

Purpose. The saline (room temperature) test for antibody detection and identification is used to detect or identify cold-reacting (IgM) alloagglutinins (anti-M, anti-N, anti-Le^a, anti-Le^b, etc.) and autoagglutinins (anti-I, anti-IH, anti-H, etc.).

Method. If incompatibility is noted in the antibody detection test at room temperature, the panel of red cells should be set up at that temperature with the patient's serum. Since the antibodies detected in this phase are often anti-I, anti-IH, or anti-H, the following red cells should also be tested with the panel:

1. *If the patient is group O*: Patient's own red cells (autocontrol), two group O (cord) cells (one Rh+, one Rh−).
2. *If the patient is group A*: Patient's own red cells (autocontrol), one group A_1 (adult), one group A_2 (adult), two group O (cord) cells (one Rh+, one Rh−), one group A (cord).
3. *If the patient is group B*: Patient's own red cells (autocontrol), one group B (adult), two group O (cord) cells (one Rh+, one Rh−), one group B (cord).
4. *If the patient is group AB*: Patient's own red cells (autocontrol), one group A_1 (adult), one group A_2 (adult), one group B (adult), two group O (cord) cells (one Rh+, one Rh−), one group A (cord), one group B (cord).

Procedure

1. Set up the appropriate number of 10 × 75 mm test tubes, as indicated above.

2. Add two drops of the patient's serum to each tube.

3. Add one drop of panel cells to each of the appropriate test tubes and one drop of a washed 5 per cent suspension of the cells indicated above to each of the other test tubes.

4. Incubate all tubes at room temperature (22°C) for one hour.

5. Shake each tube gently and read macroscopically. (Negative readings should be checked microscopically.)

6. Grade the reactions carefully.

***Note*: The above procedure can be performed at a lower temperature (e.g., 15–18°C), which tends to enhance the reactions of many cold-reacting antibodies. This temperature can be obtained by placing the rack of tubes in a pan of cold water to which a few ice cubes have been added. If this temperature is chosen, it should be maintained while reading. This can be achieved by reading each tube directly from the water bath.**

The saline technique can also be performed at 37°C, using the same basic procedure. This will be useful for those alloantibodies that favor a warmer temperature for reaction.

Albumin (37°C)

Purpose. The albumin (37°C) test is used to detect warm-reacting (IgG and complement-binding IgG and IgM) alloantibodies and autoantibodies. This technique is particularly useful in the detection and identification of Rh antibodies, which are enhanced by the albumin medium.

Method. For all groups, panel cells and the patient's own red cells (for the autocontrol) will be needed.

Procedure

1. Set up nine 10 × 75 mm test tubes in a test tube rack.

2. Label the tubes A1 through A8 and "auto control," respectively, for an eight-cell panel. (If more cells are available on the panel, set up additional test tubes and label accordingly.)

3. Place two to four drops of the patient's serum in each tube.

4. Add one drop of each appropriate panel cell to tubes A1 through A8.

5. Add one drop of a washed, 3 to 5 per cent saline suspension of red cells from the patient to the autocontrol.

6. Add 2 to 3 drops of 22 to 30 per cent bovine albumin to each tube.

7. Mix the contents of each tube well.

8. Centrifuge immediately at 3400 rpm (1000 G) (Serofuge) for 15 seconds.

9. Read macroscopically and record results. (Results should be carefully graded.)

10. After reading, mix the contents of each tube well.

11. Incubate all tubes at 37°C for 15 to 30 minutes in heat blocks or in a waterbath.

12. Centrifuge immediately after incubation at 3400 rpm (1000 G) (Serofuge) for 15 seconds.

13. Read macroscopically and record results. Negative readings should be checked microscopically.

14. Grade all results carefully.

Indirect Antiglobulin Test (Saline and Albumin 37°C)

Purpose. The indirect antiglobulin test is used to detect warm-reacting (IgG and complement-binding IgM) alloantibodies and autoantibodies.

Method. For all groups, panel cells and the patient's own red cells (for the autocontrol) will be needed.

Procedure

1. Set up nine 10 × 75 mm test tubes in a test tube rack.

2. Label the tubes IAT1 through IAT8 and autocontrol, respectively. (If more cells are available on the panel, set up additional test tubes and label accordingly.)

3. Place 2 to 4 drops of patient's serum in each tube.

4. Add one drop of each appropriate panel cell to tubes IAT1 through IAT8.

5. Add one drop of a washed, 3 to 5 per cent saline suspension of red cells from the patient to the autocontrol.

6. If the saline antiglobulin test is to be performed, proceed to step 7. If the albumin antiglobulin test is to be performed, add 2 to 3 drops of 22 to 30 per cent bovine albumin to each tube.

7. Mix the contents of each tube well.

8. Centrifuge immediately at 3400 rpm (1000 G) (Serofuge) for 15 seconds.

9. Read macroscopically and record results. Results should be carefully graded.

10. After reading, mix the contents of each tube well.

11. Incubate all tubes at 37°C for 15 to 30 minutes in heat blocks or in a waterbath.

12. Centrifuge immediately after incubation at 3400 rpm (1000 G) (Serofuge) for 15 seconds.

13. Read macroscopically and record results. Results should be carefully graded.

14. After reading, mix the contents of each tube well.

15. Wash the contents of each tube three or four times in large volumes of normal (isotonic) saline. Decant each wash as completely as possible.

16. Add 1 to 2 drops of antiglobulin reagent to each tube.

17. Mix well.

18. Centrifuge all tubes at 3400 rpm for 15 seconds.

19. Read macroscopically and record results. Negative reactions should be checked microscopically. Results should be carefully graded.

20. Interpret results.

21. Add 1 drop of antiglobulin control cells to each tube.

22. Centrifuge all tubes at 3400 rpm (1000 G) (Serofuge) for 15 seconds.

23. Examine each tube macroscopically for agglutination.

Note: If any tubes do not show agglutination after the antiglobulin control cells have been added, the test results should be considered invalid, and the tests repeated.

Enzyme Tests (One- and Two-Stage Tests at 37°C)

Purpose. Enzyme tests serve as a "back-up" test for the detection of warm-reacting (IgG or complement-binding) allo- and autoantibodies. These techniques serve to enhance the reaction of certain Rh, Lewis, and Kidd antibodies and may also be useful in identification of those antibodies which fail to react in enzymes.

Method. The method used in enzyme tests will depend on the enzyme of choice. Both one- and two-stage techniques are available, the two-stage tests being far more sensitive than the one-stage tests.

Procedure (One-stage Test Using Papain)

1. Set up nine 10 × 75 mm test tubes in a test tube rack.

2. Label the tubes E1 through E8 and autocontrol, respectively. (If more cells are available on the panel, set up additional test tubes and label accordingly.)

3. The enzyme should be prepared according to the following method: Two grams of papain (papayotin, Merck 1:350) are ground in a mortar with 100 mL of 0.067 M-phosphate buffer, pH 5.4. After filtration, 10 mL of 0.5 M-cysteine is added and the solution is diluted with the buffer to 200 mL; it is then incubated for 1 hour at 37°C. After incubation, the enzyme is ready for use. It can be stored at −20°C for many months. For use, it is diluted 1 in 10 in buffered saline, pH 7.3.

4. Mix three volumes of diluted papain with 1 volume of serum.

5. Place one volume of this mixture in each of the test tubes.

6. Add one volume of the appropriate panel cells to each of the appropriate test tubes and one volume of the patient's red cells to the autocontrol.

7. Mix well.

8. Incubate all tubes at 37°C for two hours.

9. Read macroscopically or microscopically.

Note: If weak antibodies are encountered, or are being tested for, it is advisable to use equal parts of serum and enzyme solution.

Procedure (Two-stage Test Using Papain)

1. Prepare a papain stock solution as follows:

- a. Suspend 1 g of papain in 100 mL of 0.85% NaCl. (This solution may be kept for several months at 4°C, although the bulk of the solution is best kept at −20°C.)
- b. If desired, the suspension can be centrifuged after storage for 24 hours at 4°C with occasional agitation. The clear supernatant is slightly less active than the original suspension.
- c. For use, 1 volume of the stock solution is added to 9 volumes of 0.067 M-Sørensen phosphate buffer, pH 7.3, prepared by adding 3 volumes of 0.067 M-Na_2HPO_4 (9.46 g/L) to 1 volume of 0.067 M-KH_2PO_4 (9.07 g/L).

2. Add 2 volumes of the buffered papain to 1 volume of packed red cells (panel cells) in each tube. Add 1 volume of thrice-washed patient's packed red cells to the tube labeled autocontrol.

3. Incubate all tubes at 37°C for 10 minutes.

4. Wash the red cells three times and make to a 3 per cent suspension in saline that has been warmed to 37°C.

5. Warm the tubes to 37°C and then add 2 volumes of the patient's serum to each tube.
6. Incubate for 90 minutes.
7. Read microscopically.

The Enzyme Antiglobulin Test

Purpose. The enzyme antiglobulin test provides a sensitive back-up test for the detection and identification of warm-reacting (IgG or complement-binding) alloantibodies or autoantibodies.

Method. The method used will depend to some extent on the enzyme of choice. For all groups, panel cells and the patient's own cells (for the autocontrol) will be required.

Procedure

1. Enzyme treat the panel cells and the patient's own cells as described above (see steps 1 through 4 in the procedure for the two-stage enzyme test using papain, above).
2. Set up nine 10 × 75 mm test tubes in a test tube rack. (If more cells are available on the panel, set up additional test tubes and label accordingly.)
3. Label the tubes EA1 through EA8 and autocontrol, respectively.
4. Add 2 to 4 drops of the patient's serum to each tube.
5. Add 1 drop of the appropriate enzyme-treated panel cells to tubes EA1 through EA8.
6. Add 1 drop of a 3 to 5 per cent saline suspension of enzyme-treated patient's own red cells to the autocontrol.
7. Incubate all tubes at 37°C for 15 to 30 minutes in heat blocks or in a waterbath.
8. Centrifuge all tubes at 3400 rpm (1000 G) (Serofuge) for 15 seconds.
9. Read macroscopically and record results. Results should be carefully graded.
10. Wash all red cells three times in large volumes of normal saline. Decant each wash as completely as possible.
11. Add 1 to 2 drops of antiglobulin reagent to each tube.
12. Mix well.
13. Centrifuge at 3400 rpm (1000 G) for 15 seconds.
14. Read macroscopically and record results. Negative reactions should be checked microscopically. Results should be carefully graded.
15. Add 1 drop of antiglobulin control cells to each tube.
16. Centrifuge at 3400 rpm (1000 G) for 15 seconds.
17. Examine each tube macroscopically for agglutination.

Note: If any tubes do not show agglutination after the antiglobulin control cells have been added, the test results should be considered invalid, and the tests repeated.

Antibody Detection and Identification Using Low–Ionic Strength Solution

The rate of association of antibody with antigen is greatly increased by lowering ionic strength. This increase in the rate of association allows for a greatly reduced incubation time.

Preparation of Low–Ionic Strength Solution (LISS)

1. Dissolve 18 g of glycine in approximately 500 mL of distilled water and add 1.0 M NaOH until the pH is 6.7.
2. Add the glycine dropwise with stirring until the pH has reached 6.7. (*Note*: Approximately 0.35 mL of 1.0 M NaOH will be needed.)
3. Add 20 mL of phosphate buffer, 0.15 M, pH 6.7. (Prepared by mixing approximately equal volumes of 0.15 M Na_2HPO_4 and 0.15 M NaH_2PO_4.)
4. Add 1.79 g NaCl dissolved in about 100 mL of distilled water.
5. The mixture is then made up to 1 liter with distilled water.

Procedure

1. Wash the panel cells and the patient's own cells twice in saline and then once in low–ionic strength solution.
2. Prepare a 3 per cent suspension of all of the cells in LISS.
3. Set up nine 10 × 75 mm test tubes in a test tube rack.
4. Label the tubes LISS 1 through LISS 8 and LISS autocontrol, respectively. (If more cells are available on the panel, set up additional test tubes and label accordingly.)
5. Add 2 drops of the patient's serum to each tube.
6. Add 1 drop of each of the panel cells (suspended in LISS) to the appropriate tubes and 1 drop of the patient's own cells (suspended in LISS) to the autocontrol.
7. Incubate all tubes at 37°C for 10 minutes.
8. Wash the red cells three times in LISS.
9. Add 1 to 2 drops of antiglobulin reagent to each tube.
10. Centrifuge at 3400 rpm (1000 G) (Serofuge) for 15 seconds.
11. Read and record results. Tests should be read microscopically and the reactions graded carefully.
12. Interpret results.
13. Add 1 drop of antiglobulin control cells to each tube.
14. Centrifuge at 3400 rpm (1000 G) (Serofuge) for 15 seconds.
15. Examine each tube macroscopically for agglutination.

Note: If any tubes do not show agglutination after the antiglobulin control cells have been added, the test results should be considered invalid, and the tests repeated.

Interpretation of Results

In establishing the identity of an antibody, it is good practice to use a process of basic elimination, based on the temperature of the reactions, the techniques that give reactions, and the frequency of positive results obtained. For example, an antibody reacting strongly at 37°C and weakly or not at all at room temperature allows for the exclusion of many cold antibodies (P_1, H, IH, M, Lu^a, etc.). An antibody reacting in the indirect antiglobulin test with approximately one out of ten samples *could* be anti-K, based on frequency statistics. An antibody that causes hemolysis of the red cells *could* be a Lewis antibody or some other antibody known to cause in vitro hemolysis (e.g., anti-Jk^a). The racial origin of the patient is also often helpful, based on the frequency differences of particular antigens within that race. Note that a patient who has never been transfused or been pregnant will probably possess a non–red cell immune antibody, although this kind of interpretation must be made with caution because of the general unreliability of patient information.

In difficult interpretations, the possibility that the original tests are inaccurate should not be excluded. A set of results that defies identification can often be resolved by a fresh start with a new specimen from the patient.

The establishment of specificity of an antibody is often an arduous task. The discussion that follows is aimed at the routine laboratory worker, who will undoubtedly seek the assistance of more experienced workers when meeting a particular problem that appears to defy resolution.

The Single Specific Antibody. Once the results of an investigation are known and recorded, an attempt is made to establish a pattern of reactions in accordance with those given on the panel sheet. (See Example 1.)

The test results in Example 1 exactly duplicate the reactions on the panel sheet for the D antigen. The antibody, therefore, reacts with all Rh_o(D)-positive red cells and fails to react with all Rh_o(D)-negative red cells. The specificity of the antibody, therefore, appears to be anti-Rh_o(D). In support of this is the fact that the antibody is enhanced by albumin and enzymes, a feature that is typical of Rh antibodies.

It is important to realize that the results of the tests with a known panel do not prove *conclusively* the specificity of a particular antibody. All other possibilities must be taken into account and excluded. Several steps can be taken to exclude this possibility:

1. The patient's red cells can be phenotyped for C^w antigen status. If the C^w antigen is present on the red cells, the possible presence of the antibody can be excluded.

2. The known antibody (i.e., anti-D) can be absorbed with Rh^o(D)-positive, C_w-negative red cells, and the investigation repeated with the absorbed serum.

3. A panel of cells that are Rh_o(D)-negative, C^w-positive can be used with the patient's serum. If these cells give negative reactions, the presence of anti-C^w can be discounted.

Difficult Cases

Specific Reactions That Do Not Duplicate a Pattern of Reaction on the Panel Sheet. This is not an uncommon problem and can be caused by a number of factors:

1. *A mixture of antibodies*: This possibility should be investigated by using the methods described later in this chapter.

2. *Dosage effect*: Certain antibodies show reactions with homozygous cells only or react more strongly with homozygous than with heterozygous cells. Consider the following test results (Example 2). (*Note*: Refer to the panel sheet given with Example 1.) Note that in Example 2, only homozygous (MM) red cells are showing reaction; MN red cells show no reaction.

3. *Variation in antigenic strength*: Certain antigens (P_1, Le^a, Le^b, etc.) show great variation of strength from one individual to another. When an antibody to one of these antigens is weak in a patient's serum, red cells possessing a weak antigen of the corresponding specificity may fail to react altogether.

4. *Weak reactions*: Establishing the specificity of an antibody is difficult unless the reactions obtained are in the 1+ range or stronger. Weak reactions will often cause confusion and can defy accurate identification. Antibodies may increase in strength in certain circumstances, owing to continued stimulation (e.g., in pregnancy), and it is therefore worth testing a later sample in cases such as these before giving specificity to the reactions.

5. *Contamination*: Apparent specificity may result from contamination of the patient's serum or of the panel cells. A fresh specimen from the patient or a fresh panel will eliminate this problem.

EXAMPLE 1

Antigen	**1**	**2**	**3**	**4**	**5**	**6**	**7**	**8**
D	+	+	+	+	–	–	–	–
C	+	+	–	–	+	–	–	–
c	–	–	+	+	–	+	+	+
E	+	–	+	–	–	+	–	–
e	+	+	–	+	+	+	+	+
C^w	–	+	–	–	–	–	–	–
K	–	–	–	–	+	–	+	–
k	+	+	+	+	+	+	–	+
Fy^a	–	–	–	–	–	+	+	+
Fy^b	+	+	+	+	–	–	+	–
Jk^a	+	+	–	+	+	–	–	+
Jk^b	–	–	+	–	+	+	+	+
Le^a	+	–	–	–	–	+	–	–
Le^b	–	+	–	+	–	–	+	+
P_1	–	+	+	+	–	+	+	–
M	+	+	+	–	+	+	+	+
N	–	+	–	+	+	+	+	+
S	–	–	+	–	+	–	+	+
s	+	+	–	–	+	+	+	

Panel Sheet

Test Results

ABO Group 0 Rh Negative

Rh Phenotype ce (rr)

Direct Antiglobin Test Negative

Special Phenotype ce (rr)

	1	2	3	4	5	6	7	8
Saline (RT)	–	–	–	–	–	–	–	–
Albumin (IS)	2	2	2	2	–	–	–	–
Albumin (37°C)	4	4	4	4	–	–	–	–
Albumin AHG	4	4	4	4	–	–	–	–
Enzyme	4	4	4	4	–	–	–	–

Specificity: Anti-Rh_o(D)

EXAMPLE 2

Test Results

ABO 0 Rh Positive

Rh Phenotype CDe (R_1R_1)

Direct Antiglobulin Test Negative

Special Phenotype N

	1	2	3	4	5	6	7	8
Saline (RT)	2	–	2	–	–	–	–	–
Albumin (IS)	–	–	–	–	–	–	–	–
Albumin (37°C)	–	–	–	–	–	–	–	–
Albumin AGH	–	–	–	–	–	–	–	–
Enzyme	–	–	–	–	–	–	–	–

Specificity: Anti-M (showing dosage)

6. *An antibody not represented on the cell panel*: A rare antibody not represented on the particular panel in use may be the cause of the problem. This can sometimes be overcome with the use of a panel that is more fully phenotyped or with the use of rare cells of various specificity that might be retained by the laboratory. If specificity cannot be determined, the specimen can be referred to a consultation laboratory that specializes in this sort of investigation and that, therefore, will possess large and comprehensive exclusion panels.

7. *A new antigen-antibody system*: This is an exciting but rather remote possibility. The establishment of a new blood group system is a complicated research project and as such is beyond the scope of this text.

A Mixture of Antibodies. The identification of antibody "mixtures" often constitutes a difficult and complex serological undertaking, yet the occurrence of such mixtures is not uncommon, since individuals who produce antibodies to one antigenic stimulus quite often readily produce others.

The suggestion that a mixture of antibodies is present in a serum sample may be indicated by any or all of the following:

1. *A varying distribution of positive and negative reactions at different temperatures*: This would indicate a possible mixture of warm- and cold-reacting antibodies. This type of mixture is often relatively simple to identify, provided that there is no "carry-over" of reactions through a wide thermal range. Confirmation of results can be achieved by confining the room temperature tests to red cell samples that lack the antigen to the warm-reacting antibody. The same basic rules apply to the test performed at warm temperatures.

2. *A varying distribution of positive and negative results in different techniques*: Certain antibodies react preferentially in certain techniques (for example, anti-Fy^a, which reacts well in the indirect antiglobulin test yet fails to react with enzymes). The presence of a second antibody, reactive in enzymes or in the saline technique, would therefore not be affected by the reaction of the anti-Fy^a. Such mixtures are therefore simple to identify, even if both antibodies are reactive within the same temperature range.

3. *Varying strengths of reactions in the same technique in which dosage effect is not evident*: A serum containing, for example, anti-M and anti-Lu^a cannot be differentiated through various techniques and/or temperature ranges, since both are cold agglutinins and react in saline at or below room temperature. In cases such as this, noting the antigens on the red cells that give *negative* reactions with the given serum (if any) can aid in the identification of the components of the mixture (i.e., red cells that are M-negative and Lu^a-negative). (See Example 3. Refer to the cell panel in Example 1 for interpretation.)

Note that in Example 3 the only red cell showing a negative reaction (cell 4) is Lu^a-negative and M-negative. The same basic principle can be applied to mixtures of more than two antibodies, though in these cases additional panels (or special red cells) may be needed.

Isolating the red cells on the panel that give the *strongest* reaction can often give a clue to the identity of the antibody present. In Example 3, cells 5 and 8 give 4+ reactions, whereas all other positive reactions are 2+. It will be noted that cells 5 and 8 are Lu(a+).

EXAMPLE 3

Test Results

ABO 0 Rh Negative

Rh phenotype cde (rr)

Direct Antiglobulin Test Negative

Special Phenotype Lu(a-), M–

	1	2	3	4	5	6	7	8	A
Saline (RT)	2	2	2	–	4	2	2	4	–
Albumin (IS)	–	–	–	–	–	–	–	–	–
Albumin (37°C)	–	–	–	–	–	–	–	–	–
Albumin AHG	–	–	–	–	–	–	–	–	–
Enzyme	–	–	–	–	–	–	–	–	–

Specificity: Anti-M + Anti-Lu^a

Other Procedures Used in Antibody Identification

Phenotyping

Phenotyping of the patient can often be an invaluable aid in the identification of an antibody, especially in the process of elimination, since the presence of the corresponding antigen will usually discount the possibility of the antibody present.

Full phenotyping can also be useful in difficult cases in order to ascertain which antibodies the patient is capable of producing.

Absorption

In difficult cases, the absorption of a "known" antibody from the patient's serum can often be helpful in revealing the specificity of the remaining antibody, and in some cases it may result in the total separation of the components of a mixture of antibodies. The usual method of absorption is as follows:

1. Wash a large volume of the red cells to be used in the absorption three times in normal saline. These red cells must possess the antigen corresponding to the antibody that is to be absorbed and should lack the antigen(s) corresponding to the antibody that is not to be absorbed (i.e., that is to remain in the serum).
2. After the final wash, centrifuge the red cells so that they are tightly packed, and remove *all* of the saline from the cells.
3. Add a volume of serum equal to the volume of absorbing red cells.
4. Incubate for 30 minutes to one hour at the optimum reaction temperature of the antibody being absorbed.
5. Test the serum to ensure that absorption is complete. If not, the procedure may be repeated using another aliquot of washed packed red cells. Always test to ensure that the antibody that is to remain in the serum is sufficiently reactive before continuing with repeat absorptions.

Elution

In certain cases, an antibody in a patient's serum may be taken up by the patient's own red cells (i.e., autoantibody). In antibody investigation, this will reveal itself by a positive direct antiglobulin test with no (or little) free antibody in the serum. In such cases, elution techniques are used to remove the antibody from the red cells, with subsequent identification of the antibody in the eluate. Several methods are available for performing an elution; the following represent those that are required by the syllabus of studies of the Canadian Society of Laboratory Technologists and the American Society of Clinical Pathologists:

Heat Elution

1. Wash the red cells from which the eluate is to be made six times in large volumes of normal saline. The final wash should be performed by adding a volume of saline equal to the volume of washed packed red cells. Centrifuge and recover the supernatant and test in parallel with the eluate. This "last wash" is an important negative control that demonstrates that the residual antibody has been removed before the eluate is prepared from the red cells.
2. Add a further volume of saline (or AB serum or 6 per cent albumin) equal to the volume of washed packed red cells.
3. Place the tube in a 56°C water bath for 10 minutes. Agitate frequently and strongly during incubation.
4. Centrifuge at 3400 rpm (1000 G) (Serofuge) for 1 minute.
5. Recover the hemoglobin-stained supernatant. This is the eluate.
6. Test the eluate for the presence of antibody by standard methods.

Ether Elution

1. Wash the red cells from which the eluate is to be made six times in large volumes of saline. Recover the final wash as described above (see step 1 in heat elution method).
2. Add an equal volume of saline to the washed packed red cells and mix.
3. Add reagent-grade diethyl ether in an amount equal to the total volume of the red cells plus saline. (*Note:* The ether must be fresh; the appearance of a brown color when the ether is added indicates that the ether is oxidized and that the eluate will be useless.)
4. Stopper and mix by inversion for 1 minute.
5. Carefully remove the stopper to release the volatile ether.
6. Incubate at 37°C for 30 minutes. (*Note:* This step is optional, but it will result in a more potent eluate if included.)
7. Centrifuge at 3400 rpm (1000 G) (Serofuge) for ten minutes. The tube will then contain three layers—clear ether on the top, red cell stroma in the middle, and hemoglobin-stained eluate on the bottom.
8. Aspirate and discard the top two layers, and transfer the eluate to another tube.
9. Incubate the eluate in an unstopped tube at 37°C for 15 minutes to drive off the residual ether.
10. Test the eluate for the presence of antibody by using standard methods.

Note. Elution can be used in antibody identification for the following purposes:

1. To identify the antibody on an infant's red cells in hemolytic disease of the newborn.
2. To identify the antibody producing a positive direct antiglobulin test in acquired hemolytic anemia or in suspected transfusion reactions.
3. To produce a small amount of useful single antibody preparation after the separation of a mixture of antibodies by absorption.
4. To remove antibody from the patient's red cells so that they can be used for autoabsorption, or to render them suitable for further testing.
5. To demonstrate that the red cells have absorbed an antibody and, therefore, that they possess the corresponding antigen.

Use of 2-Mercaptoethanol and Dithiothreitol

The technique of splitting 19S IgM molecules into 7S subunits using 2-mercaptoethanol or dithiothreitol can be used in antibody identification to inactivate an IgM antibody in a mixture of IgG and IgM antibodies. The techniques are as follows.

Inactivation of IgM Antibodies by 2-Mercaptoethanol

Purpose. This technique is used to separate multiple cold and warm antibodies for the purpose of identification or to determine the immunoglobulin nature of the antibody. The latter application may be particularly useful in predicting whether an antibody is likely to cause hemolytic disease of the newborn.

Reagents Required

1. Phosphate buffer pH 7.4, prepared as follows:
   a. Dissolve 9.47 g anhydrous Na_2HPO_4 in 1000 mL distilled water.
   b. Dissolve 9.08 g crystalline KH_2PO_4 in 1000 mL distilled water.
   c. Mix 80.8 mL of Na_2HPO_4 solution with 19.2 mL KH_2PO_4 solution at room temperature.
2. 0.2 M 2-Mercaptoethanol, prepared by adding 100 mL phosphate buffer, pH 7.4, to 1.56 mL 2-mercaptoethanol. (*Note:* This should not be stored for more than one month at 4°C.)
3. Buffered saline.
4. 0.2 M iodoacetamide, prepared by dissolving 0.37 g iodoacetamide in 100 mL buffered saline, pH 7.4.

Method

1. Mix 1 mL of 2-Mercaptoethanol with 1 mL of the test serum.
2. Incubate at 37°C for 15 minutes with a control (which consists of equal volumes of isotonic saline and test serum)
3. Add 1 mL iodoacetamide to the test serum and control, or dialyze overnight (16 hours) against phosphate buffered saline.
4. Test both mixtures against appropriate red cells by saline techniques (immediate spin and room temperature), convert to high-protein test (albumin) read after immediate spin and then again after 30 minutes at 37°C, and convert to the antiglobulin technique.
5. If indicated, titer both mixtures by serial dilution in isotonic saline and test against appropriate red cells by standard procedures to measure the effectiveness of inactivation.

Interpretation

1. If no reactivity is noted in the control, this indicates dilution of the antibody and invalidates the results.

2. If no reactivity is noted in the test but reactivity is noted in the control mixture, this indicates that only IgM antibodies are present.

3. Reactivity in the test mixture only in the indirect antiglobulin test and reactivity in the control mixture indicates that IgG antibodies are present.

4. If reactivity is noted in the same phases of both the test and control tubes, titration studies should be performed.

5. A fourfold reduction of activity (two-tube difference in titer) when compared with the control indicates the presence of an IgM antibody. No reduction of activity indicates that only IgG antibody is reacting or that the 2-mercaptoethanol is not working properly.

Notes. 2-Mercapthoethanol has a noxious odor and should therefore be used under a hood. Most recent investigations show 2-mercaptoethanol to be more effective than dithiothreitol for this purpose; however, a few very potent antibodies still may not be inactivated, even with prolonged incubation. The addition of iodoacetamide is necessary to prevent false positives. If the added dilution caused by the iodoacetamide is undesirable, the 2-mercaptoethanol serum mixture may be dialyzed overnight (16 hours) against phosphate buffered saline, as described.

Inactivation of IgM Antibodies by Dithiothreitol

Purpose. This technique is used to separate multiple cold and warm antibodies for the purpose of identification or to determine the immunoglobulin nature of the antibody. The latter application may be particularly useful in predicting whether an antibody is likely to cause hemolytic disease of the newborn.

Reagents Required. 0.01 M Dithiothreitol, prepared by dissolving 0.77 g DTT in isotonic saline to a volume of 500 mL. (*Note*: The DTT solution is stable at −20°C for up to six months, but is not stable at 4°C.)

Method

1. Mix equal volumes of DTT solution and test serum.

2. Incubate at 37°C for 30 minutes with a control (which consists of equal volumes of isotonic saline and test serum).

3. Test both mixtures against appropriate red cells by saline techniques (immediate spin and room temperature), convert to high-protein test (immediate spin and 37°C), then carry to antiglobulin test.

4. If indicated, titer both mixtures by serial dilutions in isotonic saline and test against appropriate red cells by standard procedures to measure the effectiveness of inactivation.

Interpretation

1. If no reactivity is noted in the control, this indicates the dilution of the antibody and invalidates the results.

2. No activity in the test but reactivity in the control mixture indicates that only IgM antibodies are present.

3. Reactivity in the test mixture only in the indirect antiglobulin test and reactivity in the control mixture indicates that IgG antibodies are present.

4. If reactivity is noted in the same phase in both the test and control tubes, titration studies should be performed. A fourfold reduction of activity (two-tube difference in titer) when compared with the control indicates the presence of IgM antibodies. No reduction of activity indicates that only IgG antibody is reacting or that the DTT is not working properly.

Notes. DTT is not as odorous as 2-mercaptoethanol and provides a more rapid test. However, it may not be as effective as 2-mercaptoethanol when dealing with more potent antibodies.

Titration

Titration can be defined as a semiquantitative means of measuring the *amount* of antibody in a serum. A *titer*, therefore, refers to the *strength* of an antibody, measured by determining the greatest dilution of antibody-containing serum that will produce a detectable reaction with a standard volume of red cells possessing the corresponding antigen.

Titration is often used to demonstrate an increase in strength of a maternal antibody during pregnancy; however, it is most useful when comparing a particular serum against several cell samples to clarify differences in strength between alloactive and autoactive antibodies in the serum (as, for example, between cord and adult red cells in the identification of anti-I) or in the search for "least incompatible" units when crossmatching difficulties are encountered.

Before titration methods are attempted as an aid to the identification of antibodies, dosage effect must first be ruled out, since this phenomenon can obviously cause titration variation. If dosage effect has been excluded, the titration of serum containing antibodies with various selected cells may give a clue to antibody specificity, since the components of a mixture are unlikely to react at equal strengths. In these cases, however, it is important that a particular specificity be suspected, since titration with random cells will often be time consuming and wasteful of the patient's serum. A suggested basic titration technique is as follows:

1. Ten (or more) test tubes (usually 10 × 75 mm) are set up in a test tube rack and labeled 1, 2, 4, 8, 16, 32, etc.

2. One volume of saline is added to all tubes.

3. One volume of the patient's serum is added to the tubes labeled 1 and 2, using the same pipette. (A routine pasteur pipette or a volumetric pipette can be used.)

4. The saline-serum mixture in tube number 2 is mixed, and one volume is transferred to the tube labeled 4. (i. e., tube number 3).

5. The contents of the tube labeled 4 are mixed, and one volume is transferred to the tube labeled 8 (i.e., tube number 4).

6. This procedure is continued through the ten (or more) tubes, and the excess volume in the last tube is discarded (or retained for further titration). The tubes now contain "master" dilutions of serum. Two drops of each dilution may now be transferred into other appropriately labeled tubes, using a pasteur pipette, if two or more different cells are to be used in the titration of the same serum.

7. A washed 5 per cent saline suspension of red cells possessing the antigen corresponding to the antibody in the serum is added to all tubes (usually one drop to each tube).

8. The tubes are tested by the technique in which the antibody is known to react best.

TABLE 28–6 INTERPRETATION OF ANTIBODY TITRATIONS

Cell Number	*1:1*	*1:2*	*1:4*	*1:16*	*1:32*	*1:64*	*1:128*	*Titer*
	Antibody Dilutions							
1	4+	3+	3+	2+	1+	–	–	32*
2	4+	4+	4+	3+	3+	1+	w	64*
3	2+	1+	1+	w	–	–	–	4*

*Note that the titers are 32, 64 and 4, respectively, and not 1:32, 1:64 and 1:4. The latter figures are serum dilutions; titers are expressed as reciprocals of serum dilutions.

(From Bryant, N. J.: An Introduction to Immunohematology. Philadelphia, W. B. Saunders Co., 1976, p. 200.)

Interpretation of Results. Results are interpreted as shown in Table 28–6.

Tests at Selected Temperatures

In some cases in which antibody identification proves difficult, variation of the incubation temperature may provide a stronger result in instances in which the antibody reacts optimally at that temperature. Cold-reactive antibodies can be tested at 4°C and at 18°C, and warm-reactive antibodies can be tested at 30°C.

Selection and Use of Special Cells

Many commercial cell panels provide at least one "special" cell (i.e., either possessing a low-frequency antigen or lacking a high-frequency antigen). These special cells can be stored frozen for use in complicated antibody identifications rather then being used in routine situations. In this way, laboratories can develop a "library" of rare or unusual red cell specimens.

REACTIONS THAT MAY BE MISLEADING IN ANTIBODY IDENTIFICATION

Rouleaux Formation

Rouleaux formation is the clumping of red cells in such a way that they have the appearance of a stack of coins (see Fig. 28–9). It is usually seen in both control and test suspensions at room temperature. When it is heavy, rouleaux formation is sometimes difficult to distinguish from true agglutination. The formation can be dispersed or diminished by adding a drop of saline to the slide or tube *after* the reaction has taken place.

Rouleaux formation is often encountered in certain disease states—notably myelomatosis, macroglobulinemia, and other dysproteinemias. It also is caused by a raised serum globulin concentration and certain synthetic plasma expanders, such as dextran. Fibrinogen has the greatest influence on rouleaux formation, and in routine blood grouping, therefore, serum is used rather than plasma because of its lack of fibrinogen. Vigorous plasma or plasma concentrate therapy induces strong rouleaux formation because of increased fibrinogen levels in the recipient.

Panagglutination

Panagglutination is the spontaneous agglutination of red cells (irrespective of blood group) by a given serum. The phenomenon is also known as *bacteriogenic agglutination* and as the *Heubener-Thomsen phenomenon.* All red cells are agglutinated, often even the red cells from the individual from whom the serum was derived.

Panagglutination is frequently the result of bacterial action and does not usually occur when blood and sera

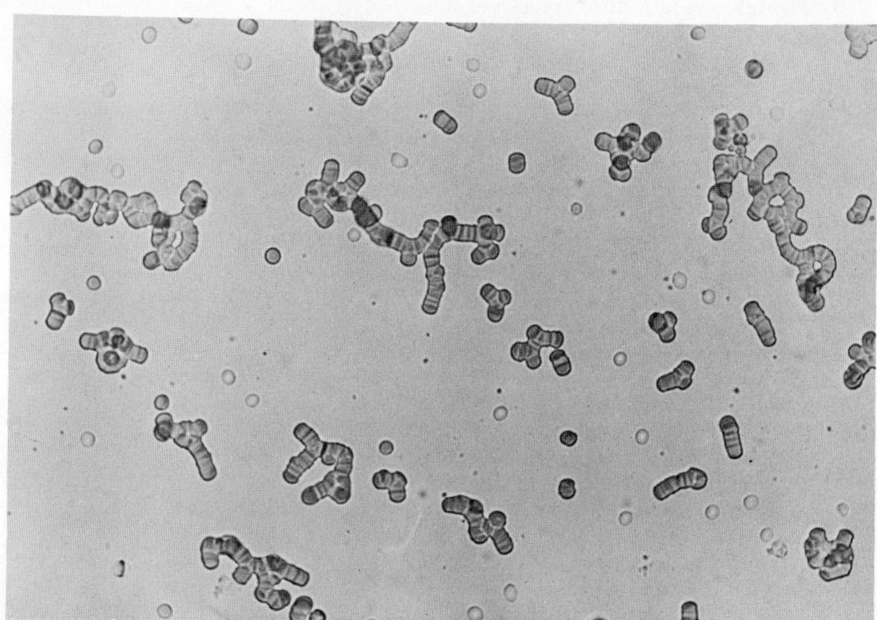

Figure 28–9 Rouleaux formation. × 300.

are fresh and sterile. The bacterial contaminant in the given serum may expose a latent receptor on the red cells known as T (see discussion under *Polyagglutination*). This receptor then reacts with anti-T in the given serum, causing agglutination of the red cells. Bacteriogenic agglutination of this kind can also occur in certain patients with sepsis whose red cells have become polyagglutinable.

Polyagglutination

Polyagglutinability (or polyagglutination) means simply that a sample of red cells is agglutinated by many samples of human serum. There are several circumstances in which red cells become agglutinable because of the exposure of antigens that form part of the structure of the normal red cells membrane but that are usually "hidden." Those situations that occur in vivo (and sometimes in vitro) include the exposure of the T, Tk, Tn, and VA antigens. Since antibodies for these four antigens are found in almost all samples of normal adult serum, the conditions are often described as polyagglutinability. Of the antigens that can be exposed, the antigen T is considered to be of greatest importance, and this will therefore be considered here.

T-Activation. The latent receptor, T, contained in all human red cells can be activated by various strains of bacteria or by enzymes derived from them. The antibody anti-T is normally present in the serum of most adults, and, therefore, T-activated red cells are agglutinated by these sera. T-activation may occur in vitro because of infection of the serum with certain enzyme-producing bacteria if it has been allowed to stand at room temperature for many hours. T-activation may also occur in vivo, in which case it is usually a transient phenomenon.

The characteristics of the reactions of T-activated red cells are as follows:

1. The red cells are agglutinated by the sera of a proportion of adults but are not agglutinated by most sera from newborn infants.
2. The reactions are strongest at room temperature; they may be weak or absent at 37°C.
3. Though agglutinates are large, many "free" cells are normally present.
4. The reactions are strongest with fresh serum; sometimes no reaction is seen with serum that has been stored frozen.
5. T-activated red cells react better with sera containing anti-A than with those that do not.
6. The red cells fail to agglutinate with their own serum, and the red cells give a negative direct antiglobulin test. At 37°C they are not sensitized to an antiglobulin serum by human sera that agglutinate them at room temperature.

T-activated red cells can usually be ABO grouped without difficulty (probably because the anti-T in commercial reagents has been diluted out in preparation). If problems are encountered, however, the tests can be performed at 37°C.

The titer of anti-T varies in different adults and is usually present in the serum by the age of six months. The antibody can be absorbed from human serum with T-activated red cells, and an anti-T lectin can be extracted from the peanut, *Arachis hypogaea.*

Most patients with T-activated red cells do not have an associated hemolytic process. Severe hemolytic transfusion reaction has been reported as a result of transfusing normal plasma to an infant with polyagglutinable red cells.

T-activated red cells are deficient in sialic acid and, therefore, are not agglutinated by polybrene (as are normal red cells). This can be useful in determining the cause of the reactions observed with polyagglutinable red cells.

Cold Autoagglutinins

Autoagglutinins represent one of the most common and harassing problems encountered in blood banking. Whereas alloagglutinins are characterized by the fact that they are produced by individuals whose red cells lack the corresponding antigen, autoagglutinins are formed *in spite of* the existence of the corresponding antigen on the individual's own red cells. The reason for the production of these autoantibodies is not clear. It appears, however, that under certain conditions or circumstances the mechanisms that control an individual's immunological tolerance to antigenic substances that are regarded as "self" appear to fail. The result is the production of an antibody against the individual's own tissues. Antibodies of this kind can also be attributed to certain drug therapy or disease states (e.g., autoimmune hemolytic anemia).

Autoantibodies can react through all thermal ranges, though they are most commonly encountered in the saline phase at or below room temperature. Frequently these antibodies increase in strength as the temperature of the test is lowered and conversely decrease in strength as the temperature of the test is raised. In some instances, however, the reactions may still be evident at 37°C because of the activation of complement. Tests for autoantibodies, even if it is evident that they are cold agglutinins, should be made through a temperature range of 4 to 37°C.

Cold agglutinins often have anti-H and/or anti-I specificity. In these cases, all panel cells will show positive results. The identity of these antibodies can often be established through the reactions of the patient's serum with his or her own cells and with the selected A_1, A_2, B, and cord cells, as described under *Antibody Identification*. The method of interpreting these results is given in Table 28–7.

Note that even when the specificity of the autoantibody is established as anti-I, anti-H, or anti-IH, it is possible that another antibody is being masked by the reaction. For this reason, anti-I, anti-H, or anti-IH should be absorbed (with the patient's own red cells), and the absorbed serum retested for the presence of antibodies.

Collection of Specimens in Cases of Cold Auto-Agglutinins. When cold agglutinins are known (or suspected) in an individual's serum, two specimens of blood should be collected—one in a "dry" tube (i.e., without anticoagulant) to provide serum and a second in EDTA to provide red cells for the direct antiglobulin test and the preparation of an eluate. The blood should be collected into warm containers and transferred directly into a heated centrifuge. The serum should then be separated from the cells in the warm (i.e., 37°C). If it is not known whether the autoantibody is warm or cold, the specimen should be collected and separated at 37°C.

EDTA is the anticoagulant of choice, since if the blood

TABLE 28–7 IDENTIFICATION OF ANTI-I, ANTI-H AND ANTI-IH

	Panel	Auto-control	0 (Adult)	A_1 (Adult)	A_2 (Adult)	B (Adult)	0 (Cord)	A (Cord)	B (Cord)
Anti-H									
1 Patient group A	4+	Neg (Mi)	4+	1+	3+	0	4+	2+	0
2 Patient group B	4+	Neg (Mi)	4+	0	0	1+	4+	0	1+
3 Patient group AB	4+	Neg (Mi)	4+	1+	3+	1+	4+	2+	1+
Anti-I (all groups)	4+*	3+†	4+	4+	4+	4+	Neg‡	Neg‡	Neg‡
Anti-IH									
1 Patient group A	4+	1+ or neg	4+	2+	4+	0	1+	Wk (Mi)	Wk (Mi)
2 Patient group B	4+	1+ or neg	4+	0	0	2+	1+	Wk (Mi)	Wk (Mi)
3 Patient group AB	4+	1+ or neg	4+	1+	3+	2+	1+	Wk (Mi)	Wk (Mi)

*Variation of antigen strength may cause varying reactions in the panel.

†This reaction may be weaker than 3+ in some cases and even negative. This is caused by the fact that the antigen receptors are "blocked" with antibody, and none is available to proceed to the second stage of agglutination.

‡With a powerful anti-I, these reactions may be positive, and dilution or titration may be necessary to demonstrate weaker reactions with cord cells than with adult cells.

O = Test not performed.

(From Bryant, N. J.: An Introduction to Immunohematology. Philadelphia, W. B. Saunders Co., 1976, p. 196.)

is cooled to below body temperature, it will prevent the binding of complement to the red cells by cold antibody or cold auto-agglutinins such as anti-I.

Cold Autoabsorption. As mentioned, cold autoagglutinins may mask the presence of another antibody. For this reason, the autoagglutinin should be absorbed with the patient's own red cells (autoabsorption), and the absorbed serum retested for the presence of antibodies.

The two cold autoabsorption techniques commonly used are described below. *Note*: For better absorption results, fresh blood samples should be obtained, as follows:

Serum for Absorptions: Draw a clotted specimen and immediately place it in an ice bath; allow clot formation under refrigerated conditions; remove the serum from the clot, maintaining iced conditions.

Cells for Absorptions: Draw an anticoagulated specimen and immediately place it in a 37°C environment; allow the cells to settle by gravity; remove the plasma; wash the remaining cells three times with warm (37°C) saline.

Method 1: Using Untreated Red Cells

1. Wash the red cells three times in isotonic saline. (This can be omitted if specimens have been collected as described above.)

2. Completely remove the supernatant saline after the last wash.

3. Add 1 volume of undiluted serum to 1 volume of washed packed red cells.

4. Mix and incubate in an ice bath or refrigerator for 30 to 60 minutes. Mix frequently during the incubation for maximum absorption.

5. Centrifuge and immediately harvest serum.

6. Test the absorbed serum against autologous cells to ensure that absorption is complete. If absorbed serum is still reactive in the autocontrol, absorption is not complete and should be repeated with a fresh aliquot of washed red cells.

Method 2: Using Enzyme-treated Red Cells

1. Add 1 volume of enzyme solution to 1 volume of washed, packed, autologous red cells.

2. Mix and incubate at 37°C for 15 minutes.

3. Wash red cells several times. Mix cells by inversion on each saline wash to ensure complete removal of the enzyme solution.

4. To 1 volume of washed, packed, enzyme-treated red cells, add 1 volume of patient's serum.

5. Mix and incubate in an ice bath or refrigerator for 15 to 60 minutes. Mix frequently during incubation for maximum absorption.

6. Centrifuge and immediately harvest serum.

7. Test absorbed serum against autologous cells to ensure that absorption is complete. If autologous control is still positive, the procedure should be repeated.

The Use of Monospecific Anti-IgG. In certain instances the cold agglutinin present in a patient's serum will readily bind complement (e.g., anti-I). As the temperature of the test is raised, the antibody elutes from the red cells, leaving complement *alone* on the red cells. A positive reaction will therefore be seen with broad-spectrum antiglobulin reagents, the reaction being between the complement on the red cells and the anticomplement in the antiglobulin serum. To prove this, monospecific anti-IgG and anticomplement antiglobulin serum can be used. If no reaction is seen with monospecific anti-IgG and a reaction is seen with monospecific anticomplement, then the presence of IgG antibody on the patient's red cells can be discounted.

Warm Autoagglutinins (Associated with Warm Autoimmune Hemolytic Anemia)

Autoagglutinins of the warm type are so called because they react as well or better at 37°C than at lower temperatures. These warm autoantibodies are usually associated with autoimmune hemolytic anemia of the warm-antibody type.

Collection of Samples in Cases of Warm Autoagglutinins. As with cold autoagglutinins, two specimens of blood should be collected from the patient—one in a "dry" tube (without anticoagulant) to provide serum and the other in EDTA to provide red cells for the direct antiglobulin test and the preparation of an eluate. It is good practice to collect the specimens and separate them at 37°C.

The Detection of Warm Autoagglutinins. Although the direct antiglobulin test provides useful information in cases of warm autoagglutinins, the definite diagnosis of autoimmune hemolytic anemia is dependent upon the characterization of antibodies present in the patient's serum and in the red cell eluate. If the direct antiglobulin test is positive it is essential to remove the antibody from the red cells (i.e., elute) in order to determine the specificity. Occasionally, red cells with a negative direct antiglobulin test will provide a strongly positive eluate. Complement components causing a positive direct antiglobulin test will result in a negative eluate; however, if IgG is present on the red cells, it can be eluted by standard methods and identified by testing the eluate against a panel of phenotyped red cells.

If the direct antiglobulin test is positive because of IgG sensitization but the eluate shows no activity against normal red cells, then drug-induced autoimmune hemolytic anemia can be suspected (see further discussion below).

The panel of red cells used for identification should be set up with both the eluate and a sample of the patient's serum. It is important that the nature of the autoantibody be identified (if possible) and also that the specificity of alloantibodies be identified in case a transfusion becomes necessary. It is desirable to *titrate* the serum and the eluate and to test the dilutions against the panel cells, because the specificity of the antibody sometimes becomes apparent only after the "nonspecific" element has been diluted out.

The warm autoabsorption technique most commonly used is as follows.

Method

1. Collect a sample of the patient's red cells in anticoagulant.

2. Wash a volume of the patient's red cells six times with warm (45°C) normal saline. (*Note*: The volume of packed red cells should be at least twice the volume of serum to be tested.)

3. Suspend the washed patient's red cells in saline at a 1:1 ratio. Divide the diluted sample into two aliquots of equal volume.

4. Elute the antibody by constant agitation of the cells at 56°C for 3 to 4 minutes (or at 44°C for 60 minutes if red cells are very fragile). *Note*: The eluate may be reserved for tests to define specificity of the autoantibody, but these should not replace testing for the presence of antibody activity in an eluate prepared by ether or digitonin techniques.)

5. Wash each sample four times in warm saline.

6. Spin and remove excess saline.

7. Add one-half to one volume of Bromelase to each volume of packed red cells.

8. Incubate at 37°C for 30 minutes.

9. Wash three or four times with saline to remove enzyme, and decant the last wash as completely as possible to minimize serum dilution.

10. Add an equal volume of patient's serum to one aliquot of the enzyme-treated red cells.

11. Incubate at 37°C for 30 to 60 minutes, mixing occasionally.

12. Centrifuge immediately and recover serum.

13. Add the once-absorbed serum to the second aliquot of Bromelase-treated red cells.

14. Repeat steps 11 and 12.

15. Test serum for antibody reactivity by performing either an antibody screen, a panel, or a compatibility test.

16. If the autoantibody reactivity has not been completely removed, the procedure should be repeated.

Specificity of the Autoantibody in Warm Autoimmune Hemolytic Anemia. The associated antibodies in autoimmune hemolytic anemia of the warm antibody type often show a relationship to Rh. Some examples are specific for one particular Rh antigen, such as e or D. Others react more strongly with e-positive than with e-negative red cells. In some cases, the antibody has been found to react well with all red cells except those of type Rh_{null} and this led Wiener and Vos to classify their cases according to whether they reacted with D-positive red cells (ndl = not deleted), with Rh-positive red cells that were "partially deleted" (pdl = partially deleted, e.g., -D-), or with both of these types of cells and also with red cells that are deleted (dl = deleted, i.e., Rh_{null}).

In 1967, Celano and Levine concluded that three specificities could be recognized:

1. Anti-LW.
2. An antibody reacting with all samples except Rh_{null}.
3. An antibody reacting with all samples including Rh_{null}.

There remains some uncertainty as to whether the specificity of antibodies that react with all red cells including Rh_{null} (i.e., anti-dl) is related in any way to the Rh structure.

A minority of warm antibodies that at first appear to have the specificity of an Rh alloantibody can be absorbed completely by red cells lacking the corresponding antigen. It has been suggested that the specificity of these antibodies is anti-Hr or anti-Hr_o.

Several other specificities have been associated with warm autoimmune hemolytic anemia, and the list appears to be far from complete. These include autoanti-Jk^a, autoanti-K, autoanti-U, autoanti-I^T, autoanti-A, autoanti-N, autoanti-Ge^a, and many others.

Wharton's Jelly

Wharton's jelly is present in varying amounts in cord samples that have been collected by transecting the umbilical cord and allowing the blood to drain from the umbilical veins into the collection tube. Samples contaminated with excessive amounts of Wharton's jelly will agglutinate spontaneously. If a cord blood sample

TABLE 28–8 PROZONE PHENOMENON

Dilutions of Serum							
1/1	1/2	1/4	1/8	1/16	1/32	1/64	1/128
–	–	–	1+	2+	2+	1+	–

is believed contaminated with Wharton's jelly, three to five saline washes will usually eliminate this spurious reaction. If Wharton's jelly contamination is a common problem, eliminate the problem by advising the delivery room to collect cord blood samples from the umbilical vein using a syringe and needle rather than allowing the blood to drain from the cord into the collection tube.

Prozone Phenomenon

This is a phenomenon observed at times in titration of antibodies in which the antibody apparently reacts more strongly when the serum is diluted than when it is undiluted. (See Table 28–8.)

The phenomenon has often been attributed to the lack of optimal proportions between antigen and antibody (see p. 559), though it may actually occur in either of two ways:

1. It may be due to the use of fresh serum containing complement. This can be proved by inactivating the serum and retitrating, whereupon the prozone disappears.
2. It may be due to the presence of both IgM (agglutinating) and IgG (blocking) antibodies in the same serum. This prozone will disappear if the tests are carried out in a high-viscosity medium (human AB serum, bovine albumin, etc.) in place of saline.

A prozone phenomenon is occasionally seen in the antiglobulin technique as a result of partial neutralization of the antiglobulin reagent.

Antigen or Antibody Deterioration

Both antigens and antibodies undergo a diminishing of reactivity on storage. For antigens, the rate of deterioration differs from one antigenic determinant to another and is dependent, to some extent, on the medium in which the red cells are stored.

Studies by various workers show that the reactivity of the antigens D, c, P_1, Jk^a, S, and Lu^a, when stored at 4°C in CPD, decreases by an average of 12% in the first week, 15% during the second week, and a further 10% during the third week. Antigenic determinants for Kell and Duffy show less deterioration during storage. It has been shown that red cells stored in CPD, ACD, and modified Alsever's solution give similar results. Clotted specimens, however, show much more rapid deterioration; in fact a 40% reduction in activity has been noted after only 14 days of storage.

The deterioration of antibodies is dependent on the specificity of the antibody and the length and method of storage. Saline-reactive antibodies deteriorate most in the first month of storage, then appear to become relatively stable. IgG antibodies, with a few exceptions, are stable. Complement-binding antibodies deteriorate owing to complement inactivation and/or the fact that at −25°C serum may acquire certain anticomplementary properties.

Dosage Effect

When the genes at a particular locus on homologous chromosomes are identical (i.e., homozygous), the gene is said to be expressed in "double dose." When they are different (i.e., heterozygous) or when the allelic gene is amorphic, the gene is said to be expressed in "single dose."

In antibody identification, certain antibodies will react with red cells expressing antigens in double dose *only* or will react more strongly with red cells expressing antigens in double dose than with red cells expressing antigens in single dose. (See Example 2 on p. 597.)

Variability of Antigen Strength on Test Cells

Certain antigens (e.g., P_1 and I) have variable strength on the red cells of different individuals. In antibody identification, the results can therefore give the appearance of a mixture of antibodies, because reactions of varying strength will be noted. Some commercial panels give a grading on the antigen profile, which aids in identification.

Drug-Induced Hemolytic Anemia

Many drugs cause a positive direct antiglobulin test and autoimmune hemolytic anemia by various mechanisms.

Alpha-Methyldopa (Unknown Mechanism). The drug alpha-methyldopa (Aldomet) is the most important of the drugs that can cause hemolytic anemia due to an unknown mechanism. Of patients who take this drug for several months, 15% develop a positive direct antiglobulin test and 0.8% develop hemolytic anemia. An antibody can be demonstrated in these patients' sera that reacts with normal red cells. Often the antibody appears to have Rh specificity.

Immune Complexes. Certain drugs (phenacetin, quinine, quinidine, etc.) that are incapable of producing an immune response by themselves because of their low molecular weight, can become immunogenic when coupled with a plasma protein. The antibody produced is directed toward the drug and forms a drug-antibody complex. This complex is absorbed nonspecifically by the red cells, white cells, and platelets and leads to rapid red cell destruction because of the subsequent activation of complement.

Cell-bound Drug and Serum Antibodies (Penicillins). Penicillin can become bound to red cells when high doses of the drug are administered, resulting in the production of IgG antipenicillin antibodies. This causes a positive direct antiglobulin test and, in some cases, hemolytic anemia. Cephalosporin drugs can also act in the same way.

Adsorption of Protein. Cephalosporins can also cause a positive direct antiglobulin test by altering the red cell membrane, resulting in the nonimmunogenic adsorption of plasma proteins, including albumin, fibrinogen, complement, and IgG.

TRANSFUSION HAZARDS

The transfusion of blood from one individual to another always involves the risk of stimulating alloantibodies in the recipient, since no two individuals possess identical antigens on their red cells (with the exception of identical twins). When alloimmunization occurs as a result of transfusion, it has harmful consequences in future transfusions and pregnancies, as follows.

Future Transfusions. Alloimmunization requires identification of the offending antibody and screening for blood that lacks the antigen corresponding to this antibody. This involves an increased time factor, which may be detrimental to the patient in extreme emergency conditions. In addition, alloimmunization may result in the production of an antibody that, after a period of time, falls below the threshold of the tests performed in the laboratory and therefore becomes undetectable in routine testing. If the antibody is not detected, incompatible blood may be transfused, resulting in immediate or delayed transfusion reaction.

Future Pregnancies. Alloimmunization resulting in production of an IgG antibody may affect future pregnancies if the antibody crosses the placenta and combines with the provoking antigen on the red cells of the fetus. This may result in hemolytic disease of the newborn (see further discussion below).

Types of Transfusion Reaction

Urticarial (Allergic) Reaction. This type of reaction is commonly encountered in modern blood transfusion practice. An urticarial reaction is a type of allergic response in which wheals develop on the body during or following transfusion. A severe allergic reaction in which the patient develops laryngeal edema or bronchospasm is rare. The development of urticaria, however, is comparatively common; many observers consider the incidence to be from 1 to 3 per cent. Antihistamines are often given to treat these reactions and also to avoid allergic reactions in future transfusions.

Anaphylactic Reaction. An anaphylactic reaction is a severe type of allergic reaction that may be fatal if untreated. It is characterized by flushing, nausea and vomiting, diarrhea, and changes in blood pressure. The reaction is seen in patients without IgA. These patients have developed IgG anti-IgA antibodies and react to all products containing IgA (e.g., plasma). Patients with known anti-IgA should be transfused only with blood or plasma obtained from themselves or from other IgA-deficient donors or with extensively washed red blood cells. Although the administration of antihistamine, e.g., diphenhydramine (Benadryl), may be appropriate for mild allergic reactions, epinephrine (adrenalin) is used to treat anaphylactic reactions.

Febrile Reaction. Febrile reactions are most commonly encountered in multitransfused and multiparous patients with leukoagglutinins, and they can be avoided with the use of leukocyte-poor blood. The reaction is characterized by chills, fever, and occasionally in the severe form, a nonproductive cough, tachycardia, and dyspnea. Febrile reactions can also be caused by pyrogens. Certain commercial solutions (e.g., citrate) may be contaminated with these bacterial polysaccharides, which, when injected into human recipients, can cause febrile reactions characterized by increased blood pressure, chills, fever, nausea, headache, and back pain. Pyrogenic reactions can be controlled by the use of sterile solutions and disposable plastic blood units and sets.

Hemolytic Reaction. A hemolytic transfusion reaction is the result of an incompatible transfusion and is recognized by signs of red cell destruction following transfusion. There are two types of red cell destruction: intravascular and extravascular. Intravascular destruction is the rupture of red cells in the bloodstream with the liberation of hemoglobin into the plasma. Extravascular destruction is the removal of red cells from the bloodstream by the cells of the reticuloendothelial system.

In addition to the transfusion of incompatible blood, hemolytic-type transfusion reactions may also be due to any of the following causes:

1. The transfusion of whole blood that is passed through a bottle containing 5 per cent dextrose and 0.224 per cent saline.
2. The injection of water into the circulation.
3. The transfusion of hemolyzed blood.
4. The transfusion of overheated blood.
5. The transfusion of blood that has been frozen.
6. The transfusion of blood under great pressure.

On occasion when incompatible blood is transfused, a weak antibody in the recipient's serum may be incapable of causing rapid, immediate red cell destruction, but the transfusion, stimulating the existing antibody, may cause the rapid destruction of the transfused red cells a few days after transfusion. This is known as a *delayed transfusion reaction (hemolytic)*. It may be characterized by an increase in serum bilirubin or a failure of the hemoglobin level to be maintained after transfusion in the absence of hemolysis.

Symptoms of an acute hemolytic transfusion reaction are flushing of the face, constricting pain in the chest and lumbar region of the back, a tendency to bleed from operative wounds, or generalized oozing of blood. Signs include hemoglobinuria, hypotension, and cyanosis.

The most common cause of acute hemolytic transfusion reaction is the administration of the wrong blood to the recipient because of inadequate patient identification or clerical error.

Contaminated Blood Reaction. Reactions to contaminated blood are characterized by fever, pain, and marked hypotension. Bacteria may be introduced into the blood unit at the time of collection (from the bacterial flora on the donor's skin or directly from the bloodstream) or administration, or they may grow within the unit if it is improperly stored. Attention to technique and sterility is essential to minimize the risk during both collection and administration of blood or blood products.

Transmission of Disease. Of the diseases that are transmissible by transfusion, the most significant include syphilis, malaria, and hepatitis.

Syphilis. Blood stored at 4° C for four days or more is unlikely to transmit syphilis, because the causative organism is unable to survive under these conditions. A serological test for syphilis is standard procedure for all blood donations, and therefore the disease is rarely a problem.

Malaria. When transmitted by transfusion, malaria is a serious complication. Careful questioning of the donor is essential (see Blood Donation). An indirect fluorescent antibody test for the detection of occult malaria in blood donations has been described, but it is not in general use.

Posttransfusion Viral Hepatitis. The occasional occurrence of posttransfusion hepatitis remains a serious consequence of blood transfusion. Many blood components such as plasma, platelets, cryoprecipitate (factor VIII concentrate), factor IX concentrate, and fibrinogen are capable of transmitting hepatitis—the risk being proportional to the number of donors whose blood is used to prepare the component. On the other hand, some components (albumin, plasma protein fraction, and immunoglobulin preparations) can be regarded as "safe" derivatives, since hepatitis virus is usually inactivated or removed during preparation.

Tests for the hepatitis B surface antigen (HB_sAg) have allowed detection of most carriers of hepatitis B virus, yet it has become clear that much work and research is still required before posttransfusion hepatitis is completely prevented. Hepatitis A virus, the agent of infective hepatitis, seems to be a relatively uncommon cause of posttransfusion hepatitis; in fact, most of the cases of hepatitis now seen following transfusion with blood screened for HB_sAg by certain routine techniques (i.e., radioimmunoassay or reversed passive hemagglutination) are not caused by either hepatitis A or hepatitis B virus.

An antigen originally called Australia antigen was first recognized in the serum of an Australian aborigine. The association of the antigen with hepatitis was realized three years later. The complete hepatitis B virus consists of a 27 nm, nucleocapsid, DNA-containing core surrounded by an outer lipoprotein coat and is known as the Dane particle, which has a diameter of 42 nm (Fig. 28–10). The "Australia antigen" is now known to be unassembled viral coat, or surface antigen, and is termed HS_sAg (hepatitis B surface antigen). The core carries an independent antigen known as HB_cAg (hepatitis B core antigen). The antibodies to the surface antigen and to the core antigen are known as anti-HB_s and anti-HB_c, respectively. A soluble antigen (which is also particle associated) known as HB_cAg is found only in some sera containing HB_sAg. Its presence appears to be related to the degree of infectivity of the serum. It appears that there is a correlation between HB_cAg, DNA

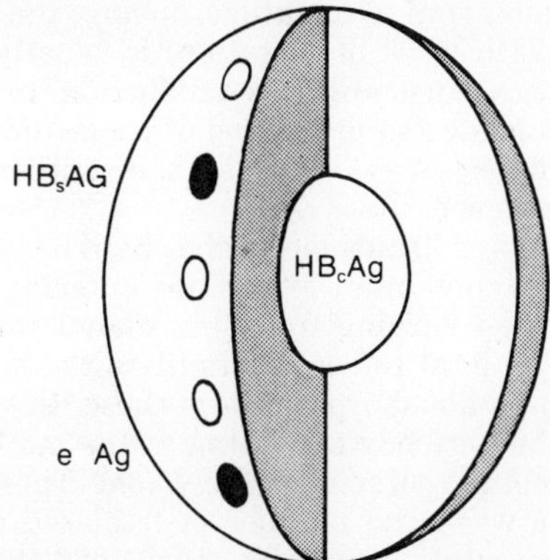

Figure 28–10 The Dane particle. (From Bryant, N. J.: An Introduction to Immunohematology, 2nd ed. Philadelphia, W. B. Saunders Co., 1982, p. 332).

polymerase (which, with double-stranded DNA, makes up the core), Dane particle count, and infectivity. Anti-HB_c occurs in a majority of sera containing HB_sAg from voluntary blood donors and can be detected, as can HB_cAg, by radioimmunoassay.

The incidence of HB_sAg among voluntary blood donors in the United States and Canada is about 0.1 per cent. Among paid donors, however, the incidence of positives is about ten times greater. This may be due to the fact that the practice of paying donors tends to attract a proportion of undesirable donors, such as alcoholics or drug addicts, in whom the risk of hepatitis B is high. The commercial blood donor also is less likely to give an accurate history of his present and past health.

Because there is currently no known, completely effective method for detecting the infectivity of all blood products capable of transmitting hepatitis, the disease remains a potentially lethal complication of blood transfusion. Of the tests available for the detection of HB_sAg, radioimmunoassay is the most sensitive.

In posttransfusion hepatitis due to hepatitis B virus, the incubation period was formerly taken as 60 to 180 days. It is now thought that cases with an incubation period of more than 120 days are rare. The average incubation period of non-A, non-B posttransfusion hepatitis has been reported to be 51 days (14 to 105 days) in one series of cases and 56 days (37 to 75 days) in another. In the occasional case due to virus A, the incubation period is about 30 days.

Although human serum albumin when heated to 60°C for 10 hours is usually incapable of transmitting hepatitis B virus, serum (and possibly plasma protein solution), when subjected to the same conditions, might still be capable of transmitting the virus, especially when heavily contaminated.

Commercially made radioimmunoassay kits are available for the detection of several components of the hepatitis B virus.* The principles of such tests are described more fully on p. 91 and may be seen in Figure 28–11.

Acquired Immune Deficiency Syndrome (AIDS). Almost 600 cases of this syndrome were reported to the Centers for Disease Control as occurring in the United States between June 1981 and September 15 of 1982. AIDS has been defined as a disease predictive of a defect in cell-mediated immunity occurring in a person with no known causes for diminished resistance to such a disease. Such diseases include *Pneumocystis carinii* pneumonia, Kaposi's sarcoma, and other conditions, as for example cryptococcosis, strongyloidosis, and candidiasis. About 75 per cent of AIDS cases occur in homosexual or bisexual males. Among the 25% of heterosexual individuals (male and female), 60 per cent used intravenous drugs. Cases have occurred in individuals with hemophilia A and in a relatively large proportion of Haitians recently entering the United States.

Although the etiology of AIDS is unknown, its pattern of occurrence suggests the possibility of an infectious agent transmitted sexually or through exposure to blood or blood products rather like that of hepatitis B. The incidence in Haitians may be connected with religious rituals related to blood.

*Abbott Diagnostics Division, North Chicago, Ill. 60064.

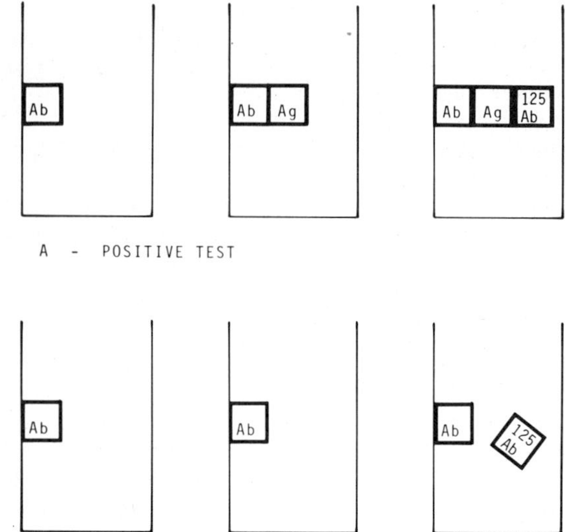

Figure 28–11 HB_sAg testing by radioimmunoassay (RIA). **A,** the antigen in the test serum is bound to the antibody coated tube. Hepatitis B antibody labeled with ^{125}I is added, reacts with the antigen, and increases the radioactivity of the sample as compared to the negative control. **B,** There is no antigen in the test serum to react with the antibody-coated tube, and therefore the ^{125}I labeled antibody does not become attached.

Investigation of Adverse Transfusion Reaction

Crossmatching specimens (unit segments, etc.) are retained for at least seven days following transfusion, so that testing may be repeated in the event of an adverse transfusion reaction. When notification of a potential hemolytic reaction is received in the laboratory, and after an appropriate clinical examination, the following procedure is suggested:

1. Check all relevant paperwork—the number of units transfused, the identity of the patient, the crossmatching results, records of previous transfusions, etc. Ensure that the transfusion was without fault through any clerical error.

2. Collect a 10-mL clotted specimen and a 10-mL anticoagulated specimen from the patient, taking particular care to avoid hemolysis resulting from the taking procedure.

3. Collect the first postreaction specimen of urine and examine it for hemoglobinuria (macroscopically). If necessary, the urine may also be examined for oxyhemoglobin and methemoglobin.

4. The patient's serum in the pre- and postreaction specimens should be examined macroscopically for hemolysis and, if necessary, the plasma hemoglobin methemoglobin and methemalbumin levels should be determined.

5. A six-hour posttransfusion specimen of blood may be required to determine serum bilirubin and hemoglobin. A lowered level of serum haptoglobin 24 to 48 hours after transfusion could suggest that intravascular hemolysis is taking place.

6. Using fluid thioglycolate, examine the remainder of the donor units for possible contamination by culture. The units should also be examined macroscopically for clots or purple discoloration.

7. The first and most important postreaction serological test is the direct antiglobulin test. This should be performed on both the pretransfusion and posttransfusion specimens. A weak positive (mixed field) direct antiglobulin test in the postreaction specimen is strongly indicative of an incompatible transfusion.

8. Repeat the crossmatch, using fresh segments from the donor pack(s). Crossmatch with the prereaction and postreaction specimens. Take special note of the results obtained in the ABO and Rh typing with respect to missing agglutinins or mixed-field reactions. Examine the posttransfusion peripheral blood film for microspherocytosis, which is also indicative of incompatibility. Regroup the donor units carefully.

9. Test the donor plasma for the presence of alloantibodies.

10. Screen the patient's serum for alloantibodies.

If it has been established from the above tests and from clinical examination that the reaction is nonhemolytic, proceed with further tests of the patient as indicated by the direct symptoms and the posttransfusion signs.

HEMOLYTIC DISEASE OF THE NEWBORN

Hemolytic disease of the newborn is a disease that starts in utero and causes jaundice, anemia, and hepatosplenomegaly in the mature infant. The degree of severity of the disease ranges from mild anemia to mental retardation, brain damage, kernicterus, or stillbirth.

The disease is caused by blood group incompatibility between the mother and the fetus. ABO and Rh antibodies, especially anti-Rh_o(D), are most commonly implicated as the cause of hemolytic disease of the newborn. Other blood group antibodies seldom cause the disease, although any IgG antibody can be responsible for it because of the ability of IgG-mediated antibodies to cross the placental barrier from mother to infant.

Mechanisms of Sensitization

In Hemolytic Disease of the Newborn. When hemolytic disease of the newborn results from anti Rh_o(D), the mother is Rh_o(D)-negative and the infant is Rh_o(D)-positive (the Rh_o(D) factor in the infant having been inherited from the father).

The first Rh-incompatible fetus is usually unaffected, since the number of fetal red cells that cross the placenta into the maternal circulation during the pregnancy (after the 24th week of gestation) is usually small and insufficient to cause antibody production. In addition to this, elevated steroid levels and other factors associated with pregnancy may suppress the mother's primary immune response.

At delivery, a transplacental hemorrhage is not uncommon, the amount of fetal blood entering the maternal circulation varying from less than 1 mL to 10 mL or more. The fetal red cells stimulate the production of anti-Rh_o(D) in about 7 per cent of these Rh_o(D)-negative mothers, the antibody appearing in the mother's serum within 6 months after delivery. (*Note:* There is a relationship between the number of fetal red cells in the maternal circulation and the chance of the appearance of the antibody.)

When pregnancy with a second Rh_o(D)-positive fetus occurs, fetal red cells crossing the placenta from about the 24th week of gestation stimulate the existing anti-

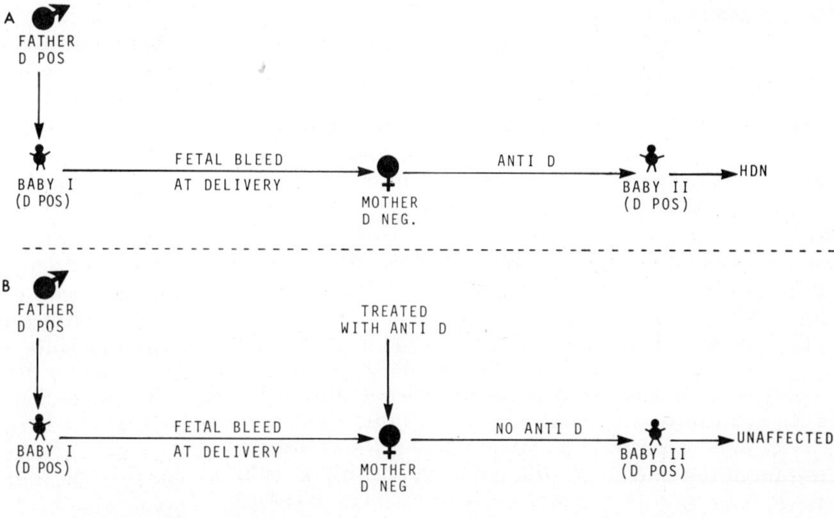

Figure 28–12 The prophylaxis of HDN: **A,** Showing the basic mechanism for HDN with production of anti D by the mother after exposure to fetal Rh(O) positive cells; **B,** Demonstrating the protective effect of Rh immune globulin (anti D). This prevents sensitization of the mother by early removal of fetal cells from the maternal circulation.

body to high titers. This is a secondary response, and therefore small amounts of red cells are capable of causing dramatic increase in the maternal antibody.

The anti-Rh_o(D) formed is IgG, and it is therefore capable of crossing the placenta into the fetal circulation, where it combines with fetal Rh_o(D)-positive red cells, leading to their destruction (see Fig. 28–12).

In ABO Hemolytic Disease of the Newborn. The mechanisms of hemolytic disease of the newborn caused by ABO incompatibility are similar to those of Rh incompatibility (i.e., the passage of fetal red cells into the maternal circulation provokes an immune response in the mother). Unlike Rh hemolytic disease of the newborn, however, the ABO form can and often does occur in the first pregnancy, since anti-A and anti-B are already present and therefore readily stimulated. Since anti-A,B in group O subjects is often partly IgG, the mother is invariably group O. (Anti-A and anti-B in group B and A subjects, respectively, is usually IgM.)

The ABO form of the disease is rarely severe, although mild forms are more common than the Rh form. The ABO form of the disease is between two and six times more common in blacks than in whites.

The Influence of ABO Incompatibility on Rh Immunization

In pregnancy, immunization resulting from Rh_o(D) is less common when the fetus is ABO incompatible with the mother. It is believed that this is because the Rh_o(D)-positive fetal red cells are destroyed by existing maternal ABO alloantibodies immediately upon entering the maternal circulation. Once the mother becomes immunized to the Rh antigen, further ABO-incompatible infants in the family are not protected.

PRENATAL AND POSTNATAL TESTING

Testing the Mother

A mother's first prenatal specimen should be taken at or before the 13th week of pregnancy (i.e., the first obstetrical visit). Routine laboratory testing should include ABO grouping, Rh typing, and antibody screening. Antibody screening should be performed using enzyme and antiglobulin techniques. Anti-Le^a, anti-Le^b, anti-IH, anti-H, and anti-I are relatively common during pregnancy but do not cause hemolytic disease of the newborn (being IgM). Treatment of the serum with 2-mercaptoethanol or dithiothreitol will aid in distinguishing IgM from IgG antibodies.

If the mother is Rh_o(D)-positive or D^u-positive, a further specimen should be taken at 32 weeks' gestation to ensure that antibodies of other specificities have not been formed.

If the mother is Rh_o(D)-negative the following should be done:

1. Test for the D^u variant.
2. Repeat the antibody screening at 26 and 32 weeks' gestation if the original screen is negative.
3. Identify the antibody if the original screen is positive.
4. Monitor all significant antibodies monthly.
5. Titrate the antibody by using doubling dilutions, employing the technique in which the antibody reacts best. Titrate in parallel with the previous sample. A change in titer of more than two tubes (more than fourfold) is significant. The correlation of the titer of maternal antibody and the severity of the disease is often inaccurate; however, titration does serve to identify those women who are candidates for amniocentesis.

Testing the Father

If the mother is Rh_o(D)-negative with no antibodies, testing the father may be helpful in establishing the risk of immunization and in predicting the outcome of future pregnancies. If the father is also Rh_o(D)-negative, hemolytic disease of the newborn resulting from Rh can be discounted. If other antibodies are involved, test the father to determine if he is homozygous or heterozygous for the gene producing the immunizing antigen (if possible).

Testing the Infant

Immediately after birth, a clotted sample of blood is taken from the placental vein, and the following tests performed:

ABO Grouping. Anti-A and anti-B do not usually develop until a few months after birth, therefore such agglutinins in the cord serum are probably of maternal origin. The ABO group of the baby is therefore based on forward (cell) grouping. Note that if the baby has received repeated intrauterine transfusions, erroneous results may be obtained in ABO grouping, Rh typing, and the direct antiglobulin test.

Rh Typing. In addition to the causes of false positive and false negative $Rh_o(D)$ typing discussed earlier, the presence of Wharton's jelly in the sample and the coating of Rh-negative red cells with antibody other than anti-$Rh_o(D)$ may cause false positive reactions, and the saturation of the cord cells with maternal anti-$Rh_o(D)$ may cause false negative reactions because of a blocking effect.

Direct Antiglobulin Test. The direct antiglobulin test is usually strongly positive in Rh and other forms of hemolytic disease of the newborn, but it may be weak or negative in the ABO variety.

Elution and Identification of Antibodies. Whenever the results of the direct antiglobulin test are positive, identification of the antibody in the eluate of cord red cells must be performed, using standard techniques.

Other Tests

The Acid Elution Test. The acid elution test of Kleihauer and Betke is performed on a prepartum and a postpartum blood film of the mother to determine the volume of the fetomaternal hemorrhage and therefore the amount of Rh immune globulin to be administered (see later discussion).

The principle of the test is related to the observation that fetal hemoglobin is resistant to acid elution, whereas adult hemoglobin is not. When a thin blood film is exposed to an acid buffer, the adult red cells lose their hemoglobin into the buffer so that only the stroma remains. Fetal red cells are not affected and retain their hemoglobin. The percentage of fetal red cells in the maternal blood film is used to calculate the approximate volume of the fetomaternal hemorrhage by multiplying the percentage of fetal cells by 50. For example, if 2000 cells are counted in acid elution and they reveal 1.2 per cent fetal cells, $1.2 \times 50 = 60$ mL fetomaternal hemorrhage. Either clotted or anticoagulated blood may be used for this test.

Amniocentesis. Amniocentesis is the technique of withdrawing amniotic fluid (which surrounds the fetus in utero) through the mother's abdominal wall for laboratory analysis. As a result of red cell destruction, excess bilirubin-like pigment is cleared from the fetal circulation via the placenta and amniotic fluid, which causes the latter to be stained yellow. The intensity of this yellow color can be measured spectrophotometrically, giving an indirect indication of the degree of red cell destruction and therefore of the severity of hemolytic disease of the fetus.

The main indications for amniocentesis are:

1. An antiglobulin titer of 32 or higher for a significant antibody.
2. A history of hemolytic disease of the newborn.

Amniocentesis should not be performed without clear indications because of the inherent risks associated with the procedure. Amniocentesis is never indicated in ABO hemolytic disease of the newborn.

RH IMMUNE GLOBULIN

The initial experiments revealing that passively administered anti-Rh could interfere with primary Rh immunization were performed by Stern and colleagues in 1961, although it had previously been postulated that fetal red cells in the maternal circulation might be destroyed by the administration of a suitable antibody.

It is now well known that an adequate dose of IgG anti-$Rh_o(D)$ is usually successful in preventing Rh immunization if given within 72 hours of delivery (Fig. 28–12). The following are candidates for this prophylaxis:

1. All Rh-negative and D^u-negative mothers who have no detectable anti-$Rh_o(D)$ in their serums and who have an Rh-positive or D^u-positive infant.
2. Women who have had abortions.
3. Women who have had first-trimester amniocentesis.
4. Women who have had antepartum hemorrhage.
5. Women who have had an ectopic pregnancy.

Rh-immune globulin is not given to Rh-negative women who deliver Rh-negative infants or whose serum contains anti-$Rh_o(D)$. It is also not given to Rh-positive or D^u-positive women.

The usual recommended dose of Rh immune globulin is about 300 µg, which is believed to offer protection against a fetomaternal hemorrhage of 30 mL or less. Larger doses can be given when a massive fetomaternal hemorrhage is suspected or confirmed (by the acid elution test).

After injection of Rh immune globulin, anti-$Rh_o(D)$ and any other antibodies in the preparation can usually be detected in the mother's serum for from 12 to 60 hours, and they may continue to be detectable for as long as five months.

Since primary Rh immunization occurs *during* pregnancy in at least 0.78% of Rh-negative women carrying an Rh-positive fetus, several workers now administer Rh immune globulin both prenatally and postnatally, and it has been shown that this combined prenatal-postnatal treatment is more effective than postnatal treatment alone in suppressing Rh immunization. Although it may appear that the injection of anti-$Rh_o(D)$ into an $Rh_o(D)$-negative woman carrying an $Rh_o(D)$-positive fetus is potentially dangerous (the antibody being IgG and therefore capable of crossing the placenta), practical experience has shown this not to be so. The reason for this is that, even if the antibody does cross the placenta, IgG is transferred relatively slowly, and not more than 30 µg of a 300-µg dose will reach the infant, most having been catabolized by the mother by the time that equilibrium is reached.

Following abortion or miscarriage, $Rh_o(D)$-negative women should be given Rh immune globulin (unless the father of the child is known to be Rh-negative), because the $Rh_o(D)$ antigen has been demonstrated on fetal red cells as early as 38 days after conception.

SELECTION OF BLOOD IN CASES OF HEMOLYTIC DISEASE OF THE NEWBORN

Exchange Transfusion

Exchange transfusion is performed for the following reasons:

1. To lower the serum bilirubin concentration.
2. To remove the infant's red cells, which have been sensitized with antibody.
3. To provide substitute compatible red cells with adequate oxygen-carrying capacity.
4. To reduce the amount of irregular antibody in the baby.

To meet these objectives, donor blood should lack the red cell antigen corresponding to the maternal antibody and should be less than five days old.

In ABO hemolytic disease of the newborn, group O red cells of the same Rh type as those of the baby should be used (as concentrated red cells or frozen deglycerolyzed red cells in combination with compatible plasma).

In Rh and other forms of hemolytic disease of the newborn, blood of the same ABO group as that of the baby can be used when the mother and baby are ABO compatible. If the donor unit is prepared before delivery, a group O $Rh_o(D)$-negative unit that lacks the corresponding antigen to the causative antibody is selected in cases of hemolytic disease of the newborn due to antibodies other than anti-$Rh_o(D)$. Alternatively, group-specific blood may be given if the infant's ABO and Rh group have been determined. In cases in which exchange transfusion is required more than once, subsequent units should be of the same ABO and Rh type as the first unit. Antibodies that do not cross the placenta may be ignored. If the antibody is reactive against a high-frequency antigen and compatible blood cannot be found, the mother's siblings can be tested for suitability — a unit of blood can be collected from the mother (the plasma being removed and the red cells suspended in AB plasma before transfusion) — or incompatible blood may be used (in extreme emergency situations, i.e., when withholding blood will result in the death of the infant).

Intrauterine Transfusion

Intrauterine transfusion is the technique of introducing red cells (which find their way into the fetal circulation) into the fetal peritoneal cavity while the fetus is still in utero.

Group O $Rh_o(D)$-negative blood (packed red cells), crossmatched against the maternal serum, is usually used. The amount of fresh blood transfused is dependent on the size of the fetus. Intrauterine transfusion is not performed later than the 34th week of pregnancy. At birth, infants with hemolytic disease of the newborn caused by anti-$Rh_o(D)$ who have received intrauterine transfusion often type as $Rh_o(D)$-negative with a negative direct antiglobulin test, since 90% of the blood in the baby's circulation may be that of the donor.

CHAPTER 28 — REVIEW QUESTIONS

1. Describe the clinical applications of stored plasma.
2. Describe the mechanisms of sensitization in cases of Rh hemolytic disease of the newborn, and briefly describe the influence of ABO incompatibility on Rh immunization in such cases.
3. In the saline (room temperature) test for antibody identification, certain cells are required to demonstrate the presence of anti-I, anti-IH, or anti-H. List which red cells are required in the case of a patient of group AB.
4. Describe Wharton's jelly as it affects the blood transfusion laboratory, and explain how the problems it causes can be eliminated.

REFERENCES FOR IMMUNOHEMATOLOGY SECTION

1. Bellanti, J. A.: Immunology. Philadelphia, W. B. Saunders Co., 1979.
2. Bryant, N. J. : An Introduction to Immunohematology, 2nd ed. Philadelphia, W. B. Saunders Co., 1982.
3. Erskine, A. G., and Socha, W. W.: The Principles and Practices of Blood Grouping, 6th ed. St. Louis, C. V. Mosby Co., 1978.
4. Herst, R., and Shepherd, F. A. (eds.): Clinical Guide to Transfusion—Products and Practices, Toronto, The Canadian Red Cross Society Blood Transfusion Service, 1979.
5. Issitt, P. D., and Issitt, C. H.: Applied Blood Group Serology, 2nd ed. West Chester, Pa., Biological Corp. of America, 1979.
6. Mollison, P. L.: Blood Transfusion in Clinical Medicine, 6th ed. Oxford, Blackwell Scientific Publications, 1979.
7. Moore, B. P. L.: Serological and Immunological Methods of the Canadian Red Cross Blood Transfusion Service, 8th ed. Toronto, Canadian Red Cross Society, 1980.
8. Petz, L. D., and Garratty, G.: Acquired Immune Hemolytic Anemias, New York, Churchill Livingstone, 1980.
9. Race, R. R., and Sanger, R.: Blood Groups in Man. 6th ed. Oxford, Blackwell Scientific Publications, 1975.
10. Technical Manual of the American Association of Blood Banks, 8th ed. Washington, D. C., the Association, 1981.
11. Zmijewski, C. M.: Immunohematology, 3rd ed. New York, Appleton-Century-Crofts, 1978.

Section IV

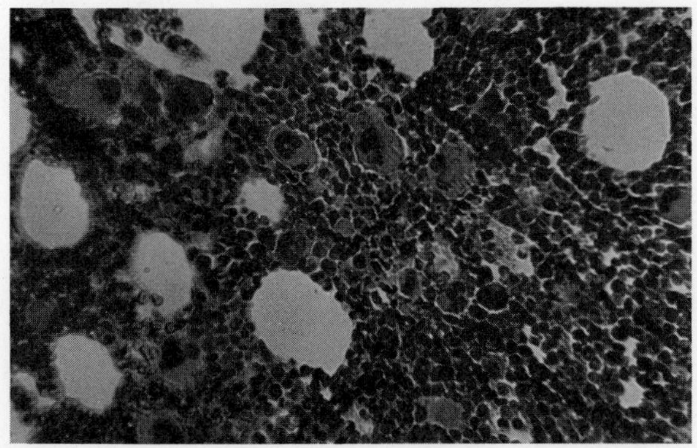

HEMATOLOGY

29 PRINCIPLES OF HEMATOLOGY

INTRODUCTION

The purpose of this chapter is briefly to introduce the reader to the mechanisms responsible for the function of the cells found in the blood, namely the erythrocytes (red cells), leukocytes (white cells), and platelets suspended in plasma. In healthy individuals there is a constant balance between the rates of formation and destruction of these cells. Disturbance of this critical balance, in terms of either changes in rates of formation, disordered formation, or increased utilization and destruction, is essentially responsible for the final pathologic condition.

HEMATOPOIESIS

There has been much debate over the years as to the actual nature of hematopoiesis. Although many questions remain unanswered, the following points are generally accepted by hematologists.

1. There is a multipotential cell that gives rise to all blood cells.
2. From the multipotential cell arise committed stem cells. Because these cells will form colonies in vitro, these cells are known as colony-forming cells (CFC). Under the influence of humoral factors, the CFCs will proliferate and differentiate into the different cell lines (Fig. 29–1).
3. Monocytes and neutrophils appear to develop from the same CFC.
4. Under the influence of the primary lymphoid organs, two types of lymphocyte are produced. B lymphocytes (equivalent of those produced in the bursa of fowl) are concerned with humoral immunity, while T lymphocytes (thymus mediated) are involved in cell-mediated immunity.

THE BONE MARROW

In the embryo the blood cells, excluding lymphocytes, are derived from embryonic connective tissue, the mesenchyme. The first cells are primitive erythroblasts in the yolk sac blood islands, but by the second month of gestation, the liver has become a center for hematopoiesis and granular leukocytes have made their appearance. In the fourth month, the bone marrow becomes a major center for the production of blood cells.

The bone marrow is found within the cavities of all bones and may be present in two forms: (1) The yellow marrow is inactive bone marrow composed mostly of adipose tissue which may be converted into active marrow in the event of abnormal demand. (2) The red marrow is active marrow producing the myeloid, erythroid, and megakaryocytic cells.

During the first few years of life, the marrow of practically all bones is red and cellular. Between the ages of 3 and 7 years, fat cells begin to appear, and with progressive age the active marrow gradually recedes from the distal parts of the skeleton to the trunk. By the age of 18, red marrow is found only in the vertebrae, ribs, sternum, skull bones, and innominate bone of the pelvis, and to some extent in the proximal epiphyses of the femur and humerus.

In certain circumstances the spleen, liver, and lymph nodes revert back to their fetal role in that they start to produce erythrocytes, granulocytes, and megakaryocytes, suggesting that the undifferentiated reticulum cell is present in these areas and is able to proliferate if an appropriate stimulus is given. This reaction is termed extramedullary hematopoiesis, and clinically it is classically seen in myelofibrosis with myeloid metaplasia (see p. 667). However, this mechanism is largely brought into operation either when the bone marrow is ablated or when it is unable to meet the demands placed on it (e.g., hemolytic anemia).

STRUCTURE OF THE BONE MARROW

Essentially, this tissue comprises the developing blood cells (hematopoietic tissue), blood vessels, fat cells, and a matrix of cancellous bone with attached osteocytes and osteoblasts. The cancellous bone provides a basic structural foundation upon which the blood vessels and cells are arranged.

The blood vessels arise from the nutrient vessels of the bone and rapidly divide into a fine network of thin-walled dilated vessels which connect the arterial and venous circulations. These are the marrow sinusoids, and as they are attached to the bony cage they are permanently dilated and represent the site at which the mature marrow cells gain access to the intravascular space. A fine network of reticulin fibers is attached to the endosteum of the bone and is adherent to the endothelial cells of the blood sinusoids. Attached to this reticulin are the reticulin or undifferentiated reticulum cells which form the nidus for the hematopoietic tissue.

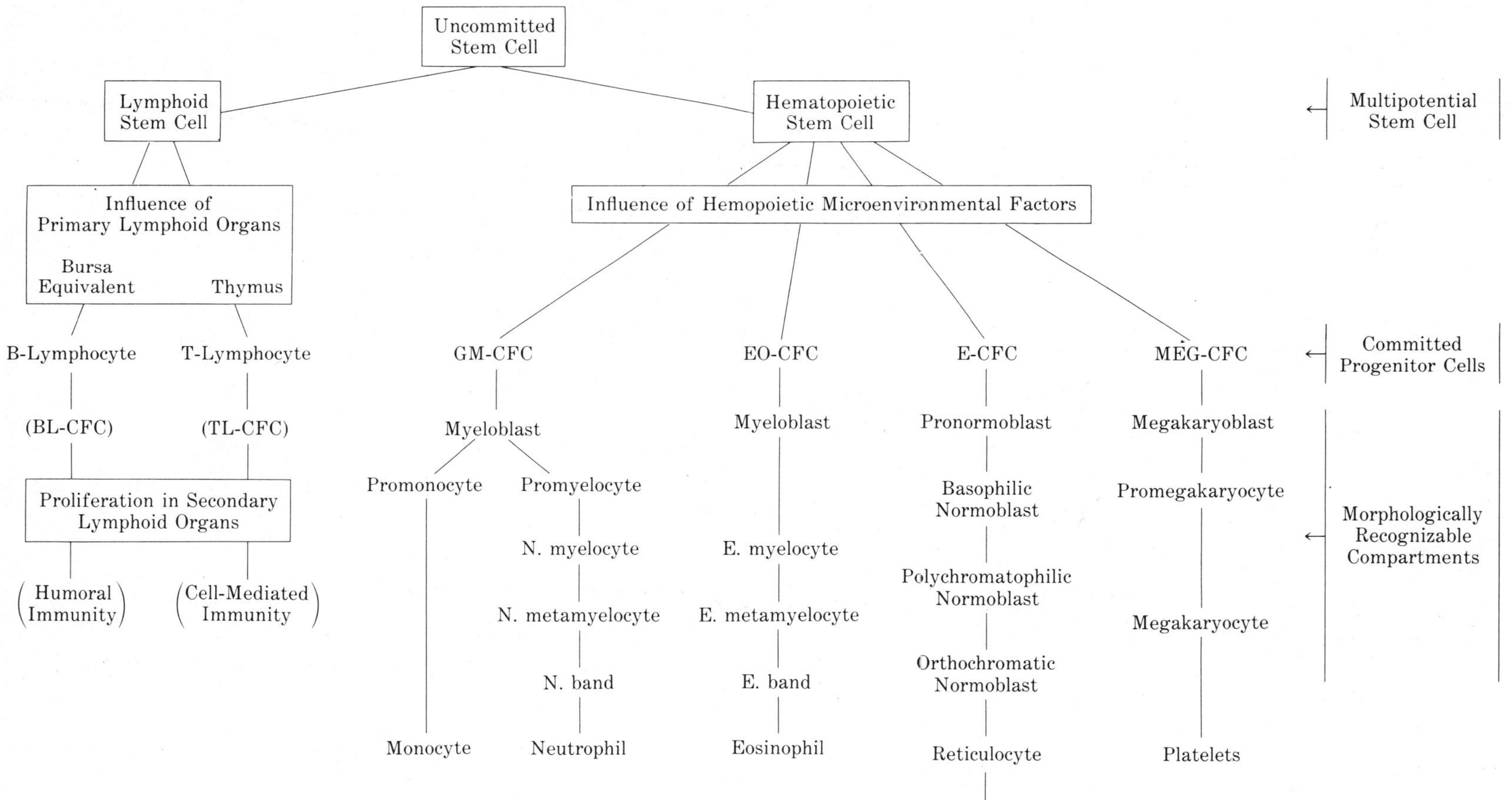

Figure 29–1 Hypothetical scheme of hematopoiesis as discussed in text. Local or short-range factors (or "influences") act on the multipotential stem cells to produce committed progenitor cells. GM-CFC, granulocyte-monocyte colony forming cell; EO-CFC, eosinophil colony forming cell; E-CFC, erythrocyte colony forming cell; MEG-CFC, megakaryocyte colony forming cell; BL-CFC, B-lymphocyte colony forming cell; TL-CFC, T-lymphocyte colony forming cell.

Though lymphocytes can be induced to grow in colonies, these CFC's are not analogous to the committed progenitor cells of the myeloid lines. The latter respond to specific hormones (e.g., erythropoietin for E-CFC, GM-CSF for GM-CSF for GM-CFC) by proliferation and differentiation into mature cells of the particular series. (From Henry, J. B. (ed.): Todd-Sanford-Davidsohn Clinical Diagnosis and Management by Laboratory Methods, 16th ed. Philadelphia, W. B. Saunders Company, 1979, p. 920.)

Hematopoiesis is concentrated in the spaces between the sinusoids and the endosteum, lying freely in the reticulin fibers and adjacent to the undifferentiated reticulum cells. Interspersed throughout are fat cells which, depending upon their number, decide whether the bone marrow is primarily red (active hematopoiesis) or yellow (inactive). In general, fat comprises approximately 25% of active tissue and the volume of active marrow is approximately 1500 to 2000 ml in the adult. In times of stress the yellow marrow reverts back into active use, and in certain congenital hemolytic anemias the demand on the bone marrow may be such as to cause distortion or thinning of the bony cortex, e.g., sickle cell anemia.

Cell maturation is usually in the form of cell nests, i.e., the developing cells form small aggregates of the same cell series with the cells in varying degrees of maturation. The normoblasts are characteristically seen in this form and are analogous to the lymphoid follicles which are scattered through a normal marrow.

CELLULAR MORPHOLOGY IN THE BONE MARROW

Successful interpretation of a large number of hematologic conditions depends upon an accurate assessment and identification of the bone marrow cells. For this reason considerable emphasis will be given to describing the cells in this organ. The reader is referred to the atlases of hematology listed at the end of this section, which provide an excellent visual appreciation of these cells. Methods for aspiration, biopsy, and preparation of the bone marrow are described on pp. 684, 767 and 789.

Stem Cell

The morphology of the multipotential stem cells and committed stem cells is unknown. It was once thought that the reticulum cells of the bone marrow were the stem cells. There is no experimental evidence that reticulum cells have any hematopoietic potential, and the term should probably be reserved for those cells which form the network in which the hematopoietic cells and fat cells are embedded. Stem cells are thought to vary in size and morphology from large forms like the hemocytoblast to small forms that resemble a transformed lymphocyte.

Hemocytoblast. This cell is found in the marrow, lymph nodes, spleen, and liver. It is a large cell (25 to 35 μm). Its nucleus, which is oval to round, almost fills the cell. The chromatin is fine and regular, and one to four pale blue nuclei may be seen in it. The nucleus is surrounded by a thin rim of blue cytoplasm. Many of these cells show some identifiable features of the cell series to which they are destined to give rise and, indeed, all transition stages between hemocytoblast and definitive blast cells may be recognized.

The "blast" (primitive or parent) cells of all blood cells have certain broadly similar characteristics:

1. They are relatively large cells (up to 20 μm in diameter). Maturation to definitive types always involves a reduction in size.
2. The cytoplasm is small in amount relative to the size of the nucleus. As the cell matures the proportion of cytoplasm increases.
3. The cytoplasm is deeply basophilic, i.e., stains a deep royal blue with Romanowsky stains. This is the result of a high content of ribonucleic acids. As the cells mature, this basophilia is lost as the result of the action of specific enzymes (ribonuclease and deoxyribonuclease), because protein synthesis for growth and division is not required by the mature cell.
4. The cytoplasm of blast cells does not contain granules.
5. The chromatin of the nuclei is relatively free. As the cell matures the chromatin becomes coarser and more densely staining.
6. The nuclei of blast cells contain small, usually well-defined, pale bodies called nucleoli. These are present only in blast cells, although their remains may be seen in cell stages following the blast form.

In addition to the common features just enumerated, the "blast" cell precursors of each cell series have certain peculiar characteristics that help the experienced hematology worker to identify them. As each cell series is described, the more marked specific features of the "blast" cells will be briefly outlined for each group.

Myeloid Series

Myeloblast. The precursor cell is the myeloblast; its chromatin is fine, dustlike, and evenly distributed, and it does not show condensed masses at the nuclear membrane. Nucleoli vary in number from two to five and are generally more numerous and more irregular in outline than those in the lymphoblast. The cytoplasm of myeloblasts is uniformly deep blue in Romanowsky-stained smears and does not show the pale or clear crescent or halo that is commonly present around the nucleus of lymphoblasts. The outline of the nucleus is round or oval, although slight or shallow indentations may occasionally be seen. Such indentations are common in leukemic myeloblasts. Normally, myeloblasts amount to 0.5 to 3% of nucleated marrow cells.

Promyelocyte. This is the next stage of maturation after the myeloblast. The basophilia of the cytoplasm is much reduced and granules are present in it. The nucleus is relatively smaller, eccentric, and oval or slightly indented. Nucleoli can still be seen but are indistinct. Promyelocytes make up 1 to 8% (average 5%) of normal marrow cells.

Myelocyte. This derives from the promyelocyte by further maturation in the form of reduction in the size of the nucleus, which also comes to lie more eccentrically in the cell and is less regular and often somewhat indented on the side of the greatest amount of cytoplasm. In the latter, granules are now more numerous and specific. Whereas in the promyelocyte the granules are often faintly azurophilic, in the myelocyte stage the granules assume the definite and specific staining characters of the definite granulocytes into which they are destined to develop—neutrophil, eosinophil, and basophil. In normal marrow, myelocytes make up some 5 to 20% (usually about 10%) of nucleated cells. Of these myelocytes the vast majority are neutrophilic; eosinophil myelocytes constitute 0.5 to 3% (average, 1.5%), and basophilic myelocytes less than 0.5% of all nucleated marrow cells.

Metamyelocyte. Further maturation of the myelocyte gives rise to this form in which the nucleus is much smaller, and indented or boomerang-shaped, and its chromatin is condensed and more deeply stained than that of the myelocyte. At this stage ameboid movement is first shown by the granulocyte series. Metamyelocytes make up 10 to 30% (average, 20%) of nucleated cells of normal marrow. Of these the eosinophil and basophil metamyelocytes account for only a small fraction, as outlined under Myelocyte.

Polymorphonuclear Leukocyte *(Segmented Granulocyte).* This is the final mature form of the granulocytic series of cells. The nucleus is composed of coarse, dense chromatin which stains a purplish color with Wright's or Leishman's stain. The youngest form is the "stab" or "band" cell, thus named because its nucleus is in the form of a curved rod. As the cell ages, the nucleus becomes segmented into lobes which are joined together by narrow chromatin threads. Thus, the older the polymorphonuclear neutrophil or polymorph, the greater the number of lobes in the nucleus. A shift to the left is defined as the presence of more than 5% band forms and/or the presence of any metamyelocytes, while a shift to the right indicates the presence of over 5% neutrophils with 5 lobes or any neutrophils with six or seven lobes. Maturation in the bone marrow (myeloblast to stab cell) takes some 4 to 6 days, and 6 to 8 mitoses. Mature polymorphonuclear leukocytes probably spend only about 8 hours in the circulating blood and then migrate into various tissues, where they may live for some 2 to 4 days. Eosinophil polymorphonuclear leukocytes are believed to have a longer life span.

The cytoplasm of the polymorphs is pale pink in Romanowsky-stained smears and contains specific granules. In the neutrophil polymorphs, which constitute the vast bulk of segmented granulocytes, the granules are fine, evenly scattered, and violet in color. In eosinophil polymorphs the granules are larger, uniformly spherical, and bright salmon-pink; they are more numerous than in the neutrophil polymorph and usually obscure the nucleus, which rarely has more than two lobes. In the basophil polymorphs the granules are abundant, large, and purplish black, and they usually almost completely obscure the nucleus. The granules of neutrophil polymorphs are peroxidase-positive. In the case of segmented neutrophil and eosinophil leukocytes, the specific granules in the cytoplasm are lysosomes.

All segmented leukocytes are motile; the neutrophils are particularly so, the eosinophils only slightly. Motility is connected with phagocytic activity, i.e., the ability of the cell to ingest foreign particles, bacteria, and so forth.

In size the segmented granulocytes average 10 to 12 μm; i.e., they are approximately one and a half times the size of erythrocytes. They make up 10 to 30% of the nucleated cells of normal marrow. The segmented neutrophil is the predominant nucleated cell in the peripheral blood after the age of 4 years.

The nuclei of female polymorphs have drumstick appendages and these have been found to be related to the presence of the inactivated X chromosome. All females (that is normal XX females) have at least 6 drumstick appendages in 500 neutrophils, while males rarely possess such appendages (Fig. 29–2).

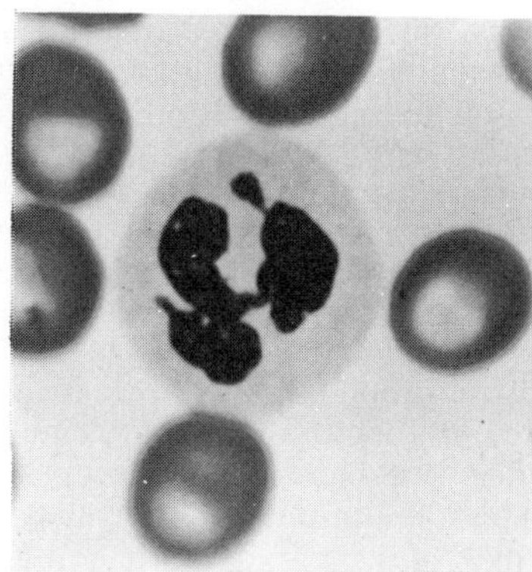

Figure 29–2 Typical drumstick projection found in female polymorphonuclear cell nuclei.

Lymphocyte Series

Recent work in immunology has added to our knowledge of the life history of the lymphocyte. Closely connected with the development of the small lymphocyte is the thymus. By the ninth week of intrauterine life, lymphocytes are seen developing in the region of the thymus, by the twelfth week, they are seen in the blood, and in 16 to 20 weeks they are found in the spleen and lymph nodes. It has been shown in experiments using labeled thymic lymphocytes that the lymphocytes go out and populate lymph nodes. Currently it is believed that lymphocytes leave the thymus and populate lymphoid tissue, and possibly the thymus produces a hormone-like substance that activates lymphocytic production in the lymphoid sites.

Lymphocytes enter the circulation mainly through the thoracic duct. About 80 to 90% are small and the remainder are large. Large lymphocytes may show mitotic figures if they are examined fresh in the lymph, and almost all of them will divide if cultured in vitro. With radioactive markers, two types of lymphocytes are identified, those with a life of 100 to 200 days (possibly years) and considered to be B lymphocytes, and those that survive only 2 to 3 days (probably T lymphocytes). It is believed but not proved that the former are identical with the small lymphocytes, and the shorter-lived lymphocytes are identical to the large type. Lymphocytes originate mainly in lymph nodes, and as a practical point it is worth noting that the finding of lymphoblasts in the bone marrow is abnormal.

As has been described in Chapter 26 and alluded to in the section on lymphoproliferative disorders, two populations of lymphocyte are now evident. The thymus or T lymphocyte is directly related with cellular immunity, while the B or bone marrow lymphocyte is responsible for humoral or antibody immunity. The genesis of the B lymphocyte is not necessarily within the bone marrow but is shared by the lymphoid tissues throughout the body, including the thymus. The B appellation more appropriately refers to the mass of lymphoid tissue in birds known as the bursa of Fabricius and the site responsible for the production of antibodies in birds. To confuse the situation it is becoming more apparent that the progenitor cell for these lymphocytes arises in the bone marrow; experimental evidence supports this concept, particularly in cases of childhood lymphocyte depletion syndromes that have been treated successfully with HL-A matched bone marrow.

The fate of the lymphocytes is probably variable. Some are believed to circulate, and then after a period in lymph nodes, recirculate; others are destroyed in lymph nodes; and a third group are transformed into other cell types. The latter include those that give rise to the plasma cells. Whether the morphologic change has been observed is, at the moment, debatable, but certainly all evidence points to lymphocytes as the origin of plasma cells.

Lymphoblast. This is a large cell (15 to 20 μm) having a large nucleus, with heavier, coarser, and denser chromatin than the myeloblasts. The nucleoli very rarely number more than two and are sharper and more nearly spherical than in the myeloblast. In Wright's stain the nucleus presents a distinctly mahogany-like appearance (dense and homogeneous). The narrow rim of clear blue cytoplasm often shows a pale crescent-like area next to the nucleus. The cytoplasm of the lymphoblast is very homogeneous, whereas that of the myeloblast is often "smoggy."

Prolymphocyte. This cell closely resembles the lymphoblast except that nucleoli are indistinct, and the nucleus is smaller in relation to the mass of cytoplasm, which is less blue.

Mature Lymphocyte. The mature lymphocyte is normally seen in two forms in the peripheral blood: the small lymphocyte and the less numerous large lymphocyte. This differentiation is mainly descriptive, depending mostly on the relative bulk of cytoplasm, although the nucleus of the large lymphocyte is also less dense and more often shows some indentation. The small lymphocyte (10 μm) has a dense nucleus which stains a deep purple with Wright's stain. The nucleus is usually spherical but may show a slight indentation on the side of the greater mass of cytoplasm. The latter is a clear sky blue and is small in amount, forming only a narrow rim about the relatively large nucleus, which is always slightly eccentric. The cytoplasm, which is the bluest (most basophilic) of all normal peripheral blood cells, is usually devoid of granules. However, some cells may contain a few azurophil (purplish red) granules in their cytoplasm. Large lymphocytes measure up to 15 to 20 μm. Transitional forms of lymphocytes are noted in conditions promoting an immune response, and these are described on p. 655.

Plasma Cell Series

Up to 2% of the nucleated cells of normal bone marrow are plasma cells, but they do not normally occur in peripheral blood. The plasma cell is probably the most easily identified of all marrow cells. It is a medium-sized (about 15 μm) cell, usually oval in outline and having abundant cytoplasm which stains a more intense royal blue than any other marrow cell. Under electron microscopy the cytoplasm is shown to consist of a complex endoplasmic reticulum. The nucleus is equally distinctive; it is markedly eccentric, less than half the diameter of the cell in size, and composed of dense masses of chromatin arranged in cartwheel-and-spoke fashion. A paler area is often seen in the cytoplasm near the nucleus on the side of the greater cytoplasmic mass. Vacuoles may be seen in the cytoplasm. Eosinophilic (acidophilic), smooth (hyaline) spherical bodies (Russell bodies) are present in the cytoplasm of some plasma cells. These bodies are composed mainly of gamma globulin.

Other forms of plasma cells, usually associated with abnormal conditions, are Mott and flame cells. The former resemble a clear honeycomb-like cytoplasm and the latter have a pyrinophilic cytoplasm, both reflecting active immunoglobulin synthesis.

Plasma cells possess several functional and structural features similar to those of lymphocytes, and are primarily responsible for the synthesis of antibodies, i.e., immunoglobulins. Once formed in the bone marrow, probably from an undifferentiated reticulum cell (although transformation from the lymphocyte has not been discounted), the mature plasma cell migrates to preselected tissues depending upon its immunoglobulin secretion. Plasma cells synthesizing IgA migrate to the gastrointestinal tract, while cells producing IgG and IgD often seek tonsillar tissue.

Plasmablast. This cell is rarely seen except in plasma cell myeloma. Its descriptive features are broadly similar to those of the plasma cell, but it is somewhat larger and has a larger and paler nucleus in which one or two indistinct nucleoli may be seen. The cytoplasm is a deeper blue than the somewhat greenish blue of the normal plasma cell. However, in multiple myeloma all types of plasma cells and precursors may be seen, from apparently normal cells to giant forms (up to 30 μm) having two or even three nuclei. (*Note:* Normal plasma cells that have two nuclei may occasionally be seen, especially in sites of chronic inflammation.)

Monocyte Series

The monocyte series produce the monocyte of the peripheral blood which is capable of differentiating into a histiocyte when confronted with a suitable inflammatory stimulus. Its partners are the fixed tissue macrophages which are found in the spleen, liver, lungs, and other organs, including the bone marrow. The phagocytic histiocytic (reticulum) cells of the bone marrow are involved in iron storage and transfer; because of this function they are often seen surrounded by a collection of normoblasts. The analogy has been stated that the histiocyte is a nurse cell surrounded by a nest of normoblasts.

The origin of the monocyte has been hotly debated. It almost certainly derives from the reticuloendothelial system of cells, but some have claimed that it arises also from myeloblasts (e.g., Naegeli), and others have claimed a kinship to the lymphocytic series. It is certainly related to the tissue macrophage (histiocyte), which may occasionally be found in peripheral blood smears and closely resembles the monocyte; however, it is larger and more oval, and has a more regular, paler, spongy nucleus and a cytoplasm that is a deeper color (pale violet-blue) than the monocyte. Fine azure granules are also present in the histiocyte. In normal marrow, monocytes make up approximately 2% of nucleated cells; primitive reticulum cells (indistinguishable from histiocytes) account for some 0.2% of cells.

The most notable function and feature of monocytes are their pronounced ameboid motility and phagocytic activity. These may be of help in differentiating certain cases of leukemia of doubtful cell type. Electron microscopy studies suggest that the monoblast, i.e., a monocyte with nucleoli, can indeed be a monocyte which is undergoing transformation to a macrophage.

Monoblast. Like many "blast" cells, this is positively identifiable by association (by the company it keeps), i.e., when it is numerous and when many of its progeny are also present (e.g., in cases of monocytic leukemia). It is a medium-sized to large cell (15 to 20 μm), and its outline is often irregular because of marked ameboid characteristics. The cytoplasm is a murky gray-blue or even gray, and it may often be vacuolated and contain extremely fine azure granules. The nucleus is rarely regular but usually shows some indentation or evidence of convolution. The chromatin forms a fine lacework, and one or two large irregular nucleoli are usually present.

Promonocyte. The features of this cell are intermediate between those of the monoblast and mature monocyte.

Monocyte. This is the largest (15 to 20 μm) cell found in normal peripheral blood and forms 4 to 8% of the normal differential WBC count (200 to 800 per μL, or 0.2 to 0.8 × 10^9/L). The nucleus is large, slightly eccentric, irregular, and deeply indented or horseshoe-shaped, and suggests an aerial view of a mountain range. The chromatin forms a delicate violet-brown, open meshwork. The cytoplasm is abundant, is of pale gray-blue, ground-glass appearance, and usually contains fine dust-like, lilac-colored granules. When, as occasionally happens, the nucleus of the monocyte is almost (although never quite) round, differentiation from a large lymphocyte will be facilitated by the paler, more delicate nuclear chromatin and the "frosted-glass" appearance of the cytoplasm of the monocyte.

Megakaryocyte Series

Platelets are produced by the fragmentation of the largest cells seen in the normal bone marrow, namely the megakaryocytes. In the fetus they appear first in the yolk sac and become evident in the marrow at approximately 12 weeks gestation. The megakaryocytic series is characterized by several unusual features in that the youngest cell is generally smaller than the adult; repeated nuclear division takes place without cellular division so that the cell becomes polyploid; ultimately, the functional final form, the blood platelet, is a cytoplasmic fragment. It has been suggested that the multilobulated nature of the mature megakaryocyte is directly related to its degree of ploidy. This observation has yet to be settled, but in general the degree of lobulation is related to maturity, with the megakaryoblast usually being unilobular.

Megakaryoblast. This is approximately 30 μm in size and has scanty basophilic cytoplasm with blunt extrusions. The nucleus is usually round or oval, with delicate chromatin and two to six indistinct nucleoli.

Promegakaryocyte. The size has increased to approximately 40 to 50 μm, and the cytoplasm is more obvious with less basophilia and fine azurophilic granulation present. Early platelet formation may be evident on the periphery. Indistinct nucleoli may be evident.

Megakaryocyte. These are the cells that give rise to the blood platelets. Normally, they make up approximately 0.5% of nucleated cells of bone marrow, but they may also be found in the lung and spleen. They are extremely large cells (40 to 100 μm) of irregular shape, having a central cluster of large nuclei linked together in the form of a lobed ring representing a cluster of balloons. No nucleoli are present. The cytoplasm is abundant and is of a pale gray-blue color with many very fine azurophil granules. Active platelet formation may be seen at the periphery of the cytoplasm. Megakaryocytes push out cytoplasmic pseudopodia between the cells lining the blood sinusoids in the marrow. These pseudopodia are then pinched off and become free platelets in the blood plasma.

Platelet. These tiny (2 to 4 μm) cytoplasmic, nonnucleated bodies are present in the blood in numbers normally ranging from 150,000 to 500,000 per μL or 150 to 500 × 10^9/L. In smears stained by Wright's or Leishman's technique they show as hyaline (glassy), light purplish blue to sky-blue, round, oval, or irregular bodies containing numerous azure granules. Large peripheral blood platelets (over 2.5 μm in diameter) are named megathrombocytes, and increased numbers can reflect increased megakaryopoiesis. They provide a useful index if platelet consumption is suspected.

The role of platelets is chiefly in hemostasis (stopping bleeding). To fit them for this function they contain many very active chemical factors. Their content of 5-hydroxytryptamine (serotonin), epinephrine (adrenaline), and norepinephrine undoubtedly aids in promoting constriction at the site of injury. Another outstanding property of platelets is their tendency to agglutinate and to adhere to injured tissue. This agglutination and adherence are quickly followed by breaking up and dissolution of the platelets, thus leading to liberation of active chemical factors. This agglutination and dissolution are prevented by intact nonwettable surfaces and, to some extent also, by anticoagulants (heparin, citrate, or EDTA). The participation of the platelet in the hemostatic mechanism with a fuller explanation of its physiologic role is discussed in Chapter 31.

Erythrocyte Series (Erythron)

The development of the mature erythrocyte has probably attracted the most attention over the years, mainly as a result of the ease with which the final cell product can be isolated, and the morphologically distinct normal and abnormal development. As in many other areas of hematology, there has been considerable confusion with regard to nomenclature and individual cell names. The terms erythroblast, normoblast, megaloblast, and rubriblast have been used interchangeably, and in this instance it is proposed that erythroblast be used as a generic term; normoblast to describe normal erythropoiesis; and megaloblast to imply abnormal development due to vitamin B_{12}, folic acid, or other deficiencies. Normoblastic erythropoiesis is first evident as the pronormoblast, which continues on to develop into a series of normoblasts. These may be described in order of maturation as basophilic, polychromatic, or orthochromatic, depending upon the degree of hemoglobinization. Alternatively these same three stages can be referred to as A, B, and C, or early, intermediate, and late. Such terminology reflects the process of normoblastic maturation which has been described as follows:

1. A progressive diminution in cell size.
2. Ripening of the cytoplasm. In Romanowsky-stained preparations this is accompanied by a change in color from deep blue to pink, owing to the progressive formation of acidophil staining hemoglobin and the simultaneous decrease of the ribonucleic acid which is responsible for the basophilia of the cytoplasm.
3. Ripening of the nucleus. This is manifest by loss of nucleoli, decrease in total size and size relative to cytoplasm, progressive clumping and condensation of the chromatin, and deepening in color. Thus the large reddish-purple open network nucleus of the pronormoblast is converted to the small deeply staining blue-black structureless nucleus of the orthochromatic normoblast.

Figure 29–3 attempts to show these relationships, and also the orderly progression of mitosis which is epitomized by this cell type. It may be appreciated that day-to-day needs are met by mitotic division of the young cells and not the primitive forms; this is described as homoplastic development and is reflected by a marrow composed mainly of relatively mature cells, e.g., normoblasts. If requirements are increased there will also be multiplication of the younger precursors, so-called heteroplastic development. Normoblastic erythropoiesis can therefore be summarized by stating that with maturation both DNA and RNA content decrease, so that when the mature red cell emerges from the marrow into the circulation, it is completely lacking in nucleus, mitochondria, ribosomes, and endoplasmic reticulum, and is a self-sustaining, nonmitotic cell containing hemoglobin.

Pronormoblast. This is a medium-sized cell (average 15 μm) somewhat resembling the myeloblast, although the nuclear chromatin is generally coarser than in the myeloblast and takes on a strandlike arrangement as the pronormoblast ages. Nucleoli are usually prominent, and there is a thin rim of deep blue homogeneous cytoplasm. In normal marrow these cells make up about 5 to 10% of nucleated erythrocyte precursors.

Early (Basophilic) Normoblast. The nucleoli of the pronormoblast have disappeared and the chromatin has a definite coarse network or strandlike pattern. This cell makes up some 15 to 20% of nucleated erythrocytes in normal marrow.

Intermediate (Polychromatic) Normoblast. The whole cell is now reduced in size (12 μm), but the reduction in size of the nucleus has been relatively greater than that of the cytoplasm. The chromatin has become much coarser, forming dark chunks. In the cytoplasm the first traces of hemoglobin appear next to the nucleus.

Late (Acidophilic or Orthochromatic) Normoblast. As hemoglobin formation progresses, basophilia disappears, and the cytoplasm of this cell usually resembles slightly dull copper. The nucleus may still be capable of mitotic division, but it soon shrinks to a dense blackish brown mass of chromatin (pyknotic degeneration) and is often irregular in shape (side buds are common). The nucleus may finally break up but, in any case, it is generally lost from the cell by extrusion. The late normoblast is slightly larger than the mature erythrocyte and makes

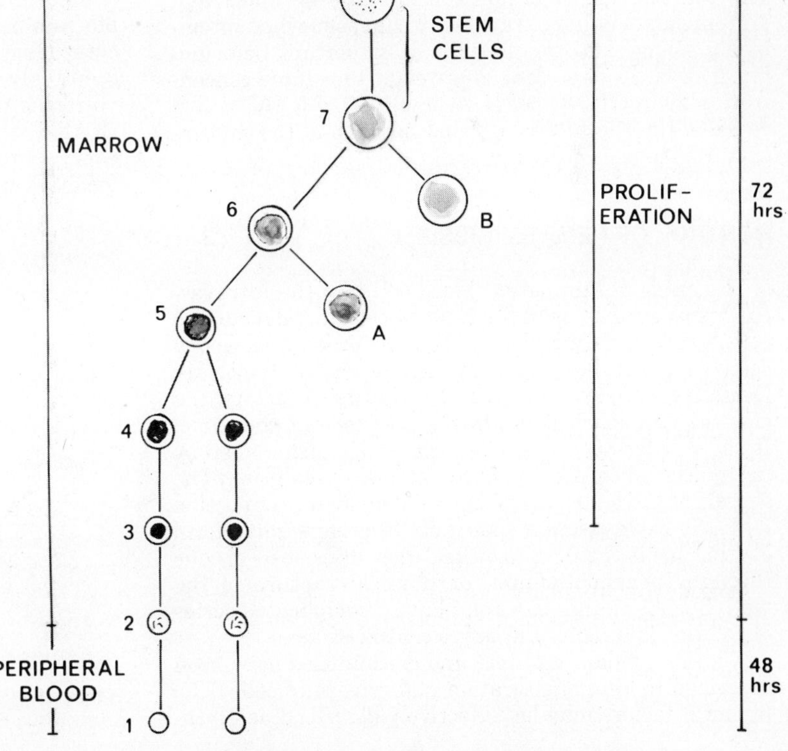

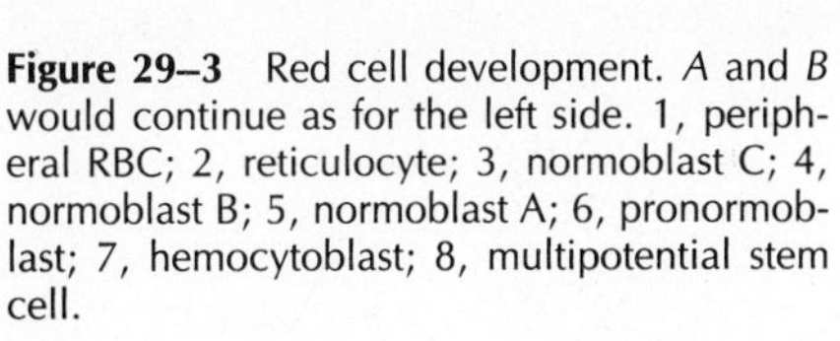
Figure 29–3 Red cell development. *A* and *B* would continue as for the left side. 1, peripheral RBC; 2, reticulocyte; 3, normoblast C; 4, normoblast B; 5, normoblast A; 6, pronormoblast; 7, hemocytoblast; 8, multipotential stem cell.

up some 50% of nucleated erythrocytes of normal marrow.

Reticulocyte. This young red blood cell, which normally accounts for 0.5 to 1.5% of circulating erythrocytes, is formed when the nucleus of the late normoblast is lost by extrusion or dissolution. Its name derives from the fact that it contains a network of basophilic material that is demonstrable by supravital dyes such as brilliant cresyl blue. Physical conditions affect the appearance of this reticular material; e.g., in ordinary Romanowsky preparations the reticular material is not precipitated or shown as a network, but its presence is manifested by a faint diffuse basophilia (polychromasia). Generally speaking, the younger the reticulocyte the more diffuse and marked is the network of reticular substance. As the cell matures this is reduced, tends to be clumped near the center of the cell, and finally is seen only as scattered granules. This maturation of the reticulocyte normally takes 2 to 4 days. Reticulocytes are slightly larger than mature red blood cells, and their number in the peripheral circulation is an indication of erythropoietic activity. Thus, high reticulocyte counts are found in the first days of life, after blood loss or hemorrhage, and following treatment of deficiency anemias with specific substances, e.g., vitamin B_{12} in pernicious anemia, folic acid in the megaloblastic anemia of sprue, and iron in hypochromic (iron-deficient) anemias. The intensity of reticulocyte response in these conditions is, generally speaking, directly proportional to the severity of the anemia.

Mature Erythrocyte *(Red Blood Cell)*. Maturation of the reticulocyte by loss of the basophilic reticular substance gives rise to the intensely acidophilic (eosinophilic) mature erythrocyte. This is a circular, nonnucleated, highly flexible, biconcave disc, averaging 7.2 μm in diameter and 2.1 μm in thickness, with an average volume of 87 fL (MCV range = 76 to 96 fL). The red cell has a complex membrane of lipids and protein surrounding a framework that somewhat resembles a sponge and contains the all-important hemoglobin. The latter is present in a weight to volume concentration averaging 34 per cent, or 340 g/L (MCHC = 320 to 360 g/L). The physiology and function of the mature erythrocyte is discussed later.

CONTROL OF HEMATOPOIESIS

The entry of the mature blood cell into the intravascular space relies upon the multiplication of developing cells, gradual maturation, and finally orderly release of cells from the bone marrow. All of these stages are regulated to varying degrees by a series of factors, the character of which is not well understood at this time. It is of interest to consider the mechanism whereby newly formed cells are released into the circulation. The vessels of the sinusoid system have no direct connection with the extravascular space, and therefore some form of stimulus is required to either allow diapedesis of cells through the endothelium, or physical rupture of the wall. Such a mechanism must have a complicated series of cellular and molecular servo-control systems.

A large number of factors and mechanisms have been described to effect maturation and release of cells. The humoral factors may be collectively described as erythropoietin, thrombopoietin, and possibly leukopoietin controlling erythrocyte, platelet, and leukocyte production, respectively. These, combined with a number of important physical factors, produce the finely balanced control of hematopoiesis.

Control of Erythropoiesis

The major factor controlling the rate of erythrocyte production is the oxygen content of the blood. Hypoxia provides the strongest stimulus, as is evident with the compensating erythrocytosis seen in individuals living at high altitudes, e.g., Andean Indians. Hypoxia does not have a direct control on the marrow, because the drive is mediated by a polypeptide hormone, erythropoietin. Erythropoietin is released primarily by the kidney in response to the decrease in tissue oxygen. The sequence of events would appear to be as follows: a decrease in arterial oxygen content is followed by a decrease in tissue oxygen; in time, erythropoietin is released from the kidney (site yet to be established), and erythropoiesis is stimulated by causing the transformation of the undifferentiated reticulum cell to the pronormoblast stage. Subsequently the increased red cell mass will increase the amount of hemoglobin available to deliver oxygen, thereby increasing the tissue oxygen level. This line of reasoning is correct but oversimplified, in that other organs can also produce erythropoietin-like substances as shown in anephric patients who are still able to maintain red cell production, although at a reduced level. (See Fig. 29–4.)

Control of Leukopoiesis

The study of leukocyte kinetics is in no way as definitive as that of erythropoiesis, mainly because of the difficulty in concentrating and detecting the various leukocyte types and tissue compartments. A considerable number of factors promoting and releasing leukocytes have been described, all or any of which can have seemingly profound effects on leukopoiesis. One observation is undoubtedly real, and that is the cyclic biorhythm which affects neutrophils, and appears to cycle every 14 to 23 days; it has been explained in terms of a feedback mechanism.

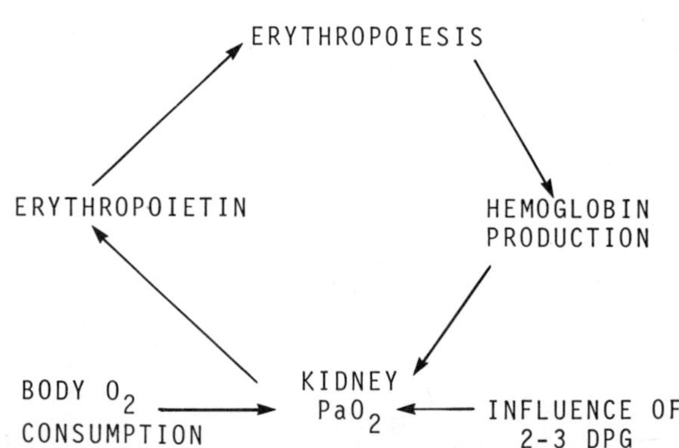

Figure 29–4 Feedback control of erythropoiesis via hemoglobin level, tissue PaO_2, and subsequent release of erythropoietin.

Control of Thrombopoiesis

The observation that plasma from individuals with idiopathic thrombocytopenic purpura (immune thrombocytopenia) was able to stimulate platelet production in other individuals led to the suggestion that a humoral agent termed thrombopoietin was present. Subsequently, a number of thrombocytopenic patients have been described who, after an infusion of normal plasma, respond with a thrombocytosis. This is not de facto evidence to suggest the presence of a humoral stimulating substance, but has provided fertile grounds for speculation. The role of the spleen has also been implicated in producing an inhibitory substance owing to the beneficial effects of splenectomy in certain individuals. Certainly at this time it is evident that some form of control is exerted on platelet production, but whether it is a uni- or multifactorial mechanism remains to be decided.

THE ERYTHROCYTE

Composition and Structure

For normal erythrocyte production the following are required:

1. Protein as a source of amino acids
2. Iron
3. Vitamin B_{12}
4. Folic acid
5. Vitamin B_6
6. Trace metals (e.g., cobalt, nickel)

The more common abnormalities in erythropoiesis arise due to a lack of any one or more of these factors. Protein deficiency is common in third-world countries. Anemia due to deficiencies of iron, folic acid, and the B vitamins is common in all countries.

The mature erythrocyte, although possessing no nucleus or organelles, is not an inert body but a self-supporting cell which is capable of existing in the intravascular circulation for up to 120 days. During this time not only is it subjected to a constant change in shape as it moves through the microcirculation, but at the same time, through the medium of its main constituent hemoglobin, it performs extremely complex and important homeostatic maneuvers. It has a deceptively simple structure in that it possesses only a membrane, internal stroma, and the cell contents which are 90% hemoglobin. Its biconcave shape (see p. 622) allows for maximal surface area and greatest flexibility. The membrane is a typical bimolecular layer of lipid covered on either side by a layer of protein. As a result, the lipid-to-protein ratio is approximately 1:1.6, the majority being lipoproteins. Functionally, it is semipermeable, allowing for water and ions to be transferred, either on an active or passive basis, but remaining impermeable to hemoglobin. Blood group antigens are strategically located either on the outer surface or within the membrane itself, and are in the form of oligosaccharides and glycoproteins.

The stroma is the innermost structure and is primarily composed of lipids and proteins in the form of a fibrous protein. The lipids are cholesterol, lecithin, and cephalins, while the proteins are primarily albuminoid, lipoproteins, and stomatin. As in other body cells, the potassium content is far in excess of the sodium. Glucose and the intermediate compounds of the Embden-Meyerhof pathways and pentose phosphate shunt are present.

Erythrocyte Metabolism

The Embden-Meyerhof and pentose phosphate shunt pathways provide 89% and 11%, respectively, of the energy derived from anaerobic and aerobic glycolysis.

When these pathways are blocked, or inefficient, the life span of the cell is reduced or, to put it another way, the cell is prematurely aged. Expressed in a relatively simple form, the process of hemolysis is favored when the pathways fail to provide sufficient reduced glutathione (which protects other elements in the cell from oxidation) or sufficient energy-providing substances such as NADH (reduced nicotinamide-adenine dinucleotide), NADPH (reduced nicotinamide-adenine dinucleotide phosphate), or ATP (adenosine triphosphate), which supply energy for vital cell functions. About 20 enzymes are involved in the pathways; only those of clinical importance are shown in Figure 29–5 and described on p. 641.

In the commonest enzyme deficiency, G-6-PD deficiency, which is found in about one-third of patients with hereditary nonspherocytic hemolytic anemia, there is disturbance of the reduction of NADP to NADPH and consequent limitation of the reduction of glutathione. With lack of reduced glutathione, the cell becomes more vulnerable to oxidative damage. Methemoglobin reduction also depends on the presence of reduced pyridine nucleotides (NADH and NADPH) and the regeneration of these substances may be decreased in the failure of carbohydrate metabolism. Certain drugs act as oxidizers and produce an excess of H_2O_2 in the cell, which favors the persistence of physiologically inert methemoglobin and the absence of reduced glutathione, and may directly damage cell stroma and membrane. In the normal cell this excess of H_2O_2 is easily handled by catalase and by other intact reducing mechanisms. As indicated, these reducing mechanisms are disabled in the absence of G-6-PD. Vitamin E deficiency may also make the cell more sensitive to the effects of increased H_2O_2. An important product of erythrocyte catabolism is 2,3-diphosphoglycerate (2,3-DPG), which has a profound effect on oxygen dissociation (vide infra).

Erythrocyte Survival and Destruction

Approximately 1% of the total erythrocyte mass is replaced every day, since the average life span of an erythrocyte is 120 days. Thus the total red cell mass is turned over every four months, and this mechanism is remarkably efficient in maintaining constant erythrocyte levels and being responsible to increased demands, e.g., hypoxia or changes in oxygen dissociation.

Senescent erythrocytes are removed from the circulation, primarily by the spleen, which is able to sense the subtle changes which characterize older cells, e.g., slight decrease in size and more variation in shape. Within the reticuloendothelial cells the ring structure of the heme is opened, iron is then split off, and the globin is liberated. The resultant iron-free nonprotein-

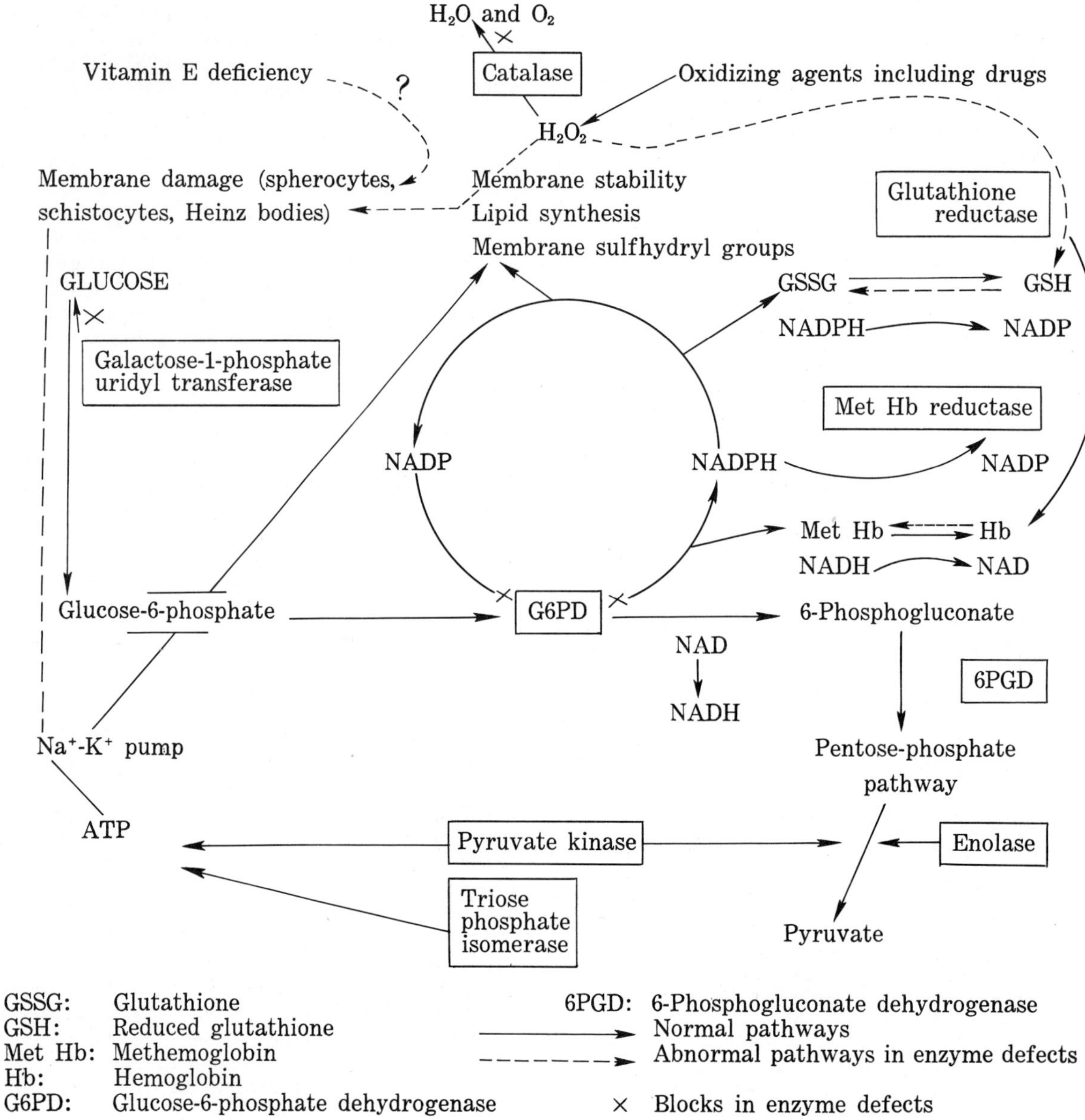

GSSG: Glutathione
GSH: Reduced glutathione
Met Hb: Methemoglobin
Hb: Hemoglobin
G6PD: Glucose-6-phosphate dehydrogenase
6PGD: 6-Phosphogluconate dehydrogenase
——→ Normal pathways
- - - -→ Abnormal pathways in enzyme defects
× Blocks in enzyme defects

Figure 29–5 Enzyme systems in red cells and results of defects (greatly simplified). Defects in G-6-PD will affect secondary reactions shown around the central circle.

containing residue is biliverdin, and this is reduced to bilirubin. This bile pigment is carried in the blood in loose combination with the plasma proteins (chiefly albumin). In the liver cells the bilirubin is set free from the protein and is bound to glucuronic acid to form water-soluble bilirubin diglucuronide, which is excreted in the bile (see Fig. 29–6).

Hemoglobin

The most important agent in the red cell is hemoglobin. This, like its quarter brother, myoglobin of muscle, the cytochrome, peroxidase, and catalase enzymes, is a

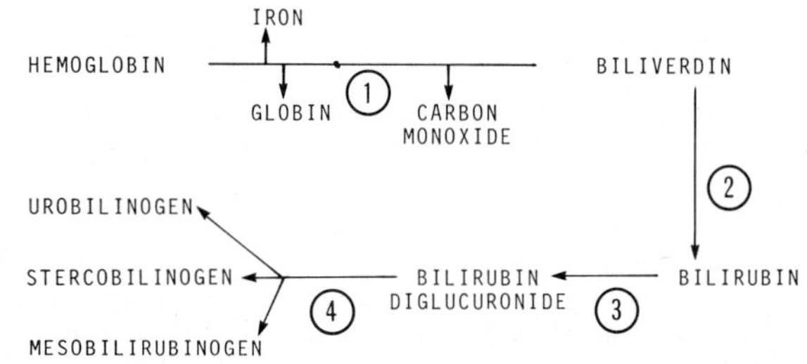

Figure 29–6 Heme catabolism. *1,* Cleavage of hemoglobin; *2,* bilirubin reductase in RE system; *3,* glucuronyl transferase in liver; *4,* reducing enzymes of intestinal bacteria.

Pyrrole ring

Globin

Heme (an iron porphyrin)

Figure 29–7 Iron porphyrin nucleus. Four such heme groups are present in each hemoglobin molecule, united to the protein globin.

hemoprotein. The protein part, known as globin, is colorless and consists of four peptide chains arranged in loops. The hemoglobin molecule has the heme group surrounded by two pairs of polypeptide chains. Normal adult hemoglobin (HB A_1) has two pairs of chains, alpha and beta. The alpha chain has 141 amino acids in a strict sequence commencing at valine and ending with arginine. The beta chain has 146 amino acids also starting at valine but ending at histidine. In the adult there is also a small amount of fetal hemoglobin (Hb F), in which the two beta chains are replaced by gamma chains. The amount of Hb F is normally high in infancy and is increased in some pathologic states. Another minor component in the adult is Hb A_2, in which the beta chains are replaced by delta chains. The peptide chains are bent in helical fashion, giving a spherical structure to the molecule. Attached to the peptide chains are four ferroporphyrin (heme) groups. The peptide-heme linkage is effected by histidine, the imidazole group of which plays a most important part in ionic buffering. Heme itself is an iron porphyrin, i.e., a cyclic compound of four pyrrole rings bound together by CH bridges and linked to iron by their N atoms. The resultant hemoglobin molecule is roughly spherical and has a molecular weight of 68,000 (see Fig. 29–7).

The heme molecule is one of the end products of porphyrin anabolism, by which the complicated structure is built up from relatively simple substances—initially succinyl coenzyme A and glycine. Deficiency of iron or abnormalities in globin will cause a decrease in hemoglobin production, and these are discussed on pp. 632 and 644.

Functions of Hemoglobin

The functions of hemoglobin are: (1) the transport of oxygen from the lungs to the tissues and of carbon dioxide in the reverse direction; and (2) assisting in acid-base regulation by eliminating CO_2 in the lungs and by the buffering action of the imidazole histidine groups of hemoglobin.

In the lungs, oxygen diffuses across the delicate walls of the air spaces and capillaries and is avidly taken up by the reduced hemoglobin: $O_2 + Hb = HbO_2$. As the blood reaches the tissues, where oxygen tension is low, the oxyhemoglobin dissociates, and oxygen diffuses into the tissue cells. At the same time the tension of CO_2 is high in these cells and in the fluid surrounding them. Within the erythrocytes an enzyme, carbonic anhydrase, drives the reaction CO_2 plus $H_2O \rightarrow H_2CO_3 \rightarrow H^+$ plus HCO_3^- very rapidly. The reduced hemoglobin (it has just given up its oxygen to the tissues) has a very powerful buffering action and neutralizes the H^+ ions liberated in the reaction just outlined. The resultant HCO_3^- ions diffuse out of the red cell to unite with Na^+, while the Cl^- ions from the plasma NaCl diffuse into the red cell and balance the HCO_3^- which has diffused out ("chloride shift"). In this way, some 70% of the CO_2 produced in the tissues, having been converted to HCO_3^- by the erythrocytes' carbonic anhydrase, is carried in the plasma as bicarbonate without upsetting the pH of the blood. In addition, some 20% of the CO_2 is carried as a compound with reduced hemoglobin (carbamino-hemoglobin). Once the blood arrives back in the lungs the whole process is reversed; the carbonic anhydrase of the red cells splits H_2CO_3 (carbonic acid) to CO_2 and H_2O. "Feeding" this reaction, HCO_3 from the plasma diffuses into the red cells, and chloride (Cl^-) diffuses out; the hemoglobin gives up H^+; the carbamino-hemoglobin is dissociated; and the reduced hemoglobin is free to take up oxygen again. One gram of hemoglobin combines with approximately 1.34 mL O_2 (Hüfner factor).

Hemoglobin and O_2 Dissociation

Mention has already been made of the ability of hemoglobin to take up oxygen at a high Po_2 (lungs) and to release it at a lower Po_2 (cellular level). The dynamics of hemoglobin make it a particularly suitable O_2 carrier, since it is able to activate sequentially each of the four heme moieties which make up hemoglobin. The reaction is rapid, as is deoxygenation, and is described by the hemoglobin dissociation curve (see Fig. 29–8), which relates percentage saturation of the O_2 carrying capacity of hemoglobin to the blood Po_2. Saturation of the first

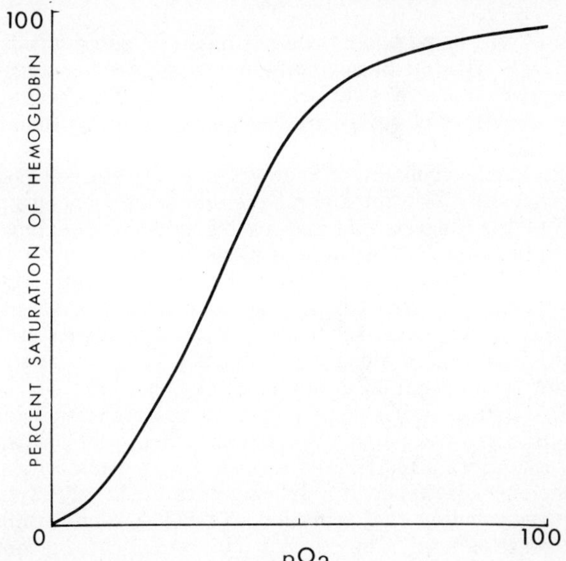

Figure 29–8 Oxygen dissociation curve of hemoglobin. At a Po_2 of 50, saturation of hemoglobin is 83.5%; a Po_2 of 30 gives a saturation of 57%.

heme on the hemoglobin molecule increases the affinity of the second heme for O_2, and so forth, so that the affinity of the fourth heme unit is many times that of the first. This shifting affinity produces the sigmoid curve. It is usual to refer to the saturation of hemoglobin when the PO_2 is at 50 mm Hg. In normal blood this is 83.5%. If the affinity of the hemoglobin for O_2 is increased (e.g., it does not release O_2 to the tissues quite as easily), the curve shifts to the left and a typical PO_2 50 might be 90%. Conversely, if the hemoglobin has less affinity for O_2, the PO_2 50 might be decreased to 75% and it will more efficiently release its oxygen to the tissues.

Up until recent times only two important conditions were thought to affect the O_2 dissociation curve: pH and temperature. A rise in temperature or a fall in pH shifts the curve to the right. The decrease in pH effect constitutes one aspect of the Bohr effect, which is an important buffer system of the body. When blood reaches the tissues where the oxygen tension (PO_2) is lower and the hydrogen ion concentration is increased by lactic acid or carbon dioxide, the Bohr shift to the right causes more oxygen to be made available.

2,3-Diphosphoglycerate and O_2 Dissociation

2,3-Diphosphoglycerate (DPG) is unique in the mammalian red cells as it is a major portion of the organic phosphate. It is produced as a late intermediate in glycolysis and binds specifically to deoxyhemoglobin in a positively charged cavity between the N–termini of the beta chains. The result, in terms of oxygen affinity, is that the higher concentration of DPG, the greater the displacement of oxygen which produces a right shift in the curve, thus facilitating oxygen transfer at the tissue level. Conversely, a decreased DPG content shifts the curve to the left, producing less available oxygen.

A number of conditions are now evident which are profoundly affected by this metabolic intermediate, and they will be mentioned briefly.

1. Fetal hemoglobin does not have the same affinity for DPG as adult hemoglobin, and therefore the oxygen dissociation curve is shifted to the left. Obvious benefits can be derived from giving fresh adult blood to anemic neonates.
2. The level of DPG falls progressively in stored blood, so that only 20% remains at the end of 14 days (see p. 577). This suggests that massive transfusion of old blood with depleted DPG content is to be avoided.
3. DPG plays an important role in anemia, with DPG levels being increased in order to maintain adequate tissue oxygen levels. Likewise, in various hypoxic states, DPG is increased along with increased red cell mass in order to maintain adequate tissue oxygenation.
4. Certain intrinsic erythrocyte defects producing anemia are associated with striking rises in DPG if the defect occurs after DPG is formed, i.e., pyruvic kinase deficiency. However, if a defect occurs in the glycolytic pathway before the formation of DPG, a considerable decrease is seen. The clinical importance can be seen with the better response to exercise in an individual deficient in pyruvic kinase as compared to a patient with hexokinase deficiency.
5. Levels of DPG are low in diabetic ketoacidosis. If the pH is rapidly restored to normal, the protective stabilization of oxygen dissociation by the Bohr effect is lost because of the low DPG, the curve shifts to the left with subsequent tissue hypoxia. Infusion of phosphate to such individuals rapidly restores DPG levels.

The above examples serve to emphasize the need to measure the functional capacity of hemoglobin and to ensure that the integrity of the hemoglobin molecule is not impaired.

MORPHOLOGY OF ABNORMAL ERYTHROCYTES

Examination of a correctly prepared and stained peripheral blood smear is of the utmost importance in hematology. Identification of morphologically abnormal erythrocytes may often enable a diagnosis to be suspected or made in a variety of disparate conditions. Classification of anemias may be made on a morphologic basis (vide infra), and the laboratory worker should be fully conversant with such changes.

In general, it is usual to describe erythrocyte abnormalities in terms of changes in size, shape, or degree of hemoglobinization (depth of staining). Changes in size and hemoglobinization can and indeed must be confirmed by the use of the appropriate erythrocyte indices (see p. 699). In this way a qualitative impression may be substantiated by quantitative data. Changes in shape are more difficult to substantiate, and here experience and a good knowledge of what constitutes normality are most important.

Artifacts produced during either sample collection or slide processing can often cause considerable confusion. Defects owing to artifacts can range from crenation of the erythrocyte membrane to changes in the density of staining. A simple rule to use in light of an unexpected finding is to repeat the examination, preferably using unanticoagulated blood. If any unexpected discrepancy is seen in size or shape, a simple wet preparation of blood examined under phase-contrast microscopy will often rule out an artifact owing to slide or stain preparation.

CHANGES IN ERYTHROCYTE SIZE

Values given for the erythrocyte indices refer to those obtained using a centrifuged rather than an extrapolated hematocrit value (see p. 697).

Normocytic. The normal erythrocyte varies slightly in size, with an MCV of between 76 and 96 fL and an MCD ranging between 6.7 and 7.7 μm. The slight variation in size should not be described as anisocytosis, but merely normal variation. A normocytic red cell does not exclude the diagnosis of anemia.

Microcytic. The microcyte has an MCD of less than 6.0 μm and an MCV of less than 76 fL. They are often present in secondary and iron deficiency anemias.

Macrocytic. The macrocyte has an MCD of greater than 8.0 μm and an MCV greater than 96 fL. It is characteristically associated with vitamin B_{12} and folic acid deficiency. Many workers make a distinction between oval and round macrocytes. The oval form is associated with vitamin B_{12} and folic acid deficiencies, while the round variety is often seen in hepatic disease.

Anisocytosis. This term refers to the pathologic variation in cell size and can often present difficulties in interpretation. It must not be confused with normal erythrocyte size variation, with increased polychromasia, or with a dimorphic blood picture. A dimorphic peripheral blood represents two separate red cell populations that are morphologically distinct, e.g., post blood transfusion. In general anisocytosis is a nonspecific feature seen in many disorders and usually reflects a change in bone marrow function.

CHANGES IN ERYTHROCYTE HEMOGLOBINIZATION

Normochromic. The normochromic erythrocyte has an evident central concavity but stains uniformly. The MCHC is between 32 to 36%, or 320 to 360 g/L, and the MCH 28 to 32 pg.

Hypochromasia. This is usually related to a decrease in hemoglobin concentration, thus giving a central pallor to the red cell. However, the same appearance may also be caused by abnormally decreased cell thickness (see target cell). The condition is usually associated with iron deficiency anemia or thalassemia, but any condition causing abnormal hemoglobin production may produce it.

Anisochromasia. This describes the morphology of cells which stain unequally with only a proportion of the cells appearing hypochromic, e.g., after blood transfusion to an iron deficiency anemia.

Hyperchromasia. Unusually deep staining of cells is not related to oversaturation of hemoglobin in the cell (maximum saturation is 36%, or 360 g/L, as indicated by the upper limit of the MCHC). It is usually seen in situations when the mean cell thickness is increased, e.g., spherocytosis. The MCH cannot be used to further define this manifestation because increased values are often seen in macrocytic anemias in which the increase in cell volume accounts for the greater weight of hemoglobin.

Polychromasia. The erythrocytes take on a slightly basophilic hue when stained with standard Romanowsky stains. This is directly relatable to reticulocytes which require supravital staining for demonstration. Any condition causing increased erythrocyte production will increase both the number of polychromatic cells and to some extent the MCV as younger cells are slightly larger than the more mature red cells.

CHANGES IN ERYTHROCYTE SHAPE

A large variety of cells may be described under this heading, and often are diagnostic for a specific condition.

Poikilocytosis. This essentially refers to variation in shape of the erythrocyte. Increased poikilocytosis usually indicates abnormal erythropoiesis owing to either a bone marrow defect (vitamin B_{12} deficiency) or abnormal erythrocyte destruction. Normally a poikilocyte will be an expression of normal erythrocyte senescence in which, as the cell ages, small parts of the membrane become pinched off. In abnormal situations the degree of poikilocytosis becomes so marked that the abnormal erythrocytes are referred to as "tear drop forms." This is very typical of extramedullary erythropoiesis.

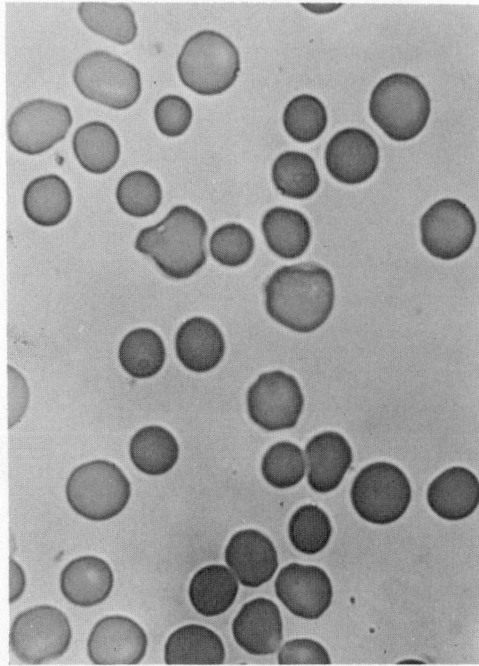

Figure 29–9 Spherocytes from a patient with congenital spherocytic anemia. × 1620.

Spherocytes. These are erythrocytes that have lost their biconcave disc profile and have assumed a spheroidal shape. This causes redistribution of the cell contents with or without a change in the diameter. Often the cells will appear smaller and very dense—so-called hyperchromic microspherocytes. The defect in shape is caused by an imbalance in maintenance of membrane function. A large number of conditions will cause this phenomenon, but classically spherocytes are seen in large numbers in hereditary spherocytic anemia. In this condition a defect in the sodium pump mechanism causes the red cell to retain sodium, increasing osmolarity and attracting further amounts of water into the cell, thus causing it to increase its intracellular volume in order to accommodate the increased volume of material. Membrane damage is associated with other hemolytic conditions, namely, immune-induced hemolysis. It is commonly seen post blood transfusion, and probably reflects contracted donor erythrocytes.

Crenation. Crenated erythrocytes typically have regular, smooth-tipped projections all around the periphery of the cell. They are not significant for any disease state and are usually an artifact. Such an artifact is due to the red cell losing intravascular fluid, as seen in blood with an unduly increased anticoagulant-blood ratio (partially filled evacuated tube), slow drying of the blood film, and very anemic samples. However, severely dehydrated patients may exhibit this change.

Acanthocytes. These are abnormally crenated erythrocytes caused by a defect in their cell membrane. Abetalipoproteinemia, either congenital or acquired, is largely responsible for this characteristic cell picture. The projections on the cell membranes are more distorted and irregular than those seen in crenation. Furthermore, the apex of the irregularity is pointed instead of being smooth.

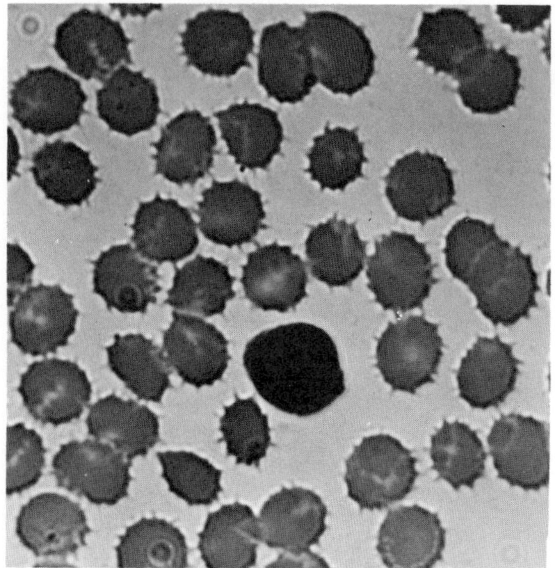

Figure 29–10 Burr cells from a patient with uremia. A small lymphocyte is also present. × 1350.

Burr Cells. These again are erythrocytes with abnormal cytoplasmic projections. In this instance they differ from both crenated and acanthocytic forms in that not only do they possess long, sharp projections, but the projections themselves assume a more regular curved or scalloped shape. Such cells are very characteristic of renal failure but may be seen in other conditions. It could well be that the burr cell is a form of schistocyte.

Schistocytes. These are red cell fragments, and they assume a wide variety of shapes and sizes. A large number of conditions are associated with their production. First, the spleen is believed to cause considerable mechanical trauma to erythrocytes as they pass through the tortuous passages of the splenic sinusoids. If erythrocytes have already sustained previous damage, e.g., hemoglobinopathy, they will not be able to maintain their integrity in the face of this repeated trauma and will fragment. The second mechanism suggests that if intravascular fibrin forms, as seen in microangiopathic hemolytic anemia, this will cause the erythrocyte to impinge itself on the strands of fibrin and, in order to release itself, cause a portion of its cytoplasm to be torn off. This leads to the formation of characteristic "helmet or triangular cells." An easily appreciated clinical condition which causes schistocytosis is the implanting of an artificial heart valve. Erythrocytes are trapped between the violently opposed mechanical surfaces, and disintegrate into various fragments, thereby inducing intravascular hemolysis. Such cells often are described as being irregularly contracted and bizarre in shape, and are synonymous with triangular or helmet cells.

Ovalocytes (Elliptocytes). These are mature red cells that have assumed an oval shape as the result of either an acquired or a congenital disorder. Normally not more than 5 to 10% of an individual's erythrocytes are oval. In dyserythropoiesis the number may become markedly increased. In congenital elliptocytosis up to 90% of the cells are elliptocytes and are responsible for a varying degree of anemia in the affected individual.

Target Cell. This describes an abnormally thin cell, and as the name implies it resembles a ringed target. Other synonyms are Mexican hat cell or leptocyte. They are associated with either abnormal hemoglobin production, hepatic disease, or absence of the spleen. In the first instance the defect is largely owing to a maldistribution of abnormal hemoglobin. In hepatic disease, as a result of the lack of the enzyme lecithin:cholesterol acyl transferase, unesterified cholesterol and phosphatidylcholine are abnormally increased within the erythrocytes; as a result these materials become incorporated into the lipid material of the erythrocyte membrane, thus decreasing the surface membrane:hemoglobin ratio. The result is a large thin cell with characteristic targeting as opposed to the small targeted cell associated with beta thalassemia. The spleen, in its role as a reticuloendothelial organ, selectively removes senescent red cells. Targeting of older erythrocytes often occurs, and if the spleen is absent they tend not to be removed but continue in the peripheral blood until poikilocytic fragmentation takes place.

Stomatocytes. These are erythrocytes with a central stoma or mouth which appears as an unstained central biconcave area, more a slit than a circle. They are a frequent artifact but can be associated with a very rare hemolytic anemia.

Sickle Cells. These abnormal erythrocytes are associated with sickle cell anemia. They are rarely seen in the heterozygous form (S/A) unless the hemoglobin is reduced with various reagents (see p. 709). In the homozygous form (S/S) the crescent-shaped cells (see Fig. 30–25) are often evident. Two forms of sickle cells appear: one is a mildly sickled, oat-shaped or holly leaf cell which reverts back to a normal shape upon exposure to oxygen; the second is a distorted filamentous form which seems irreversibly sickled. The technique for demonstrating these cells is described on p. 708.

Pyknocytes. Pyknocytes are a variety of schistocyte associated with infantile pyknocytosis, in which distorted, contracted, and densely stained erythrocytes are found in large numbers (over 6%) in the peripheral blood

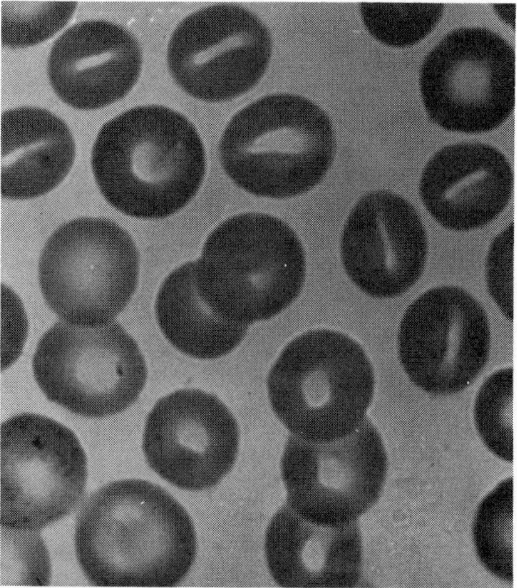

Figure 29–11 Peripheral blood smear from a patient with stomatocytosis. Wright's stain × 1840.

of newborn infants, with an associated hemolytic anemia. Some of these patients have glucose-6-phosphate dehydrogenase or pyruvate kinase deficiency, but others have no demonstrable enzyme abnormality and improve spontaneously. The defect would appear to lie not in the cells but in the milieu of the cells. There is a possibility that the disease may be related to deficiency of tocopherol (vitamin E), which has been shown to be important in maintaining the integrity of the red cell membrane by preserving glutathione in a reduced state by its antiperoxide action. A hemolytic state in premature infants deficient in vitamin E has been described.

ERYTHROCYTE INCLUSIONS

Basophilic Stippling. This is the name given to the condition in which fine or coarse gray-black granules are present in the red cell. They are usually evenly distributed and of uniform size. The "spots" or granules represent abnormal aggregates of the same basophilic ribonucleoprotein which is shown as strands in reticulocytes stained with brilliant cresyl blue and as diffuse basophilia in ordinary Romanowsky-stained smears. That is, cells showing punctate basophilia are young erythrocytes in which the basophilic "reticular" substance has been altered in some way.

Approximately 1 in 10,000 red cells of normal persons will show basophilic stippling in smears stained by Wright's or Leishman's dye. Greater numbers of stippled cells may be seen in anemias of almost all types but are very abundant in poisoning by the heavy metals, notably lead (but also silver, mercury, and bismuth). Indeed, basophilic stippling of the red cells is a reliable aid to diagnosis when symptoms or occupation suggest lead poisoning. In such cases the finding of 30 or more stippled red cells in a count of 10,000 erythrocytes is very strong evidence of plumbism. The stippling usually consists of finer granules than those seen in nonspecific stippling (anemias, and so forth).

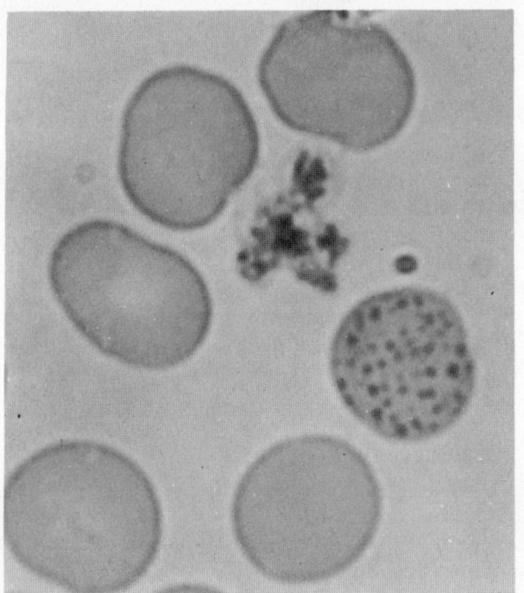

Figure 29–12 Stippling (punctate basophilia) from a patient with lead poisoning. A cluster of platelets is near top left of stippled cell. × 2250.

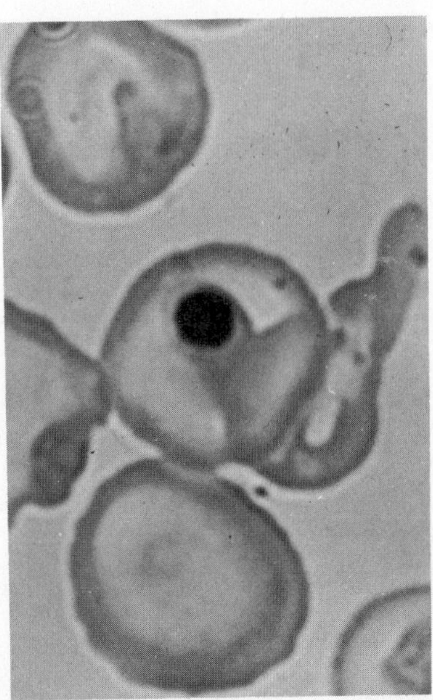

Figure 29–13 Howell-Jolly body from a patient with thalassemia major. × 2250.

Howell-Jolly Bodies. These structures are believed to represent remains of nuclear material (chromatin) within the red cell. They may be seen as bluish-purple granules measuring up to 1 μm (Howell-Jolly bodies) or similarly colored large rings (Cabot rings) in Romanowsky-stained smears. The Howell-Jolly bodies are normally removed during passage through the spleen. Consequently, if the spleen is absent on either a congenital or an acquired basis, these bodies will be evident. They are also associated with anemias caused by abnormal erythropoiesis, e.g., vitamin B_{12} deficiency. A nonfunctioning or absent spleen can often be deduced if the peripheral blood smear shows increased numbers of Howell-Jolly bodies, target cells, and fragmented erythrocytes.

Cabot Rings. Staining a red-violet with Romanowsky stains, these structures are thought to be remnants of the microtubules of the mitotic spindle. Sometimes seen in severe anemia, they appear as rings, incomplete rings, or figure-of-eight structures.

Siderocytes. These are red cells containing nonhemoglobin iron granules that stain a bright blue with the hydrochloric acid–ferrocyanide technique (Prussian blue reaction). Occasionally these iron granules are seen as basophilic grains or rods in smears stained with Romanowsky dyes and are then known as Pappenheimer bodies. As such they may require differentiation from the granules of punctate basophilia. In the latter, the granules (stipples) are generally smaller, more regular in size, and more numerous, and do not give the Prussian blue reaction. Siderocytes are most commonly and abundantly found in patients with hemolytic anemia and after splenectomy. Occasional siderocytes may be found in normal blood. The siderotic granules tend to occur in younger red cells.

Other Red Cell Inclusions. Other erythrocyte inclusions are reticulocytes (p. 701), Heinz bodies (p. 710),

Hb H bodies (p. 709), and malarial and babesial parasites (pp. 514 and 519).

ERYTHROCYTE DISORDERS

The two main disorders affecting erythrocytes are:

1. Erythrocytosis: a quantitative increase in circulating erythrocytes.
2. Anemia: a quantitative or qualitative defect in circulating erythrocytes.

Neoplastic transformation of the erythroid series is seen in myeloproliferative disorders, which are discussed on p. 666.

ERYTHROCYTOSIS

Synonyms for this condition are polycythemia or erythrocythemia. It may be defined as an increase in circulating erythrocytes which produces a manually derived hematocrit in excess of 52%, or 0.52 L/L, in the male and 47%, or 0.47 L/L, in the female. An elevated hematocrit may be classified into two major conditions: (1) absolute erythrocytosis, (2) relative erythrocytosis.

Absolute Erythrocytosis

The absolute red cell mass is increased and is associated with a normal or slightly increased plasma volume. It is associated with the following causes: (a) autonomous erythropoiesis, (b) autonomous erythropoietin production, and (c) decreased tissue oxygen saturation.

Autonomous erythropoiesis is represented by the condition polycythemia rubra vera, which is discussed on p. 666 as part of the myeloproliferative disorders.

Autonomous erythropoietin production and tissue hypoxia may be caused by a number of conditions, including local renal hypoxia (renal cortex stenosis) and production of erythropoietin by tumors, e.g., hypernephroma and hypoxia owing to either pulmonary disease, cardiac insufficiency, or abnormal hemoglobins (increased affinity for oxygen—see p. 645).

In most instances phlebotomy is the treatment of choice, unless a local lesion can be corrected, e.g., nephrectomy or increase in cardiopulmonary efficiency.

Relative Erythrocytosis

Figure 29–14 demonstrates that this is defined as a decrease in total blood volume with a normal erythrocyte volume and decreased plasma volume. This may be the result of either an acute or a chronic state. Acute plasma volume loss may be caused by: (a) marked loss of fluids, e.g., burns, diarrhea, or diuretic therapy, (b) decrease in fluid intake, (c) redistribution in body fluids, e.g., acute trauma.

A more chronic condition is seen in stress erythrocytosis, which typically presents in middle-aged individuals and is often associated with an anxiety state. The leukocyte and platelet counts are not increased, and although the individual may have the physical appearance of a polycythemic, there is no hepatosplenomegaly. Probably a significant number of patients with Gaisböck's syndrome (hypertension with erythrocytosis) possess this form of erythrocytosis.

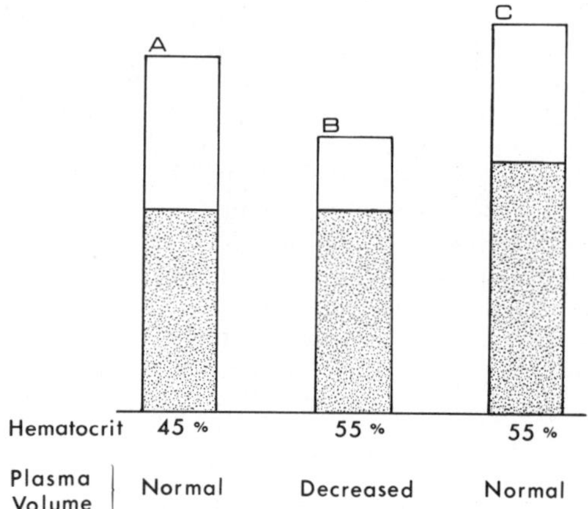

Figure 29–14 Relationship of hematocrit to plasma volume in spurious and true erythrocytosis. *A*, Normal blood; *B*, spurious or relative erythrocytosis; *C*, true erythrocytosis (note increased red cell mass).

ANEMIA

This is the most common hematologic disorder and is characterized by a multiplicity of conditions which can be complicated and confusing. Anemia is defined as a reduction in the concentration of hemoglobin in the peripheral blood which is below normal for the age and sex of the patient. This definition emphasizes the differences one should expect when evaluating probable anemia in different age groups, i.e., the infant versus the adult. Anemia must also relate to the level of hemoglobin the individual normally possesses. If an adult male usually maintains a hemoglobin of 16 g per dL, or 160 g/L, and over a period of days is noted to have decreased to 14 g per dL, or 140 g/L, this must be considered significant even though both values are within the normal range for an adult male.

Classification

Classification of anemia may be based on morphologic, physiologic, or etiologic grounds.

Morphologic classification is based on three basic erythrocyte forms: (a) microcytic hypochromic type, (b) macrocytic normochromic type, and (c) normocytic and microcytic normochromic type. The system is rigid and does not easily allow for variants.

The physiologic classification differentiates between three functional disturbances in the erythron:

1. Disorders in proliferation in which the increase in red cell precursors is less than that expected for the degree of anemia.
2. Disorders in maturation in which erythropoiesis is predominantly ineffectual.
3. Hemolytic anemia in which an increase in red cell breakdown is the major cause of anemia.

Finally, the etiologic classification suggests the following subdivisions:

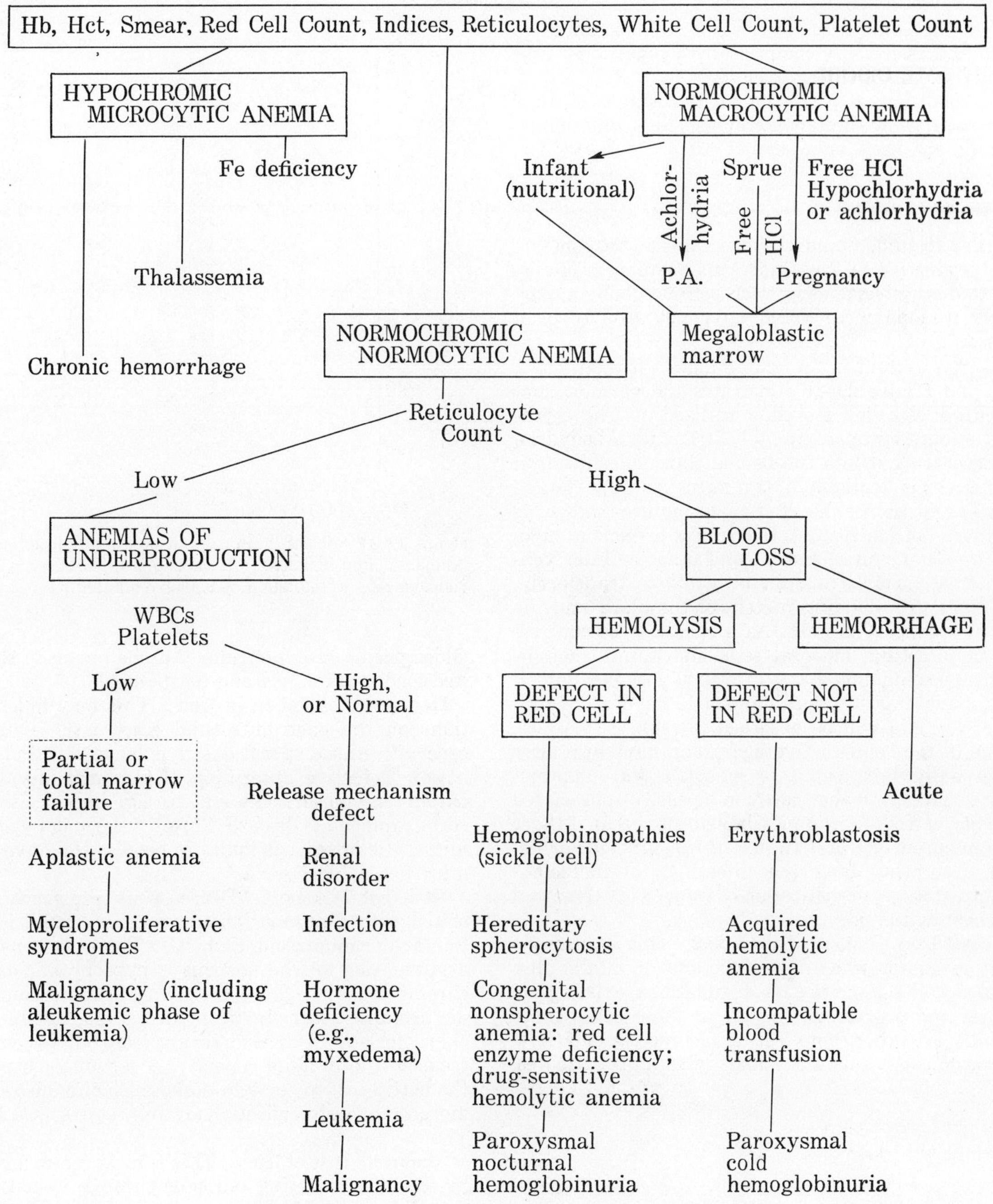

Figure 29–15 Elementary steps in the diagnosis of anemia.

1. Blood loss—either acute or chronic.
2. Impaired erythrocyte formation owing either to a predisposing condition or to a lack of factor necessary for erythropoiesis.
3. Increased erythrocyte destruction owing to intra- or extracorpuscular defects.

None of these classifications is entirely satisfactory because within each classification, the various subdivisions are not completely inclusive. It is considered that the morphologic classification is most appropriate and practical for the laboratory worker, since he or she is directly responsible for correct appraisal of erythrocyte morphology. Very often the morphologic findings will subsequently dictate what the possible etiologic causes could be. The physiologic system has much to commend it, since it describes the basic mechanisms responsible for the anemia; these mechanisms will be emphasized when discussing individual anemias.

MICROCYTIC HYPOCHROMIC ANEMIA

This is the commonest anemia seen in community practice and essentially comprises two conditions: iron deficiency anemia and thalassemia.

Other conditions may, during certain stages of their development, show similar morphology, e.g., sideroblastic anemia and beta-thalassemia trait.

IRON DEFICIENCY ANEMIA

In order to understand the mechanisms responsible for the production of this important anemia, it is necessary to discuss some aspects of iron metabolism, particularly iron balance, which have not already been described.

Total iron content in an adult ranges between 3 to 5 grams, and Figure 29–16 illustrates the various compartments it is either stored or utilized in. The erythrocytes account for approximately 70% of total body iron by incorporating it into the hemoglobin molecule. Iron in the tissues is available in two forms, namely storage and active portions. The storage forms are known as hemosiderin and ferritin. Active iron is present in myoglobin (muscle), mitochondria, and other cellular constituents. A variable amount is bound to transferrin, which is the iron-binding protein of the blood and the principal transport protein. As a result of normal renewal of intestinal mucosal cells and minute hemorrhages, approximately 1 mg of iron is lost per day. If the individual ingests a minimum of 15 mg of elemental iron daily, 1 mg will be absorbed to replace this loss. Females in the reproductive age group have a greater average daily loss owing to menstruation (approximately 2 to 3 mg). It therefore can be easily appreciated that major defects in iron metabolism can occur if there is: (a) inappropriate oral intake; (b) insufficient or defective absorption from the intestine; (c) inefficient transport, storage, or utilization of iron; or (d) abnormal loss of iron by the body.

Deficient Iron Content of the Food. This is seen especially in infants who are kept too long on a milk diet. It is also common in native populations existing on marginal and poor diets, though in these cases there frequently are other complicating factors, e.g., malaria, trypanosomiasis, kala-azar, and intestinal parasites.

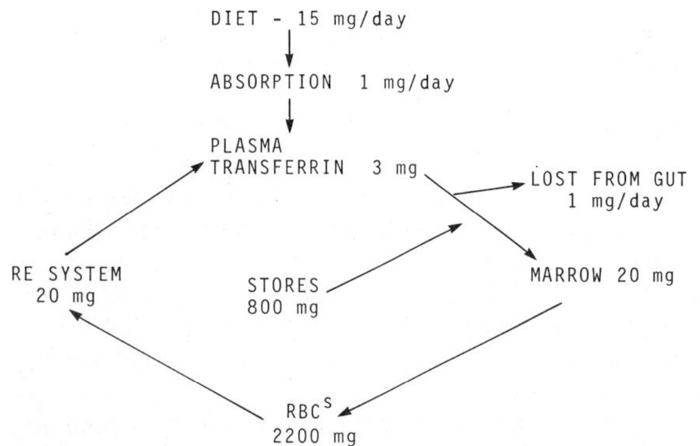

Figure 29–16 Normal iron metabolism. The amount of iron in each compartment is as for a 70 kg male.

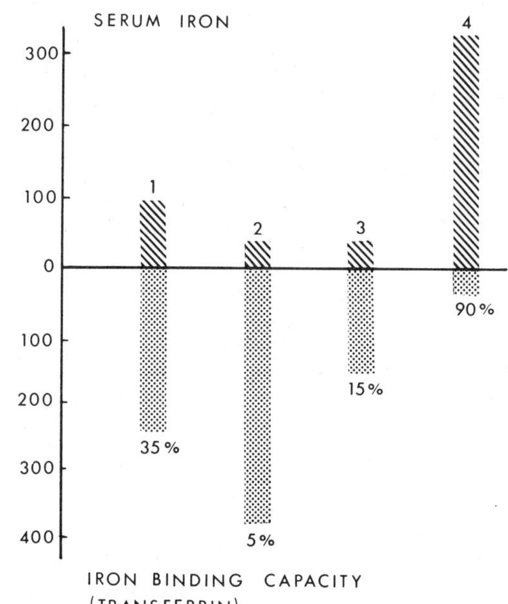

Figure 29–17 Relationship of serum iron and transferrin levels. *1,* normal; *2,* iron deficiency; *3,* infection; *4,* hemochromatosis. Percentages refer to saturation of available transferrin.

Older people are particularly prone owing to their limited food intake ("tea and toast" meals).

Deficient Absorption of Iron. This may follow operations on the gastrointestinal tract, e.g., gastrectomy, especially those operations that leave a "blind loop" of bowel. Defective absorption of iron may also occur in chronic malabsorption states, e.g, gastrocolic fistula, sprue, and celiac disease. Rarely, a form of hypochromic microcytic anemia is found in people who have a histamine-fast achlorhydria.

Deficient Transport. Decrease in transferrin is associated with a number of inflammatory conditions, particularly rheumatoid arthritis. There is considerable argument as to whether this is hypochromic or normochromic anemia. However, owing to the serum protein disturbances transferrin is decreased, producing the characteristic decreased serum iron but normal or increased iron binding capacity. A serum ferritin level is the better test to perform under such circumstances and more accurately reflects body iron stores (see Fig. 29–17).

Abnormal Loss of Iron. This is most commonly caused by loss of circulating red cells through hemorrhage or menstruation. Pathologic blood loss is a prime suspect in the male, and this can vary from simple hemorrhoids to occult carcinomas of the bowel. It is a clinical axiom that if a middle-aged male or postmenopausal female is examined and found to have an iron deficiency anemia, gastrointestinal neoplasm is a prime suspect until thoroughly excluded from the differential diagnosis. Women may lose large amounts of iron through abnormal menstrual patterns, and this is a very common cause of anemia. Hemosiderinuria is an uncommon cause and is associated with intravascular hemolysis.

Increased Physiologic Requirements. This occurs primarily in children during active growth and in pregnant women. Often, when the need for iron in the infant is

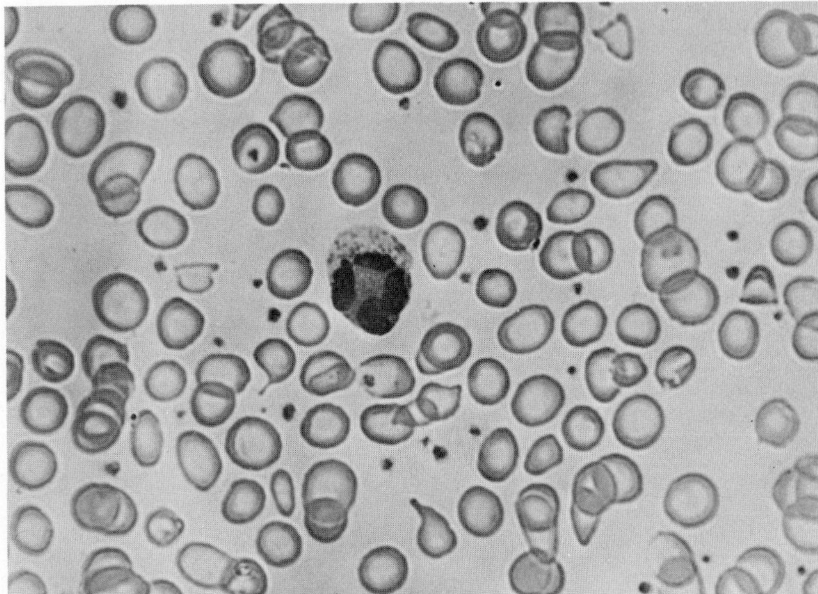

Figure 29–18 Microcytic hypochromic (iron deficiency) anemia. × 1350.

greatest, the child is fed on an iron-deficient milk diet; therefore, the anemia is common in children up to two years of age. Pregnancy places heavy demands on the iron stores of the mother, each fetus requiring approximately 500 mg of iron for full development. This requirement, associated with blood loss and interpartum menstruation, necessitates careful assessment of the female iron stores during the reproductive years.

Laboratory Findings

Laboratory diagnosis is made with the peripheral blood values, bone marrow, and biochemical findings.

Peripheral Blood. The degree of anemia varies, with the MCHC and MCH being reduced. The decreased MCHC reflects the decreased saturation of hemoglobin in the cell as a result of the lack of iron. The decreased MCH reflects not only reduced hemoglobin synthesis but also the size of the cell, which is characteristically microcytic. In severe anemia, bizarre-shaped erythrocytes will be seen with the occurrence of long elliptical or "cigar" cells. The degree of poikilocytosis may be very marked. Because the hypochromic iron deficient cells are often thinner than normal, target forms will be seen and the osmotic fragility will be decreased correspondingly. Leukocytes are not altered but a thrombocytosis is often noted, although it is not an invariable feature.

Bone Marrow. The predominant finding is an erythroid hyperplasia with a decreased M:E ratio. Erythropoiesis is abnormal in that the rate of hemoglobinization is retarded, producing an abnormal number of polychromatic normoblasts. Nuclear development is unimpeded so that a mature pyknotic nucleus is often seen, accompanied by basophilic or polychromatic cytoplasm. The margins of the cytoplasm are often irregular. The crucial observation is to demonstrate the absence of iron in marrow fragments stained with Perl's reagent (p. 805). In subclinical anemia minute amounts of iron may still be present.

Biochemical. Owing to the lack of circulating iron, the amount of transferrin available to bind any iron which may enter the circulation is increased. Therefore the serum iron is decreased (below 60 μg per dL, or 6 μmol/L) and the iron binding capacity (TIBC) is increased (up to 500 μg per dL, or 50 μmol/L). Saturation of transferrin is normally between 25 and 50%, but in this condition it is below 20%. The transferrin index or saturation is calculated by dividing the serum iron by the TIBC and expressing it as a percentage. Free erythrocyte protoporphyrin is increased to values over 60 μg per dL, or 0.60 μmol/L, red cells. Serum ferritin levels can be misleading, but a level of less than 10 μg/L, or 0.10 μmol/L, is diagnostic.

Figure 29–17 demonstrates the relationship between the serum iron and TIBC in a variety of conditions. Using these two tests, one is able to differentiate between iron deficiency anemia and secondary anemias, both of which present with a low serum iron. High serum iron with a corresponding reduced TIBC and increased saturation of transferrin indicates the presence of increased iron stores associated with hemochromatosis.

The degree of change in the biochemical, blood, and bone marrow values will depend upon the severity of the anemia. The iron stores are depleted (bone marrow), followed by changes in the serum iron and TIBC, and only when all available iron is exhausted will changes in the erythrocytes become evident. Treatment is concerned with the replacement of iron using either oral or parenteral routes. A reticulocytosis is evident after approximately one week of therapy.

Thalassemia

Although this characteristically presents with a hypochromic microcytic anemia, it will be discussed along with the hemoglobinopathies in the hemolytic anemia section.

TABLE 29–1 CLASSIFICATION OF THE MACROCYTIC ANEMIAS

Megaloblastic		Nonmegaloblastic
B_{12} Deficiency	*Folic Acid Deficiency*	*Not B_{12} or Folic Acid Deficiencies*
Inadequate oral intake: vegans, diet	Inadequate oral intake: poverty, alcoholism	Hemolytic anemias
Intrinsic factor deficiency: pernicious anemia, gastritis or gastrectomy, nonfunctional forms of IF	Intestinal disorders: gastrectomy, steatorrhea and diarrhea, surgery and neoplasm	Posthemorrhagic anemia
Small intestine disease: malabsorption—general, malabsorption—specific for B_{12}, intestinal parasites	Drugs: phenytoin, oral contraceptives, antibiotics	Associated with malignancies, protein and general vitamin deficiency, dyserythropoietic or refractory anemias, liver disease, and leukemia
Impaired utilization: hepatic and renal disease, protein deficiency, alcohol	Impaired utilization: chemotherapy, vitamin B_{12} deficiency, hepatic disease, and alcohol	
Increased requirements: hemolysis, infancy, pregnancy, malignancy	Increased requirements: pregnancy, infancy, malignancy	

Secondary and Sideroblastic Anemias

These will present on occasion with hypochromic forms, but will be discussed in the section on normochromic normocytic anemias.

MACROCYTIC ANEMIA

This constitutes an important and treatable group of anemias. The main group is the megaloblastic macrocytic anemias caused by either individual or combined deficiencies of vitamin B_{12} or folic acid. Table 29–1 attempts to classify these anemias into the diagnostically important groups of megaloblastic macrocytic and normoblastic macrocytic anemias.

MEGALOBLASTIC MACROCYTIC ANEMIA

Caused by a deficiency of either vitamin B_{12} or folic acid, these anemias constitute by far the largest group. After describing how folic acid and B_{12} interrelate with each other, the laboratory features will be presented, followed by a description of the individual anemias.

Vitamin B_{12}

Vitamin B_{12} (cyanocobalamin) is an exceedingly complex molecule having a central cobalt nucleus surrounded by a porphyrin-like ring to which, in turn, are attached a nucleotide and aminopropanol. It is found in a wide variety of foodstuffs and, until its isolation, had been known as the extrinsic factor. In order to be absorbed from the intestine it must combine with a glycoprotein-like substance which is secreted in normal saliva and gastric juice, and is known as the intrinsic factor. The requirement of vitamin B_{12} is very small (1 μg daily). It is stored in the liver and its main biochemical function in the body appears to be concerned with the formation of labile methyl groups necessary for the proper elaboration of thymidine. Hence, deficiency of vitamin B_{12} leads to impaired synthesis of nucleic acids and, therefore, to defective maturation of cell nuclei and cells generally.

Folic Acid

The name "folic acid" is given to a group of chemically related substances. Folic acid itself is pteroylglutamic acid, but the biologically active agent is probably folinic acid (citrovorum factor: 5-formyl-5,6,7,8-tetrahydrofolic acid). In the conversion to the active form, there is first a conversion to tetrahydrofolic acid, which then undergoes an exchange reaction with formiminoglutamic acid (FIGLU) to form folinic and glutamic acids. Folic acid–like substances are widely distributed in nature and are especially abundant in liver, yeast, and leafy green vegetables. The role of folinic acid appears to be that of utilization of single carbon units (formaldehydic groups) in the manufacture of the thymidine of nucleic acids. Hence, deficiency of folic acid leads to a condition very similar to that occurring as a result of lack of vitamin B_{12}. However, deficiency of vitamin B_{12} is associated with certain additional findings not seen in simple folic acid deficiency: degeneration of certain nerve pathways in the spinal cord (combined system disease) and atrophy of the mucosae of the tongue, mouth, and pharynx.

Role of Vitamin B_{12} and Folic Acid in Erythropoiesis

Megaloblastosis is characterized biochemically by defective DNA synthesis. The megaloblast presents with nuclear immaturity because of its inability to double the amount of nuclear DNA in order for the cell to divide. One pathway particularly affected is concerned with the de novo synthesis of DNA thymine, specifically the pyrimidine nucleotide (dTMP) from deoxyuridylate (dUMP). This pathway involves an interaction between B_{12}, folic acid, and pyridoxine, each of which may be associated with megaloblastic anemia. This interrelationship is shown in Figure 29–19.

As a result of a basic defect in DNA synthesis, not

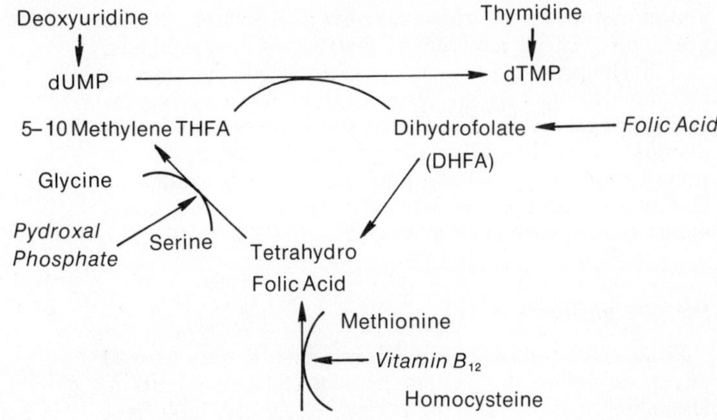

Figure 29–19 Relationship of B_{12}, folic acid, and pyridoxine to DNA synthesis.

only is erythropoiesis affected in B_{12} deficiency, but also other basic body tissues. In severe deficiency, atrophy of tissue occurs (glossitis), degeneration commences (subacute combined degeneration of the spinal cord), and a profound effect is seen in the well-being of the individual (confusion, anorexia, malaise, and general muscle weakness). Folic acid does not have such a profound systemic effect, and this probably is a reflection of the difference in pathogenesis between folic acid and vitamin B_{12} deficiencies. Owing to the accumulation of B_{12} stores, the deficiency states require an extended period of time to become apparent. Conversely, folic acid balance is marginal and with small stores may become depleted within a few months, as opposed to probably several years for B_{12}. Nevertheless, the defect in erythropoiesis is the same, namely, megaloblastosis.

Laboratory Findings

The diagnosis of megaloblastic erythropoiesis is made on the characteristic bone marrow findings. Megaloblasts are not present in normal individuals and their presence dictates a pathologic situation.

Bone Marrow

In megaloblastic maturation the cells are all larger than their normal counterparts; the chromatin of the nucleus is much finer, arranged in a delicate mesh pattern, and stains a lighter lilac than in the normal series. A most distinctive feature is the maintenance of this meshwork and the lack of the tendency of the chromatin to clump into dark masses. The stages of maturation are designated promegaloblast, early megaloblast, intermediate (polychromatic) megaloblast, late megaloblast, and macrocyte (mature erythrocyte). When the deficiency of essential factors is slight to moderate, the type of red cell maturation seen in the marrow may be in between normoblastic and megaloblastic, and is then called intermediate megaloblastic.

Very often there is a marked maturation arrest within the megaloblast series and up to 50% of the series may be either promegaloblasts or early megaloblasts. Mitosis is common and Howell-Jolly bodies are prominent. The degree of hemoglobinization is increased disproportionately to the level of nuclear maturity. The exact opposite relationship occurs in iron deficiency.

Megaloblastic marrow is characterized by: (1) the ease

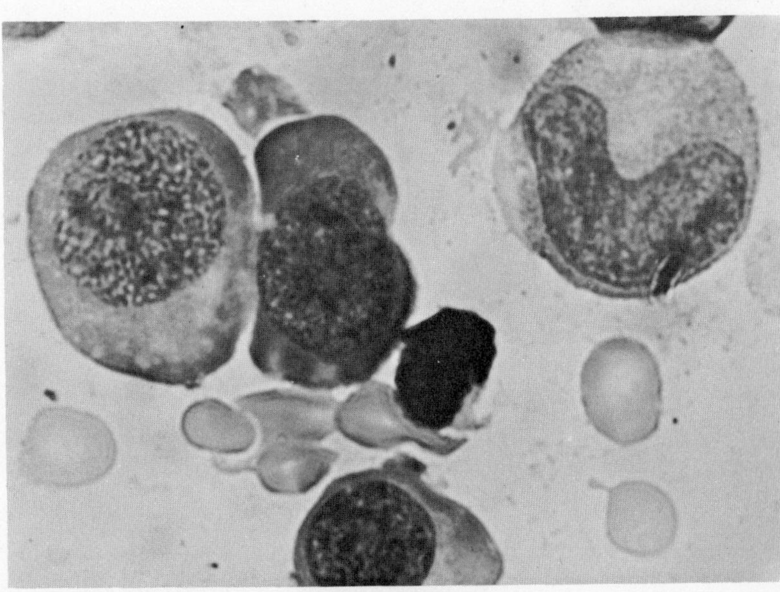

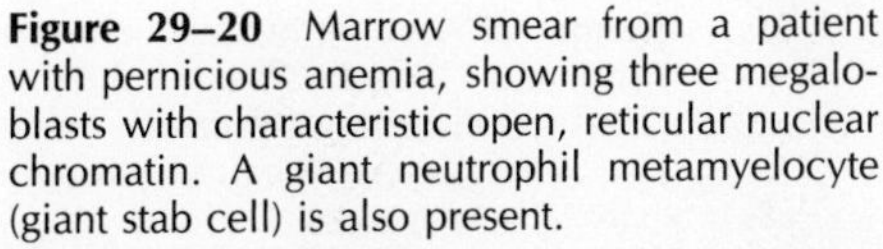

Figure 29–20 Marrow smear from a patient with pernicious anemia, showing three megaloblasts with characteristic open, reticular nuclear chromatin. A giant neutrophil metamyelocyte (giant stab cell) is also present.

and abundance with which marrow is aspirated; (2) the presence of large numbers of distinctive megaloblasts; and (3) the presence or evidence of arrested granulocytic cell development in the form of giant metamyelocytes and giant stab cells. Naturally, the percentage of megaloblasts will depend on the degree of deficiency; in severe cases megaloblasts may amount to as much as 50% of all nucleated marrow cells. Iron stores are characteristically normal or increased.

Peripheral Blood

Since the anemia is of insidious onset, it may be well advanced before the patient presents for investigation. Hemoglobin levels of 3 to 4 g per dL, or 30 to 40 g/L, are not uncommon in such cases. The MCV is increased (above 96 fL); the MCHC is normal (32 to 36%, or 320 to 360 g/L) or very slightly reduced; and the MCH is increased (above 32 pg) because the cell is larger. The large size, coupled with the fact that the MCHC is normal, leads to the appearance of these cells in smears as being more hemoglobinized than normal; hence the older designation macrocytic, hyperchromic. In addition to the large size, in stained smears there is also evident a tendency to oval shape, well-marked anisocytosis, and moderate poikilocytosis. In untreated patients the reticulocyte count is low (usually less than 50×10^9/L). The deficiencies also affect the maturation of leukocytes and platelets, and leukopenia and moderate thrombocytopenia are generally present. Leukocyte counts of 0.5 to 3.5×10^9/L are usual; the platelet count may be as low as 70.0 to 100.0×10^9/L. The changes are most evident in the granulocytic series of cells; nuclear hypersegmentation and large cell size characterize the polymorphonuclear cells ("macropolycytes"). In advanced cases if smears, especially of buffy coats, are carefully searched, occasional megaloblasts usually will be found. Often the plasma will be noted to be slightly icteric and this reflects the increased serum bilirubin, which in turn is related to an increase in hemoglobin catabolism.

Biochemical Findings

Certain tests are abnormal in both B_{12} and folic acid deficiencies, namely increased lactic acid dehydrogenase, serum iron, FIGLU, and serum bilirubin. Specific tests have been derived for the differentiation of B_{12} from folate deficiency; such a difference is of the utmost importance both on clinical and diagnostic grounds. If folic acid is given to a person with pernicious anemia and neurologic symptoms, although a reticulocytosis will occur, the severity of the neurologic condition may be accelerated.

Tests for Vitamin B_{12} Deficiency

Serum Vitamin B_{12} Level. This test is described on p. 712. Overt deficiency is very unlikely if levels are over 100 pg per mL, or 100 pmol/L. Elevated levels are seen in myeloproliferative disorders and hepatitis. This is owing to changes in transcobalamin I and II, which are the B_{12}-binding proteins in the blood. Transcobalamin I (alpha globulin) binds B_{12} avidly and is responsible for the endogenous serum B_{12} level. Transcobalamin II (beta globulin) is responsible for delivery of the B_{12} to the cell. B_{12} binding and delivery defects have been described.

Gastric Juice Examination. Achlorhydria is a feature of most adult pernicious anemias. The use of pentagastrin has largely replaced histamine in an attempt to produce maximal stimulation of the gastric mucosa with minimal systemic effects (see p. 229). Intrinsic factor may be assayed using suitable radioactive assay methods. Two types of antibodies have been described against intrinsic factor. One is directed against the intrinsic factor combining site for B_{12} and is referred to as Type I or combining site antibody. The second antibody impairs the ability of intrinsic factor to facilitate the absorption of complexed intrinsic factor–B_{12} (Type II or binding antibody). Approximately 35% of patients have Type I antibody, another 35% Types I and II, and the remainder have neither antibody. Isolated Type II an-

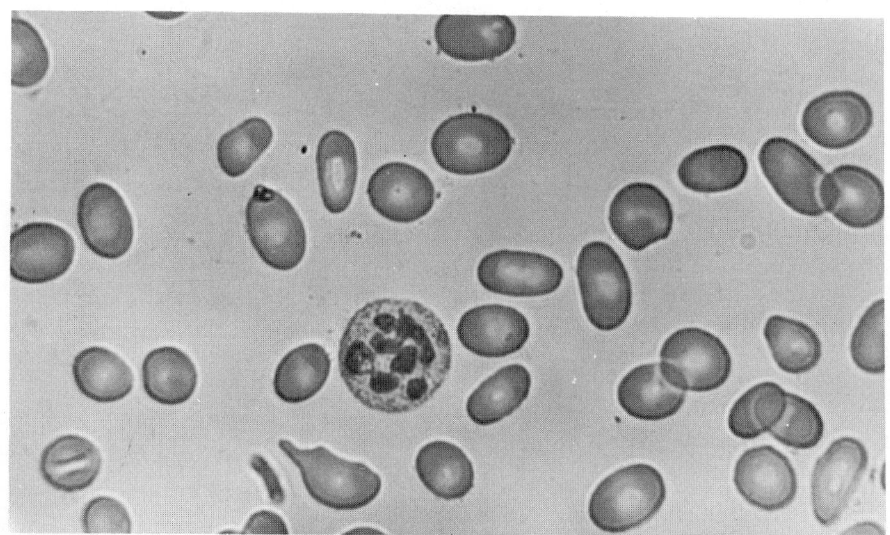

Figure 29–21 Pernicious anemia. Peripheral blood smear, showing large, well-hemoglobinized, rather oval red cells. A typical "macropolycyte" is also present. × 1350.

tibodies are rarely found. Antibodies to gastric parietal cells are also present and approximately 90% of adult patients with pernicious anemia are shown to possess them, in contrast to approximately 10% of the general population. The presence of parietal and intrinsic factor antibodies with an achlorhydria and megaloblastic bone marrow constitutes strong evidence for the diagnosis of pernicious anemia.

Vitamin B_{12} Absorption. The urinary excretion test described by Schilling using ^{60}Co as a radioactive tracer (p. 712) is used with or without intrinsic factor and is considered the diagnostic test for either pernicious anemia (lack of intrinsic factor) or terminal ileum disease (inability to absorb B_{12}–immune factor complex).

Tests for Folic Acid Deficiency

Serum and Red Cell Folate Assay. This is described on p. 712. In the genesis of folate deficiency the serum level is first reduced, followed by an increase in FIGLU and finally reduced red cell folate which initiates megaloblastic erythropoiesis. Serum folate levels are usually below 3 μg per mL, or 3 nmol/L. Red cell folate levels can also be decreased in B_{12} deficiency, so that it is of limited value if performed as a single test when endeavoring to characterize the specific defect in a megaloblastic anemia.

Therapeutic Response

Following the institution of specific therapy, especially in pernicious anemia, the first and most dramatic response is experienced by the patient who, within 24 to 48 hours of initiation of therapy, volunteers a new physical well-being and a dramatic increase in appetite. The response may be followed hematologically by changes in the reticulocyte count, the red cell count, and hemoglobin estimation. The rise in the reticulocyte count may be seen as early as 48 hours after parenteral (by injection) administration of vitamin B_{12}. From then on the reticulocyte count climbs steeply to maximal reticulocyte response (200×10^9/L or greater) with a subsequent return to basal rate with the return of the hemoglobin level to normal limits. The rise in hemoglobin lags 1 to 2 days behind the rise in red cells and then increases by approximately 0.1 g per dL, or 1 g per L, per day for 2 to 3 weeks, after which the rate of increase gradually slows down. Coincident with the rise in the reticulocyte count there is an increase in the blood and urine levels of uric acid (end product or purine metabolism from nuclei of maturing red cells). With the greatly accelerated increase in erythrocyte production, iron stores will become rapidly depleted and an iron deficiency state may be induced after several weeks of B_{12} or folic acid therapy and be responsible for a suboptimal hemoglobin level response.

MEGALOBLASTIC ANEMIAS CAUSED BY B_{12} DEFICIENCY

Pernicious Anemia

This is the most important megaloblastic anemia caused by B_{12} deficiency. It is caused by a failure of the stomach to secrete the intrinsic factor necessary for the absorption of cyanocobalamin. Usually the neurologic signs do not appear until the anemia is well advanced. However, in a minority of cases spinal cord changes may develop before anemia becomes obvious, and in such cases exact diagnosis is of the greatest importance.

The diagnosis of pernicious anemia (often called Addisonian anemia) rests firmly on the demonstration of a decreased vitamin B_{12} level, megaloblastic bone marrow, lack of intrinsic factor, achlorhydria, atrophy of gastric mucosa, and the presence of antibodies to parietal and intrinsic factors.

Other Causes of B_{12} Deficiency

Diet. This is a most unusual cause because such small amounts of B_{12} are required to maintain a satisfactory balance (1 μg per day).

Gastrointestinal Disease. Patients with a total gastrectomy will develop B_{12} deficiency within 2 to 7 years and therefore require parenteral therapy, as for pernicious anemia. Gastric carcinoma and other neoplasms are associated with a deficiency state. Diseases of the small intestine, particularly idiopathic steatorrhea, regional ileitis, blind loop syndrome, and various malabsorption diseases can all produce B_{12} deficiency, but are often accompanied by folate deficiency. If the terminal ileum is solely involved, e.g., surgical resection, a pure deficiency can result and on this basis the serum B_{12} level has been referred to as a specific test of function for the terminal ileum. Various intestinal parasites, e.g., *Diphyllobothrium latum*, compete for B_{12} and in severe infestation will produce deficiency. Various drugs, particularly para-aminosalicylic acid, have produced B_{12} deficiency.

MEGALOBLASTIC ANEMIAS CAUSED BY FOLIC ACID DEFICIENCY

This condition is more frequently diagnosed than B_{12} deficiency, for reasons stated earlier.

Dietary deficiency is a very common finding in the folate-deficient patient and, as opposed to B_{12} deficiency, constitutes an important cause for the deficiency. Folic acid content is highest in the citrus fruits, red meats, and in various vegetables and milk. All of these foods are commonly neglected by the elderly, infirm, alcoholic, or ignorant.

Alcoholism would appear to be responsible on a number of counts for folic acid–induced megaloblastic anemia. The combination of poor diet, direct effect of alcohol on erythropoiesis, and hepatic disease all tend to make this individual very prone to the condition. However, it has been demonstrated that macrocytic anemia can exist in alcoholics which is not associated with megaloblastic changes or a decrease in folic acid or B_{12} values. The erythrocyte defect reverts to normal once alcohol ingestion is stopped.

Disorders of the gastrointestinal tract ranging from malabsorption syndromes to multiple diverticula of the small intestine, surgical resection, and regional ileitis are all associated with folic acid deficiency. Chronic illness and malignancy also play an important role, although dietary factors must be considered in this instance.

A number of drugs will induce this deficiency. Phenytoin (Dilantin) and oral contraceptive combinations have been implicated. They both inhibit intestinal folate conjugase activity, thus preventing folic acid absorption.

The use of trimethoprim-sulfamethoxazole antimicrobial combinations is common antimicrobial therapy. However, owing to its antagonism of folic acid metabolism, the use of such a drug should be carefully monitored, particularly in the elderly and in pregnant women. The use of folic acid antagonists in cancer chemotherapy, e.g., methotrexate, is an obvious cause of anemia.

Increased demand for folic acid is associated with pregnancy and abnormal demands on erythropoiesis, e.g., in hemolytic anemias. The pregnant mother is particularly susceptible to the deficiency, especially if her folic acid stores are marginal, and this possibility must be investigated in all cases of anemia of pregnancy.

MEGALOBLASTIC ANEMIAS CAUSED BY SOURCES OTHER THAN B_{12} OR FOLIC ACID

These present a confused group of conditions, and in many instances they have yet to be fully characterized. Vitamin E has been implicated in the formation of megaloblastic anemia in infants. Some forms of pyridoxine-responsive sideroblastic anemias may often have megaloblastic erythropoiesis.

NONMEGALOBLASTIC MACROCYTIC ANEMIAS

This distinction is of great practical importance, because if the bone marrow does not show megaloblastic erythropoiesis even though a macrocytic anemia is present, B_{12} or folic acid deficiency cannot be implicated.

As Table 29–1 shows, the main conditions responsible for this presentation are hemolytic anemia, posthemorrhagic anemia, and less commonly a large number of anemias of disordered erythropoiesis, including bone marrow infiltration, anemia of hepatic disease, ethanol ingestion, endocrine conditions, and protein deficiency. In the first two conditions the macrocytosis is owing to the presence of young erythrocytes and reticulocytes. The latter conditions, by disruption of bone marrow function, cause the production of abnormal sized normoblasts, which have been referred to as a macronormoblast formation (see p. 651).

Differentiation from true B_{12} and folic acid deficiencies is based on: normal levels of serum B_{12} and folic acid, the erythrocyte MCV is rarely above 110 fL, oval macrocytosis is seldom seen, macropolycytes are absent, and bone marrow erythropoiesis is normoblastic or macronormoblastic.

HEMOLYTIC ANEMIAS

Table 29–2 attempts to classify these anemias in terms of congenital and acquired defects. It probably would be more appropriate to discuss these anemias in terms of intra- and extracorpuscular defects, but the traditional classification has been continued because family history has a very tangible relationship to all these conditions. They all share certain common characteristics which relate to the shortened erythrocyte survival time. These basic mechanisms and tests for general hemolysis will be discussed, followed by a description of the individual disease states.

TABLE 29–2 A CLASSIFICATION OF THE HEMOLYTIC ANEMIAS

Congenital	Acquired
Hemolytic disease newborn	Paroxysmal nocturnal hemoglobinuria
Hereditary spherocytosis	Paroxysmal cold hemoglobinuria
Hereditary elliptocytosis	Infectious agents
Hereditary stomatocytosis	Chemical agents
Hereditary acanthocytosis	Microangiopathic hemolytic anemia and physical trauma
Hereditary hemoglobin defects: thalassemia and hemoglobinopathies	Immune hemolytic anemia
	Miscellaneous

Mechanisms of Hemolysis

The exact cause or mode of hemolysis has still to be established for a variety of hemolytic conditions. Nevertheless, despite convenient classifications using etiologic, pathologic, or morphologic parameters, there are basically few mechanisms whereby the erythrocyte may undergo premature removal from the intravascular space. Three basic conditions have been proposed which encourage or predispose toward hemolysis:

1. Abnormalities of hemoglobin influencing the flow properties of erythrocytes, e.g., aggregation of sickle cell hemoglobin or denaturation of hemoglobin.
2. Exposure of erythrocytes to inordinate physical trauma, e.g., microangiopathic hemolytic anemia.
3. Abnormalities of the erythrocyte membrane.

Extravascular hemolysis accounts for the majority of erythrocyte hemolytic anemias. Intravascular hemolysis is usually associated with either physical trauma, e.g., artificial heart valves, march hemoglobinuria, or the action of complement, e.g., paroxysmal nocturnal hemoglobinuria. Extravascular hemolysis is mediated by the reticuloendothelial system, which traps and disrupts the abnormal cell. The spleen is particularly efficient in this respect, followed by the liver. Therefore it is not surprising that splenomegaly is a common finding in hemolytic disease. Since most hemolytic anemias only cause a minimal defect in the erythrocyte, if it were not for the efficiency of the spleen in detecting such cells they would probably have a near normal survival time, e.g., congenital spherocytosis postsplenectomy.

Abnormalities of hemoglobin, that is, abnormal hemoglobin function and Heinz body formation, cause the erythrocyte to lose its plasticity, with the result that when it is required to traverse through the microcirculation its membranes are unable to flex sufficiently, and this leads to its being trapped and destroyed.

An intrinsic ability of the erythrocyte membrane is to reseal itself after having either a portion removed or an opening made in it. This may be important in the extrusion of nuclei, in the "pitting" or removal of inclusion bodies by the spleen, or in cell fragmentation caused by a variety of physical traumas. The appearance of schistocytes, contracted, helmet, or triangular forms can be the result of such trauma, whether it is the guillotine-like action of fibrin strands, the sudden compression in march hemoglobinuria, or the violent turbulence created by artificial heart valves. A similar injury is probably inflicted by antibody-induced hemolysis, particularly when complement is involved.

If the erythrocyte membrane cannot be maintained using its normal intrinsic energy sources, a variety of structural defects will occur. This, in turn, will alter erythrocyte plasticity, viability, and structure, thus enabling the spleen and liver to sense such cells and remove them from the circulation. Obviously any defect which interferes with the energy source (glycolytic enzyme deficiencies), or with the stability of the erythrocyte membrane (hepatic diseases), or with its structure (spherocytosis) will cause rapid elimination. In fact often all three aspects are interrelated, as seen in hereditary spherocytosis. Basically the membrane is at fault, and this leads to elevated hemoglobin concentration and changes in viscosity. These factors impair the cell and slow its passage through the spleen, thereby stressing the capacity of the cell to maintain the integrity of its membrane. As ATP stores decline, the cell loses more membrane and becomes more spheroidal. This renders it more liable to removal by the spleen. Such observations would explain why splenectomy is of such benefit in the treatment of patients with hereditary spherocytosis and other forms of hemolytic disease associated with red cell membrane loss.

Intravascular versus Extravascular Hemolysis

In terms of laboratory findings, severe membrane damage is associated with intravascular hemolysis occurring with the release of the erythrocyte contents into the circulation. This will saturate the haptoglobin-hemopexin systems. Once saturation has occurred, methemoglobin will appear and hemosiderinuria will ultimately result if such hemolysis continues indefinitely. Overt and overwhelming hemolysis, e.g., ABO incompatible blood transfusion reactions, will overwhelm the binding system and produce gross hemoglobinemia, hemoglobinuria, and, on occasion, renal damage (see Fig. 29–22).

If the reticuloendothelial system is able to cope with the abnormal erythrocytes and remove them from the circulation before hemolysis, evidence of this will be seen by an increase in the products of hemoglobin catabolism, e.g., carbon monoxide, unconjugated bilirubin, and fecal urobilinogen. Haptoglobins may be slightly depleted, but other evidence of intravascular hemolysis is usually absent (see Fig. 29–22).

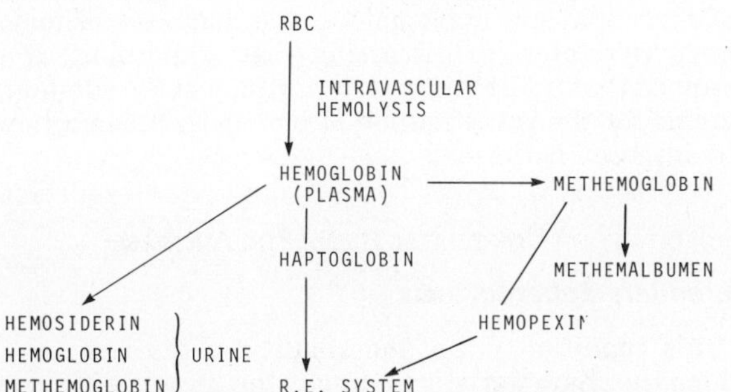

Figure 29–22 Intravascular hemolysis. Disposal of free hemoglobin from the plasma.

Hematologic and Biochemical Findings

When erythrocytes are destroyed the liberated hemoglobin is split into globin and iron. In the normal adult the average red cell survival time is 120 days, so that each day approximately 6 g of hemoglobin, corresponding to 200,000,000,000 (2×10^{11}) red cells, are broken down. This yields approximately 20 mg (3.58 μmol) of iron and 200 mg (3420 μmol) of bilirubin per day. The iron is bound to form ferritin and stored as such or as hemosiderin, and is used over and over for new hemoglobin and erythrocyte production. Naturally, it follows that in a normal adult approximately 6 g of hemoglobin are manufactured anew and incorporated into some 2×10^{11} young red cells each day.

The reticuloendothelial cells convert the non–iron-containing porphyrin into biliverdin, which is reduced to bilirubin and carried in the blood in loose combination with plasma proteins. This bilirubin is not water-soluble and is unable to couple directly with diazotized sulfanilic acid, so that it gives a negative direct van den Bergh reaction. For the same reason, it is not excreted in the urine. In passing through the liver, however, it is converted to a water-soluble diglucuronide, which gives a direct van den Bergh reaction and which, if reabsorbed into the blood (because of obstruction of the bile channels), is excreted in the urine. It follows that in hemolytic anemias, provided the liver and bile channels are normal, bilirubin does not appear in the urine. It will be evident, too, that in hemolytic anemia there will be an increased level of bilirubin in the plasma (above 0.8 mg per dL, or 13.7 μmol/L), and that this will be indirect reacting as regards the van den Bergh test.

The bacterial flora of the intestine converts bilirubin to three types of urobilinogen: *d*-urobilinogen, stercobilinogen, and mesobilirubinogen. The urobilinogens are colorless chromogens which are easily oxidized to urobilin and stercobilin. Some urobilinogen is normally absorbed from the intestines and is re-excreted in the urine. In a normal adult the daily excretion of urobilinogen is 0.5 to 3.5 mg, or 0.84 to 6.0 μmol, in the urine, and approximately 50 to 300 mg, or 84 to 507 μmol, in the feces. In hemolytic disease these values are increased as much as tenfold, or twentyfold in severe hemolytic anemia, and roughly quantitative Ehrlich and Schlesinger tests are most useful in detecting this (Schlesinger's test, p. 209).

In severe hemolytic disease associated with intravascular hemolysis, other helpful diagnostic urinary findings are the presence of hemoglobinuria during the acute process and hemosiderinuria accompanying chronic intravascular hemolysis. When the level of free hemoglobin in the plasma rises above 70 to 140 mg per dL, or 0.7 to 1.4 g/L (the renal threshold for hemoglobin), hemoglobinuria occurs and may be suspected from the dark, smoky amber color of the urine, and the presence in the urinary deposit of golden brown granular casts. Under similar conditions of chronic hemolysis, hemosiderin may also be present in the urine as dark bronze granules. The urine in both hemoglobinuria and hemosiderinuria will give a positive orthotoluidine test; the hemosiderin granules are demonstrated by staining a centrifuged deposit with Perl's reagent.

In the blood plasma, in addition to indirect reacting bilirubin, methemalbumin may be detected in the presence of intravascular hemolysis. Methemalbumin results from the combination of the iron-protoporphyrin, hematin, with albumin. It has a faint absorption band at 624 nm but is rarely detectable by direct spectroscopy of plasma. Its presence is more readily demonstrated by Schumm's test (p. 280).

Since free hemoglobin in the plasma is rapidly taken up by the reticuloendothelial system, it is only in severe intravascular hemolytic crises that it is present in sufficient concentration in the plasma to be detected (by spectroscopy or a chemical test), and even then it is not detectable for longer than a few hours.

Serum haptoglobins are reduced or absent in acute intravascular hemolysis and are useful in detecting chronic hemolysis, provided that the rate of hemolysis exceeds the production of unbound haptoglobin (see p. 275).

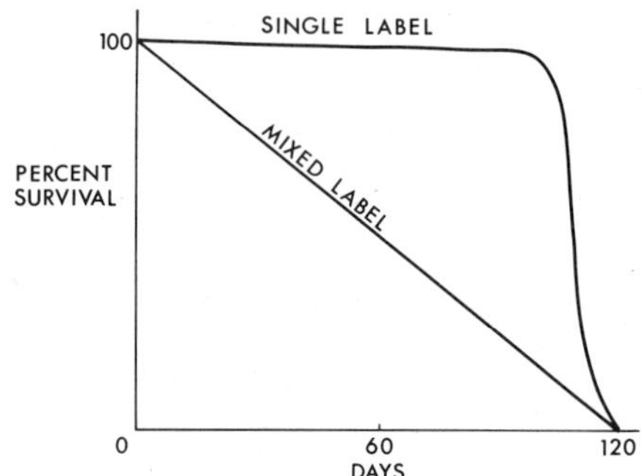

Figure 29–23 Red cell survival using labeled red cells. The mixed label refers to ^{51}Cr labeling. The single label is using ^{75}Se, a cohort label.

Peripheral Blood Morphology

Since the normal healthy adult bone marrow operates at only one-fifth to one-tenth of its full potential capacity, obviously it is capable of compensating for a considerable degree of blood destruction by expanding its red cell–producing capacity, especially if, as in hemolytic anemia, most of the essential building materials of hemoglobin are conserved. Thus, if the life span of the red cell is reduced to 60 days, a twofold expansion of marrow will be sufficient to compensate for the increased blood destruction. Evidence of this will be seen in the blood smears in the form of increased numbers of polychromatic red cells and poikilocytosis. In severe chronic hemolytic anemia this may be very marked and reticulocyte counts of greater than 350 × 10^9/L are not uncommon. In such severe crises, nucleated red cells may be present and even abundant in the smears. Other morphologic abnormalities may be found depending on the type of hemolytic anemia. Spherocytes are a common finding in antibody-mediated hemolysis as well as in the hereditary and nonhereditary spherocytic anemias; sickle cells are seen in sickle cell anemia and schistocytes are common in several different hemolytic anemias, most notably the microangiopathic forms. The morphologic appearances of the different anemias are discussed on page 633.

Bone Marrow Morphology

In hemolytic anemia the erythron is hyperplastic, i.e., the myeloid erythroid ratio (average normal adult ratio lies between 3 and 4 to 1) often reaches parity, and occasionally nucleated red cells may predominate over all other marrow elements. The hyperplastic erythron in these patients is virtually always normoblastic, unless the increased demand uncovers a relative deficiency of vitamin B_{12} or more commonly folic acid compounds, when the maturation of the red cell series may be of intermediate megaloblastic type. Sections of bone marrow from patients with hemolytic anemia, when stained for hemosiderin, will almost invariably show excessive iron deposition.

Red Cell Survival Methodology

Evidence of erythrocyte destruction can be considered either direct or indirect. The biochemical, peripheral blood, and bone marrow findings are all indirect methods, while the only direct method is to measure erythrocyte survival time.

Direct erythrocyte survival may be measured using either cohort or random tagging. Cohort or single labeling (Fig. 29–23) involves the incorporation of a radioactive substance, essential for erythropoiesis, which is incorporated into newly formed red cells. Examples of such substances are ^{15}N-glycine and ^{75}Se-methionine. It produces a characteristic plateau-type survival curve in contrast to random tagging.

Random tagging allows for the binding of radioactive ^{51}chromium (Cr) to the circulating erythrocytes. By incubating a sample of test erythrocytes with the isotope, approximately 90% of the erythrocytes are tagged by ^{51}Cr entering the cells and binding to the hemoglobin. Excessive labeling is prevented by the addition of ascorbic acid, since ^{51}Cr can induce erythrocyte injury. After reinjection of the tagged patient cells, samples are removed at frequent intervals, lysed, and counted in a scintillation counter. The slope of radioactivity decline reflects elution of the label from intact erythrocytes (at approximately 1% per day), and active destruction of the labeled cells. The usual red cell half-life ($T\frac{1}{2}$) using a mixed label technique is 25 to 35 days, varying with individual laboratories. External scanning of body organs will localize possible sites of erythrocyte sequestration, and examination of the feces will provide a means of estimating gastrointestinal bleeding.

CLASSIFICATION OF HEMOLYTIC ANEMIAS

Emphasis in this section will be on theory and resultant tests that are applicable to the diagnosis of major hemolytic states. In discussing these conditions, it is assumed that preliminary tests outlined in the summary scheme for the investigation of hemolytic anemia have already been performed.

HEREDITARY OR CONGENITAL HEMOLYTIC ANEMIAS

Hereditary Spherocytosis

This condition is an abnormality of the red cell in which the characteristic finding is the presence of spherocytes in the peripheral blood (see Fig. 29–9 and p. 627). The disease is present from birth and may be particularly severe in young children. Splenectomy is indicated in severe cases. The red cells remain spherocytic after splenectomy, although the disease is cured. (See p. 629 for postsplenectomy erythrocyte changes.) The definitive test is the red cell fragility test; hemolysis begins at 0.5 to 0.7% and may be as high as 0.8% sodium chloride. If there are not many spherocytes present, it may be necessary to incubate sterile heparinized blood at 37° C and repeat the fragility test; this makes the defect more pronounced. Mechanical fragility is also increased, but this test is difficult to standardize and is not recommended as routine method. Abnormal red cell fragility may be found in a variety of disorders, and other hemolytic syndromes must be eliminated before a firm diagnosis is made.

Hereditary Elliptocytosis (Ovalocytosis)

This is an uncommon disorder, inherited as a dominant characteristic and with a variable clinical presentation. The affected individuals, like those with hereditary spherocytosis, may be asymptomatic, have evidence of a balanced hemolytic process (no anemia), or may display frank hemolytic anemia. The peripheral blood shows between 25% and 90% of elliptical cells and these must be distinguished from macro-ovalocytosis in macrocytic anemias and elliptocytosis of iron deficiency anemia.

Hereditary Stomatocytosis

This is a rare congenital anemia inherited as a recessive autosomal pattern. Ten to thirty per cent of red cells show a mouth-like linear pallor (Fig. 29–11) instead of the normal central round pale area. Osmotic fragility is increased and the clinical course of the condition mimics hereditary spherocytosis and ovalocytosis. The syndrome must not be confused with the finding of stomatocytes in the peripheral blood as the result of artifactual circumstances (p. 628).

Hereditary Acanthocytosis

This is caused by an absence of beta-lipoprotein and produces the characteristic acanthocyte (see p. 627). The condition is associated with plasma lipid abnormalities, including low total lipid, cholesterol, and phospholipid. Marked autohemolysis occurs, which is enhanced in the presence of EDTA. Differentiation must be made from burr cells of renal failure and crenated cells.

Erythroblastosis Fetalis

This is fully discussed on p. 608.

Erythrocyte Enzyme Defects

Synonyms for this condition are congenital nonspherocytic hemolytic anemia and hereditary enzymopathies.

Since the mature erythrocyte has no nucleus or ribosomes, it must depend on the quota of enzymes obtained during its infancy when it possessed these structures. Presumably because all enzymes have a limited life span, it is usually the older erythrocytes that are destroyed or lysed when a genetically determined relative or absolute deficiency of some enzyme exists. Since the mature erythrocyte has no mitochondria, it lacks the Krebs tricarboxylic acid cycle and the cytochrome system of enzymes, and thus it is without the benefits of oxidative phosphorylation.

Only two sources of energy, therefore, remain to the red cell. It obtains 90 to 95% of its energy from the anaerobic glycolytic pathway and 5 to 10% from the oxidative pentose phosphate (phosphogluconate) shunt. For maintaining its hemoglobin iron in the reduced ferrous state, for the continued integrity of its wall, and for the maintenance of its shape, metabolic milieu, and osmotic homeostasis by means of the cation pump, the adult erythrocyte is dependent upon the correct functioning of the various steps in these two energy providing metabolic pathways. Since the discovery of G-6-PD deficiency in the mid-1950's, an increasing number of red cell enzyme defects have been found to be associated with congenital hemolytic anemia that is of nonspherocytic type.

In the glycolytic pathway, for each mole of glucose metabolized there is a net gain of 2 moles of ATP, which is the ultimate energy store that drives the cation pump and enables the red cell to perform those other functions necessary for maintaining itself as an intact functioning unit for 120 days. In the process of ATP synthesis from ADP, diphosphopyridine nucleotide acts in turn as hydrogen acceptor and donor. If there is a defect of an enzyme that catalyzes an essential step in the anaerobic glycolytic pathway, the erythrocyte will not have the energy to keep house and will lyse because of failure of the cation pump or will be sequestered in and destroyed by the spleen.

In the phosphogluconate shunt, 2 moles of reduced triphosphopyridine nucleotide (NADPH) are produced for every mole of glucose that is metabolized via the shunt. The pentose formed is further catabolized by joining the glycolytic pathway through the action of the enzymes transketolase and transaldolase. This shunt pathway is of major importance to the red cell in providing NADPH, which donates the H^+ that maintains glutathione in the reduced state. The precise mode of action of reduced glutathione (a tripeptide, γ-glutamylcysteinylglycine) is unknown, but it has been amply proved that it is essential for the prevention of hyperoxidative damage to the red cell. Since glucose-6-phosphate dehydrogenase (G-6-PD) occupies a strategic position at the entry to the shunt by catalyzing the conversion of glucose-6-phosphate to 6-phosphogluconolactone, it is not surprising that deficiency of this enzyme should lead to oxidative damage to the red cells (Heinz body anemia) in the presence of oxidative drugs such as primaquine. In the same ultimate way, deficiency of glutathione itself or of glutathione reductase is associated with drug-induced hemolysis. It may be noted that when one red cell enzyme is deficient, the activities of many others are often greatly increased because of a younger mean age of the red cell population. Many of these enzymes are much more active in reticulocytes than in average-aged erythrocytes.

Defects in the enzymes controlling erythrocyte metabolism may therefore be conveniently divided into the following groups.

1. Defect in Embden-Meyerhof pathway caused by defects in: (a) hexokinase, (b) triose isomerase, (c) py-

ruvic kinase, and (d) others, including phosphoglucoisomerase, phosphofructokinase, aldolase, glyceraldehyde-3-phosphate dehydrogenase, and phosphoglycerate kinase.

2. Defect in hexosemonophosphate pathway owing to defects in: (a) glucose-6-phosphate dehydrogenase, (b) glutathione reductase, peroxidase, and synthetase.

3. ATP deficiency and other very rare causes, the significance of which have yet to be firmly established.

Laboratory Diagnosis

These can be exceedingly difficult anemias to characterize, and often a diagnosis is arrived at by excluding other hemolytic conditions.

If oxidative damage is suspected, a Heinz body test stressing the erythrocyte with acetylphenylhydrazine will often prove positive. However, Heinz bodies are often absent in unstressed blood if the spleen is present. Conversely, if active hemolysis is taking place, red cells with low enzyme concentrations often are selectively destroyed (e.g., pyruvic kinase deficiency). The autohemolysis test can be useful in that addition of ATP will correct increased hemolysis in Embden-Meyerhof pathway defects. Screening procedures for G-6-PD deficiency are easily performed, since this is by far the most common disorder (see p. 704). However, it must be remembered that other defects in the pentose-phosphate shunt or in glutathione sythesis will also give an abnormal screening test. The procedures used in these situations and the theoretical and practical applications are described on p. 705.

Embden-Meyerhof Defects

Hexokinase Deficiency. This converts glucose to glucose-6-phosphate, and subsequently there is no abnormality of the pentose-phosphate shunt and erythrocyte stability is normal. Adenosine is more effective than glucose in correcting the autohemolysis test. This rare defect is inherited in an autosomal recessive pattern.

Triose Isomerase Deficiency. Again rare and inherited as a semirecessive autosomal characteristic, this deficiency usually presents as a mild anemia shortly after birth and is profoundly increased during infections. The defect is present in both leukocytes and erythrocytes, and the suggestion has been made that this renders the individual more sensitive to infections. Increased autohemolysis is corrected by addition of glucose, adenosine, and ATP, thus resembling hereditary spherocytosis.

Pyruvic Kinase Deficiency. After G-6-PD deficiency (which is by far the commonest), pyruvate kinase deficiency, although rare, would seem to be the next most frequent cause of congenital nonspherocytic (hemolytic) anemia.

In pyruvate kinase deficiency, phosphoenol pyruvate is not converted to pyruvate, and as a result of this there is a lack of formation of ATP from ADP in the glycolytic pathway. The defect is transmitted through an autosomal recessive gene: the red blood cells of homozygotes show about one-tenth of normal pyruvate kinase activity, while those of carriers (heterozygotes) have approximately one-half the normal activity of this enzyme. In the autohemolysis test the marked hemolysis of pyruvate kinase–deficient cells is greatly reduced if ATP is added. This serves as a useful screening procedure. Osmotic fragility is normal.

Other Defects. These are listed in the classification and are very rare in occurrence. The defect is usually suspected because of an abnormal autohemolysis test, and no other cause has been found for the hemolytic anemia. Specific identification requires the services of a specialized laboratory.

Defects of the Hexosemonophosphate Pathway

Glucose-6-Phosphate Dehydrogenase Deficiency. G-6-PD deficiency is a complex heterogeneous disorder which is ubiquitous and is the most common defect seen in this group of enzyme-deficient hemolytic anemias. From its beginning as a hemolytic anemia induced by primaquine or fava bean, it has evolved into a condition characterized by multiple abnormal variants of the basic enzyme. Using a large number of different chemical procedures, including electrophoresis, heat stability, and affinity for substrate, many different forms of the enzyme have been discovered, the main variants being:

a. Normal G-6-PD is designated Type B and is the most common form encountered.

b. Type A G-6-PD is another variety of normally active G-6-PD seen in approximately 30% of American Negro males.

G-6-PD Type A− is the most common, clinically significant abnormal form found mainly in the American Negro population. Approximately 10% of Negro males are affected, with their erythrocytes containing only 5 to 15% of normal G-6-PD activity.

G-6-PD Type Mediterranean is the most common defect affecting the Caucasian population. Its frequency varies from as low as 0.01% in the general population to 50% in Kurdish male Jews. The enzyme activity in affected individuals is as low as 1% of normal activity.

Many other variants have been described.

The deficiency is inherited as a sex-linked recessive characteristic with males fully expressing the defect and female carriers, depending upon the degree of lyonization of the affected X chromosome, having variable expression. Usually the enzyme has to be reduced to below 25% activity before it becomes clinically evident.

The mode of hemolysis is still not fully understood, although it is greatly accelerated by drug ingestion, infection, and infancy. The drug-induced hemolysis is generally accompanied by Heinz body formation (see p. 710), which reflects the cell's inability to withstand any form of oxidative injury. Normal red cells are capable of withstanding such injury by reducing glutathione through the glutathione reductase pathway. However such reduction requires NADPH (see p. 624), and G-6-PD cells cannot supply sufficient NADPH. Therefore glutathione cannot be reduced, denaturation of hemoglobin occurs, and Heinz bodies form within red cells. Subsequently these cells are selectively removed by the spleen and a hemolytic anemia results.

The peripheral blood is of no assistance except to show evidence of increased erythrocyte turnover. G-6-PD assays are the method of choice (see p. 704), although it is important not to perform these after an acute episode or a false normal level may be obtained owing to destruction of the abnormal cells. This is more a problem in the carrier female, in whom the proportion of normal cells may be variable.

A large number of drugs have been implicated in inducing hemolysis. Traditionally primaquine was one of the first drugs involved, but since this initial observation the sulfonamides, chloramphenicol, antimalarials, naphthalene, nitrofurantoin, acetanilid, and others have all been implicated. Typically hemolysis commences 1 to 3 days after administration of the drug, Heinz bodies appear, and hemolysis is apparent. If severe enough, intravascular hemolysis may become apparent.

Characteristically, infections will often precipitate a hemolytic crisis in G-6-PD–deficient individuals. The neonate is also susceptible, and hemolysis may be severe enough to cause kernicterus. Other forms behave more like the other enzyme-deficient hemolytic anemias. In most instances the anemia is mild although continuous, as opposed to the typical G-6-PD deficiency which usually only shows hemolysis under stress.

In general, prognosis is reasonable for most affected patients, particularly the A–variety; however, patients must avoid conditions or drugs known to stress the G-6-PD deficient erythrocyte.

Glutathione Stability

Glutathione Peroxidase. This catalyzes the reaction between hydrogen peroxide and reduced glutathione. Usually a mild anemia occurs if it is reduced or absent.

Glutathione Deficiency. This is very rare and could well be caused by a lack of glutathione synthetase.

Glutathione Reductase. This can produce quite a wide range of abnormalities. It catalyzes the reduction of glutathione by TPNH from the first step of the hexose monophosphate shunt. Hemolysis is usually mild but pancytopenia can occur.

HEMOGLOBINOPATHIES

This important group of hemolytic anemias comprises conditions in which a molecular defect in the globin chains of the hemoglobin molecule has occurred. This is in contrast to the thalassemias, in which a quantitative deficiency of globin chains occurs.

Changes in the molecular configuration of hemoglobin will have a profound effect on the physiochemical properties and produce changes in the patient which are often quite disparate in their expression; e.g., thrombosis, cyanosis, anemia, and erythrocytosis are all reflections of abnormal hemoglobin function.

Nomenclature

Reference has already been made to the structure of hemoglobin. It is made up of four subunits which consist of two pairs of globin chains bound to heme groups, each chain having its own group. There are a number of different normal globin or polypeptide chains which form 2 pairs of chains in various combinations. The normal chains are α, β, γ, and δ (alpha, beta, gamma, and delta); an embryonic chain ε (epsilon) is also present during the first three months of fetal life.

Since each functioning hemoglobin unit is made from four chains, the following combinations are possible.

Hemoglobin	Nomenclature	Structure
Adult	$\alpha_2A\beta_2A$	2 alpha and 2 beta
Fetal	$\alpha_2A\gamma_2F$	2 alpha and 2 gamma
Adult (A_2)	$\alpha_2A\delta_2A_2$	2 alpha and 2 delta
Gower (Embryonic)	$\alpha_2A\epsilon_2$Gower	2 alpha and 2 epsilon

Initially, the various forms of hemoglobin were given capital letter prefixes in relation to their electrophoretic mobility, e.g., Hb S, C, E, etc. However, it rapidly became obvious that this system would not be capable of sustaining the innumerable mutations which became apparent. Many of these original mutants affected the alpha and beta chains, but more gamma and delta variants are being characterized. As the original system became too unwieldy, the abnormal hemoglobin was designated by the geographic area it was discovered in, e.g., Hb Memphis, or by its relative electrophoretic mobility, e.g, Hb M Saskatoon. It was finally decided to identify the abnormal hemoglobin by specifying the name of the mutated amino acid and its position along the involved chain, with the amino terminal position being number one. Thus Hb S is $\alpha_2A\beta_2^{6\ \mathrm{valine}}$; the 6 position on the beta chain, which is normally occupied by glycine, has been replaced by valine. Likewise Hb C is $\alpha_2A\beta_2^{6\ \mathrm{lysine}}$, where glycine on the beta chain has been replaced by lysine.

Classification

Table 29–3 gives a brief classification of the various abnormal hemoglobins. This classification has been arranged in order to emphasize the changes in function which abnormalities in chain structure will cause. Changes in structure will affect hemoglobin solubility (Hb S), stability of hemoglobin (Hb Zurich), production

TABLE 29–3 DIFFERENTIATION OF THE HEMOGLOBINOPATHIES ON THE BASIS OF THEIR FUNCTIONAL DIFFERENCES

Function Defect	The Hemoglobinopathies
Normal hemoglobin	Hb A (A_1 and A_2), Hb F, Hb Gower
Abnormal Hb causing change in solubility or structure	Hbs, S, C, E, D
Combinations of abnormal globin genes and/or thalassemia gene	Hb S/thal, Hb E/thal, Hb S/C, Hb S/D, etc.
Abnormal Hb causing unstable hemoglobin	Hb Zurich, Köln, Sydney, Hammersmith, etc.
Abnormal Hb associated with methemoglobin	Hb M Boston, Milwaukee, Wales, etc.
Abnormal Hb with changes in oxygen dissociation	Hb Capetown, Chesapeake, Bristol, Seattle, etc.
Abnormal Hb mutations without clinical significance	

of methemoglobinemia (Hb M), and changes in oxygen dissociation (Hb Chesapeake). These will be discussed under individual headings.

Laboratory Investigations

The clinical presentation of the patient will largely determine what laboratory testing needs to be performed. Obviously the patient who presents with bone pain, anemia, and sickle cells in the peripheral blood will require a different laboratory approach than an individual presenting with erythrocytosis and cyanosis. Both of these presentations are attributable to abnormal hemoglobins.

The basic techniques required to differentiate most common clinical problems in this area are described on p. 706. The backbone of the investigation is contained within peripheral blood morphology, hemoglobin electrophoresis, Heinz body and hemoglobin inclusion body detection, and estimation of methemoglobin. These, combined with solubility and stability tests, will provide immediate recognition of a large variety of conditions.

More definitive procedures are aimed at analyzing the abnormal amino acid substitutions, and this requires complicated equipment in order to attempt ion-exchange chromatography, finger printing of hemoglobin digests, and isolation and recombination of the globin chains. Other texts should be consulted for details of such techniques.

Normal Hemoglobins

Normal Adult A_1 Hemoglobin ($\alpha_2\beta_2$). Each alpha chain has 141 amino acids and each beta chain 146 amino acids.

Hb A_2 ($\alpha_2\delta_2$). This is best measured by separation through a DEAE cellulose column and is normally present in concentrations of up to 3% of total hemoglobin. Beta thalassemia will cause an increase in Hb A_2 owing to a lack of available beta chains.

Hb F ($\alpha_2\gamma_2$). This differs from adult Hb A because it is not denatured by alkali, is not eluted from erythrocytes suspended in an acid buffer, and has other different physiochemical properties. Normal adult blood has less than 2% Hb F, but increased levels are found in a variety of hematologic conditions including thalassemia, sickle cell anemia, hereditary persistence of Hb F, childhood myeloid leukemia, and a large variety of neoplasms. Hb F is the predominant hemoglobin in the fetus (accompanied by Hb Gower), but at birth the infant's blood contains approximately 10 to 30% adult hemoglobin, and this rapidly rises so that by six months Hb F has largely disappeared.

ABNORMAL HEMOGLOBINS ASSOCIATED WITH SOLUBILITY AND STRUCTURAL CHANGES

Hb S Sickle Cell Disease

This important condition is the most common hemoglobinopathy seen in North America. Like the vast majority of hemoglobinopathies, it is inherited as a Mendelian dominant and although it occurs mainly in blacks, it has been detected in other parts of the world. Although inherited in a dominant pattern, it can be considered a recessive characteristic in that it requires a homozygous state to produce clinically evident symptoms; parental carriers are asymptomatic. The homozygous state is seen in approximately 2% of those with a positive sickling test, and approximately 10% of blacks are thought to be carriers. The abnormality of the hemoglobin has been located on the beta chain, where in the 6 position, glutamyl is replaced by a valyl residue. The homozygote produces the characteristic sickle cells when oxygen tension of the blood falls. Smears taken in a normal manner will show varied numbers of sickle cells with target cells, hypochromasia, and poikilocytosis. The sickling is caused by the low solubility of the abnormal hemoglobin in its reduced state, with the production of semicrystalline bodies (tactoids), which distort and elongate the cells to produce the deformity (see also p. 708). Markedly sickled cells are irreversibly changed and are removed from the circulation. Sickled cells may also block small vessels and capillaries, promoting further reduction of oxygen tension and producing a vicious circle.

In the sickle cell trait (heterozygotes), the smear shows no sickle cells, but reduced oxygen tension will cause such cells to appear, although in smaller numbers than in the homozygotes.

Electrophoretic studies show that in the homozygous condition, Hb S accounts for nearly all the hemoglobin and the balance is Hb F. In heterozygotes, Hb S constitutes 50% or less of the hemoglobin, and the balance is Hb A.

Those with the sickle cell trait (heterozygous) are asymptomatic. Those with sickle cell anemia (homozygous) suffer from anemia, hemolytic crises, leg ulcers, abdominal pains, and many other symptoms.

Hemoglobin S may be found in combination with other abnormal hemoglobins including, in decreasing order of clinical severity, thalassemia and hemoglobins C, D, E, and G. Hemoglobin D has the same electrophoretic mobility as Hb S but may be distinguished by its greater solubility (vide infra).

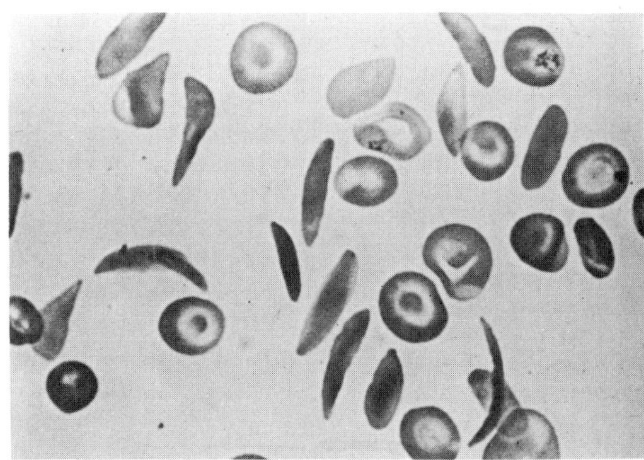

Figure 29–24 Obvious sickle-shaped cells in the peripheral blood of an individual with homozygous (S/S) sickle cell anemia. Note the presence of target cells. × 1850.

Hb C Disease

The defect is in the sixth position of the beta chain, with lysine replacing glutamine. It is found mainly in West Africa, and American blacks show an incidence of 2 to 4%.

It is present in either a trait (heterozygous) or in a homozygous form as in sickle cell disease. The trait is clinically asymptomatic, with characteristic target cells in the peripheral blood, no anemia, and approximately 40% Hb C.

Homozygous disease is rare and accompanied by moderate chronic anemia and mild constitutional symptoms (bone pain, myalgia, abdominal pain, etc.). Diagnosis is by a peripheral blood showing marked target cell formation and up to 90% Hb C. Since Hb C is relatively insoluble, if affected erythrocytes are left in a 3% sodium citrate solution for up to 12 hours, typical flat-sided intraerythrocytic crystals may be seen in wet preparations.

Hb D Disease

This is a very rare defect and laboratory identification may be very difficult. It has the same electrophoretic mobility as Hb S but is distinguished from it by having a different solubility (see p. 709). Heterozygotes are asymptomatic, while homozygotes have few symptoms. The erythrocytes in the homozygous state show targeting and spherocytic forms. The defect resides in the beta chain in a variety of amino acid positions.

Hb E Disease

This occurs most commonly in Southeast Asia, which is its major differentiating feature from the other hemoglobinopathies. It is a beta chain mutation, $\alpha_2\beta_2^{26}$ $_{\text{Glu-Lys}}$. Heterozygotes are asymptomatic and have approximately 40% Hb E. Homozygotes have a mild anemia with microcytosis and target cells.

Other Hemoglobinopathies in this Group

These constitute a large number of different mutants, many of which are asymptomatic if heterozygotes.

Combinations of Abnormal Globin Genes

Many of the above hemoglobinopathies may also combine within themselves or with the thalassemia mutant genes. This produces a variety of mixed genetic defects which can often lead to a wide variety of clinical symptoms and confusing laboratory data.

Hb S Combinations

S/C Disease. The disease syndrome is similar to S/S disease, but symptoms and onset are usually of a less severe nature. Fifty per cent of each hemoglobin type is present with target and hypochromic cells predominating; sickle cells are sparse.

S/D Disease. This has a relatively benign course with occasional crisis episodes, but not gross hemolysis. Sickle cells, target cells, and "cigar"-shaped cells are present.

Thalassemic Combinations. In S/thalassemia combinations the disease may be variable, depending upon the degree of beta chain suppression. If the S gene is combined with the beta thalassemia gene causing complete suppression of beta chain synthesis, the condition runs a severe course similar to sickle cell anemia (up to 80% of the hemoglobin may be in the S form). If beta chain synthesis is only partially suppressed (an A_1 hemoglobin concentration of approximately 25%), the clinical course is milder. Family studies are usually very helpful to avoid severe S/thalassemia patients being classified as S/S disease.

Hb C/thalassemia again has a variable expression. Many target forms and intraerythrocytic crystals may be seen. The level of Hb F is usually proportional to the severity of the clinical state. Hb A_2 can be differentiated from Hb C on ordinary electrophoresis by comparing band concentrations.

Hb E/thalassemia has been found predictably in the Far East. The clinical condition can be severe with the peripheral blood showing striking anisocytosis, poikilocytosis, and target and elliptocytic forms.

Other Hb/thalassemia combinations have been described, and such combinations must always be considered when making a diagnosis of hemoglobinopathy/thalassemia. Family studies are often the only way in which a final diagnosis can be arrived at.

Unstable Hemoglobins

If the amino acid substitution caused by the mutation impinges on or affects the structure of the heme group and the globin chain, denaturation of the heme grouping will occur far more rapidly than with normal hemoglobin. Heme-depleted globin chains are probably responsible for Heinz body formation and the abnormal heat stability test characteristic of these conditions. The sulfhydryl groups surrounding the heme pocket are also endangered in a number of variants (e.g., Hb Shepherds Bush $\alpha_2\beta_2^{26\ \text{Gly-Val}}$).

A large number of variants have been found, all named after the location in which they were detected. This accounts for such names as Köln, Zurich, Gun Hill, Hammersmith, etc. They all reflect some degree of hemolysis at a clinical level. The Heinz body test (see p. 710) is positive after incubation, and the heat stability test provides for differentiation from the other Heinz body hemolytic anemias. Hemoglobin electrophoresis is not usually helpful, although elevated levels of Hb F are often found. Other evidence of hemoglobin instability may be shown by spontaneous methemoglobinemia, excretion of hemoglobin pigments in the urine (produces a brown urine), and increased sensitivity to oxidizing drugs (e.g., Hb Zurich).

Treatment is often only on a symptomatic basis; however, splenectomy has proved useful in those syndromes which produce multiple inclusion bodies (e.g., Hb Köln).

Abnormal Hemoglobins and Methemoglobinemia

Methemoglobin has already been described (p. 275) and is derived from hemoglobin in which the ferrous grouping has been converted to the ferric form. Methemoglobin is a nonfunctioning form of hemoglobin and therefore encourages tissue hypoxia and clinical cyanosis.

It is important to differentiate between primary and secondary forms of methemoglobinemia.

Primary. (1) DPNH diaphorase or TPNH diaphorase deficiency. (2) M hemoglobins.

Secondary. A large variety of chemicals including the nitrates, nitrites, phenacetin, nitrobenzenes, etc., precipitate acute episodes of cyanosis, hypoxia, weakness, etc.

DPNH and TPNH Diaphorase Deficiencies

Both of these enzymes are methemoglobin reducing in action and prevent an abnormal build-up of methemoglobin within the erythrocyte. DPNH diaphorase produces significant disease in homozygous patients. TPNH diaphorase produces no clinically evident symptoms but can cause difficulty in interpreting G-6-PD dye reduction screening tests, since it gives a positive test.

M Hemoglobins

Amino acid substitutions on either the alpha or beta chains (mainly the beta) allow stabilization of the ferrous heme into the ferric form, thus producing methemoglobinemia. The majority discovered to date, M Boston, M Saskatoon, etc., involve substitution of tyrosine for proximal or distal histidine residues, and this prevents reduction of the ferric ion by the normal methemoglobin reducing mechanisms.

Hemoglobins with Abnormal O_2 Dissociation

These conditions present with evidence of either increased or decreased oxygen affinity, and clinically the cases with evidence of compensatory erythrocytosis arouse the most curiosity.

In essence the major defect involves abnormal interactions between the alpha and beta chains, thus producing changes in the oxygen dissociation characteristics of the hemoglobin. These abnormalities are known as $\alpha_1\beta_2$, and β–β interface or contact mutations.

The erythrocytosis caused by increased oxygen affinity of the mutant hemoglobin results in decreased release of oxygen to the tissue. This leads to tissue anoxia, production of erythropoietin, and subsequent secondary erythrocytosis. The laboratory diagnosis is arrived at by initially excluding other causes of primary and secondary erythrocytosis. Subsequently abnormal blood gas levels, erythropoietin levels, and abnormal oxygen dissociation curves in the presence of an electrophoretically abnormal hemoglobin all indicate the possibility of this condition.

THE THALASSEMIAS

Thalassemia was the first hemoglobinopathy for which a familial incidence was recognized. There are many biochemical and three main clinical varieties. The disease is not a single entity but a group of biochemically related disorders united by abnormal hemoglobin synthesis and microcytic hypochromic anemia. Over the years it has been described by a variety of terms: Cooley's anemia, Mediterranean anemia, hereditary leptocytosis, microdrepanocytic anemia, and so forth. Thalassemia is now the accepted term, and the basic defect resides in the production of globin chains.

Classification of the disease has been difficult because of the variable expression of the disease both clinically and chemically. Tables 29–4 and 29–5 divide the thalassemias into two independent groups: the alpha and beta thalassemias. The more common beta thalassemia is characterized by an increase in Hb F and/or A_2 owing to loss of normal Hb A. Because of loss of alpha chains, alpha thalassemia produces equal depression of Hb A, F, and A_2. The two conditions are separate because of the independent inheritance of the alpha and beta genes as dominant characteristics. However, the beta and delta genes appear to be closely linked, and a series of abnormal hemoglobins, the Lepore group, result from gene interaction. There are at least two loci for alpha, beta, delta chains; one gene is inherited from each parent, although considerable controversy still exists concerning gene loci and products.

Beta Thalassemia

Characteristically this anemia is found in the Middle East and Mediterranean areas, with approximately 5% of the Greek population showing evidence of the disease. However, it is becoming apparent in many other parts of the world, e.g., Africa and the West Indies, and is present in immigrant populations from these areas and from the Mediterranean littoral.

The lack of adequate numbers of beta chains in these patients will cause a decreased amount of Hb A, and

TABLE 29–4 Classification of Beta Thalassemia

Type of Thalassemia	Hemoglobins	Other Findings
Minor: heterozygous	Mostly A and A_2 Rarely F	Hypochromic microcytic Variable mild anemia
Intermedia: either mild homozygous or severe heterozygous	Mostly F Variable A and A_2	Hypochromic microcytic cells Anemia present
Major: beta	Mostly F Variable A and A_2	Hypochromic microcytic cells Anemia severe Frequent transfusions

TABLE 29–5 CLASSIFICATION OF THE ALPHA THALASSEMIAS

Type of Thalassemia	Hemoglobin Present	Other Findings
Silent (heterozygous)	A	Normal
Alpha trait (heterozygous)	A ? decreased A_2	Variable erythrocyte morphology
Hemoglobin H (probably homozygous)	A 5–30% H	Abnormal morphology anemia
Fatal form (homozygous)	No A Barts and H	Hydrops fetalis or neonatal death

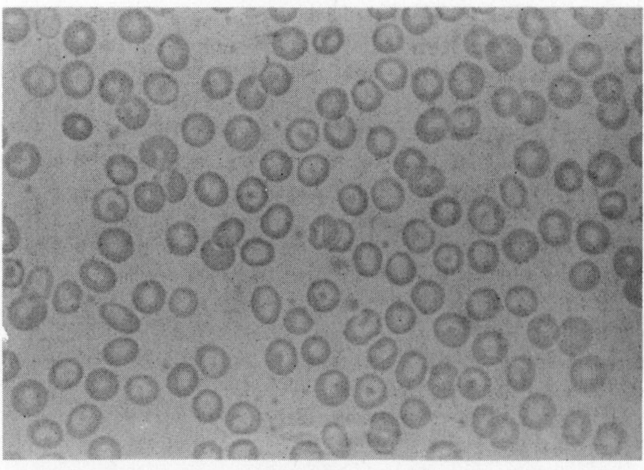

Figure 29–25 Peripheral blood from a beta thalassemia trait patient. Note the uniform microcytosis and target cells. No increased polychromasia is apparent. × 1350.

therefore they will have varying degrees of anemia which is microcytic and hypochromic in type. In an attempt to compensate, excess gamma chains will be formed to make Hb F and excess delta chains will be formed to produce Hb A_2.

Heterozygous Beta Thalassemia

These are people with thalassemia trait or thalassemia minor. They are asymptomatic and rarely have pronounced anemia. The peripheral blood shows typical microcytosis, hypochromasia, and small target forms. The microcytosis is almost diagnostic if the MCV is below 65 fL and has been used to good effect in screening populations for this condition. Iron deficiency must be excluded but prognosis is good for this group, although family studies and genetic counseling are required. Page 708 provides further details for identifying this condition.

Thalassemia Intermedia

This clinical expression would appear to be the result of either a mild homozygous or severe heterozygous condition. Patients have mild to moderate anemia, abnormal peripheral blood with increased A_2, and F hemoglobins. This type of presentation is often seen in beta thalassemia associated with abnormal hemoglobin, e.g., Hb C/thalassemia, etc.

Homozygous or Beta Thalassemia Major

This is a severe condition with insidious onset, often becoming apparent early in life and showing all the signs of chronic severe hemolytic disease, e.g., bone changes and pain, splenomegaly, ulcers, gallstones, etc.

The anemia is severe, being as low as 3 g per dL, or 30 g/L; the erythrocytes are hypochromic, microcytic with polychromasia, circulating normoblasts, and often a leukocytosis. The MCV and MCH are reduced, but the MCHC does not reflect the morphologically evident hypochromia. This is because the erythrocytes are abnormally thin and therefore target forms are evident. Osmotic fragility is characteristically decreased and the bone marrow reflects the degree of hemolysis. Hb F is predominant with variable A_2 levels.

Treatment is by blood transfusions and eventual splenectomy. Repeated transfusions encourage hemosiderosis, while folic acid is required because of ongoing hemolysis. Even with adequate treatment many patients die in adolescence.

ALPHA THALASSEMIA

Although this condition is associated with the lack of alpha chain production, the nature of the genetic defect is still not completely known. In the heterozygous forms, the patients are generally asymptomatic. In severe cases tetramers of beta chains (Hb H) and gamma chains (Hb Barts) form, causing either severe disease or death in utero. If the two gene theory is accepted, a mild $alpha_2$ or more severe $alpha_1$ gene is responsible for alpha

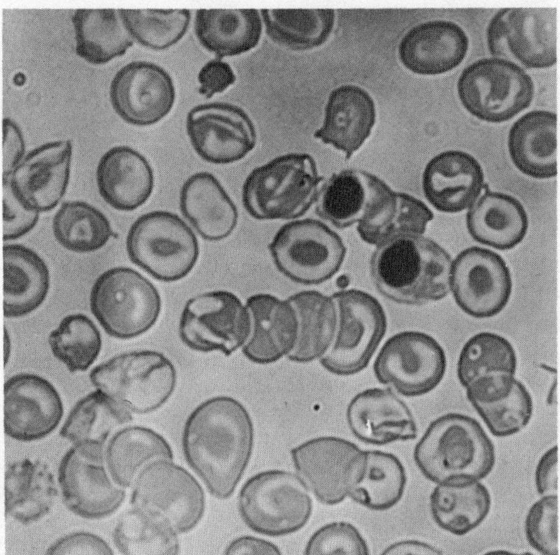

Figure 29–26 Thalassemia major. Peripheral blood smear, showing numerous target cells and two nucleated red cells. (There were 130 nucleated red cells per 100 leukocytes in the smear.) × 1350.

thalassemia inheritance, thus explaining the variable nature of the disease. However, this theory has yet to become fully accepted. As in beta thalassemia a number of different forms of varying clinical severity are apparent.

Heterozygous Alpha Thalassemia

This is represented by the silent carrier (alpha$_2$ trait) and the slightly more severe alpha$_1$ trait. As with Hb E it is more common in the Far East, including Hong Kong and Thailand. In general it is symptomless and is very difficult to detect in the adult. In the infant increased amounts of Hb Barts (gamma 4) will be noted, with the characteristic microcytosis (MCV $<$ 65 fL) seen.

Homozygous Alpha Thalassemia

Two forms are included in this group.

Hb H Disease. This probably represents a double heterozygosity for the alpha$_1$ and alpha$_2$ genes and as alpha chains are greatly diminished, large amounts of Hb H (beta 4) are formed. Mild to moderate anemia is seen with anisocytosis, poikilocytosis, hypochromasia, and polychromasia. Hb H is present in amounts up to 20 to 30% of the total hemoglobin and can be demonstrated by incubation with a suitable supravital stain (see p. 709). Because Hb H precipitates in the circulating red cells they are usually only spontaneously demonstrable if splenectomy has been performed.

Major Form. This is probably an alpha$_1$ homozygote and is usually incompatible with life, either being delivered as a hydrops fetalis or expiring shortly after delivery. This is owing to the high levels of Hb Barts (gamma 4), which has a high oxygen affinity and therefore produces general tissue hypoxia. Variable amounts of Hb H may be present.

ACQUIRED HEMOLYTIC ANEMIAS

Table 29–2 indicates the major groups for these important hemolytic disorders. The discussion is not organized around order of severity or incidence. The autoimmune and drug-induced groups are probably the common forms.

Paroxysmal Cold Hemoglobinuria

This is a rare condition in which hemolysis occurs on return to warm conditions after exposure to cold or chilling. Exposure of the hands and feet for ½ to 1 hour to temperatures below 50°F, or 10°C, may be sufficient to produce an attack. Most cases are associated with syphilis.

Paroxysmal cold hemoglobinuria is caused by the presence of an autohemolysin in the patient's plasma. This becomes attached or fixed to the red blood cells at reduced or colder temperatures only. On warming again the sensitized red cells are lysed by the action of complement. This is the basis of the Donath-Landsteiner test (see p. 705), which is positive in such cases. Anti P+P$_1$ has been shown to be responsible for the antibody in the nonsyphilitic cases of paroxysmal cold hemoglobinuria. These patients sometimes have raised gamma globulin levels, and cryoglobulins may also be present. (These should be suspected if the plasma or serum becomes very viscid or gels at room or cooler temperatures and becomes normally fluid again on warming to 37°C.) The direct antiglobulin test is positive during hemolytic attacks but is negative between these unless the cells are sensitized at lower temperature.

Paroxysmal Nocturnal Hemoglobinuria

This is a rare acquired condition in which the cell surface becomes abnormal and more sensitive to complement-mediated hemolysis. PNH has a complex relationship to aplastic anemia, myelofibrosis, and myeloblastic leukemia. For this reason it is important to exclude these and other systemic conditions. Since it is accompanied by chronic intravascular hemolysis with resultant hemosiderinuria, a not uncommon presentation is as an iron deficiency anemia with mild reticulocytosis which shows evidence of increased hemolysis upon initiating appropriate iron therapy. The hemolysis is probably the result of new "complement sensitive" erythrocytes entering the circulation from the bone marrow.

Toxic Chemicals and Drugs

Apart from conditions predisposed to hemolysis by oxidant drugs, e.g., G-6-PD deficiency, unstable hemoglobin, etc., a number of agents have been implicated in causing hemolysis on either an immune or a nonimmune basis.

Immune Drug Reaction. Three mechanisms have been implicated in causing drug-induced immune hemolytic anemia.

1. The drug combines with the erythrocyte and an IgG antibody is formed against the hapten-like combination. A direct antiglobulin test result is seen, with the erythrocytes being hemolyzed on an extravascular basis. Penicillin is a common offender in this regard.
2. Drug-induced antibodies form immune complexes with the offending drug, which, in turn, after binding complement, attaches itself to circulating erythrocytes. The immune complex activates the complement, which in turn causes hemolysis of the erythrocyte, mainly within the intravascular compartment. It is important that the antiglobulin reagent used in this instance has an avid anticomplement activity (see p. 589). Quinidine and quinine are frequent offenders in this instance.
3. The drug induces the formation of an IgG autoantibody which has specificity for the drug itself. Indeed, the drug-induced antibody often has a specificity for Rhesus antigens on the hemolyzed erythrocytes. The antihypertensive drug alpha-methyldopa was the first drug associated with this type of reaction and is an important cause of a direct antiglobulin test result, without necessarily being implicated in a clinically evident hemolytic event. It is now apparent that levodopa, a medication used to treat Parkinson's disease, has a similar effect.

Nonimmune Reactions. Although a large number of chemicals have been individually implicated in this instance, lead-induced hemolytic anemia is an increasing problem. Other heavy metals, various gases, and aniline dyes are frequent offenders. Lead poisoning is seen most frequently in children who have ingested paint containing lead (by biting or chewing painted surfaces). The lead interferes with mitochondrial and ribosomal function, as well as inhibiting several enzymes involved in hemoglobin synthesis. In severe cases, this commonly results in a slight to moderate hypochromic microcytic anemia with punctate basophilia of the red cells (p. 629). Diagnosis is confirmed by urine and blood lead levels and often by a characteristic clinical presentation.

Infectious Hemolysis

A number of microorganisms and parasites cause hemolysis. *Clostridium perfringens* and *Bartonella bacilliformis* are classically associated with hemolysis. Malarial parasites are associated with gross intravascular hemolysis and hemoglobinuria.

Fragmentation Hemolysis (Microangiopathic Hemolytic Anemia)

This term was introduced to describe hemolytic anemia associated with abnormally contracted erythrocytes, including burr cells, triangular or helmet cells, and schistocytes. Similar syndromes had been described using a variety of terms, e.g., thrombotic purpura, hemolytic-uremic syndrome, red cell fragmentation syndrome, and so forth.

It was suggested that the erythrocyte changes were brought about by damage associated with their passage through distorted or diseased blood vessels. Fragmentation with intra- and extravascular hemolysis occurred and thrombocytopenia was frequently associated with the syndrome.

Since the original description, it is now evident that a number of mechanisms can cause this phenomenon:

1. Vasculitis or microcirculatory damage such as that associated with malignant hypertension, thrombotic thrombocytopenic purpura (Moschowitz syndrome), and so forth.
2. Mechanical trauma, particularly artificial cardiac valves, will fragment the red cell, causing intravascular hemolysis.
3. Formation of intravascular fibrin as seen in disseminated intravascular coagulation will cause erythrocytes to impinge themselves on the strands of fibrin and thus cause fragmentation of the red cell. Deposition of the intravascular fibrin may be initiated by a variety of mechanisms (see p. 731).

Diagnosis is often made on the basis of the typical peripheral blood morphology of fragmented erythrocytes in association with thrombocytopenia, intravascular hemolysis, and a predisposing condition.

AUTOIMMUNE HEMOLYTIC ANEMIA

This is a common cause of hemolytic anemia and occurs in a wide range of age groups and in all grades of severity. It often accompanies primary disease process, e.g., chronic lymphocytic leukemia, and variability in the clinical condition is mediated by the type of antibody involved. Three basic forms are recognized: (1) warm or IgG type, (2) cold or IgM type, and (3) cold IgG or paroxysmal nocturnal hemoglobinuria. This last condition has already been discussed on p. 648.

Warm Type

This is usually an acute variety, with mainly extravascular hemolysis. Spherocytosis is present, with polychromasia and occasional fragmented forms. The degree of spherocytosis is not only a hallmark of this disease, but it may be mistaken for hereditary spherocytosis if severe hemolysis is present. It often accompanies other autoimmune diseases, e.g., systemic lupus erythematosus and lymphoproliferative disorders.

The antibody is IgG in type, it often has blood group specificity (particularly in the Rhesus system), and complement is not usually involved in the immune reaction. The direct antiglobulin test is positive using broad spectrum and anti IgG serum.

Cold Type

This is more often a disease of older age, with mild to moderate degrees of anemia. Intravascular hemolysis may be marked if complement is involved. The patient often complains of cold intolerance, with Reynaud's phenomenon and hemoglobinuria on occasion. It is associated with certain infections, i.e., mycoplasmal pneumonia, and lymphoproliferative disorders.

The antibody is an IgM, reacting best at 4°C, and has anti I or anti i specificity. Complement is often fixed so that the direct antiglobulin test often gives a positive reaction with broad spectrum and anti C′ (complement) serum. Elution reveals both IgM and complement components.

Characteristically, few spherocytes are seen in the peripheral blood smear. Differentiation from paroxysmal cold hemoglobinuria may be made on the basis of the antibody in PCH being IgG with $P + P_1$ specificity and major intravascular hemolysis if exposure to the cold occurs. See pp. 602 and 705 for techniques involved in investigating these conditions.

Summary for Investigation of Hemolytic Anemia

A complete clinical history is necessary. (See also Table 29–6.)

Preliminary Tests (Screening)

1. Hemoglobin, hematocrit, peripheral blood smear (spherocytes, target cells, schistocytes, sickle cells, acanthocytes, malarial parasites, evidence of infection, leukemia, marked rouleaux), reticulocyte count.
2. Urinary urobilinogen, urobilin, Perls' test for hemosiderin.
3. Spectroscopic examination of plasma for hemoglobinemia and hemoglobin compounds.
4. Direct and indirect serum bilirubin and haptoglobins if possible.
5. Direct and indirect antiglobulin test.
6. Red cell survival tests if necessary.

TABLE 29–6 HEMOLYTIC ANEMIAS

	Erythroblastosis Fetalis	Hereditary Spherocytosis	Acquired Hemolytic Anemia	Sickle Cell Anemia	Thalassemia	Drugs		Malaria	Infections	Paroxysmal Cold Hemoglobinuria	Paroxysmal Nocturnal Hemoglobinuria	G-6-PD
						Toxic	Sensitive					
Heredity	Blood Groups	Mendel dom'nt	–	Homozygous S Hb	T. major homozygous	–	Maybe	–	–	–	–	Sex-linked
Spherocytes	– Rh + ABO	++	±	–	–	–	±	–	±	Rare	–	–
Osmotic fragility	N Rh Inc ABO	Inc	Inc or N	Dec	Dec	N	N or Inc	N	N or Inc	N	N	N
RBC survival												
Patient's cells in normal	Dec	Dec	Dec or N	Dec	Dec	N	Dec	–	N or Dec	N	Dec	Dec
Normal cells in patient	N or Dec	N	Dec	N	N	N	N	–	N or Dec	Dec if cold	N	N
Heinz bodies	–	–	–	–	–	+	++	Maybe	–	–	–	Beutler test +
Hemoglobinemia	–	–	±	±	±	+	+	+	±	+	+	+
Methemalbuminemia	–	–	±	±	±	+	+	+	±	+	+	+
Methemoglobinemia	–	–	–	–	–	+	+	–	–	–	–	–
Hemoglobinuria	–	–	±	±	±	+	+	±	±	+	+	+
Hemosiderinuria	–	–	±	±	±	+	+	+	±	+	+	+
Direct Coombs	+ Rh ± ABO	–	+ Most	–	–	–	–	–	±	+ Cold	–	–
Indirect Coombs	+	–	±	–	–	–	–	–	–	+	–	–
Warm agglutinins	±	–	–±–	–	–	–	–	–	–	Cold	–	–
Cold agglutinins	– Rh ± ABO	–	±+	–	–	–	–	–	±	– D-L ++	–	–
Autohemolysins	–	–	±	–	–	–	–	–	±	++	–	–
Acid hemolysis	±	–	±	–	–	–	–	–	±	–	Ham ++	–
Glucose-6-phosphate dehydrogenase		N	N	N	N		Absent			N		Absent
Sucrose hemolysis test	–	–	–	–	–	–	–	–	–	–	+	–

Note: N = Normal; Inc = Increased; Dec = Decreased.

Upon completion of these studies, it should be possible to state not only whether or not a hemolytic process is present but also if hemolysis is primarily intra- or extravascular.

Specific Tests

If hereditary or congenital anemia is suspected:

1. Osmotic fragility on a fresh specimen and after incubation at 37°C for 24 hours.
2. Autohemolysis test.
3. G-6-PD test.
4. Glutathione stability.
5. Hemoglobin electrophoresis and Hb F.
6. Heat stability tests.
7. Heinz body and Hb H staining.

If an autoimmune hemolytic process is suspected:

1. Direct and indirect antiglobulin tests using broad spectrum IgG and C′ sera.
2. Tests for antibodies in patient's serum, including cold agglutinins and hemolysins.
3. Elution of antibodies from patient's cells.
4. Donath-Landsteiner test.
5. Test for PNH.
6. Serum protein electrophoresis and immunoelectrophoresis.
7. Serologic tests for syphilis.

Many of the tests are described in Chapter 30 on hematologic techniques.

THE NORMOCHROMIC NORMOCYTIC ANEMIAS

Several conditions will be described in this section which do not always present with this type of erythrocyte morphology.

Aplastic Anemia

The use of the term aplastic anemia is not as clear as it should be. The term aplastic anemia is best reserved for cases with a truly aplastic or hypocellular marrow.

Peripheral Blood Picture. There is a normocytic or possibly slight macrocytic normochromic anemia and leukopenia, thrombocytopenia, few or no reticulocytes, and absence of immature erythroid or granulocytic cells. The severity of each deficiency may vary from patient to patient and from time to time.

The causes of aplastic anemia are as follows:

1. Chemicals: aminopyrines, benzol, carbon tetrachloride, DDT (and other insecticides), nitrogen mustards, sulfonamide drugs, chloramphenicol, and many others.
2. Ionizing radiation: gamma rays, neutrons.
3. With tumors of the thymus: these cases are not necessarily cured by thymectomy.
4. Idiopathic (without apparent cause).
5. Associated with viral hepatitis.

The disease is not common but is important because a high proportion of cases are fatal and because some cases are iatrogenic.

Pancytopenia

Pancytopenia is a condition characterized by a reduction in all three elements of the blood and can result from a wide variety of causes. These include aleukemic leukemia, bone marrow infiltration for a variety of reasons, e.g., malignancy, myeloma, etc., hypersplenism, and autoimmune disease.

The peripheral blood and bone marrow can vary widely in appearance owing to the disparity in the originating conditions, and for that reason alone a full investigation must be performed in order to define the primary condition.

Anemia of Hemorrhage

Acute hemorrhage is not immediately followed by a decrease in hemoglobin and hematocrit because both the erythrocyte and plasma ratios are still in the same proportions. As plasma enters the intravascular space to restore blood volume, the anemia becomes evident and progresses to maximum within 24 to 48 hours. After this time increased bone marrow regeneration is noted with polychromasia, leukocytosis, and increased reticulocytes. Severe hemorrhage often causes immature myeloid cells and the occasional normoblast to be released. Chronic blood loss is characterized by an iron deficiency anemia.

Anemia of Chronic Disorders

This is a mild anemia, not progressive in severity, which is characterized by decreased plasma iron, decreased total iron-binding capacity, normal saturation of transferrin with iron, decreased bone marrow sideroblasts, normal or increased reticuloendothelial iron, and normal ferritin level.

This type of anemia is ubiquitous, commonly seen in a hospital population and associated with such conditions as malignancy, rheumatoid arthritis, collagen vascular diseases, long-term surgical patients, generalized inflammatory conditions, and many others. In general, it may be said to parallel the course of the disease and this is particularly evident in rheumatoid arthritis, in which the serum iron is inversely proportional to the sedimentation rate and directly proportional to the albumin level.

The pathophysiology of the condition would indicate that the prime mechanism is undue mobilization of iron to the reticuloendothelial system, with a defect in release to the erythropoietic tissues. However, decreased erythrocyte survival times, impaired bone marrow response to anemia, and negative nitrogen balance are also implicated.

The peripheral blood is most frequently normocytic normochromic and less frequently hypochromic; if this occurs microcytosis is evident. Diagnosis is by those parameters mentioned in the definition. Treatment is essentially alleviating the primary condition causing the anemia.

Malignant Disease

In malignant disease, anemia may also occur from hemorrhage, infection, interference with nutrition, X-irradiation, or chemotherapy, occasionally from an acquired hemolytic anemia, and not uncommonly from metastases to bone marrow. In the latter instance, there may be a leukoerythroblastic anemia characterized by the presence of primitive red and white cell precursors in the peripheral blood. There may be thrombocytopenia. Malignant cells may be found on bone marrow examination.

Endocrine Disease

Myxedema is a rare cause of anemia, since thyroxine is involved in marrow function and activity. The anemia is normochromic and normocytic or mildly macrocytic; white cells and platelets are normal. The anemia responds specifically to thyroid administration. Hypopituitarism, such as occurs in Simmond's disease, is often associated with normocytic normochromic, possibly macrocytic or hypochromic anemia, which also responds to hormonal therapy. Addison's disease follows a similar pattern.

Sideroblastic Anemia

This has been classified as another form of dyserythropoietic anemia similar to the anemia of chronic disorders. The anemia is associated with a wide range of conditions and may be congenital or acquired. To date no specific mechanism has been implicated, except to suggest that pyridoxine is involved, since response to pyridoxine administration is noted with a subgroup of the anemia.

Apart from the congenital forms the acquired variety is associated with drugs, chronic nutritional problems, e.g., alcoholism and malabsorption, and hemopoietic malignancies.

The peripheral blood morphology may vary widely in its appearance. A dimorphic picture of normochromic normocytic cells with other more microcytic hypochromic erythrocytes is considered characteristic of the condition. However, the erythrocytes may also be macrocytic in some patients and hypochromic in others.

The bone marrow is usually hyperplastic, with the typical diagnostic appearance of ringed sideroblasts.

These are different from normal sideroblasts (up to 20% in normal bone marrow), in that increased numbers may be evident and increased granulation is present. The granules are larger than normal and form a ring around the nucleus. A similar appearance may be seen in thalassemia and represents the degree of dyserythropoiesis present.

Diagnosis rests firmly on the appearance of the ringed sideroblasts, and response to treatment is generally unsatisfactory or "refractory." Pyridoxine probably causes a response in a proportion of acquired anemias, but other forms of therapy have been largely unsuccessful, e.g., steroids, anabolic agents, and so forth.

Congenital Dyserythropoietic Anemias

These anemias have been defined as a therapy-resistant anemia with ineffective erythropoiesis which manifests itself in the first 15 years of life and is sometimes complicated by a moderately increased peripheral erythrocyte turnover. There is a disturbance of iron metabolism with a general siderosis.

Characteristic morphologic alterations of the erythroblasts are seen and on this basis three types have been identified.

Type I: with megaloblastoid erythroblasts and erythroblastic internuclear chromatin bridges.

Type II: with erythroblastic multinuclearity and a positive acidifed serum test (HEMPAS type).

Type III: with erythroblastic multinuclearity and gigantoblasts.

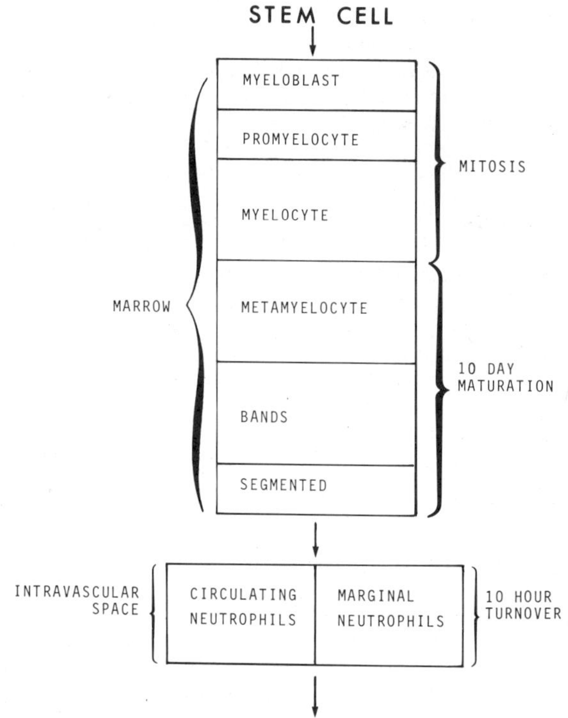

Figure 29–27 Maturation and kinetics of leukocytes.

LEUKOCYTES

PHYSIOLOGY AND FUNCTION

Leukocyte function differs from that of erythrocytes for a variety of reasons. There is more than one cell type circulating at any one time, their functions are numerous and diverse, and their presence in the bloodstream is merely a matter of convenient transportation. In contrast to erythrocytes, their function is primarily in the extravascular compartment and their ability to traverse the endothelial barrier is greatly superior to that of the erythrocyte. Therefore changes in either function or number of leukocytes will reflect the leukocytes' response to systemic conditions and so provide a valuable diagnostic index.

NEUTROPHIL LEUKOCYTE

Figure 29–27 indicates that the neutrophil is found in at least three body compartments. The marrow compartment is the largest and is composed of mitotic and postmitotic pools. The morphology of these two pools, although arbitrary, is identifiable. Mitosis under normal circumstances would appear to stop at the myelocyte level. Segmented forms are preferentially released but in times of stress, e.g., infection, large numbers of band forms and occasional metamyelocytes are found in the peripheral blood. Abnormal proliferation will allow for uncontrolled mitosis with the appearance of immature myeloid cells such as myeloblasts in the peripheral blood, e.g., leukemia.

Band and segmented neutrophils make up approximately 60% of the total postmitotic neutrophil pool in the marrow and since this is approximately 15 times the blood pool, it constitutes a large reserve. When stress is placed on the system as the result of either physiologic or pathologic mechanisms, these compartments act in a predictable manner.

After tissue injury and increased metabolic activity, neutrophils accumulate in marginal positions on the walls of capillaries and venules. In normal circumstances there is always a certain number of neutrophils in this position (approximately 50%), and they constitute the marginal pool. They are in the intravascular space but are immobile and not reflected in the total leukocyte count. With the appropriate stress they are mobilized along with the mature cells from the bone marrow, converge on the affected areas, cross the endothelial barrier by diapedesis, and start to form an exudate. The turnover of mature neutrophils in the blood and bone marrow can be increased to the point that there is a definite leukocytosis. In turn, if the demand is so great, e.g., in septicemia, the accelerated production is not sufficient to meet the needs of the body and a neutropenia will result with the disappearance of mature neutrophils (usually considered a grave sign).

The mature neutrophil is similar to the erythrocyte in that it is incapable of further mitosis. In order to sustain itself during its life span (approximately 10 to 14 days), it requires an endogenous energy supply. This is accomplished using an active glycolytic process, primarily aerobic, utilizing large amounts of glycogen, which acts as a source of energy.

Neutrophil Function

The neutrophil is the most important cell in the cellular defenses of the body against acute bacterial infection and is the most important factor in the killing of invading bacteria. The killing of bacteria by the polymorphonuclear leukocyte is the result of a complex process involving a sequence of activities utilizing both the cell and many plasma factors. It is the most actively mobile peripheral blood cell, and by a process of chemotaxis is attracted to bacteria in order to phagocytose them. A vacuole forms around the organism and the cell kills it by releasing the contents of its cytoplasmic granules into the vacuole. The offending material is subsequently digested and removed by the reticuloendothelial system. This oversimplified description suggests a number of different areas in which function may become impaired: namely, in defects of number of neutrophils, motility, phagocytosis, and killing ability.

Motility. When moving out on a glass surface, polymorphs have a very typical appearance when viewed under phase microscopy. Although the movement can be described as ameboid, the actual mechanism is still shrouded in controversy. Defects in this area are still related to the chemotactic mechanism.

Chemotaxis. Experimental evidence is now available to suggest that the neutrophil can move toward bacteria in a purposeful motion. A number of different techniques are available to demonstrate this phenomenon, and they all share the basic principle of having a two compartment system; neutrophils are separated from the stimulus (bacteria), and the neutrophil is shown to be directly atracted to it. A number of conditions are now shown to be related to defects in this mechanism, e.g., Chédiak-Higashi syndrome, patients with rheumatoid arthritis, and recurrent infections.

Phagocytosis. Electron microscopy has greatly increased knowledge in this area. It is first necessary for the neutrophil to adhere to the bacterium. Subsequent to adhesion the bacterium is surrounded by the cell membrane, which in turn fuses to itself to form two layers. Separation of the cell membrane is followed by fusion of the neutrophil granules and release of their contents into the vacuole. Observations on living polymorphs suggest that the two events of phagocytosis and degranulation occur simultaneously. Again a significant number of clinical conditions have been noted. The opsonins are humoral factors that are collectively either antibacterial or antifungal antibodies, components of complement or other heat-labile factors. Absence of this factor(s) results in significant defects in phagocytosis and resultant clinical conditions. The actual killing of intracellular organisms would appear to depend upon myeloperoxidase and other enzymes, and families have been described which lack these.

LYMPHOCYTES

Currently, the specific interest engendered in this remarkable cell series is related to the function of the two main cell types, namely the T (thymus) and B (bone marrow) cells.

It is now becoming apparent that not only do these two cell types have largely different functions—that is, the T cell is mainly related to cellular immunity and the B cell to humoral immunity—but that they are present in different proportions in various hematologic conditions other than the immunologic and autoimmune disorders.

Infectious mononucleosis is considered a self-limited lymphoproliferative disorder associated with abnormal lymphoid cells, mostly of T cell origin. Chronic lymphocytic leukemia generally represents a clonal proliferation of B cells; the T cells appear remarkably reduced. In Waldenström's macroglobulinemia the abnormal marrow proliferating cells (B type) appear to be carrying the same surface immunoglobulin as is found in the serum. In lymphocytic leukemia with the Sézary variant, the abnormal cells are T type and suggest that this form of lymphocytic leukemia does not originate from the bone marrow. Likewise, some cases of acute lymphoblastic leukemia are associated with T cell proliferation.

MONOCYTES

The peripheral blood monocyte is usually thought of as being a circulating phagocytic leukocyte that plays a prominent role only in certain infections. It is capable of motility and phagocytosis, and because of large amounts of lipase appears quite able to attack those bacteria with a lipid capsule, e.g., *Mycobacterium tuberculosis.* As previously mentioned, the monocyte is produced in the bone marrow, has a peripheral blood circulation time of approximately 24 hours, and then randomly leaves the circulation to become a fixed tissue macrophage.

While in the peripheral blood, monocytes have the ability to respond to inflammatory and cellular immune stimuli. It is now apparent that the macrophages, because of their attraction to areas of inflammation, play a unique role in antigen processing and immunity.

Monocytes share with neutrophils the ability to ingest and destroy cells coated with complement-fixing antibody. However, monocytes also have a membrane receptor for Fc and IgG immunoglobulin, which allows them to bind and destroy cells coated with noncomplement fixing antibodies, as occur in autoimmune hemolytic anemia.

In cellular immunity monocytes assume a "killer" role in that they are activated by sensitized lymphocytes to phagocytose offending cells or antigen particles. This property of monocytes is becoming important in the area of tumor immunology where the monocytes, if specifically activated, apparently are able to destroy neoplastic cells.

Increasing attention is now being focused on this ubiquitous cell in regard to its ability to synthesize a number of biologically important products, including transferrin, complement, interferon, pyrogens, and certain growth factors.

EOSINOPHILS

Until recently, it was thought that the eosinophil was a variety of polymorphonuclear neutrophil, and apart from sharing similar functions was particularly involved in the allergic reaction as a carrier of histamine and was markedly dependent on hormonal control. It is now evident that such an appreciation is superficial and does not reflect the total role of the cell in the body.

The eosinophil is a hardy cell, completing its life cycle intact and morphologically unchanged. After 4 days of maturation in the bone marrow the eosinophil spends only 3 to 4 hours in the bloodstream before it seeks a tissue site, where it remains to complete a life cycle of approximately 8 to 12 days. Therefore, any meaningful studies on eosinophil number and function must not merely rest on peripheral blood studies, but must also encompass the tissue level. A further differentiation between the eosinophil and the neutrophil is now evident in that the eosinophil has a unique leukocyte basic protein and that chemical differences exist between the neutrophilic and eosinophilic myeloperoxidase.

In the immune conditions the eosinophil is attracted to the abnormal area by a series of eosinophil chemotactic factors (ECF) which are dependent on a variety of stimuli, i.e., complement fragments, antigen-stimulated leukocytes, and anaphylaxis. The last-named mechanism also produces histamine, which independently allows circulating eosinophils to escape from the intravascular space.

In nonallergic conditions eosinophils may still be actively involved by molecular aggregates of proteins, polysaccharides, and endotoxins. There may also be loss of regulatory control of the eosinophil in situations characterized by functional defects in beta-adrenergic receptors and in the endocrine organs.

BASOPHIL

The basophil, although initially thought to be a blood mast cell, is still a cell of considerable mystery. The physiology and function of the cell are still undefined. It undoubtedly plays a role in acute systemic allergic reactions in releasing histamine and probably heparin. Binding of IgE antibody with its corresponding antigen is another shared responsibility with its fixed tissue partner. Such observations as increased numbers in chronic myeloid leukemia in relapse probably also indicate an immunologic role yet to be defined.

MORPHOLOGIC ABNORMALITIES IN LEUKOCYTES

Congenital Defects

There are five main conditions: (1) Alder-Reilly syndrome, (2) Chédiak-Higashi syndrome, (3) familial amaurotic idiocy, (4) Pelger-Huët anomaly, and (5) May-Hegglin anomaly.

Abnormal Granulation of Polymorphs

These are extremely rare, mainly familial abnormalities in which there may be marked azurophil granulation of all leukocytes but especially the granulocytes (Alder's granulation anomaly). Giant peroxidase granules, together with large red inclusions, may be seen chiefly in the granulocytes but also in the lymphocytes and less commonly in the monocytes. These represent abnormal lysosomes. A similar condition has been recognized in mink and cattle. The condition, Chédiak-Higashi syndrome, appears to be caused by the inheritance of an autosomal ecessive gene from each parent.

In familial amaurotic idiocy (both the Batten and Tay-Sachs varieties), coarse light blue to purple granules up to 2 μm in diameter have been found in the cytoplasm of both granulocytes and monocytes. They are not distinguishable from Alder's granules.

Inclusions similar to Döhle bodies are seen in the May-Hegglin anomaly. These bodies are found in all the leukocytes, including lymphocytes. Unlike the Döhle bodies, they persist during the patient's lifetime. In addition, there is an associated gigantism of platelets, with thrombocytopenia.

Pelger-Huët Abnormality

This is a rather rare, dominant, nonsex-linked hereditary abnormality of nuclei and chromatin. It gives rise to "dumbbell" polymorph nuclei that do not segment further and to coarse chromatin in these and other cells. Its chief importance lies in differentiating it from a "shift to the left" owing to infection or other cause.

Acquired Abnormalities

The following abnormalities are associated with a variety of pathologic conditions:

Döhle-Amato Bodies

These are acquired, frequent, and easily recognizable neutrophil cytoplasm structures. They are associated with a variety of infections, trauma, burns, neoplasm, and pregnancy, although originally they were thought to be associated only with scarlet fever. They are pale blue, approximately 1 to 2 μm in diameter, usually located at the periphery of the cytoplasm, and slightly refractile. They may be either single or multiple in number.

Toxic Granulation and Vacuolation

Toxic granulation is seen when fine to coarse, markedly basophilic (dark purple to purplish black) granules are in the cytoplasm of neutrophil polymorphs in severe infections. When they are abundant there may be few or no normal granules present in the cytoplasm and, corresponding to this, the peroxidase reaction may be reduced or absent. Toxic granules may be mimicked by overstaining. In severe infections and toxemias the cytoplasm of the polymorphs, in addition to toxic granules, may also contain small to medium-sized vacuoles.

Macropolycytes (Hypersegmented Neutrophils)

Macropolycytes are abnormally large (15 to 25 μm) neutrophils with multilobed nuclei. They are associated with either vitamin B_{12} or folic acid deficiency, and are often present before other clinical or hematologic features of the disease are apparent. They represent a generalized metabolic defect, since all bone marrow

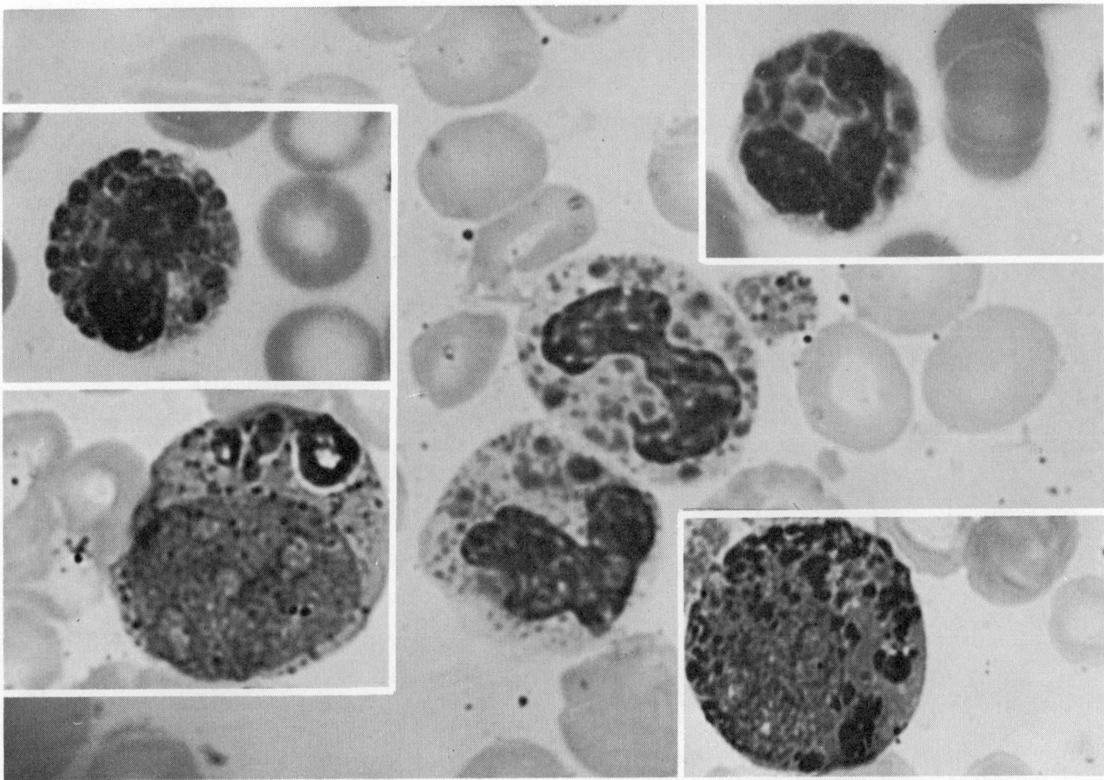

Figure 29–28 Chédiak-Higashi syndrome: Composite photograph, showing cells seen in peripheral blood and bone marrow. *Top left*: Eosinophil. *Lower left:* Pale red inclusions in early myeloid precursor. *Top right:* Severely affected neutrophil. *Lower right:* Basophil myelocyte with inclusions. *Center*: Two neutrophils with abnormalities of granulation and inclusion-like bodies. × 1840.

precursors are enlarged, e.g., as in megaloblastic anemia (see Fig. 29–21).

Reactive Lymphocytes

Hyperbasophilic medium-sized lymphocytes, plasma cells, and primitive lymphoid cells appear in the blood after immunization, infection, hypersensitivity reactions, and onset of autoimmune disease. There is now considerable evidence that these cells represent a circulating population of lymphoid cells derived from lymphoid tissues responding to antigenic stimulation. The primitive lymphoid cells or "immunoblasts" which appear after immunization are large pyroninophilic blast cells which are present in the blood for only a short time before going to the lymph nodes to disseminate the immunologic message. The cell of infectious mononucleosis is a modified reactive lymphocyte.

Terminology is confused for this group of cells, and although there have been attempts to classify such cells, probably the term reactive lymphocyte is perfectly acceptable, provided that an explanation is given if they are present in numbers exceeding 500/μL, or 0.5 × 10^9/L.

LEUKOCYTOSIS

This designates an increase in leukocytes above the normal range. Usually values in excess of 10.0 to 12.0 × 10^9/L are taken as representing leukocytosis. Many factors, apart from disease, may cause a leukocytosis. Thus, strenuous exercise (work, childbirth, epileptic seizures), epinephrine (adrenaline) injections, anxious emotional reactions, pain, and anoxia all tend to produce leukocytosis. Normally, there is a slight leukocytosis during pregancy. Also, diurnal variation of leukocyte counts is the rule in normal, healthy people, the count being lowest in the morning and rising gradually (about 2.0 × 10^9L) in the course of the day, and after meals.

An increase in all types of circulating leukocytes, called a balanced leukocytosis, is seldom seen except in acute hemoconcentration. It is more usual to see an increase in one cell type only, and this forms the basis for this section. The more obvious causes, as seen in leukemia and myeloproliferative syndromes, will be discussed separately.

NEUTROPHIL LEUKOCYTOSIS (NEUTROPHILIA)

This usually implies neutrophils in excess of 6.0 × 10^9/L in the adult. The more common stimuli which cause this are inflammation, necrosis, or metabolic disturbances as shown in Table 29–7.

This reaction occurs in many general and extensive local infections caused by pyogenic organisms, and also in those caused by many organisms that are, strictly speaking, not pyogenic. Total white cell counts in such conditions generally range from 12.0 to 25.0 × 10^9/L (and may reach 30.0 to 40.0 × 10^9/L), and there may be

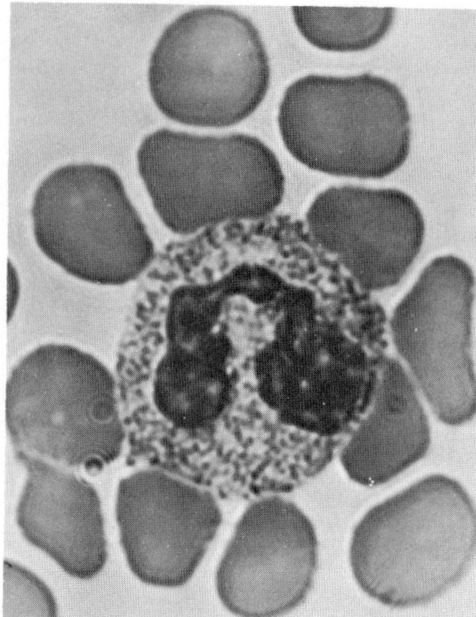

Figure 29–29 Neurtrophil granulocyte showing early toxic granulation. The granules are coarser than normal and tend to be of a dark purple color in Romanowsky-stained smears. × 2250.

up to 90% neutrophil polymorphs. Examples of such conditions are pneumonia (caused by pneumococcus, *Streptococcus,* and *Staphylococcus*), boils, abscesses, osteomyelitis, tonsillitis (caused by *Staphylococcus, Streptococcus,* and other organisms), and general and local infections caused by bacteria and certain viruses, e.g., septicemia, pyemia, endocarditis, scarlet fever, peritonitis, appendicitis, cholecystitis, salpingitis, rheumatic fever (acute), purulent meningitis, otitis media, diphtheria, and chickenpox.

In severe acute infections with good response there is a marked "shift to the left" in the lobe count of the neutrophil polymorphs, and some metamyelocytes and myelocytes may be seen in the smears. In severe infections in infants (first month or two of life) immature leukocytes and red cells (normoblasts) may be found in the peripheral blood (leukoerythroblastic reaction) as a result of intense stimulation of the marrow by the products of infection. Not infrequently in very severe infections toxic granulation of the neutrophil polymorphs will be seen. Rarely, the infection is so overwhelming that leukocytosis is slight, or leukopenia may actually occur; toxic granulation is then prominent and may be of diagnostic significance. As infection subsides or is overcome, the output of cells by the marrow drops, and the nuclear lobe count gradually shifts to the right; in fact, in the recovery phase a large number of polymorphs may have four to six lobes but are normal in size. These "polycytes" must be distinguished from "macropolycytes," seen in vitamin B_{12} and folic acid deficiencies. In the recovery stage following an infection that has led to a high leukocytosis and, indeed, during the height of the infection, degenerate neutrophil polymorph cells may be seen in abundance in smears of peripheral blood. These are known as "basket" cells and are seen as a loose basketwork (meshwork) of pale lilac or brown-staining material (Fig. 29–33). It is probable that most such basket and ruptured cells represent segmented leukocytes that were old, effete, or toxic to begin with, and that the trauma of making the smear accounts for most of them. Smaller numbers of such cells are found in wet preparations made in such conditions. Basket cells may be found abundantly in chronic myelogenous (granulocytic) leukemia, and also in small numbers in all bone marrow smears. The corresponding damaged lymphocyte is known as a "smudge" cell, although many workers use the terms "basket," "smudge," or "smear" interchangeably for all types of damaged white blood cells.

TABLE 29–7 CAUSES OF PATHOLOGIC NEUTROPHILIA

Acute infections	Either localized or generalized.
Inflammation	Owing to necrosis in a variety of conditions, e.g., neoplasm, burns.
Metabolic	Uremia, acidosis, drugs, chemicals, and allergic reactions.
Others	Hemorrhage, hemolysis, leukemia.

At the height of an inflammatory or infective leukocytosis, eosinophils are reduced in number and may be absent altogether (stress reaction), and as recovery and convalescence set in their numbers increase again in the peripheral blood, and a mild absolute eosinophilia is then common (as a result of fall in output of adrenocortical, cortisone-like hormones).

Neutrophil leukocytosis also occurs under the following pathologic conditions: within a few hours of moderate to severe hemorrhage, either internal or external; in burns of any extent (even before infection sets in); in extensive tissue injury, damage, or destruction (accidents, after operations, coronary thrombosis), and, generally, after the initial phases of shock or acute stressing episode (burns, coronary thrombosis after severe hemolytic reaction, and after a foreign protein reaction); associated with rapidly growing and widely invading cancers; in metabolic intoxications (diabetic coma, uremia, acute attacks of gout, eclampsia); and in many cases of Hodgkin's disease, in polycythemia vera, and in myelogenous leukemia. In general, the degree of leukocytosis is proportional to the severity of the infection or inciting cause.

EOSINOPHILIC LEUKOCYTOSIS (EOSINOPHILIA)

Eosinophilia (more than 400 per μL, or 0.4×10^9/L) occurs in infestation by many parasites; in tropical eosinophilia and Löffler's syndrome; in allergic conditions; in certain extensive skin diseases; in a few infections (scarlet fever especially); in the recovery stage of many infections; in some cases of Hodgkin's disease; in chronic myelogenous leukemia; and in some malignant neoplasias when the tumor invades serous surfaces (pleura, peritoneum).

Parasitic infestation is more likely to produce eosinophilia when the parasites actually invade the tissues, e.g., trichinosis, the larval migratory stage of ascariasis, cysticercosis, visceral larva migrans, and echinococcosis. In such states there may be over 50% eosinophils in total counts ranging to 40.0×10^9/L and over. In intestinal parasitism (pinworm, ascariasis, hookworm, tapeworm, whipworm) eosinophilia is less constant and less marked.

Basophilic Leukocytosis (Basophilia)

Basophilia (in excess of 0.1 to 0.2 × 10^9/L) is rarely seen. Although it has been noted as an isolated event in a number of inflammatory diseases, it is mainly associated with polycythemia rubra vera and chronic myeloid leukemia. Diffuse tissue infiltration occurs in a variety of conditions, but difficulty is then experienced in defining a tissue mast cell versus a blood basophil. Systemic mast cell disease is the result of diffuse infiltration of the tissues. In a variant, mast cell leukemia, the bone marrow and peripheral blood contain free mast cells.

Monocytosis

Absolute monocytosis (more than 0.8 × 10^9/L) may be found in chronic tuberculosis, brucellosis, subacute bacterial endocarditis, typhus, kala-azar, rickettsial infections, and malaria, and in the recovery phase of infections that cause leukocytosis. A slight monocytosis may result from overexposure to x-rays. *Listeria monocytogenes* causes monocytosis in laboratory animals but its hematologic consequence in man is less specific.

An increase in monocytes may also be found in some cases of Hodgkin's disease.

Lymphocytosis

Lymphocytosis is natural and normal in infants and young children (up to 9.0 × 10^9/L). It probably results from the relatively small production of adrenocortical hormones at this period of development, and the same cause may underlie the lymphocytosis seen in later childhood in such generally debilitating conditions as undernutrition, rickets, and scurvy. Absolute lymphocytosis is characteristic of a number of conditions seen in both children and adults. They are, in general terms, (a) acute viral infections, particularly infectious mononucleosis and infectious lymphocytosis, (b) whooping cough—pertussis infection, (c) brucellosis, and (d) lymphocytic leukemia.

Whooping Cough. In whooping cough, leukocyte counts as high as 100.0 × 10^9/L with 80 to 90% lymphocytes may be seen, and one may have to differentiate it from lymphocytic leukemia, especially if the characteristic cough has not developed (or has been slight and missed). Helpful hematologic signs indicating pertussis include absence of anemia, although at the usual age of pertussis patients a mild anemia is not uncommon; no reduction in platelets; and, although there is an enormous lymphocytosis, rare occurrence of lymphoblasts (while lymphocytic leukemia at this age is usually acute lymphoblastic in type).

Infectious Lymphocytosis. Acute infectious lymphocytosis is a mild condition that chiefly affects children and in which there may be a very marked lymphocytosis. The cells concerned are normal-looking adult lymphocytes, of which there may be 80% of leukocyte counts up to 100.0 × 10^9/L or greater. The Paul-Bunnell (heterophil agglutination) test is negative, and there may be eosinophilia. The absence of blast cells and marrow examination will differentiate the condition from leukemia. Some doubt the clinical homogeneity of the syndrome.

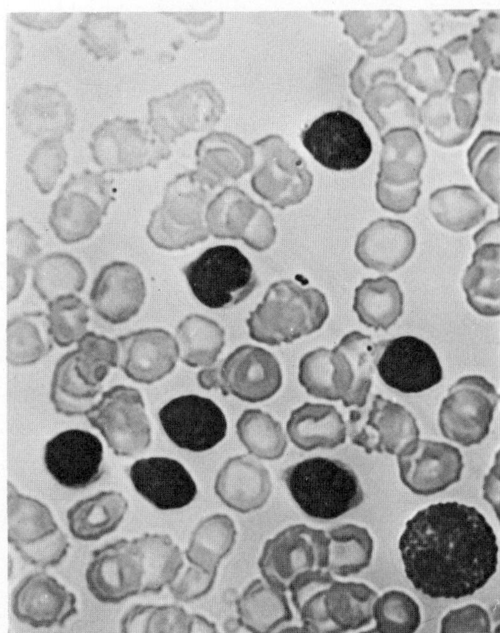

Figure 29–30 Peripheral blood smear from a child suffering from whooping cough (pertussis). Many mature small lymphocytes are present. × 1350.

Other infections in which absolute lymphocytosis may occur are tuberculosis and rubella. In rubella (German measles) leukopenia is the rule (leukocytes 3.0 to 6.0 × 10^9/L) and moderate neutropenia is usual, with relative or slight absolute lymphocytosis. Reactive lymphocytes characteristic of rubella are present and range from 4 to 12% in the differential count.

Infectious Mononucleosis

Classically this important condition has been considered an acute infectious disease, viral in origin and represented by the following relatively well-defined hematologic picture. The total leukocyte count varies between 10.0 and 20.0 × 10^9/L in about two-thirds of cases. In some cases it may be higher, but in about 10% of cases there may be leukopenia. While in the first week there may be a neutrophilia, by the end of this time in over 75% of cases there is a decided mononucleosis (50 to 80% of cells being mononuclears). Although normal lymphocytes and monocytes are both increased, the characteristic cell of infectious mononucleosis is a characteristic reactive lymphocyte. This is a large lymphocyte whose nucleus is often indented or irregular. The cytoplasm is sky blue and is characteristically "moth-eaten" because of the presence of numerous tiny (0.25 to 1 μm) clear vacuoles (Fig. 29–31). The Paul-Bunnell test is positive. The blood changes commonly persist for 1 to 2 months (sometimes as long as 4 to 6 months) after the illness. Rarely, meningoencephalitis, jaundice (resulting from hepatitis), hemolytic anemia, and immune thrombocytopenia may be precipitated by infectious mononucleosis. In most cases, however, the platelet count is normal.

Diagnosis is discussed on pp. 544 and 691 and has

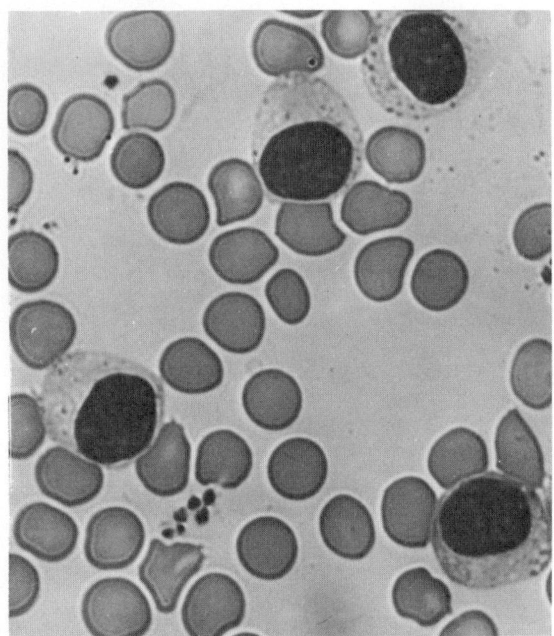

Figure 29–31 Peripheral blood smear from a patient with infectious mononucleosis. The smear was taken when the heterophil titer of the serum was 1280 (after guinea pig kidney absorption). Four large lymphocytes are seen, with numerous tiny vacuoles in their (sky-blue) cytoplasm. × 1350.

rested mainly upon the clinical presentation and a positive heterophil test.

It is now evident that a virus is responsible for this condition. Evidence has been obtained by a number of methods, the most important of which has been isolation of the Epstein-Barr virus and characterization of the immune response.

The Epstein-Barr virus is a human herpes virus which has now been isolated with increasing regularity from cases of infectious mononucleosis. It is linked with a number of other conditions, including Burkitt's lymphoma and nasopharyngeal carcinoma. It is clearly a potent stimulator of lymphoproliferation during infectious mononucleosis and may indeed have oncogenic potential. Similar peripheral blood morphology may be seen in other virally mediated disorders, including cytomegalovirus disease (see p. 476).

The antibodies found in infectious mononucleosis fall into three distinct groups: (a) heterophil antibodies (Paul-Bunnell), (b) Epstein-Barr (EB) virus antibody, and (c) multiple autoantibodies, isoantibodies, and heteroantibodies. The heterophil antibodies are agglutinins reacting particularly to sheep and horse erythrocytes. They have characteristic absorption patterns and are mainly or exclusively IgG globulins showing little or no IgM-IgG conversion during convalescence. The antibody is detected by the Paul-Bunnell test. The other antibodies apart from the EB virus antibody are diverse in nature, tend to appear transiently during the acute phase, are mainly IgM or IgM-IgG complexes, and are not specific for the condition. Clinically, the most important is anti i, which is present in most patients in low titer but occasionally is responsible for a hemolytic anemia. Rheumatoid factor, antinuclear factor, Donath-Landsteiner cold hemolysin, lymphotoxins, and antibodies against T and B lymphocytes have all been reported. Given all this intense antibody production it is not surprising that increased amounts of immunoglobulin, particularly IgM, are detected.

LEUKOPENIA

This signifies a reduction below normal in the number of leukocytes. Values below 4.0 × 10^9/L in the adult constitute leukopenia. Similar to leukocytosis, a reduction in all the types of leukocyte represents a balanced leukopenia, Uusually only one type of cell is involved and this is more exactly defined as neutropenia, eosinopenia, or lymphopenia. Deficiencies in basophils and monocytes do not appear to be clinically significant, while neutropenia is the most important syndrome.

Neutropenia

Synonyms for this condition are acute agranulocytosis or agranulocytic angina. It is associated with an acute onset of malaise, fever, chills, and classically a gangrenous ulceration of the oral cavity, nasopharynx, and throat. If a patient develops an acute sore throat while on any new form of drug therapy, a leukocyte count must always be performed to exclude neutropenia. The mortality rate can be high, despite treatment, with the bone marrow showing varying degrees of cellularity. Most drug reactions causing this complication probably represent a hypersensitivity reaction. Discontinuing the drug will reverse the condition.

The main conditions that cause this complication are infection, hypersplenism, deficiency in maturation factors (e.g., vitamin B_{12}), replacement of marrow by malignant tissue, bone marrow aplasia, and physical agents (e.g., radiation). Chronic neutropenia can be related to immune disorders (e.g., lupus erythematosus) and familial or idiopathic "cyclic" conditions.

Eosinopenia

Endogenous or exogenous increase in ACTH or adrenocortical steroids are the usual cause of this problem. Eosinopenia in stress situations or Cushing's disease reflects increased adrenocortical activity.

Lymphopenia

Lymphopenia is a common response to stress and to the administration of corticosteroid. It is generally defined as a lymphocyte count of less than 1.5 × 10^9/L in adults and less than 3.0 × 10^9/L in children. In general the conditions associated with such a decrease are immunodeficiency disorders, physical agents (e.g., radiation, drugs including the adrenocorticoids), and immune-mediated conditions (e.g., lupus erythematosus).

LEUKEMIAS

Leukemias are diseases characterized by malignant proliferation of the cells of the blood and bone marrow (and of the lymph nodes in the case of the lymphocytic varieties). Any cell type may be involved; hence they may be classified as follows:

Myelocytic (granulocytic)—involving the granulocytes and their precursors.

Lymphocytic—involving the lymphocytes and their precursors.

Monocytic—involving the monocytes and their precursors.

Plasmacytic—involving plasma cells and their precursors.

Erythroblastic—involving red cell precursors.

Any variety may be acute or chronic, with intermediate grades of subacute and subchronic. Generally, the acute forms are fatal within 6 months if untreated, and blast cells are numerous in the peripheral blood. In the chronic forms the disease may not kill for several years, and the blood picture is characterized by more differentiated, i.e., less immature, cell types. The acute leukemias are seen mainly in children and young adults; the chronic forms are more characteristic of middle life and old age. However, many cases of chronic leukemia end in a subacute or acute phase.

The end result in all varieties is practically the same: replacement of normal marrow elements by uncontrolled growth of malignant cells. Infiltration of certain organs, e.g., liver and spleen, is common. Anemia, thrombocytopenia, and hemorrhages are usual and result from replacement of marrow elements. However, the anemia of leukemia frequently also has a hemolytic component. The term "aleukemic" is applied to those cases in which there is little alteration in the white cell picture in the peripheral blood; i.e., the total count may be normal or actually reduced (leukopenic), and abnormal (immature or blast) cells are scanty, although they are usually to be found on careful examination, especially if buffy coat smears are employed. As many as one-quarter of all acute leukemias are aleukemic at some phase, but only 10% of chronic leukemias are aleukemic. The greatest incidence of acute leukemia is in the first 5 years of life, and the lymphoblastic variety predominates. Past middle age chronic lymphocytic and chronic granulocytic varieties are about equally frequent, although some believe that the lymphocytic type is slightly more common.

The leukemias appear to have increased in frequency over the last few decades. The increase may reflect better diagnosis and reporting and may be related to the increased life expectancy of the population. Etiologically, ionizing radiations are well-documented leukemia-inducing agents. The incidence of leukemia in children with Down's syndrome is no less than 20 times the frequency one would expect on a chance basis. Such children are often born to women late in their reproductive period.

Epidemiologic studies of "cluster" outbreaks occurring unexpectedly in limited geographic areas may yield more information. Viruses have been implicated in many animal leukemias, and "clustering" of a few human childhood cases has suggested an infectious agent.

ACUTE LEUKEMIAS

As already mentioned, these are found more frequently in children, and the vast majority of them occur in those under the age of 20 years. They usually run a rapidly fatal course, often with an abrupt onset, fever, rapidly developing anemia, thrombocytopenia, and hemorrhages (petechiae and purpura in skin or mucous membranes). Rarely does the disease last long enough to produce very appreciable enlargement of liver, spleen, or lymph nodes. Generally, the white cell counts are less than $100.0 \times 10^9/L$.

Acute Lymphocytic (Lymphoblastic) Leukemia

Of the two common leukemias of childhood, i.e., lymphoblastic and myeloblastic, the lymphoblastic type is probably the more common, although in many cases it is difficult to be certain of the cell type. In lymphoblastic leukemia the leukocyte count is generally in the range of 30.0 to $130.0 \times 10^9/L$, but as many as 25% of patients are aleukemic. Usually in excess of 50% of the cells are lymphoblasts, i.e., round cells approximately 1½ times the size of adult lymphocytes, with a narrow rim of basophilic cytoplasm and sometimes a clear perinuclear crescent. There is a distinct nuclear membrane, and the chromatin is rather heavy and solid with one or two distinct, round, pale nucleoli. As intimated, in the more acute forms it may not be possible to be certain of the cell type. Smudge cells are often abundant in the peripheral blood smears, and thrombocytopenia is the rule. Normoblasts are usually also seen in smears. Autoimmune hemolytic anemia may develop but is much commoner in chronic lymphocytic leukemia. The bone marrow is invariably infiltrated with the same blast cells seen in the peripheral blood.

It is important that a specific diagnosis be made, rather than merely labeling the leukemia an acute stem cell variety. This is necessary because the treatment of the condition should become very optimistic if sufficiently aggressive therapy is instituted. Up to 80% of children who have received optimal treatment should survive for at least five years.

Acute Myeloblastic Leukemia

This is probably slightly less common than the lymphoblastic variety. the cell counts are of the same order as found in the lymphoblastic type, although they tend to be slightly higher on average. In the peripheral blood up to 90% of nucleated cells are blast forms. These have a cytoplasm that is blue, but generally not so clear a blue as that of the lymphoblast. Not infrequently the cytoplasm shows small vacuoles, and in some cases this vacuolation is very pronounced. The nuclei are round, but occasionally slight irregularities in outline are seen. The chromatin is finer and less dense than that of the lymphoblast, and several (two to five) fairly distinct and sometimes large nucleoli are evident. A small number of these immature cells may be found to contain a few granules in their cytoplasm (promyelocytes), and an occasional myelocyte and metamyelocyte may also be seen. In a small proportion of cases small myeloblasts are the predominant cell type seen in the blood.

Azurophilic, rod-shaped bodies, measuring approximately 0.1 to 2 μm in breadth and 3 to 6 μm in length, may be found in the cytoplasm of the myeloblasts. These are Auer bodies (Fig. 29–35). They have been found also in hemohistioblasts and in monoblasts but do not occur

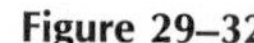

Figure 29–32

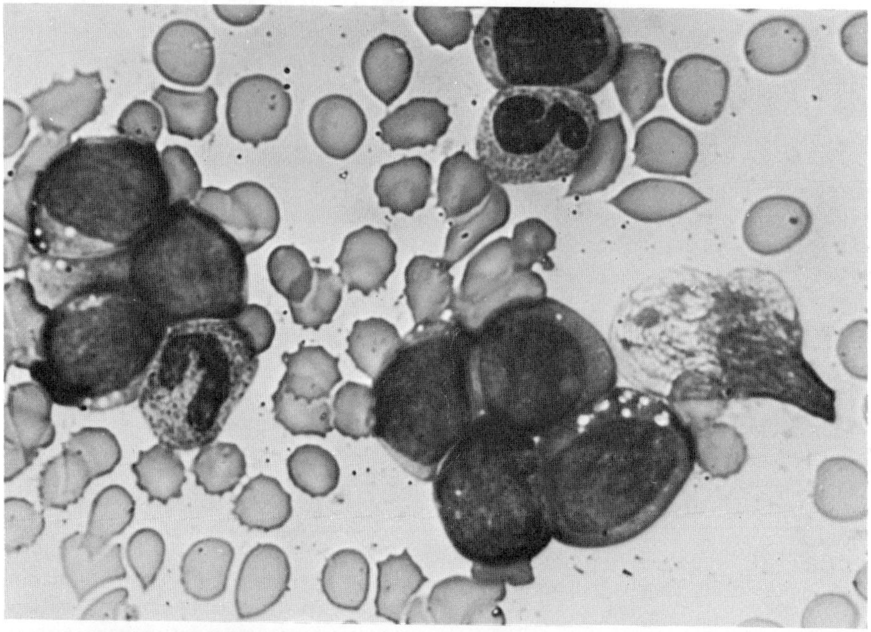

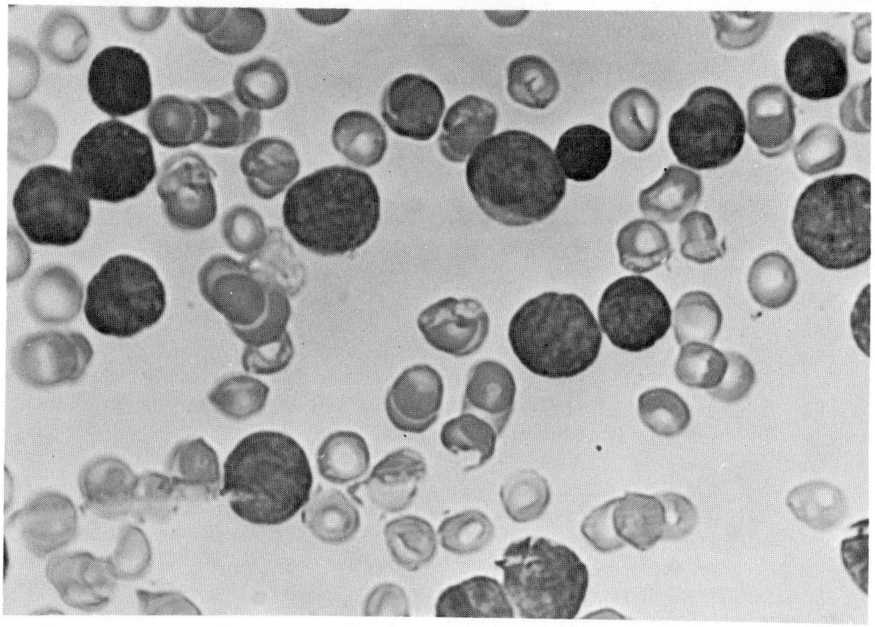

Figure 29–33

Figure 29–32 Acute lymphoblastic leukemia. Of the 15 cells depicted, 12 are lymphoblasts. Peripheral blood smear (boy, age 3½ years). × 1350.

Figure 29–33 Acute myeloblastic leukemia. Cytoplasmic vacuolation is seen in many of the myeloblasts. A "basket" cell is shown on the left. Peripheral blood smear (child, age 2 years). × 1350.

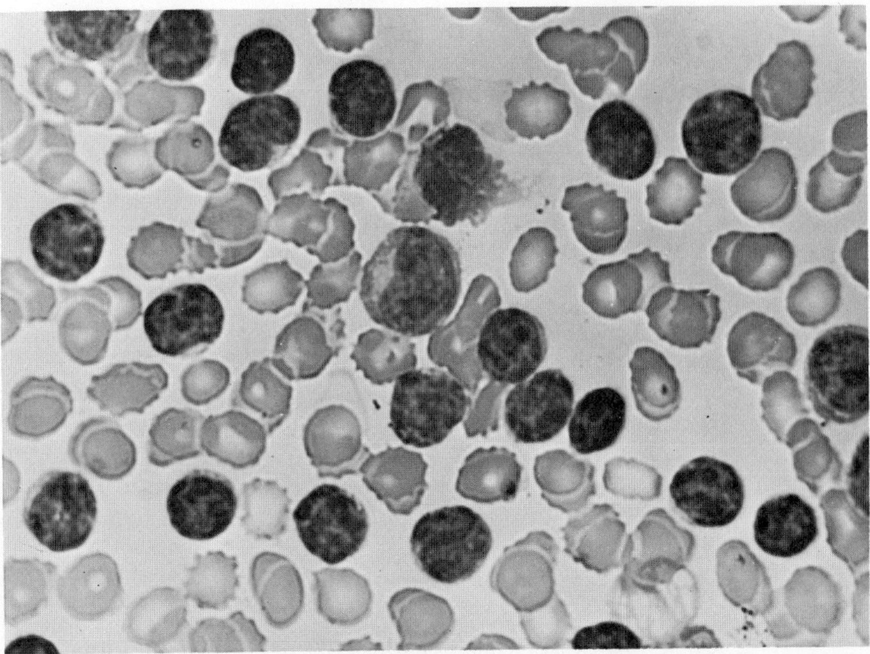

Figure 29–34 Chronic lymphocytic leukemia. One lymphoblast is present near the center and above it is a smudge cell. Peripheral blood smear from a man aged 47 years; white cell count 420 × 10^9/L. × 1350.

in lymphoblasts. A morphologic classification of the various subtypes of acute myeloid leukemia has been established. Known as the FAB classification (as it was the result of French-American-British collaboration), it identifies the subtypes as follows:

Morphologic Cell Type	FAB Classification
Myeloblastic (AMbL)	
Undifferentiated	M-1
Myeloblastic	M-2
Promyelocytic (APL)	M-3
Myelomonocytic (AMML)	M-4
Monocytic (AMoL)	M-5
Erythroleukemic (AEL)	M-6

In acute myeloblastic leukemia the platelet count is generally below 100.0 × 10^9/L. Nucleated red cells are usually to be found in the peripheral blood smears, and anemia is generally more severe than in lymphoblastic leukemia.

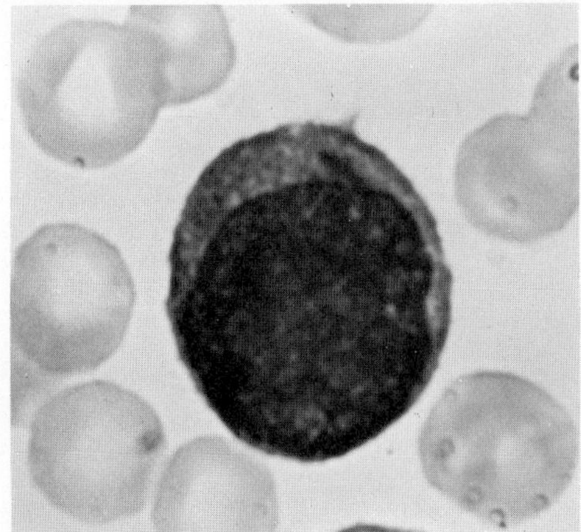

Figure 29–35 Auer body in the cytoplasm of a leukemic myeloblast (rodlike body to right of top pole of nucleus). × 2250.

Chronic Leukemias

These occur in later life, especially from middle age onward. Chronic lymphocytic leukemia tends to occur at older ages than the chronic granulocytic variety. In both types the onset is usually gradual (insidious), and the first complaint is often one of weakness and easy fatigability resulting from anemia.

Anemia is usually slow to develop and may be very slight or absent in the early stages. The anemia may become hypochromic if there has been blood loss, e.g., gastrointestinal hemorrhage; otherwise, it is mainly normocytic and normochromic. Platelets are usually reduced in chronic lymphocytic leukemia, but they may actually be increased in the early phases of the granulocytic variety. In this connection it is worth remembering that some cases of polycythemia vera develop into chronic myelogenous leukemia. In both types severe platelet reduction usually does not occur until the late stages. About 10% of chronic cases are aleukemic or subleukemic. Terminally, many patients show a more acute blood picture with numerous blast cells. In addition to the general findings just mentioned, more specific aspects to be noted in the peripheral blood are as follows.

Chronic Lymphocytic Leukemia

Average leukocyte counts range from 15.0 to 250.0 × 10^9/L. Up to 95% of cells are small lymphocytes with dense nuclei and almost no cytoplasm. Only a few (0 to 5%) blast cells are seen until the later stages, when lymphoblasts may become abundant. Prolymphocytes are always to be seen (5 to 40% of cells); these are larger and paler than the predominant adult lymphoblast.

Smudge cells are usually abundant. The bone marrow is similarly infiltrated with large numbers of small lymphocytes with only very occasional blast cells.

Hemolytic anemia is often associated with this condition, and a positive reaction to the antiglobulin test is owing to fixation of IgG and sometimes complement onto the red cells. Immunoglobulins are generally decreased, and a reduction in serum protein level has always been associated with a grave prognosis. Monoclonal immunoglobulin "spikes" of either the IgG, IgM, or IgA type are seen in approximately 5% of cases.

Chronic lymphocytic leukemia may often be a protracted, relatively benign condition lasting up to 20 years before causing the demise of the patient.

FAB Classification of Lymphocytic Leukemia

L1	Small cells predominant. Nucleus regular; occasional cleft from nucleoli not visible or inconspicuous. Slightly basophilic cytoplasm.
L2	Large, heterogeneous in size. Nuclear shape irregular, clefting common. One or more large nucleoli present. Cytoplasm may be variable or deeply basophilic.
L3	Large and homogeneous in size. Nuclear shape regular—oval to round. Nucleoli are prominent. Cytoplasm deeply basophilic with vacuolation often prominent.

Chronic Myeloid (Granulocytic) Leukemia

Chronic granulocytic leukemia gives the highest leukocyte counts encountered, although these are very variable from patient to patient. Counts may range from normal to 1000.0 × 10^9/L, but in most cases are between 100.0 and 400.0 × 10^9/L. Of the cells in the peripheral blood, 30 to 70% are neutrophil polymorphs, 10 to 40% are neutrophil myelocytes and metamyelocytes, and 0 to 10% are myeloblasts; basophils usually range from 2 to 20%, and eosinophils from 2 to 10%. Rarely, patients are seen in whom the eosinophils preponderate, and such cases have been designated "eosinophilic leukemia," though they are merely varieties of the granulocyte type. Not infrequently, granulation is poorly developed in chronic granulocytic leukemia, and such agranular cases may cause difficulty in differentiation from monocytic leukemia. However, the presence of some definitive granules, the nuclear pattern, and evidence of maturation to segmented granulocytes usually suffice to make the diagnosis. Occasionally, there may be difficulty in deciding whether the picture in the peripheral blood represents leukemia or merely a pronounced leukocytosis or leukoerythroblastic reaction caused by infection (see p. 665). In such cases the leukocyte alkaline phosphatase reaction may be of considerable help; in chronic myeloid leukemia, the neutrophil phosphatase activity is greatly reduced or absent altogether, whereas in normal neutrophils it is well marked or even pronounced.

In 1960 a chromosome abnormality was noted in cells obtained from chronic myeloid leukemia. The Philadelphia chromosome is a group G chromosome, number 22, which has lost a portion of its long arms. In most patients, the missing portion is found translocated to chromosome number 9, although translocations to other chromosomes have been found. The Philadelphia chromosome is present in approximately 90% of patients with chronic myeloid leukemia and is absent from other myeloproliferative variants which can mimic this condition. The erythroid and megakaryocytic cell lines share the abnormal chromosome. Various family studies have proved that it is an acquired defect and is found to persist even when the patient is in remission or has relapsed into an acute blast crisis. Successful treatment will often cause its disappearance until relapse, and chromosome analysis has been used as an indicator for therapy.

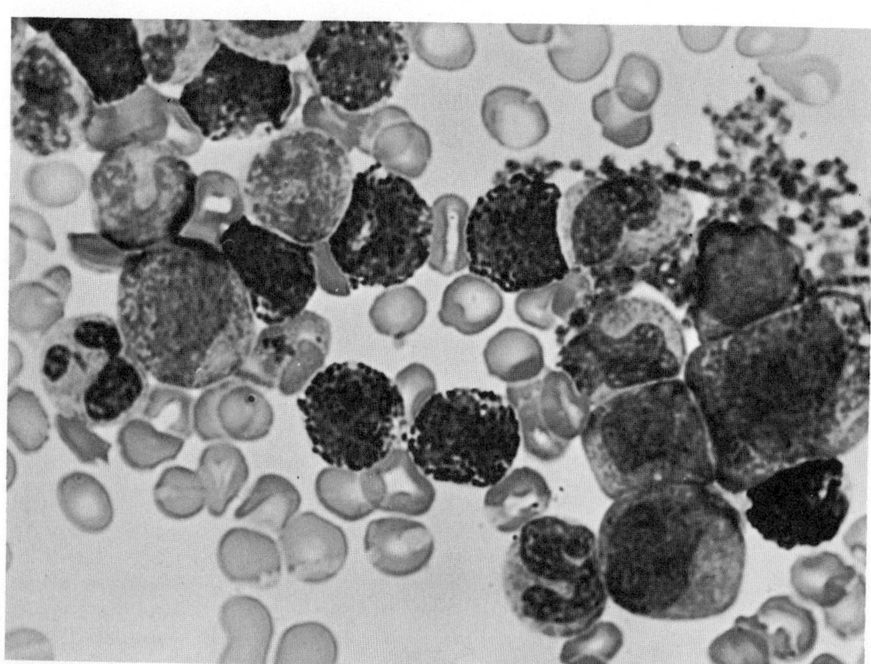

Figure 29–36 Chronic granulocytic leukemia. Peripheral blood smear showing numerous myelocytes and basophils. Platelets are also abundant (top right). Woman, age 55 years; white cell count, 500 × 10^9/L. × 1350.

Chronic myeloid leukemia therefore has two distinct markers, i.e., decreased leukocyte alkaline phosphatase activity (see p. 687), and the presence of the Philadelphia chromosome. Apart from clinically evident syndromes such hyperuricemia and thrombocytosis high levels of vitamin B_{12} are often seen, and this is related to the increased levels of a transcobalamin-like binding protein in the abnormal neutrophils which is released into the plasma upon death of the cell.

Monocytic Leukemia

This variety constitutes about 10 to 15% of all leukemias. Both types are very rare in the young age groups and characteristically occur after middle age. The acute form often has a dramatic onset with fever, headache, ulceration of mouth and gums, and bleeding from the mouth or nose.

The onset of chronic monocytic leukemia is generally gradual and insidious. Most often the diagnosis is made in the course of investigation for anemia. Not infrequently the clinical picture suggests pernicious anemia. The duration of life from the time of onset (itself very difficult to determine) of chronic monocytic leukemia is very variable and ranges from 6 months to 5 years, with an average life expectancy of about 1½ years. Chronic cases frequently terminate with more acute manifestations. In both varieties of monocytic leukemia, enlargement of lymph nodes and spleen is slight and may not be detectable.

Acute Monocytic Leukemia

Leukocyte counts vary from 15.0 (or less) to 100.0 × 10^9/L. Promonocytes and monoblasts make up 25 to 75% of cells. The leukemic monoblast frequently has, in Romanowsky smears, a muddy or smoggy gray-blue cytoplasm which contains tiny granules. Small cytoplasmic protrusions (pseudopodia) are common, and the cells vary considerably in outline. The nucleus usually shows some irregularity in the form of indentation. The chromatin shows a rather reticulogranular appearance, and one to five indistinct, irregular, and sometimes very large nucleoli are seen. In the acute variety platelets are generally severely reduced, and nucleated red cells may be seen.

Chronic Monocytic Leukemia

Leukocyte counts tend to be low and vary from 3.0 to 70.0 × 10^9/L. Many cases are leukopenic for considerable periods, the only abnormal findings being anemia and an increase in large, mature monocytes with convoluted, indented, irregular nuclei which possess a lace-pattern, delicate chromatin. The cytoplasm possesses sparse to abundant, very fine lilac granules, and pseudopodal protrusions are rather characteristic. Platelets are moderately reduced, but severe thrombocytopenia may appear in the terminal phases.

The blood picture just described is that of the classic Schilling type of monocytic leukemia. The designation Naegeli type has been applied to those cases in which myelocytes are abundant. Naegeli believed that monocytes derived from myeloblasts and would not recognize monocytic leukemia as an entity. It is indeed questionable whether the Naegeli type exists as an entity at all.

Other Forms of Leukemia

Since leukemia is a disease of the bone marrow, any hematopoietic cell can be affected. The following variants of the main types of leukemia are probably related either to each other or to the forms described, but because they often present with unique morphologic or clinical features, they will be discussed separately.

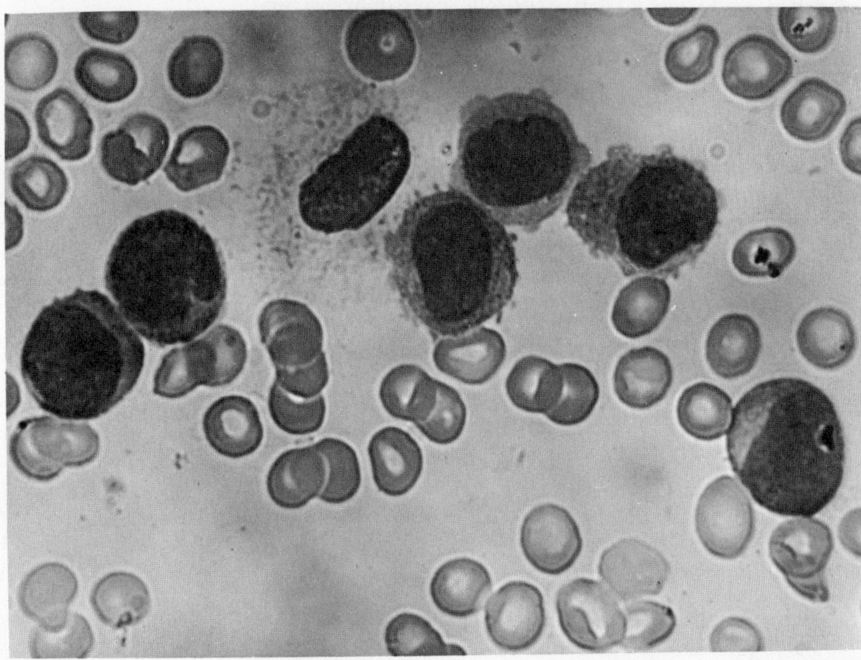

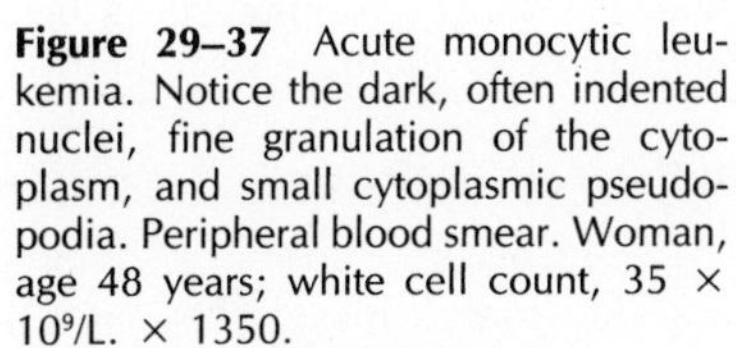

Figure 29–37 Acute monocytic leukemia. Notice the dark, often indented nuclei, fine granulation of the cytoplasm, and small cytoplasmic pseudopodia. Peripheral blood smear. Woman, age 48 years; white cell count, 35 × 10^9/L. × 1350.

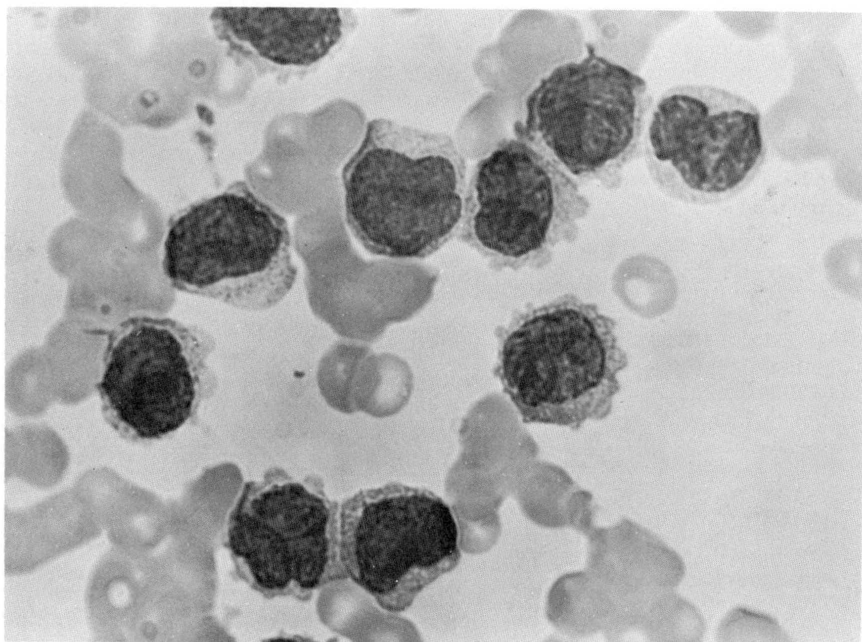

Figure 29–38 Chronic monocytic leukemia. Notice the indentations, foldings, and "lobulation" of the nuclei, fine granulation of the cytoplasm, and small cytoplasmic pseudopods. Peripheral blood smear. (Man, age 50 years.) × 1350.

Stem Cell Leukemia

In some acute leukemias the cell type is so primitive and undifferentiated that it is impossible to classify. Probably the majority are made up of highly malignant forms of hemohistioblastic and monoblastic leukemia. In the peripheral blood most of the cells are hyperchromatic (heavily staining) blast cells with dense nuclei and a small amount of murky cytoplasm. Stem cell leukemia occurs mainly in children.

Promyelocytic Leukemia

This leukemia is characterized by an accumulation of atypical promyelocytes in both the bone marrow and peripheral blood. Patients with this condition often present with bleeding episodes and often die as a result of disseminated intravascular coagulation. Presumably the abnormal cells release thromboplastin-like material into the circulation which initiates intravascular coagulation (see p. 731). Patients respond poorly to therapy and have a rapidly fatal course. An interesting feature is that if remission is achieved the hemostatic defect is reversed, only to recur when the patient relapses.

Eosinophilic Leukemia

Characteristically, patients present with pulmonary and cardiac involvement. Large numbers of eosinophilic immature myeloid cells are seen in the peripheral blood and bone marrow which can regress into an acute leukemic picture. It is a very rare variant and is considered analogous to myeloid leukemia, although usually there is no Philadelphia chromosome present.

Mast Cell Leukemia

This is probably the rarest form of leukemia, and is part of the spectrum of mast cell disorders. The leukemic phase may be related to a generalized mastocytosis, with the patient presenting with evidence of bone marrow involvement as well as other organ spread. The clinical features are very interesting because of the symptoms related to the release of histamine from the proliferating mast cells. Mature and immature mast cells may account for up to 50% of the circulating leukocytes, and anemia and thrombocytopenia are invariably present. Mast cells are easily identified, but cellular specimens have to be handled extremely carefully owing to the fragile nature of the cells. They can usually be distinguished from basophils, but toluidine blue staining will demonstrate the typical metachromatic nature of the mast cell granule.

Plasma Cell Leukemia

This rather rare condition occurs from middle age onward. The leukocyte count ranges from 15.0 to 100.0 $\times 10^9$/L, and up to 90% of the cells may be plasma cells, some of which may show two or even three nuclei. Rouleaux formation is pronounced, and there is usually an increase in the immunoglobulins with associated light chains in the urine. Plasma cell leukemia is best regarded as a leukemic form of myeloma (see p. 669).

Leukemic Reticuloendotheliosis (Hairy Cell Leukemia)

This disease accounts for approximately 2% of all leukemias, and although it has a characteristic morphologic appearance, diagnosis is not always straightforward. It is characterized by the presence in the bone marrow and usually in the blood of a "hairy" cell. Recent evidence suggests that the cell is of lymphocytic origin, having surface-bound immunoglobulin and B lymphocyte characteristics.

The condition usually presents as an anemia of obscure origin, with normal or low leukocyte counts. Oc-

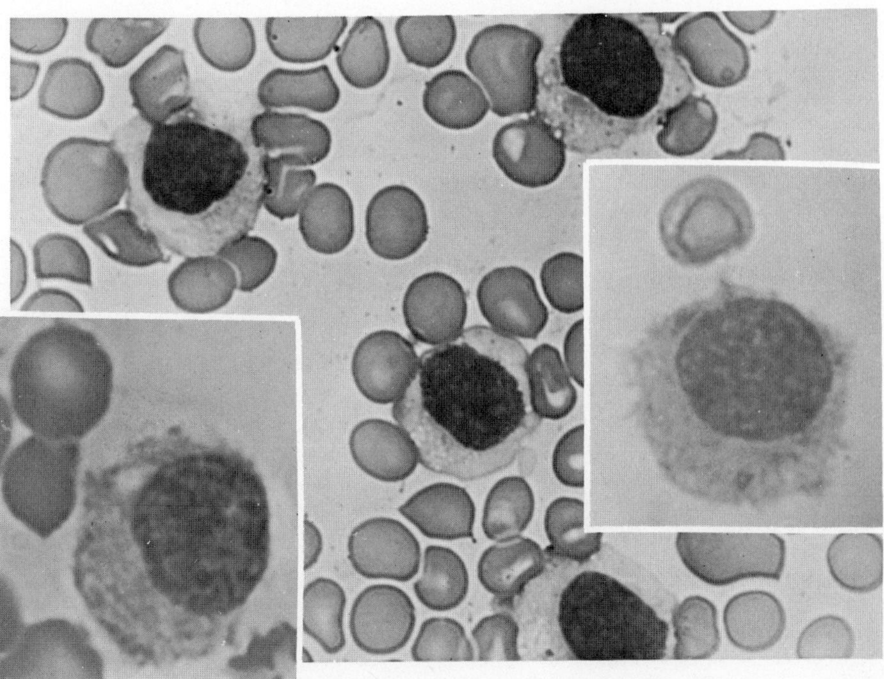

Figure 29–39 Histocytic or reticuloendothelial cell leukemia (hairy cell leukemia). Four abnormal cells in a buffy coat smear of peripheral blood. (Man, age 53 years; white cell count, 3.8 × 10^9/L. × 1350. Inset, lower left and midright, are two similar cells from another patient (× 2250). Notice the wispy cytoplasm, which is free of granules and stains a mauve color with Romanowsky dyes. This type is quite distinct from monocytic leukemia, with which it is often confused in the literature.

casionally, the leukocyte count is moderately raised. Even experienced workers may miss the condition, but a careful examination of smears, especially of buffy coat, will reveal 10 to 60% of nucleated cells to be abnormal, large, irregularly oval cells (15 to 25 μm), having a small to moderate amount of gray-mauve cytoplasm in which no granules are present. The edge of cytoplasm is often wavy, and tiny pseudopods may be present. The nucleus is round to oval and large, and fills two-thirds to five-sixths of the cell mass. Chromatin is abundant, reticular, and lilac-brown in Romanowsky smears. One to five irregular, indistinct, and sometimes large nucleoli may be seen. As in all leukemias, smears of aspirated marrow will be found to contain a large (20 to 60%) number of the abnormal cells.

Leukemoid Reactions

In leukemoid reactions the peripheral blood picture is such as to raise the suspicion of leukemia. The leukocyte count is usually elevated, and immature leukocytes and erythrocytes are present. Granulocytes, lymphocytes, or monocytes may be involved. Severe infections, tuberculosis, hemolytic anemias, carcinomatosis, and heavy infestation with *Trichinella spiralis* are causes of leukemoid reactions of the granulocytic type. Another example is the leukoerythroblastic reaction often associated with severe infections in infancy and widespread carcinomatosis in later life.

In the leukemoid reaction the total leukocyte count is rarely much above 50.0 × 10^9/L; myelocytes rarely make up more than 10 to 15% of nucleated cells in the peripheral blood; and only an occasional myeloblast is seen. Few, if any, basophils will be found in the smears, and toxic granulation of the segmented neutrophils may be noted. In marrow smears from patients with a granulocytic leukemoid reaction it will be seen that, although the cells of the granulocytic series make up 60 to 80% of nucleated cells, less than 6% will be myeloblasts. Causes of neutrophilic, lymphocytic, and monocytic leukocytosis have been discussed in preceding sections of this chapter.

Identification of Leukemia Using Special Stains

The majority of the chronic leukemias may be diagnosed from peripheral blood and bone marrow preparations with routine staining. However, in the acute leukemias, the problem is more difficult, since the distinction between the various types of "blast" cells is not easy.

Using a conventional Romanowsky stain along with PAS, Sudan black B, and alkaline phosphatase techniques (see p. 687), it is possible to ensure a more accurate diagnosis. The following reactions are typical for the three types of "blast" cells seen in acute leukemia.

Lymphoblast. The PAS stain shows clumps of positive material around the periphery of the cell; Sudan black B is negative, and the alkaline phosphatase score is, in the neutrophils, normal.

Myeloblast. The myeloblast has no positive PAS material but may impart a faint magenta color throughout the cytoplasm. Sudan black B gives a negative reaction and the alkaline phosphatase score is invariably reduced. Myeloblasts and monoblasts can be differentiated by esterase staining.

Monoblast. As described before, there are two forms of monoblastic leukemia. In the Schilling type, the PAS reaction yields a dust-like particulation over a small portion of the cell cytoplasm and the Sudan black gives a similar result. The neutrophil alkaline phosphatase is normal. The Naegeli type is more difficult to interpret. As may be expected, a picture similar to that of the myeloblast is obtained, except that the alkaline phosphatase score is at the low end of normal.

Confidence in interpretation can come only with experience. Careful appreciation of the information in Romanowsky-stained films must always be utilized.

The use of these stains not only aids in differentiation of the leukemia, which is necessary for optimum treatment, but in general contributes to a greater understanding of the acute leukemia. The use of electron microscopy, microdensitometry, and immunologic methods are all valuable and progressive methods of identification. Immunopathology is now allowing specific identification of T and B lymphocyte–derived cells in association with other chemical markers.

LABORATORY MONITORING OF LEUKEMIA

The use of multiple drug progams and sophisticated radiation and immunotherapy techniques has caused the role of the laboratory to be emphasized during the management of leukemic patients. The oncologist now relies to a very large degree on the laboratory findings in order to ascertain the effectiveness of therapy. The majority of chemotherapeutic agents, although very effective in destroying the malignant cells, can have a profound effect on the normal hemopoietic cells. For this reason the laboratory must maintain a system of recording serial results of peripheral blood examination in order that cumulative data may be arranged in an appropriate manner. It has been demonstrated that if the laboratory data are presented in such a manner, therapy can be modified in order to prevent overaggressive use of drugs and to monitor the course of disease. Calculation of the rate of cell count decline can be used to assess the effectiveness of therapy and to forecast remission or relapse.

During induction of multiple chemotherapy, bizarre changes may be seen in individual cell morphology along with changes in the actual counts. It has been emphasized that a rapid recovery of the neutrophil count is often preceded by the appearance of large numbers of atypical monocytoid cells. Occasionally a large number of lymphocytes may be seen during active remission, and this usually implies slower response of the neutrophil count. The bone marrow may show bizarre changes with erythroid hyperplasia, depressed granulopoiesis, and atypical mononuclear cells accounting for up to 20% of the bone marrow population. These changes should not be interpreted as a relapse, but as a manifestation of regeneration by the bone marrow under stress.

MYELOPROLIFERATIVE DISORDERS (Table 29–8)

This term covers a group of conditions that are related in that they show hyperplasia or neoplasia of one or more hematopioetic derivatives in bone marrow or extramedullary sites. Reactive hyperplasia of red cells occurring after hemorrhage and polymorphonuclear proliferation during infection is not included. The myeloproliferative disorders occur without apparent physiologic or reactive cause.

Controversy still exists as to the genesis of this group of diseases and as to whether they can properly be classified together. However, such a concept has brought some degree of order into a group of disease states which were confused by a wide range of synonyms and clinical descriptions. Extramedullary hematopoiesis, which frequently occurs in this syndrome, not only caused clinical confusion but gave rise to a large number of titles that still confuse the hematologist; i.e., it can be variously described as myeloid metaplasia, agnogenic myeloid metaplasia, aleukemic myelosis, chronic nonleukemic myelosis, myelophthistic splenomegaly. aleukemic hepatosplenic myelosis, and leukoerythroblastic anemia.

TABLE 29–8 CLASSIFICATION OF THE MYELOPROLIFERATIVE SYNDROMES ACCORDING TO THE DEGREE OF CELLULAR PROLIFERATION

	RBCs	WBCs	Platelets	Fibroblasts	EH*
Polycythemia	+++	++	+++	+	++
Erythroleukemia	+++	+++	±	+	±
Thrombocythemia	±	±	+++	±	++
Myelofibrosis	−	++	+	+++	+++
Chronic granulocytic leukemia	−	+++	++	+	++

***Extramedullary hematopoiesis; − = Absent; + = Normal; ++ and +++ = Increased.**

The following descriptions are, by necessity, oversimplified but serve to demonstrate that the bone marrow, as the result of an abnormal stimulus, will respond in an abnormal manner involving any one or all of its cell lines. Chronic myeloid leukemia has already been described on p. 662.

POLYCYTHEMIA RUBRA VERA

This is a disease of middle age characterized by erythrocytosis with hemoglobulin up to or greater than 20 g per dL (or 200 g/L), plethora, and pruritus. In the peripheral blood, in addition to the erythrocytosis, there is leukocytosis and thrombocytosis. The marrow is hyperplastic, and the granulocytic, erythroid, and megakaryocyte systems share in the hyperplasia. The disease is chronic, and many patients die of cardiovascular and thrombotic disease. Of those who survive these diseases, many develop myelosclerosis with myeloid metaplasia or granulocytic leukemia. There is some evidence that the incidence of leukemia is related, in this condition, to X-ray therapy or treatment with ^{32}P.

The condition is not to be confused with secondary erythrocytosis or stress erythrocytosis, which is discussed on p. 630. The diagnosis of polycythemia rubra vera rests firmly on the demonstration of an increase in erythrocytes, leukocytes (myeloid series), and platelets.

ERYTHROLEUKEMIA (DI GUGLIELMO'S SYNDROME)

Characteristically the disease has three phases, although in the individual case the phases may not be apparent or well delineated. In the first phase, there is preponderant erythroblastic proliferation with abnormal forms demonstrating gigantism, polyploidism, and bizarre neoplastic features. In the second phase, myeloblasts become more prominent in the marrow and the condition may be regarded as erythroleukemia. The last stage is frank myeloblastic leukemia. The picture in the peripheral blood will of course be determined by the marrow pattern. The cytoplasm of the erythroblast and proerythroblast of the Di Guglielmo syndrome is PAS-positive. The only other conditions in which this has been described are iron deficiency anemia and thalassemia major.

Thrombocythemia

This condition must not be confused with a reactive thrombocytosis. In some cases that have been described, the platelet count is over 5000 × 10^9/L, and there is polymorphonuclear leukocytosis, hypochromic anemia, and chronic bleeding from mucous membranes. On the peripheral smears the platelets are often in aggregates and giant irregular forms are seen (megathrombocytes). It should be noted that the platelet count is notoriously inaccurate when counts are above 1000 × 10^9/L, particularly when using automated counters (p. 678). The hematocrit will show a greatly increased layer of platelets, not to be confused with the leukocyte layer. It usually poses no diagnostic problem, and indeed the triad of an extremely high platelet count, leukocytosis, and hypochromic anemia (owing to blood loss) is virtually diagnostic. The paradoxical bleeding is due to the platelet having defective function in addition to abnormal morphology.

Myelofibrosis

The disease occurs typically in the middle years, and is characterized by fibrosis of the marrow, gross enlargement of the spleen owing to active extramedullary hematopoiesis, and leukoerythroblastic anemia. There is nearly always leukocytosis, with circulating primitive cells, which may reach 100 × 10^9/L. Thrombocytosis is also nearly always present, and there may be several million platelets. The condition may be confused with granulocytic leukemia. A high leukocyte alkaline phosphatase score would exclude leukemia, and the presence of a Ph^1 chromosome would exclude myelofibrosis. Histologically, the myelofibrosis may be quite patchy; however, bone marrow biopsy will often demonstrate this. The hallmark of the process is seen in the peripheral blood, in which the erythrocytes are characteristically misshapen, with many teardrop forms and at times gross ovalocytosis (see Fig. 29–40). The appearance can be so striking that a tentative diagnosis may be made. Histologic appearance of the mandatory bone marrow biopsy shows characteristic greatly increased amount of reticulin material.

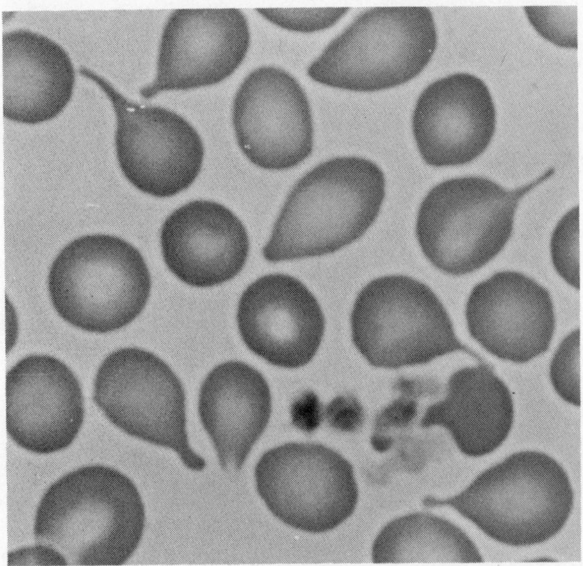

Figure 29–40 Peripheral blood smear from a child with myelosclerosis. Several "tear-drop" poikilocytes are seen.

LYMPHOMAS

Up until recent times lymphomas have been a poorly classified heterogeneous group of diseases characterized by a proliferation of one or more kinds of cells which ordinarily reside or originate in the lymphoid tissue. As the result of intensive clinical and histologic studies a number of distinct disease entities are now apparent, each of which has a definitive histologic appearance and reacts in a predictable clinical pattern. The cell types involved, namely primitive reticuloendothelial cells, histiocytes, and lymphocytes, give rise to several different conditions. The major subdivisions are the malignant lymphomas (histiocytic and lymphocytic), Hodgkin's disease, and two rarer variants, mycosis fungoides and Burkitt's lymphoma. The plasma cell tumors and macroglobulinemias originating from the lymphoid system are discussed further in this chapter.

Table 29–9 provides a general classification for the malignant lymphomas and Hodgkin's disease groups. The hematologic picture for all these neoplasms is by no means specific, but they comprise an important segment of patients being referred to the laboratory because of the need to monitor the radiotherapy and chemotherapy so necessary to control these conditions.

Hodgkin's Disease

This is a malignant lymphoma, involving proliferation of the cellular elements of lymph nodes. It may begin in

TABLE 29–9 Classification of Hodgkin's Disease and Malignant Lymphoma

Hodgkin's Disease	Malignant Lymphoma*
Lymphocytic predominant	Undifferentiated
Nodular sclerosis	Histiocytic
Mixed cellularity	Mixed cell
Lymphocytic depletion (diffuse fibrosis)	Lymphocytic (poorly differentiated)
Lymphocytic depletion (reticular)	Lymphocytic (well differentiated)
	Hodgkin's disease

*Each of these may appear in either a nodular or a diffuse form.

Note: Advances in immunology and electron microscopy have expanded the recognizable varieties of lymphoma. Currently, at least six classifications are proposed. Time will tell which of these is the most practicable, acceptable, and useful.

one or several groups of lymph nodes, e.g., neck, mediastinum, or mesentery. As in almost all malignant lymphomas, the erythrocyte sedimentation rate is increased. Mild to moderate anemia of normocytic type is common, but hemolytic anemia may occur. Although some patients have a leukopenia, most have relatively normal leukocyte counts, and about 25% show a mild to moderate leukocytosis (15.0 to 20.0 × 10^9/L) with an absolute neutrophilia. About 20% of patients show a moderate eosinophilia in the peripheral blood at some time, and in a few this may be extremely high. Careful differential counts, especially if performed on buffy coat smears, may reveal abnormal mononuclear cells. Involvement of the bone marrow can often be patchy, with characteristic Reed-Sternberg cells being found in the bone marrow biopsy rather than in aspiration material.

The treatment of this condition has markedly improved since staging procedures and multiple chemotherapy have evolved. Staging is a procedure whereby the clinician, using a variety of diagnostic procedures, endeavors to locate all areas of the body that are involved with active disease. If active disease is found in only one site, on one side of the diaphragm, in the absence of systemic symptoms this represents a Stage IA which, if correctly treated with radiotherapy, should provide for a complete cure. Conversely, if disease is found on both sides of the diaphragm, involving organs other than the lymph nodes in the presence of systemic symptoms, this constitutes a Stage IVB which entails aggressive chemotherapy. It is of considerable importance to note that if abnormal cells are seen in the bone marrow, i.e., Reed-Sternberg cells, this automatically places the patient in a Stage IV group; bone marrow examination using aspiration and biopsy techniques is therefore a very valuable part of the staging procedure.

Malignant Lymphoma

Malignancies of lymphoid tissue are broadly divided into two groups—the leukemias and the malignant lymphomas. While the lymphocytic leukemias primarily affect the blood and bone marrow, the lymphomas are often localized as solid tumors in the body. However, certain lymphomas can give rise to abnormal cells in the peripheral blood which are morphologically similar to leukemic lymphocytic cells. Morphology can range from the histiocytic undifferentiated forms to the well-differentiated lymphocytic type. As in Hodgkin's disease, staging is based on clinical and morphologic findings, the undifferentiated type being more serious than the well-differentiated variety.

Mycosis fungoides and Sézary's disease are specialized forms of lymphoma and are mentioned here because abnormal lymphoma cells are seen in the peripheral blood. The Sézary cell has a large nucleus, pseudopodia, and vacuoles in an irregularly dense cytoplasm. Examination of the buffy coat preparation will often demonstrate these cells with greater reliability and ease than the peripheral blood film.

IMMUNOPROLIFERATIVE DISORDERS

These disorders have in common a proliferation of immunoglobulin-secreting cells with the resultant increase in either complete or incomplete immunoglobulin molecules. Classically, the proliferating cells have been of the plasma cell type and for this reason the condition generally has been termed a plasma cell dyscrasia. Other synonyms describe the abnormal immunoglobulin production, namely, monoclonal gammopathy, dysgammaglobulinemia, and dysproteinemia.

It is now apparent that all plasma cell tumors appear to be B lymphocyte cell in origin. Table 29–10 shows a presumptive relationship between this class of conditions and the lymphomas and Hodgkin's disease. They are probably related by virtue of their T or B cell origin, and the immunoproliferative conditions are classified as a separate group because of their propensity to produce abnormal amounts of immunoglobulin. The emphasis

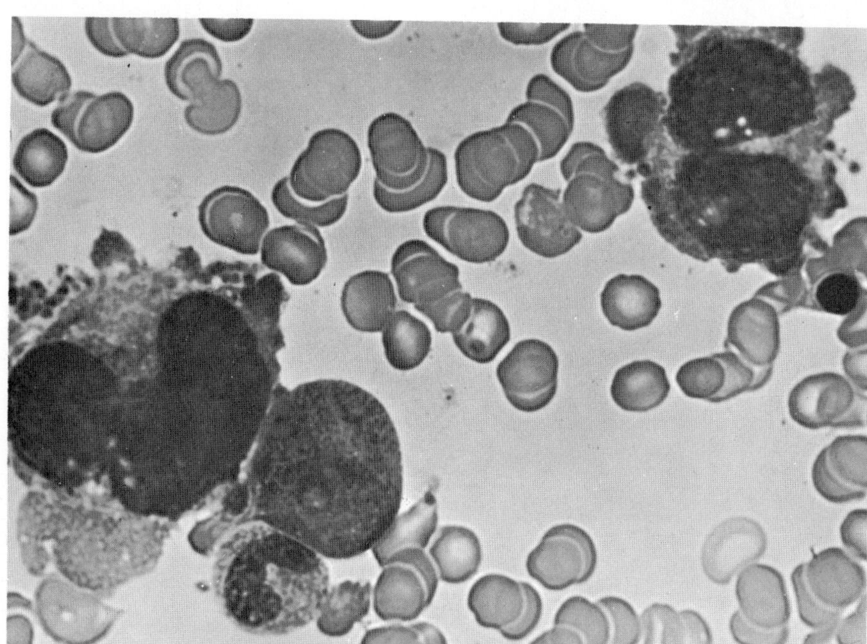

Figure 29–41 Smear of aspirated marrow from a patient with Hodgkin's disease, showing two Reed-Sternberg giant cells. × 1350.

TABLE 29–10 Lymphocytic Origins in the Lymphoreticular Neoplasms

Disease	Lymphocyte Type
Acute lymphocytic leukemia	Some T, rare B, commonly indeterminate
Chronic lymphatic leukemia	2% T, 98% B
Hodgkin's disease	?
Follicular lymphoma	B
Lymphocytic lymphoma (intermediate and well-differentiated)	B
Lymphoblastic lymphoma (poorly differentiated)	T
Hairy cell leukemia	B
Burkitt's lymphoma	B
Multiple myeloma	B
Macroglobulinemia (Waldenström's)	B
Heavy chain disease	B

should therefore be placed not only on the morphologic appearance of these conditions, but also on their functional patterns, and the following classification allows for this.

a. Plasma cell myeloma (multiple myeloma, solitary plasmacytoma, or plasma cell leukemia).
b. Primary macroglobulinemia (Waldenström's).
c. Heavy chain disease.
d. Miscellaneous, including amyloidosis, chronic inflammatory and infectious states, carcinoma, and idiopathic monoclonal gammopathy.

Table 29–11 provides a broad classification of these diseases on the basis of clinical, morphologic, and biochemical discriminants. The reader is referred to the chapter on immunology for a description of the immunoglobulins and their various fragments (Chapter 26).

Myeloma

This is the most common and important condition of this group. It may present in a variety of clinical patterns, depending upon the degree of organ involvement, pressure from plasma cell tumors, effects of the abnormal proteins, and specific metabolic complications.

The condition may be a diffuse involvement of the bone marrow which is called multiple myeloma; or discrete tumor production, a plasmacytoma, which produces local disturbances. Finally there may be a primarily hematogenous spread in which the peripheral blood is so inundated with abnormal cells it is called plasma cell leukemia. All these varieties nevertheless share aberrant B cell functions and produce immunoglobulins in varying types and amounts.

The laboratory features of this disease may be divided conveniently into two areas: blood and bone marrow; serum and urine proteins.

Hematologic Changes

In diffuse disease, anemia is seen to a variable degree and may be severe. It is normochromic normocytic, with marked rouleaux formation. The rouleaux formation may be so avid as to prevent even thin peripheral blood smears from being produced, and is accompanied by a greatly increased sedimentation rate. If the aberrant immunoglobulin is present in large amounts, the Romanowsky stained film will assume a characteristic blue appearance, similar to a film stained with an inappropriately high pH buffer solution. This is due to the metachromatic staining of the abnormal protein. Examination of a buffy coat preparation will often demonstrate abnormal plasma cells, normoblasts, and immature leukocytes. In severe disease the peripheral blood film may resemble a severe leukoerythroblastic reaction. Thrombocytopenia may be present and a func-

TABLE 29–11 Differentiations of the Major Immunoproliferative Disorders

	Multiple Myeloma	Macroglobulinemia	Heavy Chain Disease			Idiopathic Monoclonal Gammopathy
			IgG	IgA	IgM	
Distinctive clinical features	Lytic bone lesions Hypercalcemia	Hyperviscosity Bleeding tendency	Pancytopenia Lymphoma Eosinophilia	Intestinal lymphoma Malabsorption	Chronic lymphocytic leukemia Amyloidosis	Asymptomatic
Predominant cell type	Plasma cell	Plasmacytoid cell	Lymphocyte Plasma cells Eosinophils	Lymphocytes Plasma cells	Lymphocyte Vacuolated plasma cells	None
Serum electrophoresis	M spike	M spike	M spike	Diffuse hypergammaglobulinemia	Hypogammaglobulinemia	M spike
Serum abnormal protein	IgG, IgA, IgD, kappa, lambda	IgM, kappa, lambda	Fc fragment	Fc fragment	Fc fragment	Usually IgG, IgA
Urinary abnormal protein	kappa, lambda (B.J. protein)	kappa, lambda (B.J. protein)	Fc fragment	Fc fragment	kappa, lambda, (B.J. protein)	Nil

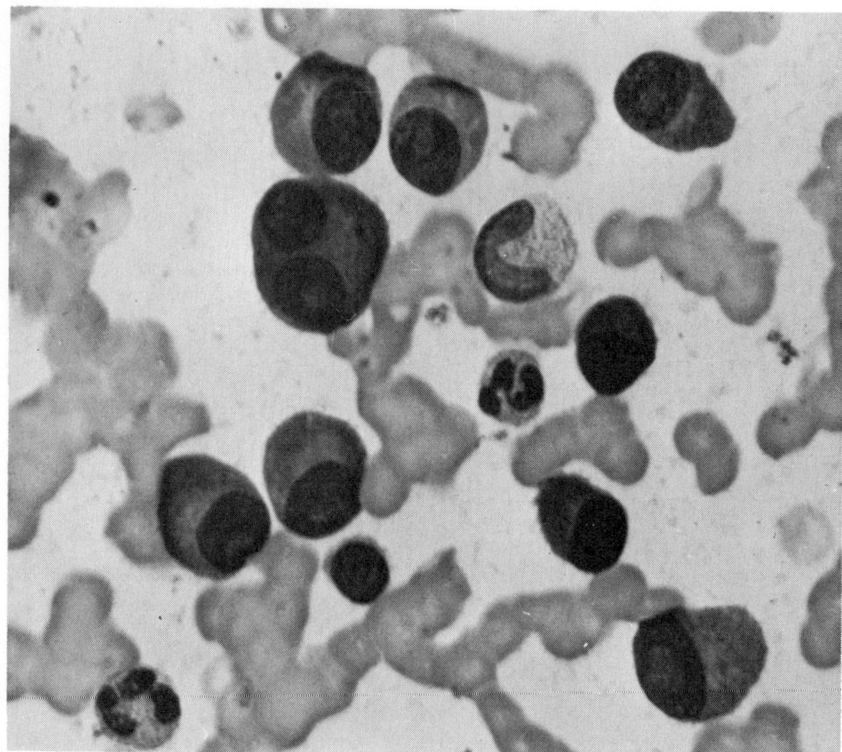

Figure 29–42 Multiple myeloma. Bone marrow smear preparation. Note the numerous plasma cells, which display eccentric nuclei and a perinuclear halo. As evidence of immaturity the nucleoli are disproportionately large and may be seen in some of the cells as lighter areas of the nucleus. A double-nucleated plasmacyte is present near the center of the field. There is strong rouleaux formation. Wright's stain × 920.

tional platelet defect may develop (see p. 731) owing to coating of the platelets with the abnormal protein.

In diffuse disease, the bone marrow characteristically shows sheets of abnormal plasma cells. A minimum of 15% of the bone marrow cells must be abnormal plasma cells before a diagnosis of multiple myeloma or other diffuse plasma cell malignancy can be established.

The abnormal cells are large (15 to 30 μm), with a round, eccentrically placed nucleus with prominent nucleoli, and may be regarded as atypical plasmablasts or proplasmacytes. Multiple vacuolations are seen in some cells (Mott cells); others have small eosinophilic bodies (Russell bodies). Some may have a crystalline protein deposit, and occasionally there are cells with brilliant eosinophilic cytoplasm (flame cells). The myeloma cells may be clumped together and are differentiated from mature cells by their large size, large nucleoli, and atypism. Bone marrow biopsy is necessary because of the discrete nature of the abnormal cell foci.

Serum and Urine Abnormalities

Chapter 26 describes the abnormal changes in the plasma of these individuals, and this information is summarized in Table 29–12. If careful examination of the serum and urine is performed, more than 99% of cases will demonstrate a monoclonal immunoglobulin in either the serum or the urine. The serum abnormal M protein is normally found in the general region of the gamma globulin on conventional protein electrophoresis. Immunoelectrophoresis will subsequently identify the specific immunoglobulin, which in over 50% of cases is IgG (see Fig. 29–43).

The urine has been classically described as having a Bence Jones protein (see p. 534); however, the chemical test for detecting this protein is highly insensitive and it is preferable to refer to the urinary protein as light chains, thereby implying that sensitive immunologic methods should be used for their detection (p. 550). The light chains of the aberrant globulin may be the only indication of disease, and it may be important to concentrate the urine before examining it (p. 89).

TABLE 29–12 DISTRIBUTION OF SERUM AND URINE PROTEINS IN MULTIPLE MYELOMA

Serum M Type Protein	Urine Bence Jones Protein (Light Chains)	Incidence %
IgG	—	52
IgG	kappa	
IgG	lambda	
IgA	—	21
IgA	kappa	
IgA	lambda	
IgD		2
IgD	†	
Mixed		
None	kappa	25
None	lambda	

*Adapted from Osserman et al., 1972.
†Variable.

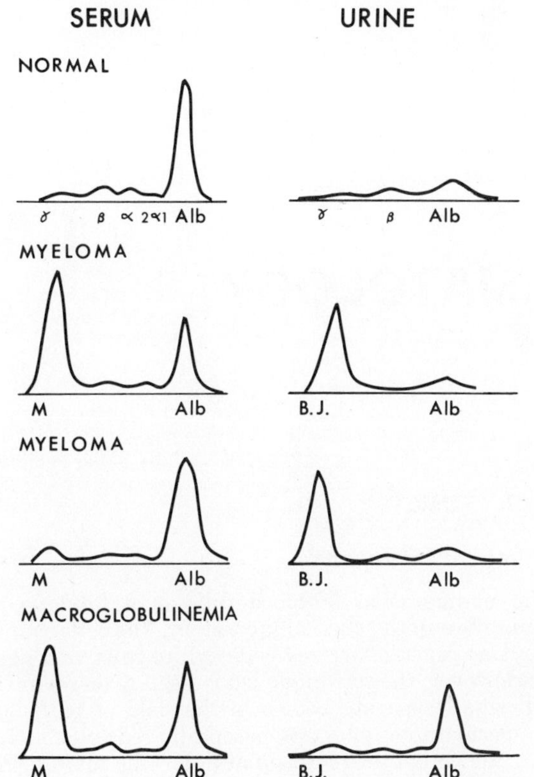

Figure 29–43 Serum and urine electrophoresis. The normal serum and urine sample show the absence of an M spike in the serum and no Bence Jones protein in the urine. The two sets of samples from cases of myeloma show a typical M spike and B.J. protein in 2. Sample 3 shows abnormal B.J. protein in the urine despite no apparent M spike in the serum. Sample 4 shows characteristic findings in macroglobulinemia.

Primary Macroglobulinemia (Waldenström's)

Macroglobulinemia (see also p. 534) is an abnormality that may occur with chronic lymphatic leukemia, lymphoma, and myeloma. With these conditions, there is circulating macroglobulin with a molecular weight of 1,000,000 or greater. About 15% of cases of macroglobulinemia are found in association with the diseases mentioned, but the rest, which may be termed idiopathic, form a clinical entity which is called Waldenström's macroglobulinemia. There is excessive macroglobulin in the serum, and the marrow is replaced with cells of an atypical lymphoid type which may be found also in lymph nodes, spleen, and liver. The patient has anemia, hemorrhagic disorders, and hemolytic anemia owing to cold antibodies. The abnormal cells are rarely found in peripheral blood. Because of the defective protein anabolism, excessive numbers of L chains may be manufactured and may spill over into the urine and appear as Bence Jones protein. This occurs in up to 30% of cases. The clinical course may be from several months to several years.

It is important to differentiate this condition from myeloma, and this usually can be done on clinical, blood, and bone marrow findings.

The peripheral blood picture is similar to multiple myeloma, except that an absolute lymphocytosis is usually present. Autoagglutination and positive direct antiglobulin tests owing to the IgM are common. Crossmatching of donor blood is occasionally a problem as a result of these last two features. The bone marrow shows an increase in lymphocytic-plasmacytic forms, with eosinophilia and mast cells occasionally present. Degenerating lymphocytes are often seen and these probably represent cells which have released their immunoglobulin (clasmatosis).

The abnormal protein is IgM, and can be present in large amounts with light chains in the urine in up to 30% of cases. The typical IgM protein has the following properties, which produce characteristic phenomena. It can behave as a cryoglobulin, and this will be evident if the blood is left at 4°C, since the plasma will gel. Indeed, if the plasma contains a particularly avid cryoglobulin, the sedimentation rate tube will gel, giving a false low result. There is greatly increased viscosity of the blood sample and occasionally the IgM can act as a pyroglobulin, in that heating the serum to 60°C will cause irreversible gelling. The specific diagnostic test is immunoelectrophoresis.

Other Immunoproliferative Disorders

Heavy Chain Disease. Associated with varying degrees of anemia, abnormal bone marrow and characteristic immunoglobulin findings.

Amyloidosis. No typical hematologic findings.

Idiopathic Monoclonal Gammopathy. No peripheral blood or bone marrow findings, but an increased monoclonal immunoglobulin is present with no other abnormalities of the serum protein.

Lupus Erythematosus (LE). Mention of this condition has already been made on p. 692 when discussing the LE cell phenomenon, i.e., the typical LE cell consisting of a neutrophil with ingested nucleoprotein material. Emphasis is given to this condition here because of the wide range of immunologic aberrations which are shared by LE with the other collagen disorders, bearing in mind that as a group they probably represent autoimmune disease in which immunologically-induced tissue injury plays a prominent role.

LE is a systemic disease which affects women most commonly and is characterized by a skin rash, fever, and renal, cardiac, and vascular lesions. The clinical presentation may be insidious, and diagnosis is possible only by the use of the specific tests mentioned on pp. 692 and 693. The hematologic abnormalities, apart from the formation of the LE cell, are also the result of autoantibodies. The anemia is often caused by a positive antiglobulin test causing a hemolytic anemia. Similarly, the leukopenia and thrombocytopenia are related to autoantibodies. Circulating antibodies also can be demonstrated against various coagulation factors, particularly factor VIII (see p. 748).

CHAPTER 29—REVIEW QUESTIONS

1. What is the normal sequence (from primitive to mature cell) of (a) erythrocytes, (b) leukocytes, and (c) platelets?
2. What is the function of (a) neutrophils, (b) lymphocyties, and (c) platelets?
3. What are the characteristic laboratory findings in (a) iron deficiency anemia, (b) pernicious anemia, and (c) sickle cell anemia?
4. What inclusions can be found in erythrocytes, and what are their significance?
5. What are the characteristic morphological differences between acute myeloblastic leukemia and chronic myeloid leukemia?

PRACTICE OF HEMATOLOGY

INTRODUCTION

As with all laboratory disciplines, the range of hematological techniques has greatly expanded in the past decade. The increasing demands placed on the hematology laboratory have necessitated the development of sophisticated automated equipment that can accurately handle large volumes of work. The application of quality control techniques ensures the reliability of results. This chapter will emphasize the more common hematological techniques required by the laboratory.

SI Units in Hematology

SI units have been replacing traditional units of measurement in hematology (p. 61). Unfortunately, the change to SI units has not progressed at the same rate in Canada and the United States, even though the majority of scientific journals published in North America have made the transition. No attempt has been made here either to provide a complete transition to SI units (e.g., banning of percentage values) or to cite values in all instances in traditional as well as SI unit form. The following table summarizes the SI units used.

Component	In SI Units
Hemoglobin	144 g/L
RBC (RCC)	4.5 × 10^{12}/L*
Hematocrit (PCV)	0.41 L/L
MCV	75–95 fL
MCH	27–32 pg
MCHC	300–350 g/L
WBC (WCC)	4.0–11.0 × 10^9/L
Platelets	150–400 × 10^9/L
Reticulocytes	25–65 × 10^9/L
Serum iron	14–29 μmol/L
Total iron-binding capacity	45–72 μmol/L
Transferrin	1.2–2.0 g/L
Serum haptoglobins (Hb binding)	0.3–2.0 g/L
Serum B_{12} (as cyanocobalamin)	160–925 pmol/L
Serum folate	3–20 nmol/L
Plasma fibrinogen	1.5–4.0 g/L

*As the normal range varies with age and sex, only one measurement in the normal range has been given as an example.

HEMOCYTOMETRY

General Considerations

The enumeration of blood cells is a fundamental examination in the clinical laboratory. The cells counted in routine practice are red cells, white cells, and platelets. However, the technique lends itself to enumeration of all small separate bodies in the field of pathology, e.g., spermatozoa, punctate basophilic red cells, eosinophils, and cells in cerebrospinal fluid. The main principles for such examinations are:

1. Selection of a diluting fluid that not only will dilute the cells to manageable levels, but will either identify them in some fashion or destroy contaminant cellular elements.
2. The use of a hemocytometer or electronic cell counter that will present the cells in such a way to the observer or to an electronic device that the number of cells per unit volume of fluid can be counted. The electronic cell counter avoids human error and by virtue of the larger number of cells counted is statistically more accurate.

Manual Hemocytometry

The counting chamber consists of a thick rectangular glass slide. In the center of the upper surface there are ruled areas separated by moats from the rest of the slide, and two raised transverse bars, one of which is present on each side of the ruled area. The ruled portion may be in the center of the central area (single chamber), or there may be an upper and lower ruled portion (double chamber). The double chamber is to be recommended, since it enables duplicate counts to be made rapidly. When an optically plane coverglass (and only such should be used) is rested on the raised bars, there is a predetermined gap, or chamber, formed between it and the ruled area. The ruled area itself is divided by lines into a pattern that varies with the type of chamber used and represents fractional portions or multiples of a square millimeter.

Dilution of the cell sample may be accomplished using either a Thoma pipette or the tube dilution system. Thoma and Sahli pipettes are illustrated in Figure 30–1, and their use in hematology will be described under the specific techniques. With tubes, larger volumes of

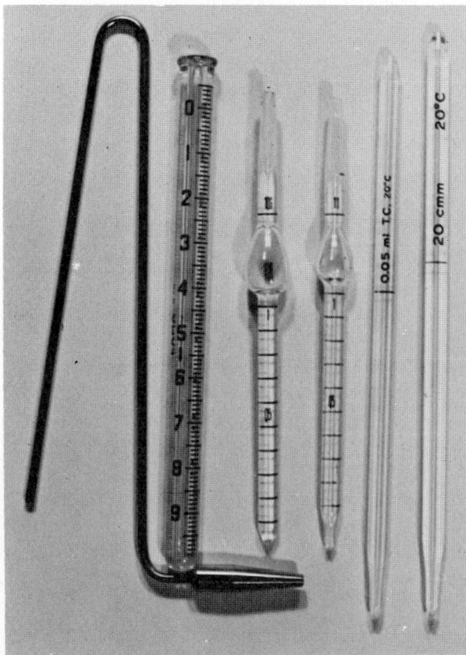

Figure 30–1 From left to right: suction cleaner and Wintrobe hematocrit tube; red cell pipette; white cell pipette; 50 μL pipette; 20 μL pipette.

blood and diluting fluid are used and the greater will be the degree of accuracy as compared with the smaller volumes used in the pipette techniques. Tubes are less expensive and easier to clean than pipettes, and their contents are easier to mix, especially when the apparatus shown in Figure 30–2 is used. Disposable, self-filling, self-measuring dilution micropipettes are commercially available.* These are easy to use, are available with a series of different diluting fluids, and in some circumstances may offer considerable advantage. Tube dilution techniques and precalibrated micropipettes have largely superseded the use of Thoma and Sahli pipettes and are to be recommended.

The diluted cells are introduced into the counting chamber and allowed to settle. They may then be counted in the designated area(s). Cells lying on or touching the upper or left boundary lines are included; those on the lower and right boundary lines are disregarded. It will be appreciated that with the dilution factor and the small area counted, an error in counting a single cell may make a considerable difference in the final count.

*Unopette, Becton, Dickinson and Co., Rutherford, N.J. 07070, and Mississauga, Ont. L5J 2M8.

Errors in Hemocytomtery

These may arise from three sources: apparatus, personal technique, and inherent error.

Apparatus. Accurate apparatus should be purchased from reputable sources. Broken pipettes (especially those with chipped tips) must be discarded. Markings on pipettes should be plainly visible. Only optically plane coverglasses should be used.

All apparatus should be thoroughly cleaned after each use. If nondisposable pipettes are used they are washed well with a sequence of water and acetone (filled three or four times with each fluid), and air is drawn through after the acetone until the inside of the pipette is thoroughly dried. Hemocytometers should be washed in water immediately after use and dried with soft paper tissue. They should be stored in such a manner as to avoid breakage and scratching of the counting surface. Many hemocytometers, when purchased, come in a plastic case that is ideal for storage and prevents dust accumulation on the instrument.

Personal Technique. Personal errors may arise in taking the sample of blood, in mixing, in filling the counting chamber, and in counting. If a capillary blood sample is taken, a free flow of blood should be ensured by puncturing only warmed fingers or ears and by not squeezing the punctured part. No matter what pipette is used, it must be filled accurately and quickly to the mark so that clotting does not occur. If the mark on the pipette is grossly overshot, it is better to start afresh using a clean pipette; expelling the excess will lead to inaccuracy because of blood clinging to the walls of the pipette above the mark, especially since any such error is multiplied by the dilution factor. Samples should be mixed well for 2 minutes before the counting chamber is filled; this also applies in the case of making dilutions from samples of whole blood. A clean, grease-free counting chamber and coverglass allow proper filling by capillary attraction. Once the chamber is filled, the cells must be allowed to settle for at least 2 minutes. A mechanical counter helps in counting.

Each technologist must be on guard against psycho-

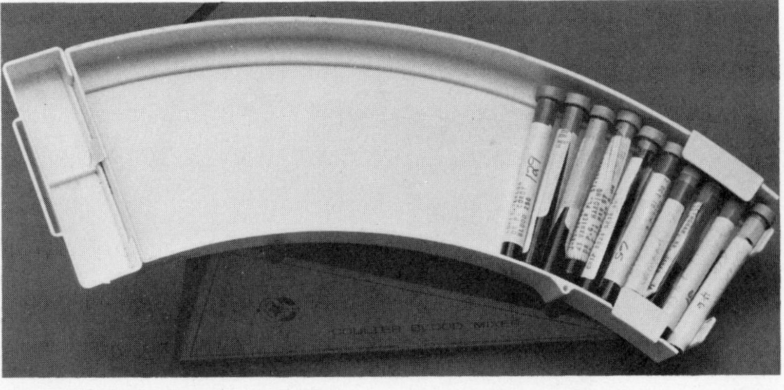

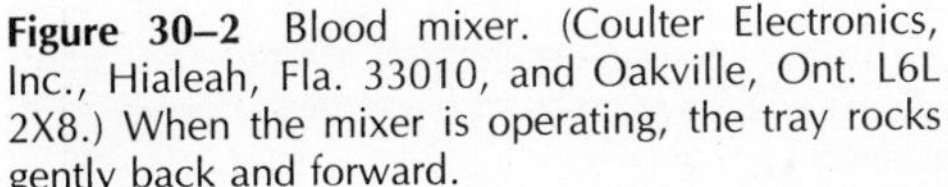

Figure 30–2 Blood mixer. (Coulter Electronics, Inc., Hialeah, Fla. 33010, and Oakville, Ont. L6L 2X8.) When the mixer is operating, the tray rocks gently back and forward.

logical factors causing error, such as starting to count in one area of the chamber and then subconsciously "fitting" counts from subsequent areas to the preconceived number.

Inherent Error. The "inherent" or "field" error depends upon the distribution of the cells in the counting chamber and therefore is unavoidable. It can be reduced by counting large numbers of cells. The standard error attributable to the distribution of cells in the area counted is proportional to the square root of the number of cells counted. Since the rate of increase of the square root is less than the rate of increase in the number of cells counted, it follows that the percentage error in counts diminishes with increase in the number of cells counted.

Commonly Used Hemocytometers

Improved Neubauer (Fig. 30–3). The depth between the lower surface of the coverglass, which is lying on the raised bars and the ruled area is 0.1 mm. Each ruled area is a square of 3 mm divided into nine large squares, each of 1 mm side. The central square of these nine is divided by engraved lines into 400 tiny squares arranged in 25 groups of 16 by triple boundary lines. Each large square is 1 mm square, each of the 25 medium squares is of 0.2 mm side (0.04 sq mm area), and each of the 400 tiny squares is of 0.05 mm side (0.0025 sq mm area).

Fuchs-Rosenthal. When the coverglass is correctly placed, the depth between its lower surface and the ruled area is 0.2 mm. Each ruled area is a square of 4 mm divided into 16 squares of 1 sq mm each. These squares are divided by triple lines. Each large square is further subdivided into 16 smaller squares. The total volume over the ruled area is 16 × 0.2 cmm = 3.2 μL.

MANUAL ERYTHROCYTE OR RED CELL COUNT

The manual red cell count is so inaccurate that it cannot be recommended. Unless automated equipment is available, red cell counts should be discouraged in favor of the more accurate hemoglobin and hematocrit.

Normal Values

Adults

Men: 4.5 to 6.2 × 10^{12}/L
Women: 4.0 to 5.5 × 10^{12}/L

Infants and Children

Birth (cord blood): 4.0 to 6.0 × 10^{12}/L
First 3 months: 4.0 to 5.5 × 10^{12}/L
3 months to 3 years: 4.0 to 5.2 × 10^{12}/L
3 years to 10 years: 4.0 to 5.0 × 10^{12}/L

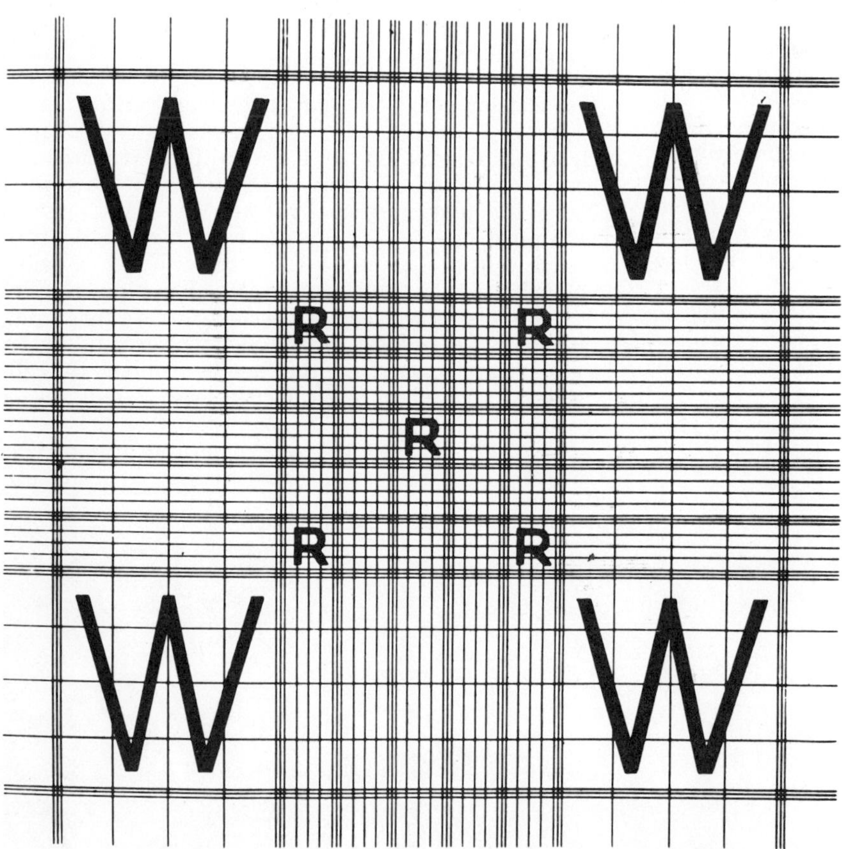

Figure 30–3 Rulings for an improved Neubauer counting chamber. The areas counted for the leukocyte count are marked W. The platelet areas are marked R.

MANUAL LEUKOCYTE OR WHITE BLOOD CELL COUNT

Principle

Blood is diluted with a fluid that causes hemolysis of erythrocytes but has no effect on leukocytes, which can then be counted in a Neubauer hemocytometer.

Reagents

2% Aqueous Solution of Acetic Acid. Gentian violet is added until the solution is a pale blue-violet color. The acetic acid solution causes erythrocyte lysis, while gentian violet lightly stains the leukocytes, permitting easier enumeration.

Method

Thoma White Cell Pipette. The long stem is divided into 10 equal parts, with "0.5" and "1" engraved on it. On the short limb just above the bulb, the mark "11" is engraved. When blood is drawn up to the 0.5 mark and diluting fluid to the 11 mark, the sample of blood (now in the bulb) is diluted 1 in 20.

Once the pipette is accurately filled to the mark, the rubber suction tube is carefully removed, with the pipette held horizontally and only one finger sealing the tip. Both ends of the pipette may then be sealed with special small rubber or plastic scaling caps or with the thumb on the tip and the middle or index finger on the other end. The pipette is shaken either mechanically or manually for at least 1 minute and preferably for 2 minutes. A bead contained in the bulb of the pipette aids in the mixing. If the shaking is done manually, the shaking motions should be varied and alternated with rotation by rolling the pipette horizontally between the palms of the hands.

The coverglass is placed on the chamber. If it is accurately placed and if the glass of the chamber is transparent, then slight pressure to the ends of the coverglass will reveal "rainbow" Newton diffraction rings. The chamber is now ready to be charged.

Once the diluted blood in the pipette has been thoroughly mixed, a few drops are expelled to discard the diluting fluid in the long stem of the pipette. Now, with the index finger forming a controlled seal over the end of the pipette, which is held almost vertically, the tip of the pipette is brought up to the edge of the coverglass. By gentle release of index finger pressure, fluid is allowed to run out slowly until the counting platform is just covered. The fluid is drawn into the chamber by capillary attraction. The chamber is placed in position on the microscope stage and is allowed to stand for 2 or 3 minutes so that the cells may settle.

Tube Technique. 0.02 mL of blood is taken and mixed with 0.38 mL of diluting fluid in a small tube or snap cap plastic vial. Tube techniques are preferable to the Thoma pipette method, because they allow greater accuracy of dilution. Unopettes (p. 673) are highly recommended for manual cell counting techniques.

Performance of the Count

The counting chamber is surveyed with a lower power objective (× 10) to ascertain whether the cells are evenly distributed. Then the number of cells in 4 large squares are counted (see Fig. 30–3).

Calculation

If x is the number of leukocytes in 4 large squares, then x WBCs are present in $4 \times 1 \times 0.1\ \mu L = 0.4\ \mu L$.

$$\therefore \frac{x \times 10}{4} \text{ WBCs are present in } 1\ \mu L.$$

But the dilution of blood is 1 in 20.

$$\therefore \text{number of WBCs in } 1\ \mu L \text{ blood}$$

$$= \frac{x \times 10 \times 20}{4} = 50x$$

Note: When the leukocyte count is low (below $4.0 \times 10^9/L$), it is advisable for greater accuracy to use a 1 in 10 dilution (i.e., take blood to the 1 mark of the pipette, or place 0.1 mL of blood in 0.9 mL of diluent). When the white cell count is very high, it may be necessary to make a higher dilution.

Normal Values

Adults. 5.0 to $10.0 \times 10^9/L$
Infants at birth. 10.0 to $25.0 \times 10^9/L$
1 year. 8.0 to $15.0 \times 10^9/L$

Sources of Error

1. Improper mixing of blood
2. Clots in blood sample
3. Improper dilutions
4. Improper filling of hemocytometers
5. Errors in calculations

Significance of Results

Leukocyte counts are commonly increased in infections and, when considered along with the differential leukocyte count, can be an indicator as to whether the infecting agent is bacterial or viral. Variations can occur in a wide variety of conditions (e.g., leukemias), making the leukocyte count an important diagnostic parameter. See p. 655.

MANUAL PLATELET COUNT

Prinicple

Blood is diluted with a diluting fluid that causes lysis of erythrocytes but has no effect on platelets, which can then be counted in Neubauer hemocytometer.

Reagents

1% Aqueous Solution of Ammonium Oxalate. The solution should be filtered before use, and fresh solution should be made frequently.

Procedure

1. Using either a Thoma WBC pipette or tube method, prepare a 1:20 dilution as for the WBC method. EDTA venous blood is preferable to capillary blood, since some platelets are unavoidably lost from the latter because they adhere to the edges of the wound; this favors falsely low values.
2. Mix for two minutes on a mechanical mixer. Then fill both sides of a Neubauer counting chamber and allow the platelets to settle for 20 minutes in a Petri dish, on the bottom of which is a moist disc of filter paper. It is essential that the preparation not be left in the pipette or tube for any undue length of time before being transferred to the counting chamber.
3. Count the number of platelets, which will appear as small refractile bodies, in 5 squares in the central ruled area of a Neubauer hemocytometer (see Fig. 30–3). It should be noted that leukocytes are not affected by the diluting fluid and will be readily visible. Leukocytes, however, are much larger than platelets and are unlikely to cause any confusion.
4. Platelet counting is facilitated by using a phase contrast microscope. Alternatively, a light microscope may be used with the condenser well down.

Calculation

Area of 5 squares in central ruled area = 0.2 sq mm
Volume of 5 squares in central ruled areas $= 0.2 \times 0.1\ \mu L$
$= 0.02\ \mu L$

Dilution of blood sample = 1:20
If R = number of platelets counted in 0.02 μL

$$\text{then number of platelets}/\mu L = R \times 20 \times \frac{1}{0.2}$$
$$= R \times 20 \times 50$$
$$= R \times 1000$$

Normal Values

Normal values are 150 to 450 $\times 10^9$/L (mean values range between 200 and 300 $\times 10^9$/L).

Sources of Error

1. Clots in sample
2. Improper dilution
3. Improper filling of hemocytometer
4. Improper calculations
5. Contamination of counting fluid
6. Clumping of platelets. Although this has been largely overcome by the use of EDTA anticoagulant, there are occasions when platelet clumping will be found.
7. It should be noted that counts on samples collected by skin puncture are usually lower than those performed on venipuncture samples. The function of platelets is to adhere to wounds and skin punctures, so inevitably there is a loss of platelets during micro collection.

Significance of Results

Low platelet counts (thrombocytopenia) can be found in a variety of conditions, either as a primary condition (ITP) or secondarily as a complication of other diseases (e.g., leukemia). High platelet counts (thrombocytosis) can be found following splenectomy and in polycythemic conditions.

Indirect Platelet Count

1. Make a good blood smear from venous blood taken into EDTA, or from a freely flowing skin puncture. Dry in the air and stain with Wright's or Leishman's stain.
2. Using an oil immersion objective, count the number of platelets per 1000 RBCs.
3. Perform an accurate red cell count.
4. Calculate as follows: If P is the number of platelets counted per 1000 RBCs, then platelets

$$= \frac{P \times \text{RBCs per } \mu L}{1000}$$

Therefore, if the red cell count is 5.0 $\times 10^{12}$/L and 60 platelets are counted per 1000 RBCs, then platelet count/μL

$$= \frac{60 \times 5{,}000{,}000}{1000}$$

$$= 300{,}000/\mu L$$

$$= 300 \times 10^9/L$$

Alternatively, the formula can be simplified as follows:

$$\text{Platelet count} \times 10^9/L = P \times \text{RBC}$$
$$= 60 \times 5.0$$
$$= 300$$

Note: A low or borderline platelet count obtained by the indirect method should be checked carefully by a count using a direct method. All thrombocytopenic results by whatever method must be confirmed before being reported. The indirect method is not recommended as a method of choice.

TOTAL EOSINOPHIL COUNT

Definition

The total eosinophil count is the determination of the number of eosinophils per liter.

Principle

Blood is diluted with a fluid that causes lysis of erythrocytes and stains eosinophils, rendering them readily visible.

Reagents

Hinkleman's fluid has the advantages of keeping well at room temperature and not needing filtering before use.

Eosin yellow	0.5 g
Formaldehyde (40%)	0.5 mL
Phenol (95% aqueous solution)	0.5 mL
Distilled water	to 100 mL

Filter after preparation. The solution will keep indefinitely at 4°C.

Method

With the solution given here, make dilutions of blood using the Thoma pipette or tube technique as described for the white cell count. A Fuchs-Rosenthal chamber is used, and counting is carried out as soon as the cells have settled. Usually 10 minutes in a moist-atmosphere Petri dish will suffice. All the cells in the ruled area are counted.

Calculation

If E is the number of eosinophils in 16 large squares (3.2 μL), then the absolute eosinophil count per μL, blood

$$= \frac{E \times 20}{3.2} = 6.25\ E$$

Note: To increase the accuracy, at least 100 cells should be counted; i.e., both ruled areas should be counted and, if the count is low, the chamber should be cleaned and refilled, average counts per ruled area being used for the calculation.

Normal Values

0.04 to 0.44×10^9/L

Sources of Error

The first five sources of error listed for the platelet count apply to the eosinophil count also.

Significance of Results

Eosinophilia is common in allergic conditions (e.g., asthma) and in parasitic infections.

AUTOMATED EQUIPMENT

A wide range of automated and semiautomated equipment is available for measuring different hematological parameters. The most useful are those that count cells. Automated cell counters count larger numbers of cells when compared to manual methods, thus allowing greater precision. The coefficient of variation using manual cell counting techniques varies from 8 to 15%, depending on the cell type being counted, whereas automated methods have been reported as having a coefficient of variation of 1 to 3%. A number of different systems are currently available.

TYPES OF AUTOMATED SYSTEMS

Coulter Counter. (Coulter Electronics Inc., Hialeah, Fla. 33010, and Oakville, Ont. L6L 2X8.) This is the system used by the authors, and it will be described in detail.

Hemalog System. (Technicon Corp., Tarrytown, N.Y. 10591.) This system measures those parameters already mentioned plus conductivity cell volume, conductivity cell volume/packed cell volume ratio, prothrombin time, partial thromboplastin time, and platelet count. The system can be expanded to include leukocyte differential counts based on the cytochemical staining reactions of different white cells. The hematocrit is measured by automatic centrifugation. Cell counts are coincidence free, and results can be displayed visually or on a digital printout.

ELT-8. (Ortho Diagnostic Instruments, Raritan, N.J. 08869, and Don Mills, Ont. M3C 1L9.) This instrument measures white cell, red cell, and platelet counts and hematocrit and hemoglobin and calculates MCV, MCH, and MCHC. As each cell flows through an 18-micron aperture created by laminar flow, a 20-micron laser beam is interrupted. The hematocrit is measured by the pulse amplitudes produced by narrow angle diffraction measurements. The hemoglobin is measured as cyanmethemoglobin.

TOA CC-800. (TOA Medical Electronics Co., Ltd., P. O. Box 1002 Kobe Central Post Office, Japan; TOA Medical Electronics (USA), Inc., Carson, Calif. 90746; Western Scientific Services, Scarborough, Ont. M1H 2X1.) This recently introduced cell counter from Japan measures white cell, red cell, and platelet counts and hematocrit and hemoglobin and calculates MCV, MCH, and MCHC. It uses the impedance method of counting cells, and hemoglobin is measured as cyanmethemoglobin.

The choice of instrument can be problematical. The multichannel instruments are very attractive for large institutions. A laboratory can very quickly become dependent on these machines so that any breakdown is a disaster. Consequently, it is necessary for each laboratory to have a backup system. This can be readily provided by the semiautomated machines. Accuracy and reliability are probably the most important requisites for any automated system. It is useful, when contemplating the purchase of such a system, to communicate with laboratories in which that system is being used. An objective appraisal can thus be obtained from workers who use the system on a daily basis. Whatever system is chosen, it is essential that the manufacturer's instructions regarding cleaning, maintenance, and servicing be followed.

COULTER METHODS

The Coulter Counter is so designed that by means of a mercury manometer, a specific volume containing particles in an electrolyte (0.9% sodium chloride) is forced through an aperture of specific dimensions. An aperture current passes between an electrode within the aperture tube and another outside the aperture. As a particle passes through the aperture it lowers electrolytic conductivity between the two electrodes, producing an impulse, the magnitude of which is proportional to the volume of the particle. The voltage pulses are fed into a threshold circuit that discriminates between pulses of different sizes, generating counting impulses for those particles that exceed the threshold level alone

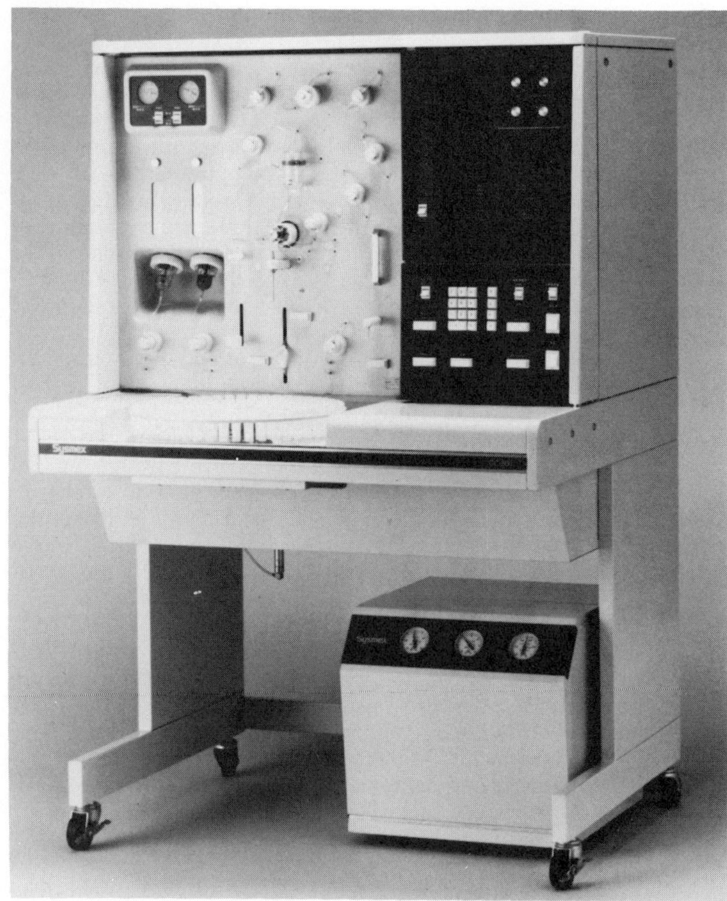

Figure 30–4 The TOA CC–800 Automated blood counter. (For manufacturer's information see text.)

and thus counting the number of particles of threshold size in passage (Fig. 30–5). The whole operation may be monitored for debris accumulation in the fluid or in the aperture orifice by inspection of the oscilloscope screen, which displays irregularities in pulse patterns, or by direct inspection of the orifice using a built-in projection apparatus. If blocking of the orifice occurs, the debris may be brushed away with a soft brush and flushed out with clean saline solution.

The saponin method for leukocyte counting permits red cell counts to be prepared conveniently from the original white cell dilution. Only capillary, EDTA-treated, or heparinized blood can be used for this technique, since oxalated blood with saponin accelerates the deterioration of white cells, decreasing the available working time. If white cells alone are to be estimated, the use of a cetrimide counting fluid is recommended.

PLATELET COUNT

Considerable problems are experienced by many laboratories in counting platelets using an automated method. This is particularly evident when enumerating counts below 50×10^9/L, and when there is wide variability in platelet size. For most routine clinical purposes the method of Bull is recommended; however, such a count must always be checked by examination of a stained peripheral smear. A number of automated counting machines specifically developed for platelet counting are available. The Thrombocounter, manufactured by Coulter Electronics, is such an example. The platelet count is one of the parameters offered by the current generation of multichannel instruments. Commercial controls are available for the quality control of platelet counts.

Method of Bull

Separation of the platelets is accomplished by transferring EDTA anticoagulated blood into a piece of polyvinyl chloride tubing 4 cm long and with a 2-mm internal bore. One end is sealed using a blood bank tubing sealer. The tubing can be prepared by sealing the tubing every 8 cm and cutting through at the seals and midway between them. Coulter Electronics has a complete kit available.

Method

1. Using well-mixed EDTA blood, the open end of the plastic tube is dipped into the container and filled by pressing the tubing flat and then allowing it to expand.

2. Remove excess blood and place the tube open end up at an angle of 45°. Allow sedimentation of the red cells to occur (this will vary with individual samples), and as soon as sufficient platelet-rich plasma is evident, remove 3.3 μL, avoiding red cell contamination, into 10 mL of 0.9% sodium chloride.

3. With the Model F counter 2 counts are taken—one at the lower threshold setting (usually 7) and one at the upper threshold setting (usually 70). The difference between the counts is the platelet population. The instrument count is converted to an actual count by means of a chart, this count being corrected by a hematocrit factor (both charts available from Coulter Electronics) to give the platelet count per μL of whole blood. The coefficient of variation of this method has been reported as being 4%. Model Z counters have dual threshold controls, enabling instrument counts to be read directly.

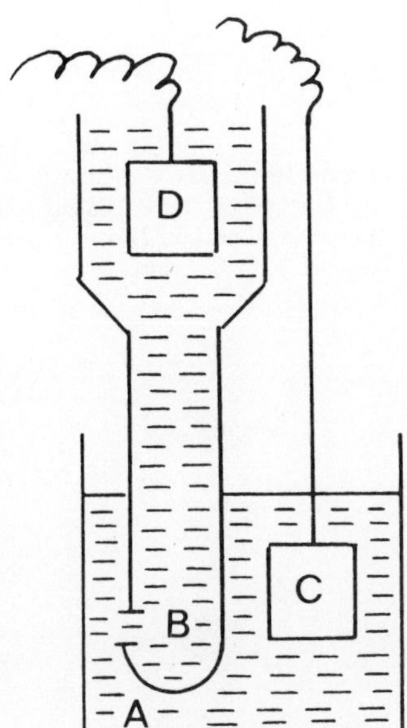

Figure 30–5 Principle of impedance counting. *A, electrolyte in counting vial; B,* 100 μ aperture—fluid and cells are drawn through for a preset time; *C,* external electrode; *D,* internal electrode. The electrical resistance between *C* and *D* as a cell is drawn through aperture *B* registers as a voltage pulse on the counter.

General Comments for Coulter Counter

The grouping of a Coulter Counter (Model F or Z), Coulter hemoglobinometer, and automatic diluter such as that in Figure 30–6 is a useful combination capable of measuring hemoglobins and leukocyte and erythrocyte counts. For large workloads, a multichannel instrument, the Coulter S, provides seven parameters: hemoglobin, leukocyte count, erythrocyte count, and MCV are measured, whereas the hematocrit, MCH, and MCHC are calculated from the resulting data. The Coulter S Plus (Fig. 30–7) also provides a platelet count, red cell distribution width (RDW), platelet volume, platelet-sizing histogram and, as an option, a visual display of the neutrophil/lymphocyte ratio.

Method of Using Coulter S Plus

Before use a check is made of the instrument to ensure that all vacuum and pressure gauges are registering according to manufacturer's specifications.

1. The sample is presented to aspirator tip, and the sampling button is pressed.

2. 1 mL of the blood sample is aspirated. 1.6 μL of blood is segmented off by the blood sampling valve for MCV and erythrocyte and platelet counts, while 42.9 μL is segmented off for a leukocyte count and hemoglobin determination.

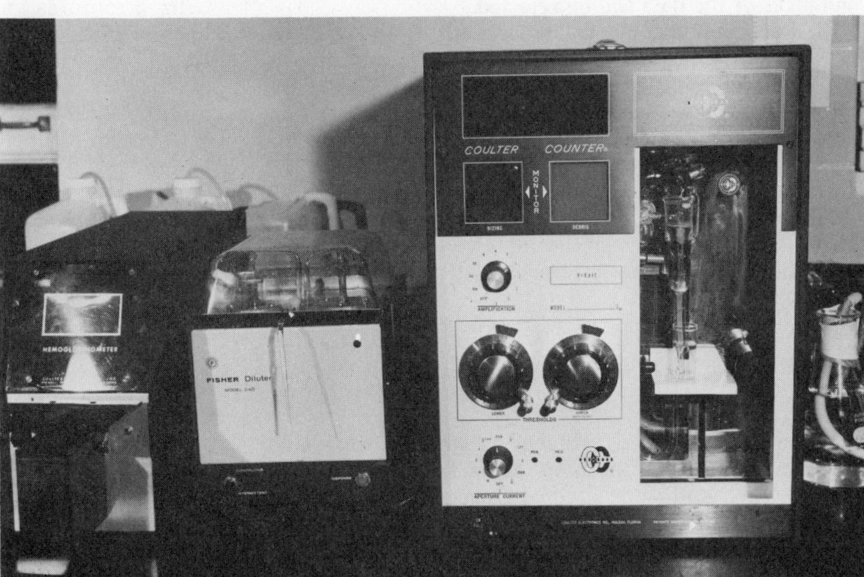

Figure 30–6 A grouping of Coulter counter, diluter, and hemoglobinometer.

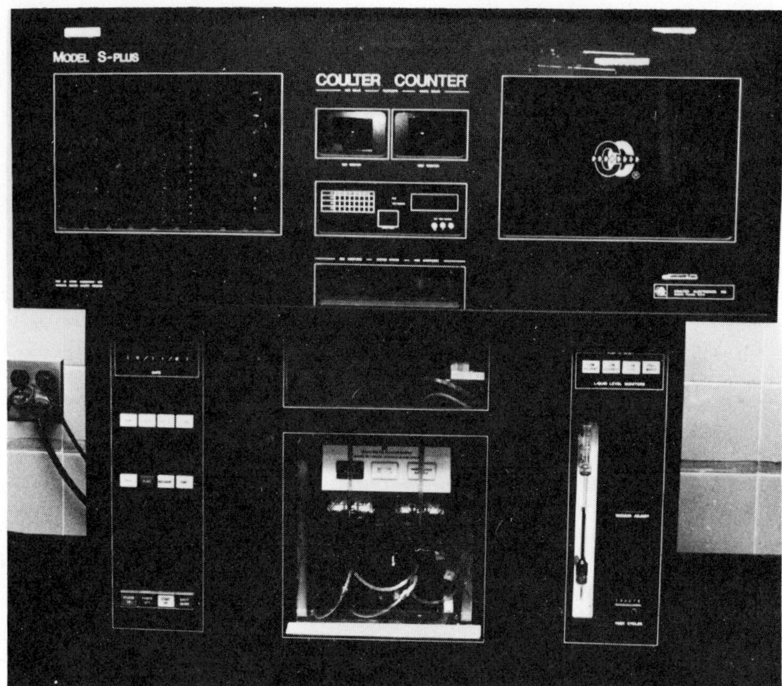

Figure 30–7 The Coulter S Plus counter. (Coulter Electronics, Inc., Hialeah, Fla. 33010, and Oakville, Ont. L6L 2X8.)

3. Each volume of blood is directed to its respective analytical bath along with 10 mL of isotonic diluent. Mixing bubbles ensure adequate mixing in the baths before counting. The final dilution in the erythrocyte bath is 1:6250. 0.77 mL of lysing agent is added to the leukocyte bath to lyse the erythrocytes before hemoglobin measurement. The final dilution is 1:251.

4. A precise volume of fluid is drawn through three apertures in each of the baths, and leukocytes, erythrocytes, and platelets are counted. The MCV is measured in the erythrocyte bath by volume displacement. The counts on at least two of the apertures must be within preprogrammed tolerances or the data will be rejected.

5. After counting, the leukocyte bath drains into the hemoglobin cuvette and the hemoglobin concentration is measured photometrically.

6. The instrument then goes through a backwash and rinse cycle, and the results obtained are printed out on the requisition. The Coulter S Plus has some preprogrammed error codes that, in the event of problems, will either be visually displayed on the instrument or printed on the requisition. These codes are useful in troubleshooting, because they give a guide to possible defects in instrument performance.

Although the Coulter S Plus is an excellent machine capable of handling large volumes of work, there are certain situations in which faulty results may be obtained.

1. Cold agglutinins. Samples in which strong cold agglutinins are present may show falsely decreased erythrocyte counts owing to agglutination of the red cells. The erythrocyte count is best performed on a Coulter Model F or Z after the sample has been diluted in diluent warmed to 37°C.

2. Hemoglobins. Falsely elevated hemoglobin levels are a problem with all automatic sampling machines. They can occur for two reasons: (a) very high leukocyte counts (in leukemic patients) may cause a turbidity that results in a false hemoglobin reading. This can be overcome by adding the lysing agent to the diluted sample (as described for Model F and Z). The diluted sample is then centrifuged to precipitate the leukocytes, and the supernatant can be transferred directly to the hemoglobinometer (e.g., Coulter hemoglobinometer). (b) Lipemic plasma may cause similar problems. This can be overcome by centrifuging the blood sample at 1500 G for 5 minutes and removing the maximal amount of lipemic plasma without disturbing the red cell layer. Note how much plasma was removed, and, using another pipette, add exactly the same volume of normal saline. Mix the sample on a rotator for five minutes and repeat the procedure until the supernatant shows no trace of lipemia. The sample can then be measured on the Coulter S Plus or any other hemoglobinometer. The use of high lipid content–hyperalimentation intravenous fluids also affects the hemoglobin estimation because of the ensuing lipidemia. Avoid taking blood samples while this intravenous material is being transfused.

3. Platelets. Using the Coulter S Plus, erroneous platelet counts can be obtained because of the presence of microcytes that are small enough to be included in the threshold range for platelet counting. This can be detected by performing a platelet-sizing histogram and by noting the presence of a very low MCV.

4. The red cell distribution width (RDW) available on the Coulter S Plus indicates, if abnormal, the presence of two difference cell populations. The normal range is 10 ± 1.5.

Reporting of Results

Most multichannel machines print results onto the original requisition form. If results have to be hand-written they should be legible and presented in such a manner that the laboratory and clinician may quickly note any changes. Cumulative reporting provides at a glance the patient's hematological status over a period of time. The laboratory copy is a useful quality control tool. Unless a transfusion has been given, an individual's hematological indices tend to vary very little from day to day. A discrepancy on a cumulative report may be the first indication that something is amiss with a technique. The most obvious and efficient way of producing cumulative reports is by using a computer. The computer can also be programmed to note abnormal results. For hospitals without laboratory computer facilities, reports can be charted in such a way as to provide a cumulative report.

In the authors' laboratory, seven individual reports can be presented in a cumulative manner on a single patient chart sheet.

QUALITY CONTROL IN HEMATOLOGY

The advent of automation in the hematology laboratory has greatly improved the accuracy and precision of laboratory results as well as improving efficiency. Machines, however, are not infallible. Electronic components can fail, mechanical parts can wear out, and laboratory results suffer accordingly. The principles of quality control and the mathematical manipulations necessary are outlined in another chapter (see p. 43).

Any quality control program should simulate the test situation as closely as possible. Cyanmethemoglobin standards are available for standardizing hemoglobinometers. These should not be confused with controls, since they merely help to standardize an instrument, not control a technique. Consequently, a whole blood sample is used to control the automated cell counters. The most convenient of these is a whole blood control (usually chicken blood), which is sold by many manufacturers.* This has the advantage of stability over a fairly long period (2 to 3 weeks), and the manufacturer supplies a chart with the values for the different parameters controlled by it. The disadvantages of such a control are:

1. It does not control a very important part of the total testing sequence, namely the venipuncture.
2. It is easily recognized as a control and may be given preferential treatment by the laboratory worker.
3. It is relatively expensive.

These disadvantages can be overcome by using a sample taken from a patient. The patient's sample is, however, unstable and is unsuitable as a control for more than a day or so. Moreover, it is not known what the patient's results are, so it is impossible to establish accuracy. Using a combination of commercial controls and patient controls provides a satisfactory basis for a quality control program. The commercial controls should be run several times a day and standard deviation charts drawn. It is important that the control should be used during the entire working cycle and not merely during a normal day shift. Duplicate samples can be taken from several patients and these samples submitted for testing. It is our practice to appoint a quality control technologist to coordinate the program. The patients' samples are submitted under fictitious names so that, as far as is possible, the technologists performing the tests are not aware that they are dealing with a control. The quality control technologist later retrieves the completed results and compares the results of the duplicate samples. The duplicate patient samples may also be used to control differential counts, peripheral blood morphology, platelet counts, reticulocyte counts, and eosinophil counts. Other useful parameters for controlling the program are the MCHC and the MCV. For most of the population these fall within narrowly defined limits. The majority of MCHCs fall between 33 to 35%, or 330 to 350 g/L, and the majority of MCVs between 86 to 94 fL. Any trend away from these values should be viewed with suspicion unless substantiated by other investigations, e.g., peripheral blood smear. If an MCHC is over 36%, or 360 g/L this must certainly imply faulty methodology unless a Coulter S Plus is being used (see p. 679). Cumulative reporting systems serve a similar function for the other hematological parameters.

Despite the most stringent quality control procedures, random errors still will occur. Quality control, however, minimizes these errors and allows greater confidence in laboratory results. The axiom must be that if there is any doubt in a result, it should be repeated using a fresh sample.

In Ontario, a comprehensive quality control program is organized by the Laboratory Proficiency Testing Program (LPTP). Samples of blood and blood smears are sent to laboratories for analysis and comment. Results are compared with those of other reporting laboratories, and each laboratory receives a report. Since its inception, LPTP has identified a number of problems in laboratory practice, thus proving the value of some form of external quality control. Many states of the U.S. have similar programs.

PREPARATION OF PERIPHERAL BLOOD SMEARS

Correct preparation and proper staining of blood or bone marrow smears is another fundamental technique in hematology. The amount of information gained from such a specimen may be of inestimable value in the care of the patient. Technologists engaged in hematology must be able to produce excellent preparations and should not be content with mediocre ones. A hallmark of a good laboratory is the quality of its blood and bone marrow smears.

Smears may be made either on slides or on coverglasses. The latter method gives a more even distribution of cells, but the former is preferred because: (1) slides are easier to handle; (2) they are less easily broken; (3) they may be more clearly labeled; and (4) they do not require mounting and can be readily filed.

*4C Plus, Coulter Electronics, Hialeah, Fla. 33014, and Oakville, Ont. L6L 2X8. CH-60, Dade Reagents, Miami, Fla. 33152.

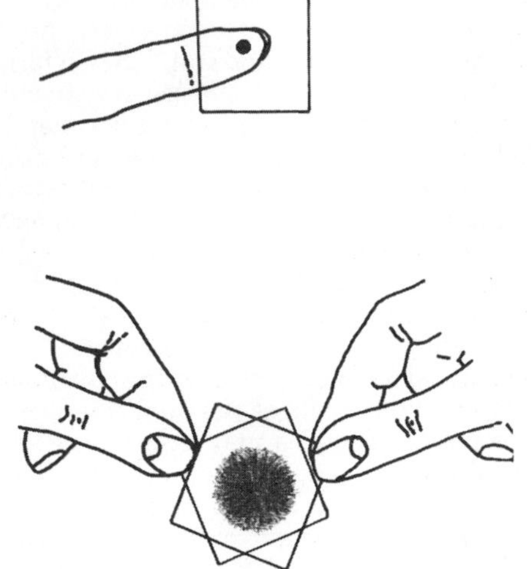

Figure 30–8 Method of making coverglass blood films.

Coverglass Smears

A clear, dry, grease-free, square coverglass (22 mm square) is held in each hand by the edges. One is held horizontally over a drop of blood welling up from a skin puncture, and the center of the glass is allowed to touch the drop of blood. The glass is removed from contact with the drop as soon as a drop of approximately 2 mm diameter has adhered to the glass, and *immediately* the other coverglass is superimposed diagonally on it. The blood begins to spread at once in a thin, even film between the coverglasses, and *just before* spreading is complete, the glasses (held horizontally by a corner of each between index finger and thumb of each hand) are evenly and smoothly drawn apart by sliding in the horizontal plane. When dry they are stained, either film side down, in watch glasses, or using special staining racks. When staining is completed and the films are dry, they are mounted with Permount (or similar medium), film side down on clean glass slides.

Slide Method

It is essential that clean, grease-free slides be used. It may be necessary to wash new slides in alcohol or in a

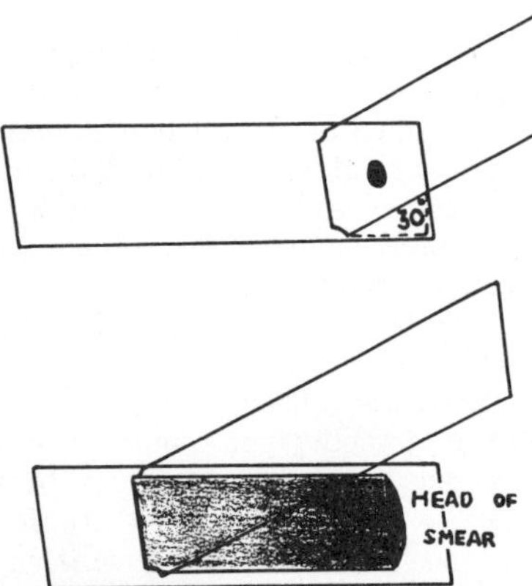

Figure 30–9 Technique of making slide blood smears.

50 to 50 alcohol-ether mixture. Dirty slides may be treated initially for 24 hours in dichromate cleaning solution (sodium or potassium dichromate, 100 g, dissolved in 750 mL of water to which 250 mL of concentrated H_2SO_4 has been added carefully). On removal from the dichromate mixture the slides are washed well in running tap water, then rinsed in distilled water, and stored in 95 or 100% alcohol. Before use they are dried and polished with a soft cloth. Some laboratories clean old blood smear slides (with warm soap and water, dichromate, and other agents), but this is a false economy and, in addition, the slides become scratched.

To make a blood smear on a slide, a drop of blood (approximately 1 mm in diameter, depending on how anemic the blood is) is placed about 1 or 2 cm from one end, and the slide is then laid on a bench top, drop uppermost. As spreader, another slide with an even, unchipped edge is taken and its corners are broken off so that the width of the spreading edge is about 4 mm less than the total slide width. This spreading edge is placed on the slide holding the drop of blood so that the spreading slide is held at an angle of about 30 degrees to the blood slide. The spreading slide's edge is then drawn backward until it just touches the drop of blood, which is in the acute angle. Immediately the drop of blood spreads along the edge of the spreading slide, which is then (still at angle of 30 degrees), smoothly, evenly, and quickly, pushed away from the drop of blood. The more rapid the movement, the thicker the resultant smear. Thickness is also affected by the angle at which the spreading slide is held; the bigger this angle, the thicker the smear.

Thick smears are desirable when searching for parasites (malaria, filaria, trypanosomes), but for routine hematological purposes moderately thin smears are desirable. Such smears will vary from frank overlap of the red blood cells in the head of the smear, through some overlap in the body, to separate red blood cells in the tail. The more slowly a smear is made, the thinner it will be and the greater will be the proportion of segmented leukocytes at the edges and in the tail section. In smears that are too thick the leukocytes appear small, proper staining is difficult, and cell identification may be impossible. In the best-made smears, however, because of differences in size, density, and other factors, the different leukocytes show certain tendencies of distribution in the smear. Thus, the larger monocytes and polymorphs tend to predominate at the margins and in the tail section of the smear, whereas the smaller lymphocytes are more evenly distributed and, by virtue of the preferential location of the other leukocytes, appear to predominate in the body of the smear. This unevenness of distribution does not occur in coverslip smears. Once made, all smears are allowed to dry in the air before staining. When dry, names of patients, numbers, and other identification may be written on the slide with a diamond marker, or on the smear with lead pencil.

Some common errors in making peripheral blood smears, and their causes, are illustrated in Figure 30–10.

Thick Blood Smear Preparation

The thick blood smear or film is widely used in the diagnosis of blood parasites, particularly malaria (see

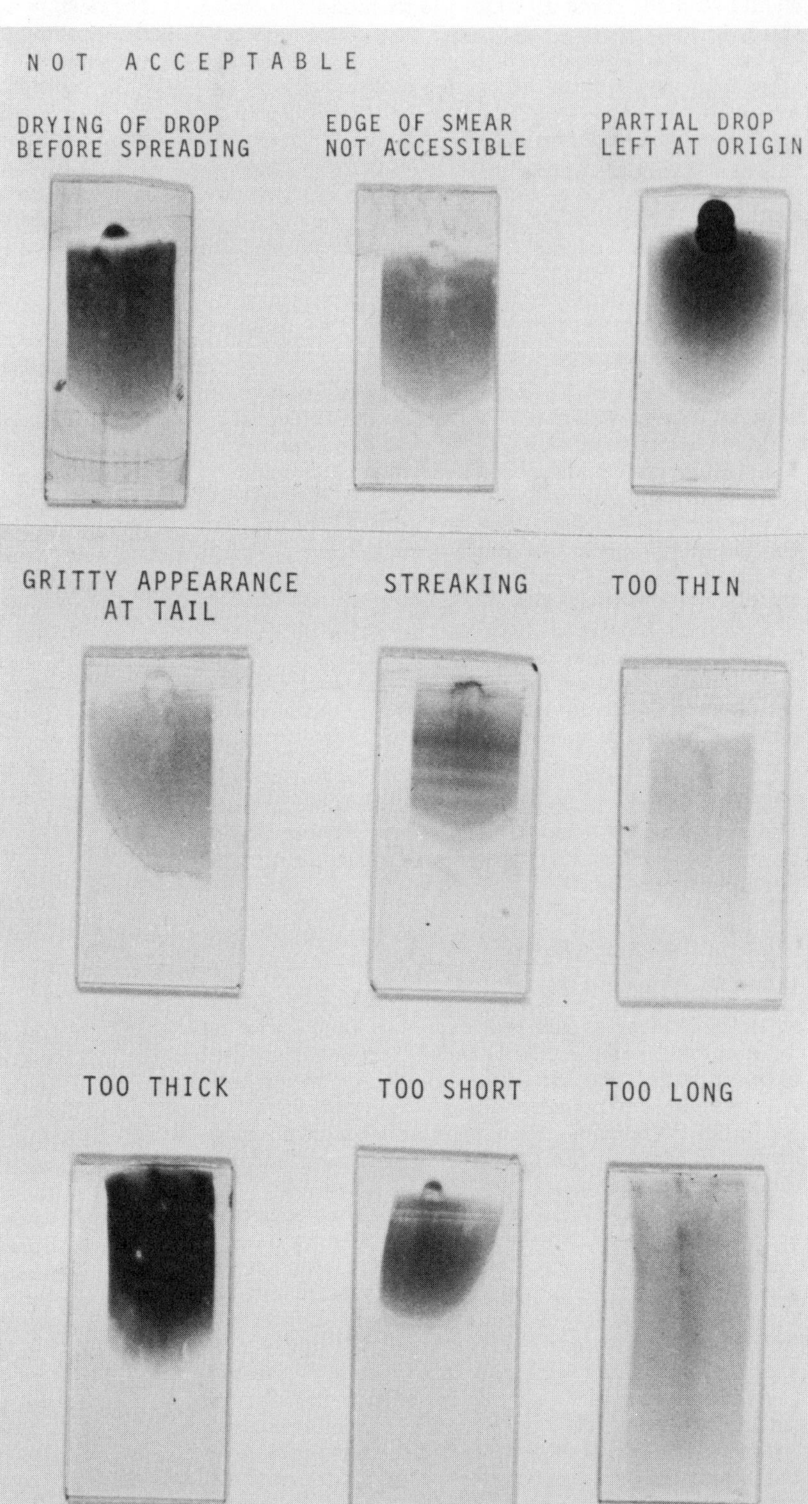

Figure 30–10 Some examples of unacceptable blood smears. The error in each is shown above the poorly made slide.

also p. 518). Some experience is required in the use of this method, which gives a higher percentage of positive diagnoses in much less time. Generally, the blood films should be made about 10 times the thickness of normal smears.

Place a good-sized drop of blood on a clean slide and spread it with the corner of another slide or with a glass rod until the hands of an average-size watch or small print are just visible through the blood smear; normally this corresponds to a drop spread over a circle of approximately 2 cm diameter. Allow the film to dry in the air, or in an incubator at 37°C.

The stains used employ the principle of destroying the red cells and staining leukocytes and parasites. The method using Giemsa's stain is very satisfactory, although Field's method has been described as a method of choice for many years.

1. Place the slides in 1 in 10 diluted Giemsa stain, using buffered distilled water at pH 6.8 as the diluent. ***Do not fix the films before immersion.*** **Leave for 30 to 60 minutes.**

2. Differentiate in distilled water for 3 to 10 minutes.

3. Air dry and examine.

A more sensitive technique is to make smears from concentrates prepared by saponin hemolysis.

1. To 2 mL of EDTA anticoagulated blood add 1.5 mL of 1% saponin in normal saline.

2. Mix for 30 seconds and centrifuge at 1500 G for 3 minutes. Transfer supernatant to a second tube.

3. Make smears from the remaining sediment.

4. Repeat the centrifugation process on the transferred supernatant for 20 minutes, and make smears from the resultant sediment.

The smears are stained with Wright's or Giemsa stain. The addition of the saponin solution is critical, and to avoid excessive treatment the use of a mixer-illuminator device is suggested.

BUFFY COAT SMEARS

Smears made from the buffy coat are extremely useful when the leukocyte count is decreased or when searching for abnormal cells, e.g., LE cells, megaloblasts, blast cells, or malignant cells and organisms. Plasma cells will be found in the peripheral blood in almost 50% of patients with multiple myeloma if buffy coat smears are examined carefully. To make such smears a number of methods are available:

Using Hematocrit. After performing a routine hematocrit the buffy coat can be removed either by using a Pasteur pipette for the Wintrobe tube method or by cutting the microhematocrit capillary tube just below the level of the buffy coat and packed red cell interface. In the latter instance the buffy coat layer is tapped onto a glass slide along with a small amount of plasma. Conventional preparations are made, ensuring that the smears are relatively thin in order to avoid excessive crowding of the leukocytes and that the buffy coat layer has been well mixed on the slide to avoid just one cell type being examined.

Using Leukocyte-Rich Plasma. Unless the worker is particularly skilled, the hematocrit method produces varying degrees of contamination with red cells. Therefore an alternate method of preparing buffy coat smears is to concentrate the leukocytes with dextran.

1. Add 1 mL of 6% dextran to 4 mL anticoagulated (EDTA, heparin, or defibrinated) blood.

2. Allow the red cells to sediment for 20 to 30 minutes. The dextran causes the erythrocytes to form rouleaux and the erythrocytes sediment rapidly, leaving the leukocytes suspended in the supernatant.

3. Transfer a sample of the supernatant into a microhematocrit tube, centrifuge as the hematocrit method, and make smears.

4. If the sedimentation rate of the blood is sufficiently increased the addition of dextran may be dispensed with, and the sample of blood allowed to separate by gravity. Inclining the specimen tube to 45° will hasten the procedure.

BONE MARROW SMEARS

Bone marrow smears are usually made at the bedside, directly after aspiration of the bone marrow. The most common fault of bone marrow smears is excess blood on the slide. This can be avoided by using the following technique.

1. Apparatus:
   (a) Clean, dust-free slides
   (b) Snap cap vial containing 10 drops of 1.8 per cent EDTA
   (c) Pasteur pipettes
   (d) Watchglass
   (e) Filter paper
2. Method:
   (a) At the bedside, 1 mL of aspirate is added to the EDTA vial, mixed well, and sent to the laboratory.
   (b) Using a Pasteur pipette (previously rinsed with EDTA solution), an aliquot of aspirate is transferred to a watchglass.
   (c) If the watchglass is gently tilted, blood will run to one side and marrow particles will be visible.
   (d) The particles are transferred to glass slides. Any excess blood can be gently blotted away using filter paper, taking care not to touch the marrow particles or contaminate one's hands with blood.
3. Three types of smear can be made.
   (a) Squash smear: squash the marrow particles with another slide and pull to the end of the marrow slide. This type of preparation often causes considerable cellular artifact.
   (b) Spread smear: the marrow particles are placed at one end of the slide and spread with another slide as for a blood smear. This allows excellent detail of individual cell morphology in the cell trails that are formed.
   (c) Coverslip preparations also may be made using the technique described for peripheral blood, and they produce excellent cellular morphology.
4. At least six smears should be made, since special stains are required and slides vary in their cellular content. The marrow in the EDTA vial can be used to prepare extra slides, if necessary, and histological sections.
5. Bone marrow smears must be completely dry before being stained, otherwise artifact will result. Allow

to dry at room temperature for one hour before staining.

6. Particles of aspirate can be fixed for histological study as follows:
   (a) Fold a Telfa pad (shiny side up) so that a pocket is formed, and place in a clean 10 mL vial.
   (b) Pour marrow aspirate into pocket.
   (c) Fold Telfa pad and secure with a paper clip. The marrow particles are now contained within the pad.
   (d) Add fixative (see p. 767) to the vial.
   The blood drains through the pad, leaving the marrow particles on the Telfa pad surface. After fixation, the pad is opened and the marrow particles collected for processing.

FIXATION OF SMEARS

All blood and marrow smears are allowed to dry in the air. With routine hematological stains fixation is accomplished in the 1-minute application of undiluted stain (by the absolute methyl alcohol used as solvent). When it is planned to use an aqueous or diluted stain, e.g., Giemsa, the air-dried smears must first be fixed by flooding for 3 to 5 minutes with absolute methyl or ethyl alcohol, or for 1 to 2 minutes in 1% formalin solution in 50% alcohol (2.5 mL commercial formalin, 50 mL alcohol, and 47.5 mL water). It should be remembered that alcohol absorbs water and so becomes a less effective fixing agent. If staining problems arise (particularly with bone marrow smears), improper fixation must be suspected. In the case of marrow smears that are excessively fatty, staining may be improved by preliminary 3 minute fixation in a 50-50 mixture of absolute alcohol and ether; then, after the smear is washed in water, prediluted Romanowsky stain is applied.

STAINING BLOOD AND BONE MARROW SMEARS

Principle

Acidic dyes unite with the basic components of the cells (cytoplasm). Conversely, basic stains are attracted to and combine with the acidic parts of the cell (nucleic acids and nucleoproteins of the nuclei). Eosin is an acidic dye; hence "eosinophilic" and "acidophilic" are used interchangeably in describing staining qualities of cell components.

History

Ehrlich was the first to use simple aniline dyes—at first in sequence and later as premixed acidic-basic stains (neutral dyes). In this way Ehrlich evolved his historic but misnamed "triacid" stain. This is a mixture of orange G, acid fuchsin, and methyl green (the three basic groups of the methyl green were believed to combine with the two acid dyes, hence the name). It is not used now.

Jenner (1889) found that the precipitate formed when eosin and methylene blue are mixed could be dissolved in methyl alcohol to form a useful stain combining certain properties of both parent dye-stuffs. Jenner's is very similar to the May-Grünwald stain.

Romanowsky (1890) found that when old (ripened and therefore "polychromed") methylene blue solution is mixed with eosin and the precipitate dissolved in methyl alcohol, a stain results that has a wider range than Jenner's stain, staining cell nuclei and platelet granules (which Jenner's mixture failed to stain).

Modern Romanowsky stains, for example, Wright's and Leishman's, are basically similar to Romanowsky's original method, the main difference being the method of polychroming the methylene blue.

ROMANOWSKY STAINS IN COMMON USE

Wright's Stain

This excellent blood stain is very widely used, especially on the American continent. In its preparation the methylene blue is polychromed by heating with sodium bicarbonate. It may be purchased in solution ready for use or as powder, 1.0 g of which is carefully dissolved in 600 mL of methyl alcohol.

Staining Method with Wright's Stain

1. Place the air-dried smear, film side up, on a staining rack (two parallel glass rods 5 cm apart).

2. Cover smear with undiluted stain and leave for 1 minute. The methyl alcohol fixes the smear.

3. Dilute with distilled water (approximately equal volume) until a metallic scum appears. Allow this diluted stain to act for 2½ to 5 minutes.

4. Without disturbing the slide, flood with distilled water and wash until thinner parts of film are pinkish red. It may frequently be found that distilled water does not give adequate differentiation. In this case a phosphate buffer (pH 6.4 to 6.5) should be used, at least for washing, but possibly also for diluting the stain (step 3).

Leishman's Stain

This is the stain most commonly used in the British Isles. In its preparation the methylene blue is polychromed by heating a 1% solution with 0.5% sodium carbonate at 65°C for 12 hours, after which a further ripening is allowed to proceed for 10 days before it is mixed with an equal volume of 0.1% eosin B. After this mixture has stood for 10 hours it is filtered and the precipitate is collected and washed with distilled water until no more color comes out in the washing. The precipitate is then dried and ground to a fine powder. To make up the stain a small knife-point of the powder at a time is ground well with 10 to 20 mL of absolute methyl alcohol and allowed to settle (1 minute), and the supernatant alcoholic solution of the stain is filtered into the stock bottle. This is repeated until 0.15 g has been dissolved in 100 mL of absolute methyl alcohol. This stain improves with age and is not satisfactory until a minimum of 3 weeks has elapsed after its preparation.

Staining with Leishman's Stain. The method is similar to that used with Wright's stain except for step 3. With Leishman's stain, dilution is effected with approximately 2 volumes of distilled water to 1 volume of stain (the best

guide is the appearance of the metallic scum). If a phosphate buffer is required for washing, one of pH 6.8 is best. This may be substituted for the distilled water when diluting the stain.

Comments on Wright's and Leishman's Stains

After staining, once the smears are washed to the desired degree of differentiation (usually up to 1 minute), they are stood on end to dry. The appearances of the cellular blood elements are quite similar with the two methods. Possibly, Leishman's stain gives better staining and contrast to the nuclear structures. With both, the red cells should be a soft pink; eosinophil granules, bright reddish pink; nuclei, varying shades of lilac to purple; and neutrophil granules, lilac in color.

If the film has a bright pink appearance to the naked eye, microscopically the erythrocytes are likely to appear vivid red, the eosinophil granules a pale incandescent pink, and nuclei a faint, washed-out blue color. This defect of staining may result from acidity of the stain or buffer or from excessive washing. Unripened Leishman's stain will also give pale nuclear staining.

Conversely, if the smear has a bluish to violet appearance on naked eye inspection, then microscopically the erythrocytes are likely to appear as muddy gray to purple, eosinophil granules have a gun-metal sheen, nuclei and polymorph granules are a deep blackish purple, and nuclear and other details are obscured. The cause of this unsatisfactory appearance may lie in overstaining, underwashing, or too alkaline a stain or wash. Washing with a buffer solution (pH 6.5 or 6.8) may improve the quality. Recently stained smears, especially those that are understained or appear washed-out (overdifferentiated), may be decolorized by a rinse in 95% alcohol, washed with distilled water, and restained.

Generally, it must be remembered that both Wright's and Leishman's stains are somewhat empirical mixtures of polychromed dyes, so that one batch may differ from another. Also, the "ripening" or polychroming continues in the stock solution of stain. If the stock stain solution becomes contaminated with water, poor results are to be expected. To avoid such poor results, it has been suggested that all films be fixed in pure methanol before staining.

Giemsa Stain

Instead of empirically polychromed dyes, this stain employs various azure compounds (thionine and its methyl derivatives) with eosin and methylene blue. It is best purchased commercially in solution. Smears must be prefixed for 3 minutes with methyl alcohol. They are dried and immersed in dilute Giemsa stain (1 volume stain plus 9 to 15 volumes of distilled water or buffer of pH 6.8) in Coplin jars for ¼ to 1 hour. They are then washed in distilled water and dried in air and are not mounted. This stain is not commonly used alone in hematology but is an excellent stain for inclusion bodies (e.g., inclusion conjunctivitis), but to show the inclusions well the smears should be allowed to stain in the dilute Giemsa stain for 12 to 18 hours.

By itself Giemsa stains red cells and neutrophil granules poorly, but azurophil granules (red) are well stained. In combination with Jenner or May-Grünwald stains it constitutes "panoptic" staining.

Panoptic Staining

This consists of the combination of a Romanowsky stain with another stain. Such a combination improves the staining of cytoplasmic granules, and other bodies. The two most popular methods employed are the Jenner-Giemsa and May-Grünwald-Giemsa methods.

Jenner-Giemsa Staining

1. Air-dried smears are fixed *10 to 20 minutes* in methyl alcohol.

2. Jenner's stain (another Romanowsky stain, i.e., eosin–methylene blue), best purchased commercially, is freshly diluted in the proportion of 1 volume of stain to 4 volumes of distilled water buffered to pH 6.8 (see end of this section). Smears are stained in this for 4 minutes.

3. The smears are not washed but are transferred to freshly diluted (same day) Giemsa stain (1 volume stain plus 9 volumes of buffered distilled water of pH 6.8) and allowed to stain for 7 to 10 minutes.

4. Wash quickly in three changes of buffered (pH 6.8) distilled water and place in a fourth change of buffered water for 3 to 12 minutes for differentiation to take place. Experience, gross appearance, and low-power microscopic examination will control the differentiation.

5. Stand on end to dry.

May-Grünwald-Giemsa

This gives slightly better results than the Jenner-Giemsa.

1. Air-dried smears are fixed 5 minutes in methyl alcohol.

2. Transfer to May-Grünwald stain (another Romanowsky dye) freshly diluted with 1 to 2 volumes of buffered (pH 6.8) distilled water. Leave 3 to 5 minutes.

3. Transfer, without washing, to fresh diluted Giemsa (see under Jenner-Giemsa) and allow to stain for 7 to 15 minutes.

4. Differentiate as for Jenner-Giemsa.

Formulas of Phosphate Buffers

(For Romanowsky and other stains.)

0.2 M KH_2PO_4 (2.722% w/v) (mL)	0.2 N NaOH (0.8% w/v) (mL)	pH
50	17.8	6.6
50	21.0	6.7
50	23.7	6.8
50	26.5	6.9
50	29.6	7.0

Alternatively, prepared capsules of buffer salts may be purchased from any reputable supply house. These are available over a wide pH range. For use, the contents of one capsule are dissolved in the stated amount (100 mL) of distilled water. (See also phosphate buffer, Appendix F, p. 822.)

Automated Staining

For large workloads, automatic stainers can process large numbers of smears with excellent results.

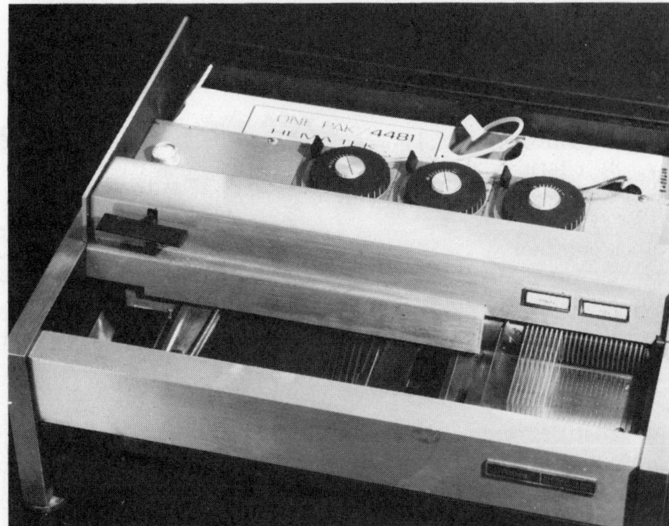

Figure 30–11 The Hematek stainer. (Ames Co., Elkhart, Ind. 46514, and Rexdale, Ont. M4C 1A7.)

Hematek* **(see Fig. 30–11).** This instrument stains smears by capillary action. The smear, moving face down along a stage, triggers delivery of reagents from a storage pack in the rear of the machine. There is a small space between the slide and the instrument stage, and the reagent fills this by capillary action. Staining and washing, followed by air drying, are accomplished before the slide drops off the stage into a collection drawer.

Shandon.† Slides held in a rack are automatically rotated around baths containing staining and buffering reagents. A significant advantage of this machine is that staining times can be varied by calibrating a timing dial, allowing greater flexibility in the use of different Romanowsky stains. The reagents have to be renewed regularly. The instrument has the advantage that it can easily be adapted for staining techniques other than Romanowsky staining, it uses laboratory prepared reagents, and it allows for complete adaptability in staining times.

CYTOCHEMISTRY

Although the examination of a properly prepared and stained peripheral blood film or bone marrow smear will produce an abundant amount of information, a number of special stains may be required for further elucidation. Such stains will be described here although they will be referred to again under specific disease headings. They apply mainly to the leukocytes. Control slides must always be used for specific staining reactions.

Peroxidase Reaction

The demonstration of peroxidase granules in certain leukocytes depends on their content of an iron porphyrin–containing enzyme (peroxidase) that promotes the oxidation of benzidine by hydrogen peroxide. Copper sulfate then forms a blue-green compound with the oxidized benzidine and thus renders the granules visible. The method of Kaplow is recommended because it uses benzidine dihydrochloride, which is less carcinogenic than benzidine.

Reagents

FIXATIVE SOLUTION	
95% ethanol	9 parts
40% formaldehyde	1 part
STAINING SOLUTION	
30% ethanol	100 mL
Benzidine dihydrochloride	0.3 g
3.8% zinc sulfate	1.0 mL
Sodium acetate	1.0 g
1N-sodium hydroxide	1.5 mL
3% hydrogen peroxide (10 vols)	0.7 mL

COUNTERSTAIN

Giemsa stain diluted 1 in 10 with buffered distilled water pH 6.8.

Method

1. Fix smears in the fixative solution for 60 seconds, then wash gently in running water.

2. Immerse smears for 30 seconds in a jar containing the staining solution.

3. Wash in running water and counterstain with dilute Giemsa for 10 to 15 minutes.

Results. Peroxidase activity is shown by the presence of green to dark blue granules in the cytoplasm. In some neutrophils and in eosinophils, rods and needle-like projections may be seen emanating from the cell margin. Basophils, lymphocytes, and erythroblasts are negative; monocytes show slight activity; myeloid cells (excepting basophils) are positive.

Leukocyte Alkaline Phosphatase

A number of techniques have been devised for this study. The method of Kaplow, modified by Hayhoe and Quaglino, has been selected because it gives reproducible results that facilitate subsequent scoring and reporting. The reaction depends on the hydrolysis of alpha-

*Ames, Elkhart, Ind. 46515, and Rexdale, Ont. M9W 1G6.

†Shandon Southern Instruments, Sewickley, Pa. 15143, and Johns Scientific, Toronto, Ont. M4C 1A7.

naphthyl phosphate by alkaline phosphatase to produce a colored precipitate with a diazotized amine.

Solutions

FIXATIVE

Absolute methanol	9 parts
40% formaldehyde	1 part

Store in freezing compartment of refrigerator.

BUFFER

Stock solution

2-amino-2-methyl propane-(1:3)-diol	10.5 g
Distilled water	500 mL

Working solution

Stock solution	25 mL
0.1 N HCl	5 mL
Distilled water	70 mL

Store at 4°C.

SUBSTRATE

Sodium alpha-naphthyl phosphate	20 mg
Brentamine-fast garnet (GBC) salt	20 mg
Working buffer (HCl in water as earlier)	20 mL

The substrate must be prepared fresh and filtered just before use.

COUNTERSTAIN. Mayer's aqueous hematoxylin, 2%.

Method

1. Using a fresh EDTA blood sample prepare blood smears, and immediately fix with the fixative for 30 seconds at 4°C.

2. Wash with distilled water and allow to air dry.

3. Leave in, or pour on, substrate and allow to remain for 10 minutes, then rinse in distilled water.

4. Counterstain for 10 to 15 minutes.

5. Drain off excess water and mount in an aqueous mounting medium (see p. 786).

Results. A red-brown precipitate in the cytoplasm indicates alkaline phosphatase activity. Control slides should preferably show high and low values, e.g., films from pregnant women and from patients with untreated myeloid leukemia. These may be stored in a fixed state for a considerable time. Small batches of slides should be stained at one time, since timing is important if scoring is to be used.

The slides should be scanned as soon as possible after preparation, since the stain tends to fade, particularly in weakly reacting cells.

Kaplow's scoring values for neutrophils are as follows:

0: Negative.
1: Barely visible diffuse staining with an occasional positively stained granule.
2: Diffuse staining with moderate granule formation.
3: Strong positive with numerous granules.
4: Very strong positive with much of the cytoplasm filled with precipitate.

One hundred neutrophils are examined, and the individual scores are added together. The normal range is from 15 to 100, although individual laboratories may seek a closer range with a carefully controlled method.

The leukocyte alkaline phosphatase test is useful in differentiating chronic myeloid leukemia from other conditions that may cause similar cellular morphology on Romanowsky staining.

Low score: Chronic myeloid leukemia.
High score: Bacterial infections, leukemoid reactions, myelofibrosis, polycythemia vera.

Periodic Acid–Schiff (PAS) Stain

Blood films should be fixed in methanol and brought to water before staining. The methodology is to be found in the histopathology section (p. 799). A positive reaction probably denotes the presence of glycogen.

PAS stain is used in differentiating acute lymphatic leukemia (ALL) from the other acute leukemias, because the blast cells of ALL usually contain large blocks of positive material in their cytoplasm.

Sudan Black

This material demonstrates lipid granules in leukocytes. It is interesting to note that there is a close correlation between sudanophilia (i.e., the presence of lipid material) and a positive reaction for peroxidase granules.

Reagents

SUDAN BLACK B. To 0.5 g Sudan black B add 100 mL absolute ethanol. Shake well over a period of 1 to 2 days until all the stain is dissolved and then filter.

SUFFER SOLUTION

Phenol (analytic-grade)	16 g
Ethanol	30 mL
0.3% aqueous $Na_2HPO^4 \cdot 12\ H_2O$	100 mL

Method. Just before use, add 60 mL of the stain to 40 mL of the buffer, mix, and filter. This is the working solution.

1. Fix air-dried films in formalin vapor for 10 minutes.

2. Place films in the working solution for 30 minutes at 37°C.

3. Wash with absolute ethanol.

4. Wash with distilled water.

5. Counterstain, if desired, with 1 in 20 Giemsa's stain for 1 hour.

6. Mount with coverglass or examine directly.

Results. Lipid particles appear dense black.

Stain for Iron Granules (Hemosiderin)

The Gomori modification of the Perls' Prussian blue reaction for hemosiderin (see p. 805) is very suitable. The blood smears are fixed in methanol and air dried before treatment with potassium ferrocyanide solution.

THE DIFFERENTIAL LEUKOCYTE COUNT

Principle

This consists of the enumeration of the relative proportions (percentages) of the various types of white blood cells as seen in stained films of peripheral blood.

Only well-made smears should be used. If the smear is too thick, differentiation of cell types, especially monocytes from lymphocytes, will be difficult or impossible. If it is too thin, the majority of polymorphs and monocytes will be located at the edges and tail; the same maldistribution occurs if a chipped or jagged-edged spreader has been used.

First, the smear should be surveyed with a dry objective (× 20 objective with × 10 or 12 eyepieces) to ascertain the quality of the smear and to assess the evenness of distribution of leukocytes. With this magnification the experienced observer can pick out abnormal cells, e.g., plasma cells, megaloblasts, normoblasts, and blast cells. Although many workers prefer to use a high-resolution, low-magnification oil immersion objective (× 54 apochromatic), a × 40 dry objective with a mounted smear provides excellent magnification for the differential count. Large numbers of cells may be quickly counted. Any abnormality in morphology can be further evaluated with higher magnification. Unmounted smears collect dust and tend to fade on storage. Smears can either be cover-slipped or dipped in a solution of Diatex* and toluene. The latter method is rapid and is highly recommended for routine scanning of peripheral blood smears, provided that adequate ventilation in the preparation area is available.

The differential count may be performed in one of two ways:

1. All the cells in a longitudinal strip from head to end or tail of the smear are counted. If enough cells are not found in this, a second strip may be counted.

2. In the exaggerated battlement method, one begins at one edge of the smear and counts all cells, advancing inward to one-third the width of the smear, then on a line parallel to the edge, then out to the edge, then along the edge for an equal distance before turning inward again.

In either method, ideally 200 cells should be counted, but certainly not fewer than 100.

Error in Differential Count. When 200 cells are counted, because of various factors (e.g., distribution), the error is of the order of ±7% (±10% if only 100 cells are counted). In general the greater the number of leukocytes counted, the smaller the error.

Automated Leukocyte Differential Counters

Two different principles are used in the current generation of automated differential counters: cytochemistry and pattern recognition.

Cytochemistry. The Hemalog D† uses peroxide, esterase, and alcian blue staining to differentiate the different type of leukocytes as shown below:

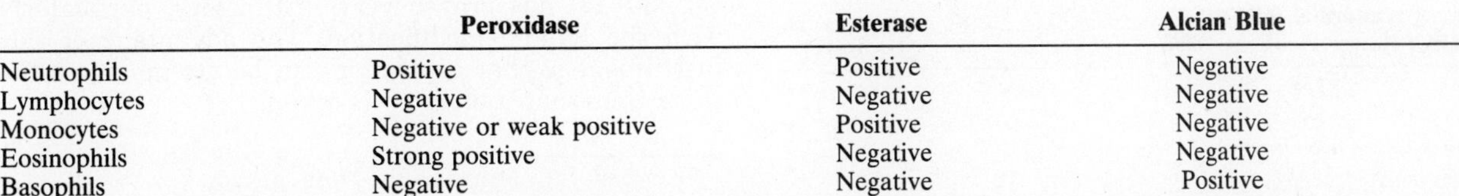

	Peroxidase	Esterase	Alcian Blue
Neutrophils	Positive	Positive	Negative
Lymphocytes	Negative	Negative	Negative
Monocytes	Negative or weak positive	Positive	Negative
Eosinophils	Strong positive	Negative	Negative
Basophils	Negative	Negative	Positive

The instrument is programmed to recognize these staining reactions, whereas the unstained lymphocyte is measured by electronic sizing. Immature cells are interpreted as large unclassified cells (LUC), and a blood smear made automatically by the instrument has to be examined for satisfactory identification. The differential count is performed on 10,000 cells, which permits good precision.

Pattern Recognition Differential Counters. Several instruments using this principle are available.* The morphological characteristics of leukocytes are programmed into a computer, and the machine recognizes them in turn as they are viewed through a scanner. The differential count is performed on 100 leukocytes, whereas cells that the instrument is unable to classify can be recalled and viewed by the operator on a microscope or monitor.

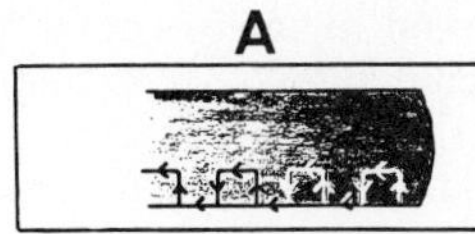

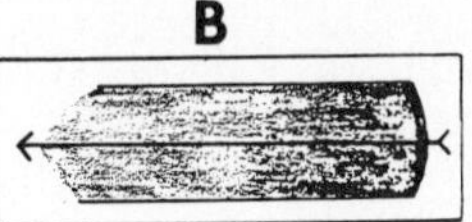

Figure 30–12 Techniques of performing differential leukocyte counts.

Normal Adult Leukocyte Differential Ranges

	Absolute Numbers/10^9/L			
	Minimum	Average	Maximum	Percentage
Total WBC Count	4.0	7.0–8.0	10.0	
Neutrophils	3.0	4.0–4.5	7.0	50–70%
Lymphocytes	1.5	2.0	3.0	25–40%
Monocytes	0.2	0.4	0.8	3–8%
Eosinophils	0.05	0.2	0.4	1–4%
Basophils	0	0.025	0.1	0–1%

Age Variations

At the outset it must be stressed that *the* important consideration is the absolute number of any type of cell. Thus, the fact that a patient may have 60% polymorphs is of little use by itself: he may have 60% of a total leukocyte count of 8.0 × 10^9/L, i.e., 4.8 × 10^9/L neutrophils, which is quite normal; but if he has 60% neutrophil polymorphs in a total count of only 3.0 × 10^9/L, then he has granulocytopenia (1.8 × 10^9/L neutrophils), which is abnormal.

At birth there is a polymorphonuclear leukocytosis

*Canadian Laboratory Supplies, Toronto, Ont. M8Z 2H4.
†Technicon, Tarrytown, N.Y. 10591.

*Honeywell, Inc., Hopkins, Minn. 55343. Geometric Data, Wayne, Pa. 19087, and Mississauga, Ont.

(and a few myelocytes may be seen in smears of peripheral blood), but this falls to about 5.0 × 10^9/L neutrophils after 7 to 14 days and thereafter remains at a level that is substantially the same as the normal adult value. On the other hand, lymphocytes increase in the first 2 weeks after birth, at the end of which time they reach a maximum value of about 8.0 to 10.0 × 10^9/L. From then on the number of lymphocytes in the peripheral blood gradually falls, and at about 4 years the number of lymphocytes and neutrophil polymorphs are approximately equal, at 4.0 × 10^9/L of each type (usually about 40% of each type in an average normal white cell count of 10.0 × 10^9/L at 4 years of age). After this—from 4 to 12 years—there is a slow, slight further fall in the number of lymphocytes and an approximately parallel increase in the number of neutrophil polymorphs until normal adult figures are reached at about 12 years of age. During these periods there is also a qualitative change in lymphocytes; the number of large lymphocytes, which predominate at first, gradually falls until the small adult-type lymphocyte predominates at 12 years. Monocytes are increased in the first 2 weeks of life and, thereafter, though reduced from the neonatal values, they remain above the normal adult figure for the first few years of life (range up to 1.0 × 10^9/L). Eosinophils and basophils undergo no significant numerical changes with age.

General Examination of Blood Smear

Each technologist must learn to observe all elements of the blood smear while performing the differential count. One must form the habit of checking the following points:

Erythrocytes. Size, shape, and degree of hemoglobinization must be observed. Is there *significant* anisocytosis, or poikilocytosis, hypochromia, microcytosis, macrocytosis, or apparent hyperchromia? Is there apparent or obvious increase in the proportion of polychromatic red cells? Are spherocytes present? Do any red cells show basophilic stippling? Are normoblasts present, and if so, how many per 100 WBCs? If normoblasts are present, the leukocyte count must be corrected. Automated cell counters count all nucleated cells and do not discriminate between leukocytes and normoblasts. The correction can be made as follows:

$$\text{Leukocyte count} = L \times 10^9/\text{L}$$
$$\text{Normoblasts} = \text{N}/100 \text{ Leukocytes}$$
$$\text{Corrected leukocyte count} = L \times \frac{100}{100 + N} \times 10^9/\text{L}$$

It is highly desirable that a uniform grading system be adopted for assessing changes in erythrocyte morphology. The following system enables standard reporting by individual technologists and allows for effective quality control using appropriate abnormal peripheral blood smears.

Average Number of Abnormal RBCs/ High Power Field (× 1000)	Score
3–6	+
7–10	+ +
11–20	+ + +
> 20	+ + + +

Platelets. Are they present in roughly normal proportions (3 to 8 platelets per 100 RBCs)? Reduction in platelets in a smear may result from the manner in which it was made, but their absence or considerable reduction in a satisfactory preparation must make one suspect thrombocytopenia. Do the platelets present look normal, or are many giant or bizarre forms seen?

Leukocytes. Are the leukocytes mature, immature, or atypical? An assessment should be made of the average number of lobes shown by the polymorphs, and also whether toxic granulation, vacuolation, and so forth are seen. Does the number of WBCs seen in the smear tally with total count?

Average Number of Leukocytes or Platelets/High Power Field (×1000)	Leukocyte Count × 10^9/L	Platelet Count × 10^9/L
1–4	2.0– 8.0	30–60
4–6	8.0–12.0	60–90
6–10	12.0–20.0	90–150
10–20	20.0–40.0	150–300

The report on the smear should include a brief mention of the appearance of the red cells, white cells, and platelets with a note on any *significant* deviation from normal. In this connection, the inexperienced tend to see far too much anisocytosis and poikilocytosis.

BONE MARROW EXAMINATION

Bone Marrow Aspiration and Biopsy

A wide variety of conditions require examination of the bone marrow for both assessment of cellular morphology and changes in microstructure. To these ends, aspiration and biopsy of marrow is a common procedure.

The sites for bone marrow aspiration are usually confined to the sternum, iliac crests, and spinous processes in the adult; the anteromedial surface of the tibia is the site of choice in the infant. Using a sterile technique and appropriate local anesthesia, the bone marrow cavity is entered using a suitable needle (see Fig. 30–13). Using minimal suction, 0.2 mL to 0.5 mL of bone marrow is aspirated, using a well-fitting 1 mL syringe. Use of greater suction or taking of larger amounts will only cause dilution and distortion of the bone marrow cells. The smears are prepared as described on p. 684.

Bone marrow biopsy is usually indicated when material cannot be obtained by aspiration (a "dry tap" as often seen in aplastic anemia, myelofibrosis, and so forth), or when a specific need for bone marrow structure is required (the lipid storage diseases or malignant conditions constitute such a reason). A closed biopsy technique is preferred to the open variety, and the posterior iliac crest is the site of choice. A number of needles and trephine devices are available to obtain a core of bone marrow. The Jamshidi biopsy needle* (see Fig. 30–14) has proved very satisfactory, particularly with the handle modification. The advantage of this instrument is that aspiration can be attempted at the same time that the biopsy is taken.

---

*Kormed, Inc., Minneapolis, Minn. 55420.

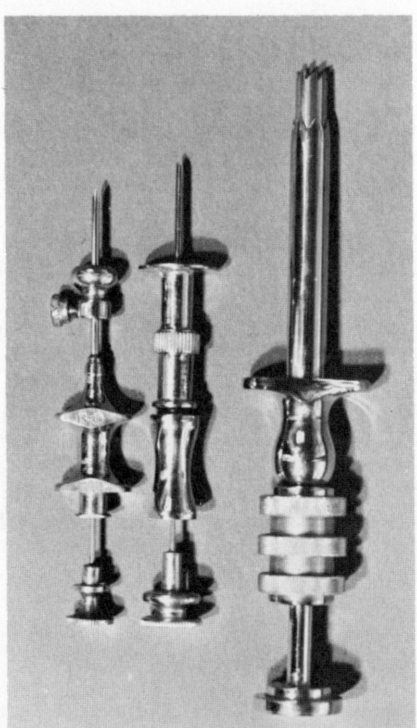

Figure 30–13 Types of bone marrow biopsy apparatus. From left to right: Salah, Klima, and trephine. Approximately natural size.

Because normal marrow cells tend to clump together and the factor of dilution with peripheral blood is not under control, quantitative counts are not usually performed on aspirated bone marrow. The degree of cellularity can be assessed within very broad limits as increased, normal, or reduced, by inspection of stained bone marrow smears. Sectioned material gives a better evaluation. Some large cells such as megakaryocytes tend to resist aspiration, or become ruptured in smearing, and appear generally in disproportionate numbers in the tail of the film.

For these reasons, and because of the naturally variegated pattern of the bone marrow, differential counts indicate so wide a range of normality that minor deviations are difficult to establish.

If counts are desired, then at least 500 cells should be counted in a highly cellular and well stained area. More reliable results may be obtained in areas occurring in the tails of smeared marrow fragments.

It is important to scan the film under low power before attempting detailed examination, to assess cellularity and to note any aggregations of atypical or abnormal cells or parasites.

Normal Ranges for Bone Marrow Differentiation

Cell	%
Reticulum cell	0.1–2.0
Hemocytoblast	0.1–1.0
Myeloblast	0.1–3.5
Promyelocyte	0.5–5.0
Myelocyte	
Neutrophil	5–20
Eosinophil	0.1–3.0
Basophil	0–0.5
Metamyelocyte	10–30
Polymorphonuclears	
Neutrophil	7–25
Eosinophil	0.2–3
Basophil	0–0.5
Lymphocyte	5–20
Monocyte	0–2.0
Megakaryocyte	0.1–0.5
Plasma cells	0.1–1.5
Normoblasts	
Polychromatic	2–20
Orthochromic	2–10

Myeloid-Erythroid Ratio

The myeloid-erythroid ratio expresses the ratio of the total myeloid cells to the nucleated erythroid cells. It is influenced by contamination with peripheral blood. Normally it is 3 or 4 to 1, but with contamination, it may be as high as 5 to 1 and still be regarded as normal.

TESTS FOR HETEROPHIL ANTIBODIES

Principle

Infectious mononucleosis (described on pp. 544 and 657) is caused by the Epstein-Barr virus (EB virus), a member of the herpes group of viruses. Antibodies to the virus are produced early in the course of the disease and can be detected by complement fixation tests or immunofluorescent techniques. The demonstration of these antibodies is beyond the scope of most routine laboratories but, fortunately, other antibodies are associated with infectious mononucleosis and are easily detected.

An antibody is produced that reacts with the cells of sheep and horses. Since it reacts with cells of another species of animal, it is known as a heterophil antibody. It has a wide thermal range but reacts best at 37°C.

Heterophil antibodies in low titer (up to 56) are present in the sera of most normal people and are known

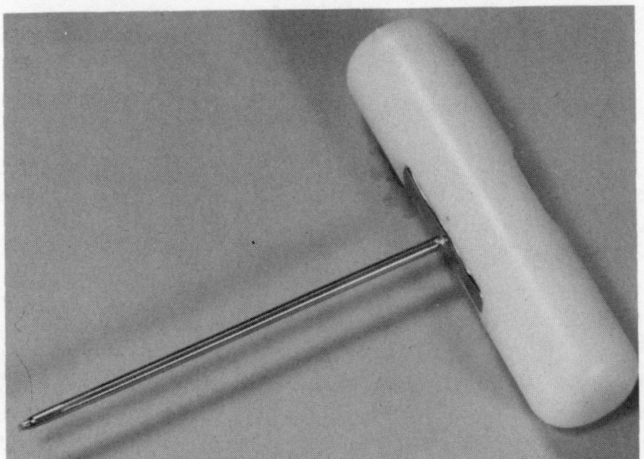

Figure 30–14 Jamshidi bone marrow biopsy needle with modified handle attached.

as Forssman antibodies. They resemble the antibodies found in infectious mononucleosis in that they agglutinate sheep erythrocytes, but they differ from them in that they are absorbed by an emulsion of guinea pig kidney, which is rich in Forssman antigen, and are not absorbed by ox cells (poor in Forssman antigen). A nonspecific rise in titer of Forssman antibodies may occur in some infections and after various immunizations.

In serum sickness (sensitization to animal—usually horse—serum) a further type of sheep cell agglutinating antibody is found and may be of high (over 224) titer. However, this again is distinguishable from the antibody of infectious mononucleosis by its being absorbed by guinea pig kidney, and from Forssman antibodies by being absorbed by ox cells.

Under normal circumstances, a screening test for heterophil antibodies is performed. Horse cells are more sensitive to the heterophil antibody than sheep cells, and screening tests that utilize horse cells are available (see p. 544).

Another antibody, anti i, may increase in strength in infectious mononucleosis. In a minority of patients, a hemolytic anemia may result. The identification of anti i is described on p. 571.

LUPUS ERYTHEMATOSUS (LE) CELL PHENOMENON

Principle

Systemic lupus erythematosus affects women most commonly and is characterized by a skin rash, arthralgia, fever, renal, cardiac, and vascular lesions, anemia, leukopenia, and often thrombocytopenia. There is a factor in the serum that has the ability to cause depolymerization of the nuclear chromatin of polymorphonuclear leukocytes, and this depolymerized material is subsequently phagocytosed by an intact polymorph, giving rise to the "LE cell." This antinuclear material may be found in other collagen disorders, in some cases of rheumatoid arthritis, and in some cases of chronic discoid lupus erythematosus, which is a relatively benign form of the disease limited to the skin. The serum factor is an immunoglobulin and may be of the IgG, IgM, or IgA class, or combinations of them. IgG is most commonly present. There does not appear to be any relationship between the immunoglobulin class and the clinical status.

Demonstration of LE Cells

A variety of methods exist, all of which can be used. The rotary technique is considered the most sensitive cellular technique. In practice, most laboratories perform a latex test and antiDNA antibody test (see pp. 532 and 536). If these are both negative, the LE cell preparation is not performed (vide infra).

Clotted Blood. This is the simplest method and gives good results. 10 mL of clotted blood is placed in the water bath at 37°C for 1 to 2 hours. After incubation the supernatant and loose cells are withdrawn (the clot may first have to be "ringed" or separated) and buffy coat smears made (p. 684).

Alternatively, the whole clotted specimen after incubation may be mashed through a fine wire sieve and buffy coat smears made from the resultant cell suspension.

Defibrinated Blood. Defibrinated blood gives good preparations. The blood is defibrinated immediately after withdrawal and the blood incubated for 2 hours at 37°C. Smears are made as with clotted blood.

Citrated or Heparinized Blood. Citrated or heparinized blood may be used and incubated, as for clotted and defibrinated blood. The preparations obtained in this manner are satisfactory, but inferior to those from clotted or defibrinated blood. Also, heparin tends to produce bluish staining.

Incubated Serum. The patient's serum may be incubated with washed normal leukocytes, even after storage of the serum at −20°C for months.

Rotary Method. Five glass beads 3 mm in diameter are added to a heparinized sample of blood. The tube is then rotated at 50 rpm for 30 minutes at 37°C. Buffy coat smears are subsequently prepared.

The LE Cell

This is usually a neutrophil polymorph (occasionally a monocyte or eosinophil) that has ingested the altered nucleus of another polymorph. The bulk of the cell is occupied by a spherical, homogeneous mass that stains purplish-brown. The lobes of the polymorph are usually seen at the periphery of the mass. The smears, especially their edges (LE cells are most numerous at the edges and end of the smear), are searched and a minimum of 500 polymorphs are counted before a negative result is given. Frequently, dead nuclei will be seen lying free; if numerous, these may heighten suspicions, but they are never diagnostic. Occasionally a group of polymorphs will collect around altered nuclear material and will form a "rosette."

With the rotary technique, free extracellular altered nucleoprotein may be seen and this again will increase the suspicion of LE cells being present. LE cells must be differentiated from "tart" cells, which are usually monocytes that have phagocytosed another whole cell or nucleus (often a lymphocyte). The ingested nuclear material is well preserved in contrast to the LE cell inclusion body, and may be found in normal people. Its significance, if any, is unknown.

Sensitivity and Specificity of LE Tests

The simplest test to perform is the latex nucleoprotein test. This test is specific when positive, but will detect only 45 to 50% of possible positives. The LE cell test is moderately sensitive and specific but both false positive and false negative results can occur. Attention to technique is important and serial examinations should be performed before a patient can be considered negative for LE. The fluorescent technique for antinuclear antibody (ANA) is a highly suitable screening procedure because of its sensitivity. It does, however, lack specificity, and positive results can be obtained in other autoimmune and collagen diseases. A negative ANA virtually eliminates a diagnosis of LE (see p. 532).

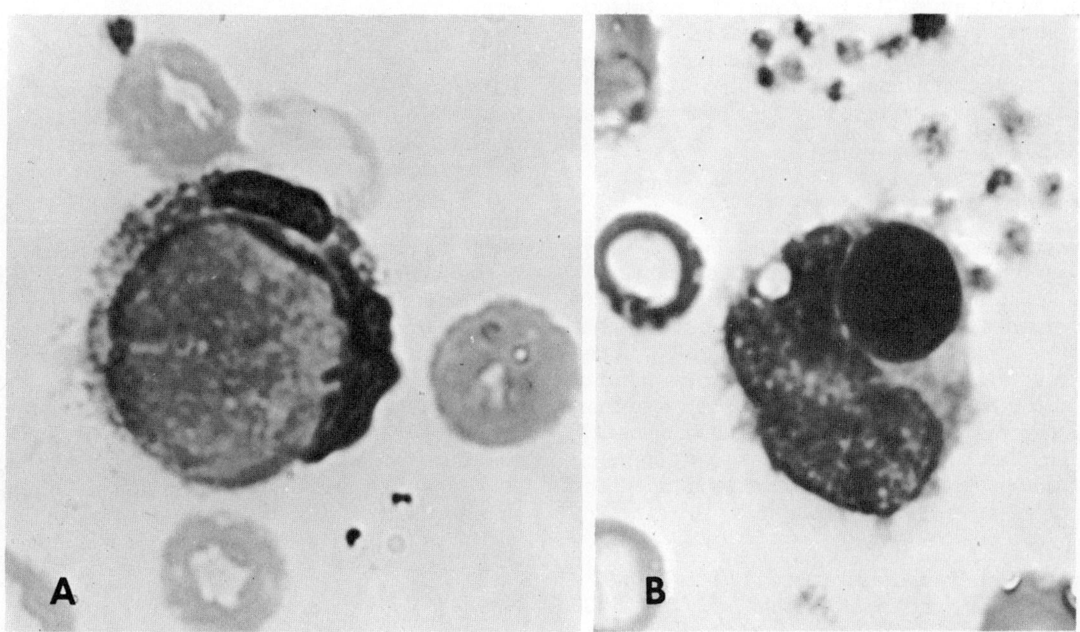

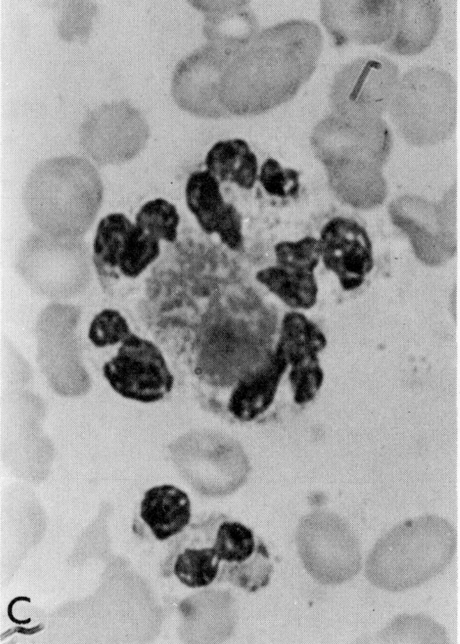

Figure 30–15 **A,** Lupus erythematosus (LE) cell. Preparation made from a patient with disseminated lupus erythematosus. The nuclear lobes of the segmented neutrophil are displaced to the edge of the cell by the phagocytosed amorphous mass of altered chromatin. × 2250. **B,** "Tart" cell, monocyte containing ingested small lymphocyte; only the nucleus of the latter is visible. × 2000. **C,** Lupus rosette. A group of polymorphs is seen surrounding and demonstrating efforts at phagocytosis of a central mass of amorphous nuclear material. Such groups are seen more rarely than the usual LE cell, but occasionally, in some cases, they are common. Wright's stain × 1500.

ERYTHROCYTE SEDIMENTATION RATE (ESR)

Principle

This simple test is universally used as an index of the presence of active diseases of many types. The test depends on the fact that in blood to which anticoagulant has been added, the red corpuscles sediment until they form a packed column in the lower part of the tube or container. The rate of this process depends on a number of factors, chief among which are (1) rouleaux formation, (2) concentration of fibrinogen in the plasma, and (3) concentration of alpha and beta globulins in the plasma.

Rouleaux Formation

Erythrocytes sediment in fluid blood because their density is greater than that of plasma. The buoyancy-producing action of the plasma opposes this tendency of the red corpuscles to settle, and this force is proportional to the surface area of the corpuscles. If a number of red corpuscles aggregate in the form of a cylindrical column, the area of the resultant "rouleaux" is much less than that of the sum of the areas of the constituent corpuscles. The result is that the action of the plasma in opposing sedimentation is greatly reduced and settling of the erythrocytes is enhanced. For example,

Surface area of individual average red cell: 140 μm^2
Surface area of 10 individual average red cells: 1400 μm^2
Surface area of rouleaux of 10 average red cells

$= \pi \times D \times H + 2\pi R_2$
$= 3.14 \times 7.2 \times 22 + 2 \times 50\ \mu m^2$
$= 498 + 100 = 598\ \mu m^2$

when D = diameter of column,
H = height of column,
R = radius of column.

This tendency to rouleaux formation is the greatest single factor leading to an increase in sedimentation rate, and itself is promoted by colloidal changes in the plasma resulting mainly from increase in concentrations of fibrinogen and of alpha and beta globulins. These factors also lead to increased viscosity of the plasma so that, broadly speaking, plasma viscosity parallels the ESR except when the former is very great.

The alignment of the sedimenting column is an important factor. If the tube is inclined from the vertical position, the ESR will be accelerated, since the RBCs have a shorter distance through which to settle and the "up-current" of plasma is along the long slope, thus bypassing the sedimenting RBCs. For this reason it is most important that the tube be held absolutely vertically, and sedimentation racks are designed for this. Extremes of temperature should be avoided.

Anemia affects the sedimentation rate, increasing the ESR by promoting rouleaux, for example. Many methods and nomograms have been devised for correcting this effect, but none is entirely free of objections. Characteristically, increased red cell mass will retard the sedimentation rate, e.g., polycythemia.

Effect of Fibrinogen Concentration

The ESR shows a linear relationship to the concentration of fibrinogen except in chronic liver disease, e.g., cirrhosis; but here the reduced albumin and increased globulins play a part in the increased ESR found and, with other factors, are more than sufficient to offset the effect of the lowered fibrinogen levels.

Alpha and Beta Globulins

Plasma albumin retards sedimentation of RBCs. In most acute infections plasma albumin tends to be somewhat reduced, whereas alpha globulins and fibrinogen are increased, and this combination enhances the ESR. Gamma globulins have little effect on the ESR. The combinations of lowered plasma albumin and increased globulins (relative and absolute) found in nephrosis and in cirrhosis account for the major part of the increase in ESR noted in these conditions. In multiple myeloma the ESR is frequently enormously increased and, indeed, spontaneous rouleaux formation may render the preparation of good blood smears impossible. Though the plasma protein picture is extremely variable in multiple myeloma, generally there is a great increase in gamma globulin fractions with moderate increase of alpha and beta globulins and a slight decrease in albumin. The changes in the latter three fractions probably account for the raised ESR found in multiple myeloma.

Stages in ESR

There are three stages in erythrocyte sedimentation: (1) an initial period of a few minutes during which rouleaux formation takes place; (2) a period of approximately ½ to 2 hours depending on the length of the tube, during which settling or sedimentation occurs at a more or less constant rate; and (3) a slower rate of fall during which packing of the sedimented red cell column occurs. The second is the most significant phase. ESR preparations should preferably be set up within 2 hours of collection, but under extenuating circumstances may be refrigerated overnight at 4°C before testing.

Methods

Generally the main methods are:
1. Wintrobe.
2. Westergren.

Wintrobe Method

Blood is collected with EDTA. It is important here as in any hematological procedure that the correct amount of blood be taken to ensure a constant anticoagulant-blood ratio.

Enough blood (1 mL) to fill a Wintrobe hematocrit tube is drawn into a Pasteur pipette having a long (15 cm) stem. The Wintrobe tube is then filled from the bottom up (so as to exclude any air bubbles) to the 100 mm mark. The tube is placed in the support in an exactly vertical position, and the time is noted. At the end of 1 hour the ESR is read as the length of the plasma column above the cells.

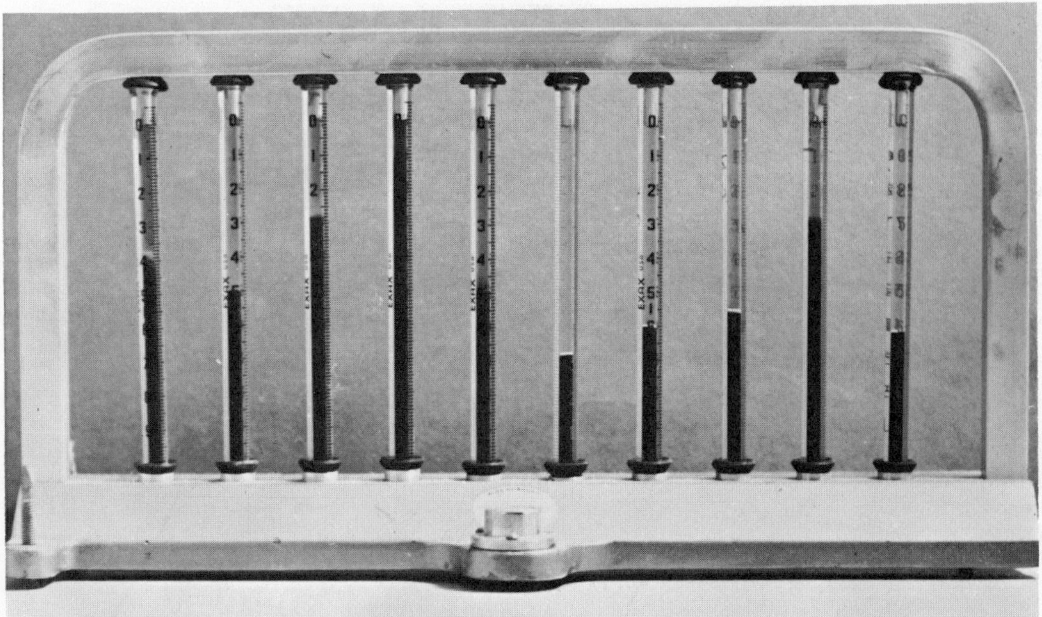

Figure 30–16 Wintrobe erythrocyte sedimentation rate tubes and stand. Some of the tubes have been centrifuged in order to show the markings and the buffy coats.

Normal Values (Wintrobe) of ESR

	Range (mm)	Average (mm)
Men	0–7	4
Women	0–15	10
Children	1–15	5–10

Advantages. The Wintrobe method is simple; it requires a small amount of blood; there is no dilution. If a disposable tube is used, contamination with extraneous blood is negligible. With the same preparation, once the ESR has been read, the hematocrit value can be determined; microbilirubin determination can be made on the supernatant plasma, and smears of buffy coat can be made. Correction for anemia can be applied from the hematocrit value, although this is not always a reliable procedure.

Disadvantages. Because of the short column and the choice of anticoagulant, the Wintrobe method is not quite so sensitive an index of systemic disease activity as the Westergren method.

Westergren Method

This is the reference method for the ESR (International Committee for Standardization in Hematology, 1973).

Anticoagulant

Trisodium citrate dihydrate ($Na_3C_6H_5O_7{\cdot}2H_2O$)	30.88 g
Distilled water	1 liter

Four volumes of blood are added to 1 volume of anticoagulant. Suitable evacuated tubes are available. If EDTA is used as an anticoagulant, the blood must be diluted with trisodium citrate before testing (i.e., 4 volumes of blood plus 1 volume of trisodium citrate). The standard Westergren tube is 300 mm in length, graduated from 0 to 200 mm, and has a 2.55 mm bore.

Procedure. The test should be commenced within two hours of taking the blood sample. The sample can be refrigerated, in which case the maximum time interval before testing is six hours. The blood-citrate mixture is mixed and drawn up to the 0 mark of a Westergren tube. It is placed in a rack in strict vertical position at room temperature. Direct drafts, sunlight, and vibration must be avoided. After one hour, the distance from the surface meniscus to the top of the column of sedimenting red cells where full density is apparent is measured and recorded in millimeters. Figure 30–17 shows a disposable Westergren system that overcomes the need to use an oral method to draw up the blood column.* Such a modification is considered mandatory if the transmission of hepatitis B is to be avoided.

Normal Westergren Ranges

	ESR Ranges	
Sex	1 Hour	2 Hours
Man	3–5 mm	7–15 mm
Woman	4–7 mm	12–17 mm

Advantages. This is probably the most sensitive ESR method for serial study of chronic disease, e.g., tuberculosis.

Disadvantages. The method requires a large amount of blood and involves dilution with its attendant sources of error.

*Dispette, Guest Medical and Dental Products A. G., 6301 Zug. Switzerland; distributed in Canada by Esbe Laboratory Supplies, Downsview, Ont. M3J 2T8.

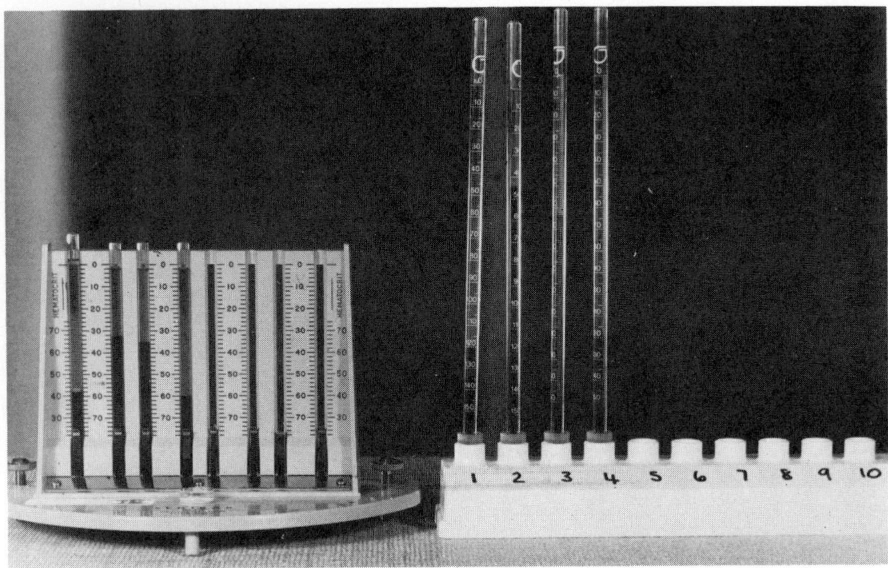

Figure 30–17 Wintrobe *(left)* and Westergren (Dispette) sedimentation rate apparatus. Note that the Westergren tube No. 1 test is technically unacceptable because of its lack of vertical position.

Sources of Error

1. Sedimentation tube not vertically aligned.
2. Vibration in the testing area. Centrifuges should not be in an area where sedimentation tests are being performed.
3. Variations in temperature.
4. Hemolysis in sample.
5. Clots in blood sample.

General Application of ESR

The chief applications and value of the ESR are:

1. As an indication of the presence of active but obscure disease processes, e.g., tuberculosis, subacute bacterial endocarditis, ankylosing spondylitis, disseminated lupus erythematosus, rheumatic carditis, malignancy, and so forth. It should be noted that the ESR may not be elevated in malignancy, but it is generally rapid when metastases or breakdown and inflammation of tumor are present.
2. As a serial control on the activity of chronic disease, e.g., tuberculosis, rheumatic carditis, rheumatoid arthritis, and ankylosing spondylitis.

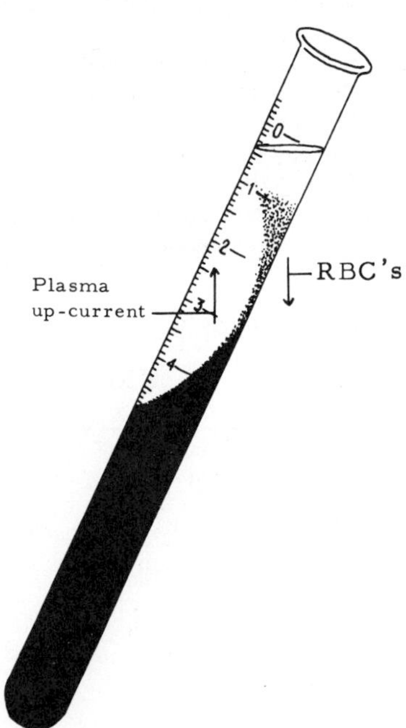

Figure 30–18 The effect of tilting sedimentation tube from the vertical.

RED CELL STUDIES

HEMOGLOBIN ESTIMATION

PRIMARY METHODS OF ESTIMATION OF HEMOGLOBIN

There are two primary methods for the estimation of hemoglobin:

Blood Oxygen Capacity. This measures the functional hemoglobin only and is inaccurate in that 2 to 12% of the normal adult hemoglobin may be of an inactive form (i.e., unable to take up oxygen), which can be regenerated and therefore should be measured.

Blood Iron Content. For all practical purposes the total iron content of blood may be regarded as being bound to hemoglobin, the serum iron level as being relatively small. All other methods require standardization by one of these methods.

Reference Values

1. Hemoglobin oxygen capacity = 1.34 mL per g (Hüfner's factor).
2. Hemoglobin iron content = 0.347 g per 100 g of hemoglobin.
3. Approximately 34% of the normal red cell is hemoglobin.
4. Approximately 85% of the dry weight of the red cell is hemoglobin.

Conversion Factors

1. $\frac{\text{Oxygen capacity in mL/dL of blood}}{1.34} = \text{g Hb/dL}$

2. $\frac{\text{Blood iron content in mg/dL}}{3.47} = \text{g Hb/dL}$

Blood Iron Estimation

(See p. 278.)

SECONDARY METHODS OF HEMOGLOBIN ESTIMATION

The methods used in the routine clinical laboratory employ photoelectric colorimetry. A method must be used that will detect all forms of hemoglobin; this consideration excludes most except the cyanmethemoglobin method.

Cyanmethemoglobin Method

In view of the standards that are available, this is the most suitable method to use; also, it estimates all forms of hemoglobin except sulfhemoglobin. Most of the current instrumentation available for the measurement of hemoglobin employs this method.

Principle. Hemoglobin is converted to cyanmethemoglobin by the addition of potassium ferricyanide and sodium cyanide. The density of the color produced is directly proportional to the amount of hemoglobin present.

Procedure. Twenty microliters (0.02 mL) of blood are diluted with 5.0 mL of reagent. After 10 minutes the density of the solution is measured photometrically at 540 nm, with water as blank. The hemoglobin level is obtained from a calibration curve prepared with the aid of the standards. (Details are supplied with the standards.)

Reagent

Drabkin's reagent	
Sodium bicarbonate	1 g
Potassium ferricyanide	0.2 g
Potassium cyanide	0.05 g
Distilled water	to 1 L

The reagent may be obtained commercially.* Other lysing agents that contain detergent may be obtained† and are useful because of their rapid lysing properties.

Controls. Commercially available standards are the most convenient method of control. Other standards for cyanmethemoglobin are available from the College of American Pathologists, Chicago, Illinois, and from the Division of Medical Research, National Research Council, Ottawa, Ontario. In 1967, the International Committee for Standardization in Hematology established specifications for a cyanmethemoglobin. It must have a molecular weight of 64,458, a millimolar coefficient extinction of 44.0, and an iron content of 0.347%.

*Ortho Diagnostics, Raritan, N.J. 08869, and Don Mills, Ont. M3C 1L9.

†Coulter Electronics, Hialeah, Fla. 33014, and Oakville, Ont. L6L 2X8.

Oxyhemoglobin Method

This is a simple and reliable method that is not affected by moderate bilirubinemia, which does interfere to a slight extent with the cyanmethemoglobin method. It does not measure all forms of hemoglobin, e.g., sulfhemoglobin or methemoglobin.

Procedure. Twenty μL of blood is diluted with 5.0 mL of N/150 ammonia solution. The density of the solution is measured at 540 nm with a water blank.

To prepare a calibration curve, carry out iron estimations on at least three specimens of blood and then use these bloods in suitable dilutions for the preparation of the curve. A variation of the oxyhemoglobin method, involving the use of 0.1% w/v aqueous sodium carbonate as diluent, is employed in some laboratories. Blood samples of known concentration must be used as controls.

Normal Range

Cord blood	136–196 g/L
1 year	113–125 g/L
10 years	120–144 g/L
Adult male	135–180 g/L
Adult female	115–164 g/L

HEMATOCRIT (PACKED CELL VOLUME, PCV)

Principle

Whole blood is centrifuged to pack the red cells. The volume of red cells can then be expressed as a percentage of the whole blood volume.

This is one of the simplest, most accurate, and most valuable of all hematological investigations. It is of far greater reliability and usefulness than the red cell count when this latter examination has to be performed manually. It, together with accurately determined hemoglobin and red cell count, enables the red cell indices to be calculated. If performed manually the resultant buffy coat serves to give a rough idea of the white cell count and is divisible into an uppermost, very thin yellowish-white (creamy) layer of platelets, and a lower, thicker layer of reddish-gray color that consists of leukocytes. In cases of marked leukopenia the buffy coat is very thin and may be little more than a delicate gray "scum" on top of the red cell column. In cases of leukemia the buffy coat may be very thick. Not rarely, leukopenia and leukemia are first suggested by the hematocrit, and every technologist should cultivate the habit of inspecting both the buffy coat and the supernatant plasma when reading the hematocrit value. The great advantages of buffy coat smears have already been referred to. They are especially valuable in cases of leukopenia, in which leukemic or other malignant cells are scanty in the peripheral blood, and in searching for LE cells and for megaloblasts. Early jaundice may be noted from inspection of the plasma column, along with other abnormalities of plasma color or clarity, e.g., hyperlipidemia. A note should always be made on the patient's report if an abnormal plasma is seen, since this is often an important clue for the physician.

Wintrobe Hematocrit Method

The Wintrobe tube (same as used for ESR) is 11.5 cm long, of 3 mm internal bore, graduated 0 to 100 in millimeters with the centimeters marked by number, both ascending and descending. The tube is filled with well-mixed EDTA-treated venous blood to the mark "0," as described under ESR, making sure that no air bubbles are trapped. It has recently been emphasized that the ratio of EDTA to volume of blood is important. The final concentration must be less than 2 mg EDTA per 1 mL of blood; otherwise discrepancies in the hematocrit will result. This is particularly important if an evacuated tube containing a fixed amount of EDTA is used, since inadequate filling of the tube will cause an increased EDTA to blood ratio. The preparation is then spun for 30 minutes at not less than 2300 G in a centrifuge of 15 cm effective radius (i.e., 15 cm from axis or center of spindle to bottom of horizontally held cup). This is important, as the relative centrifugal force (RCF) is directly proportional to the radius and square of the speed.

Example. If a centrifuge has a 15 cm effective radius (R) and it is centrifuged at 3000 rpm, the RCF would be:

$$
\begin{aligned}
& 1118 \times R(cm) \times (rpm)^2 \times 10^{-8}\ G \\
= & 1118 \times 15 \times 3000^2 \times 10^{-8}\ G \\
= & 2054\ G
\end{aligned}
$$

To obtain optimal packing of the red cells, the Wintrobe tube would require centrifuging for 45 minutes. It will be obvious from the formula that packing of the RBCs will be more complete when the hematocrit is low (anemia) than when it is high (polycythemia), because the RCF diminishes linearly up the column of cells. It goes without saying that the head of the centrifuge must allow the buckets to swing out in the horizontal plane for calculation of the RCF by the formula given. However, angle centrifuges may be used for hematocrit estimations, but the readings should be compared with those obtained under defined conditions so that the correct minimal speed for packing on the angle centrifuge may be determined.

Reading. Once packing is complete, the hematocrit is read from the scale on the righthand side of the tube, taking the top of the black band of reduced erythrocytes, immediately beneath the reddish gray leukocyte layer.

Accuracy. With proper conditions the degree of error in the hematocrit estimation should not exceed 1%. This fact makes the hematocrit the best single test for the presence and degree of anemia, polycythemia, or hemoconcentration.

Normal Hematocrit Values

Sex and Age	Range (%)	Average (%)
Men	40–54	47
Women	37–47	42
Newborn	44–64	54
1 Year		35
10 Years		37.5

Cleaning Hematocrit Tubes. In the event that disposable tubes are unavailable the stem of a long Pasteur pipette, one end of which is attached to a water suction pump, is passed to the bottom of the Wintrobe tube, which is completely immersed in water. Special U-shaped metal tubes are available and are more suitable than glass pipettes (Fig. 30–1). Periodically, the Wintrobe tubes should be filled with strong acid and left overnight so that the protein scum is cleaned off.

Microhematocrit Determination

This method, although originally designed for capillary blood samples, has now become the method of choice. It enables higher centrifugation speeds (up to 10,000 G) with consequent shorter centrifugation times and superior packing.

The collection of the blood sample is the same as described for the Wintrobe method. Capillary blood may be taken directly into heparinized capillary tubes. The tubes vary in measurement but are approximately 70 mm long and have a 1 mm bore.

Procedure. After partially filling the tube by capillary action leaving approximately 10 mm unfilled, the empty end is sealed with plastic compound.* Special racks are available to identify the tubes.* After appropriate centrifugation in a specially designed centrifuge, the packed cell column is read using a reading device that is either part of the centrifuge or separate from it.

Buffy coat smears can be made by making a glass file cut just below the red cell–buffy coat interface, snapping the tube in two, and tapping the buffy coat and suitable amount of plasma onto a glass slide.

Sources of Error

1. Incomplete packing due to insufficient centrifugation. Centrifuges should be checked regularly to ensure proper operation.
2. Incorrect reading of results.
3. Hemolysis or clotting of samples.
4. Occasionally, the red cell–plasma interface is not clear-cut, and the hematocrit may be difficult to read.

RED CELL INDICES

Although the skilled laboratory worker is able to provide a large amount of information as to the relative size, hemoglobinization, and character of the red cells, absolute measurements of various red cell parameters enable a more accurate appreciation of erythrocyte pathology.

Using the red cell count, hemoglobin concentration, and hematocrit, a series of clinically useful indices can be obtained. Up until the time of the introduction of electronic or automated counting devices, the erythrocyte count was a source of considerable inaccuracy in these values. However, now that more reliable counts are available, the routine calculation of the MCHC, MCH, and MCV is mandatory for the investigation of all anemias. It also serves as a valuable quality control procedure (see p. 681).

RED CELL VOLUME INDICES

MCV (Mean Cell Volume)

This is the volume of one red cell expressed in femtoliters.

*Clay Adams Inc., Parsippany, N.J. 07054.

$$MCV = \frac{\text{Hematocrit (L/L)} \times 1000}{\text{RBC} \times 10^{12}/\text{L}}$$

For example: basing the calculation on normal blood with an RBC count of 5 million and an hematocrit of 0.45 L/L in 1 μL of blood, this is:

$$\frac{0.45 \times 1000}{5.0} = \frac{450}{5} = 90 \text{ fL}$$

$$\text{Normal Range} = 86 \pm 10 \text{ fL}$$

The MCV is increased in macrocytic anemias and decreased in iron deficiency, thalassemia, and secondary anemia.

Mean Cell Thickness and Diameter (MCAT and MCD)

MCAT (Mean Corpuscular Average Thickness). This is a seldom used index, and the following formula assumes that the red cell is a short cylinder rather than a biconcave disc.

$$MCAT = \frac{MCV}{\pi\left(\frac{MCD}{2}\right)^2}$$

$$\text{Normal Range} = 1.7 \text{ to } 2.5 \ \mu\text{m}$$

MCD (Mean Corpuscular Diameter). The MCD is the mean cell diameter and relates to the average diameter of the red cells. Its measurement was originally reported by Price Jones, who described the distribution of cells in various diameter ranges (Price Jones curve). The original method required the diameters of 100 to 500 red cells to be measured via camera lucida or photographs. This time consuming method has been supplanted by the electronic particle counter.

Normal Range = 6.7 to 7.7 μm.

Although enlarged thin red cells are found in pathological conditions (leptocytes), the routine measurement of MDC and MCAT is not required. The MCV is the most valuable erythrocyte volume measurement.

Red Cell Hemoglobin Indices

MCH (Mean Corpuscular Hemoglobin)

$$MCH^* = \frac{\text{Hemoglobin (g/L)}}{\text{RBC} (\times 10^{12}/\text{L})}$$

For example, if Hb = 148 g/L and RBC = 5.00 × 10^{12}/L, then

$$MCH = \frac{148}{5.0} = 29.6 \text{ pg}$$

$$\text{Normal range} = 27 \text{ to } 32 \text{ pg}$$

*MCH expresses the amount of hemoglobin in one red cell. It is directly proportional to the amount of hemoglobin and also to the size of the red cell.

In macrocytic anemias there is a high MCH; because the cells are larger, they carry more hemoglobin, though the concentration of hemoglobin per unit of volume of the cell (MCHC) may be normal or even slightly reduced. In microcytic anemias (unless also spherocytic) there is a lower MCH than normal; if the anemia is also hypochromic the MCH will be lower still.

MCHC (Mean Corpuscular Hemoglobin Concentration)

This absolute value expresses the concentration of hemoglobin per unit volume of red cells.

$$MCHC = \frac{\text{Hemoglobin (g/L)}}{\text{Hematocrit (L/L)}}$$

$$\text{e.g.,} \frac{148}{0.45} = 328 \text{ g/L}$$

$$\text{Normal Range} = 320 \text{ to } 360 \text{ g/L}$$

Low values (200 to 300 g/L) for MCHC are found in iron-deficiency anemias. In macrocytic anemias the MCHC is normal or slightly reduced.

Value of Red Cell Indices

The advent of automated instruments for measuring hematological parameters has changed the emphasis placed on these indices. This change is mainly owing to the differences in measuring the hematocrit and increased reliability of the red cell count. The MCHC has a time-honored place in hematology because in the past it was calculated from two parameters that would always be measured accurately, i.e., the hemoglobin concentration and the hematocrit. The hematocrit, however, suffers the disadvantage of having plasma trapped in the red cell column. Complete packing of the red cells is impossible, especially in anemias in which the red cells may be different shapes and sizes. Nevertheless, the MCHC provides valuable clinical information. The Coulter S Plus hematocrit is computed from the individual red cell volumes and is consequently not affected by trapped plasma. The Coulter S Plus hematocrit is therefore 2.5% lower than a centrifuged hematocrit, and therefore the MCHC derived from this value is higher than the manual counterpart. This explains why hypochromic red cells are noted even though the Coulter S Plus–derived MCHC may be in excess of 320 g/L.

The hypochromia seen on iron deficient smears is probably not due solely to less hemoglobin concentration in the cells, but rather reflects the optical qualities of small, thin, red cells.

Conversely, because of the increased reliability of the red cell count, the MCV has become increasingly valuable. It is now considered the most valuable automated index and serves as probably the most effective discriminant for classification of anemias. Typical results found are as follows.

Normal	84.1 – 99.8 fL
Pernicious anemia	99.7 – 146.9 fL
Beta thalassemia minor	53.7 – 73.5 fL
Iron deficiency	56.7 – 88.8 fL

England and Fraser describe a discriminant function (DF) based on the MCV that can help differentiate thalassemia trait from iron deficiency:

$$DF = MCV - RBC - (5 \times Hb) - 3.4$$

A positive value indicates iron deficiency, a negative value thalassemia minor. This function is not applicable in pregnancy and certain myeloproliferative disorders.

RETICULOCYTE COUNTS

Principle

Reticulocytes are immature erythrocytes that contain aggregations of ribonucleic acid (RNA) within disintegrating ribosomes. The amount of RNA is greatest when the erythroblast has just discarded its nucleus, and decreases until its complete absence from the mature erythrocyte. The reticulocyte count is a very valuable index of erythropoiesis.

Method

The following technique is recommended:

Brilliant cresyl blue (water-soluble)	1.0 g
Sodium citrate	0.4 g
0.85% sodium chloride	100 mL

Dissolve the dye in saline, add the sodium citrate, mix, and filter before use. One gram of new methylene blue may be substituted for the brilliant cresyl blue and appears to give more uniform results. Different batches of brilliant cresyl blue may vary in their ability to stain reticulocytes.

Procedure

1. To 3 drops of stain in a small tube, add 6 to 8 drops of blood (capillary, EDTA-treated, or oxalated). If capillary blood is used, it is advisable to increase the amount of stain to prevent clotting.

2. Incubate at 37°C for 10 to 20 minutes. Do not overincubate.

3. Prepare slides in the usual manner, making thin smears. Counterstaining with Romanowsky stain is not advised.

Satisfactory preparations may be made on blood stored at 4°C for 24 hours.

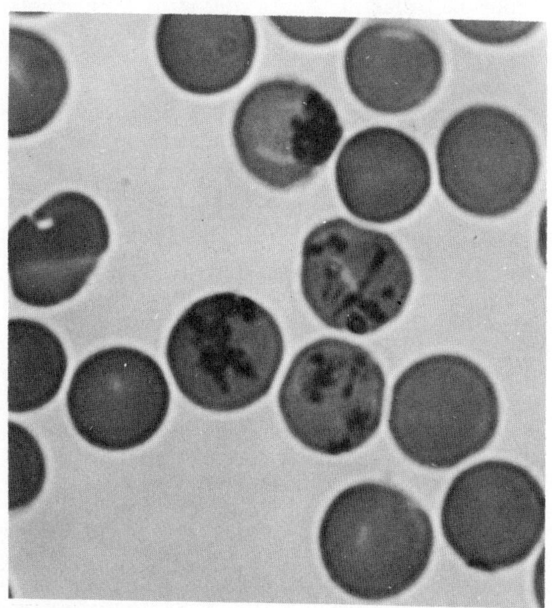

Figure 30–19 Reticulocytes. Brilliant cresyl blue counterstained with Wright's stain. × 2250.

Counting. Select a well-spread portion of the smear in which the red cells are just overlapping. An eyepiece with an adjustable diaphragm is helpful in counting the cells. The decision as to whether a cell is a reticulocyte may be difficult, since most mature reticulocytes contain only a few dots or threads of reticular material.

Dacie has shown that to obtain a 5% accuracy with a 2% reticulocyte count, 19,600 cells must be counted. In this regard it is advisable to count at least 100 reticulocytes if less than a 10% reticulocytosis is expected. The method of Dacie is recommended: Count the number of reticulocytes until 100 are counted. Note the number of fields counted to obtain this number. Count the total number of cells in every tenth field for at least 10 fields. The following example quoted by Dacie demonstrates the calculation:

Number of reticulocytes in 150 fields:	100
Total number of cells in 15 fields:	300
approximate number of cells (all types) in 150 fields:	3000

$$\text{Reticulocyte percentage: } \frac{100}{3000} \times 100 = 3.3\%$$

It is recommended that two separate individuals count two separate reticulocyte preparations. If the two values do not vary from each other by 10% or more, the average can be taken. If the values are not with these limits, a third observer should perform the reticulocyte count and an average of the two closest values should be taken. There is considerable variation between observers in reticulocyte counting, especially when increased values are obtained. Every effort must be made to make the counting process as accurate as possible.

Pappenheimer and Heinz bodies will be stained by this method.

Sources of Error

1. Insufficient number of cells counted.
2. Confusion with red cell inclusions, which may be difficult to distinguish from reticulocytes. This occurs in some types of anemia in which there are Pappenheimer bodies and/or basophilic stippling present.

Interpretation of Reticulocyte Count

Reticulocyte Percentage. The reporting of reticulocytes as a percentage of red cells counted is of little clinical significance. The normal range is 0.5 to 2%, but this is meaningless unless correlated with other hematological parameters.

Absolute Number of Reticulocytes. The absolute number of reticulocytes is of more value. The normal range is 25 to 75 × 10^9/L.

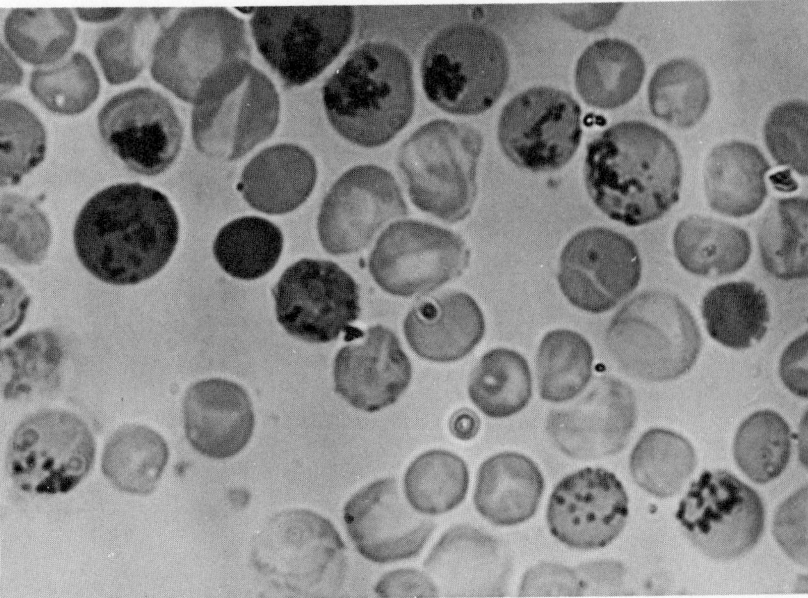

Figure 30–20 Reticulocyte crisis. Reticulocytes stained by Brecher's new methylene blue method. × 2250.

$$\text{Reticulocytes} = \left(\text{RBC count} \times \frac{\text{Retic. count}}{100}\right) \times 10^9/\text{L}$$

It is recommended that reticulocytes be routinely reported in absolute numbers along with the percentage value.

The clinical significance of this method of reporting is based on the principle of comparing the basal rate (normal range) to the maximal response that bone marrow erythropoiesis is capable of producing. The maximal rate under appropriate circumstances is considered seven times the basal rate, i.e., 250 to 350 × 10^9/L. If anemia exists and the bone marrow is not reacting at a maximal response, causes for the retarded reticulocytosis (vitamin B_{12} deficiency, folate deficiency, bone marrow invasion by malignant cells, etc.) must be investigated.

STAINING SMEARS FOR STIPPLED CELLS

Although stippled cells may be seen and counted in ordinary Romanowsky stained smears, the following stain offers a less tedious procedure:

Staining Solution

Methylene blue	1.5 g
1% Potassium alum sulfate in 50% methyl alcohol	0.5 mL
1% NaOH in methyl alcohol	0.2 mL
Methyl alcohol	100.0 mL

Procedure. **Immerse air-dried smears in the stain for 4 or 6 seconds; then wash rapidly in 0.025% sodium hydrogen carbonate in distilled water, and blot dry. An increase in stippled cells is seen in conditions in which heme synthesis is altered, most notably thalassemia and lead poisoning.**

TESTS FOR HEMOLYSIS OF RED CELLS

The following procedures are most important routine tests in solving the problem of specific reasons for decreased red cell survival. The reader is referred to the chapter on red cell disorders for their clinical application and to larger texts for information on less commonly required tests that may be used to advantage in arriving at a final diagnosis.

Osmotic Fragility of RBC

Principle

The red cell envelope is a semipermeable membrane. When red cells are placed in a hypertonic solution they lose fluid (and thereby shrink and crenate) until osmotic equilibrium is established with the surrounding fluid. When, however, the red cells are placed in hypotonic solution they imbibe fluid (and thereby swell) until osmotic equilibrium is set up or until they rupture. It follows, then, that there is a limit to the hypotonicity of a solution that normal red cells can stand. In certain hemolytic anemias, e.g., hereditary spherocytosis and acquired hemolytic anemia, the resistance of the red cells to hypotonic solutions is reduced. Although the osmotic fragility test depends upon osmosis, the actual rupture of the cell results from alteration of its shape and diminished resistance to osmotic forces rather than a change in the composition of the cell or its osmolarity; hence the use of the word *fragility*. Cells that are spherocytic rupture more easily than others and, indeed, the osmotic fragility test may be regarded as the most sensitive index of the extent and degree of spherocytosis. Conversely, increased resistance against lysis in hypotonic solution is shown by the red cells in thalassemia, sickle cell anemia, and ordinary hypochromic (iron-deficiency) anemia, probably because the cells in these conditions have a greater cell surface area to volume

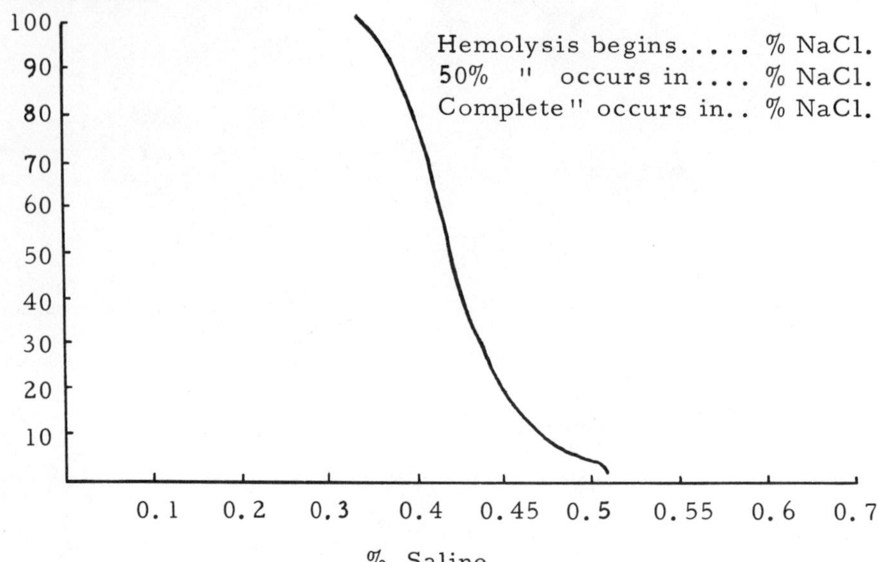

Figure 30–21 Graphic method of reporting the osmotic fragility of red cells.

ratio, e.g., target cells. Manual and automated methods are available for the estimation of red cell osmotic fragility.

Manual Method

Principle. Test and normal red cells are placed in a series of graded-strength sodium chloride solutions and any resultant hemolysis is compared with a 100% standard.

The method of Dacie is recommended:

Stock Buffered Salt Solution

Sodium chloride	180 g
Na_2HPO_4	27.31 g
$NaH_2PO_4 \cdot 2H_2O$	4.86 g

Make up to 2 liters with distilled water; store at 4°C. The solution is osmotically equivalent to 10% NaCl and will keep for many months without deterioration.

Dilutions. These may be prepared in 50-mL amounts and stored at 4°C for up to 6 months, or they may be prepared just before the test. It is convenient to make a 1% solution from the stock 10% and proceed as follows:

Tube No.	mL of 1% Buffered NaCl	mL of Distilled Water	% Buffered NaCl
1	0.5	4.5	0.1
2	1.0	4.0	0.2
3	1.5	3.5	0.3
4	1.75	3.25	0.35
5	2.0	3.0	0.4
6	2.25	2.75	0.45
7	2.5	2.5	0.5
8	2.75	2.25	0.55
9	3.0	2.	0.6
10	3.25	1.75	0.65
11	3.5	1.5	0.7
12	4.0	1.0	0.8

Procedure

1. Mix the contents of each tube before adding the blood. If dilutions have already been prepared in bulk, place 5 ml of the appropriate salt dilution in each tube. The 12 dilutions are set up in duplicate.
2. The patient's blood and a normal control specimen are taken with a minimum of stasis and trauma into wide-bore heparinized tubes. Each sample is gently rotated in the tube until it is bright red (fully oxygenated). If blood has been taken into a heparinized evacuated tube it should be transferred into a wide bore tube or a flask and oxygenated before testing.
3. To each of the 12 tubes in one row (marked test) is added 0.02 mL (accurately measured in a pipette or calibrated Pasteur pipette) of patient's blood. If the hemoglobin concentration of the blood is below 10.5 g per dL, or 105 g/L, 0.05-mL amounts are added to each tube.
4. Similar amounts of the normal control blood are placed in the second row of tubes (marked control).
5. Mix each tube well.
6. Let stand at room temperature for 30 minutes. Then remix and centrifuge at 1000 G for 10 minutes.
7. Using a spectrophotometer at 540 nm or appropriate colorimeter, measure supernatants as for a hemoglobin estimation, using tube No. 12 of the test and control as blanks for the respective rows. For the reading the supernatant of each tube must be removed carefully so as not to include any cells. Tube No. 1 in each case is the 100% hemolysis standard.

Calculation Example

Absorbance tube No. 12 (blank)	0
Absorbance tube No. 1 (100%)	0.4
Absorbance tube No. 5	0.2

Therefore, % hemolysis of tube No. 5 =

$$\frac{\text{Test reading} - \text{blank}}{\text{100\% reading} - \text{blank}} \times \frac{100}{1} = 50\%.$$

Reporting Results. The red cell fragility test is best reported as a curve on linear graph paper, always including the normal control, and indicating the salt concentrations in which (1) hemolysis begins; (2) is complete; and (3) 50% hemolysis occurs.

Normal Range of Osmotic Fragility (at 20°C and pH 7.4) (Dacie)

NaCl (%)	Hemolysis (%)
0.30	97–100
0.35	90–99
0.40	50–90
0.45	5–45
0.50	0–5
0.55	0

50% hemolysis or mean corpuscular fragility (MCF) = 0.40 to 0.44% NaCl.

Precautions Necessary in Performing Fragility Test. The sample of blood should be obtained with a minimum of stasis and trauma, and the test must be set up as soon as possible after the sample is taken. The use of anticoagulants such as oxalates, which involves the addition of osmotically active salts, is undesirable. Heparin is the anticoagulant of choice, but carefully defibrinated blood may be used. For the quantitative test outlined it will be obvious that accurate amounts of blood are added to each tube.

Care must be taken to deliver the blood directly into the saline solution in order to avoid contact with the dry sides of the tube above the fluid and subsequent increased hemolysis.

Osmotic Fragility After 24 Hours Incubation at 37°C

Incubation at 37°C for 24 hours enhances red cell fragility changes. Fragility curves that are normal on immediate testing may be abnormal if testing is done after incubation of the blood. It is therefore advisable to perform an immediate fragility and an incubated fragility on each sample submitted for investigation. Normal MCF for incubated fragility is 0.46 to 0.59%.

Significance of Results

Increased fragility indicates the presence of spherocytes, whereas decreased fragility is found in the presence of target cells and hypochromia as in thalassemia.

Fragillograph Method

An automated method of performing red cell fragilities is available. The fragillograph is an instrument that has a cuvette, the sides of which consist of a dialyzing membrane. Red cells diluted in 0.9% sodium chloride are placed in the cuvette, which is surrounded by distilled water. As the salt concentration in the cuvette decreases, the degree of lysis of the red cells is recorded as a fragility curve.

AUTOHEMOLYSIS TEST

Principle

When normal blood is incubated under sterile conditions for 48 hours, little or no hemolysis takes place. In a variety of hemolytic conditions, however, hemolysis is significantly increased. The method of Dacie is recommended.

Method

Using sterile precautions, 2 mL of defibrinated blood is added to each of four 5 mL screw-cap bottles or tubes. Another 2 mL of blood is refrigerated at 4°C. 0.1 mL of sterile 10% glucose is added to two of the bottles to provide a final glucose concentration of at least 500 mg per dL. The bottles are suitably labeled and incubated at 37°C for 48 hours. Mix gently after the first 24 hours. At the end of 48 hours, the contents of each pair of tubes are pooled, a hematocrit performed, and the two samples centrifuged to obtain serum. The supernatant serum samples are diluted 1 in 10 in 0.04% ammonia. A 1 in 10 dilution of preincubation serum is used as a blank and a 1 in 200 dilution of whole blood in 0.04% ammonia serves as a standard. The degree of hemolysis is measured in a spectrophotometer at 520 nm.

The percentage lysis is calculated as follows:

$$\%\ \text{lysis} = \frac{R_1\,(100 - \text{HCT}) \times D^1}{R_2 \times D^2}$$

When

R_1 = reading of diluted serum
R_2 = reading of whole blood
D^1 = dilution of test serum (1/10)
D^2 = dilution of whole blood (1/200)
HCT = Hematocrit

$$\text{Therefore}\ \%\ \text{lysis} = \frac{R_1\,(100 - \text{HCT})}{R_2 \times 20}$$

Normal range of lysis after 48 hours incubation:
without glucose 0.2–3%
with glucose 0–0.9%

Significance of Results

Autohemolysis is increased in hereditary spherocytosis, acquired spherocytosis, hereditary nonspherocytic hemolytic anemia, and in hemolysis owing to chemicals. The addition of glucose has a variable effect but generally reduces the degree of hemolysis. Hereditary nonspherocytic hemolytic anemia can be classified by the correction by glucose: type 1—autohemolysis 3 to 6% corrected by the addition of glucose; type 2—autohemolysis 7 to 15% not corrected by the addition of glucose.

TESTS FOR RED CELL ENZYME DEFICIENCIES

The erythrocyte obtains energy from the metabolism of glucose. Two pathways exist for this metabolism, namely the Embden-Meyerhof pathway of anaerobic glycolysis and the hexose monophosphate oxidative pathway. Many enzymes interact in these pathways to produce the energy that the erythrocyte requires to maintain its shape and its ionic equilibrium, and to maintain hemoglobin iron in its reduced state. Consequently, deficiencies of these enzymes may cause a decrease in energy in the form of ATP (adenosine triphosphate is the energy product), rendering the cell liable to lysis.

DEFECTS OF THE HEXOSE MONOPHOSPHATE SHUNT

Glucose-6-Phosphate Dehydrogenase (G-6-PD) Deficiency

Over 100 variants of this enzyme have been described, based on their electrophoretic mobilities and avidity for substrate. The two variants that most commonly cause hemolytic events are G-6-PD A-, which is found in approximately 11% of American Negroes, and G-6-PD Mediterranean, the incidence of which varies from 0.01% in Northern Europeans to 50% in male Kurdish Jews. Inheritance of the enzyme is sex linked, the gene being carried on the X chromosome. G-6-PD reacts with its coenzyme, oxidized triphosphopyridine nucleotide (NADP) to produce 6-phosphogluconolactone and reduced triphosphopyridine nucleotide (NADPH).

$$\text{G-6-PD} + \text{NADP} \rightarrow$$
$$\text{6-phosphogluconolactone} + \text{NADPH}$$

NADPH is an important intracellular reducing agent and is necessary for the reduction of oxidized glutathione (GSSG) to reduced glutathione (GSH) by the enzyme glutathione reductase. This can be summarized as follows:

$$\text{GSSG} + \text{GSSG reductase} + \text{NADPH} \rightarrow \text{GSH}$$
$$\text{NADP} + \text{G-6-PD} \rightarrow \text{6-P-gluconolactone}$$

In the absence of GSH, oxidizing drugs produce hydrogen peroxide, which oxidizes hemoglobin to methemoglobin. Excess GSSG forms insoluble complexes with hemoglobin, resulting in Heinz body formation. Heinz bodies may cause membrane damage by binding to membrane sulfhydryl groups.

G-6-PD activity decreases as cells age. Therefore, during a hemolytic episode, senescent cells are preferentially destroyed. A person suffering from a moderate G-6-PD deficiency may show normal levels of G-6-PD following a hemolytic episode, since the cells in the circulation would all be relatively young. Consequently, it is not advisable to test for G-6-PD deficiency during a hemolytic episode. Testing should be repeated on several occasions after the hemolytic event before G-6-PD deficiency can be ruled out.

A variety of tests are described, since they vary greatly in their sophistication and specificity. Brilliant cresyl blue decolorization is a convenient screening test, whereas the ascorbate-cyanide test is a very sensitive procedure. Direct assays of G-6-PD are recommended if facilities are available.

Glutathione Instability (Heinz Body) Test

Principle. This test depends on the abnormal sensitivity of G-6-PD-deficient red cells to the toxic effects of phenylhydrazine.

Procedure

Blood sample: This must be freshly drawn (under 1 hour). Either heparinized blood or that drawn directly from a skin puncture may be used.

1. Add 0.1 mL of fresh blood to 2.0 mL of 0.1% w/v solution of acetylphenylhydrazine in pH 7.6 Sorensen phosphate buffer (Appendix F, p. 822). Mix and aerate by blowing through the pipette a few times.

2. Incubate *(unstoppered)* in the 37°C water bath for 2 hours. Then repeat the aeration and continue incubation for a further 2 hours, i.e., 4 hours incubation in all.

3. Mix. Place a drop of crystal violet solution (1% w/v in 0.73% NaCl, filtered) on a clean microscope slide. Add a small drop of the incubation mixture and mix; cover with coverglass. Let stand 5 to 10 minutes. Count the percentage of cells containing five or more Heinz bodies.

Interpretation. In normal persons 30% or less of red cells will contain five or more Heinz bodies. In a patient whose red cells are "sensitized" by a drug, or in any person having a complete or considerable partial lack of G-6-PD, more than 40% of the red cells will show five or more Heinz bodies. Splenectomy can increase the number of Heinz bodies found in the test red cell. A normal (control) blood should be tested in parallel.

Cresyl Blue Decolorization Test

Blood is collected in the usual manner and with the usual anticoagulants. It may be refrigerated (4°C) for up to 1 week before testing. Packed red cells are obtained by centrifugation.

Principle. A known volume of packed red cells is lysed and incubated with measured amounts of glucose-6-phosphate and NADP. If G-6-PD is present in the red cells it will remove hydrogen from the glucose-6-phosphate. Brilliant cresyl blue serves as a hydrogen acceptor and is reduced to a colorless leuco compound by H^+.

Reagents

Glucose-6-Phosphate Solution. Dissolve 16.5 mg glucose-6-phosphate, disodium salt* in 1.0 mL distilled water. Prepare fresh.

TRIS Buffer, 0.74 M, pH 8.5. (See Appendix F, p. 824.)

NADP, 0.1%. Dissolve 5.0 mg NADP in 5.0 mL of distilled water. Prepare fresh.

Brilliant Cresyl Blue. Dissolve 0.32 g brilliant cresyl blue† in distilled water and make to 1 liter.

Procedure

1. In a test tube place 1.0 mL distilled water; add 0.2 mL of TRIS buffer. Mix and add 0.01 mL of packed red cells. Set up as a control a normal blood similarly treated.

2. Add in sequence:

0.05 mL glucose-6-phosphate solution
0.05 mL of 0.1% triphosphopyridine nucleotide
0.25 mL brilliant cresyl blue solution.

---

*Sigma Chemical Co., St. Louis, Mo. 63178.

†Harleco, Gibbstown, N.J. 08027, or BDH, Toronto, Ont. M8Z 1K5.

3. Mix well and overlay with mineral oil. Place in the 37°C water bath. Inspect (against daylight) for decolorization at 50, 75, 100, 120, and 180 minutes and at 6 hours.

Results. Normal blood (with normal G-6-PD activity) shows complete decolorization at 100 minutes. Blood that does not show decolorization in the test at 3 to 6 hours is considered as having no G-6-PD activity. Intermediate grades of decolorization of the brilliant cresyl blue are taken as indicating partial G-6-PD deficiency. Tests should be run in parallel on normal (control) blood, and all abnormal tests should be repeated. The test is essentially qualitative.

G-6-PD Assays

Probably the most informative procedure is an assay for G-6-PD activity. A hemolysate prepared from the patient's blood is incubated with excess glucose-6-phosphate and excess NADP at a constant temperature. The amount of NADPH produced is dependent on the patient's G-6-PD activity and is measured in a spectrophotometer at 340 nm. Commercial kits are available* for performing this assay and are, for the average laboratory, the method of choice.

Other Deficient States

Hemolysis caused by deficiencies of other enzymes within the hexose monophosphate pathway have been reported but are rare and of considerably less clinical importance than G-6-PD defects.

Deficiencies of 6-phosphogluconate dehydrogenase, glutathione reductase, and glutathione peroxidase have been reported, and their assay requires the services of specialized laboratories. However, the screening procedure described for G-6-PD deficiency will enable detection of these deficient states.

Detection of Defects of the Embden-Meyerhof Pathway

Pyruvate Kinase Deficiency

Deficiencies of pyruvate kinase (PK) are the commonest abnormalities of the glycolytic pathway. The defect is transmitted as an autosomal recessive characteristic. PK deficiency is probably the commonest cause of nonspherocytic hemolytic anemia and usually presents in childhood as a hyperbilirubinemic condition. The autohemolysis test is markedly abnormal and is not corrected by glucose but is corrected by the addition of ATP. The primary defect results from a failure to produce ATP because of a lack of PK:

$$\text{Phosphoenolpyruvate (PEP)} + \text{ADP} + \text{PK} \rightarrow \text{Pyruvate} + \text{ATP}$$

Assay methods are available for measuring PK, and reagents can be obtained commercially in kit form.† The pyruvate formed in the above reaction is converted to lactic acid by lactic dehydrogenase (LDH) with the oxidation of NADH to NAD. In the assay, the conversion of NADH to NAD is measured spectrophotometrically at 340 nm. The complete reaction sequence is, therefore, as follows:

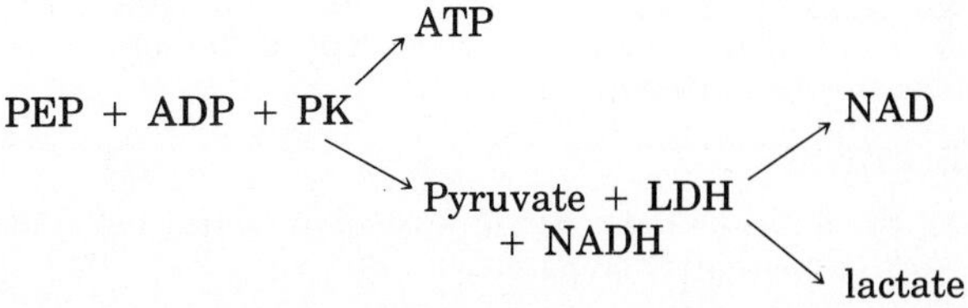

A spot screening test can be used. NADH fluoresces, whereas NAD does not. A cell suspension is added to a reaction mixture of PEP, ADP, NADH, and $MgSO_4$. A drop of this mixture is placed on a piece of filter paper at 10-minute intervals. If PK levels are normal, fluorescence should disappear between 10 and 20 minutes (i.e., all NADH is converted to NAD). Homozygote PK deficiencies continue to show fluorescence, whereas heterozygotes fluoresce longer than normal controls.

Other rare enzyme deficiencies occur, and the reference texts should be consulted for their characteristics.

Donath-Landsteiner Test for Paroxysmal Cold Hemoglobinuria

Principle. The Donath-Landsteiner antibody is both a complete agglutinating and strong hemolyzing antibody that does not require lowering of the pH (acid conditions) to cause hemolysis. It is an IgG immunoglobulin, rarely present in high titer and usually has specificity for the normal red cell antigen P in both the luetic and idiopathic cases.

Procedure

1. Two stoppered, dry, test tubes or screw-cap bottles are warmed to 37° C by standing in the 37°C bath.

2. Blood is drawn from the patient into a syringe which has been previously warmed at 37°C. With minimal delay the sample is divided between the two tubes.

3. One tube is immediately placed in a 37°C bath. It is marked W.

4. The other tube (C) is stood in a beaker of crushed ice in the refrigerator for 30 minutes.

5. The refrigerated tube C is then placed in the water bath at 37°C. Both tubes are allowed to remain undisturbed in the bath until the clots have retracted. When this has occurred, the serum of tube C will show obvious hemolytic discoloration in a positive test.

For titration of the Donath-Landsteiner antibody the patient's serum must be diluted with fresh normal AB serum (so as to provide complement). Any group O cells may be used.

Paroxysmal Nocturnal Hemoglobinuria

A variety of methods exist, all of which serve to increase the sensitivity of the defective red cell mem-

*Sigma Chemical Co., St. Louis, Mo. 63178.

†Biomedix, Princeton Biomedix Inc., Princeton, N.J. 08540; distributed in Canada by I and B Maynard Scientific, Weston, Ont. M9M 1M6.

brane to action of complement. No one test should be relied upon to detect this condition, which characteristically often requires serial testing to detect the defect.

Ham's Test

Principle. When serum is acidified, it enhances the binding of complement to red cells. Red cells from individuals with PNH are more susceptible to hemolysis under such conditions.

Procedure

1. The patient's red cells are washed in saline, and a 40 to 50% suspension is prepared.
2. To 1 mL of fresh normal serum add 0.1 mL of N/5 HCl and mix.
3. To the acidified serum add 2 drops of the patient's red cell suspension.
4. As controls, set up (a) the patient's cells with unacidified normal serum and (b) normal red cells with acidified patient's serum.
5. Mix and incubate at 37°C for 1 hour.
6. Centrifuge and examine the supernatants. A positive reaction is indicated by definite hemolytic staining of the supernatant in the test with, at most, slight staining of the supernatant in control (a), and a clear supernatant in control (b). The only other condition that gives this positive result is marked erythrospherocytosis, which will be obvious in a blood smear.

Modification. Addition of 0.003 to 0.005 M magnesium to the serum before testing greatly enhances the sensitivity of the test owing to the activation of an alternate complement pathway. 0.1 M magnesium is prepared from a stock solution of 2.8 M magnesium chloride. Add 0.1 mL of 0.1 M magnesium chloride to 1.9 mL of serum before testing.

Sucrose Hemolysis Test

Principle. The test is based on an empirical observation that erythrocytes from patients with paroxysmal nocturnal hemoglobinuria are hemolyzed when incubated with autologous or isologous compatible normal serum or plasma in low–ionic strength sucrose solutions.

Reagents

1. Sucrose, reagent grade 92.4 g
0.005 M monobasic sodium phosphate 910 mL
0.005 M dibasic sodium phosphate 90 mL
Adjust pH to 6.1 if necessary.
2. Serum. Type compatible normal serum either fresh or stored at −20°C for not longer than 2 weeks in order to retain full complement activity. The test serum is not suitable.
3. Cells. Fresh EDTA or ACD anticoagulated test blood. Wash the red cells at least three times with 0.85% NaCl and make up to a final 50% suspension.

Procedure. Set up the following tubes:

	1	2	3	4	
Sucrose	0.90	0.95	0.95		mL
Cells	0.05	0.05		0.05	mL
Serum	0.05		0.05		mL
0.04% Ammonia in distilled water.				0.95	mL

Incubate at room temperature for 60 minutes, then centrifuge to obtain cell free supernatant. Transfer supernatant and add 4 mL 0.9% NaCl to each tube and read the optical density (OD) against a water blank at 540 nm.

$$\% \text{ lysis} = \frac{OD_1 - (OD_2 + OD_3)}{OD_4 - OD_2} \times 100.$$

Over 5% lysis indicates paroxysmal nocturnal hemoglobinuria.

ABNORMAL HEMOGLOBIN IDENTIFICATION

HEMOGLOBIN ELECTROPHORESIS

The principles of electrophoresis have been described elsewhere (p. 88). Hemoglobin electrophoresis is the definitive technique for detecting hemoglobins in which the substitution of an amino acid leads to a change in electrical charge. Electrophoresis is performed on a hemolysate prepared from the red cells.

Preparation of Hemolysate

1. Centrifuge fresh EDTA anticoagulated blood and remove supernatant plasma and buffy coat.
2. Wash × 3 in saline and discard the last supernatant.
3. Add an equal volume (to the red cell volume) of distilled water and a half volume of carbon tetrachloride. Shake vigorously.
4. Centrifuge at 1500 G for 5 minutes.
5. 3 layers are obtained: on top the hemolysate, in the middle red cell stroma, on the bottom carbon tetrachloride.
6. Carefully pipette off the supernatant hemolysate, which should be clear and ruby red.
7. Adjust the hemoglobin concentration to between 70 and 100 g/L with water.
8. If the hemolysate is to be stored, add 1 drop of M/100 potassium cyanide; otherwise electrophoresis can be performed immediately.

Electrophoresis

Many media have been and are being used for electrophoresis: cellulose acetate, starch gel, agar, starch block, polyacrylamide gel, and paper.

The most efficient for routine purposes is cellulose acetate membrane, and this is the method of choice for most laboratories. Starch gel techniques require specialized facilities.

Cellulose Acetate Electrophoresis

Reagents

1. Buffer—0.025 M TRIS-EDTA-Borate pH 8.4.*
2. Fixative dye solution—Ponceau S 0.2 g in 100 mL of 5% trichloroacetic acid.
3. Rinse solution 5% glacial acetic acid in distilled water.

---

*Supreheme, Helena Laboratories, Beaumont, Tex. 77704; in Canada distributed by I and B Maynard Scientific, Weston, Ont. M9M 1M6.

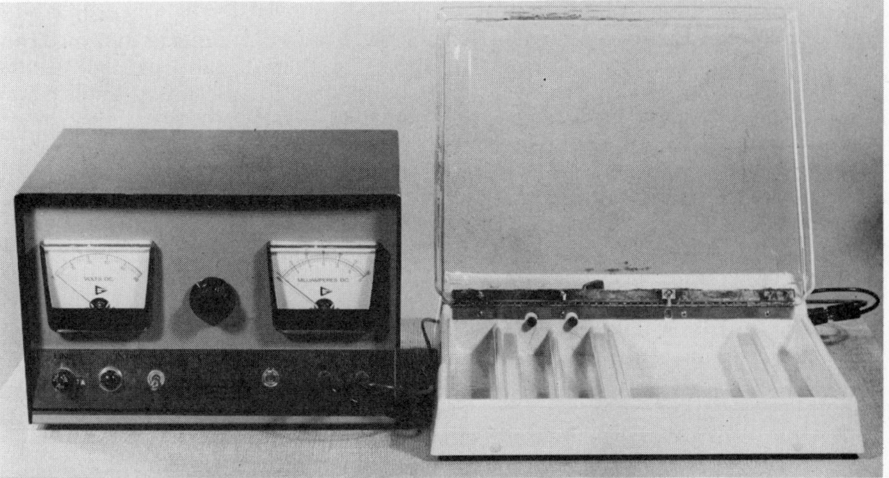

Figure 30–22 Gelman electrophoresis power supply and tank. (Gelman Sciences, Inc., Ann Arbor, Mich. 48106, and Montreal, Que. H4S 1M7.)

4. Clearing solution 12% glacial acetic acid in methanol.

Many electrophoresis chambers are available. The instrument shown in Figure 30–22 is recommended.

Technique

1. Immerse the cellulose acetate strips in buffer, taking care to avoid entrapment of bubbles on the membrane.

2. Once thoroughly soaked, remove and blot off excess buffer. DO NOT ALLOW THE STRIPS TO DRY.

3. Apply the hemolysate to the strip using a suitable applicator.* This operation is a crucial part of the procedure and requires care and practice. If inexpertly applied the hemoglobin will not separate optimally.

4. Commence electrophoresis and run for 30 minutes at 360 volts.

5. When separation is complete, remove strips from chamber and stain for 5 minutes in Ponceau S solution.

6. Remove excess stain by rinsing several times in 5% acetic acid, in order to obtain well defined separation of the hemoglobin bands.

Estimation. The concentration of hemoglobins can be measured either by elution or densitometer scanning.

Elution

1. After the strips have been rinsed, blot off excess fluid.

2. Cut out the hemoglobin bands and place in separate tubes.

3. Add 2 mL of 0.1 N NaOH to each tube. The amount can be varied, depending on the density obtained, but the exact volume added should be noted.

4. Shake vigorously to elute the stain.

5. Add 1 drop of acetic acid to each tube and read the optical densities at 525 nm.

If three hemoglobin bands were found—HbA, HbS and HbA_2—and 2 mL 0.1 N NaOH had been added to each tube, the HbA_2 concentration would be:

$$\% \, HbA_2 = \frac{OD\ A_2 \times 2}{OD\ A_2 \times 2 + OD\ HbA \times 2 + OD\ HbS \times 2} \times 100$$

If the amount of NaOH added is varied, the multiplication factor varies accordingly.

Densitometry

1. After the strips have been rinsed, immerse strips in the clearing solution for 30 to 60 seconds.

2. Roll strips onto a flat glass surface removing all air bubbles.

3. Dry quickly in a hot air oven at 60°C. The strips are then ready for scanning. Many different densitometers are available (see p. 89). Cellulose acetate strips with a plastic backing* can be obtained, and these are very convenient to use for scanning.

Interpretation

On cellulose acetate, the commonly found hemoglobins migrate as follows:

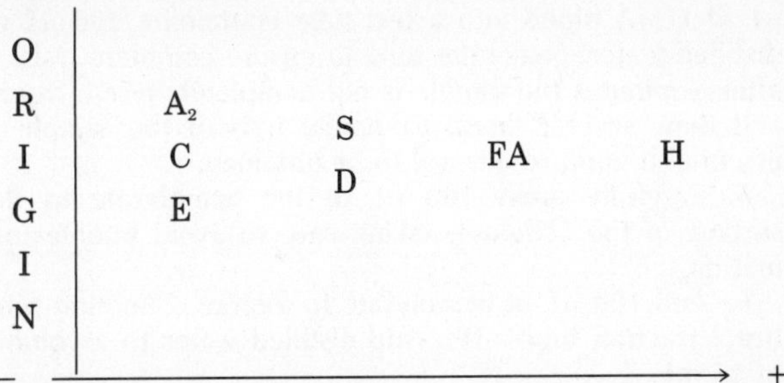

It can be seen that several hemoglobins have similar migration patterns.

*Gelman Instrument Co., Ann Arbor, Mich. 48106, and Montreal, Quebec H4S 1M7.

*Titan III, Helena Laboratories, Beaumont, Tex. 77704; in Canada distributed by I and B Maynard Scientific, Weston, Ont. M9M 1M6.

HbA_2 can be differentiated from HbC and HbE, since it never reaches the concentrations that would be found if the band were due to HbC and HbE. HbA_2 seldom exceeds 7%, whereas HbC and HbE are usually 20% to 30% in the heterozygous state and higher in the homozygous state. HbC can be differentiated from HbE by agar gel electrophoresis at pH 5.9. On this medium, HbE migrates with HbA while HbC migrates with HbS. The ethnicity of the patient may also indicate whether HbC or HbE is present. HbD and HbS can be distinguished by agar gel electrophoresis; HbD also migrates with HbA. Alternatively, the solubility test (vide infra) can be used; HbS cells give a positive result, and HbD cells a negative result. HbF and HbA migrate very closely together and are again difficult to separate. The alkali denaturation test serves to separate the two.

It is necessary to emphasize that both the elution and densitometric methods can produce variable results, particularly with HbA_2, and repeat testing may be necessary.

Quantitation of HbA_2 by DEAE Cellulose Chromatography

The most accurate method of quantifying hemoglobin A_2 uses DEAE cellulose chromatography.

Principle

Hemoglobin A_2 can be eluted from a DEAE cellulose column by treatment with 0.2 M glycine buffer. At this ionic strength, HbA remains bound to the cellulose.

Method

1. 300 mg DEAE cellulose is suspended in 0.2 M glycine buffer and allowed to settle in a column. Pasteur pipettes can be used as a column, or they can be purchased commercially.*

2. Immediately after suspension of cellulose in the column, allow the buffer to drain into a container. As the cellulose packs down, an interface will form between the cellulose and supernatant buffer. Remove the supernatant, taking care not to disturb the sedimented cellulose.

3. Place column in rack over collection tube.

4. Prepare patient sample in the following way. Place 50 μL of EDTA blood into a test tube containing 200 μL of distilled water. Shake the tube to ensure complete lysis. If after 5 minutes the sample is not completely lysed, freeze and thaw several times. Complete lysis of the sample is essential if good results are to be obtained.

5. Carefully apply 100 μL of the hemolysate to the surface of the cellulose, taking care to avoid bubble formation.

6. Add 100 μL of hemolysate to a large collection tube (total fraction tube—TF). Add distilled water to a volume of 15 mL.

7. By this time the hemolysate will have been absorbed into the cellulose. Once it is certain that this has occurred, slowly add 2 mL of 0.2 M glycine buffer. Allow the buffer to pass through the column, thus eluting the HbA_2 fraction into the collecting tube.

8. Add distilled water to the collecting tube to bring the volume to 3 mL. This contains the A_2 fraction. Mix the A_2 tube and the TF tube and record the opical density (OD against a distilled water blank at 415 nm.

Calculation

$$\% A_2 = \frac{\text{OD of } A_2 \text{ tube}}{5 \times (\text{OD of TF tube})}$$

Normal Range = 1.3 to 3.5%

Values between 3.5% and 8% are indicative of β-thalassemia minor. Values above 8% are indicative of hemoglobins that will elute from the column in the same manner as HbA_2 (HbS, C, E, etc.). If such values are found, cellulose acetate electrophoresis must be done to identify the presence of hemoglobins other than hemoglobin A_2.

Hemoglobin S (HbS)

A variety of methods are used to detect this hemoglobin and the following tests are convenient screening procedures that can be confirmed by electrophoresis.

Demonstration of Sickling Principle

Sickling of HbS containing red cells is hastened by the reduction of the hemoglobin and the pH.

Reagent. 2% sodium metabisulfite. This is best freshly prepared at the time of the test.

Method

1. Place a drop of fresh anticoagulated blood on a slide.

2. Mix with a drop of 2% sodium metabisulfite and coverslip.

3. Place in a wet chamber for 30 minutes and examine microscopically (see Figs. 30–23 to 30–25).

Results. Homozygous HbS causes complete sickling of the cells when deoxygenated by the sodium metabisulfite. The heterozygous cells show less severe changes and may show a prickly "holly leaf" effect.

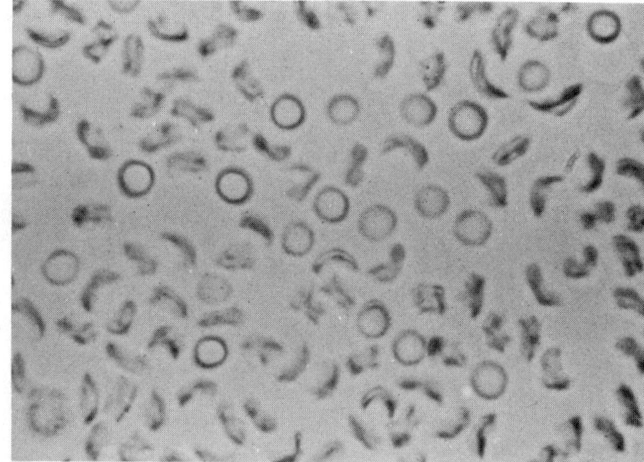

Figure 30–23 Sodium metabisulfite preparation: sickle cell anemia. Note the typical sickle shaped cells as opposed to occasional normal shaped erythrocytes.

*Helena Laboratories, Beaumont, Tex. 77704.

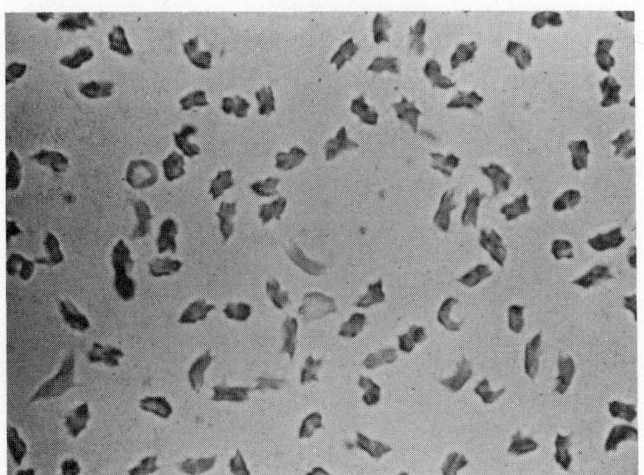

Figure 30–24 Sodium metabisulfite sickling preparation demonstrating the "holly leaf" effect produced by a sickle cell trait sample (S/A).

Solubility Screening

Hemoglobin S is more insoluble than normal hemoglobins. The testing reagent consists of a reducing substance, a lysing reagent, and a strong inorganic buffer. When cells containing HbS are added to the reagent mixture, a turbidity occurs owing to the insolubility of the reduced HbS. Normal hemoglobins are more soluble and show a clear end point. This is the most sensitive screening test available; commercial tests are available.*

Solubility Test for HbS

Reagents

1. Buffer 2.24 M, pH 6.7

Dipotassium hydrogen phosphate (K_2HPO_4)	220.3 g
Potassium dihydrogen phosphate (KH_2PO_4)	132.45 g
Saponin	5.0 g

Distilled water to 1 liter.

2. Reducing Reagent

Sodium dithionite. Place 20 mg in bottom of a test tube before adding buffer solution. The exact quantity is not critical.

Method

1. Dissolve reducing agent in 2 mL buffer solution. This is the test solution.

2. Add 0.02 mL of blood to test solution and mix by inversion.

3. Allow to stand for 3 minutes at room temperature.

4. Read the test by holding in front of a black and white lined background. The lines will be visible with a negative result, and not visible with a positive result.

Notes

1. The concentration of hemoglobin in the test is critical. Patients with hemoglobin values of less than 70 g/L should have a double aliquot of blood added to the test solution. Otherwise false negatives may result. On the other hand, if the concentration of hemoglobin added is too high, a false positive may result. It is advisable to use specimens with hemoglobin concentrations between 100 and 140 g/L.

2. Positive and negative controls must be run with each batch of tests.

3. Reading before the 3 minutes waiting period may result in a false positive result.

4. *Any* detection of the lined background should be considered a negative result, providing the hemoglobin concentration of the specimen is adequate, because some normal specimens will not become completely clear.

5. If batches of test solution are made up, they may be stored at 4°C for one month before the reducing agent loses its activity. When this happens, a false negative result may occur.

6. The buffer solution must be stored at 4°C. If it becomes contaminated with mold, new solution should be prepared.

7. Results should be confirmed by hemoglobin electrophoresis.

HEMOGLOBIN INCLUSION BODIES

Inclusion bodies are found in the HbH disease and are tetramers of beta chains. They are also seen in Hb-Zurich disease after therapy with sulfonamides and other medications and, in this instance, appear to be composed of denatured hemoglobin (Heinz bodies). Hemoglobin inclusion bodies are not demonstrable with Romanowsky stain.

Reagents

1. Citrate-Saline Solution

Sodium citrate	3 g
Normal saline	100 mL

2. Staining Solution

Brilliant cresyl blue	1 g
Citrate-saline solution	100 mL

*Sickledex, Ortho Diagnostics, Raritan, N.J. 08869, and Don Mills, Ont. M3C 1L9.

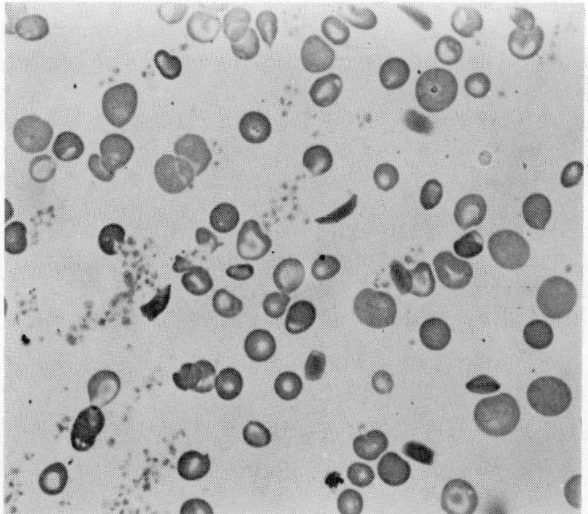

Figure 30–25 Peripheral blood film in sickle cell anemia. Several drepanocytes are present in this field, which also shows anisocytosis, poikilocytosis, and hypochromia. One normoblast is also present. × 675.

Method

1. Mix equal volumes of blood and stain.
2. Incubate at 37°C for 2 hours.
3. Make smears and search for HbH inclusions.

Very careful examination of the smear is necessary, since the inclusions can be very scanty. Usually in HbH disease, however, the majority of cells show multiple blue-green spherical inclusions. They can be distinguished from reticular material which also stains with brilliant cresyl blue by counterstaining with a Romanowsky stain. The inclusion bodies disappear while the reticular material retains its blue color.

Detection of Unstable Hemoglobins

Normal hemoglobin and the common abnormal hemoglobins remain soluble at 50°C. Several rare abnormal hemoglobins, however, are unstable and precipitate when heated to 50°C. These hemoglobins are associated with hemolytic anemia and Heinz body formation.

Heat Stability Test

Reagent

Tris Buffer

Tris-2 amino-2 (hydroxymethyl)-
1-3 propandiol — 12.1 g
0.1 N HCl — 125.0 mL
Distilled water to 1 liter. Adjust pH to 7.4.

1. Prepare a red cell hemolysate.
2. Add 3 mL of hemolysate to 3 mL Tris buffer pH 7.4.
3. Incubate at 50°C for 2 hours.

Results. Unstable hemoglobins (Hb Zurich, Hb Köln, etc.) show a moderate to heavy flocculation while normally no or little precipitate forms.

Detection of Hemoglobins with Abnormal Heme Function

Demonstration of HbM

The hemoglobin M diseases are characterized by methemoglobin formation. Amino acid substitution occurs near the site of the heme group in either the alpha or beta globin chain. The charge on the abnormal chain probably bonds with heme iron, and, by electron transfer, the iron becomes trivalent (methemoglobin formation). The demonstration of HbM by electrophoresis identifies the condition. For identification, the hemolysate should be converted to cyanmethemoglobin before electrophoresis. HbM can also be detected by its abnormal spectral characteristics. It shows a peak at 630 nm and a depression at 600 nm.

Demonstration of Heinz Bodies

Heinz bodies can be produced in the red cells as a result of unstable hemoglobins or a wide variety of medication or exogenous poisons affecting the red cell enzyme systems.

Reagent. 0.5% methyl violet in 0.9% sodium

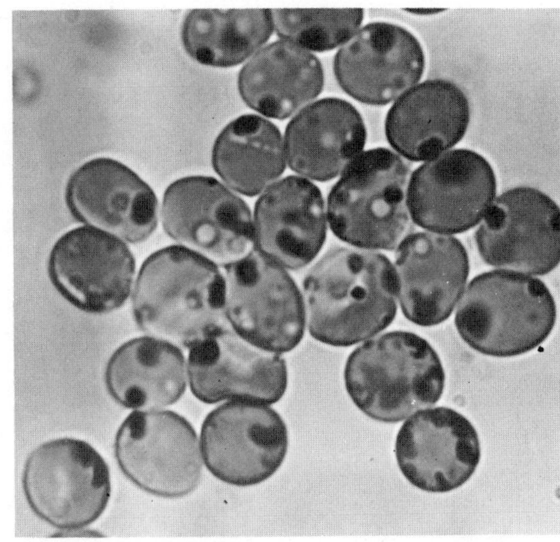

Figure 30–26 Heinz bodies, from glutathione instability test on normal blood. × 2250.

Method

1. One volume of blood in any anticoagulant is added to four volumes of stain.
2. Leave at room temperature for 10 minutes.
3. Make smears and examine for Heinz bodies, which stain as intense purple and are often located near the periphery of the cell.

Hemoglobin F (Fetal)

This may be estimated by either direct chemical analysis or by identifying peripheral blood erythrocytes that contain HbF.

Qualitative

Principle. Fetal hemoglobin resists alkali denaturation.

Procedure

1. Place a disc of filter paper flat on the top of a funnel. Onto the center of the paper pipette 4 drops of 1% aqueous NaOH.
2. Without delay, place 1 drop of a 1 in 2 dilution (in isotonic saline) of the test blood in the center of the hydroxide-moist patch. Read result within 1 or 2 minutes.

Result. Adult hemoglobin gives a green brown stain spreading out from the center. Fetal hemoglobin gives a pink color. This is a very useful method for distinguishing fetal cord blood from adult blood samples.

Quantitative Alkali Denaturation

Principle. Fetal hemoglobin resists denaturation by alkali, whereas adult hemoglobin is quickly denatured.

Procedure. *Note.* The test should be performed within the temperature range of 18 to 25°C.

1. Wash a sample of the patient's red cells three times in three to five times its volume of normal saline.

2. To the washed, packed cells add an equal volume of distilled water and 0.4 volume of carbon tetrachloride. Stopper and shake for 5 minutes, or until hemolysis is complete. Freezing and thawing will accelerate lysis.

3. Centrifuge at 2000 G for 20 minutes.

4. Filter supernatant through two layers of Whatman No. 1 filter paper (5 cm diameter, and moistened with distilled water so as to minimize loss of hemoglobin.)

5. Estimate hemoglobin in filtrate and adjust to approximately 100 g/L.

6. To a test tube containing 3.2 mL of 1/12 N sodium hydroxide add 0.2 mL of the oxyhemoglobin solution. Mix well and let stand exactly 1 minute.

7. Add 6.8 mL ammonium sulfate solution (38 g of $(NH_4)_2SO_4$ per 100 mL distilled water and 0.25 mL of 10 M HCl added). Mix by repeated inversion. Let stand 1 minute.

8. Filter through Whatman No. 42 paper. If the filtrate is clear, no hemoglobin F is present (the ammonium sulfate precipitates the denatured adult, A, hemoglobin). If the filtrate is pinkish, the amount of HbF present is measured by comparing the filtrate in a spectrophotometer at 540 nm with a mixture of 0.1 mL of the oxyhemoglobin solution (step 5) in 5.0 mL of 1% ammonia water.

Result. More than 4% of HbF is significant; below this level, the significance is dubious.

RBC Acid Elution Test (Kleihauer)

Principle. Adult hemoglobin is readily eluted from red cells by an acid phosphate buffer; fetal hemoglobin resists such elution.

Reagents

1. ***Fixative.*** 80% ethanol.

2. ***Acid Phosphate Buffer.*** Solution A—NaH_2PO_4—28.4 g; distilled water to 1 liter. Solution B—Citric acid 19.2 g; distilled water to 1 liter. These solutions can be stored at 4°C. For use, mix 14.25 ml of solution A with 35.75 mL of solution B. The pH must be 3.2.

3. ***Counterstain.*** 0.5% eosin.

Procedure

1. Thin smears are prepared using capillary or EDTA venous blood. Dilute blood 1 in 3 with isotonic saline to ensure very thin even smears.

2. Fix slides with 80% ethanol.

3. Place slides in the acid buffer previously heated to 37°C. Leave for exactly five minutes, agitating gently during that time.

4. Wash in distilled water for approximately 30 seconds and counterstain for 3 minutes. Wash well and stand to dry.

Results. On microscopic examination the fetal red cells stand out as dark refractile bodies against the unstained ghost forms of the adult erythrocytes. This method will also detect the presence of hemoglobin F in certain hemoglobinopathies, including hereditary persistence of hemoglobin F.

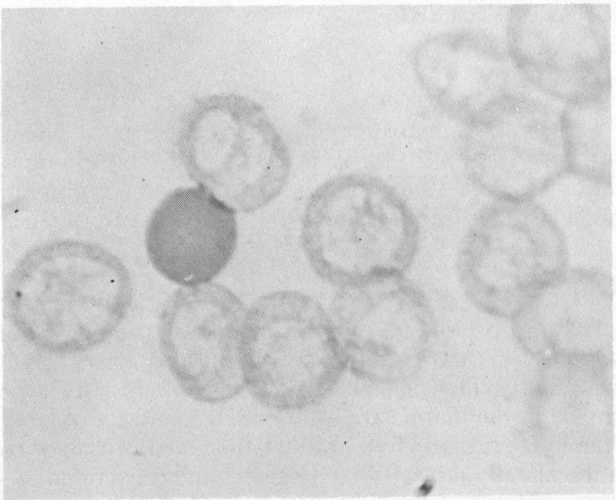

Figure 30–27 The Kleihauer technique. The cell that has retained its hemoglobin is of fetal origin, and the surrounding cells from which the hemoglobin has been eluted are of adult origin. × 2300.

Detection of Fetal Hemorrhage into Maternal Circulation

Almost 20% of pregnancies are believed to be associated with bleeding from the fetus into the maternal circulation. Occasionally, however, massive transplacental hemorrhage may occur and will result in the birth of a severely anemic infant. The detection of fetal cells in the maternal circulation has also gained increasing importance in the prophylaxis of hemolytic disease of the newborn (see p. 609). The size of the fetal bleed can be estimated as follows:

1. Count the number of fetal cells in 100 high power fields (hpf). Estimate the number of maternal cells in 5 hpf.

2. Calculate the percentage of the fetal cells:

$$\frac{\text{Average number of fetal cells/hpf}}{\text{Average number of maternal cells/hpf}} \times 100$$

3. Assume maternal blood volume is 5000 mL. Fetal bleed = % fetal cells × 5000/mL.

E.g., number of fetal cells seen in 100 hpf = 40.
Average number of fetal cells in 1 hpf = 0.4.
Number of maternal cells in 5 hpf = 1000.
Average number of maternal cells in 1 hpf = 200.

$$\% \text{ fetal cells} = \frac{0.4}{200} \times 100 = 0.2\%.$$

$$\text{Fetal bleed} = 0.2\% \times 5000 = \frac{0.2}{100} \times 5000 = 10 \text{ mL}$$

When ABO incompatibility exists between mother and child, the fetal cells may be destroyed by the maternal antiA or antiB, resulting in misleading estimates of the fetal bleed.

SCHILLING'S TEST

Principle

This is the most commonly performed test for ascertaining vitamin B_{12} absorption. It involves giving the patient radioactive vitamin B_{12} and determining how much of the vitamin is eventually excreted in the urine.

Method

1000 μg of nonradioactive vitamin B_{12} is injected intramuscularly. This is known as a "flushing dose," and it ensures that the vitamin B_{12}–binding proteins (transcobalamins) in the plasma are saturated. 0.5 to 2 μg of labeled vitamin B_{12} is then given orally. If absorbed, it cannot bind to the already saturated binding sites and is excreted in the urine, which is collected for 24 hours thereafter. In pernicious anemia, recovery of radioactive vitamin B_{12} is markedly reduced. The test can then be performed with radioactive B_{12} plus intrinsic factor, in which case patients with pernicious anemia will show normal recovery of radioactive B_{12}.

In practice, ^{58}Co-labeled B_{12} and ^{57}Co-labeled B_{12} bound to intrinsic factor can be given simultaneously, and the ratio of ^{57}Co to ^{58}Co vitamin B_{12} in the urine can be ascertained. This helps to overcome the problems of renal disease and incomplete collection of urine, which may cause inaccurate results with the traditional Schilling test.

Results

Diagnosis	Per cent Excreted: ^{57}*Co* (*B_{12} + IF*)	Per cent Excreted: ^{58}*Co*	^{57}Co/^{58}Co Ratio
Normal	10–42%	10–40%	0.7–1.3
Pernicious anemia	6–12%	0–7%	> 1.7
Malabsorption syndromes other than PA	6%	6%	0.7–1.3

FOLIC ACID AND VITAMIN B_{12} ASSAYS

Serum vitamin B_{12}, serum folate, and red cell folate are commonly ordered tests for the assessment of anemia. Deficiencies in B_{12} and folate result in megaloblastic erythropoeisis and macrocytic erythrocytes in the peripheral blood. In the past, vitamin B_{12} and serum folate were assayed by microbiological assay techniques, *Lactobacillus casei* being used for folate and *Euglena gracilis* or *Lactobacillus leichmanii* for vitamin B_{12} assays. These bacteria required the appropriate compound for growth; thus the degree of growth in the test system was proportional to the amount of vitamin B_{12} or serum folate in the patient's serum. These microbiological techniques have given way to radioisotopic techniques using the principle of saturation analysis.

Vitamin B_{12} Assay

Measured amounts of patient's serum, buffer, cyanide, and radioactively labeled vitamin B_{12} (^{57}Co) are mixed and heated. The action of heating and cyanide on the mixture causes various forms of vitamin B_{12} to be dissociated from the serum-binding proteins (transcobalamins) and converted to cyanocobalamin. The mixture is then incubated with intrinsic factor. The labeled and unlabeled vitamin B_{12} in the mixture compete for intrinsic factor on the basis of their concentrations. The more unlabeled vitamin B_{12} the mixture contains, the less labeled vitamin B_{12} will bind to intrinsic factor. Following incubation, the free vitamin B_{12} is absorbed with charcoal. Thereafter, either the bond fraction or free fraction may be counted. The serum vitamin B_{12} level is determined by ascertaining the degree of inhibition of binding of labeled vitamin B_{12} by unlabeled vitamin B_{12} and comparing this to a previously made standard curve.

Normal Range. 200 to 800 pmol/L.

Serum Folate and Red Cell Folate

The same principle is used in serum folate assays. A measured amount of serum or whole blood is mixed with folate-protecting buffer and a radioactively labeled folate derivative ^{125}I (PGA). Heat causes the folate-binding proteins to be inactivated while the folate is stabilized by the buffer. A measured amount of folate-binding is stabilized by the buffer. A measured amount of folate-binding protein is added, and the labeled and unlabeled folate compete for binding sites on the basis of their concentration. The more unlabeled folate the mixture contains, the less labeled folate will be able to bind. Once the bound and unbound folate are separated, the serum folate or red cell folate can be ascertained by comparing the degree to which the binding of labeled folate is inhibited to a previously prepared standard curve.

Newer assays offer the ability to perform vitamin B_{12} and serum folate simultaneously.

Normal Ranges

Serum folate: 1.9 to 14 nmol/L
Red cell folate: 100 to 550 nmol/L whole blood

SEMINAL ANALYSIS

Principle

A fresh sample of seminal fluid is examined for liquefaction and for number, motility, and morphological appearance of spermatozoa. Abnormalities may cause infertility.

Collection of Sample

Patients should be asked to abstain from sexual intercourse for three days before sample collection. The most satisfactory sample is that collected by masturbation in the clinical laboratory. If this is impossible, patients should bring the sample to the laboratory within two hours of collection, protecting it from extremes of temperature. It should be collected in a widemouth plastic or glass container but not in condoms, which may contain spermatocides.

Elements of Analysis

1. Liquefaction. Freshly ejaculated semen is a viscid, opaque, white coagulum. Incubate the sample at 37°C for 30 minutes, and examine for liquefaction of the semen. Normal semen should be completely liquefied.

2. Volume. Normally the volume of seminal fluid ranges from 1.5 to 5 mL with a mean of 3.5 mL. Infertile males often have an increased volume of seminal fluid with a diminished sperm count.

3. pH. Normally the pH does not vary much, and it is usually between 7.7 and 8.0. Values below 7.0 are usually associated with semen consisting primarily of prostatic secretion.

Sperm Count

Reagent

Sodium bicarbonate	5 g
Formalin	1 mL
Distilled water	100 mL

Method

a. Pipette 0.02 mL of well-mixed seminal fluid into 0.38 mL of diluting fluid in a test tube.

b. Mix and charge a Neubauer hemocytometer chamber. Allow to settle for two minutes.

c. Count two of the large squares (2 sq mm), and multiply the figure obtained by 100,000 to obtain the number per mL. When counting, constantly focus up and down so as to see spermatozoa that may be in different focal planes. Normal values range from 60 to 150 million per mL of seminal fluid. Values of less than 20 million per mL are associated with infertility.

5. Sperm Motility. To evaluate motility, place a drop of seminal fluid on a slide that has been prewarmed to 37°C. Examine under a × 40 objective and determine the percentage of motile spermatozoa. Also note whether the sperm are actively or feebly motile. Normally more than 70% of spermatozoa show active motility within one hour of ejaculation.

6. Sperm Morphology. A smear of the seminal fluid is made and stained by the Papanicolaou technique. At least 200 sperm are examined under oil immersion, and the percentage of abnormal forms is reported. Normally fewer than 30% are abnormal forms. In addition, the number of leukocytes or red cells should be noted; leukocytes should not exceed 2000/μL, and 5000/μL is considered definitely pathological. Immature germ cells may also be seen.

Other characteristics may be measured. One of these is sperm viability, and it may be estimated by eosin staining. Only dead spermatozoa will take up the dye, and such measurements may be of value in cases in which simpler measurements have yielded confusing results. Fructose is produced by the seminal vesicles and is absent in the semen of those with congenital absence of these structures. The spermatozoa mature in the vesicles, and absence of fructose in the semen may explain those rare causes of sterility that are caused by congenital absence of the seminal vesicles. Clumping of sperm in the semen may indicate sperm agglutinins in the blood, which may be sought by appropriate serological means.

CHAPTER 30—REVIEW QUESTIONS

1. What is the significance of red cell indices, and how are they calculated?
2. What are the advantages of automated over manual cell counting?
3. What factors influence the erythrocyte sedimentation rate?
4. What tests can be performed to demonstrate the presence of hemoglobin S?
5. What method is used to demonstrate LE cells?

31

HEMOSTASIS: PRINCIPLES AND PRACTICE

In this chapter the normal mechanisms by which the body is able to contain blood within the intravascular space (hemostasis) will be described, followed by a description of the abnormal conditions involving this mechanism and the tests used to make a laboratory diagnosis. It is particularly important for the laboratory worker to understand the complexities of these physiological and pathological processes, since they have a very real effect on the information to be derived from the laboratory tests. Like other hematological problems, this type of investigation requires a logical approach for laboratory investigation, and therefore a brief section is devoted to a description of the screening procedures used in the investigation of hemostatic dyscrasias.

HEMOSTATIC MECHANISM

Hemostasis is the entire mechanism by which bleeding from an injured blood vessel is controlled and finally stopped. The process is far from simple, and must be looked upon as a progression or chain of physical and biochemical changes normally initiated by injury to the tissues and blood vessels, and culminating in the transformation of fluid blood into a solid thrombus or clot that effectively seals the torn vessels. The entire mechanism is divisible into three parts: extravascular phenomena, vascular phenomena, and intravascular phenomena.

Extravascular Phenomena

These consist of: (1) the physical effect of the surrounding tissues, e.g., skin, muscle, and elastic tissue, in tending to close and seal the rent in the injured blood vessel; and (2) the biochemical effects of substances released from the injured tissues and reacting with plasma and platelet factors. This latter or "extrinsic system" of coagulation possibly may play some role in promoting the activation of the "intrinsic" clotting mechanism of the blood itself in the case of in vivo trauma and hemorrhage.

Vascular Phenomena

The damaged blood vessel constricts almost instantaneously. This process is known as vasoconstriction, and is important in the early control of hemorrhage following injury to a vessel. This reflex nervous vasoconstriction tends to pass off within a relatively short, though variable time, but it is possibly enhanced and prolonged by local release of vasoactive amines, e.g., serotonin. These substances are released from platelets as these adhere or stick to the margins of the injury or defect in the wall of the vessel; it promotes a local, direct, biochemically stimulated narrowing of the torn blood vessel and of intact vessels in the immediate vicinity.

Intravascular Phenomena

These consist of the enormously complex sequence of physiochemical reactions which transform fluid blood into a firm fibrin clot. This process requires the initiation of a platelet plug, followed by reinforcement with fibrin derived from the activation of the intrinsic coagulation system. Simultaneously, a complex interplay of various natural inhibitors and accelerators is brought into action.

Normal Hemostatic Sequence (See Figs. 31–1 and 31–2)

1. Blood vessel and tissues injured; bleeding begins through transected and injured vessels.
2. Nervous vasoconstriction of injured vessel occurs.
3. The torn endothelium of the vessel retracts or curls up.
4. Thromboplastic substances are released from damaged tissues.
5. Plasma (blood) flows over the damaged tissues. As it does so, Factor XII (contact factor) is activated and this triggers the activation of the intrinsic system. Factor VII of the plasma activates the tissue thromboplastic substances (extrinsic thromboplastic system is activated).
6. The activated extrinsic thromboplastin(s), in the presence of Ca^{++}, then interact with Factors V and X, thus forming definitive thromboplastin, which converts some of the plasma prothrombin to thrombin.
7. In the meantime, platelets have begun to adhere to the damaged endothelium of the vessel. The thrombin produced by the extrinsic thromboplastin system and ADP now comes into contact with the platelets adhering to the subendothelial collagen, causing them to aggre-

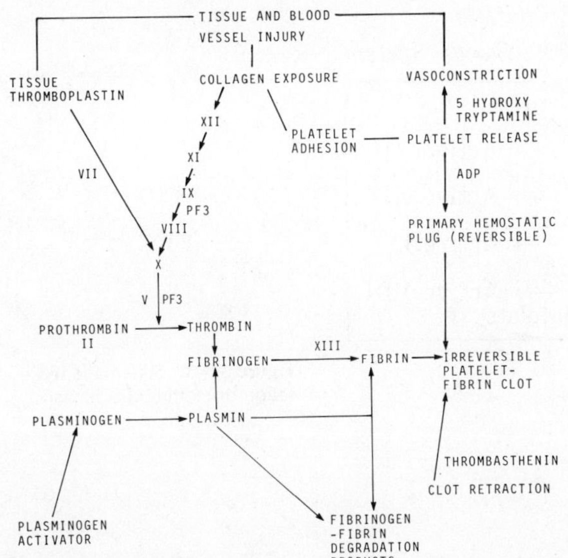

Figure 31–1 Schematic diagram of the hemostatic mechanism. Normal hemostasis is a complex and balanced interplay of the vascular, platelet, procoagulant and fibrinolytic mechanisms. If any or a combination of these main mechanisms is interrupted or unduly activated, a hemostatic defect will result.

gate into a plug (see p. 722 for full explanation of this phenomenon).

8. The platelets release a number of substances that encourage further aggregation of platelets and laying down of fibrin to reinforce the platelet plug.

9. The hemostatic platelet plug thus grows continuously until it seals the defect in the vessel.

10. During this time the platelets in the plug are using glucose metabolism to manufacture high-energy adenosine triphosphate (ATP), which triggers an actomyosin-like protein in the platelets to contract. This contraction of platelets is promoted by relatively high concentrations of thrombin.

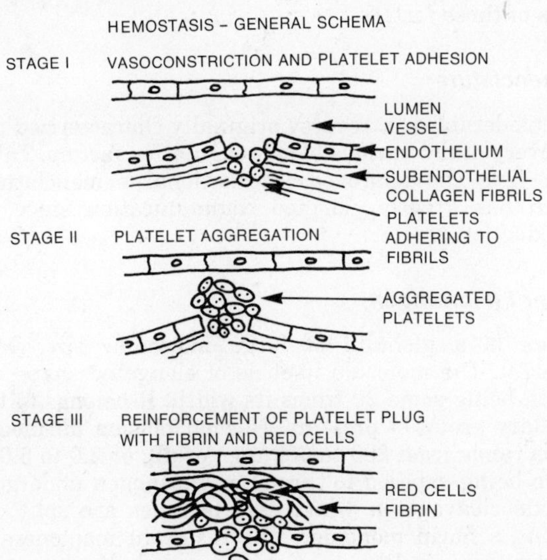

Figure 31–2 A schematic diagram showing the main stages in the formation of a hemostatic plug.

11. In the meantime, the intrinsic thromboplastin mechanism has been activated, leading to the production of relatively large amounts of thrombin.

12. The thrombin thus produced converts fibrinogen to fibrin. The fibrin absorbs much of the excess thrombin, and the remainder is neutralized by antithrombins.

13. The fibrin latticework so produced between and on the framework of the platelet plug polymerizes and contracts, thus effectively anchoring the platelet plug and sealing the defect in the vessel.

14. The endothelium of the vessel grows over the fibrin plug, and any clot that has formed within the lumen of the vessel is gradually recanalized or is lysed by the action of plasmin so that continuity of the lumen is established. The fibrin is slowly converted to collagen, contracting still further until only a small scar marks the site of injury in the wall of the vessel.

EXTRINSIC AND INTRINSIC COAGULATION OF BLOOD

Since the vast majority of clinical conditions involve the intrinsic coagulation system, emphasis will be given to this aspect. After the nomenclature and theory of coagulation are dealt with, each factor will be discussed in detail.

The three main mechanisms involved in this phenomenon are: (1) intrinsic and extrinsic procoagulant action, (2) platelet interaction through the hemostatic plug, and (3) the fibrinolytic system.

Procoagulant Action

Classic Theory of Morawitz

In 1905–06, P. Morawitz published his theory of blood coagulation. This theory provided a satisfactory basic working hypothesis that remained more or less unchanged for 40 years. Morawitz divided coagulation into two phases: in the first stage prothrombin was converted to thrombin by an enzyme (thrombokinase) in the presence of calcium ions; the second stage consisted of the conversion of fibrinogen to fibrin by the thrombin produced in stage 1.

Stage 1:

$$\text{Prothrombin} \xrightarrow[\text{Ca}^{++}]{\text{Thrombokinase}} \text{Thrombin}$$

Stage 2:

$$\text{Fibrinogen} \xrightarrow{\text{Thrombin}} \text{Fibrin}$$

Morawitz's theory has been proved basically correct. The great increase in our knowledge of the complexity of this mechanism brought to light in recent years has developed along the lines of elaboration of what the "thrombokinase" action consists of and how it is activated; in short, recent advances have concerned thromboplastin generation and thromboplastin activity.

Modern Concept of Blood Coagulation

Stage 1: Generation of thromboplastin activity ("extrinsic" and "intrinsic")

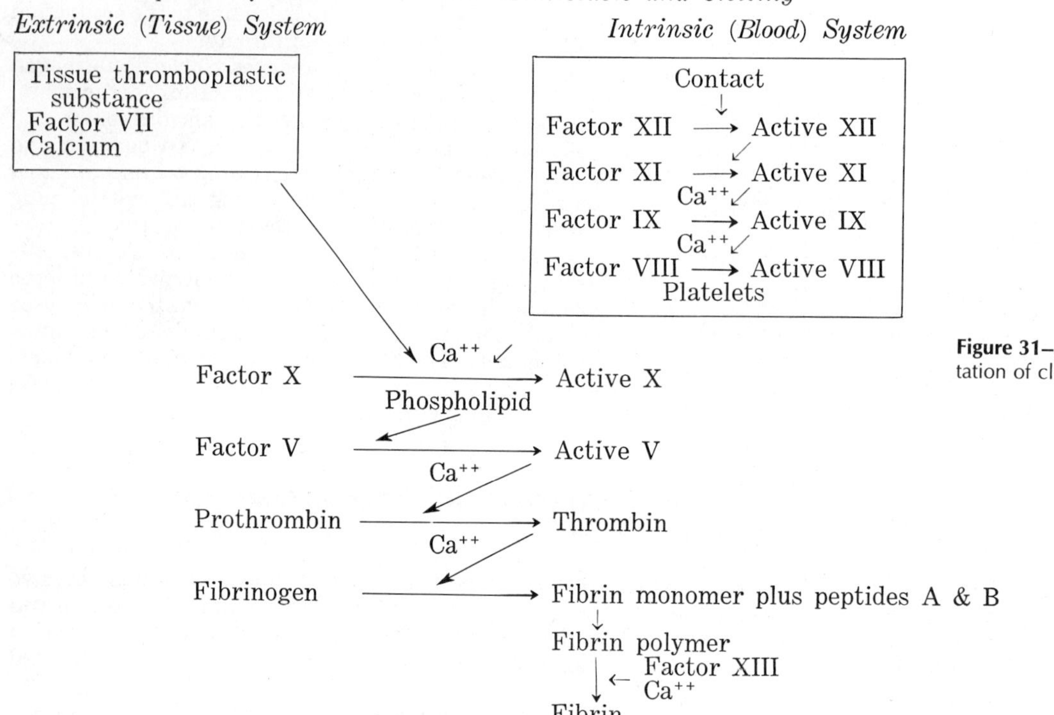

Figure 31–3 Schematic representation of clotting mechanism.

Stage 2: Conversion of prothrombin to thrombin by "thromboplastin" in the presence of Ca^{++}.

Stage 3: Conversion of fibrinogen to fibrin by thrombin.

Cascade Theory of Coagulation. From Figure 31–3 it can be seen that the blood clotting factors are present in an inactive form, which if stimulated becomes an active form. This has been proposed to account for the phenomena seen in coagulation studies. It has been postulated that this "cascade" of enzyme action permits a very great amount of material to be changed, by amplification of the initial surface contact activation, to the final product fibrin. A simplified diagram of the process may be as follows (a indicates activated form):

Surface contact
↓
XII → XIIa
XI → XIa
IX → IXa
VIII → VIIIa
X → Xa
Tissue damage
VII
←V plus Phospholipid
Prothrombin (II) → Thrombin............... Platelets
Fibrinogen → Fibrin

The cascade or waterfall hypotheses are not entirely acceptable, because not all the factors have been isolated in their inactivated or activated forms (e.g., activated Factor VIII). Nevertheless, they have gained popular approval because they explain the enormous amplification of thrombin production and are a suitable framework for explaining the action and use of many of the laboratory procedures.

The Coagulation Factors

Table 31–1 presents some of the laboratory characteristics of these factors.

Nomenclature

Considerable controversy originally characterized the discovery of the various blood coagulation factors. Table 31–1 lists the approved international nomenclature, which has greatly clarified communication since its introduction.

Factor I (Fibrinogen)

This is a globulin of large molecular size (MW 341,000). The molecule itself is of elongated shape, its length being some 20 times its width. It belongs to the fibrillary group of proteins. Normal plasma fibrinogen levels range from 200 to 500 mg per dL, or 2.0 to 5.0 g/L. On being exposed to thrombin, fibrinogen undergoes peptide cleavage in which two peptides are split off, leaving a fibrin monomer. The resultant monomers of fibrin undergo polymerization to form a bulky insoluble hydrogen bonded aggregate. Further modification of the strandlike molecules of fibrin then takes place, possibly

TABLE 31–1 NOMENCLATURE OF THE VARIOUS COAGULATION FACTORS*

Roman Numeral	Name	Synonym
I	Fibrinogen	
II	Prothrombin	
III	Thromboplastin	
IV	Calcium	
V	Proaccelerin	Labile factor, Ac globulin
VII	Proconvertin	Stable factor, SPCA
VIII	Antihemophilic factor (AHF)	Antihemophilic globulin (AHG), antihemophilic factor A
IX	Plasma thromboplastin component (PTC)	Christmas factor, antihemophilic factor B
X	Stuart factor	Prower factor
XI	Plasma thromboplastin antecedent	Antihemophilic factor C
XII	Hageman factor	Glass or contact factor
XIII	Fibrinase	Clot or fibrin stabilizing factor

***The Roman numeral is the preferred form. Note that no Factor VI is recognized at present.**

by means of cross S—S linkages. This final strengthening of the polymerized fibrin is effected by Factor XIII (fibrin-stabilizing factor), which forms covalent bonds within the fibrin polymer.

Fibrinogen is manufactured by the liver, and severe liver disease may lead to a moderate lowering of plasma fibrinogen levels, though rarely to a degree sufficient to cause hemorrhage. About 50% of transfused fibrinogen disappears from the circulation in 48 hours, and 75% by the sixth day.

Factor II (Prothrombin)

This is a stable protein of alpha$_2$ globulin type (MW 63,000), containing some 18 amino acids, including the sulfur-containing amino acids. It is normally present in the blood in a concentration of approximately 20 mg per dL, or 0.2 g/L. In the presence of ionized calcium it is converted to thrombin by enzymatic action of thromboplastins from both extrinsic and intrinsic sources. It is also slowly activated by high citrate concentration. It is manufactured in the liver under the influence of fat-soluble vitamin K. Prothrombin is related to Factor VII (proconvertin), which is also manufactured in the liver. It has a half-life of approximately 60 hours, and approximately 70% of this is consumed during the clotting process.

Thrombin. The active principle derived from prothrombin is a powerful proteolytic enzyme that can clot many hundreds of times its own weight of fibrinogen. It is a potent platelet-aggregating substance. It has been isolated in relatively pure form with a MW of approximately 40,000. The unit of thrombin is the amount that will coagulate 1 mL of standard fibrinogen solution in 15 seconds at 28°C. During the conversion of fibrinogen to fibrin much of the thrombin is consumed; this results, at least in part, from adsorption onto the fibrin.

Factor III (Thromboplastin)

This is the name given to any substance capable of converting prothrombin to thrombin.

In blood coagulation, two initially separate mechanisms are involved, the extrinsic thromboplastin-generating mechanism and the intrinsic thromboplastin-generating mechanism. Although these two mechanisms are initially separate, they progress through the same final pathway reactions with Factor V and Factor X to produce the definitive thromboplastin. This, in turn, causes the conversion of prothrombin to thrombin and subsequent conversion of fibrinogen to fibrin, i.e., clotting.

Factor IV (Calcium)

Ionized calcium is necessary for the clotting mechanism at three points: (1) in the final elaboration or activation of thromboplastin by interaction of the thromboplastic products of the extrinsic or intrinsic systems with Factor V and Factor X; (2) for the enzymatic conversion of prothrombin to thrombin by active thromboplastin (thrombokinase); and (3) for the formation of fibrin. Of the normal blood calcium approximately half is ionized, and since only very small amounts of ionized calcium are required in the clotting mechanism, defects are not seen clinically except after massive transfusion with citrated blood, when other factors besides depression of ionized calcium are involved.

Factor V (Proaccelerin)

This is a globulin, intermediate between beta and gamma globulins, that is labile, deteriorating rapidly in

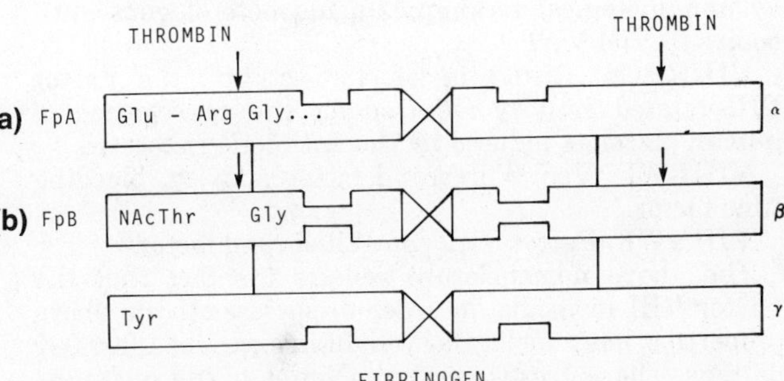

Figure 31–4 Schematic diagram of the fibrinogen molecule. The action of thrombin to produce fibrin monomer is shown by the arrows splitting: *a,* The Arg-Gly bond, producing fibrinopeptide A (FpA); *b,* the Thr-Gly bond, producing fibrinopeptide B (FpB).

plasma, especially oxalated plasma (not so quickly in citrated plasma). Even in frozen (−20°C) plasma, Factor V activity decreases over a period of weeks. It is consumed in the clotting process and is therefore not found in serum. The liver is the site of its manufacture. Factor V is essential to the later phases of thromboplastin formation; i.e., the thromboplastic products of both the extrinsic and intrinsic mechanisms seem to react with Factor V (and probably also Factor X) in the presence of ionic calcium. It is not adsorbed by barium sulfate ($BaSO_4$) or aluminum hydroxide gel ($Al(OH)_3$). Its half-life is approximately 16 hours.

Factor VII (Proconvertin)

Factor VII is not destroyed or consumed in the clotting process, so it is present in both plasma and serum (even in serum left at room temperature for up to 3 days). It appears to be a beta globulin and is removed from plasma or serum by adsorption with $Al(OH)_3$ or $BaSO_4$. The action of Factor VII consists of (1) activation of tissue thromboplastins and (2) acceleration of production of thrombin from prothrombin. It does not form an essential component of the intrinsic thromboplastin-generating mechanism. The concentration of Factor VII (and to a lesser extent, that of prothrombin, Factor IX, and Factor X) is reduced by vitamin K antagonists. Its half-life is approximately 4 to 6 hours.

Factor VIII (Antihemophilic Factor)

Traditionally this factor is described as being consumed during clotting and therefore not found in serum. It is an extremely labile factor: 50 per cent of Factor VIII activity is lost within 12 hours in fresh ACPD anticoagulated blood stored at 4°C. Its life within the body, in vivo survival, is no longer than this: 50 per cent loss in the posttransfusion level occurs within 8 to 12 hours following transfusion. It is more stable in fresh frozen plasma stored at −30°C to −70°C. Lyophilization will preserve it indefinitely with small loss of activity. It is not removed from plasma by adsorption with $Al(OH)_3$ or $BaSO_4$. It is the factor that is deficient in classic hemophilia (p. 724).

It is now evident that this description is inadequate, and this is reflected in the current nomenclature for describing Factor VIII function, namely:

VIIIC. Factor VIII procoagulant activity as measured by clotting assay techniques.

VIIICAg. Factor VIII procoagulant antigen as measured by immunological techniques using homologous antibodies to Factor VIIIC.

VIIIRAg. Factor VIII–related antigen as measured by immunological techniques using heterologous antibodies to VIII/VWF.

VIIIRRCo. Ristocetin-cofactor activity, the Factor VIII–related activity required for the aggregation of human platelets induced by the antibiotic ristocetin.

VIIIRWF. Von Willebrand factor activity, bleeding time factor.

VIII/vWF. Factor VIII/Von Willebrand factor.

The above nomenclature reflects the fact that the Factor VIII molecule, in order to possess all the above properties, has a molecular weight in excess of 1,000,000 daltons. There are two major moieties to the molecule. The high–molecular weight moiety (HMW) possesses the vWF/VIIIRRCo/VIIIRAg properties. A low–molecular weight portion (LMW) possesses the VIIIC and VIIICAg properties. The total molecule is composed of both of these fractions and is described by the nomenclature VIII/vWF.

The HMW portion is under the control of an autosomal gene and is required to be present before the LMW can be induced under the control of a sex-linked (X) gene. Therefore in most circumstances an individual with classic hemophilia (Factor VIII deficiency) has an intact HMW moiety and a deficient procoagulant portion (LMW). This produces an hemophiliac with normal amounts of VIIIRAg, VIIIRRCo, and VIIIRWF and decreased VIIIC and VIIICAg. Using more traditional terms this translates to a sex-linked disorder of procoagulant synthesis with decreased Factor VIII clotting assay results and a normal bleeding time (p. 724). Conversely, severe Von Willebrand's disease has an decreased HMW moiety, and because of this the LMW moiety is also decreased. This produces an individual with decreased amounts of all of the Factor VIII–related activity. In traditional terms an individual who is severely affected with Von Willebrand's disease inherits in an autosomal dominant fashion and has a prolonged bleeding time, defective platelet aggregation to ristocetin, and defective adhesiveness, accompanied by reduced Factor VIII procoagulant levels (p. 731).

It is now evident that the molecular defects in the Factor VIII molecule are manifold, and the above explanation reflects a very crude appreciation of the complexity of both the molecular and inherited defects that can accrue from both autosomal and X chromosome transmission.

Factor IX (Plasma Thromboplastin Component)

This is a stable protein factor. It is not consumed during clotting and is not destroyed by aging, i.e., it is present in both plasma and serum, and there is probably no significant loss of the factor in blood or plasma stored at 4°C for 2 weeks. It is adsorbed by $Al(OH)_3$ and by $BaSO_4$. Factor IX is an essential component of the intrinsic thromboplastin generating system, in which it influences the amount rather than the rate of thromboplastin formation. It has a half-life of approximately 20 hours.

Factor X (Stuart Factor)

This is a relatively stable factor that is not consumed in the clotting process; i.e., it is found in both plasma and serum. It is adsorbed by $Al(OH)_3$ and $BaSO_4$. In its activity it appears to be related to Factor VII. Together with Factor V in the presence of calcium ions, it forms the final common pathway through which the products of both the extrinsic and intrinsic thromboplastin-generating systems work to form the ultimate thromboplastin(s) that convert prothrombin to thrombin. It is an alpha globulin that requires vitamin K for its synthesis in the liver. It has a half-life of approximately 40 hours.

Factor XI (Plasma Thromboplastin Antecedent)

This beta globulin is only partly consumed during clotting. Only small amounts of Factor XI are adsorbed from plasma by $Al(OH)_3$ and $BaSO_4$. Since it is only partly consumed during clotting, it is present in serum. It is essential for the intrinsic thromboplastin-generating mechanism. Factor XI and Factor XII constitute the two "contact" factors of the clotting system. The half-life of Factor XI following transfusion is in some doubt and may be only a few hours.

Factor XII (Hageman Factor)

This is a stable globulin that is not consumed in the clotting process. It is not adsorbed from plasma by $Al(OH)_3$ or $BaSO_4$, but is adsorbed onto powdered glass, Celite, or bentonite.

When Hageman factor comes in contact with glass, it is converted from an inactive to an active form. The natural counterpart to glass is not certain, but damaged endothelium or platelets could well be implicated in this primary activation process. Since glass, Celite, and bentonite are all negatively charged, it is presumed that a reaction occurs with positively charged amino acid residues of Hageman factor. This sequence of events is greatly accelerated by two other plasma proteins, the Fletcher and Fitzgerald factors. These two factors accelerate the conversion of Factor XI to Factor XIa by Factor XIIa. The active form of Fletcher factor is identical to a plasma kallikrein, which releases biologically active polypeptide kinins, e.g., bradykinin from kininogens. Fitzgerald factor is considered to be a high–molecular weight kininogen, which causes optimum conversion of prekallikrein to kallikrein (Fletcher factor) and Factor XI to its activated form.

Factor XIII (Fibrinase)

Thrombin (T) splits four arginyl-glycine bonds of fibrinogen (F) to produce two peptides A, two peptides B (together labeled P), and a fibrin monomer (labeled f). The latter polymerizes and forms intermediate fibrin polymer (labeled fn). Fibrin clot results from further polymerization. With purified reagents, a so-called fine clot (fibrin I) results that is soluble in 5M urea and 1% monochloroacetic acid. If calcium and a serum factor are added, a coarse clot results (fibrin II) that is insoluble in urea or acetic acid. The serum factor is called Factor XIII or fibrinase.

The relationship of the various factors may be illustrated as follows:

Proteolysis	$F \xrightleftharpoons{\text{Thrombin}} f + P\ (\text{A and B})$
Polymerization	Many $f \rightleftharpoons$: fn
Clotting	Many fn $\rightleftharpoons$: Fibrin I
	$\text{Fibrin I} \xrightarrow[\text{Factor XIII + Calcium}]{} \text{Fibrin II}$

Anticoagulants and Inhibitors

It is easily appreciated that if blood is to remain fluid, deposition of intravascular fibrin must be avoided. Various mechanisms are available to contain or control the activation of thrombin.

The pathological or acquired anticoagulants are discussed on p. 746, the therapeutic anticoagulants on p. 734, and artificial anticoagulants on p. 29. Attention is given in this section to the natural anticoagulants or inhibitors of procoagulant action. This will be followed by a description of the plasminolytic mechanism, which is activated in a variety of circumstances to combat fibrin deposition.

Antithrombin System

The term *antithrombin* has been applied collectively to the blood's ability to neutralize thrombin activation.

Antithrombin III. This is the most important of several poorly defined entities and has been relatively well characterized. It is found in the plasma or serum, and reacts with thrombin to form metathrombin. Antithrombin III disappears slowly, since it inactivates thrombin, and is referred to as a progressive antithrombin. There is still confusion as to whether antithrombin III is heparin cofactor identical to antithrombin II. This confusion is not helped by the observation that three separate proteins make up antithrombin III activity. The first is an $alpha_2$ globulin, the second a much larger $alpha_2$ macroglobulin, and the third an $alpha_2$ antitrypsin. The second factor is heparin cofactor. Decreased levels of antithrombin III have been associated with repeated thromboembolism and liver disease. A large number of methods exist for its estimation, using a variety of biological and chemical principles.

Heparin

This material is discussed on p. 734. It has been suggested that owing to endogenous mast cell activity, heparin plays a role in physiological control of coagulation by potentiating anti Xa.

THE PLASMINOLYTIC MECHANISM

Owing to a number of pathological circumstances, fibrin may become deposited either intravascularly or extravascularly; obviously, intravascular deposition has serious consequences (see p. 731). The body has provided a powerful proteolytic enzyme, plasmin, which has the ability to digest not only fibrin but also fibrinogen and other coagulation factors, e.g., Factors VIII and V. Under normal circumstances, plasmin is activated without appreciable plasmin activity appearing in the circulation. In pathological situations overwhelming plasmin action may be initiated and the other clotting factors rapidly destroyed, e.g., the defibrination syndrome.

Figure 31–5 is a simplified concept of how plasmin is elaborated. Under a suitable stimulus plasminogen is activated to form plasmin. Plasmin, in turn, can selectively or nonselectively digest fibrin, fibrinogen, other clotting factors, and activate the kinin system. The last-mentioned system is a complex mechanism whereby certain humoral factors are elaborated during pathological stimulation (e.g., bradykinin, a potent vasodilator),

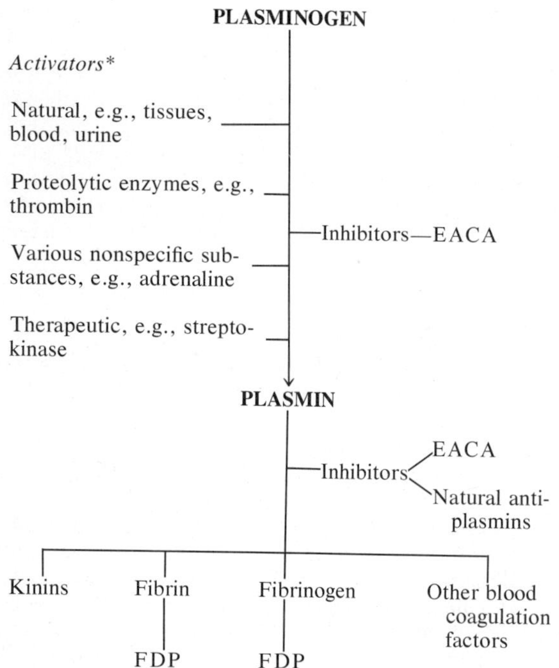

Figure 31–5 The plasminolytic mechanism. *A number of proactivators have been described, particularly the system involved with streptokinase, i.e., proactivator + streptokinase = activator. *EACA*, epsilon amino caproic acid; *FDP*, fibrinogen-fibrin degradation products.

and a feedback mechanism exists to activate the procoagulant system through Factor XII.

Plasminogen activators are found in most tissues and are probably localized inside lysosomes. Endothelial cells of the blood vessels are particularly rich in activator, which can be secreted directly into the bloodstream. As Figure 31–5 suggests, other proteolytic enzymes are capable of activating plasminogen, and again another feedback mechanism is available through thrombin when excessive production causes the reflex activation of the plasminolytic mechanism. Streptokinase, elaborated by streptococci, has been used along with urokinase (isolated from urine) as a therapeutic substance. That is, the plasminolytic system is purposely activated to encourage controlled fibrinolysis and dissolution of intravascular thrombus, e.g., arterial thrombi (see p. 731). Plasminogen activators are released in a variety of nonpathological circumstances, such as emotional stress and exercise. Their release frequently accompanies surgical operations, trauma, hypoxia, etc. Therefore tests that are sensitive to plasminogen activator, i.e., the euglobulin lysis time, will often reflect such activation without pathological plasminolysis having occurred. Plasminogen activator, being released by hypoxia, is therefore increased in blood specimens obtained with the protracted use of a tourniquet and this is responsible for the rule that blood samples being collected for plasminolytic studies should be taken without the use of a tourniquet.

Once plasminogen has been activated, it is transformed to plasmin, which is then able to dissolve or lyse fibrin or other proteins.

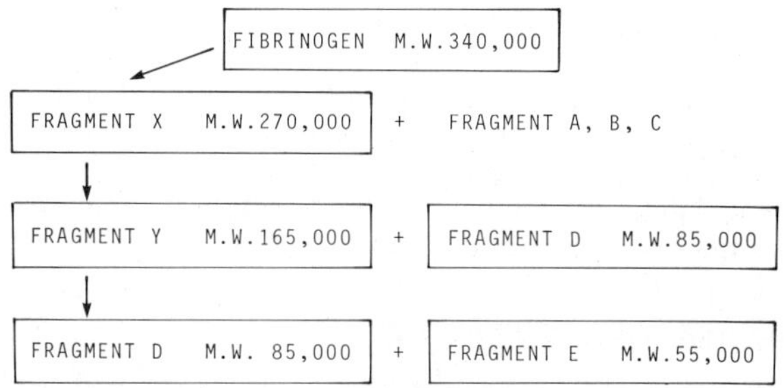

Figure 31–6 Products of plasmin digestion of fibrinogen.

Formation of Fibrinogen-Fibrin Degradation Products (FDP)

The proteolytic digestion of fibrinogen has been thoroughly investigated. Figure 31–6 demonstrates that the progressive digestion of fibrinogen results in a number of fragments; fragments X and Y are larger products that appear transiently during the initial stages of the sequential degradation process. Fragment X has a molecular weight in the range of 240,000 to 265,000, is thrombin clottable, and is derived from the action of plasmin on the alpha and beta chains of fibrinogen. Fragment X is further degraded (at the alpha, beta, and gamma chains) to yield fragments Y and D with respective molecular weights of 155,000 and 83,000. The remnants of alpha, beta, and gamma chains of fragment Y are further and finally degraded into fragments D and E, E having a molecular weight of 41,000. Fragments Y, D, and E are nonclottable with thrombin. A similar degradation occurs with fibrin, although minor differences have been reported.

A considerable degree of confusion has resulted from the terminology of these new biological compounds. It has been suggested that fibrinogen degradation products be labeled FDP, whereas those derived from fibrin be described as fdp. Similarly, because current methods do not distinguish between fibrin and fibrinogen, it has been suggested that they be termed fibrinogen-related antigens. Other synonyms are fibrinogen-derived degradation products and fibrinogen split products.

The physiological properties of FDP are still to be fully elucidated. The anticoagulant properties of fragment X and particularly fragment Y are thought to be caused by their formation of nonclottable complexes with fibrin monomer. These have been referred to as soluble fibrin monomer complexes (SFMC), and the various combinations are shown in Figure 31–7. This reduces the amount of fibrin monomer available for polymerization into fibrin and results in an inadequate thrombus. Fragment D also inhibits fibrin-monomer polymerization, whereas fragment E appears to be a competitive inhibitor of thrombin. FDP also interferes with platelet function and plays an important role in the positive feedback mechanism regulating fibrinogen metabolism. Even the small molecular weight peptides (A, B, and C) have been incriminated in histamine and bradykinin release. Clearance of FDP is usually rapid unless liver or renal function is impaired.

The techniques used to detect these products are described on p. 749; the majority of them rely upon immunological principles. None of the routine methods

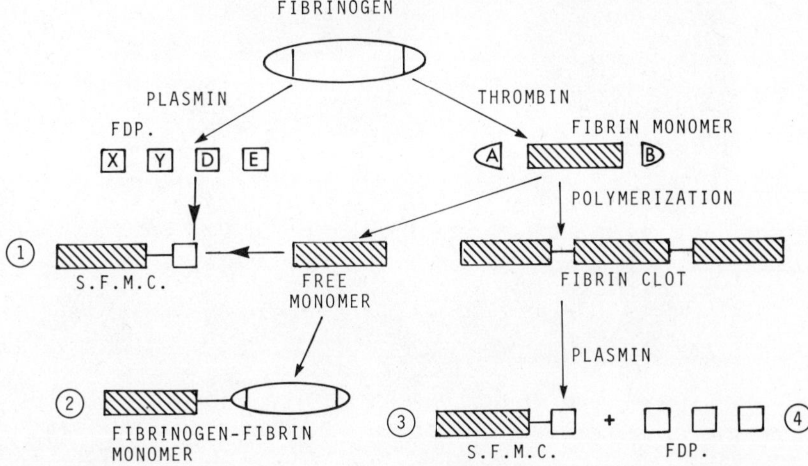

Figure 31–7 Showing the relationship between the action of plasmin on fibrin and fibrinogen, and thrombin on fibrinogen. The main products are *1* and *3*. Soluble fibrin monomer complexes: *2*, fibrinogen-fibrin monomer clot; *4*, fibrinogen degradation products (FDP).

can differentiate between fibrinogen or fibrin degradation products, although the radioimmune assays show promise in this area. If the protamine sulfate test is positive in association with increased FDP, it is assumed that fibrin products are also present owing to the presence of SFMC (see p. 749).

Classically, increased FDP levels have been associated with disseminated intravascular coagulation or thrombosis (DIC—see p. 731). However, it is important to realize that the conditions associated with increased plasminolysis produce FDP without fibrin deposition's necessarily being implicated. Not only are increased levels associated with exercise and stress, but any serious illness or surgical maneuver will cause increases compatible with nonspecific plasminolytic activation.

Inhibitors of Plasminolysis

Various substances are capable of inhibiting the plasminogen-plasmin system. Present in the blood are large amounts of alpha globulins with antiplasmin activity of two types: immediate and slow-acting. Platelets also appear to inhibit plasmin. There are also a number of substances that inhibit plasminogen activators. Two compounds are used therapeutically in this instance: epsilon amino caproic acid and tranexamic acid. Both are useful in conditions in which primary plasminolysis is diagnosed. They are contraindicated in the majority of conditions associated with gross plasminolysis, because this is invariably a reflection of DIC, and neutralization of the system can lead to uncontrolled intravascular fibrin deposition.

Primary Versus Secondary Plasminolysis

This will be discussed further in the classification of hemostatic defects, but it is important to recognize that when free plasmin is present in the circulation, it can be the result either of primary activation of the plasminogen-plasmin system or of activation of plasminolysis secondary to intravascular fibrin formation.

Conditions classified as primary plasminolysis disorders are related to excessive plasminogen activator release, such as occurs in anoxia or shock, and the blood of such patients not only shows all the signs of fibrinogen proteolysis, but an acute abnormality of hemostasis results. Secondary plasminolysis is associated with fibrin formation and is rightly considered a reflection of localized or generalized fibrin deposition. The tests used to discriminate between these two conditions are discussed on p. 748.

THE PLATELET SYSTEM

Platelets fulfill a vital role in hemostasis and are now recognized as being responsible for a series of complex maneuvers that initiate the primary hemostatic plug (platelet plug) and so afford the first line of defense in normal hemostasis. Platelet defects not only cause functional or numerical deficiencies with pathological bleeding, but they are often responsible for the formation of abnormal intravascular thrombi.

The normal function of platelets may be summarized as follows:

1. Maintenance of normal endothelial integrity.
2. Formation of the primary platelet plug.
3. Release of vasoactive substances, e.g., vasoconstriction of injured blood vessels by serotonin.
4. Promotion of initial stages of blood coagulation by membrane-mediated factors, and subsequent involvement through phospholipid production.
5. Production of clot retraction protein (thrombosthenin).
6. Release of other substances that have a wide variety of physiological or pathological effects, e.g., histamine.

Structure and Contents of the Platelet

The formation of platelets has already been described on p. 620, and Figure 31–8 shows typical platelet morphology. The trilaminar membrane is covered by an amorphous surface coat that may be related to the innate stickiness of the activated platelet. The microtubular system acts as a form of submembranous skeleton and maintains the cell in a discoid state. Cytoplasmic or submembranous fibrils are seen and may participate in clot retraction. The interior of the cell consists of a variety of organelles, including mitochondria, permit

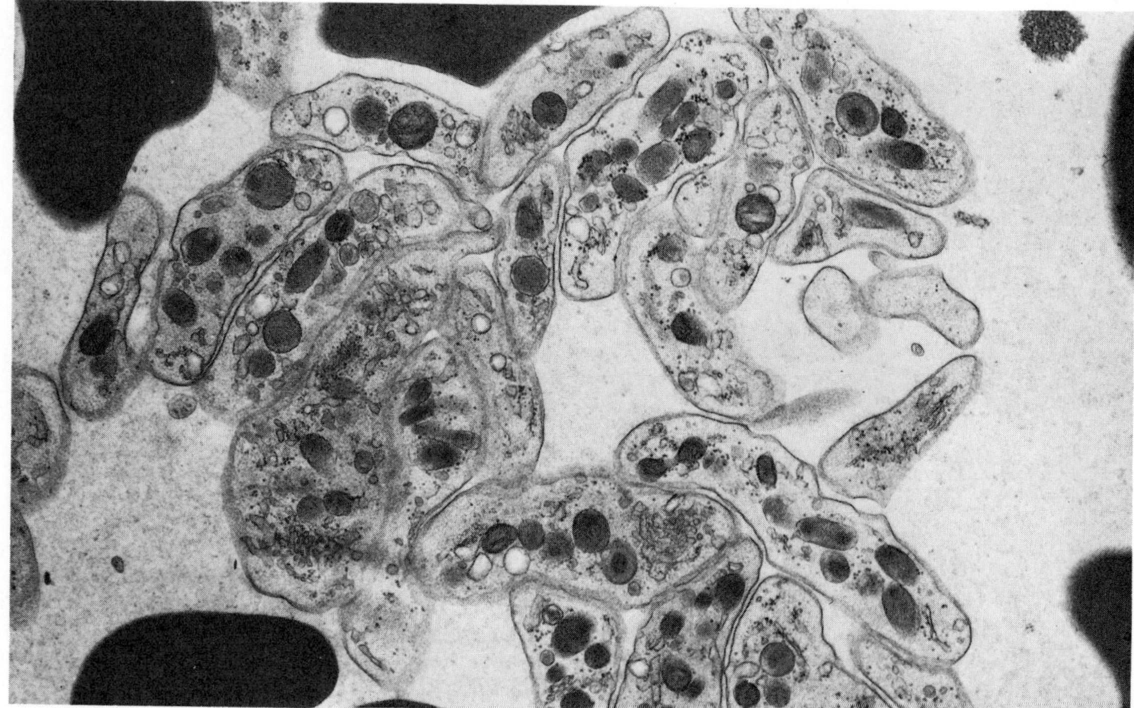

Figure 31–8 Electron micrograph of platelets in a hamster cheek pouch vessel showing a primary aggregate with the majority of the platelets not having undergone a release reaction.

ting oxidative phosphorylation and alpha granules which contain fibrinogen, ATP, ADP, and a number of enzymes, including Platelet Factor 3. The dense bodies contain epinephrine, serotonin, and norepinephrine, which are released during secondary aggregation. A canalicular system representing tubelike invaginations of the cell cytoplasm is often present. Vacuoles are present in varying number and size, along with glycogen particles.

A number of platelet factors involved in intrinsic and extrinsic coagulation have been described, although there are still some discrepancies in terminology among workers. Platelet Factor 1 (PF 1) is absorbed Factor V; PF 2 is a thrombin accelerator. PF 3 is found in the alpha granulomeres as well as in the surface membrane. It appears to be intimately involved in intrinsic coagulation, acting as a prothrombin activator by catalyzing the reaction between Factors Xa, V, and calcium. It is released by platelet aggregation and is equivalent to the phospholipid platelet substitutes. PF 4 has been described variously as an inhibitor of heparin and having Factor XIII activity.

Adhesion and Aggregation

It is now recognized that a wide variety of agents will cause initial adhesion followed by aggregation and irreversible changes in platelet morphology. These agents include a wide variety of damaged tissues, viruses, antigen-antibody complexes, collagen, ADP, thrombin, and foreign surfaces. Platelets do not normally adhere to intact endothelium.

Whatever the stimulus required to cause adhesion of platelets in a given area, it is the sequelae that determine the course of events leading to the production of a permanent platelet plug. Adhesion is followed by the "release reaction" in which various agents are selectively released by the platelet. The secreted substances include epinephrine, adenine nucleotides, serotonin, calcium, potassium, PF 4, and the other various coagulant factors. PF 3 does not reside in the soluble substance expelled into the plasma but represents an alteration in the platelet membrane, making phospholipid available for intrinsic coagulation.

The release reaction occupies a central position in platelet function, since it accounts for the complex effects of platelet adhesion and subsequent aggregation. Many stimuli, besides surface interactions, will induce the release reaction. Epinephrine, ADP, and serotonin, once released, continue to induce further release and so become self-perpetuating until the platelet has undergone irreversible aggregation. The release of ADP is particularly important, since it not only causes platelet swelling and transformation from thin discs to spiculated spheres, but increases platelet stickiness and aggregation. Collagen, epinephrine, and thrombin are potent aggregating agents but each acts by causing platelets to release endogenous ADP stores, which in turn promotes further aggregation.

Once aggregation has been induced, the subsequent release reaction converts the reversible primary aggregates of readily dissociable platelets into an irreversibly bound platelet plug. The platelet membrane becomes irregular, and interdigitation of adjacent platelet pseudopodia occurs. As Figure 31–9 indicates, the internal structure of the platelet changes drastically, with the

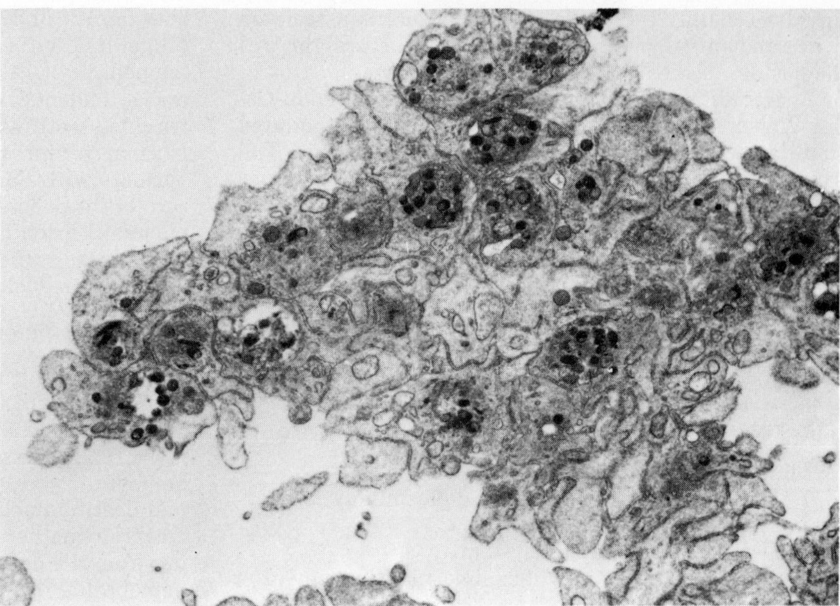

Figure 31–9 Electron micrograph of human platelets aggregated with *Trimeresurus okinavensis* snake venom. It shows the compactness of the final irreversible platelet aggregate with loss of discoid shape, formation of irregular surfaces, and granule fusion.

granules moving to the center of the cell and discharging their contents into the canalicular system. With the release of the previously mentioned substances, activation of the coagulation mechanism also occurs with the final laying down of fibrin to reinforce the platelet plug.

The thrombus requires a final function from platelets, namely, clot retraction, and this is mediated through the platelet contractile protein thrombosthenin. This is a fibrillar protein with a periodic structure similar to that of actomyosin, and it would appear to be the largest component of the platelet microfibrils and tubules. The stimulus for contraction is unknown, but it is ATP and calcium dependent and occurs in the pseudopods of the activated platelets causing consolidation of the clot.

Mention must be made of the mechanism by which platelets are either prevented or encouraged to aggregate. The common factor mediating this reaction is the universal "hormone messenger" 3′5′ cyclic adenosine monophosphate (CAMP). It has now been demonstrated that if the level of CAMP is increased within the platelet, aggregation does not take place and vice versa. Epinephrine, thrombin, ADP, and collagen all decrease CAMP and are potent aggregating agents. Dipyridamole, papaverine, caffeine, and prostaglandin E_1 (PGE_1) all increase CAMP levels and inhibit platelet aggregation

Tests of platelet function must be able to reflect the ability of the platelet to adhere, aggregate, and form a hemostatic plug. The range of tests required is described on p. 750, whereas defects in these functions are described on p. 730.

It is now evident that prostaglandin synthesis and various intermediate compounds resulting from such synthesis occupy an important role in the mediation of platelet action. Prostacylin contained in the vessel wall (prostaglandin 1_2) is a vigorous deaggregating agent, and thromboxane produced within the platelet is an equally active aggregating agent. The balance between these antithetical agents is maintained by other prostaglandin intermediates and metabolites. Similarly, various converting enzymes, e.g., cyclooxygenase, play an important role in determining whether thromboxane or prostacyclin is produced; e.g., ASA will inhibit cyclooxygenase, causing the platelet to become deficient in thromboxane and less liable to aggregate if the platelet activates its release mechanisms.

Classification of Abnormal Bleeding Tendencies

From the foregoing description of the hemostatic mechanism, it follows that abnormal bleeding tendencies may result from defects in any one of the three main hemostatic mechanisms: extravascular, vascular, or intravascular (blood). The following classification, therefore, may be useful, though it should be emphasized that the bulk of abnormalities requiring technological elucidation fall into the third category, i.e., abnormalities of the intravascular system or clotting of blood.

Extravascular and Vascular Defects

1. Atrophy of elastic tissues: e.g., senile purpura, seen as ecchymoses (diffuse bruising) in the loose tissues of the backs of the hands and feet of elderly persons.
2. Hyperlaxity of the skin: e.g., Ehlers-Danlos syndrome (rare).
3. Unusual "fragility": susceptibility to trauma on the part of the skin, e.g., in Cushing's syndrome or steroid administration.
4. Local pressures: e.g., tight garments or elastic bands (anoxia is involved in addition to local trauma).
5. Vitamin C deficiency: in clinical scurvy loss of vascular integrity is characterized by a positive tourniquet test and a distinctive clinical picture. It often causes diagnostic problems, and it is important to exclude other, more serious conditions, e.g., leukemia.
6. Allergic purpura: Henoch-Schönlein purpura is part of a widespread disease that probably represents an immune complex process. The characteristic rash

involves mainly the limbs and trunk and is associated with abdominal pain, hematuria, and arthralgia. All hemostasis screening tests are usually normal.

7. Hereditary hemorrhagic telangiectasia: Rendu-Osler-Weber disease is a condition of multiple dilated capillaries that present a typical telangiectasia. The condition is dominantly inherited and usually becomes evident and increases in severity with age. Bleeding presents from the skin and mucosal surface, particularly the gastrointestinal tract, and may be very severe.

8. Miscellaneous: a number of chronic diseases are associated with vascular abnormalities with bruising and abnormal capillary structure. Infections and liver disease are examples.

Intravascular Defects

The main defects are:

1. Defects of the coagulation and plasminolytic mechanisms.
2. Defects of the platelet system.
3. Acquired defects in which abnormalities may exist in all three systems.

DEFECTS OF COAGULATION MECHANISM

The associated conditions are:

1. Defects of thromboplastin formation: Factor XII deficiency, Factor XI deficiency, Factor IX deficiency, and Factor VIII deficiency.
2. Defects of second stage coagulation: Factor X deficiency, Factor V deficiency, Factor VII deficiency, and Factor II deficiency.
3. Defects of fibrin formation: Factor I deficiency and Factor XIII deficiency.

Factor XII Deficiency

This is inherited as an autosomal recessive and, like Fletcher and Fitzgerald factor deficiencies, is not associated with any hemorrhagic manifestation. It is usually detected by accident, e.g., routine preoperative screen. Laboratory diagnosis is by use of a specific assay after an abnormal APTT is found.

Factor XI Deficiency

The deficiency is inherited as an incomplete recessive autosomal (i.e., not sex linked), and the trait affects both males and females. Deficiency thus inherited is congenital and leads to a mild hemophilia-like condition (hemophilia C) that manifests itself as a slight to moderate tendency to excessive bleeding following cuts, trauma, teeth extraction, tonsillectomy, and so forth. Normal serum, normal plasma, and also plasma from patients with Factor VIII and Factor IX deficiency will correct the deficiency, as will $Al(OH)_3$ or $BaSO_4$-adsorbed plasma. Frozen or refrigerated stored plasma (up to 14 days old) is sufficient to control the bleeding. The effect of such transfusion wears off in about one week.

TABLE 31–2 CLASSIFICATION OF THE MAJOR HEMOSTATIC DEFECTS

Vascular and extravascular defects
Intravascular defects
Coagulation defects:
Factor deficiencies
Defects in the plasminolytic system
Platelet defects:
Quantitative
Qualitative functional
Mixed defects (acquired):
Disseminated intravascular coagulation
Hepatic disease
Miscellaneous

Factor IX Deficiency (Christmas Disease)

This congenital deficiency was first described in a family living in Canada named Christmas, and, coincidentally, the report appeared during the week of Christmas, 1952. Heredity plays the same role as in classic hemophilia, i.e., the condition is a sex-linked recessive, manifesting itself in half the sons; half the daughters of a carrier mother become carriers. The condition resulting from the deficiency is indistinguishable from classic hemophilia. In the laboratory the defect leads to delayed thromboplastin generation and is correctable by the addition of small amounts of either fresh or aged normal plasma or serum (but not by $Al(OH)_3$- or $BaSO_4$-adsorbed plasma or serum). Of final diagnostic importance, the defect is corrected by addition of plasma from patients with Factor VIII deficiency or of plasma from persons deficient in Factor XI.

A number of variants of this condition now exist, the most common being hemophilia B^M. This has the unusual property of giving a prolonged one-stage prothrombin time using ox brain thromboplastin.

Treatment of patients deficient in Factor IX is determined by the degree of severity. Up until recent times the infusion of fresh or stored plasma was the only material available. However, a number of prothrombin complex concentrates containing Factor IX are available (see p. 578).

Factor VIII Deficiency (Classic Hemophilia)

This has the same clinical presentation and inheritance as Factor IX deficiency, in which recurrent bleeding into joints (hemarthroses) and bleeding from mucous membranes, kidneys, and other organs may be crippling or fatal. The reason only very few female hemophiliacs are found probably lies in the lethal character of the double-dose inheritance. At least some of the females who have been described as true hemophiliacs have since been shown to be of chromosomal male type. As in any sex-linked inheritance, various family patterns are possible. The following provide examples of possible matings:

HEMOPHILIAC MALE AND NORMAL FEMALE:

Father		Mother	
X^HY		XX	
XX^H	XX^H	XY	XY
Carrier Daughters		Normal Sons	

NORMAL MALE AND CARRIER FEMALE (most common):

Father		Mother	
XY		$X^H X$	
XX	XX^H	XY	X^HY
Normal Daughter	Carrier Daughter	Normal Son	Hemophiliac Son

HEMOPHILIAC MALE AND CARRIER MOTHER (very rare):

Father		Mother	
$X^H Y$		$X^H X$	
$X^H X^H$	$X^H X$	$X^H Y$	XY
Hemophiliac Daughter	Carrier Daughter	Hemophiliac Son	Normal Son

The incidence of hemophilia A is approximately 1 per 10,000 live male births, but it does vary slightly from area to area. Before the introduction of Factor VIII concentrates, the life expectancy of severe hemophiliacs was very poor. However, they now can be expected to live relatively normal lives provided they receive prompt and expert treatment as soon as there is any evidence of bleeding. In general, hemophiliacs with a Factor VIII level of below 1 per cent are severely affected, whereas levels above 10 per cent are not associated with spontaneous hemorrhages.

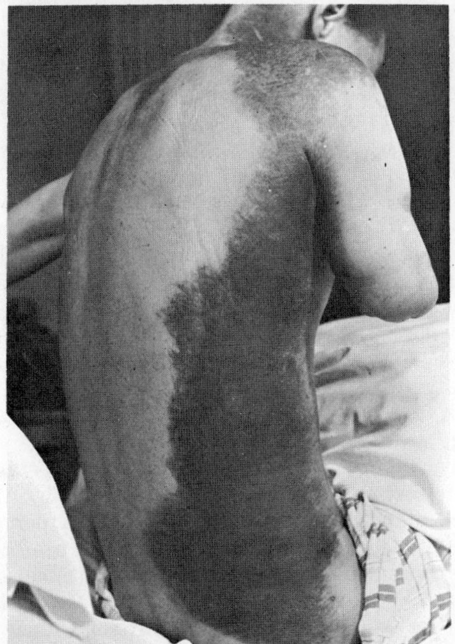

Figure 31–10 Extensive bruising (in a patient with classic hemophilia) caused by a minor fall. The patient has been hospitalized many times before because of severe bleeding episodes. A previous minor injury led to the loss of his right forearm.

Diagnosis. Diagnosis of Factor VIII and IX deficiencies is by the usual parameters of family history (e.g., sex-linked versus autosomal), clinical presentation, and laboratory tests. The PTT will be prolonged, with a normal one-stage, prothrombin time. Occasionally, in very mild cases (e.g., 30 per cent Factor VIII level), the PTT may be normal, and one must be guided by the clinical assessment and still use the usual confirmatory tests. These are Factor VIII assays; correction of deficient plasma with $Al(OH)_3$-absorbed plasma and Factor IX–deficient plasma. Differentiation from von Willebrand's disease can be confusing (see p. 731). The level of antigenic Factor VIII is normal compared to the abnormally low clottable Factor VIII (see p. 718).

Treatment. The treatment of such individuals is now governed by the availability of suitable concentrates. Cryoprecipitated Factor VIII and lyophilized concentrates are the materials of choice (see p. 579). The administration of these products has now become simplified enough to justify the use of home treatment programs.

It is important to achieve hemostatic levels of Factor VIII as quickly as possible; this is usually accepted as being approximately 30 per cent Factor VIII. Once this level has been achieved it may be maintained by frequent infusions. If levels are allowed to drop to below therapeutic values, further hemorrhage is to be expected. This approach is of the greatest importance when performing surgical procedures on hemophiliacs, e.g., tooth extractions. The use of EACA (epsilon amino caproic acid, an antifibrinolytic substance) has been advocated by a number of workers in order to stabilize the friable hemophiliac's clot. To date the main indication for its use is in oral surgery, and the therapy is not without complications.

Inhibitors. Inhibitors to Factor VIII have become an increasingly difficult problem in treating hemophiliacs. Since the use of specific therapy, it has become evident that some severely affected hemophiliacs become resistant to therapy. Examination of plasma from such individuals shows the presence of antibodies to Factor VIII. Approximately 10 per cent of hemophiliacs will produce antibodies, and that antibody production is probably related to therapeutic Factor VIII infusions either in plasma or concentrated form. They occur primarily in severely affected individuals and therefore constitute a serious complication.

Detection of such antibodies can be accomplished by a variety of methods. It is suggested that such assays use the principle of mixing the test plasma containing the suspected antibody with a plasma of known Factor VIII level. After suitable incubation at 37°C, the mixture is reassayed to ascertain whether there has been a greater decrease in Factor VIII as compared to the control.

Treatment of hemophiliacs with inhibitors is by no means stabilized. A number of different approaches have been used, namely:

1. Use of minidoses of Factor VIII aimed at reducing the degree of hemorrhage but not encouraging stimulation of the antibody.

2. Use of overwhelming doses of Factor VIII material (as much as 20,000 units of Factor VIII in one infusion) to overwhelm the circulating antibody and establish a therapeutic level of Factor VIII.

3. Use of various immunosuppressive agents in combination with Factor VIII material. Agents such as cyclophosphamide, corticosteroids, 6-mercaptopurine, and azathioprine have all been used with varied degrees of success.

4. Use of activated prothrombin complex concentrates that bypass Factor VIII and directly activate Factor X or other factors.

5. Use of Factor VIII derived from animal sources (e.g., porcine), which does not react with the human Factor VIII antibody.

Factor X Deficiency

This rare congenital deficiency leads to a clinical state characterized by excessive bruising and nosebleeds and is very similar to Factor VII deficiency. The blood of persons deficient in Factor X gives an abnormal partial thromboplastin time and one-stage prothrombin time. The defect is correctable by the addition of small amounts of normal serum or of serum from Factor VII–deficient patients. The Russell viper venom test is often abnormal. Clinically, bleeding may be controlled by transfusion of blood, plasma, or serum. Inheritance appears to be controlled by an incompletely recessive autosomal gene, and carriers (heterozygotes) may display mild bleeding tendencies. Factor X levels are decreased in hepatic disease and during oral vitamin K antagonist therapy.

Factor V Deficiency

This rare congenital deficiency leads to a tendency to excessive bleeding from mucous membranes, and nosebleeds and menorrhagia can be fatal. Inheritance appears to be through a recessive autosomal gene. Although heterozygotes do not suffer from excessive bleeding, their plasma may be shown to be relatively deficient in Factor V (levels of 20 to 60 per cent of normal are usually encountered). Stored plasma (especially if oxalated) will fail to correct the prolonged prothrombin time, but small amounts of fresh normal plasma or of adsorbed normal plasma will completely correct the abnormal results. Affected persons who are bleeding must receive a transfusion of fresh whole blood or fresh plasma. Since the effect of transfused blood does not last much longer than one day, it may be necessary to repeat the transfusions daily or every second day until the bleeding is controlled. Acquired Factor V deficiency may occur in severe liver disease or may result from circulating anticoagulant activity.

Factor VII Deficiency

This congenital deficiency state shares common features with Factor V deficiency in that it has similar patterns of inheritance and clinical presentation. However, it is characterized by a normal APTT, abnormal one-stage prothrombin time, and correction of the defect by aged serum. The thromboplastin generation test is also normal in most circumstances.

Factor VII levels are also decreased in vitamin K antagonist therapy and liver disease. Treatment is with either stored plasma or appropriate plasma concentrate.

TABLE 31–3 CONSUMPTION, AGING, AND ADSORPTION CHARACTERISTICS OF CLOTTING FACTORS

Factor Substance	Present in Normal Plasma: Fresh	Present in Normal Plasma: Aged	Present in Normal Serum	Adsorbed by $BaSO_4$ or $Al(OH)_3$
Factor VII	Yes	Yes (3 days)	Yes	Yes
Factor IX	Yes	Yes	Yes	Yes
Factor VIII	Yes	No	No	No
Factor XI	Yes	Yes	Yes	No (partly)
Factor XII	Yes	Yes (but adsorbed by glass)	Yes	No
Factor V	Yes	No	No	No
Factor X	Yes	Yes	Yes	Yes
Prothrombin (Factor II)	Yes	Yes (but gradually falls)	20% or less	Yes
Fibrinogen (Factor I)	Yes	Yes	No	No

Factor II Deficiency

Primary or idiopathic deficiency is exceedingly rare and only a few cases have been reported. Deficiency is usually acquired and results from conditions that impair either the absorption of vitamin K from the gut or utilization of this vitamin by the liver. Vitamin K is present in green vegetables, but most of the vitamin absorbed is manufactured by bacteria in the intestine. Suppression of the bacterial flora of the gut (e.g., by antibiotics) for a long enough period may lead to a deficiency, since the vitamin is not stored by the body. Vitamin K is fat soluble, and its absorption from the gut parallels that of fats. Hence, conditions that lead to impairment of fat absorption are likely to lead to deficient supplies of the vitamin and therefore to deficiency of prothrombin. Major examples of such conditions are obstructive jaundice (lack of bile, which causes malabsorption of fats) and steatorrhea. Severe liver diseases, e.g., infectious hepatitis and advanced cirrhosis, lead to depression of plasma prothrombin levels as well as Factors VII, IX, and X, because the disordered liver cells appear unable to use vitamin K adequately. The oral anticoagulant drugs in normal therapeutic dosage depress plasma prothrombin levels only moderately, but overdosage with these drugs may lead to severe prothrombin deficiency. In newborn infants, prothrombin levels and also levels of Factor VII, Factor IX, and Factor X tend to be lower than normal but rise gradually with age.

Laboratory findings are a prolonged one-stage prothrombin test and APTT, both not corrected by $Al(OH)_3$-adsorbed plasma, aged serum, or Russell viper venom. The two-stage prothrombin assay is often used to identify the condition, although absolute identification may be exceedingly difficult. A circulating anticoagulant must be excluded as for any of the rare deficiency states.

Factor I Deficiency

This deficiency is now characterized by three modes of presentation: (a) congenital afibrinogenemia, (b) congenital dysfibrinogenemia, and (c) acquired hypofibrinogenemia.

Congenital Afibrinogenemia. This is transmitted as a non–sex-linked recessive character. Not infrequently, parents of affected persons are blood relations. In many cases the defect is not absolute, i.e., approximately 5 mg of fibrinogen per dL, or 0.5 g/L, of blood is present. The condition is likely to manifest itself as unusual bleeding from wounds affecting larger vessels, e.g., at birth, from the umbilical cord, and in later life, following extensive trauma or surgery.

Laboratory identification rests firmly on a quantitative fibrinogen assay, although all clotting tests show an infinite prolongation owing to the absence of clottable material. However, in tests that use normal substrate plasma (thromboplastin generation test) the results show normal thrombin formation. Platelet function is generally normal, with small amounts of platelet fibrinogen being demonstrable.

Treatment is usually in the form of plasma or the same cryoprecipitate that is used to treat Factor VIII deficiency (which contains Factor VIII and fibrinogen).

Congenital Dysfibrinogenemia. Congenital dysfibrinogenemia is characterized by the presence of functionally defective forms of fibrinogen, although conventional assays may indicate normal levels of clottable protein. In the majority of cases reported, the mode of inheritance is by an autosomal dominant gene. The clinical presentation is varied in that individuals may be asymptomatic or may have a bleeding diathesis or recurrent thromboembolism.

In the laboratory the usual abnormality is a prolonged thrombin time, variable results with a reptilase clotting test, and quantitative assays that may vary from low to normal to raised.

Acquired Hypofibrinogenemia. This will be discussed under the headings of disseminated intravascular coagulation and primary plasminolysis.

Defects of the Plasminolytic Mechanism

Mention has been made of the disturbances that occur in this system (see p. 719). Defects or changes in the system are as follows: (1) physiological changes, (2) primary plasminolysis, (3) secondary plasminolysis, and (4) iatrogenic plasminolysis.

Physiological Changes. It must again be emphasized that release of plasminogen activator is a normal event in a number of circumstances. Slight elevation of FDPs or a decreased euglobulin lysis time without diminution of fibrinogen must not be construed as a pathological state.

Primary Plasminolysis. Primary plasminolysis is associated with conditions in which there is gross activation of the plasminolytic system with subsequent fibrinogen and other coagulation factor digestion. The important clinical and laboratory distinction is that there is no evidence to suggest fibrin deposition; therefore a DIC (disseminated intravascular coagulation) event may be excluded. Not only is this distinction valuable in terms of patient management, but more important, the modalities of treatment are radically different for the two conditions.

Primary plasminolysis occurs when large amounts of plasminogen activator enter the intravascular space as a result of tissue trauma, surgical operations, and malignant conditions. However, all these conditions are also associated with DIC in which the plasminolytic reaction is secondary and protective (vide infra). Since both conditions often produce precipitous generalized bleeding, distinction between the two rests essentially on the demonstration of fibrin formation. Clinically, the conditions classically associated with primary reactions are thoracic and prostatic surgery, carcinoma of the prostate, and hepatic disease.

TABLE 31–4 Laboratory Differentiation Between a Primary and Secondary (DIC) Plasminolytic Event

Tests	Primary	Secondary (DIC)
PT	Decreased	Decreased
PTT	Decreased	Decreased
TCT	Decreased	Decreased
Fibrinogen	Decreased	Decreased
FDPs	Increased	Increased
Protamine sulfate test	Negative	Positive
Microangiopathic blood morphology	No	Yes
Platelet count	Normal	Reduced

Laboratory diagnosis is summarized in Table 31–4.

Once a satisfactory diagnosis has been made, the abnormal plasminolysis may be modified by the use of plasminogen-plasmin inhibitors, i.e., EACA (epsilon amino caproic acid) and tranexamic acid. If there is any doubt as to whether plasminolysis is secondary, these agents must not be given or diffuse or localized organ thrombosis may result.

Secondary Plasminolysis. This is discussed on p. 731 under DIC or the defibrination syndrome.

Iatrogenic Plasminolysis. Page 736 discusses the use of streptokinase and urokinase as inducers of therapeutic defibrination.

PLATELET DEFECTS

Thrombocytopenia

Table 31–5 shows the major classification for the platelet disorders. A physiological classification has been used in an attempt to localize the defect either at the bone marrow, peripheral blood, or cellular level. Page 750 discusses the platelet function tests used in the investigation of these conditions.

Decreased Production

A number of conditions are implicated in a decrease in megakaryopoiesis. They are: (a) congenital, (b) drug-induced, (c) malignant disease, and (d) megaloblastic anemia.

Lack of thrombopoietin has been reported as causing thrombocytopenia. However, it is a very rare disorder and the nature of thrombopoietin is unknown at this time. More commonly, decreased production is owing to acquired conditions, namely, aplastic anemia, marrow infiltration by neoplastic cells, carcinoma, acute and chronic leukemia, and other malignant conditions. Often use of antineoplastic drugs, e.g., cystosine arabinoside, and the alkylating agents will cause profound thrombocytopenia.

TABLE 31–5 CLASSIFICATION OF PLATELET DISORDERS

Thrombocytopenia	Thrombocytosis	Functional
Decreased production due to bone marrow failure Increased destruction and utilization due to: Immune mechanisms Hypersplenism Endothelial damage DIC	Myeloproliferative disorders Inflammation Postsplenectomy Neoplasia	Thrombasthenia Thrombocytopathy Drug-induced Uremia Dysgammaglobulinemia

Nutritional deficiencies (e.g., vitamin B_{12} and folic acid deficiencies), if severe enough, will show striking thrombocytopenia.

The congenital thrombocytopenias are rare and associated with Fanconi's syndrome, Wiskott-Aldrich syndrome, and the May-Hegglin anomaly.

Laboratory Diagnosis

This usually depends on (1) examination of the bone marrow, which shows evidence of decreased or abnormal megakaryopoiesis along with the presence of obvious bone marrow disease, e.g., leukemia, and (2) a decreased platelet count, with a low megathrombocyte index.

INCREASED DESTRUCTION OR UTILIZATION

Excessive Consumption or Utilization of Platelets. (1) Activation of the hemostatic mechanism, (2) endothelial cell damage, and (3) hypersplenism (excessive trapping of platelets in the spleen).

Immune Mechanisms. (1) Idiopathic thrombocytopenic purpura, (2) autoimmune disease, (3) infections, (4) drug-induced.

Transfusion-Induced. (1) Dilutional, (2) immune, and (3) extracorporeal circulation.

EXCESSIVE CONSUMPTION OF PLATELETS

Activation of Hemostatic Mechanism

This is described in detail on p. 714, but it is important to note that in some conditions platelets appear to be selectively utilized on either a generalized basis, i.e., endotoxemia, or on a local basis, i.e., giant hemangioma (Kasabach-Merritt syndrome).

Endothelial Cell Damage

A variety of conditions are related to endothelial cell damage. Clinically these are referred to as vasculitis syndromes, e.g., lupus erythematosus and thrombotic thrombocytopenic purpura. A major requirement is that the vessel wall is damaged, causing adhesion and aggregation of platelets to the damaged vascular segments. The platelets will then either undergo a fibrinoid change or become the focus for fibrin deposition.

Hypersplenism

This is a hematological term describing premature destruction of the blood cells by the spleen, usually with consequent anemia, leukopenia, or thrombocytopenia. The four signs of hypersplenism are cytopenia, corre-

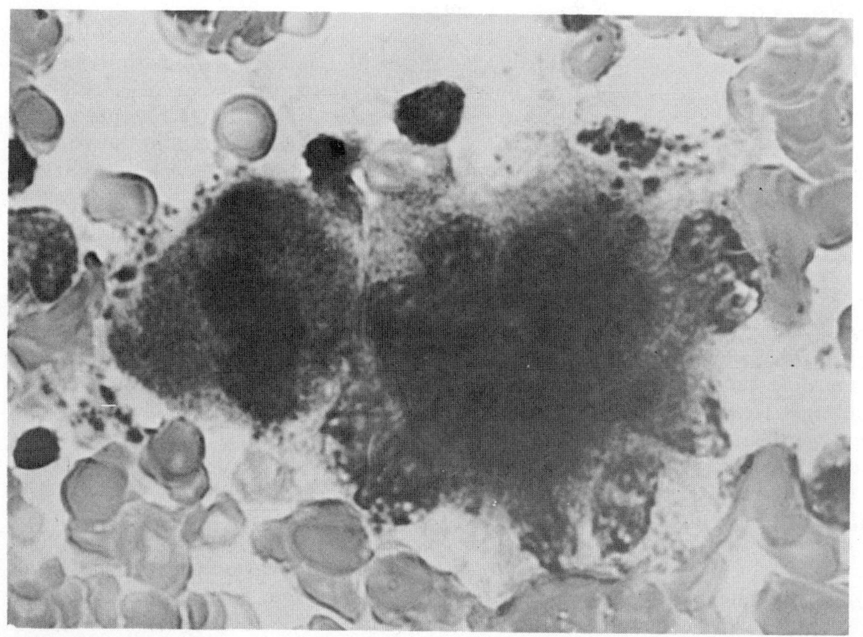

Figure 31–11 Normal megakaryocyte in a smear of aspirated marrow. Platelets are being formed in the peripheral cytoplasm and are separating off from the edges of the cytoplasm. The nucleus is large and multilobed. × 1350.

sponding hyperplasia in the bone marrow precursor cells (e.g., thrombocytopenia with increased megakaryocytes), splenomegaly, and the relief of the cytopenia by splenectomy. Differentiation has to be made from the immune thrombocytopenias in which an excessive number of platelets are removed because of an immune-mediated mechanism. Diagnosis can be difficult and is usually one of exclusion.

Laboratory Diagnosis of Excessive Platelet Consumption

The following general tests are of use:

1. Bone marrow to prove adequate megakaryopoiesis.
2. Megathrombocyte index is usually increased, i.e., platelets larger than 2.5 μm as a percentage of all platelets exceeds a normal value (usually up to 20%).
3. Platelet survival studies with organ scanning demonstrate decreased platelet survival with increased uptake by the spleen or liver, or both.
4. A hemostatic survey must exclude DIC.
5. Platelet antibody tests (platelet-associated IgG) must exclude an immune process, e.g., normal or elevated levels.

IMMUNE THROMBOCYTOPENIA

Idiopathic Thrombocytopenic Purpura (ITP)

Until recent years this was the term given to any thrombocytopenia that produced purpura and for which no reason could be found. It is now apparent that this disease is antibody mediated, owing to the production of a specific antiplatelet antibody. Serological demonstration of antiplatelet antibodies has been difficult, since they do not uniformly fix complement or react in standard immunological tests. However, with the introduction of radioimmune isotope and other assays the detection of platelet-associated IgG is now feasible. As a result, ITP is now more appropriately referred to as *idiopathic immune thrombocytopenia,* provided that elevated levels of platelet-associated IgG are demonstrated.

Acute, chronic, and recurrent forms of the disease have been described with a predilection of the chronic form for females. Most of the patients with acute disease give a history of an antecedent infection in the week preceding the onset of purpura. For this reason it is entirely possible that many acute cases of immune-mediated thrombocytopenia are viral mediated. Most patients with the acute form clear spontaneously. Chronic ITP is often a difficult disease to treat, and there is a variable response to splenectomy and steroid or immunosuppressive therapy.

Infections

Reference has already been made to the ability of viruses to induce an immune thrombocytopenia. It is difficult to ascertain whether sequestration is mediated by a viral antibody complex's being absorbed onto the platelet or whether infections cause spontaneous aggregation of platelets owing to the production of toxins (as in endotoxemia). The suggestion has been made that megakaryocytes may also undergo structural damage, and as a result, the thrombocytopenia is compounded by decreased megakaryopoiesis. The course of the disease is invariably acute and self-limiting, and it responds to the treatment of the bacterial or viral infection.

Drug-Induced Thrombocytopenia

Immune-mediated drug-induced thrombocytopenia is not to be confused with thrombocytopenia secondary to drug-induced bone marrow depression. A number of mechanisms appear responsible for such a situation:

a. Immune complex disease. In its simplest terms the drug becomes attached to the circulating serum antibody, which in turn becomes fixed to the surface of the platelet, causing its elimination by the reticuloendothelial system.

b. Hapten formation. The drug becomes attached to the platelet, and the subsequently formed antibody attacks both components.

c. The antibody produced against the drug may have cross specificity with certain platelet antigens.

Most investigations support the immune complex theory, because complement fixation is assisted by an immediately available cellular membrane, in this instance the platelets. Many drugs are responsible for this condition, and they bear a strong association with drug-induced hemolytic anemias. Quinine and quinidine are frequent offenders, with digoxin, phenytoin, isoniazid, phenylbutazone, penicillin, sulfa drugs, etc., all being incriminated.

Laboratory Diagnosis of Immune Thrombocytopenia

These are the same general criteria as outlined previously with the presence of a positive platelet-associated IgG test that is either drug related or idiopathic.

TRANSFUSION-INDUCED

This is also discussed in the blood transfusion section (p. 579).

Dilutional

This is a common problem, and it relates to the transfusion of large amounts of stored blood deficient in viable platelets. It often requires 72 to 96 hours until the platelet count returns to normal, owing to the lag in megakaryopoiesis and the demands made on the production system during the bleeding episode.

Immune

Posttransfusion purpura (PTP) is a rare but well-defined syndrome in which severe thrombocytopenia develops one week after blood transfusion. In each case a platelet isoantibody has been present that usually reacted with the transfused donor platelets but not the patient's own platelets (such individuals are almost invariably multiparous or have been previously transfused with blood products).

Extracorporeal Circulation

The use of heart-lung bypass or extracorporeal circulation exposes the blood to large foreign surface areas and gas bubbles. As a result, platelets are often selectively removed, owing to adhesion to these surfaces. Postbypass thrombocytopenia should therefore be treated with appropriate transfusion therapy. The newer biological materials reduce the incidence of this complication (e.g., heparin-impregnated surfaces).

Thrombocytosis

Thrombocytosis or primary thrombocythemia has already been discussed on p. 667 as part of the myeloproliferative disorders. Secondary thrombocytosis often accompanies hemorrhage, hemolysis, splenectomy, malignant disease, inflammatory disease, or dyserythropoietic anemias (iron deficiency). Although primary thrombocytosis is associated with a bleeding diathesis, secondary thrombocytosis is relatively free of such complications, although excessive thromboembolism has been associated with postsplenectomy thrombocytosis in association with hemolysis and other postoperative complications.

Functional Platelet Defects

These constitute a rapidly evolving series of conditions, the classification of which is by no means complete. A practical classification, considered most suitable at this time, follows:

1. Primary: defective collagen aggregation, defective release, and thrombasthenia.
2. Secondary: drugs, miscellaneous.
3. Von Willebrand's disease.

Primary

Defective Release. Within this very heterogeneous group are a large number of conditions associated with abnormal bleeding. Various synonyms are and have been used, e.g., thrombocytopathy, thrombopathy, and thrombocytopathia. Abnormal platelet release can be considered the result of any one of three defects: failure of platelets to adhere to collagen; failure to release platelet constituents after adhesion; or the amounts of constituents released being quantitatively or qualitatively inadequate.

On this basis any platelet defect that demonstrates an abnormality in platelet aggregation and/or platelet Factor 3 (PF 3) should be considered a member of this group. Therefore the laboratory investigation of these disorders must include a bleeding time, aggregation, and PF 3 storage and release studies (see p. 750).

Thrombasthenia. Thrombasthenia is an hereditary disorder, initially characterized by a prolonged bleeding time, poor clot retraction, and a normal platelet count. The differentiating feature of this condition is its complete failure to aggregate in the presence of ADP. Platelet adhesiveness, PF 3, and platelet fibrinogen have all been reported to be subnormal.

Secondary Platelet Dysfunction

Drugs. These constitute the largest single cause of secondary platelet dysfunction. Acetylsalicylic acid (ASA) is the most common offender, with other nonsteroidal anti-inflammatory drugs being implicated. The action of ASA is uncertain and probably inhibits release by acetylating the platelet membrane. Figure 31–12 shows the effect of a single dose of ASA on collagen, epinephrine, and ADP-induced aggregation. Such an effect persists for at least four days, i.e., it appears to permanently affect those platelets exposed to a transient circulating blood level of ASA. Many other drugs inhibit platelet aggregation, and for this reason any patient with a bleeding diathesis should avoid taking any drug that interferes with platelet function (antihistamines, analgesics, etc.). For similar reasons, any patient to be

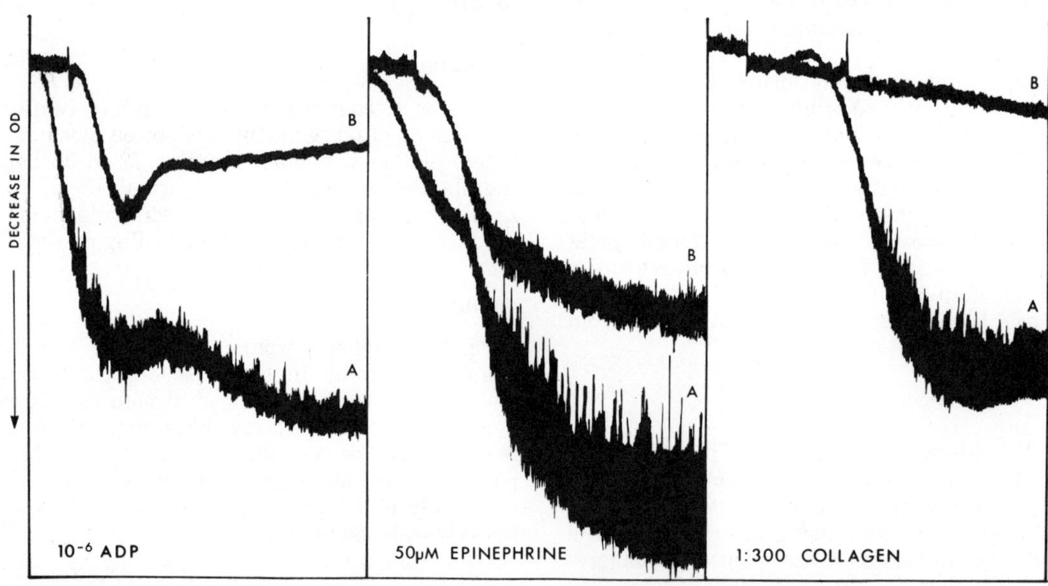

Figure 31–12 Typical platelet aggregation curves obtained before and after the ingestion of aspirin. *A* is before and *B* after aspirin ingestion. Note the loss of second phase aggregation with ADP and adrenalin, with complete abolition of collagen response.

investigated for platelet function must refrain from any form of drug ingestion, including smoking and alcohol, for a minimum of four days before testing.

Other conditions causing platelet dysfunction include uremia (prolonged bleeding time and defective aggregation correctable by dialysis), dysproteinemia (coating of platelet membrane and interfering with release), dextran administration, and myeloproliferative disorders.

Von Willebrand's Disease (VWD)

Von Willebrand's disease (VWD) is defined as an autosomal dominant bleeding disorder accompanied by a variety of symptoms attributable to a platelet-vascular pattern of bleeding of varying severity. In severely affected individuals, hemarthroses and intramuscular hemorrhages can also occur.

Laboratory diagnosis was originally made on the basis of a prolonged bleeding time, low Factor VIII procoagulant activity, and defective platelet adhesion to glass. With increased knowledge of the Factor VIII molecule (p. 718) it is now evident that these laboratory observations require revision for the following reasons:

1. Milder cases of VWD often show only minor changes in the above tests that will fluctuate on a day-to-day basis.
2. Many variants of VWD have now been described that do not have the above characteristics.
3. Measurement of the VWD factor is more accurately performed using other test procedures.

For these reasons laboratory diagnosis is now made using the following criteria (refer to p. 718 for explanation of the nomenclature):

1. Individuals having a decrease in all Factor VIII–related activities have Type I disease. This is exhibited as decreased Factor VIII clotting and antigenic assays, prolonged bleeding time, decreased platelet glass retention, and ristocetin-induced platelet aggregation.
2. Individuals with a normal or only slightly reduced VIIRAg or VIIIC but more severely decreased VIIIRRCo and abnormal electrophoresis of the molecule (crossed immunoelectrophoresis) are designated Type II. These individuals have normal Factor VIII clotting and antigenic levels as compared to Type I individuals.
3. Individuals with a variety of changes in their VIIIRRCo factor can often present to the routine laboratory with an intermittently prolonged bleeding time and an equivocal family or bleeding history. This group is the subject of considerable research activity at this time.

Treatment of these individuals relies upon replacement of the missing Factor VIII–related activities, particularly the bleeding time (platelet)–dependent VIIIRRCo factor. Either fresh frozen plasma or cryoprecipitate will provide effective therapy, with the patient's condition being monitored using a bleeding time rather than other, more complex tests reflecting adequate platelet/VIII factor activity, e.g., platelet ristocetin-induced aggregation and Factor VIII antigenic levels. A curious phenomenon in the severely affected VWD patient occurs when transfusions cause the circulating VIIIC levels to rise rather than naturally decrease following transfusion, as is seen in the Factor VIII deficient hemophiliac. This is probably due to the ability of the high–molecular weight moiety of the transfused Factor VIII to induce Factor VIIIC activity from the recipient's own sources. Needless to say, without the additional transfused platelet-related Factor VIII factors, bleeding would commence even in the presence of adequate levels of VIIIC.

Mixed Hemostatic Defects

These are a series of complicated acquired conditions that will be discussed under the following headings: (1) disseminated intravascular coagulation (DIC), (2) hepatic and gastrointestinal disease, (3) circulating anticoagulants, and (4) massive blood transfusion.

Disseminated Intravascular Coagulation (DIC)

Synonyms for this condition include defibrination syndrome, disseminated intravascular thrombosis, secondary fibrinolysis, and consumption coagulopathy. The multiplicity of names indicates the confusion this condition has caused clinicians and laboratory investigators in endeavoring to decide its common characteristics. The condition has, by necessity, been defined in a variety of ways, and probably a reasonable definition is an acute or chronic event that complicates a variety of clinical conditions, any of which produces activation of the hemostatic mechanism, laying down of intravascular fibrin, and secondary fibrinolysis. It is important to recognize that DIC accompanies, rather than causes, the primary pathological condition. However, when initiated it precipitates a wide variety of serious complications.

Classification of the syndrome in terms of initiating events indicates the predisposing conditions or causes of DIC: (1) intravascular hemolysis, (2) tissue procoagulant, (3) other procoagulant sources, (4) endothelial cell damage, (5) vascular stasis, and (6) miscellaneous.

Intravascular Hemolysis. Any condition that causes large amounts of free hemoglobin to be released into the intravascular compartment causes erythrocytic thromboplastin material to activate the intrinsic coagulation mechanism. This causes fibrin deposition with platelet consumption and secondary fibrinolysis. Incompatible blood transfusion will often be a prime cause for such an event, with malaria, paroxysmal nocturnal hemoglobinuria, and other conditions being implicated. Removal of the source of hemolysis prevents further activation of the hemostatic system.

Tissue Procoagulants. Obstetrical problems, including amniotic fluid embolism, abruptio placentae, toxemia, and retained dead fetus are all associated with a precipitous DIC. Probably related to tissue thromboplastin derived from the placenta entering the maternal circulation. The term *acute defibrination* has often been applied to this condition, owing to the sudden and massive depletion of fibrinogen as a result of coagulation activation and resultant overwhelming fibrinolysis. Neoplasms (adenocarcinoma and promyelocytic leukemia) have been associated with similar episodes. Removal of the offending tissue, e.g., placenta, relieves the condition.

Other Procoagulant Sources. Included here are the bacterial, viral, and rickettsial infections that primarily promote platelet aggregation and subsequent activation of the coagulation system. This may be a severe syndrome; thrombocytopenia may be severe and life threatening. Fat embolism associated with bony fractures has a similar onset, as does air embolism. Treatment of the infection or condition restores normal hemostasis.

Endothelial Cell Damage. This encompasses all the conditions in which a vasculitis exists, along with heat stroke and other more unusual causes. Again the platelets are primarily activated, with subsequent activation of the hemostastic mechanism (p. 728). Restoration of endothelial integrity returns the hemostatic defect to normal.

Vascular Stasis. This implies that as a result of shock, congenital heart disease, and vascular malformations (giant hemangioma, Kasabach-Merritt syndrome), stasis of blood occurs, with subsequent anoxia, endothelial damage, deposition of platelets, and activation of the coagulation mechanism. Restoration of intravascular flow and adequate perfusion of vital organs, e.g., liver, restores normal hemostasis.

Miscellaneous Conditions. These include immune complex disease, which activates platelet release reactions. Local DIC can occur, as in renal homograft rejection phenomena. Liver disease promotes DIC owing to nonclearance of activated coagulation factors. Snake bite will often produce profound defibrination. Purpura fulminans seen in young children probably initially represents a localized form of DIC.

Pathophysiology. As can be appreciated from the preceding necessarily brief classification, any abnormal stimulus of a continuing nature may precipitate DIC, with inadequate clearance of activated clotting factors by the reticuloendothelial system having a similar effect. In the first instance removal of the stimulus arrests the condition; in the second instance increased reticuloendothelial efficiency, i.e., restoration of hepatic function, achieves the same result. Prevention of fibrin, or platelet thrombi, or both, is the objective.

Laboratory Diagnosis of DIC

Considerable difficulty is often experienced in deciding whether a DIC event is occurring. Clinically it presents as a generalized bleeding diathesis with bleeding from intravenous sites, gastrointestinal tract, mucous membranes, etc. Earlier in the condition all these signs may not be present, even though laboratory evidence suggests platelet and fibrin deposition.

Similarly, the laboratory tests may be taken at a time when either only minimal changes have taken place or only one part of the hemostatic mechanism has been activated, e.g., overwhelming fibrinolysis but minimal platelet consumption. The laboratory tests must therefore reflect all aspects of the disturbed hemostatic mechanism that identify DIC, namely:

Increased Platelet Consumption. A decreased platelet count and increased megathrombocyte index will provide this information. An increased bleeding time reflects the decreased platelets and a possible functional defect owing to their being coated with FDPs.

Increased Coagulation Factor Consumption. A PTT, PT, and thrombin time will enable all stages of the intrinsic and extrinsic coagulation mechanism to be evaluated. Specific assays will detect changes in the consumption factors, particularly Factors I, V, and VII. The PTT may not reflect the degree of factor consumption owing to the increase in activated factors, producing a false low clotting time (see p. 744).

Increased Plasminolysis. The most useful test is fibrinogen-fibrin degradation product (FDP) estimation. The euglobulin lysis time may often appear prolonged beyond normal because of plasminogen exhaustion.

Increased Erythrocyte Fragmentation. A microangiopathic hemolytic anemia may occur owing to intravascular fibrin formation (see p. 649).

Evidence of Fibrin Deposition. The demonstration of SFMC (see p. 749) using the protamine sulfate test or other paracoagulation tests is probably the most important test of all, because these complexes indicate the presence of intravascular fibrin monomer, i.e., uncontrolled thrombin generation.

If certain trends are seen, e.g., a decreasing platelet count in the face of an increasingly prolonged PTT and increasing FDPs, this provides more definite evidence for DIC.

The diagnosis of the condition is nevertheless fraught with problems. Emphasis has already been given to the differentiation of primary from secondary plasminolysis (see p. 721).

Treatment

It has already been emphasized that removal of the offending agent or condition will reduce the potentiation of the accompanying DIC and allow for the replacement of depleted hemostatic factors. In some cases (hepatic failure, multiple trauma, burns, etc.) it may not be possible to remove the initiating cause except over a period of time. In these situations the continuing deposition of fibrin must be avoided and life-threatening hemorrhage caused by factor depletion must be corrected. The use of heparin and judicious transfusion would appear to be indicated. This paradoxical situation of giving anticoagulant to an already thrombocytopenic, factor-depleted individual is not without its dangers, but the principle is that if the foreign procoagulant can be prevented from activating the hemostatic mechanism, further consumption of factors will cease. The various factor levels including fibrinogen will then start rising, the formation of intravascular fibrin will be prevented, clinical bleeding alleviated, and various concentrated factors, i.e., platelets and factor concentrates, given with safety. By interrupting the vicious cycle of hemostatic activation, factor depletion, and fibrin deposition, the patient is also spared the serious complications of organ damage (caused by disseminated thrombosis) and hypotension (caused by blood loss and kinin activation).

Hepatic and Gastrointestinal Disease

A variety of defects may be attributable to disease of these organs.

Defect in Vitamin K–Dependent Factor Synthesis

Vitamin K deficiency occurs in malabsorption syndrome owing to interference with the absorption of the fat-soluble vitamins, e.g., vitamins A, D, E, and K. Obstructive jaundice will lead to impaired absorption owing to lack of bile salts. Malabsorption syndrome, pancreatic disease, and other conditions have a similar effect. The use of parenteral therapy and antibiotics in hospitalized patients greatly accelerates a vitamin K–dependent state. It is also associated with a bleeding diathesis of the newborn (hemorrhagic disease of the newborn), whose lack of vitamin K is owing to a variety of causes: liver immaturity, lack of bacterial synthesis of vitamin K, and so forth.

Diagnosis is made on the basis of a prolonged PT and PTT, which assay analysis will show to be caused by a deficiency in Factors II, VII, IX, and X. Treatment is parenteral injection of vitamin K_1 and infusion of II, VII, IX, and X plasma concentrates (see p. 579). Response to intravenous vitamin K_1 is usually apparent within six hours, and reflects adequate liver function.

Hepatic Disease

A variety of hemostatic defects accompany hepatic disease other than vitamin K–dependent states. The defects may be summarized under the headings of synthesis, fibrinolysis, thrombocytopenia, and DIC. Defects in synthesis are usually associated with all types of hepatic disease, whereas acute DIC and fibrinolysis are restricted to severe and acute liver damage, e.g., acute hepatitis and hepatic necrosis.

Defects in Synthesis. The vitamin K–dependent Factors II, VII, IX, and X are the first to be affected, followed by Factor V, and then fibrinogen. Treatment is as for vitamin K deficiency, and it may be necessary to use plasma concentrates and fresh plasma. If a significant decrease in fibrinogen is seen DIC must be excluded, since the liver has an enormous reserve capacity for fibrinogen production.

Plasminolysis. Severe disease may greatly impair the production of antiplasmin and the inactivation of plasminogen activator, which is being continuously released by the vascular tissue. Primary plasminolysis results; however, it is a rare event, usually restricted to individuals who have undergone hepatic shunt procedures, and again DIC must be excluded.

Thrombocytopenia. Alcohol injury, and the effects of increased portal pressure (hypersplenism) rather than a specific liver effect could contribute to a platelet decrease. It is again important to exclude DIC.

DIC. Mention has already been made of the involvement of the liver in DIC (p. 732). The lack of activated factor clearance would appear to be the main contributor to its initiation. It may appear as an acute or chronic condition, with the added difficulty of discriminating it from superimposed vitamin K deficiency.

Blood Transfusion–Induced Disease

Diagnosis is usually evident if the patient is relatively healthy. However, in the seriously sick patient, who may have undergone surgery, the diagnosis may be both obscure and difficult to make (see p. 577).

Circulating Anticoagulants

The significance of these substances has already been alluded to on pp. 719 and 725. However, apart from the natural anticoagulants and those related to hemophilia, a number of pathological inhibitors have been associated with other conditions. The characterization of these inhibitors has yet to be fully established. A number of them, particularly those associated with such conditions as lupus erythematosus, rheumatoid arthritis, pregnancy, and the immunoproliferative syndromes appear to be largely reversible, have either specific or nonspecific factor antagonism, and are active in either a PTT or PT system. As such they present great difficulty in diagnosis. Page 746 describes the test systems necessary for the detection of such anticoagulants.

INVESTIGATION OF A BLEEDING DIATHESIS

Clinical History

This is most important. An accurate clinical and family history will often give invaluable and time-saving clues as to the nature of the underlying disorder. Generally, cutaneous purpura or superficial bruises, especially over commonly injured surfaces, suggest an abnormality of the vascular aspect of hemostasis. Deeper, large bruises, hematomas, bleeding into joints, and prolonged or continuous bleeding from mucous membranes, cuts, and wounds suggest a defect in the blood coagulation system itself.

If the patient is a male, and there is evidence of bleeding into a joint or other abnormal hemorrhage, and if there is a positive familial history of brothers or uncles having been similarly affected, classic hemophilia or Factor IX deficiency is suggested; Factor XI deficiency is also possible although less likely. Bruising or bleeding in a jaundiced person, in a person being treated with coumarin drugs, or in a severe chronic alcoholic is often caused by deficiency of the vitamin K–dependent factors, i.e., II, VII, IX, and X. Excessive bleeding following delivery or associated with retention of a dead fetus, hemothorax, or prolonged oozing following extensive surgery or trauma will all suggest the possibility of fibrinogen depletion. Finally, it should never be forgotten that "common things commonly occur," e.g., nosebleeds are not uncommon in normal children; excessive menstrual loss is more often caused by gynecological conditions than attributable to defects in the hemostatic mechanism; and ulcers, cancers, polyps, and piles are common causes of gastrointestinal bleeding. Also, trauma will cause bruising in anyone, and often the incident is forgotten.

The patient should be closely questioned regarding previous surgical operations. If a person has had a tonsillectomy or a tooth extraction without bleeding, this often suggests that a serious hereditary defect is not present. Bleeding at childbirth can often be minimal in spite of a defect being present. In the platelet-vascular defects it is often surprising that abdominal surgery has been performed, e.g., appendectomy, with no abnormal hemorrhage, while a simple tooth extraction may present major bleeding problems.

The occasional patient will be seen who presents with a significant history of bleeding, but no abnormal tests are found. It is wise not to discount the history but to repeat the tests again at a later date and not to rely simply upon the screening tests. It may be necessary to use definitive procedures in the event of normal screening tests. A common example is the suspected von Willebrand's patient (see p. 731).

Basic Screening Procedures

A precise and orderly routine should be followed, if only to save the patient from needlessly repeated venipunctures. Only well-trained, experienced technologists should undertake the investigation, to which they must be free to give their undivided attention. Preferably, the investigation should begin early in the morning so that it can be completed in one day. The lability of some of the factors involved explains why this is necessary. Keeping specimens overnight, even if they are properly deep-frozen, is to be discouraged. Precise temperature and pH control is most important in the investigation of most clotting factors.

Taking of Blood Samples

Although atraumatic venipunctures are necessary under any circumstances, the need in hemostasis is particularly important. If any difficulty whatsoever is experienced in performing the venipuncture, the attempt must be abandoned and a fresh site and apparatus chosen.

Many workers suggest using two plastic syringes for collecting blood for hemostatic investigations. The venipuncture is performed using a 19-gauge thin-wall butterfly needle with attached plastic tubing; 2 to 3 mL of blood is withdrawn and the partially filled syringe replaced with another, which is then filled with the required amount of blood. If a Vacutainer system is used, the first tube is discarded. All apparatus preferably should be plastic or siliconized, and the blood transferred into the required anticoagulants as quickly as possible (clotted blood samples are an exception).

Capillary blood samples should be avoided for coagulation studies. It is very important for the patient to avoid taking medications, particularly platelet active agents (see pp. 730 and 737).

Screening Hemostasis Tests

The following screening tests are suggested for investigating a potential hemostatic defect. It must be emphasized that if the screening tests are normal but there is a significant clinical history, it is necessary to perform more definitive procedures (vide infra).

1. Bleeding time—preferably the standardized Ivy or template method.
2. Peripheral blood examination including platelet count and morphology.
3. Thrombin clotting time.
4. One-stage prothrombin time.
5. Partial thromboplastin time.

If there is any suspicion of disseminated intravascular coagulation or excessive plasminolysis occurring, the following should be added:

6. Fibrinogen-fibrin degradation products.
7. Protamine sulfate or other test for fibrin monomer complexes.

Samples required: (1) EDTA sample for peripheral blood hematology; (2) citrated sample for procoagulant tests and platelet-rich plasma; (3) citrated sample with added EACA and thrombin for FDP-monomer tests (see p. 749).

A whole blood clotting time is used by some laboratories as a source of serum, and it provides ancillary information. Process all samples as quickly as possible; while awaiting testing, keep all samples at 4°C.

Table 31–6 aids in identification of the more common disorders using the screening tests.

CONTROL OF ANTICOAGULANT THERAPY

The use of antithrombotic drugs is gaining increasing importance, and with this increase has come an increasing responsibility on the part of the laboratory to provide techniques that aid the physician in controlling a form of drug therapy that has very real hazards. If the degree of anticoagulation is not sufficient, rethrombosis, extension, or embolism from existing thrombus can occur. Overenthusiastic use of such agents can result in fatal hemorrhage. The therapeutic balance is maintained by using suitable laboratory procedures and appropriate patient selection.

There are five main classes of antithrombotic agents: (1) heparin, (2) vitamin K antagonists, (3) fibrinolytic agents, (4) fibrinogenolytic agents and (5) antiplatelet drugs.

All of the above are controlled by laboratory procedures; however, heparin and the vitamin K antagonists are the most important agents.

Heparin

Heparin, a potent organic acid, is a mixture of sulfate-containing mucopolysaccharides with molecular weights ranging between 8000 and 15,000. Because of its strong electrostatic charge, heparin combines with a wide variety of proteins. Approximately 20 per cent can be recovered intact excreted in the urine, and the remainder is apparently degraded by the liver. It does not cross the intact placenta.

It has a number of anticoagulant actions:

1. It prevents activation of Factor IX.
2. It inhibits the formation of thrombin in conjunction with a plasma cofactor.
3. It augments the antiactivated Factor X inhibitor (synonymous with antithrombin III or "heparin cofactor").
4. It interferes with platelet function to a variable degree.

It is therefore used either to prevent thrombus formation or further extension onto an existing thrombus. In the first instance, small doses are given to individuals who are predisposed to thrombus formation, particularly during the postoperative period. This prophylactic approach is being used with increasing frequency and would appear to be relatively free from side effects owing to the small doses of heparin used. However, laboratory control is recommended. Usual doses are in the order of 5000 units every 8 hours, given subcutaneously. Therapeutic heparin is used to prevent an existing thrombus from extending or embolizing, and in this instance larger doses of heparin (up to 60,000 units every 24 hours) are given intravenously either on an intermittent or continuous basis. Irrespective of the method of administration, it is important to maintain a reasonably constant level.

TABLE 31–6 RESULTS OF SCREENING TESTS IN COMMON BLEEDING ABNORMALITIES

Defect or Disease	Bleeding Time	Platelet Count	Thrombin Clotting Time	Prothrombin Time	Partial Thromboplastin Time
Vascular Phase					
Hereditary telangiectasia	N	N	N	N	N
Scurvy	±A	N	N	N	N
Thrombocytopenia	A	A	N	N	N
Thrombopathy	N	N	N	N	N
1st Stage Clotting					
Factor VIII deficiency	N	N	N	N	A
Factor IX deficiency	N	N	N	N	A
Factor XI deficiency	N	N	N	N	A
Circulating anticoagulant	N	N	N	N	A
Factor VII deficiency	N	N	N	A	N
2nd Stage Clotting					
Factor V deficiency	N	N	N	A	A
Factor X deficiency	N	N	N	A	A
Factor II deficiency	N	N	N	A	A
3rd Stage Clotting					
Factor I deficiency	N	N	A	±A	±A
Factor XIII deficiency	N	N	N	N	N
Miscellaneous					
von Willebrand's disease	A	N	N	N	±N
Plasminolysis (acute)	N	N	A	±A	±A
Disseminated intravascular coagulation (acute)	A	A	A	A	A

A = Abnormal; N = Normal; ± Result depends upon severity of condition.

Probably it is more important to emphasize the need to monitor the dose in order that sufficient heparin be given rather than too much.

A variety of laboratory techniques are available to monitor heparin therapy.

Whole Blood Clotting Time. This has been the time-honored method, but has been largely superseded by other, more convenient methods. However, it still offers relatively precise control if performed correctly or used as an activated whole blood clotting test. Therapeutic value is usually two times the preheparin clotting time.

Partial Thromboplastin Time. Use of this test has increased within recent times, probably because blood can be taken and the test performed at the convenience of the laboratory. The PTT is usually kept prolonged at approximately two and a half times the preheparinization value. Although simple to perform, the test is not without its defects, and it is important that a laboratory perform a careful evaluation of the sensitivity of their PTT to heparin before using it for heparin control.

Thrombin Clotting Time. The great advantage of this method of heparin control is that it is not influenced by oral anticoagulant therapy if given concomitantly with heparin. Similarly, it is not affected by the factors that give spuriously high or low PTT values in the presence of heparin, e.g., altered levels of coagulation factors, activated products, differences in sensitivity of PTT reagents to heparin. It is the method of choice if a clotting test is desired, provided that the laboratory performs regular heparin sensitivity assays.

Other Methods. A variety of assay procedures are available, all of which are too complicated for simple screening procedures. Recently, a number of whole blood tests have been described; these essentially are whole blood PTT tests that can, if necessary, be performed at the bedside. The BART and HAREM tests are examples of such tests. A rational method would be to report heparin levels rather than the indirect coagulation tests. However, heparin assay methods are still technically complicated and difficult to interpret.

The specific antidote to heparin is protamine sulfate, a highly basic substance that forms an irreversible complex with heparin. Usually it is given in a dose of 1 mg for every 100 units of heparin to be neutralized.

A considerable degree of controvery surrounds the need for continuous versus intermittent heparin administration. If continuous administration is required, a loading dose of heparin is given followed by continuous infusion. (A suitable initial dose is a 5000-unit bolus followed by 1000 units of heparin per hour as a continuous infusion.) Repeated testing is required during this initial period in order to achieve satisfactory anticoagulation. Once a steady state degree of heparinization is attained, daily testing is usually appropriate in the absence of clinical complications or interruptions of the intravenous access. If the intermittent intravenous method is used (5000 units every 4 hours after a suitable loading dose), the PTT has to be taken approximately 30 minutes before the next dose is due in order to assess whether there is an undue or negligible heparin effect.

Whatever method is used, the laboratory has the responsibility of using a method that has a proven sensitivity to heparin (this may not be the optimal method for coagulation factor deficiencies) and is capable of providing quick results to the clinician.

Vitamin K Antagonists

The coumarin drugs were first discovered to have an effect on the blood coagulation factors after Link's discovery of the material in spoiled sweet clover. This fortuitous association with hemorrhagic disease in cattle has led to the use of these vitamin K antagonists in anticoagulant therapy, particularly as a means of treating the patient with an oral medication, as opposed to heparin, which requires parenteral administration. The form most used in North America is sodium warfarin.

Vitamin K reaches the liver after absorption through the gut to cause synthesis of Factors II, VII, IX, and X, the so-called vitamin K–dependent clotting factors. If sufficient quantities of warfarin are given, synthesis of these factors is blocked, possibly by interfering with the metabolism of vitamin K. Synthesis of the four procoagulants ceases and they disappear from the blood in proportion to their individual degradation rates. Factor VII, with a half-life of 5 hours, disappears first, followed by Factors IX and X with half-lives of 20 and 30 hours, respectively. Factor II is the last factor to disappear, since it has a half-life of approximately 60 hours.

It follows that warfarin therapy requires approximately 48 to 72 hours before sufficient depression of the clotting factors has occurred to give abnormal laboratory tests. Such a depression may not be synonymous with protection, since the levels of Factor II will be relatively unaltered in that time period. Considerable controversy has raged over the years as to the most suitable laboratory test for oral anticoagulant control. However, there is little doubt that in North America the one-stage prothrombin test is considered the method of choice.

One-Stage Prothrombin. This method of control works well despite criticisms that it does not reflect changes in Factor IX concentration and is relatively insensitive to Factor VII levels. As has been mentioned elsewhere (see pp. 741 and 742), it is very important not only that the thromboplastin reagent be sensitive to Factors VII, X, and II, but that it give reproducible results from one laboratory to another in order that the degree of anticoagulation be kept constant for any one patient. This has led to the formulation of various standard thromboplastins. The European concept would support a standardized thromboplastin reagent, whereas North American opinion recommends the use of standard plasma controls.

The basis of control with this method is to prolong the PT to two or three times the pretreatment PT of the patient. A great number of variables affect the response of the patient to the drug, particularly interactions with other drugs. These interactions can either increase the metabolism of warfarin (decrease the PT; a frequent offender is barbiturate), or cause an increase in warfarin availability. This is made possible by many drugs that displace warfarin from albumin (aspirin does this as well as interfering with platelet function, thus becoming a doubly dangerous agent). It is therefore very important that any any radical change in the PT of a patient receiving oral anticoagulants be reported to the physician without delay. Excessively prolonged times can be corrected with the judicious use of vitamin K, which is the treatment of choice in bleeding associated with this treatment. Identification of the patient who is being treated with warfarin is recommended, since this will alert any laboratory if bleeding is associated with a prolonged PT. In cases of severe bleeding, replacement with fresh blood and rarely, in acute emergencies, II, VII, IX, and X plasma concentrate may also be required.

Thrombotest. This test was introduced by Owren in 1959 in order to assess not only Factors II, VII, and X, but also IX, which is not estimated by the PT. The Thrombotest reagent contains cephalin, thromboplastin, and all the coagulant factors except the vitamin K–dependent ones. It also has the advantage of being capable of using blood up to 24 hours old (samples can be mailed). Therapeutic range is in the 7 to 15% range, compared to a normal control.

PTT. The PTT should be able to detect significant changes in Factors II, IX, and X, but not VII. Its use has been advocated by a number of workers, but it has yet to meet with any universal acceptance.

Fibrinolytic Therapy

An ideal fibrinolytic agent should induce reproducible thrombolytic activity capable of dissolving pathological thrombi and emboli rapidly. The two examples currently used for this purpose are streptokinase and urokinase. The first is derived from the beta hemolytic streptococcus; the second is obtained from human urine. Both agents activate plasminogen to form plasmin, which can either digest the offending fibrin clot from the outside or from within via the retained plasminogen. The therapy is not without its dangers, particularly in regard to massive hemorrhage.

The laboratory performs several roles in the use of these agents. It is first necessary to measure the degree of natural "resistance" to these agents in order that a correct loading dose be given. Subsequently, a maintenance dose of 100,000 units is given per hour, and the patient is monitored to assess effective activation of plasminogen but prevention of systemic defibrination. In practice a thrombin time is considered adequate in that, once circulating plasminogen has been quickly exhausted and continuing activation of endogenous plasminogen started, this test reflects fibrinogen levels. If the thrombin clotting time starts to increase, the dosage is reduced accordingly.

Fibrinogenolytic Therapy

A number of substances, notably snake venoms, have the ability to act as thrombin-like substances and cause the conversion of fibrinogen to an ineffective fibrin monomer that is rapidly cleared from the circulation by reactive fibrinolysis. The anticoagulant effect is caused mainly by fibrinogen depletion's preventing either extension onto existing clots or the formation of fresh thrombus.

Venom from the Malayan pit viper *(Agkistrodon rhodostoma)* is used for therapeutic fibrinogenolysis and is available as ancrod.* Its specific action is to remove only

*Arvin, Connaught Laboratories, Willowdale, Ont. M2M 3Y8.

fibrinopeptide A from fibrinogen rather than fibrinopeptides A and B, which are both removed by thrombin.

Monitoring of the therapy is again accomplished using some form of fibrinogen assay, in this instance trying to achieve maximum fibrinogen depletion but not affecting platelet function.

Antiplatelet Therapy

A number of agents are known to have antiplatelet activity, principally aspirin, dipyridamole, sulfinpyrazone, clofibrate, etc. After intensive clinical testing during the past decade it is difficult to prove that such agents are clinically effective. Laboratory monitoring using conventional platelet function tests, i.e., adhesiveness and aggregation, serve as useful in vitro observations but do not aid in establishing in vivo effectiveness. The platelet survival test is becoming more useful in this regard.

TECHNIQUES FOR INVESTIGATION OF HEMOSTATIC DEFECTS

As for any other branch of laboratory science, tests of hemostasis require scrupulous attention to methodology, quality control, and apparatus. The elucidation and assay of any hemostatic defect depends upon the complex interplay of enzyme systems with various labile plasma proteins. Probably the most important aspect of these points is the ability of a laboratory to develop a testing procedure that will provide constant reproducibility and exact results for the specific phenomena being investigated. A quality control system will partially assist in this respect, but it is equally important that there be adequate liaison between the laboratory and clinical services, so that the results of the hemostasis test can be correlated with the clinical situation.

The methods to be described in this section have proved themselves useful and adequate in our laboratory. Nevertheless, small differences in reagent preparation will make a considerable difference in the final result, e.g., using a different platelet substitute for the PTT. Therefore, it is advised that the worker not accept any procedure at face value until it has proved itself capable of performing all the functions required of it, e.g., proof that the PTT is not only capable of showing differences in stage one factor levels, but that it also provides a good index for heparin control without being overly sensitive to activated clotting factors.

Once a method has been evaluated and the final procedure decided upon, it is most important that the exact method be followed as described. Small changes in technique can often result in considerable differences in the final result, i.e., the temperature deviating from 37°C, or the pH of the buffer not being exactly pH 7.4.

Quality Control

The principles of quality control have been described elsewhere in this book (see Chap. 3), and may be applied to certain tests of hemostatic function. Conventionally, normal limits are set for laboratory tests and results related to these values. However, in setting normal limits, it is important to decide what will constitute the normal population. The sole use of laboratory personnel, although convenient, should not be encouraged because for certain age groups of patients, e.g., the newborn, the normal values have to be related specifically to this group. Likewise changes in normal pregnancy cannot be equated to normal values obtained from a sample of healthy male laboratory technologists.

Once normal limits have been established for a given group of patients, the other vexing problem is to establish day-to-day control for the test procedures. For most other laboratory procedures this entails the use of standard normal and abnormal blood or serum samples, setting acceptable limits of variation, e.g., ±2 SD, and running these controls before the test samples.

The procoagulant procedures can be conveniently monitored using such abnormal and normal plasma samples. However, it is wise to remember that the whole procedure should be monitored from the instant the blood is collected, since considerable changes may ensue if blood collection and subsequent storage are not adequate. Therefore, some form of laboratory prepared plasma or serum control is advised (vide infra) in order to assess the efficacy of blood sample taking and sample preparation and storage.

The tests for plasminolysis and platelet function are considerably more difficult to assess using normal samples. For example, the bleeding time can only be compared to the normal values in other population groups, and in the event of an abnormal result, it can then only be related to the cause of the possible abnormality, e.g., thrombocytopenia. Platelet function tests can only rely upon one or two normal samples being run simultaneously with the test. The source of the normal samples is invariably the laboratory staff, and in this instance it is preferable to have only one or two members of the staff selected for this function in view of the wide range of normality for these procedures. Tests for fibrinolysis have similar restrictions, although the assay of FDP and plasminogen lends itself to conventional control procedures. The advice given to cover these situations must be dictated by the clinical situation and the need to repeat abnormal results with fresh samples or procedures.

To illustrate this point, let us assume that a euglobulin lysis time is abnormally short, e.g., 15 minutes, while the FDP, fibrinogen, plasminogen, and plasmin levels are normal. This would suggest that no pathological fibrinolysis is ensuing, even though the ELT test is abnormal. Such a conclusion can be made only after investigating how the sample was obtained, the clinical situation, and repeating the tests. The dictum must be that when an abnormal result is discovered and quality control procedures cannot be fully utilized, the procedure must first be repeated before the initial result is accepted.

Apparatus

A glass or Lucite bath is used for manual methods so that tubes may be seen without being removed from the water (Fig. 31–13). The temperature must not be allowed to vary from 37°C ± 1°C. The use of "dry" conduction wells is recommended only when the instruments have some means of monitoring the temperature.

All glassware must be scrupulously clean and kept separate from other laboratory stock. A very mild detergent is advised for cleaning purposes, and washing

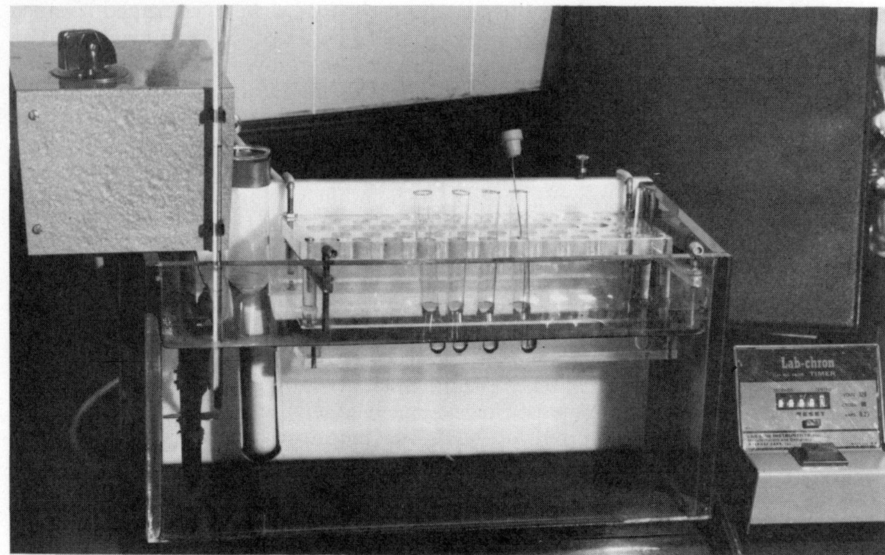

Figure 31–13 A Phipps-Bird water bath (Richmond, Va. 23205). Note the Nicrhome loop and easy visualization of the tubes. The back panel is illuminated.

should be followed by thorough rinsing in distilled water. Badly scratched glassware must be discarded. The use of plastic tubes and syringes can be recommended when siliconized equipment is required. The use of disposable glass tubes is recommended, provided the laboratory user can be assured that they are received from the supplier chemically clean; otherwise they must be thoroughly washed before use. It is further suggested that once a particular brand of tubes has proved satisfactory, no change be made in the supplier. Alternatively, siliconization of equipment may be done with Siliclad.* Seventy-five by 10 mm tubes are used unless otherwise stated.

The routine 0.1 and 0.2 mL pipette should be short so that the delivery time is fast. The use of automatic delivery pipettes is strongly recommended. Examples are shown in Figure 31–14.

To time the clotting of plasma, which is usually the end point of a test, a number of different methods may be used.

Automatic Clot Timers

The automatic sensing of clot formation has been accomplished using a variety of physical principles. The two most common principles that have stood the test of time and utility are:

1. A change in light transmission either through absorbance or changes in optical density versus time (Coagamate system†).

2. Conduction or impedance of an electrical current by fibrin (Fibrometer system‡).

Other principles that have been or are still being used include clumping of iron oxide particles within the fibrin clot, arrest of a steel ball bearing within the clot, and determination of the kinetic reaction involved in clot formation.

*Clay-Adams, Parsippany, N.J. 07054.

†General Diagnostics, Morris Plains, N.J. 07950 and Toronto Ont. M1K 5C9.

‡Becton, Dickinson and Co., Cockeysville, Md. 21030 and Mississauga, Ont. L5J 2M8.

Coagamate System. This instrument employs either a single- or a dual-channel system with printout and automatic delivery of reagents into prefilled plasma sample trays on a turntable. Such a system allows for the processing of large numbers of samples in duplicate for either the more common procoagulant tests (e.g., PT, PTT, and TCT) or the more complicated factor assay techniques.

When the test button is activated the reagents are added in correct sequence using constant-volume delivery pumps. After appropriate mixing and incubation on an incubator test plate the electro-optical sensing circuit is activated. The clot is detected by the rate of change in absorbance of light that exceeds a predetermined threshold over a specific period of time (see Fig. 31–16).

As with any instrument of this kind, it is important to avoid any contamination of the optical system, an unstable work surface, high humidity, or direct sunlight. The pump delivery system must be checked frequently and a constant feed voltage maintained. The instrument requires daily calibration.

Fibrometer System. This is a semiautomatic instrument using an automatic reagent delivery system but not having a printout or constant plasma delivery process. The system is very rugged, with a mechanical system of clot detection and a series of interchangeable modules that allows for considerable flexibility of operation (see Fig. 31–15). The essential modules are the automatic pipette, heating blocks, and Fibrometer probe units.

After appropriate filling and incubation of the disposable plastic reaction cups the final reagent is delivered via the pipette system, which coincidentally triggers a digital readout timer and the probe unit. The probe unit is composed of two electrodes and a probe foot. When triggered, the probe foot activates the moving electrode. The other electrode is fixed and is responsible for creating an electric potential between it and the moving electrode. A detection circuit is activated when a fibrin strand is formed between the two electrodes, thus completing the circuit. This circuit activation will stop the timer and prevent further movements of the moving electrode.

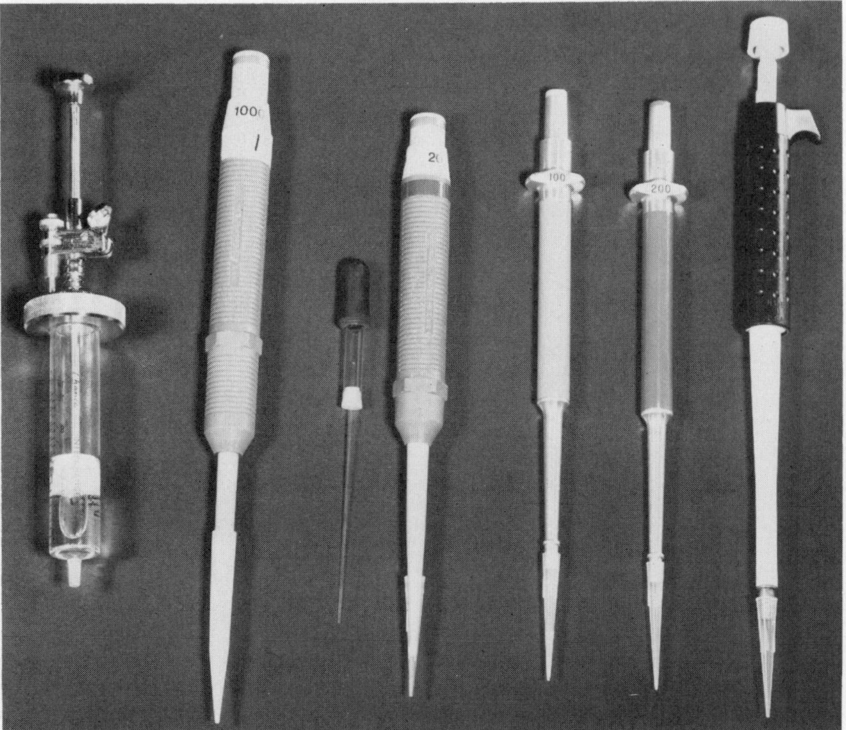

Figure 31–14 A series of automatic pipettes commonly used in hemostasis laboratories. From left to right: spring loaded syringe; 1.0 mL Eppendorf (Brinkman Instruments Inc., Westbury, N.Y. 11590); 20 μL micropipette; 0.2 mL Eppendorf; 0.1 mL M.L.A. (Dow Diagnostics, Toronto, Ontario); 0.2 mL M.L.A.; and 0.2 mL Oxford (Oxford Laboratories Inc., Foster City, Calif. 94404). Note the disposable tips for pipettes 2–7.

Again, it is important to avoid contamination with dust and debris and to avoid protein buildup and sample contamination of the electrodes; one should never attempt to oil any of the moving parts. Maintenance is minimal because of the sealed timer unit: there are no controls to calibrate or day-to-day adjustments to be made. Conversely it does not have the sophistication of a fully automated process.

Selection of an Instrument. In general the selection of an instrument will depend upon the number of tests to be performed, the type of tests, and the service facilities available. It is important to recognize that one machine may function better for a particular test when compared to a competitive system. It is also necessary to have the appropriate experience to assess and evaluate the end-point readings of abnormal samples, as this can result in wide variations using different instruments. Thus it is imperative to use both normal and abnormal plasma samples when evaluating and comparing instrument performance.

Manual Methods

The Wire Loop Technique. This involves gently stirring the coagulating plasma substrate with a Nichrome or platinum wire loop as used in bacteriology. When this technique is used with a transparent water bath, there is no need to remove the tube from the water bath. Great care should be taken to keep the loop clean between tests.

The simple visual technique of observing the clot forming with the naked eye can be recommended only when the tube is observed in the water bath by an underwater source of light, and then only by an experienced technologist. Nevertheless, in the case of "wispy" end points it can give excellent end-point reproducibility.

Stopwatches. At least three are required. They should be mounted on bench stands and should be foot-operated if possible. Foot-operated electronic digital readout second counters are very convenient and are the equipment of choice.

STANDARD REAGENTS

Anticoagulants

The anticoagulant of choice is 3.2% w/v of trisodium citrate in distilled water. Nine parts of blood to one part

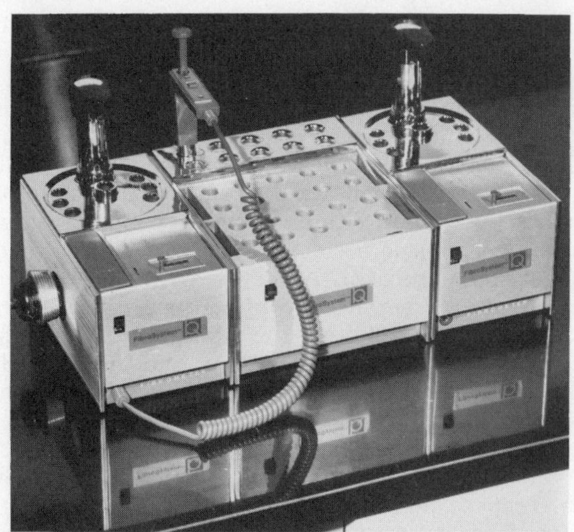

Figure 31–15 Dual Fibrometer System (Becton, Dickinson, and Co., Rutherford, N.J. 07070); automatic clot timer.

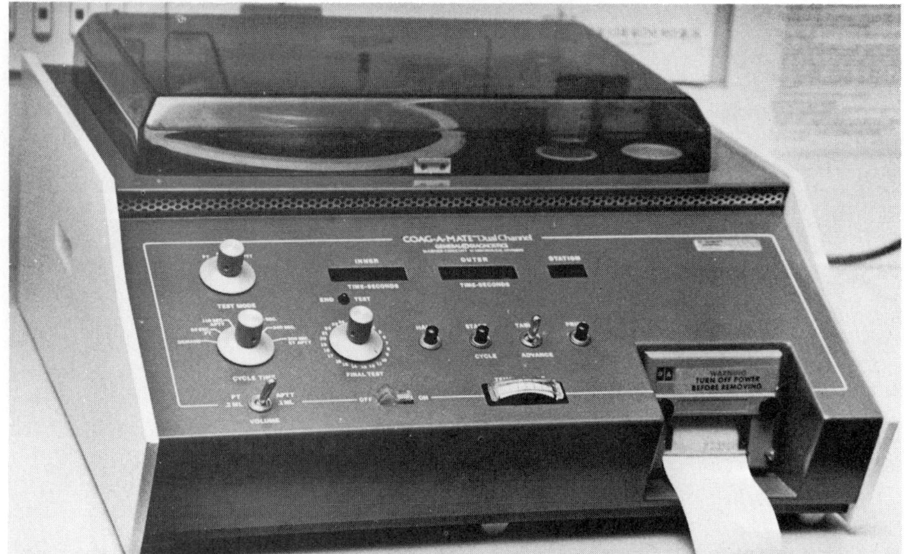

Figure 31–16 Coag-a-Mate clot timer with automatic feed turntable and print-out of results. (General Diagnostics, Morris Plains, N.J. 07950, and Toronto, Ont. M1K 5C9.)

of anticoagulant is usually used. If the hematocrit of the patient is greatly reduced or increased from the average figure of 45%, then the amount of anticoagulant should be adjusted to correspond to the amount of plasma. Once an anticoagulant is selected for routine use, a change cannot be made unless methods are recalibrated. Oxalate anticoagulants generally do not preserve Factor VIII as well as citrate. The use of acidified sodium citrate anticoagulant, pH 6.8, is recommended if samples are to be frozen. All anticoagulant solutions should be stored at 4°C and renewed regularly.

Once a blood sample has been taken into anticoagulant, it must be centrifuged, preferably at 4°C, to produce platelet-free plasma and tested at once. If a delay is unavoidable, then the plasma should be stored at 4°C or deep frozen at −20°C. Plastic tubes are highly recommended for holding plasma samples, since they produce minimal contact activation.

Normal Plasma

This is used not only as a means of quality control, but also as a suitable normal plasma substrate for various tests. Two sources are available:

Commercial. A wide variety are available and they provide a suitable means of checking the performance of day to day tests. However, some may be unsuitable for setting normal limits and as substrate sources, particularly for two-stage thromboplastin generation tests. Careful selection is necessary, and a reputable manufacturer should be used.

Laboratory-Prepared Pool. This preparation has the advantage of reflecting the method of blood sample taking, the choice of anticoagulant, and the method of plasma preparation. The following procedure is recommended:

1. Take citrated plasma samples from at least 24 individuals who should be regular donors for this purpose. Prepare platelet-poor plasma by centrifuging at 4°C for a minimum of 20 minutes at 3000 G. Perform a PTT and PT on each sample. If the control for the PTT for the laboratory is set for 40 seconds, take all samples with this value and mix. Plasmas with values above and below this figure are mixed in varying proportions to ensure that the final plasma pool provides the required clotting time, e.g., 40 seconds. The PT does not normally give wide ranges with normal samples, and random sampling often provides a constant plasma clotting time. Divide the pool into small aliquots, deep freeze at −70°C in plastic or siliconized containers, and do not refreeze samples after use. Under correct conditions of storage such samples can be stored for up to two months without loss of potency. This method of pooling normal plasma usually allows for a relatively constant level of coagulation factors, particularly Factor VIII.

Normal Serum

This is obtained from blood allowed to clot for at least 6 hours at 37°C and then for 18 hours at 4°C in the presence of glass beads or broken glass to allow maximal contact activation. It is stored in the same way as normal plasma. It is assumed to contain factors VII, IX, X, XI, and XII; Factors VII and IX appear concentrated.

Adsorbed Normal Plasma

Adsorption of plasma yields a fluid containing Factors I, V, VIII, XI, and XII, especially Factors V and VIII. The plasma is adsorbed by either aluminum hydroxide or barium sulfate. The potency of a plasma adsorber may vary from manufacturer to manufacturer and even from batch to batch, so that careful testing of the product is necessary.

Aluminum Hydroxide Adsorption. To 9 vol of citrated plasma add 1 vol of $Al(OH)_3$ gel suspension (1 g of gel* in 4 mL distilled water). Mix well, and incubate for 5 minutes at 37°C. Centrifuge at 2000 G to obtain a clear supernatant and perform a one-stage prothrombin test. If adsorption is satisfactory, the time should be more than 60 seconds.

*British Drug Houses, Ltd., Toronto, Ont. M8Z 1K5.

Barium Sulfate Adsorption. To 1 mL of plasma add 50 mg of $BaSO_4$.* Place at 37°C for 15 minutes with frequent mixing, and test as for aluminum hydroxide adsorption. Always use immediately after preparation.

Diluting Solutions and Buffers

For most purposes a buffered diluting fluid is indicated, since most coagulation and platelet reactions are pH dependent. The following two buffers are recommended, particularly the TRIS buffer. If 0.85% w/v sodium chloride is used it must be fresh and have a pH of approximately 7.2.

TRIS Buffer, pH 7.4. Prepare a 2.43% w/v aqueous solution of hydroxymethyl aminomethane. Place 25 mL of this in a 100-mL volumetric flask; add 40 mL of 0.1N HCl; make to volume with distilled water and mix. Check the pH before use and adjust by addition of 0.1N HCl or TRIS as indicated.

Veronal Buffered Saline, pH 7.35. To 570 mL of 0.1M sodium diethyl barbiturate add 430 mL of 0.1N HCl and 5.67 grams of sodium chloride. Just before use 200 mL of the buffer is added to 800 mL of 0.9% saline and 700 mg of potassium monohydrate is added to the mixture.

M/40 (0.025 M) Calcium Chloride. A variety of methods exist for preparing this seemingly simple reagent. The essential part of the procedure is to ensure that the molarity of the stock or working solution is correct, since anhydrous calcium chloride may contain appreciable quantities of water. Therefore, if titration facilities are not available, purchase a commercial source.†

1. Stock solution (0.2 M calcium chloride). First method: Dissolve 22.2 g of anhydrous reagent-grade calcium chloride in 1 liter of distilled water. Store at 4°C and dilute to 0.025 molar with distilled water before use, filtering if necessary.

2. Working solution. Second method: Dissolve 0.277 g of anhydrous reagent-grade calcium chloride in distilled water and make up to 100 mL. Store up to one month at 4°C.

As with any reagent used in hemostatic investigations, it is recommended that a small amount of reagent be taken from the stock bottle at the beginning of the day's work and discarded after use.

Abnormal Control Samples

The crux of any coagulation deficiency investigation is proof that the patient's plasma remains uncorrected by addition of plasma that has been previously diagnosed as having the suspected deficiency. Fresh samples are desirable, but deficient plasmas may be stored as normal plasmas and may be of considerable help on occasion. A file of patients with known deficiencies should be kept so that they may be followed and contacted if a control sample is needed.

Platelet Reagent

Platelet reagent may be obtained either from normal platelets or from platelet substitutes. Normal platelet suspensions are difficult to prepare and may contain adsorbed coagulation factors (such as Factor VIII), but such suspensions must be used in cases in which platelet factor deficiency is suspected.

Platelet Suspension. Centrifuge 10 mL of citrated blood in a plastic or siliconized tube for 5 minutes at 1000 G (exact time will depend on the centrifuge). Transfer the supernatant platelet-rich plasma to another plastic tube and centrifuge at 2000 G for 15 minutes. Remove the supernatant plasma (which may be used as plasma) and wash the deposited platelets with saline, breaking up the platelet button with an applicator stick. Resuspend the washed platelets in saline so as to obtain a final concentration of about 1.5×10^6 platelets per µL or restore the volume with saline to about one-third the original plasma volume. The suspension may be stored at −20°C for several weeks without apparent loss of potency.

In cases in which platelets are presumably normal, platelet substitutes may be used in the coagulation study. These substitutes are commercially available and may be used with confidence.*

Activators. One of the problems associated with coagulation studies is the variable amount of contact activation of the plasma samples under test. To obtain a standardized degree of activation, a synthetic activator is recommended when thromboplastin formation is part of the sequence. Commercially, activators such as kaolin or celite may be combined with the platelet substitute† or may be added separately. Kaolin may be used; 10 mg kaolin‡ is suspended per 1 mL saline. This may be stored frozen at −20°C for periods of up to 1 month.

Fibrinogen. The source of fibrinogen is important, since the preparation must be completely free of thrombin contamination. Human fibrinogen (Grade L) obtained from Kabi, Stockholm, Sweden is recommended. Meticulous preparation is required. Storage in a 1% concentration at −70°C is permissible, provided more dilute concentrations are made up freshly and discarded after use.

Thromboplastin. Thromboplastin is obtained from animal or human brain. Commercially available thromboplastins are widely used, but if desired the substance may be made as follows: The meningeal membranes are removed, and the brain is washed under tap water. The brain stem is usually discarded, since it is a poor thromboplastin source. Portions of brain are then emulsified in a blender with acetone until the brain appears "flaky." Decant the supernatant acetone into water and repeat the emulsification until the water does not become milky when the acetone is added, indicating that all acetone-soluble lipids have been removed. Spread the residual brain material on dry paper towels and allow to dry at room temperature. The dried material should be powdery and pale tan, and it may be stored at 4°C in airtight containers; it keeps indefinitely. For use, 0.5 g of dried brain powder is suspended in 10 mL saline and incubated at 37°C for 15 minutes with gentle mixing, and then the coarse particles are allowed to settle out. Control one-stage prothrombin times are

*Merck & Company, Inc., Rahway, N.J. 07065.
†British Drug Houses, Ltd., Toronto, Ont. M8Z 1K5.

*Platelin, General Diagnostics, Morris Plains, N.J. 07950 and Toronto Ont. M1K 5C9.
†Platelin with Activator, General Diagnostics, Morris Plains, N.J. 07950 and Toronto Ont. M1K 5C9.
‡Matheson, Coleman and Bell, Norwood, Ohio 45212.

performed to obtain the range of normal values, which should fall in the range of 11 to 14 seconds.

Thromboplastin with optimal amounts of calcium added has proved popular for the one-stage prothrombin test.*

It has been apparent for a number of years that different thromboplastin preparations have different specificities for the various coagulation factors. This causes considerable discrepancies to occur when comparing results of one-stage prothrombin times using different thromboplastins. Attempts have been made to standardize the activity of this reagent, notably the British comparative thromboplastin.

Thrombin. The main sources of this reagent are human† or bovine.‡ Solutions of thrombin are not stable, and it is suggested that once the lyophilized solution is reconstituted it should be discarded after use. Aliquots may be stored at −20°C for several days, provided that refreezing is not attempted.

METHODS FOR INVESTIGATING DISORDERS OF HEMOSTASIS

Many of the methods set out here have already been referred to and described in principle. Certain additional methods have been added that, although not essential in the valuation of most defects, have the sanction of popularity. Others are included that help in the isolation or differentiation of specific defects. Footnotes to individual methods describe their application if this has not already been dealt with. If automated methods are used instead of the manual procedures, the individual manufacturer's instructions must be followed carefully.

COAGULATION TESTS

WHOLE BLOOD CLOTTING TIME

Method of Lee and White

Principle. Whole blood is delivered using a carefully controlled venipuncture and collection process into standardized glass tubes. The clotting time of the blood is timed and expressed in minutes. It is prolonged in defects of intrinsic and extrinsic coagulation and in the presence of certain pathological anticoagulants and heparin. It is grossly unreliable for the detection of mild or moderate procoagulant defects and is therefore not recommended as a screening test. At a gross level it will provide useful ancillary information regarding clot retraction and plasminolysis. It is still useful for control of heparin, provided that the test is carefully performed.

Procedure

1. Venous blood is withdrawn using normal precautions, and a stop watch is started the moment blood appears in the syringe. The blood coagulation time is recorded from that moment.
2. Deliver 1 mL of blood into each of four 10 by 1 cm dry, chemically clean glass tubes, which have previously been placed in a container of water maintained at 37°C.
3. After 3 minutes have elapsed, keeping the tubes out of the water for as short a time as possible, tilt them individually every 30 seconds. Avoid unnecessary agitation, since this may prolong the clotting time. The clotting time is taken when the tube can be inverted without its contents spilling. The clotting time of each tube is recorded separately, and the coagulation time is reported as an average of the four tubes. The normal clotting time is 4 to 10 minutes.

Note. The test is a rough measure of the efficiency of the intrinsic blood clotting mechanism, and normal values do not exclude major defects. It is most important that standard technique and equipment be used; in borderline cases the test should also be run on a normal control. Siliconized tubes may provide a more sensitive index; normal values are then prolonged to 18 minutes.

By keeping the tubes in the water bath for another hour, a gross estimate can also be obtained as to the degree of clot retraction, the size of the clot, and whether the clot undergoes rapid lysis. Such observations are crude and cannot be used in place of the more definitive procedures.

The clotting time still provides a simple method for heparin control (vide infra). However, it has been superseded by other methods, e.g., the PTT, mainly because such methods are more convenient.

Dale and Laidlaw's Capillary Clotting Time (Modified)

This method is insensitive and unreliable, and should be used only if venous blood cannot be obtained. It is essential to obtain a rapid, free flow of blood, requiring no squeezing or manipulation of the puncture wound. If manipulation is required, the test must be abandoned.

Procedure

1. A warmed ear or finger is punctured to a depth of 3 mm with a sterile disposable lancet. A stopwatch is started as soon as the puncture wound is made.
2. The first drop of blood is gently wiped off, and the ensuing flow is collected by capillary attraction into two lengths of capillary glass tubing, each measuring 10 to 15 cm by 1.5 mm.
3. After 2 minutes have elapsed, small pieces (approximately 1 to 2 cm long) are carefully broken off the tubing with the aid of a glass file. The watch is stopped when a thin string of fibrin can be seen when two broken ends are gently drawn apart. The coagulation time is expressed as the average of the times for the two tubes. When reporting the result it must be specified that this method was used. The normal clotting time is up to 4 minutes.

ONE-STAGE PROTHROMBIN TIME (PT)

Principle. An excess of preformed extrinsic thromboplastin is added to the test plasma in the presence of calcium, and the clotting time is determined. Factors XII, XI, IX, and VIII and platelets are bypassed, and the test thus depends upon the activity of Factors VII, V, X, II and I. Deficiency of any of these factors may only cause 3 to 4 seconds' prolongation in the test, and

*Simplastin, General Diagnostics, Morris Plains, N.J. 07950 and Toronto, Ont. M1K 5C9.

†Ortho Diagnostics, Raritan, N.J. 08869 and Toronto, Ont. M3C 1L9.

‡Parke, Davis & Co., Detroit, Mich. 48232.

it is therefore most important to carefully control the reagents used. Considerable attention has been given to the sensitivity and reproducibility of the thromboplastin reagent because of the importance of the one-stage prothrombin time for the control of vitamin K antagonist (oral anticoagulant) therapy. Specific assays or differential tests must be done in the presence of an abnormal test.

Reagents

Citrated Test Plasma.
Citrated Normal Plasma.
*Thromboplastin Reagent with Added Calcium.**

Procedure

1. Allow the test reagents to warm up at 37°C for 5 minutes. Do not use large amounts of reagent, and keep the stock to be used in melting ice at the side of the water bath.

2. To a tube containing 0.1 mL normal plasma add 0.2 mL of calcium-thromboplastin by blowing it in from a pipette as quickly as possible, with the tip of the pipette just above the surface of the plasma, and start a stopwatch at the same instant.

3. Stop the stopwatch as soon as the first strand of fibrin appears. If the Nichrome loop technique is used, the loop is swept through the mixture at approximately 2 sweeps a second until the first strand of fibrin is seen. If one is directly observing the clot the appearance of fibrin may well become evident by the sudden formation of a clot as the tube is tilted in the water bath at the same rate.

As with any of the tests described in this section, the use of direct clot observation or a loop technique can provide different end points. This is particularly evident in the abnormal tests in which fibrin formation is retarded. Once a laboratory decides on one technique, it must not be used interchangeably with another owing to the preferences of different technologists. A standard loop or tilting technique is vital and serves to emphasize the need to control fine details so necessary in techniques of hemostatic function.

4. Perform the test in replicate with test plasma. Results should be within 1 second of one another. Continue similarly with other test plasmas. For control purposes, the clotting time of normal plasma should be within the specification of the manufacturer of the thromboplastin (always less than 15 seconds). Plot the results of normal and diluted plasmas each day; if the results are not acceptable, repeat the determination with freshly prepared thromboplastin.

TABLE 31–7 RESULTS OF ONE-STAGE PROTHROMBIN TIME TEST

Prolonged in:	*Normal in:*
Factor VII deficiency	Factor VIII deficiency (hemophilia)
Factor V deficiency	Factor IX deficiency (Christmas disease)
Factor X deficiency	Factor XI deficiency (hemophilia C)
Factor II deficiency	Von Willebrand's disease
Factor I deficiency	
Circulating anticoagulants (active against Factors V and VII or thromboplastin)	

*Simplastin, General Diagnostics, Morris Plains, N.J. 07950 and Toronto, Ont. M1K 5C9.

Control of Procedure. The one-stage prothrombin time is probably the most common coagulation procedure performed in the laboratory. The control of this procedure has been given a considerable degree of attention in the past few years and has resulted in a proposal for a standard thromboplastin reagent. Most laboratories use both pooled normal and abnormal plasmas in order to control this very important procedure. As mentioned in the section on quality control, it is necessary to ensure that the thromboplastin is sensitive to all the second- and third-stage clotting defects. It is probably the most easily controlled test in hemostasis, but nevertheless presents numerous pitfalls for the inexperienced worker.

Reporting Results. There is little doubt that the most informative method of reporting is to report the "prothrombin time" in seconds as follows:

Mr. J. B.	Prothrombin time	25 seconds
	Control	13 seconds

Other methods are:

Prothrombin index: This expresses the clotting time of the control plasma as a percentage of the test plasma clotting time, i.e.,

$$\frac{\text{Control time (seconds)}}{\text{Patient's time (seconds)}} \times \frac{100}{1}$$

Prothrombin activity: This is estimated from a graph constructed by diluting normal plasma, with the undiluted plasma regarding as having 100% activity. This method of reporting presents no advantage and may be misleading.

Abnormal one-stage prothrombin times may be given by deficiency of Factor II (prothrombin), Factor I (fibrinogen), V, VII, or X. (See Table 31–7.)

Abnormal and normal plasma controls* are commercially available and may be used to great advantage for controlling this procedure.

Qualitative Test for Factors V, VII, and X

1. Addition of normal plasma: To 9 vol of patient's plasma add 1 vol normal plasma. Repeat the one-stage prothrombin test on this mixture. If the time is corrected, then a definitive factor deficiency should be suspected.

2. Addition of $Al(OH)_3$-adsorbed normal plasma: To nine parts of the patient's plasma add one part of $Al(OH)_3$-adsorbed normal plasma. Perform the one-stage prothrombin test and if the time obtained is significantly shorter than the original time, then there is a possible Factor V deficiency.

3. Addition of normal serum: To 9 vol of the abnormal plasma add 1 vol of normal serum. Perform a one-stage prothrombin test; a significant reduction in time from the original indicates a Factor VII or X deficiency. Factor X deficiency may be assumed in the latter instance if the PTT or thromboplastin generation test is abnormal.

4. If available, plasma lacking Factor V, VII, or X may be added in the ratio of 1 to 9 to the patient's plasma. Failure of this addition to correct the defect identifies the deficient factor.

*General Diagnostics, Verify I and II, Morris Plains, N.J. 07950 and Toronto, Ont. M1K 5C9.

ACTIVATED PARTIAL THROMBOPLASTIN TIME (APTT)

Principle. Platelet substitute, in the form of a partial thromboplastin prepared usually from rabbit brain, is incubated with a contacting agent to provide optimal activation of the intrinsic coagulation factors. The clotting time is determined after the addition of an excess of calcium.

Its use in conjunction with a one-stage prothrombin time provides a simple method for differentiating between Stage 1 intrinsic defects and other factor deficiencies. The APTT is abnormal in Factor XII, XI, X, IX, and VIII deficiencies, whereas the PT is normal with the exception of Factor X. Factors I, II, and V provide abnormal PT and PTT tests. The PTT is also sensitive to various specific and nonspecific circulating anticoagulants.

As a screening test for procoagulant deficiencies the APTT shares the same problem as the PT, namely a lack of sensitivity to mild defects. Therefore, the same considerations hold in the interpretation of normal PT, and an APTT results in a clinically symptomatic individual. APTT is widely advocated as the test of choice for the control of heparin therapy (see p. 735).

Reagents

M/40 Calcium Chloride.

Citrated Test Plasma.

Citrated Normal Plasma.

Platelet Substitute. Preferably with added activator; the method described uses an activator. An unsensitized test may be used, or sensitization may be performed with separately added kaolin. The platelet substitute acts as a "partial" thromboplastin and is more sensitive to the absence of factors involved in intrinsic thromboplastin formation than the more "complete" tissue thromboplastins.

Method

1. Prewarm reagents at 37°C.

2. Add 0.1 mL of platelet substitute with activator to 0.1 mL of normal plasma. Leave at 37°C for 5 minutes after mixing.

3. Blow in 0.1 mL of M/40 $CaCl_2$ and start stop watch immediately.

4. Mix, and leave undisturbed for 20 seconds.

5. Gently tilt the tube to observe the end point or use a Nichrome loop if desired. The end point is the appearance of fibrin strands and is usually sharp.

6. At the appearance of the strands, stop the stop watch and note the time.

7. Repeat the test with the test plasma.

8. It is advisable to replicate all tests.

Results. If commercial reagents are used, the normal times proposed by the manufacturers should be adhered to.

If laboratory-prepared reagents are used, then each batch of reagents should be standardized with a range of known normal plasmas. Acceptable times for the test are: activated partial thromboplastin time, up to 44 seconds; unactivated partial thromboplastin time, up to 100 seconds. The test will detect deficiencies of Factors II (prothrombin), V, VIII, IX, X, XI, and XII, but is relatively insensitive to lack of Factor VII.

Qualitative Tests

Using exactly the same dilution of test plasma and reagents as described under the one-stage prothrombin time, it is possible to obtain an indication of the type of deficiency revealed nonspecifically in the partial thromboplastin time. This applies particularly to Factor VIII and Factor IX deficiencies: partial thromboplastin time corrected by $Al(OH)_3$-adsorbed plasma indicates a possible Factor VIII deficiency; correction with normal serum suggests Factor IX deficiency. Various combinations of abnormal plasmas may further elucidate the problem, but formal factor assays must be performed to substantiate the deficiency (Table 31–5).

THROMBIN CLOTTING TIME (TCT)

Principle. A known concentration of human thrombin and calcium is added to the test plasma. The clotting time is a direct measure of the amount of fibrinogen present, the function of the fibrinogen, and the presence of antithrombins, e.g., heparin. Therefore a prolonged thrombin clotting time is usually considered to be due to either a decrease in fibrinogen concentration, the presence of a dysfunctional fibrinogen, or the presence of heparin or high concentrations of fibrin-fibrinogen degration products, which prevent the formation of the fibrin clot. The test is particularly useful if other screening tests are prolonged, e.g., PT, APTT. Estimation of the fibrinogen level, neutralization of the plasma for heparin presence, and a FDP test will usually provide the necessary explanation for the prolongation of all three screening tests. Conversely, if the TCT is normal with prolonged PT and APTT, defects of Stage *I* and *II* clotting factors should be suspected.

Reagents

Thrombin Solution. Reconstitute 1 vial of 50-unit lyophilized human thrombin with 1 mL distilled water.* Allow to stabilize at room temperature for 5 minutes. Cover the vial top with parafilm and mix gently. Remove the entire contents of vial with a pasteur pipette and add to 9 mL 0.1 M $CaCl_2$ to give a working solution of 5 units of thrombin per mL. Rinse the vial with the $CaCl_2$/thrombin mixture to ensure that all the thrombin has been removed, and store at 4°C. Make fresh daily.

0.1M Calcium Chloride. Make an accurate 1:10 dilution of 1 M calcium chloride, which is kept as a stock solution. (See p. 741 for preparation of calcium chloride.)

Method

Using either a manual or automatic clot timer:

1. Warm 0.2 mL of test plasma for 3 minutes at 37°C.

2. Add 0.1 mL of 5-unit thrombin/calcium solution, and time clot formation. The thrombin calcium mixture should be previously warmed to 37°C for a minute, using a small amount of the working solution.

3. Test each plasma in duplicate in association with appropriate normal and abnormal controls.

Normal Range. Approximately 8 to 10 seconds. As for any other clotting test, the normal range will depend upon the method and choice of normal control plasmas.

---

*Fibrindex, Ortho Diagnostics, Raritan, N.J. 08869 and Don Mills, Ont. M3C 1L9.

Fibrinogen Estimation

A variety of methods are used to estimate fibrinogen concentration. The final choice for the laboratory will depend upon the need for a result in emergency conditions versus a more exact physicochemical analysis. The majority of tests used for the routine determination of fibrinogen use an excess of thrombin and relate the time of clot formation to the amount of fibrinogen present. This thrombin-based technique has superceded the paracoagulation, turbidity, and salting out methods.

Fibrinogen Estimation Using Thrombin

Principle. An excess of thrombin is added to a diluted test plasma sample. The clotting time is compared to a standard calibration graph relating thrombin clotting times to fibrinogen concentration. The test is very similar to the TCT (p. 744), but because an excess of thrombin is used, the clotting time should not give spuriously prolonged results with the presence of heparin, excess fibrin-fibrinogen degradation products, or a dysfunctional fibrinogen. It provides an excellent method for emergency situations.

Reagents

Thombin Solution. 100-unit human or bovine thrombin is freshly prepared using either a lyophilized human or bovine preparation (see p. 742).

0.85% Sodium Chloride—pH 7.4.

Citrated Plasma Samples—Normal and Test.

Calibration Chart. Using a suitable lyophilized source of fibrinogen,* a series of dilutions ranging from 50 mg to 800 mg/dL is prepared and a straight-line calibration graph constructed relating clotting times to fibrinogen concentration.

Method

1. Use either a manual or an automatic clot timer. The fibrometer method is particularly useful for this technique.

2. Make a 1:10 (0.1 mL of plasma + 0.9 mL of saline) dilution of the citrated normal or test plasmas.

3. Transfer 0.2 mL of this dilution to 37°C for 3 minutes.

4. Add 0.1 mL of thrombin solution and record the clotting time.

5. Refer to the calibration graph and read off the fibrinogen level.

Note

1. Very high fibrinogen values (greater than 800 mg/dL, or 8 g/L). Such values produce a very short clotting time, and it will require diluting the plasma 1:20 rather than 1:10 in order to ensure that the linear capability of the calibration graph is maintained. Read the value from the graph and multiply the result by the dilution factor of 2.

2. Very low fibrinogen values (lower than 0.5 g/L). Conversely, low values will give a very prolonged clotting time. Prepare a 1:5 dilution, dividing the final result by a factor of 2. No clotting of a 1:2 dilution of the patient's plasma suggests a fibrinogen concentration below 0.15 g/L.

Normal Values. 1.5 to 4.0 g/L. This range will vary according to the age and condition of the patient. Characteristically the normal pregnant mother has increased levels. Postoperative and septic individuals often have raised levels. A value below 2.0 g/L in the pregnant mother must be interpreted with caution, and it is reasonable to perform sequential studies to rule out a fibrinogen consumption state (p. 732).

*General Diagnostics, Morris Plains, N.J. 07950 and Toronto, Ont. M1K 5C9.

Two-Stage Assay for Prothrombin

Principle. Thromboplastin (brain extract) is added to plasma. Calcium is then added and the thrombin formed is measured by determining the time taken by subsamples (taken at short intervals) to induce clotting in a solution of fibrinogen. The thromboplastin may be used as in the one-stage test, although the test is easier to perform if the thromboplastin is diluted with saline so as to give a one-stage prothrombin time of 25 to 30 seconds with a normal plasma.

In prothrombin deficiency thrombin is generated, but in greatly reduced quantities. Deficiencies of Factors V and VII cause a more prolonged peak of thrombin production. (See Fig. 31–17.)

Method. The reader is referred to one of the reference texts.

Prothrombin Consumption Test

Principle. If serum is examined 1 hour after a normal blood sample has clotted, little or no prothrombin is found. If, however, there is deficiency of blood coagulation, some of the prothrombin will not be utilized. Thus the amount of prothrombin left in the serum is in some measure proportional to the severity of the defect.

This is an extremely *sensitive* although nonspecific test, and may be positive even when the deficiency is not definable by more specific methods.

Abnormal results are obtained in factor deficiencies, circulating anticoagulants, platelet number or function defects, or any condition producing inadequate intrinsic coagulation function. Considerable variation in results is to be expected.

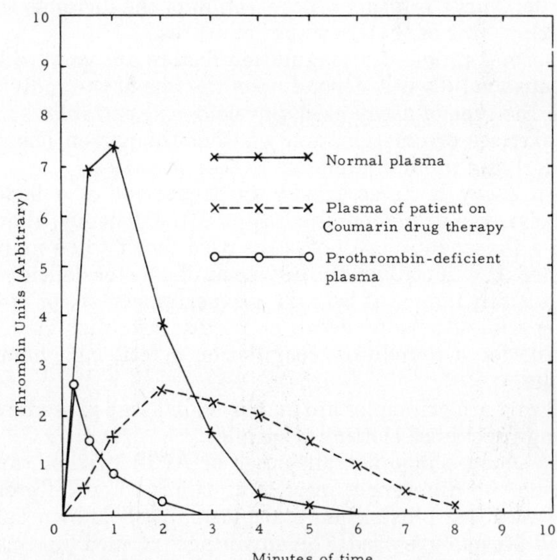

Figure 31–17 Two-stage prothrombin estimation.

Test for Fibrinase (Factor XIII) Deficiency

Principle. Factor XIII renders a fibrin clot insoluble to the lytic action of 5 M urea or 1% monochloracetic acid. In Factor XIII deficiency, contact with these reagents will cause lysis of the test clot.

Reagents

Citrated Normal Plasma.
Citrated Test Plasma.
TRIS Buffer, pH 7.4.
M/40 Calcium Chloride.
5 M Urea in TRIS Buffer.
1% Monochloracetic Acid in TRIS Buffer.

Method

1. Dilute the two plasmas by adding 0.6 mL of plasma to 0.3 mL of TRIS buffer.

2. Add 0.3 mL of normal plasma to each of two tubes, and 0.3 mL of test plasma to each of two other tubes.

3. To all four tubes, add 0.2 mL M/40 $CaCl_2$, and incubate at 37°C for 30 minutes.

4. Add 3.0 mL of 5 M urea to one tube of each plasma clot, and 3 mL of 1% monochloracetic acid to the other tube of each plasma clot.

5. Shake, and leave at room temperature for 24 hours.

Results. If Factor XIII is absent, the test plasma clot will be completely lysed in both tubes; the normal control will be unaffected.

If no Factor XIII activity is seen, the addition of cysteine to a final concentration of 0.02 M will detect whether the factor is present in an unactivated form or is completely absent. (Cysteine will activate it by donating sulfhydryl groups.)

Procoagulant Factor Assay Procedures

Theoretically all blood coagulation factors may be assayed to provide their concentration in blood, which is usually expressed as a percentage of normal or as units per mL of plasma. The percentage or units of activity are extrapolated from the clotting times of various test plasma mixtures after reference to a calibration curve relating concentration of the factor to the clotting time of their reaction mixtures.

Normal ranges for coagulation factors are very wide, because values will depend upon the age of the individual, the type of assay used, physiological variables such as exercise or emotion, and whether the person has an underlying inflammatory or neoplastic process.

An assay is necessary in the treatment of a factor deficiency, e.g., hemophilia Factor VIII deficiency, allowing a therapeutic level of transfused factor to be maintained. It will confirm the diagnosis of a factor deficiency as initially indicated by mixing experiments (see p. 744). In special situations it can be used to establish carrier status for a hereditary coagulation defect, e.g., hemophilia.

Two main principles are employed in assay procedures using functional clotting principles:

1. Using a modified one-stage or APTT method, and noting the differences in clotting times when different ratios of test plasma, normal plasma, and known deficient plasma are used. The advantages of such an assay are speed and simplicity using a well-appreciated method. However, the problems affecting the APTT are reflected in the assay procedure, namely the presence of activated clotting factors producing spurious high assay results, the presence of nonspecific inhibitors producing a spurious low assay result, and wide variability of APTT reagents that prevents consistent assay results.

2. Using a two-stage method similar to that used in the two-stage prothrombin assay or thromboplastin generation test. To avoid the problems of the one-stage assay an incubation mixture of test plasma, platelet substitute, and a substrate plasma containing all but the factor to be assayed is incubated. The resulting generation of "prothrombin converting principle" is used to clot a normal plasma in the presence of additional calcium. It is a technically difficult assay to perform and is not without interpretation difficulties. The one-stage assay is currently the procedure of choice for most laboratories, and the following principle is used for the assay of Factor VIII.

Principle of Factor VIII Assay (One Stage)

This assay uses an APTT procedure and measures the ability of dilutions of patient plasma to correct a known Factor VIII–deficient plasma. A well-characterized Factor VIII–deficient plasma and known Factor VIII standard is essential for the assay.

Normal plasma obtained from a suitable pool of normal donors (see p. 740) is diluted 1:5, 1:10, and 1:20. Each dilution is incubated with a mixture of Factor VIII–deficient plasma, calcium, platelet substitute, and contacting agent, used in the appropriate order. It is particularly important that the normal plasma pool not contain individuals who have elevated Factor VIII levels, e.g., those with inflammatory diseases or those using a birth control medication. Similar dilutions of test plasma are made and tested with the same mixture.

A calibration curve (see Fig. 31–18) is prepared using single logarithmic paper. It is important that the test and normal plasma lines be parallel; otherwise the procedure must be repeated, because the assay has doubtful linearity in all the test dilutions used. Results are expressed either as a percentage of normal (50 to 200%) or in units per mL of plasma (0.5 to 2 units/mL). A unit of Factor VIII is arbitrarily defined as that amount contained within 1 mL of pooled normal plasma. International standards are available, and it is important for any laboratory performing this procedure to regularly calibrate its normal plamsa—either laboratory or commercially prepared—with such a standard.

This type of assay procedure appears deceptively simple. However, long experience has demonstrated that attention to a large number of small but very important details (e.g., type of glass tubes, incubation temperature, individual lots of reagents, and an experienced technologist) is necessary if reproducible results are to be obtained.

Demonstration of Circulating Anticoagulants

The most common forms of circulating anticoagulants interfere with the normal action of factors essential to intrinsic thromboplastin formation. Prolongation of the commoner screening tests (e.g., PT, APTT, TCT) is not uncommon in the laboratory. The technologist has to

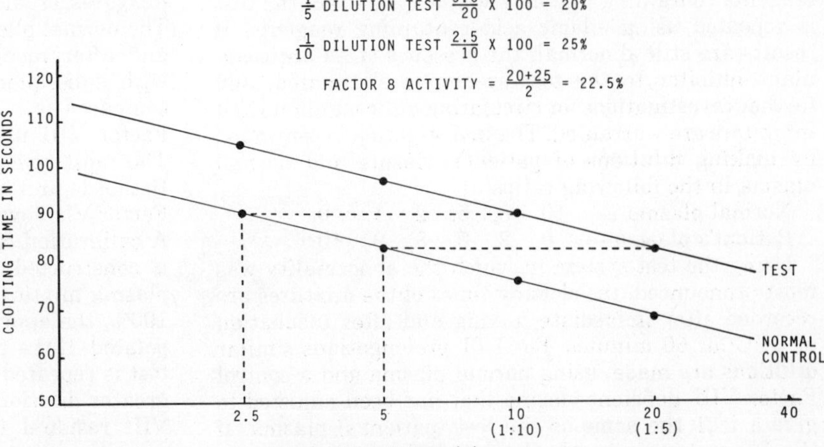

Figure 31–18 A typical semilogarithmic plot for a one-stage Factor VIII assay. See the text for further details.

determine whether such a prolongation is due to a deficiency or to the presence of an anticoagulant or factor inhibitor. An anticoagulant is any substance that will interfere with the normal clotting of blood or plasma in a laboratory test, whereas the term *inhibitor* is reserved to describe an effect on a particular factor (or factors), usually immune mediated, that in turn causes a prolongation of the test or tests that measure the activity of the factor(s) being inhibited.

The most confusing part of this process occurs when a nonspecific anticoagulant effect is demonstrated rather than a specific inhibitory effect. In the latter, the factor(s) being inhibited will demonstrate a decreased or absent factor level(s) in addition to a prolonged screening test(s). A common example is the formation of a Factor VIII inhibitor in a multitransfused Factor VIII–deficient hemophiliac. In this instance, the individual will have a prolonged PTT not only because of the low Factor VIII level, but also because of the added effect of the Factor VIII inhibitor (see p. 725). The nonspecific inhibitor or anticoagulant will produce a prolonged screening test, but when assays of the specific factors involved in that test are performed, they are all normal. An example is a prolonged PTT with normal Factor VIII, IX, XI, XII, and X assays. Very often such non–factor-specific but test-specific anticoagulants are directed to the reagents used in the test rather than the procoagulant factors. Therefore, individuals with spuriously prolonged APTT tests due to nonspecific inhibitors will very likely not have a clinically evident bleeding syndrome, and can have surgical procedures without risk of intraoperative or postoperative hemorrhage. Differentiation of such defects is therefore of the greatest importance for the subsequent welfare of the patient.

The investigations are often time consuming, demanding considerable experience and close cooperation with the clinician. Further procedures, such as immunological characterization of the inhibitors (antibodies) with appropriate in vivo survival studies, are necessary if a precise diagnosis is to be made.

NEUTRALIZATION OF HEPARINIZED PLASMA

It is often necessary to neutralize heparin in plasma in order to decide whether the prolonged procoagulant test(s) is due to heparin or an underlying coagulation factor(s) deficiency. Herparinization of the sample may be the result of either inadvertent contamination (removing blood sample from a previously heparinized indwelling venous catheter) or therapeutic heparinization. The following method is recommended.

Reagents

*Protamine Sulfate,** 100 μg in 100 mL of 0.85% saline. Dilute the protamine sulfate solution as follows:

Dilution	Protamine Sulfate Dilutions (mL)	85% NaCl (mL)	Final Concentration of Protamine Sulfate
1	0.1	0.9	10 μg
2	0.5 of 1	0.5	5 μg
3	0.5 of 2	0.5	2.5 μg
4	0.5 of 3	0.5	1.25 μg
5	0.5 of 4	0.5	0.625 μg
6	0.5 of 5	0.5	0.3125 μg

Method

1. Add 0.05 mL from each dilution to 0.2 mL of test plasma.

2. Perform an APTT or TCT (see p. 744).

3. Select the dilution that gives the shortest APTT or TCT, and use it for subsequent testing.

Note. It is important not to use an excess of protamine sulfate, otherwise paradoxically prolonged clotting times will result.

A commercial heparin neutralizer† is available that uses an ion exchange procedure with the added advantage of being in a convenient, stable tablet. The tablet is added to the test plasma, mixed, and subsequently centrifuged, and the supernatant plasma is used.

Circulating Anticoagulant Demonstration

The test showing prolongation is repeated using different reagents to ensure that the abnormality found is not reagent dependent. For example, if the activated partial thromboplastin time (APTT) is abnormal when

*E. Lilly and Co., Indianapolis, Ind. 46206; Sigma Chemical Co., St. Louis, Mo. 63178.

†Heparsorb, General Diagnostics, Morris Plains, N. J. 07950 and Toronto, Ont. M1K 5C9.

reagents containing micronized silica are used, the test is repeated using ellagic acid–containing reagents. If results are still abnormal, the presence of an anticoagulant/inhibitor to the test system is eliminated, and further investigations for circulating anticoagulants and inhibitors are warranted. The investigation is continued by making dilutions of patient's plasma and normal plasma in the following ratios:

Normal plasma — 10, 8, 5, 2, 1, 0.
Patient's plasma— 0, 2, 5, 8, 9, 10.

Using the test system in which the abnormality was most pronounced, the clotting times of the mixtures are recorded after immediate mixing and after incubation at 37°C for 60 minutes. For PTT prolongations similar dilutions are made, using normal plasma and a control Factor VIII–deficient plasma that has been adjusted to give a PTT the same as the test (patient's) plasma. If the PT system is involved, plasma from a patient receiving warfarin treatment would be used to the same effect. Incubation of the test and factor-deficient plasma is performed to rule out if the plasma anticoagulant/inhibitor is time dependent, e.g., requires time to interact with factors in the normal plasma.

The use of a factor-deficient control plasma provides the technologist with a series of clotting times reflecting a clotting factor deficiency rather than an inhibitor/anticoagulant. It would be expected to require more normal plasma to correct an anticoagulant/inhibitor–prolonged PTT than that required for correcting a factor-deficiency defect.

Interpretation of the test results take a great deal of experience and must be done in conjunction with previously mentioned clinical information. The following combinations are usually expected:

1. If the correction of the clotting time back to 50% of the difference from the median of the normal range to the abnormal test time requires more than 20% added normal plasma, an anticoagulant/inhibitor is suspected.
2. If the minimum amount of normal plasma required to correct the specific factor–depleted plasma back to the upper range of normal is exceeded by the amount of normal plasma to correct the test (patient's) plasma, an inhibitor/anticoagulant is suspected.
3. If the defect is markedly potentiated by incubation for 1 hour at 37°C, an inhibitor is suspected.

With very avid or high titer inhibitors it may be necessary to adjust the mixtures of plasma. Nonspecific inhibitors are most often associated with either test-specific (reagent) dependent prolongations or autoimmune disorders (lupus erythematosus, neoplasms, etc.). It is very important that such observations be repeated and followed up to judge whether they are of a transient or permanent nature—the latter being more suggestive of a pathological state. Factor-specific inhibitors are pathological entities, often associated with severe bleeding disorders and disorders of immunity (e.g., postpregnancy, lupus erythematosus, collagen vascular disorders). Treatment is different and may require immunosuppressive medications or special replacement therapy (see p. 725).

Factor VIII–Specific Inhibitor Assay (Bethesda)

The test is the same method as the Factor VIII assay, with the exception that it is performed on various mixtures of the patient's plasma and normal plasma. The normal plasma Factor VIII level is measured before and after incubation with the test plasma dilutions, with subsequent diminution of the Factor VIII level compared to a suitable control of normal plasma. The Factor VIII inhibition strength is expressed in units. The most common unit used in North America is the Bethesda unit, which is the loss of 50% of normal plasma Factor VIII level after mixing with the patient's plasma. A calibration curve using the various plasma dilutions is constructed, and provided that the loss in the test plasma mixture Factor VIII activity is between 25 and 100%, the appropriate units of inhibition can be interpolated. If the residual Factor VIII is less than 25% the test is repeated using incubation mixtures containing a greater dilution of the test plasma to give final Factor VIII residual levels within a 25 to 75% range. For example, if the test (patient's) plasma is diluted 1:5, the residual Factor VIII after incubation is 35%, which equals 1.5 Bethesda units. Because the plasma was diluted 1:5, the final inhibitor strength is $1.5 \times 5 = 7.5$ Bethesda units/mL plasma.

Normal values are difficult to interpret, because normal levels may indicate a low titer of inhibitor; if the inhibitor is quiescent (e.g., has not been recently challenged with Factor VIII–containing transfusion materials), a normal result does not guarantee that an anamnestic response will not occur. Therefore, appropriate in vivo Factor VIII survival must be performed in parallel with repeat inhibitor examination approximately 14 to 21 days after the transfusion challenge. If an inhibitor level of less than 0.6 units is found no inhibitor is present.

TESTS FOR PLASMINOLYSIS

Primary and secondary plasminolysis are important physiological and pathological mechanisms (see p. 719). Any laboratory method that is to demonstrate such processes must be able to reflect that plasminogen activator has been released and has subsequently converted plasminogen to plasmin, which in turn is able to vicariously digest fibrinogen or remove offending intravascular fibrin. Because of the inability of plasmin to differentiate between fibrin or fibrinogen (its trypsin-like effect) the beneficial fibrin digestion may be complicated by bleeding caused by a concomitant fibrinogen digestion (secondary fibrinogenolysis).

Laboratory methods for plasminolysis are therefore divided into three major categories.

1. Clot digestion—the ability of the test plasma to digest its own or a normal fibrin clot.
2. Fibrin-fibrinogen degradation products—identification of the products of fibrin-fibrinogen digestion by plasmin.
3. Plasminogen-plasmin levels—changes in level or activity of plasminogen activator, plasminogen, plasmin, or antiplasmins.

Tests in category three generally are difficult for the nonspecialized laboratory to perform, have ephemeral levels, and cause difficulties in interpretation because of the presence of concomitant pathological states. Tests in category one are simple to perform but are relatively insensitive and lack specificity, with resultant low clinical predictiveness. Category two tests have become popular because of the availability of commercially produced kits. The principles of tests from category one and two, e.g., euglobulin lysis in category one and FDP tests in category two, will be described.

Euglobulin Lysis Time

Principle. Euglobulin, a mixture of plasminogen and its activators in association with fibrinogen and cold insoluble globulins is precipitated from the patient's plasma using 1% acetic acid. The precipitated euglobulin has its supernatant discarded by centrifugation and is clotted with an excess of thrombin. This clot is observed for lysis at 37°C.

A normal range of 90 to 360 minutes is associated with normal plasminolysis. Unfortunately the number of variables associated with the principle and performance of the test makes interpretation of the final result very difficult. The time of lysis is directly related to the level of fibrinogen, plasminogen activators, and plasminogen in the test plasma (antiplasmins are not precipitated). Therefore, a decrease in fibrinogen will produce a spuriously decreased time, whereas a decrease in plasminogen activator or plasminogen will produce a falsely prolonged time. A low fibrinogen level as a cause of a short test result (positive) can be excluded if a fibrinogen assay is performed.

Fibrinogen-Fibrin Degradation Products (FDP)

Principle. When human fibrinogen and/or fibrin is digested by plasmin a number of large and small degradation products are produced (p. 720). These products are further catabolized by the liver and excreted by the renal system. Nevertheless, if such products are present in increased amounts in an individual with normal hepatic and renal function, it is assumed that a recent plasminolytic event has taken or is taking place. Unfortunately the FDP tests that are currently available for routine purposes are unable to distinguish between the products of fibrin and fibrinogen digestion. Therefore a raised FDP test does not necessarily indicate that intravascular fibrin has been deposited, merely that the release of plasmin has occurred or is occurring. Tests that would differentiate fibrin from fibrinogen degradation or digestion are required to demonstrate the production of fibrin monomer soluble complexes (protamine sulfate test) or the presence of fibrinopeptides A and B (using radioimmune methods). The former test is nonspecific and the latter highly specific.

The tests that have been developed to determine FDP concentrations include:

1. Agglutination tests, e.g., the staphylococcal clumping test.
2. Tanned red cell tests, using antifibrinogen-coated red cells as indicator cells for the presence of FDPs.
3. Immunoprecipitin tests, e.g., using an agar plate system.
4. Latex particle tests.

This latter group of tests is now popular because of their simplicity of use in emergency situations, high sensitivity, and specificity, using a principle that is common to the other methods, e.g., the use of an indicator substance or cells to provide a reaction with FDPs. Latex particles are sensitized with a rabbit-derived antihuman FDP antibody. The sensitized latex particles become macroscopically agglutinated in the presence of FDPs. Since the coated particles are unable to differentiate between FDPs and fibrinogen, it is necessary to use a special collecting tube for the original blood sample. An excess of thrombin ensures complete clotting of all residual fibrinogen in the sample, leaving the FDPs free in the resultant serum. An antiplasminolytic substance, e.g., tranexamic acid is used to prevent further ex vivo digestion of fibrinogen or fibrin monomer complexes, which would result in a falsely high FDP test. Dilutions of the treated serum are made in association with appropriate negative and positive controls. The results are expressed in μg FDP per mL of serum. Most latex tests are capable of detecting FDP to a level of 2.5 μg/mL, i.e., the last dilution of the serum that produces agglutination of the latex particles. If the test dilution of the serum that produced the last agglutination reaction were 1:10 the final result would be $2.5 \times 10 = 25$ μg/mL.

Normal values are considered to be less than 20 μg/mL, depending upon the pathological process and the condition of the patient. The postoperative patient, the pregnant mother, and the individual with an acute febrile illness are all examples in which raised FDPs are found in the absence of any laboratory or clinical hemostatic abnormality. Therefore interpretation of isolated FDP results must be done with great caution.

Test for Fibrin Monomer

A variety of procedures are available to demonstrate the inappropriate presence of intravascular fibrin monomer. The protamine sulfate methods are the most practical for routine clinical purposes.

Serial Dilution Protamine Sulfate Test—PST

Principle. The addition of protamine sulfate to plasma results in the formation of fibrin strands or gelling (paracoagulation) in the presence of fibrin monomer or early fibrin degradation products (Fragment X⁰). It appears insensitive to fibrinogen or fibrinogen degradation products, and therefore probably reflects the formation of excessive amounts of endogenous thrombin, e.g., in disseminated intravascular thrombosis.

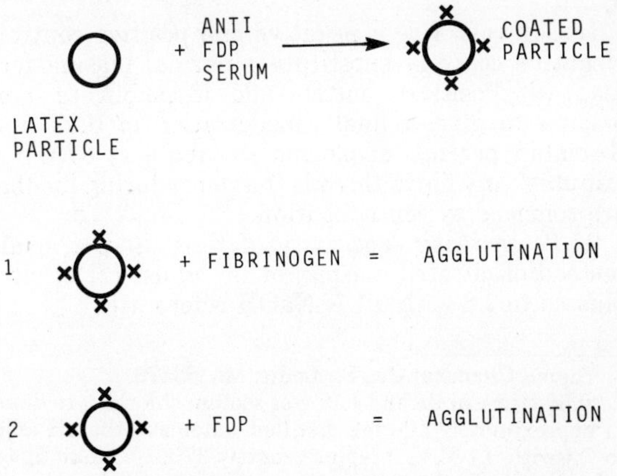

Figure 31–19 Principle of the latex agglutination test for FDPs and fibrinogen. Either fibrinogen or its derivatives will cause agglutination of the coated latex particles.

Reagents

*1% Protamine Sulfate.** Freshly prepared in distilled water; adjust to pH 6.5.

0.85% Sodium Chloride.

Citrated Plasma. Add 0.1 mL EACA (250 mg/mL) to anticoagulant before use.

Method

1. Prepare the following dilutions of protamine sulfate in saline: 1:5, 1:10, 1:20, 1:40, 1:80, in 0.2-mL aliquots.

2. Add an equal volume of plasma.

3. Shake gently and allow to stand at room temperature for 30 minutes.

4. Read with direct light and a nonreflective background.

Reading

g = Gel = Solid white clumps.
fs = Fibrin strands = Fine strands white material.
+ = Coarse precipitate.
± = Fine precipitate.
− = Clear solution.

Note. g and fs indicate the presence of fibrin monomer and early FDP. A positive result may occur in any of the dilutions.

Protamine Sulfate and 1-Tube Test—PST

Principle. The principle for this test is the same as that for the serial dilution method. However, only one dilution is used, along with a different buffering and reading system.

Reagents

Fresh Citrated Plasma. Collected as for FDP analysis.

*Protamine Sulfate.** 1% in imidazole buffer† pH 7.8. Store at 4°C. Make fresh solution weekly.

Method

1. Prewarm 1 mL of plasma to 37°C.

2. Add 0.1 mL of 1% protamine sulfate.

3. Mix and incubate at 37°C for 3 minutes.

4. Read against indirect lighting and a black background. Grade the results as for the serial dilution test.

Notes

1. Controls: Use a negative and positive control. (a) Negative control—substitute a normal plasma for the test. (b) Positive control—add thrombin to normal plasma to give a final concentration of 0.02 unit of thrombin per mL of plasma. Incubate at 37°C for 30 minutes. Any fibrin threads that form during incubation are removed by centrifugation.

2. To increase sensitivity of test: (a) Use oxalated instead of citrated plasma, or (b) adjust pH of citrated plasma to 7.8 with 0.1 N NaOH before use.

*Sigma Chemical Co., St. Louis, Mo. 63178.

†0.68 g imidazole and 1.17 g of sodium chloride are dissolved in approximately 100 mL distilled water and the pH adjusted to 7.3 with 0.1 M HCl (approximately 37 mL). Make up to 200 mL with distilled water.

TESTS OF PLATELET AND VASCULAR FUNCTION

This section describes tests used to detect abnormalities in the vascular and platelet systems. In general they are difficult procedures to standardize, and the results reflect the degree of effort expended in obtaining consistent technique.

Bleeding Time Determination

This test provides an estimate of the integrity of the primary hemostatic plug and thus measures the interaction between the microvasculature (capillaries) and platelets. Hence it is abnormal in a variety of quantitative or qualitative platelet defects and occasionally in vascular disorders. It represents a cornerstone in assessing the hemostatic integrity of the platelet-vascular axis in that if a normal result is correctly obtained, it indicates that there is no clinically significant platelet-vascular defect that would cause catastrophic hemorrhage, particularly if the individual being tested requires a surgical procedure. Nevertheless it is not always positive in platelet function defects, either because of the mildness of the defect or the variability of the condition, e.g., von Willebrand's disease. Therefore, if the clinical history is suggestive of a platelet vascular defect, even though the bleeding time is normal, further tests would be indicated (p. 733).

Principle

The test requires that an atraumatic subcutaneous incision be made without transecting vessels larger than subcutaneous capillaries. The depth and length of the incision requires careful control, as does the removal of blood welling from the incision. It is vital to remove all blood from the incision, otherwise fibrin formation (assuming a normal procoagulant system) may produce a spuriously low bleeding time. The position of the extremity on which the incision is made will interfere with the intracapillary pressure; therefore most methods now recommend that this be stabilized using an exterior pressure cuff (sphygmomanometer cuff) and a constant pressure of 40 mm of mercury if an upper extremity is used. The end point of the test is reached when all bleeding ceases, and this is most conveniently detected for routine purposes using a filter paper to blot away the surplus blood. When the filter paper remains clean, the end point is reached.

Two methods are recommended:

1. Ivy Method. It is important that the lancet and lancet holder be carefully designed in order to provide a standard incision.

2. Template Method. This provides an incision of similar precision; it is not so deep as that of the Ivy method, but it has a longer incision. Each method has its own merits. In general, they are difficult tests to perform but provide consistently reproducible results. Attention to detail, site preparation, and patient cooperation are essential prerequisites.

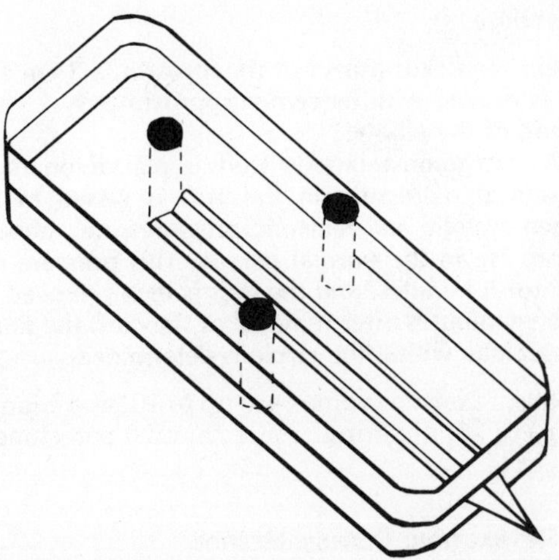

Figure 31–20 Lucite holder for standardized Ivy bleeding time. This simple device ensures that an incision of standard depth and width is made.

Ivy Method

Materials

1. Disposable lancets (Red Label*) producing a 2 mm long and 3 mm deep v-shaped incision.
2. Plastic template to control incision depth and length (see Fig. 31–20).
3. Sphygmomanometer cuff.
4. Number 42, 11-cm filter paper discs.
5. Three stopwatches.

Method

1. Prepare the patient by explaining the procedure. Allow him to relax in a comfortable position, with the test arm supported in an extended position. Require him to have arrived in the building at least fifteen minutes before the test, and avoid testing excessively cold or sweating extremities. Question the patient regarding recent use of medications, and note the responses on an appropriate form, e.g., recent ASA use. Have a pretest platelet count performed—if this is less than 60,000 further advice should be obtained from a supervisor before proceeding.
2. Examine the volar surfaces of both forearms, and choose the extremity with the fewer surface veins. Inflating the pressure cuff to 70 mm Hg if necessary will assist in this procedure.
3. Wash the forearm well. Mark three potential incision sites with a small-tip marking pen.
4. Wipe the site with a 70% alcohol swab and allow to dry.
5. While waiting, insert a red disposable lancet into the plastic holder.
6. Only when ready, inflate a well-fitting, appropriate-size pressure cuff to 40 mm Hg, and maintain this at a constant reading during the entire test period.
7. Make three incisions at 15-second intervals, starting a separate stopwatch for each incision. It is important to tense the skin by pulling on redundant forearm tissue with one hand and using the other for the lancet. This also serves to momentarily separate the lips of the incision, so allowing blood to escape. A vertical or horizontal incision can be made provided the same direction is used for all incisions at all times.
8. Using a separate filter paper disc for each incision, remove the blood at 30-second intervals by gently touching the filter paper to the *edge* rather than the site of the incision. It may be necessary to perform this at 15-second intervals if the bleeding is unusually brisk and prolonged. The interval is important only to avoid unnecessary interference with the flow of blood and provided that each incision is treated in exactly the same manner.
9. The end point is reached when only a miniscule trace or no blood is picked up on the filter paper. Make a note of the elapsed time and record it on the filter paper. Alternatively, the number of drops of blood on the filter paper can be counted and the necessary calculations made.
10. An average of the three times is the bleeding time. Occasionally one incision will bleed for an inordinately long period of time compared with the other two. Under these circumstances, take an average of the two incision times and note this and the discrepant result in the workbook. This aberrant result is usually due to inadvertently transecting a large subcutaneous vessel.
11. Release the pressure cuff and wash the forearm with soap and water. Avoid interfering with the bleeding sites. Place a sterile dressing over the incision, which can be removed in 24 hours. Prolonged bleeding times may require a pressure dressing and an adhesive dressing to prevent secondary hemorrhage (vide infra).

Normal Range. This will depend upon individual laboratory results. In our experience any time greater than 5.5 minutes is abnormal until proven otherwise. The range, however, will depend upon individual technique, and the technologist must standardize for individual idiosyncrasies to avoid undue variation. The use of a lancet holder is mandatory if this method is to give reproducible results.

Template Method

This method was introduced to avoid inadvertent transection of larger subcutaneous vessels and to standardize the length of the incision. The original technique produced an incision 10 mm long and 1 mm deep. This has subsequently been modified to a 5-mm and, in some cases, a 3-mm incision.

The method, if correctly performed, produces excellent reproducibility, but all the considerations regarding preparation and performance of the Ivy method as previously described are still necessary. Major problems of the original Mielke method were undue scarring, particularly of children's arms, and the need for custom-designed template materials that required considerable practice to permit the technologist to become suitably adept. The introduction of spring-loaded disposable materials has eliminated these disadvantages, and these are the materials of choice.

Materials. These are similar to those of the Ivy Method, except for replacement of the lancet and holder

*Becton, Dickinson and Co., Rutherford, N.J. 07070 and Mississauga, Ont. L5J 2M8.

with a disposable spring-loaded blade that produces an incision 1 mm deep and 5 mm long.*

Method

1. Steps 1 through 6 of the Ivy method are used.

2. The incisions are made using the spring-loaded plastic template and blade. The same precautions cited for the Ivy method are necessary regarding placing of incisions and manipulation of the skin and arm. Follow any additional instructions of the manufacturer carefully.

3. Determine bleeding times in exactly the same manner as the Ivy method.

4. Care of the incision is slightly different in that it is recommended that the incisions be carefully cleaned of any excess blood with soap and water, dried, and then dressed with a small sterile adhesive dressing to ensure that the incisions' edges are in close approximation.† This avoids, to a large degree, the possibility of excessive scar (keloid) formation.

Normal Values. The same comments apply as for the Ivy method. Expected normal values are 2.5 to 9.5 minutes.

Notes

1. It is recommended that bleeding times not be performed on thrombocytopenic individuals (< 100,000), unless there is a clinical need. For example, in immune platelet consumption states, a paradoxically normal bleeding time is obtained in a severely thrombocytopenic individual because of the population of depleted platelets' being juvenile and therefore very active.

2. ASA and other medications are known to prolong the bleeding time. This has been used to advantage in the ASA tolerance test. Bleeding times are performed before and after a 600-mg oral dose of ASA. Prolongation of the pre-ASA bleeding time by greater than 100% after ingestion of ASA indicates an underlying platelet function defect.

3. It bears repeating that attention to detail is so important. Once your method has been standardized, do not deviate from it in any way. A simple example would be changing the type of pressure cuff to one of a different width, thus changing intracapillary pressure. Remember that obese individuals require a wider cuff and children narrower cuffs to avoid false high or low pressure readings.

Tourniquet Capillary Resistance Test

Principle. This test measures the resistance of the capillaries to the increased intraluminal pressure and partial anoxia caused by a carefully controlled tourniquet on the proximal aspect of the upper extremity. Abnormalities are found in defects of the supporting tissues (e.g., senile purpura), defects in capillary endothelial integrity (e.g., scurvy), and defects in platelet number and function (e.g., thrombocytopenia). Because of its widely varying sensitivity and specificity, it is seldom used for routine hemostasis screening.

Procedure

1. On the flexor aspect of the forearm, a 3 cm diameter circle is drawn, with its center approximately 2 cm below the bend of the elbow.

2. A sphygmomanometer cuff is placed on the upper arm, and the pressure in the cuff is raised to midway between systolic and diastolic pressures, i.e., about 80 to 100 mm Hg in the normal person. This pressure is maintained for 5 minutes, and the cuff is then removed.

3. Five minutes after removal of the cuff, the number of the petechiae within the circle is determined.

Results. Normal values are up to 10 petechiae; equivocal, 10 to 20; abnormal, more than 20 petechiae in the 3-cm circle.

Clot Retraction: Classic Method

Principle. Clot retraction is a measure of: (1) the amount of fibrin formed and its subsequent contraction, (2) the number and quality of platelets, since platelets have a protein similar to actomyosin that causes clot retraction. Since the fibrin clot enmeshes the cellular elements of the blood, a limit is set to the extent fibrin contracts by the volume of red blood cells (hematocrit). Hence, the smaller the hematocrit, the greater the degree of clot retraction. Clot retraction is directly proportional to the number of platelets and inversely proportional to the hematocrit and fibrinogen levels. When fibrinolysis is very active, the fibrin may be dissolved almost as quickly as it is formed, and clot retraction will be impaired.

Procedure

1. Place 5 mL of venous blood into an unscratched graduated centrifuge tube. Insert a coiled wire in the bottom of the tube (1 mm thickness wire, with a 3 cm diameter coil).

2. Place at 37°C for 1 hour after clotting has occurred.

3. Gently lift the wire and allow the attached clot to drain for 1 or 2 minutes.

4. Read the volume of fluid remaining in the tube (some red cells will also be present). Express this volume as a percentage of the original volume of whole blood placed in the tube. Normal values are 48 to 64% (average 55%).

Screening Test for Clot Retraction

A simple screening test consists of keeping the tubes from the Lee and White coagulation time at 37°C for a further hour, then "ringing" the tubes and withdrawing the clots. If clot retraction is normal, approximately 0.5 mL of serum should remain, i.e., half of the original total volume.

Platelet Adhesiveness

Principle. A wide variety of methods exist to measure the ability of platelets to adhere to a variety of material. The most common adhesive foreign surface is glass in the form of small beads; this gives rise to the term *glass retention index*. Under a constant pressure or vacuum, unanticoagulated blood is passed through a column of standard dimension containing a known weight of glass

---

*Simplate. General Diagnostics, Morris Plains, N.J. 07950 and Toronto Ont. M1K 5C9.

†Steristrip. 3M Medical Products Division, St. Paul, Minn. 55101 and Toronto, Ont. M3C 2V3.

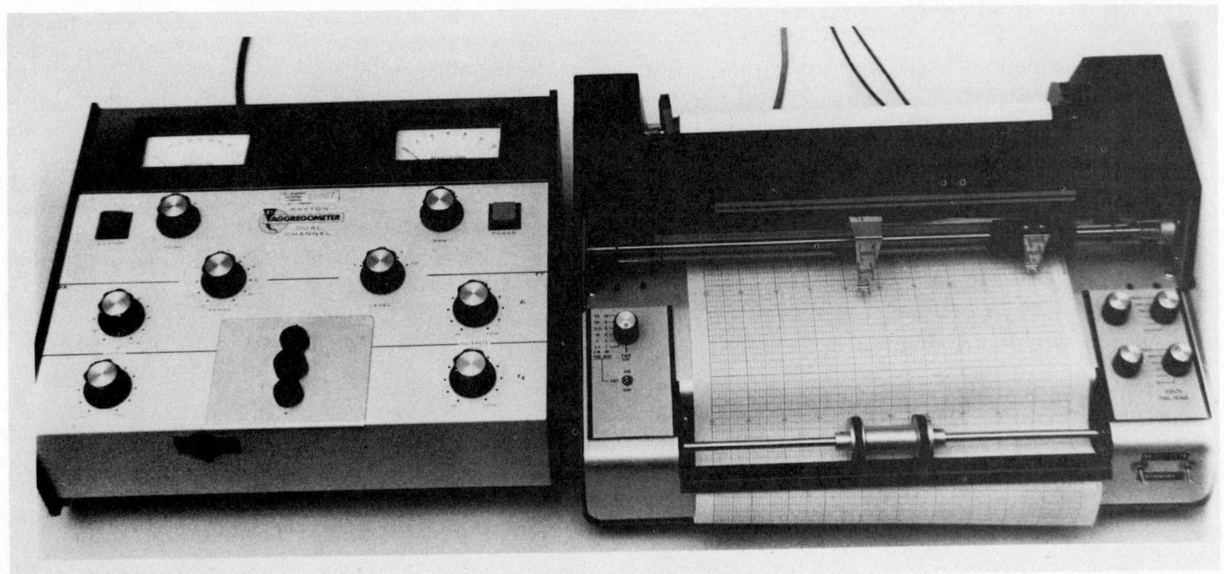

Figure 31–21 Payton dual-channel aggregometer with recorder.

beads. A sample of prepassage and postpassage blood is anticoagulated in EDTA, and platelet counts are performed. Platelet-glass adhesiveness or retention is expressed as a percentage of the initial platelet count minus the final platelet count divided by the initial platelet count.

Classically the results are reduced in von Willebrand's disease and other platelet function disorders, including the results for ASA-treated platelets. Normal results have such a wide range of variability (20 to 85% retention) that the test can be performed with confidence only by using a series of estimations over a number of days and a very refined technique.

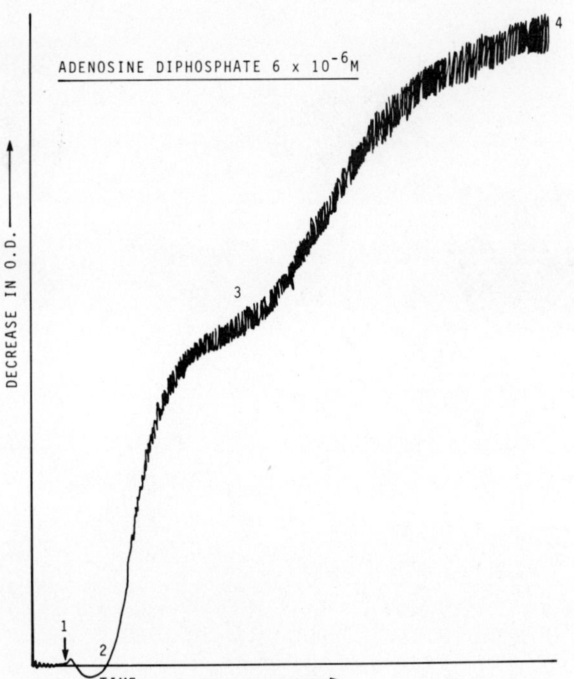

Figure 31–22 A typical platelet aggregation curve with ADP showing: (1) addition of ADP, (2) initial swell reaction, (3) second phase aggregation, (4) maximal response.

Platelet Aggregation

A variety of methods have been described to assess this phenomenon. A photometer connected to a pen recorder is probably the most representative method available. (See Fig. 31–21.)

Principle. A sample of platelet-rich plasma is placed in a cuvette and the instrument calibrated to a zero base line. Aggregating agent is added, and with continuous stirring of the suspension the reaction is monitored on the pen recorder. According to the type of aggregating agent used, e.g., ADP, adrenalin, and collagen, a curve is obtained that can be used to assess platelet function.

The curve reflects the changes in optical density of the platelet-rich plasma as the platelets become aggregated; platelet aggregation increases light transmission through the cuvette and gives a positive deflection in the pen recorder. This can be seen macroscopically as the platelet-rich plasma changes from a turbid to a granular and slightly opalescent appearance.

A wide variety of instruments for performing platelet aggregation are available. Instruments manufactured by Bryston Manufacturing* and Payton Associates† are recommended. The Payton instrument has the advantage of having dual modules. Any 10-mV potentiometric pen recorder may be used; however, it is wise to accept the manufacturer's recommendations regarding a particular instrument. Matched cuvettes and stir bars are specifically designed for a particular instrument. Both should be regularly siliconized and carefully handled.

*Bryston Manufacturing, Rexdale, Ont. M9V 4M3.

†Payton Associates, Buffalo, N.Y. 14202 and Scarborough, Ont. M1S 3R2.

CHAPTER 31—REVIEW QUESTIONS

1. What screening tests would be useful in the investigation of a possible hemostatic defect?
2. What is the difference between a sex-linked inherited disorder and an autosomal-dominant inherited disorder? Give examples of hemostatic disorders showing each type of inheritance.
3. What tests would you perform in the investigation of disseminated intravascular coagulation?
4. What differences are there between the intrinsic and extrinsic pathways of coagulation?
5. Describe the reagents to be used and technical precautions to be taken in the performance of an activated partial thromboplastin time.
6. Describe principles for two automatic clot timers; cite their advantage and disadvantage in a routine laboratory, and give a short description of their operation.
7. Describe the principle, reagents used, and method for performing a thrombin clotting time? What are the principle advantages for using this test?
8. How would you organize a quality control (assurance) program for a hemostasis laboratory?

REFERENCES FOR HEMATOLOGY SECTION

Beck, W., ed. Hematology. Cambridge, Mass.: M.I.T. Press, 1981.

Bessis M. Blood Smears Reinterpreted. New York: Springer International, 1977.

Biggs R. Human Blood Coagulation, Haemostasis and Thrombosis. Oxford: Blackwell Scientific Publications, 1972.

Bloom AL, and Thomas DP. Haemostasis and Thrombosis. New York: Churchill-Livingstone, 1981.

Dacie JV, and Lewis SM. Practical Hematology, 5th ed. Edinburgh: Churchill-Livingstone, 1975.

Hayhoe FGH, and Quaglino D. Haematological Cytochemistry. Edinburgh: Churchill-Livingstone, 1980.

Hirsh J, Brain EA, and Skov KC. Concepts in Hemostasis and Thrombosis. Hamilton, Ont.: McMaster University, 1976.

Hirsh J, Senton E, and Hull R. Venous Thromboembolism. New York: Grune and Stratton Inc., 1981.

McDonald GA, Dodds TC, and Cruickshank, B. Atlas of Haematology. Edinburgh: Churchill-Livingstone, 1978.

Platt WR. Color atlas and textbook of Hematology, 2nd ed. Philadelphia: JB Lippincott Co., 1979.

Simmons A. Technical Hematology, 3rd ed. Philadelphia: JB Lippincott Co., 1980.

Thomson JM. Blood Coagulation and Hemostasis. New York: Churchill-Livingstone, 1980.

Williams WJ, Beutler E, Ersler AJ, and Rundles RW. Hematology, 2nd ed. New York: McGraw-Hill, 1977.

Wintrobe MM, Lee GR, Boggs DR, Bithell TC, Foerster J, and Athens JW. Clinical Hematology. 8th ed. Philadelphia: Lea and Febiger, 1981.

Section V

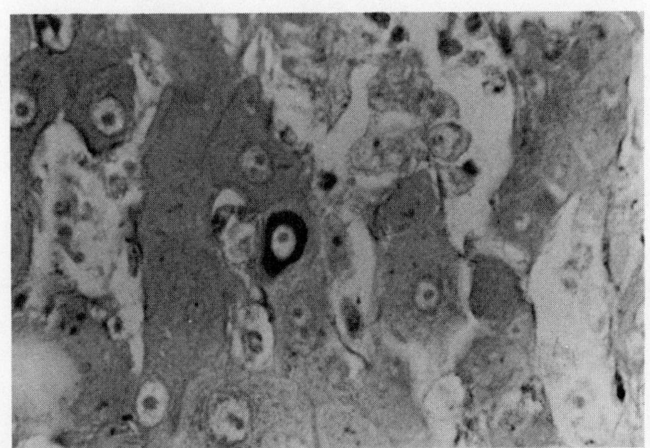

HISTOTECHNOLOGY

32

PROCESSING TISSUES FOR HISTOTECHNOLOGY

INTRODUCTION

Histological technique deals with the preparation of tissues for microscopic examination. Briefly, this is accomplished by submitting the total or a selected part of the tissue presented for examination to a series of processes, namely, fixation, dehydration, clearing, embedding, cutting, and staining.

As soon as a tissue is removed from the body or cut off from its blood supply, it begins to decompose. This results from the deprivation of oxygen and essential metabolites, from the accumulation of carbon dioxide and other products of cell metabolism, and from the action of various enzymes (autolysis). The same processes begin in all tissues of the body as soon as death occurs, and the speed of decomposition appears to be proportional to the natural metabolic activity of the tissue; e.g., it is rapid in the convoluted tubules of the kidney and the liver, and especially rapid in the pancreas if death occurs within a few hours of eating, because this gland then contains large amounts of digestive enzymes that are activated and released by tissue death. To preserve as nearly as possible the natural state of the tissue cells, it is essential to check these processes of decomposition with a minimum of delay. To this end the tissue should be placed in an adequate bulk of a suitable fixing solution as soon as possible after removal by the surgeon. However, many pathologists like to examine the gross tissue before it is placed in fixative solution, because the natural color and appearance are altered by even short periods of fixation. For this reason, many larger institutions provide cooled receptacles on trolleys in which excised tissues are placed for the few hours elapsing between removal by the surgeon and gross description and selection of blocks for sectioning by the pathologist. With most specimens, however, it is very doubtful if the gain accruing from this practice adequately offsets the drying and deterioration in cell structures entailed thereby.

There are a number of other reasons for fixation's being an essential first step in routine histological procedure. Most cells consist of an outer complex membrane containing the fluid protoplasm, which is a mixed, true and colloidal, solution of salts, proteins, carbohydrates, lipids, organic acids, and enzymes. Were the cells not "fixed," many of these substances would be lost by simple solution, dialysis, or osmotic swelling and rupture of the cells in the processing that must precede the cutting and staining of sections. Again, and largely to the same ends, fixation must be thoroughly effected before dehydration can be accomplished.

On microscopic examination, autolyzed tissues show changes in, and finally disappearance of, nuclei while the cytoplasm becomes cloudy and loses its usual staining affinities. Surface cells are lost by desquamation. Bacterial colonies appear and may produce disruptive gas. Fine intracellular structures such as mitochondria are lost in a very short period if material is left unfixed.

PRESERVATION OF TISSUES

The aim of good histopathological technique is to produce microscopic preparations of tissue, usually stained, that represent as closely as possible their structure in life. Although the aim of ideal fixation is to preserve the tissue in as lifelike a manner as possible, only the very rapid freezing of small pieces of tissue in isopentane in liquid nitrogen ($-160°C$) will actually achieve this end, and then only while it is maintained in a frozen state without any loss of water. It may then be dried in a special freeze-drying apparatus and immediately embedded in wax. Sections of such blocks may be used for enzyme, carbohydrate, and lipid demonstrations but usually must be fixed before being mounted. Chemical fixation represents a compromise in that, although not all tissue constituents can be preserved in a reactive state with a single fixative, by a suitable combination of the latter (together with the use of cryostat sections) all constituents can be preserved and demonstrated.

DEFINITION OF FIXATION

This is the process by which the constituents of the cells, and therefore of the tissues, are fixed in a physical, and partly also in a chemical, state so that they will withstand subsequent treatment with various reagents with a minimum of loss, significant distortion, or decomposition. Most fixatives act by denaturing or precipitating proteins, which then form a sponge or meshwork, tending to hold the other cell constituents. Ideally, a fixative should penetrate a tissue quickly, be rapid in action, be isotonic, cause a minimum loss and minimum physical and chemical alteration of the tissue and its components, and be cheap, stable, and safe to handle. It should not bind those reactive groups upon which specific staining of the tissue elements will depend.

Effects of Fixatives on Tissues

Most fixatives produce some tissue hardening, which helps in the cutting of sections, but this hardening effect will be reinforced by the action of the alcohols used during the process of dehydration. Certain fixatives act as mordants for certain stains; e.g., after the use of mercuric fixatives the staining of the tissue constituents with many dyes is enhanced. Also, fixatives usually increase the optical differentiation of cell and tissue components, at the same time rendering the cells insensitive to hypo- and hypertonic solutions used subsequent to fixation. Since microorganisms are composed of protein and so forth, they will also be fixed (and killed), preventing putrefactive changes in the tissues and minimizing the risk of infection for those who handle them.

The Ideal Fixative

The ideal fixative would

1. Prevent autolysis and bacterial decomposition.
2. Preserve tissues in their natural state and fix all components (protein, carbohydrate, fat, etc.).
3. Make the cellular components insoluble to liquids encountered in the tissue processing.
4. Preserve tissue volume.
5. Avoid excessive hardness of fixed tissue.
6. Allow enhanced staining of tissues.
7. Be nontoxic and nonallergenic.

The fact that there are so many fixatives indicates that the ideal has not been found. We tend to use fixatives that are adequate for the end result we require. Thus we use fixatives that preserve protein substances and conserve structure in the way to which we have become accustomed but that are inadequate for lipids and carbohydrates, since these are generally of minor significance. Other fixatives are used should these latter substances, enzymes, or antigens become critical for diagnosis.

GENERAL PRINCIPLES IN HANDLING AND FIXATION OF SPECIMENS

Amount of Fixing Fluid

This should be approximately 10 to 20 times the volume of the specimen, except when osmium tetroxide is used.

Surgical Specimens

These should be placed in an adequate amount of fixative as soon as possible after removal. Bacteriological studies of surgical specimens should be encouraged. The surgeon should be encouraged to place representative portions of lymph nodes, and indeed of any other lesions, in separate, sterile, small, screw-cap bottles. These may then be subjected to immediate bacteriological study in the laboratory or kept frozen until the pathologist decides whether such study is necessary.

Autopsy Material

For reasons outlined previously it is preferable that the autopsy examination be performed as soon after death as possible. Therefore, if a delay is unavoidable, the body should be placed in the mortuary refrigerator (4°C), or arterial embalming should be carried out without delay, provided that toxicological or microbiological examinations are not indicated. Such embalming, well done, is most advantageous and gives excellent preservation. Slices of organs taken at autopsy should be thin to facilitate fixation.

ROUTINE FIXATIVES

Formaldehyde; Formalin

Commercial formaldehyde (formalin) is a saturated solution of formaldehyde (H · CHO) gas in water, approximately 40% gas by weight. For purposes of designating strengths of diluted solutions it is customary to regard the saturated solution as 100% formalin, and it will be so designated throughout this section. Thus, a mixture of 10 mL formalin with 90 mL of water or saline is known as 10% formalin. Commercial formalin often becomes turbid, especially if stored in a very cold place, because of the formation of paraformaldehyde resulting from polymerization of H · CHO. This may be removed by filtration, but almost all commercial formaldehydes contain 11 to 16% methanol, which tends to inhibit the formation of paraformaldehyde.

Traces of formic acid are normally present in commercial formaldehyde and tend to form in all formalin-containing solutions by oxidation. This acidity reduces the quality of routine staining, particularly nuclear, leaches out hemosiderin, and promotes the formation of formalin pigment; it must be guarded against by some form of buffering. This may be effected simply (though not thoroughly) by the use of formol-saline to which is added a handful of calcium carbonate, the mixture then being shaken well and stored in a jar containing a layer of marble chips. This, however, gives only approximate neutrality.

Nature of Formalin Action

The aldehyde (H · CHO) group in formalin permits many and complicated reactions with tissue components. Probably chief among these is the polymerizing action, i.e., the formation of additive compounds and complexes by development of links (methylene bridges) between protein molecules. These reactions naturally produce alterations in cell physicochemistry and will, of course, alter the reactivity of the tissues to certain histochemical stains. However, many of these changes appear to be reversible by washing in water, and in routine tissues, which are processed after only 6 to 24 hours in formalin, the changes do not progress to any great extent.

Formalin Fixation and Temperature

A block of average tissue (not fatty) up to 4 mm thick will be adequately fixed in 10 to 20 times its volume of buffered neutral formalin in about 8 hours at room temperature, and 4 hours may suffice with agitation. These times may be shortened 25 to 40% if the fixative's temperature is raised to 45°C, and although there is some loss of quality, this maneuver is currently in use.

Advantages of Formalin

Among these are the facts that formalin is cheap, easy to prepare, and relatively stable (especially if buffered), and that its use allows the subsequent application of most staining techniques without special preliminary procedures. In addition, frozen sections can be prepared with great ease from formalin-fixed material. Staining for fat can easily be carried out on tissues fixed in formalin and, indeed, some tissue enzymes can be studied after its use. It penetrates tissues reasonably well and does not cause excessive hardening or render them brittle, and natural tissue colors can be restored with no great difficulty after formalin fixation. Unless they have been in formalin for long periods, blocks do not require washing before processing. Formalin is the best fixative for the nervous system.

Disadvantages of Formalin

Handling of formalin may lead to troublesome dermatitis of the hands in some workers, and its fumes are irritating to the nostrils. It may also cause asthma in some allergic individuals. However, skin contact with it is not necessary, and its irritant effect on the nostrils may be minimized by handling tissues (gross description and block selection) in a well-ventilated area. The National Institute for Occupational Safety and Health (NIOSH) in the United States recommends that no worker be exposed to more than 1 part per million (ppm) of formaldehyde for any 30-minute period. Industrial exposure has been reported to cause a reduction in pulmonary ventilating capacity, and experimental exposure has produced nasal cancers in rats, but no excess of cancer deaths has occurred in embalmers, morticians, or manufacturers of formaldehyde, who are often subject to its fumes.

In tissues containing much blood (e.g., spleen) unbuffered formalin leads to the formation of dark-brown artifact pigment granules. These granules consist of acid formaldehyde hematin and are doubly refractile. Reagent-grade formaldehyde solutions contain 10% methanol as a preservative to retard decomposition to formic acid. Methanol has a denaturing effect on proteins, and this factor renders formalin unsuitable for the critical fixation required in electron microscopy. Pure formaldehyde, however, is suitable.

Removal of Formalin Pigment

Removal of pigment is relatively simple and is achieved by either of the following:

Kardasewitsch's Method.

1. Bring sections down to water.

2. Place the sections, for 5 minutes to 3 hours, depending on amount of pigment, in a mixture of

70% ethyl alcohol	**100 mL**
28% ammonia water	**1 or 2 mL**

3. Wash thoroughly in water.

Lillie's Method. **After bringing down to water, place the sections for 1 to 5 minutes in a mixture of**

Acetone	**50 mL**
3 vol hydrogen peroxide	**50 mL**
28% ammonia water	**1 mL**

This should be followed by washing in 70% alcohol and then in running water.

Picric Acid. **Place sections (after bringing to water) in a saturated alcoholic solution of picric acid for 5 minutes to 2 hours. Then wash for 10 to 15 minutes in running tap water.**

Routine Formalin Fixatives

Traditionally formol-saline (usually buffered) has been the most commonly used fixative in pathology.

10% Formol-Saline

Water (preferably distilled)	900 mL
Sodium chloride	8.5 g
Formalin	100 mL

For better results, however, one should use buffered neutral formalin as recommended by Lillie.

10% Buffered Neutral Formalin

Water (distilled)	900 mL
NaH_2PO_4 (anhydrous)	3.5 g
Na_2HPO_4 (anhydrous)	6.5 g
Formalin	100 mL

For the hydrated salts the quantities are:

$NaH_2PO_4 \cdot H_2O$	4.02 g
$Na_2HPO_4 \cdot 12H_2O$	16.37g/L

Storage of specimens in 10% buffered formalin is suitable for most routine purposes, but the use of 70% ethyl alcohol or 10 to 20% diethylene glycol in water is considered better because, even with buffered formalin, there is gradual loss in basophilic staining of the cytoplasm and nucleus, together with loss in reactivity of myelin to the Weigert iron hematoxylin method.

Formalin and Lipids

Formalin is largely inert toward lipids. It fixes some complex and unsaturated lipids, but neutral fats are unaltered, and phospholipids tend to diffuse slowly into the fixative. Formol-mercuric chloride is better. Calcium, cobalt, or cadmium ions help prevent phospholipid loss by forming complexes (coacervates) between phospholipids and large molecules such as proteins and polysaccharides. Chromation after use of calcium-cobalt will cause even more lipids to be retained in paraffin sections.

Formalin is a medium-speed fixative: for routine diagnostic purposes blocks of average tissue density not thicker than 4 mm are adequately fixed in 4 to 6 hours with agitation, but complete fixation requires 12 to 24 hours at room temperature. Owing to its polymerizing action, formalin tends to reduce the PAS positivity of reactive mucins.

Secondary Fixation (Postmordanting)

Some laboratories use this technique for special purposes, e.g., metachromasy, trichrome staining, and for the chromaffin reaction.

Secondary Fixation. Blocks that have been in formalin for 1 to 4 hours are placed for 4 to 6 hours in Helly's fluid, or *preferably*, for 4 to 16 hours in *formol-mercuric chloride*:

Mercuric chloride	30 g
Distilled water	900 mL
Formalin	100 mL

Note: The formaldehyde should be added just before use, because the completed formula is unstable, with the formaldehyde reducing the $HgCl_2$ to HgCl and Hg (white and gray precipitates, respectively).

Mordanting in $HgCl_2$. Alternatively, though this method is not as good as secondary fixation in formol-mercuric chloride, dewaxed and hydrated sections are mordanted for 1 hour in saturated aqueous $HgCl_2$ before staining.

Metallic Fixatives

Mercury Fixatives

Of the metallic fixatives, those containing mercury are most commonly used. The mercuric ions act chiefly by combining with the acidic (carboxyl-COOH) groups of proteins and form especially strong combinations with the sulfur (thiol) radicals.

Formulas of Mercuric Salt Fixatives

ZENKER'S

Mercuric chloride ($HgCl_2$)	50 g
Potassium dichromate	25 g
Sodium sulfate (often omitted)	10 g
Distilled water	1000 mL

Add 50 mL (5 mL/dL stock) of glacial acetic acid just before use.

After treatment with Zenker's fixative the potassium dichromate deposit should be removed by washing the tissue in running water for at least an hour (preferably overnight) before dehydration and the removal of the mercuric deposit. The tissue blocks are then placed in 70% ethanol.

SCHAUDINN'S "SUBLIMATED ALCOHOL"

Mercuric chloride	3 g
Distilled water	50 mL

Dissolve the $HgCl_2$ in the water by shaking, and then add 25 mL of absolute ethyl alcohol. This is probably the most useful fixative for making smears of loose cells on a slide, following which they are less likely to detach during staining than with any other fixative.

Fixation Times in Mercury Fixatives. In Zenker's at room temperature small blocks 2 to 4 mm thick will be fixed in 2 to 6 hours; tiny specimens, such as needle biopsies of liver or kidney, require only 30 to 60 minutes, and average-sized blocks (2½ by 1½ cm and 4 mm thick) fix in 6 to 15 hours, depending on texture.

Advantages of Mercurial Fixatives. These tend to give better staining of nuclei and connective tissues than do other fixatives; trichrome staining is particularly good. Cytoplasmic staining with acidic dyes is enhanced and nuclear chromatin is shown in fine detail. Mercurial fixatives give the best results with metachromatic staining and are the routine fixatives of choice for preservation of detail for photography.

Disadvantages of Mercurial Fixatives. These are excellent but slightly troublesome fixatives. Solutions of mercuric chloride corrode all metals except the nickel alloy Monel. The complete solution (after addition of acetic acid or formalin) deteriorates rapidly. However, with modern reagent-grade acetic acid, which is free of methanol and acetone, Zenker's formula is stable for several months. Zenker's solution causes considerable lysis of red blood cells and removes much iron from hemosiderin. Mercuric chloride causes marked shrinkage; mainly to counteract this, most formulas prescribe addition of acids. All fixatives containing $HgCl_2$ reduce the amount of demonstrable glycogen. With all mercurial fixatives, penetration beyond the first 2 to 3 mm is very slow. If the tissues are left in these fixatives for more than 1 to 2 days they become unduly hard and brittle. Cutting of frozen sections on tissues fixed in mercurial solutions is extremely difficult. Mercurial fixing solutions lead to the formation in the tissues of diffuse black granules, and these mercury deposits must be removed before staining. With small pieces of tissue this can be accomplished by adding to the initial alcohol used in dehydration enough of a saturated solution of iodine in 96% alcohol to confer upon it a rich brown color. The coloration of the tissues caused by the iodine is removed during the treatment with the absolute alcohol in the later stages of dehydration.

Large pieces of tissue are best treated in a similar manner but followed by a repetition of the process when the sections are on the slide. The idea is to remove gross mercuric chloride deposit before sectioning so as to save the knife edge; once the section has been cut, the finer precipitate that remains is easily and rapidly removed by the following method:

1. Place section in 70% alcohol to which saturated solution of iodine has been added to confer a brown color (approximately 0.5 mL of USP tincture of iodine per 100 mL of the alcohol). Leave 1 to 2 minutes to remove the mercurous chloride (HgCl) deposit:

$$2HgCl + I_2 = HgCl_2 + HgI_2$$

2. Rinse in water and place in 5% w/v sodium thiosulfate 1 to 2 minutes to remove iodine:

$$2\ Na_2S_2O_3 + I_2 = 2\ NaI + Na_2S_4O_6$$

3. Wash sections in running tap water for 2 to 5 minutes to remove the sodium thiosulfate crystals, and then stain.

Chromate Fixatives

Chromium salts in water form Cr-O-Cr complexes that have an affinity for the COOH and -OH groups of proteins, so that complexes between adjacent protein molecules are formed. This leads to disruption of the internal salt linkages of the protein, increasing the reactive basic groups and thereby enhancing acidophilia in staining.

Orth's Fluid

2.5% Potassium dichromate ($K_2Cr_2O_7$), aqueous	100 mL
Sodium sulfate (optional)	1 g
Add, just before using, Formalin solution	10 mL

Regaud's (Möller's) Fluid

3% Potassium dichromate	80 mL
Add, just before using Formalin	20 mL

Fixation of average blocks in chromate fixatives takes from 24 to 48 hours. Tissues should therefore be thin. Chromate fixed tissue must be washed for at least an hour, and preferably overnight, to avoid formation of a lower oxide. This will appear as a black precipitate in the tissues if the chromate is allowed to interact with alcohol during processing.

Advantages of Chromate Fixatives. Chromate fixatives are recommended for the demonstration of chromaffin tissue, e.g., adrenal medulla, mitochondria, Golgi apparatus, mitotic figures, colloid-containing tissues, and red blood cells. The combination of mercury, chromate, and formalin, as in Helly's fluid, gives better and faster tissue preservation than either mercuric chloride or chromate alone. Chromate-containing fixatives tend to preserve phospholipids in paraffin sections; because of oxidation (chromation) they are rendered less soluble in routine dehydrating and clearing agents.

Disadvantages of Chromate Fixatives. Chromate-formaldehyde solutions darken on standing because of acidity. Prolonged fixation in chromate solutions tends to bleach all tissue pigments, e.g., melanin, as a result of oxidation.

Glycogen preservation is usually poor; indeed, chromate-containing fixatives are generally contraindicated for carbohydrates. Because of oxidation, they reduce the intensity of the PAS reaction and also lessen the basophilia of acidic polysaccharides. However, this effect can be used to advantage in preserving PAS-reactive lipid substances; e.g., chromation of formalin-fixed tissue blocks will increase the intensity of the PAS reaction in Gaucher's and Niemann-Pick's storage cells.

PICRIC ACID FIXATIVES

In practice, only strong solutions are used. The solubility of picric acid is such that 1.17 g will just dissolve in 100 mL of distilled water at 15°C. Chemically, picric acid is 2, 4, 6-trinitrophenol, $C_6H_2\ (NO_2)_3OH$. It forms protein picrates, some of which are water-soluble until treated with alcohol. It is said to give better preservation of glycogen than any other fixing agent.

Bouin's Fluid

1.2% w/v (saturated) aqueous picric acid	75 mL
Formalin	25 mL
Glacial acetic acid	5 mL

Advantages of Bouin's Fluid. This is a good fixative for the demonstration of glycogen. It penetrates rapidly and is a good fixative for most purposes, except for work with mammalian kidney, which it fixes badly. As a result of their picking up the yellow color, small fragments of tissue are easily identified. It is very suitable for Mallory's, Heidenhain's, and Masson's aniline stains. Shrinkage is slight. Depending on the size of the block, fixation takes about 1 to 12 hours. The complete Bouin's formula is a stable solution.

Disadvantages of Bouin's Fluid. It lyses (lakes) red blood cells and reduces the amount of demonstrable ferric iron. Tissues should not be allowed to remain in the fluid longer than 12 to 24 hours (depending on their size), as they become hard and brittle and are difficult to section. Lipids are both altered and decreased. Bouin-fixed material should not be placed in water until the water-soluble picrates have been rendered insoluble by the action of two or three changes of 70% ethyl alcohol, which also removes the excess picric acid. After fixation stock tissues should be stored in 70% ethyl alcohol.

The yellow color of the sections on the slide can be removed subsequently by one of the following methods:

1. Place the section in a saturated solution of lithium carbonate in 70% ethyl alcohol for some minutes.
2. Treat the sections with ethyl alcohol followed by 5% sodium thiosulfate. Then wash in running water.

Brasil's Alcoholic Picro-Formol Fixative

The following is a modified Brasil formula:

Formalin	2040 mL
Picric acid (BDH: 50% water)	80 g
Ethanol or isopropyl alcohol	6000 mL
Trichloroacetic acid	65 g

Brasil's fixative is better and less "messy" than Bouin's and is used routinely by many workers for surgical specimens. Automated overnight schedules may employ three or four changes of Brasil's fixative, each of 1½ or 2 hours, and these are succeeded directly by absolute alcohol. The first container of fixative is discarded each day, the others are moved up, and fresh fixative is placed in the third (or fourth) container. It is one of the best routine fixatives for glycogen, but it shares some disadvantages of Bouin's.

ALCOHOLIC FIXATION

Alcohol denatures and precipitates protein, possibly by disrupting hydrogen and other bonds. Methyl alcohol, 80 to 100%, is an excellent fixative for smears, either wet or dry, but in concentrations below 80% it causes lysis of cells. Ethyl alcohol is used as a fixative for enzymes, but only Carnoy's fluid is generally used in pathological histology, and then only for specific purposes.

Disadvantages of Alcohol Fixatives

Unless used at 0°C or colder, alcohol causes severe shrinkage. It tends to harden tissues excessively and always distorts morphology. At −5 to −20°C it preserves some enzymes well, e.g., alkaline phosphatase. Although it is a good fixative for glycogen, polarization (streaming of protoplasm to one pole of the cell) is marked unless very cold temperatures (−70°C) are used. Alcohol-containing fixatives are contraindicated whenever lipids are to be studied.

Carnoy's Fixative

Absolute ethyl alcohol	60 mL
Chloroform	30 mL
Glacial acetic acid	10 mL

Advantages of Carnoy's Fluid. This is very suitable for small tissue fragments, e.g., curettings, which it fixes well in ½ to 2 hours. It also initiates dehydration and is a good fixative for glycogen; nuclear staining and carbohydrate preservation are good.

Disadvantages of Carnoy's Fluid. It lakes red blood cells and causes considerable shrinkage if left too long.

Lipids and myelin are dissolved by it. Though it is a good fixative for glycogen, it leads to "polarization" because of streaming of the glycogen granules to one pole of the cells.

Acetic Acid (CH_3COOH)

This is never used by itself, since it fixes only nucleoproteins by precipitation and causes tissues to swell, especially collagen. Because this swelling counteracts the shrinkage effect of fixing agents such as mercury salts, alcohol, and formalin, acetic acid is included in many compound fixatives. All mucins except the gastric variety are precipitated by acetic acid.

SPECIAL FACTORS AFFECTING FIXATION

Apart from the size and thickness of the piece of tissue to be fixed, certain other considerations are of importance. Thus, tissues containing, or covered by, a large amount of mucus fix slowly and poorly because the mucus prevents penetration of the fixative. Whenever possible, e.g., in the case of pseudomucinous cysts of the ovary, it is advisable to remove as much of the mucus as practical by washing with normal saline. The same applies to tissue covered by blood; organs containing very large amounts of blood, e.g, lungs, may with advantage be flushed out (by arterial cannulization) with saline before fixing. Fatty and lipomatous tissues fix slowly, and the blocks of such tissues should be thin and may require longer than average in fixative. Like all chemicophysical reactions, fixation is accelerated by agitation, and this is one of the advantages of the mechanical tissue processors. Moderate heat (37 to 56°C) will accelerate fixation, but it also hastens and accentuates autolytic changes in the deeper parts of the tissue block before the fixing agent gains access to these regions. Also, even with good fixatives, tissue damage roughly parallels the rise in temperature.

Osmotic Considerations in Fixation

An ideal fixative should not cause swelling or shrinkage of cells due to osmotic factors. In practice, few fixatives are isotonic and only with very few are the observed effects attributable to osmotic forces. In general, heavy metal fixatives and those that act mainly as protein precipitants, e.g., picric acid, cause shrinkage whatever the osmotic pressure of their solutions is. Acetic acid, 5%, although it is markedly hypertonic in relation to body fluids, leads to swelling of tissues, especially of collagen. Formaldehyde, because of its small, freely diffusible organic molecule and polymerizing action, must be used in as nearly isotonic solution as is possible; if the solution is hypotonic, swelling will result.

COMPATIBILITY AND INCOMPATIBILITY OF FIXATIVES AND STAINS

Few fixatives permit the use of all stains. One and the same fixative may act as a mordant for one group of dyes and an inhibitor for another set of stains. In the case of certain tissues and investigations the types of stains to be used must be considered when choosing the fixative. In general, however, buffered neutral formalin, Zenker's, Helly's, Bouin's, and Carnoy's fluids permit the use of a broad spectrum of staining methods. With some fixatives, e.g., Zenker's and Helly's fluids, the fixative must be thoroughly washed from the tissues before many stains may be used to best advantage. Formalin is not the best fixative for aniline dyes (trichrome stains), and prolonged formalin fixation tends to inhibit eosin. Mercurial fixatives enhance nuclear staining and cellular detail in general and are the best (apart from Bouin's) for trichrome stains. Osmic acid (OsO_4) makes counterstaining almost impossible, and the combination of chromium and osmic acid fixation depresses hematoxylin avidity (especially Ehrlich's hematoxylin). Buffered neutral formalin is the best fixative for the demonstration of iron pigments and for elastic fibers, which generally do not stain well after Zenker or chromate fixatives.

POSTCHROMATION

This is used when chromation (oxidation) is desired in tissues that have already been fixed in other fixatives, e.g., for chromaffin tissue or in Weigert's method for myelin. The tissues are placed in 2.5% potassium dichromate for 4 to 8 days.

This particular secondary fixation renders phospholipids more resistant to extraction by dehydrating and clearing agents; but chromation also acts as a mordant for subsequent staining.

SOFTENING HARD TISSUES

This is occasionally necessary, e.g., in the case of cervix, fibroids, some hyperkeratotic skin lesions, and fingernails. Lendrum's method consists of washing the tissue in running tap water overnight so as to remove the fixative. The tissue is then placed for 1 to 3 days in 4% aqueous phenol, after which it is processed in the usual manner. The use of benzene or chloroform instead of xylene will reduce hardness.

FIXATION OF TISSUES FOR ELECTRON MICROSCOPY

General Principles

Because of the high resolution obtainable with electron microscopes, it is desirable that tissues be preserved with a minimum of alteration from their state in vivo. Ideally, the nearest we can come to this is by arterial perfusion of experimental animals, e.g., with aldehyde fixatives. But even in this case, for best results, fragments of the tissues required should be removed as soon as possible after death, minced, and subjected to further fixation, e.g., in OsO_4. Absence of osmotic effects is also important, and whenever possible, isotonic media should be used and drying avoided at all costs. In the case of human tissues removed at operation, if it is not convenient to start definitive fixation immediately on removal of the tissue from the patient, drying on the way to the laboratory may be prevented by placing thin razor slices of the specimen into buffered glutaraldehyde or formalin. Subsequently, the tissue may be minced and subjected to further fixation. *Fixation for electron microscopy should be carried out at 4°C in the refrigerator.*

The commonly used fixatives are osmium tetroxide and the aldehydes, since they particularly preserve cellular structure and need only a short time to fix small fragments. The latter property is important, since there is little time then for autolysis and in a short while little extraction of cytoplasmic components is possible. Osmium tetroxide gels protein by forming bridges between molecules via SH, C, NH_2, and OH groups. With lipids OsO_4 forms monoester and diester linkages. Its virtue in electron microscopy is that it rapidly fixes tissue and also stains tissue structures. The staining results from the reduction of the fixative with deposition of gray deposit to various tissue components in proportion to their content of reactive and reducing groups. Glutaraldehyde also forms cross-linkages between tissue molecules and gives good preservation of structure, since extraction of cytoplasmic components is minimized.

Freeze-Drying

There is a method of rapidly freezing (quenching) the tissues at −150°C that forms only tiny ice crystals in the tissues, crystals that do not cause any morphological damage. The ice is removed by sublimation in a vacuum at −40° to −70°C. When dry, the material is brought to room temperature and may be either fixed and processed or embedded in wax directly and sectioned. The prepared material may be used for the demonstration of hydrolytic enzymes, for fluorescent antibody studies, autoradiography, identification of protein, and other techniques that are generally regarded now as in the field of research. The methodology avoids the chemical alteration of cellular components, denaturation of protein, destruction of enzymes, and loss of tissue constituents that occurs in the usual histological processing.

DECALCIFICATION

The cutting of thin sections by ordinary methods is impossible in the case of bone, teeth, some teratomas containing bony tissue, and also many pathological lesions that have become partly calcified, e.g., tuberculosis foci, some abscesses (especially those following injections), and arteries that are affected by calcified atheroma. Such tissue must be treated to remove the calcium and phosphate salts that are deposited in them. Almost all the methods commonly used for decalcification involve the use of acids, in which the bone salts are dissolved. All such acid solutions are injurious to the organic ground substance of the bone or other tissue, which must, therefore, be protected by adequate fixation before decalcification is begun. Fixation is best accomplished by selecting suitable blocks 2 to 4 mm thick with the aid of a fine hacksaw, jig saw, or fret saw (a high-speed band saw gives good results) and placing them in buffered neutral formalin for 2 to 4 days, or in Helly's fluid or Zenker for 15 to 24 hours. The longer time is required in formalin so that the nucleic acids will become resistant to the hydrolytic action of acids used in decalcification; chromate-containing fixatives confer this resistance in a much shorter time.

When it is desired to study only cancellous bone or its content, e.g., marrow, the process of decalcification may be expedited by cutting off the outer dense or ivory bone. This may, in most cases, be done without too great distortion before decalcification has been started, but it may be easier when the process has advanced somewhat. This discarding of the outer hard bone will protect the more delicate cancellous bone and its contained marrow, as the latter will usually be severely damaged by the time the outer hard bone has been sufficiently decalcified. The narrow zones of cellular distortion and impacted bone sawdust adjoining the saw cuts may be eliminated by cutting off a thin slice with a sharp scalpel or razor blade once decalcification has been completed. In the case of bone marrow (hemopoietic) it is most important that fixation be started as soon as possible after death and removal from the body and that it be prolonged to completion; otherwise, enzymes will continue to act and destroy many cellular details, a state that will also be brought about by excessive action of any mineral acid.

Effects of Heat, Agitation, and Vacuum

Heat will accelerate the process of demineralization, but it also promotes the destructive action of acids on matrix and, for this reason, is better avoided altogether. When heat is used in expediting decalcification, subsequent nuclear staining is considerably reduced, as are the effectiveness of trichrome and van Gieson stains, and the PAS technique may be completely vitiated. If heat is to be used at all, one should confine it to the 37°C range and remember that the time required at 37°C is nearly half that required for demineralization at room temperature. Agitation of the tissue in the acid solution has little if any accelerating effect, and the same holds for decalcifying in partial or complete vacuum, although it may have a beneficial effect in that it removes bubbles. Processes employing electrolysis will accomplish little more than to provide heat.

Hemosiderin will be removed particularly by acids or by Versene, but more hemosiderin remains after treatment with formic acid. A method to preserve hemosiderin in tissues to be decalcified is as follows:

Fix the bone and marrow in 10% formalin to which 2% yellow ammonium sulfide has been added. After fixation, decalcify with 5% formic acid (Lillie and Fullmer, 1976).

Routine Acid Techniques: General Remarks

For routine purposes only acids are recommended, viz., formic and nitric acids. Nitric acid is almost twice as fast as formic, but formic acid provides better tissue preservation and staining.

The volume of decalcifying solution used should be at least 1 oz per g of tissue and should be changed once or twice a day until decalcification is completed. Glass jars of 4 and 8 oz size suffice for most specimens. It is advantageous to arrange a gauze platform supported by a glass rod frame in the jar so that the bone block rests at, or a little below, the middle of the fluid.

Tests for Completion of Decalcification

Decalcification may be tested for in a number of ways, e.g., by touch, pliability, and resistance to fingernail, by needling, by x-ray, or by chemical testing of the decalcifying fluid. The physical methods are not recommended, because they damage the tissue. X-ray is good but not always convenient, and it cannot be used when radiopaque metallic salts such as $HgCl_2$ have been used in fixation. The chemical test is favored:

1. In a clean test tube place 5 mL of decalcifying fluid that has been in contact with the bone block for 3 to 12 hours.
2. Alkalinize to litmus paper by carefully adding strong ammonia water, shaking after each addition.
3. Add 0.5 mL saturated aqueous ammonium oxalate: mix and let stand 15 to 30 minutes (some workers use 1% sodium oxalate).

Results. If fluid remains clear, decalcification is completed. If cloudiness develops, it is owing to calcium oxalate and means that decalcification is not complete. (*Note:* if the bone is grossly underdecalcified, the fluid may contain so much calcium that a cloud of $Ca(OH)_2$ forms when strong ammonia is added. When this happens the bone obviously requires further decalcification.) The test as outlined can be used with almost all methods using acids, except Perenyi's fluid. After each chemical testing, the decalcifying fluid must be decanted and the jar rinsed well with water before new decalcifying fluid is placed in it.

Formic Acid

As purchased, the concentrated reagent consists of 90% formic acid (sp. gr. 1.2), and for purposes of calculating percentages in mixtures this is regarded as 100%. It is recommended for use in either of the following two ways:

Aqueous Formic Acid

1. Place well-fixed 2 to 5 mm thick bone blocks in:

Concentrated formic acid	5 to 25 mL
Distilled water	to 100 mL
40% Formaldehyde *(optional)*	5 mL

2. Change fluid daily until decalcification is completed (1 to 7 days for average bone blocks, depending on concentration of acid).
3. Replace fluid with 5% sodium sulfate overnight.
4. Wash for 12 to 24 hours in running tap water. (This is best done by placing the bone block in a closed metal capsule, such as is used in automatic tissue processers, in a 4 to 12 oz jar beneath tap; larger blocks are placed in jars covered by gauze or wire mesh.)
5. Dehydrate in graded alcohols, clear in chloroform or toluene, and embed in wax.

Formic Acid–Sodium Citrate

Stock citrate solution:	
Sodium citrate ($Na_3C_6H_5O_7{\cdot}2H_2O$)	100 g
Distilled water	500 mL
Stock formic acid:	
Concentrated formic acid	250 mL
Distilled water	250 mL

1. Place well-fixed bone blocks in a mixture of equal parts of the stock citrate and formic acid solutions. Change fluid daily until decalcification is completed (1 to 2 days for average blocks).
2. Wash in running water for 4 to 8 hours.
3. Dehydrate, clear in chloroform or toluene, and embed in wax.

Comments on Formic Acid Decalcification

For several reasons this has proved to be one of the most popular methods. Since it is gentler on tissues than, say, nitric acid, there is a wider latitude as regards time; also, it is safer to handle than nitric acid. It spares hemosiderin to a greater degree than do other acid decalcifying agents. Addition of citrate probably accelerates decalcification by chelating the calcium as it is liberated from the bone. Some workers place a ½-inch layer of ion-exchange resin (e.g., ammonium-sulfonated polystyrene) on the bottom of the jar. This also sequesters the liberated calcium, so that the end point of decalcification has to be checked with x-rays. Used resin is regenerated by two washings with N/10 HCl, followed by three or four washings with distilled water.

Nitric Acid

1. Fix the selected block of bone for 2 to 3 days in buffered neutral formalin.
2. Place in a mixture of 95 mL distilled water and 5 mL nitric acid (sp. gr. 1.4).
3. Change the nitric acid solution daily until bubbles cease to evolve from the tissue (1 to 3 days, depending on the size and consistency of the bone block).
4. Wash in 3 changes of 90% alcohol.
5. Dehydrate, clear in xylene or benzene, and embed in paraffin. It is important that the time in the nitric acid be kept to the absolute minimum; otherwise staining will suffer severely.

Comments on Nitric Acid Decalcification

Undoubtedly, this is the fastest decalcifier, but the end point has to be carefully watched for; otherwise, progressive tissue damage occurs and staining is severely impaired. Nitric acid undergoes spontaneous yellow discoloration owing to formation of nitrous acid; this accelerates decalcification but also stains and damages the tissues. Formation of nitrous acid may be checked temporarily by addition of 0.1% urea to the concentrated nitric acid. When decalcification is complete, the acid must be removed by three changes of 70 to 90% ethanol, since washing in watery solutions leads to excessive swelling and deterioration of tissues. When the sections are cut, the slides are brought to water and placed in 1% aqueous lithium carbonate for 1 hour, washed in water for 15 minutes, and then stained. Alternatively, the tissue may be placed in a solution of lithium carbonate overnight following its decalcification, rinsed subsequently in water, and then replaced in fixative with other tissues in the automatic processor. A particularly useful nitric acid formula is that of De Castro, especially if one wishes to use silver impregnation for nerve fibers and other tissues subsequently, although we have found it to be a good routine decalcifying agent.

De Castro's Fluid. Dissolve 20 g chloral hydrate in 250 mL distilled water; then add 250 mL of 95% ethanol, followed by 20 mL nitric acid (sp. gr. 1.41).

Versene (EDTA)

Ethylenediaminetetraacetic acid combines with calcium, forming a soluble nonionized complex (hence its use as an anticoagulant and water softener). It is used in amounts of about 2 to 4 oz per g of bone, as a 5 to 7% solution of the disodium salt buffered to pH 7.0 to 7.4 with phosphate buffer (Appendix F) or, more simply, with NaOH. The solution is changed every 2 to 4 days. Depending on the bone block, decalcification will take 4 days to 8 weeks; i.e., it is a very slow decalcifying agent. However, it does not interfere with staining, does not distort tissues with gas bubbles, and does not destroy enzymes. It is a potent chelating agent and also removes all other metals, e.g., iron, magnesium, and lead.

Greater speed may be achieved by a continuous change of EDTA solution, using a transfusion set to give a slow drip, in a closed container with an overflow. This will decalcify all but dense bone in 1 to 2 days and give excellent staining even with Wright's or Leishman's stain.

PARAFFIN SECTIONS OF ASPIRATED BONE MARROW

Bone marrow is usually obtained by aspiration with a sternal puncture needle. In all cases, as soon as smears have been made from the freshly aspirated material, whatever remains over should be placed in 50 to 100 mL of fixative.

Fixative for Aspirated Bone Marrow

Formaldehyde (40%)	200 mL
Glacial acetic acid	165 mL
Sodium sulfate	60 g
Distilled water to	1000 mL

Not infrequently sections of bone marrow will reveal conditions that may easily escape detection in examination of Romanowsky stained smears, e.g., secondary malignant deposits, Hodgkin's disease, tuberculosis, brucellosis, sarcoidosis, and occasionally isolated or small deposits of lymphocytic lymphoma or plasma cell myeloma. In addition, sections will give confirmation of such conditions as aplastic anemia, myelosclerosis, and polycythemia vera, and may help in cases of occult hemolytic anemia (iron deposits shown by hemosiderin stain).

Processing of Aspirated Fragments

1. Place the aspirated fragments in 50 to 100 mL of fixative. Mix by inversion or by figure-of-8 motion. Allow to fix for 30 to 60 minutes.
2. Pour off the bulk of the supernatant fixative and place the remainder, together with the marrow fragments, in a Petri dish on a black background.
3. With the aid of a Pasteur pipette select all the marrow fragments (white) and place in a test tube (a 17 by 55 mm flat-bottomed test tube is suitable). As soon as the fragments have settled, aspirate the remainder of the fixative with the pipette.
4. Fill the tube to within ½ cm of the top with 50% ethyl alcohol. Stopper and mix by inversion. Let stand 20 minutes; pipette off the supernatant.
5. Replace with 70% alcohol; let stand 20 minutes; pipette off the supernatant.
6. Replace with 90% alcohol for 15 minutes.
7. Replace with absolute alcohol for 15 to 20 minutes.
8. Replace with fresh absolute alcohol for 15 to 20 minutes.

Note. If the time schedule precludes taking the specimen through completely in the same day, the fragments may be left overnight in the 90% alcohol without too much harm. Alternatively, and actually better, by dou-

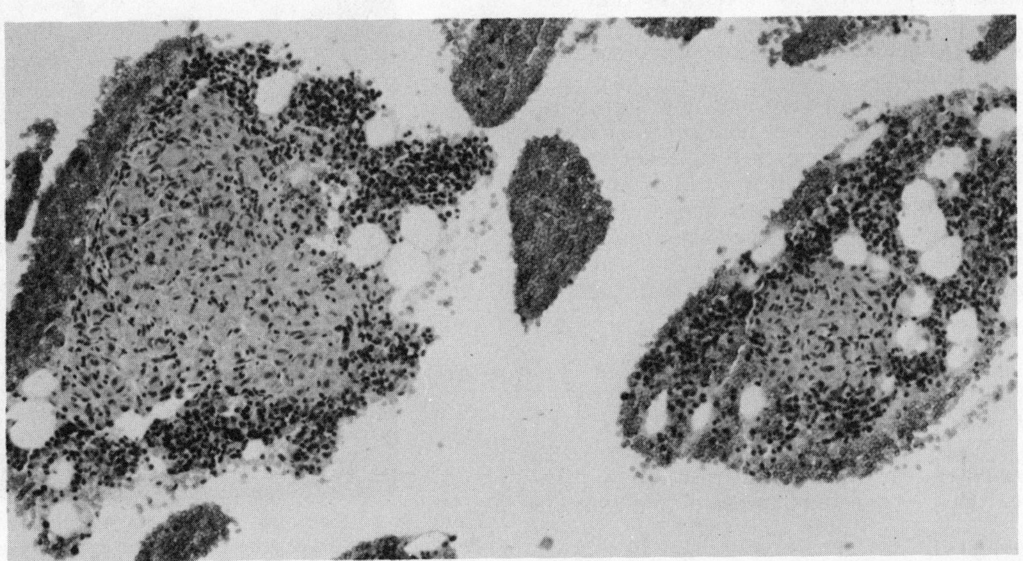

Figure 32–1 Sarcoidosis diagnosed in a section of a aspirated bone marrow. Two fragments showing the characteristic lesions. Hematoxylin-eosin × 115.

bling the number of alcohol changes in each step from steps 4 to 8, inclusive, the total time for each step can be halved.

9. Replace the alcohol with xylol or toluene. Stand 1 hour.

10. Replace with fresh xylol. Let stand 1 to 2 hours.

11. Pipette off the xylol. Place the tube in the wax oven and fill with molten wax (56°C). Let stand 1 hour in the oven.

12. Replace with fresh wax and allow to remain in the wax oven for 1 to 2 hours more.

13. Replace with fresh embedding wax; remove from the oven and allow to set.

14. Immerse for 5 minutes in cold tap water to harden.

15. Carefully break the tube, removing all fragments of glass. Mount the block ready for sectioning.

Bag Method of Processing Bone Marrow Fragments

Immediately after aspiration the marrow fragments are fixed in buffered formalin in a test tube. Subsequently, the contents of the tube are poured into a paper-fiber bag* that retains the tiny tissue fragments. The bag is then folded to fit the usual tissue processing capsule and to prevent the escape of the fragments. The specimen is then treated in the same way as other small surgical specimens.

AUTOMATED TISSUE PROCESSING

Dehydration, clearing, and preparation for embedding usually are accomplished by the use of one of the many automatic tissue processors. Most of these work on the principle of a central, rotating spindle that carries a "basket" suspended from the outer end of a horizontal radial arm. An electrically operated clockwork device rotates a notched clockface card on the circumference of which a spring-balanced "tooth" (pawl) rides. Notches are cut to suit the time schedule desired. When the tooth falls into one of the notches, a motor is activated and elevates the central spindle, which, by a fixed helical screw, automatically rotates as it rises so that the "bucket" arm is swung over the next beaker of solution. The spindle then is automatically lowered, bringing the basket into the solution.

A short, repetitive, up-and-down motion of the entire head assembly or arm, or a separate motor on the basket-carrying arm, continuously moves the basket in the solutions. This movement is most important, as it has the effect of speeding up the interchanges between chemicals and tissues. Two metal beakers or containers hold the wax, which is kept molten and at a constant temperature by thermostats within the walls of the beakers.

TIME SCHEDULES FOR DEHYDRATION, CLEARING, AND WAX IMPREGNATION

These depend on many factors, but especially on the thickness of the tissue being processed, the type of fixative used, and the degree of urgency, e.g., whether surgical or autopsy tissues are being processed.

*Templefiber Disposable Tissue Bags, Temple T Co., Philadelphia, Pa. 19115.

16-Hour Schedule

An example of a 16-hour schedule follows:
Starting time: 4 P.M.

10% Buffered neutral formalin (changed daily)	4 hr
70% Ethyl alcohol	1 hr
80% Ethyl alcohol	1 hr
95% Ethyl alcohol	1 hr
100% Ethyl alcohol	1 hr
100% Ethyl alcohol	1 hr
100% Ethyl alcohol	1 hr
Toluene or chloroform	1 hr
Toluene or chloroform	1 hr
Toluene or chloroform	1 hr
Wax, Paraplast	1 hr
Wax, Paraplast	2 hr

Rapid Schedules: Autotechnicon Ultra

The Technicon Company,* pioneer in this field for almost 40 years, has marketed a thermostatically con-

*Tarrytown, N.Y. 10591 and Montreal, Que. H4T 1P5.

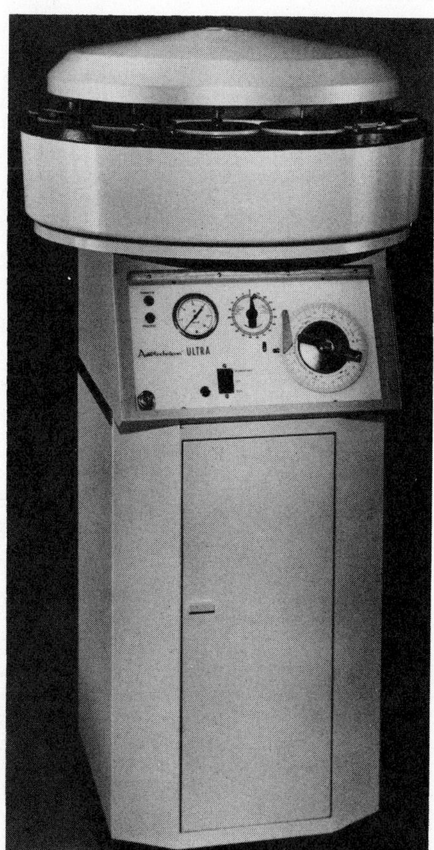

Figure 32–2 The Autotechnicon Ultra, an automated tissue processing machine that combines controlled heat and vacuum with the traditional features of automated processing. (Courtesy Technicon Instruments Corp., Tarrytown, N.Y. 10591.)

trolled vacuum Ultra model. It combines the expediting advantages of reciprocal up-and-down agitation (10/min), controlled temperature of all fluids (e.g., 45°C), and vacuum, which is automatically applied to each metal beaker shortly after the receptacle-carrying basket is immersed in that beaker and released shortly before the basket rises from the beaker. The entire cycle, from fixing to wax impregnation inclusive, for blocks up to 3 mm thick can be completed in as little as 1 to 2 hours, but any longer schedule may be selected by suitably notching a timing disc. This use of both heat and vacuum is not good for delicate tissues, but many laboratories find it satisfactory for routine use.

Maintenance of Automated Processor

The machine should be placed, if possible, in an area separate from the place in which technologists work. Failing that, it should be provided with an adequate exhaust ventilating system so that the various fumes that may periodically be released (formalin and toluene) do not unnecessarily pollute the working atmosphere. The electrical supply should be ensured, as is that of the blood bank or operating room, by an automatic switch to an emergency generator in the case of a power failure. All beakers should be kept filled, with correct strength fluids, to correct levels and checked to see that they are firmly in place. Any spillage should be cleared immediately. Plugs into paraffin wax baths are checked daily to ascertain that the current is flowing and that the wax is molten and at the correct temperature.

Selection of Tissue Blocks For Sections

This is usually done by a pathologist, who describes the gross specimen, the description being recorded by someone who also numbers the gross specimens and prepares a small tag (filing card or similar quality paper) on which the number is inscribed in pencil (not ballpoint ink, which is soluble in alcohol). This tag is placed in the perforated "button" along with the tissue block (see also the Tissue-Tek system, p. 772). Blocks may be up to 3 by 2½ cm in area but should not be more than 4 mm thick (preferably 2 to 3 mm). The technologist records the number of blocks taken, and whether or not the whole specimen (e.g., curettings) has been embedded, and secures the "snap" cover on the "button." The remainder of the gross specimen is returned to its container, which is stored for as long as there is a possibility that further material may be required. Appropriate entries are made giving all pertinent information (consecutive laboratory number, name of patient, ward and room number, doctor's name, age of patient, nature of specimen, date, number of sections taken, and clinical diagnosis).

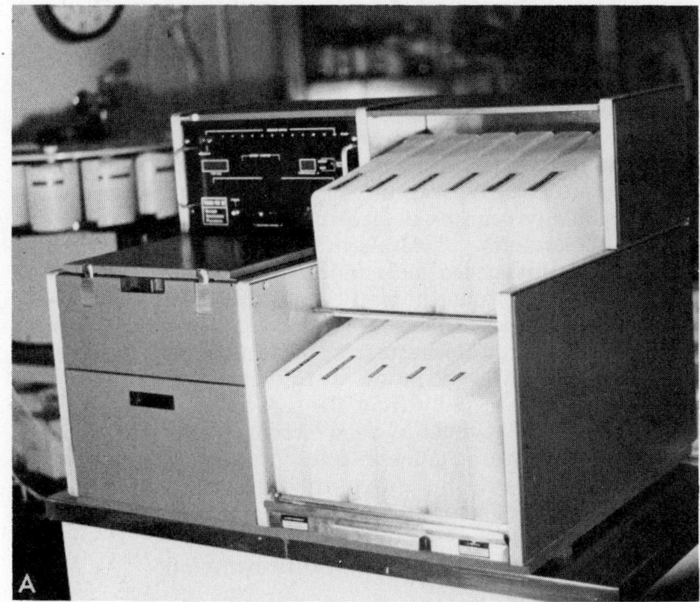

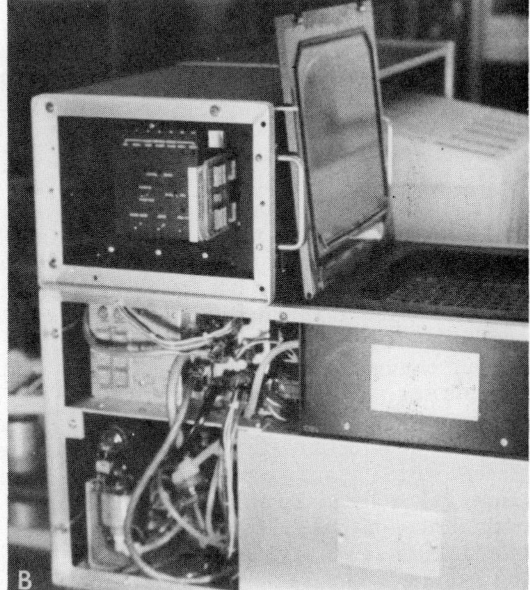

Figure 32–3 Tissue-Tek III VIP. **A,** Frontview. **B,** Side view. This tissue processor will accommodate 300 specimens in individual cassettes at one time. They are placed in the retort, which is seen opened in *B*. Fluids in the plastic containers seen in *A* are brought in turn to the retort by atuomated solid state electronic controls that are easily reached in the side of the machine *(B)*. The fluid within the retort may be programmed to be under alternating vacuum and pressure every 3 minutes. This aids speedy infiltration. Paraffin wax (2 gallons, or 7.6 L) is kept at 60°C below the retort and is used for impregnation in the last stage of the cycle. If desired, the other fluids may be maintained in the retort at 40°C to speed these stages of processing. A control panel (left upper in *A*) displays the stage of the cycle reached, the temperature of the retort and paraffin oven, and a series of warning lights that come on in case of malfunction. Besides other advantages, the machine avoids hazardous fumes, which are charcoal scrubbed before venting. To the left of the Tissue-Tek machine in *A,* a more common type of tissue processing machine employing a central spindle and a basket of tissues that enter beakers of processing fluids and wax is seen. (Tissue-Tek, Miles Laboratories, Naperville, Ill. 60540; distributed in Canada by Canlab, Toronto, Ont. M8Z 2H4.)

DEHYDRATION

Tissues contain large amounts of water, both intracellular and extracellular. This water must be removed so that it may be replaced by wax. This process of water removal is called dehydration. Naturally, it must be carried out by the use of some reagent that mixes with and has a certain affinity for water so that it may penetrate easily between the tissue cells. The best agent is undoubtedly ethyl alcohol, which has the advantage of not being poisonous. Dehydration is best accomplished by the use of graded alcohols, beginning with 70%. Transfer of tissue directly from formalin to higher grades of alcohol, e.g., 85 or 95%, is risky, since it is liable to lead to distortion of the tissues. In the case of delicate tissues, e.g., brain, embryos, and insects, dehydration should be even more gradual, beginning with 50% alcohol. If good-grade absolute ethyl alcohol is not easily available (it should be at least 99.7% pure, and freedom from water should be checked by adding a small amount of dried, powdered, white copper sulfate: if water is present the copper sulfate will again become tinged with blue), isopropyl alcohol should be used.

Acetone may be used. Acetone is a good dehydrant and is cheap but, unfortunately, very volatile and flammable (though not much more so than alcohol). It hardens tissues more than ethanol does, and a much greater volume of it is necessary than is required with ethanol. Four to six changes of acetone should be used. In the case of both alcohol and acetone, about twice each week (depending on the load of tissues going through) the jars should be "moved down," i.e., the first (70% alcohol) should be discarded, the second jar becoming first, and so forth, and fresh 100% alcohol or acetone should be placed in the last beaker. Whatever agent is used, its amount in each stage should not be less than 10 times the volume of tissue to be dehydrated.

Other substances that may be used as dehydrants are methyl alcohol, isopropyl alcohol, ethylene glycol monoethyl ether (cellosolve), and dioxane (diethylene dioxide). Of these, dioxane is remarkable in that it is miscible with water, alcohol, xylol, balsam, and paraffin wax. From many fixatives (except chromate) it is possible to take the tissue directly into dioxane (three or four changes of dioxane), then into a mixture of dioxane and wax, and then into pure wax. The dioxane can be recovered by removing the water with calcium chloride or quicklime (CaO). Tissues that have been treated with a fixative containing a chromate must be thoroughly washed in running water before treatment with alcohol or dioxane to remove the chromate. After mercurial fixatives, iodine crystals should be added to the dioxane to remove the mercurial deposit. However, dioxane is a dangerous substance with little warning odor and a cumulative toxic action, and it is not recommended for routine use. Isopropyl alcohol does not harden or shrink tissues as much as ethanol does, and it may be less expensive if tax has to be paid on the latter. A few clearing agents also act partially as dehydrants, e.g., aniline oil can follow 70% alcohol, cedar oil can follow 95% alcohol, and oil of bergamot can follow 90% alcohol.

Dehydration is also essential before stained sections can be mounted.

CLEARING (Dealcoholization)

This has to be accomplished so that the alcohol in the tissues is replaced by a fluid that will dissolve the wax with which the tissue must be impregnated. Among the paraffin wax solvents used are benzene, xylene, toluene, petroleum ether, chloroform, carbon bisulfide, cedar oil, carbon tetrachloride, and aniline oil. Other clearing agents are clove oil, oil of bergamot, terpineol, phenol in alcohol, creosote, carbolxylol, and dioxane. The word *clearing* is used because, in addition to removing alcohol, many of these substances have the property of making tissues transparent. They effect this by virtue of their high index of refraction and the resultant optical changes when the clearing agents penetrate between the highly refractile tissue elements; i.e., the refractive index of clearing agents is approximately equal to that of the tissues. However, not all dealcoholization agents can act as clearing agents, and vice versa. Good clearing agents should remove alcohol quickly and clear quickly without overhardening and should not dissolve out aniline dyes or evaporate too quickly in the wax baths. They should be used in amounts not less than 10 times the volume of tissue.

Xylene (Xylol). This is an excellent and true "clearing" agent but it tends to make tissues excessively hard and brittle, and tissues should never be left in it longer than 3 hours; otherwise, section cutting is apt to be difficult. When dehydration is not complete, the xylene becomes milky when the tissue or section is added to it. Xylene is unsuitable for brain and lymph nodes, as it makes them far too brittle. They are best cleared in chloroform. Xylene is cheap and can be used with celloidin sections but tends to cause excessive shrinkage of tissues.

Toluene (Toluol). In general properties toluene is similar to xylene but is preferable because it does not harden tissues nearly so much. It is somewhat slower than xylene or benzene in clearing. Its fumes may be toxic.

Chloroform. Chloroform is excellent for nervous tissue, lymph nodes, and embryos, as it causes little shrinkage and does not harden tissues excessively. It is probably the most widely used clearing agent, is one of the best for large blocks, and is not flammable. With average caution and ventilation its toxicity is not a factor. It evaporates rapidly from the wax bath. It is relatively expensive. It must be used in tightly closed containers, since it absorbs much moisture from the atmosphere.

Histoclear.* Recently introduced, this nontoxic derivative of food-grade materials has much promise.

Applications of Clearing in Histopathology

1. For dealcoholization of tissues preparatory to wax impregnation as already outlined.
2. For dealcoholization of stained sections before mounting in Permount, Clarite, Canada balsam, etc.
3. For the purpose of making tissues, embryos, and parasites transparent so that their internal structure is demonstrable to the naked eye. This is done by impregnating them with a clearing agent whose refractive index is close to that of the tissues themselves. For this

*National Diagnostics, South Somerville, N. J. 08878; Diamed, Mississauga, Ont. L4X 2E6.

purpose oil of wintergreen (methyl salicylate) and xylene are used, oil of wintergreen being the slower and better of the two for this purpose.

Tissue Factors in Clearing

Chloroform gives the widest latitude and is the best of the traditional clearing agents for routine use; it is also best for nervous tissue, lymph nodes, granulation tissue, and fetal and other delicate, highly cellular specimens, all of which tend to become distorted and to break up on sectioning if cleared in xylene, toluene, or benzene.

IMPREGNATION AND EMBEDDING

This process involves the impregnation of the tissues with a medium that will fill all natural cavities, spaces, and interstices of the tissues, even the spaces within the constituent cells, and that will set to a sufficiently firm consistency to allow the cutting of suitably thin sections without undue distortion and without alteration of the spatial relationships of the tissue and cellular elements. An additional physical advantage in the handling of small specimens, and indeed of all specimens, is provided by surrounding the specimen with a mass or block of embedding material, thus allowing the specimen to be handled and fixed to the microtome block without damage to the actual tissue. In histology two methods of embedding are used: paraffin wax embedding and celloidin (collodion) embedding. Of these, the paraffin wax method is the simpler, more commonly used, and by far the better for routine use. The celloidin method is suitable for specimens containing large cavities or hollow spaces which tend to collapse, e.g., eyes, and for larger embryos, but it is slow and tedious and does not allow serial sections to be obtained with any ease or certainty; also, sections cannot be cut as thin as they can with paraffin wax embedding. However, celloidin causes much less shrinkage and distortion than paraffin wax, which shrinks about 10% on cooling.

Volume. Generally speaking, the volume of the impregnating medium should be at least 25 times the volume of tissue.

Paraffin Wax Embedding

Tissues, having been completely dehydrated and cleared, are impregnated with paraffin wax or Paraplast by immersion in a succession of molten wax baths; this is usually achieved with agitation on an automatic tissue processor (e.g., Autotechnicon). Following impregnation, tissues are embedded in a wax block that enables them to be cut into thin sections (2 to 8 microns thick) on a microtome.

Generally speaking, blood and markedly congested tissues, muscle, and fibrous connective tissue tend to become excessively hard if left more than 3 hours in wax. On the other hand, brain, skin, dense bone, and blocks from female breasts having a large amount of retained secretions in dilated ducts require longer times in wax. This is impractical in routine work involving bulk processing but may be circumvented by selecting from such tissues blocks that are not thicker than 3 mm and ensuring that these are thoroughly fixed before processing.

Paraffin waxes are hydrocarbons, and they are obtainable in a variety of melting point ranges.

Care and Selection of Waxes

At one time it was thought that waxes of differing melting points (MPs) should be used, depending upon the prevailing temperature of the locale of the laboratory; this is not true. If the temperature in the laboratory is high, then blocks may be cooled in the refrigerator before cutting and further cooled with ice blocks during cutting; a low temperature in the laboratory will be an aid to cutting; therefore an MP of 56°C will be found adequate for use anywhere. In the past, various admixtures, e.g., paraffin wax plus 10 to 20% beeswax, have been used to give extra hardness in very warm environments. A mixture of one part paraffin wax (MP 52°C) and one part ceresin (MP about 72°C) (made by melting and blending in a container placed in heated water and then filtering) gives excellent results and a firm embedding medium. Ceresin also has the advantage of changing the physical structure of the wax to a microcrystalline one. The type of microtome has some bearing on the type of wax chosen; for fixed-knife microtomes a relatively hard wax is desirable, and the heavier knives take a harder wax than the lighter ones. Many authors say that mixtures of waxes of different melting points give better results than a single wax. The need for such mixtures has been largely obviated by the introduction of Paraplast. Paraffin wax does not deteriorate with age; indeed, an older wax shows less tendency to crystallize during setting.

Substitutes for Paraffin Wax

*Paraplast**

This mixture of highly purified paraffin wax and several synthetic plastic polymers is a distinct advance in tissue embedding. Its MP is 56 to 57°C. Regardless of the rate of setting, the blocks it gives are more uniform than those obtained with any other medium. There is no need for rapid cooling or embedding; indeed, sections may be cut without cooling the block face, though we find the ice cube still advantageous. With Paraplast, ribbon sectioning is easy, and it does not tend to crack like other paraffin wax substitutes. It is more resilient than paraffin wax and permits large blocks and dense bone blocks to be cut with relative ease, thus avoiding tedious double embedding. Naturally, when employed it must be used in all phases, i.e., both impregnation baths and embedding.

Embeddol.† This largely synthetic wax substitute is similar to Paraplast and is thought by some to be as good. Its melting range is 56 to 58°C. Bioloid is another semisynthetic wax that is used for embedding eyes.

Carbowax

Higher alcohols, e.g., those with 12 or more carbon atoms, are solid at ordinary room temperatures. Those with 18 to 22 (approximately) carbon atoms in their molecules have physical characteristics that are suitable for tissue embedding. The polyethylene glycols (Carbowax) are used for this purpose. In this connection,

*Sherwood Medical Industries Inc., St. Louis, Mo. 63103.
†Hartman-Leddon Co., Inc., Philadelphia, Pa. 19142.

however, certain peculiarities of Carbowax must be borne in mind. It is soluble in and miscible with water, so that embedding may be done directly from the watery fixation phase, i.e., without dehydration and clearing. For routine tissues, four changes of Carbowax (70%, 90%, and two times in 100%) at 56°C are used, the length of time in each being, respectively, 30 minutes, 45 minutes, and 1 hour (with agitation). The specimens are then blocked out in fresh Carbowax at 50°C, and blocks are immediately and rapidly cooled in the refrigerator. (Note: The blocks must not be allowed to come into contact with water or ice, since the Carbowax is very hygroscopic. For the same reason, blocks and unstained sections must be stored in dry, airtight containers coated with paraffin wax in a cool atmosphere, or in a desiccator.) Difficulty may be experienced in obtaining good sections because of the tendency of the Carbowax to crumble, although this is less marked with some of the softer grades. Because of the water-soluble properties of Carbowax, sections cannot be floated out on water; they must be floated out in one or other of the following solutions:

PEARSE

Diethylene glycol	40 parts
Distilled water	50 parts
Strong (40%) formaldehyde	10 parts

BLANK AND MCCARTHY. A mixture of equal parts of 0.02% gelatin and 0.02% potassium dichromate, boiled for 5 minutes in full daylight, and then cooled and filtered.

Preferably, the sections should be mounted on slides coated with the following glycerin-gelatin mixture (Pearse):

Granular gelatin	10 g
Distilled water	60 mL
Glycerin	50 mL
Phenol	1 g

Advantages of Carbowax

1. It eliminates dehydration and clearing.
2. Because of this, it does not remove such substances as lipids and neutral fats, thus allowing these substances to be demonstrated in thin sections.
3. The processing time is reduced.
4. The technique is good for many enzyme histochemical studies.
5. It reduces shrinkage and distortion.

Precaution Against Overheating. If Carbowax is overheated, various polymers of higher molecular weight are formed, and these tend to make the blocks more "crumbly" in section cutting.

Resin-Paraffin Additives

A number of resins have been introduced in recent years that increase the hardness of wax media and facilitate the cutting of thinner sections. A number of these resins are available commercially, among which the author has some experience with Piccolyte S 115.* This is used in the following formula for embedding after infiltration by wax in automatic processing:

Paraplast	2200 g
Piccolyte	300 g

The Paraplast is melted, and small amounts of Piccolyte are added until the requisite amount is dissolved. When resin-paraffin sections are floated on the water bath, the surface tension must be reduced by the addition of 3 or 4 drops of liquid soap, and the temperature must be kept to 45°C. Sections may be cut as thin as 2 μm, and sections of eyes and bone are obtained with fewer crushing artifacts.

BLOCKING OUT MOLDS (SHAPES, CUPS)

These may be of many types:

1. Leuckhart's embedding irons. These consist of two L-shaped pieces of heavy brass or similar metal, a base being formed by a piece of ⅛ inch thick copper or brass, about 3 by 2 inches square, or a piece of plate glass. The L-shaped sides may be purchased in pairs of various sizes. They have certain advantages—they give even blocks with parallel sides, they provide fairly rapid initial setting of the wax, and they are adjustable to give a wide variety of block sizes. They are, however, somewhat cumbersome and too slow for a busy laboratory.
2. Trays or cups made of thin or stout paper are sometimes used, but waxed paper cups are more suitable.
3. Tissue-Tek system.* This convenient system comprises stainless steel base molds in which the tissue block is embedded. A plastic mold is then placed on top and filled with wax; it is left in place and fits the chuck of the microtome. The metal base molds are precoated with a release compound in alcoholic solution so that the wax does not adhere to them. The Mark II Tissue-Tek system employs the same basic principle as that just described, and offers additional advantages. White plastic cassettes (2.5 × 4, sloping to 3 cm at top, and 5 mm deep), with detachable, perforated stainless steel hinge-and-snap-on lids, are used to hold the tissue specimen throughout fixation, dehydration, clearing, and wax impregnation. The number of the specimen is written on the one sloping side of the cassette with a graphite pencil. After processing, the tissue is embedded in one of five sizes of stainless steel molds (7 × 7; 15 × 15; 24 × 24; 30 × 24; and 37 × 24 mm—all 5 mm deep). While the embedding wax filling the mold is still molten, the base of the cassette used in processing the tissue block in question is placed on the mold, perforated bottom-side down, and filled with wax. The assembly is then cooled on a refrigerated plate. For sectioning, the metal mold is removed and the block is mounted by gripping the plastic cassette in the jaws of the microtome clamp. The Mark II uses about one-third less wax than the Mark I system, and the blocks occupy much less storage space.
4. Very convenient are the Peel-A-Way† disposable thin plastic embedding molds, which come in three sizes, 22 by 22 mm, 22 by 30 mm, and 22 by 40 mm; small

*Hercules Chemical Co., Wilmington, Del. 19899; Charles Tennant and Co., Weston, Ont. M9M 2G8.

*Lab-Tek Products, Naperville, Ill. 60540.

†Peel-A-Way Scientific, South El Monte, Calif. 91733.

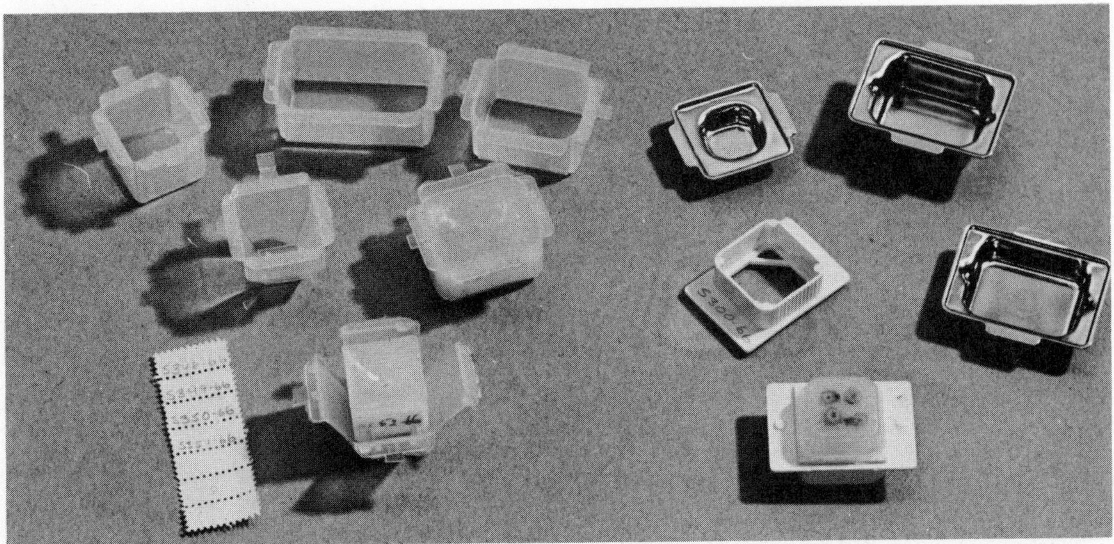

Figure 32–4 Two widely used blocking out systems: on the left, Peel-A-Way molds and strip labels; on the right, Tissue-Tek molds (Mark I).

number tabs (in pads of 50 perforated sheets, 200 tabs per sheet) are embedded in the still molten wax, block number facing out against the transparent plastic. As the name implies, once the wax has solidified, the plastic walls are simply peeled off one at a time, giving perfect blocks requiring no trimming. Also, they may be placed directly in the chuck of the microtome.

5. TIMS tissue processing and embedding system.* This complete system offers many advantages. The molded plastic capsules or "buttons" come in two sizes (1 × 1 inch and 1 × 1½ inch), each in two bottom depths (⅛ inch and ¼ inch). Each consists of three pieces: a perforated bottom, a frame center piece, and a perforated lid, all three snapping together to form a capsule in which the tissue block may be fixed, dehydrated, cleared, and embedded, the identifying number being written on the center frame. When wax impregnation has been completed, the capsules are drained; slight cooling seals the perforations in the floor of the bottom piece; the lid is removed and the tissue is embedded by adding fresh wax to the still united bottom and center frame mold. When cooled and ready for cutting the assembly is mounted so that the microtome clamp or chuck grips the center frame piece. The bottom is then removed and the block is ready for sectioning. When the sections have been cut the bottom is replaced so that the block surface is protected in storage.

PROCEDURE. The wax used for embedding into blocks must be of high grade (as indeed should all of the wax). The wax is kept molten in a wax oven kept at 2°C higher than the melting point of the wax used. The final wax beaker on the automatic tissue processing machine is moved to the sit-down work bench, where it may be plugged into an electrical outlet so that the wax is kept molten. The small perforated metal buttons containing the tissues are "fished out" of the beaker one at a time. The button is opened, the number is noted, and a suitable mold is chosen and marked with the block number (or a number tab is prepared). The mold is then filled with wax to within a few mm of its top, the tissue is picked out of its metal button by a pair of blunt forceps that have been slightly heated in a Bunsen burner flame, and the tissue is placed in the mold of molten wax. The side of the tissue from which it is desired to take sections is placed face down, and all other tissues must be carefully oriented so that the plane of sectioning will be correct; e.g., walls of cysts must be embedded edge down and biopsies of skin must be embedded so that the plane of the skin surface is vertical to the bottom of the mold. It is often necessary to press down the tissue specimen in the mold for a few seconds until it is held by the cooling wax; also it will be found necessary to flame the forceps periodically to prevent wax and tissue from adhering to its points. When the tissue blocks have been thus embedded, and as soon as the wax has become partly solid, the cups should be placed in a basin of cold water (10 to 18°C) or in the refrigerator to cool. This method of cooling lessens the tendency of some waxes to crystallize when allowed to set at room temperature and gives blocks of uniform, smooth, and solid consistency.

Wax Dispensers. These are a great convenience in the busy laboratory. The market offers a variety.

*Lab-Line Instruments Inc., Melrose Park, Ill. 60160.

TRIMMING OF BLOCKS

When the blocks have hardened in the cold water they are removed, the number is noted, and the mold is removed. If necessary, excess wax is cut off (in thin slices to prevent the block from cracking), so that the block forms a four-sided prism or truncated pyramid, the opposite sides being parallel (this is most important if serial sections are desired). At least 2 mm of wax should surround the tissue block. The small paper tag bearing the tissue number may then be affixed to the block with the aid of a hot spatula, or, if metal block holders are not used, a suitable fiber or wooden block may be selected and the number written on its side with a grease pencil. To attach the block to the fiber or wooden block holder, heat a flat spatula (1 to 2 inches wide blade) in a Bunsen flame; place the bottom of the

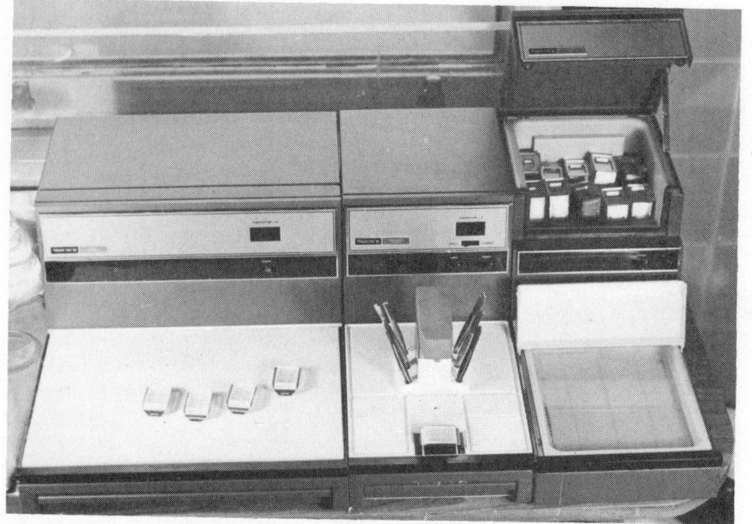

Figure 32–5 Tissue-Tek III Embedding Console System. The system has three modules under electronic control. On the right, the thermal console stores and warms (50° to 70°C) base molds in the back and holds specimens in cassettes awaiting paraffin embedding in the heated front chamber. Centrally, there is a 2-liter paraffin chamber that dispenses paraffin into the molds under control of a hand or foot switch. A "cold spot," also in this module (at 15°C), will solidify the paraffin when the tissue is sufficiently well oriented. To the left is a refrigerated plate, kept at -5°C, on which the embedded specimens are kept cool until sectioned. (Tissue-Tek, Miles Laboratories, Naperville, Ill. 60540; distributed in Canada by Canlab, Toronto, Ont. M8Z 2H4.)

wax block on the spatula and, as soon as the bottom of the wax block is molten, slide it onto the serrated surface of the fiber block so that the sides of the block are parallel to those of the fiber or wooden block, press the wax block down firmly, and allow to harden.

Cleaning of Tissue Buttons

Excess wax may be flamed off, and the buttons, when cool, immersed in a beaker of used xylene, where they may remain until required again. They are thoroughly dried before use.

VACUUM EMBEDDING

Vacuum embedding or, more accurately, embedding under reduced pressure, is of use for certain purposes, e.g.:

1. Lung or other tissue that contains much air.
2. Dense pieces of tissue, e.g., skin, and embryos, and certain other tissues, e.g., blood clot and spleen, which tend to become excessively hard in routine processing.
3. Any work in which prolonged heat is to be avoided, e.g., for certain silver impregnation methods and enzyme studies.
4. When time is of importance.

Advantages

1. The embedding time is approximately one-third to one-half that of the routine wax embedding method.
2. Any air in the tissue is extracted.
3 Clearing agents are rapidly eliminated.

Disadvantages

1. Embedding requires the care and personal supervision of the technologist as compared to the now widely used automatic tissue processor. However, the Technicon Ultra and the Tissue-Tek III V.I.P. incorporate automatic vacuum.
2. Care must be taken when dealing with pieces of lung by this method, as too rapid evacuation of air is liable to rupture the lung alveoli, which, when examined microscopically, may then simulate pulmonary emphysema.

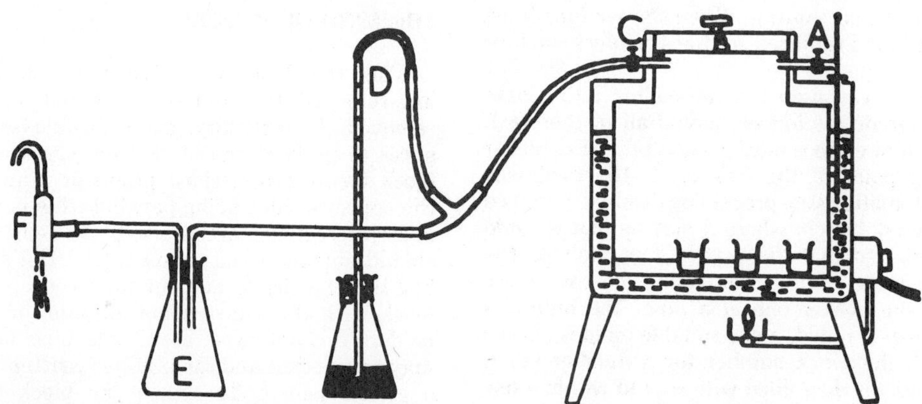

Figure 32–6 Vacuum embedding. *A*, Air inlet; *C*, exhaust outlet; *D*, mercury manometer; *E*, trap; *F*, water vacuum pump.

Apparatus

The apparatus required consists of a thermostatically controlled vacuum embedding bath, of which there are two main types, gas and electric, both of which work on the same principle. The door or lid of the bath must be fitted with a well-fitting rubber washer and, when evacuated by either a mechanical or water pump, must be able to maintain a vacuum. The degree of vacuum is controlled by the use of a gauge on the electric model or a mercury manometer on the older gas model. There should be a trap between the water evacuation pump and the manometer to prevent a backflow of water directly into the oven should the water supply be inadvertently turned off before the exhaust tap on the oven has been closed.

Procedure (for Use with Either the Gas or Electric Model)

Close the door or lid and exert slight pressure on it during the initial part of the evacuation. Close the air intake valve, open the exhaust valve, and turn on the evacuation pump.

Slowly reduce the pressure until a reduction of 400 to 500 mm of mercury is obtained.

Close the exhaust valve and turn off the pump.

To *admit air,* slowly open the air intake valve until the pressure within the oven equals that of the atmosphere.

For larger specimens and blocks this process has to be repeated two or three times, with the wax changed on each occasion and the specimen left in the wax under "vacuum" for 30 to 45 minutes each time.

SECTION CUTTING

Microtomes

These are machines or instruments designed for the accurate cutting of thin slices (sections) of tissue. Depending on the type of work, the nature of the tissue preparation and embedding, and other factors, many types of microtomes are used, certain types being best adapted for special work. Generally, there are five classes of microtomes: (1) sliding, (2) rotary, (3) rocker, (4) freezing, and (5) ultrathin section microtomes for electron microscopy work. These may be further subdivided according to whether the knives move or are rigidly fixed or whether the plane of cutting is vertical or horizontal.

Rotary. This was invented by Minot in 1885–1886 and independently by Pfeiffer (a mechanic at Johns Hopkins) in 1886. The rotary microtome is probably the most popular microtome in the North American continent—a fact that is sufficient testimony to its merit. In the rotary microtome, only a relatively small length of knife is available for use, and the knife is dangerously placed (blade up); also, it is complex in design and construction, and this complexity leads to high initial cost. It is not suitable for cutting large blocks as is the sliding microtome, nor for celloidin sections, but is more convenient for cutting serial sections and for large numbers of routine blocks.

Freezing. See p. 781.

Microtome Knives

Today most knives used in section cutting are wedge-shaped. The sides of the wedge knives are inclined at an angle of approximately 15 degrees, and the surfaces of these are highly polished so that sections will not adhere to them but will move on the surface, thus minimizing folding, distortion, and sticking, and facilitating good ribbon formation. The actual cutting part of the knife forms a very small area, the sides of which (cutting facets) are more acutely inclined toward each other than the sides of the knife proper; the angle formed between the cutting facets where they meet at the cutting edge is known as the "bevel angle," and is normally about 27 to 32 degrees. The angle of these facets is kept constant for each knife by the provision of a slide-on back for use on each knife during the processes of honing and stropping. Each knife and its back should be marked with corresponding numbers and the back of

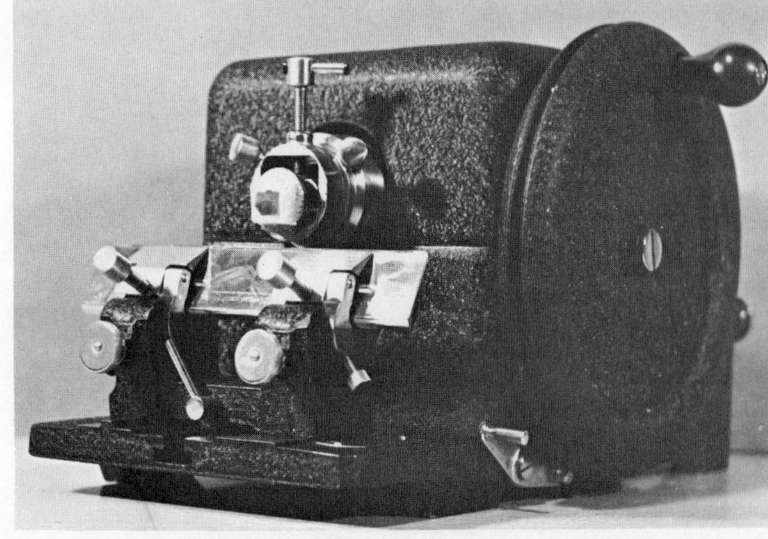

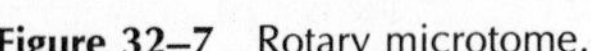
Figure 32–7 Rotary microtome.

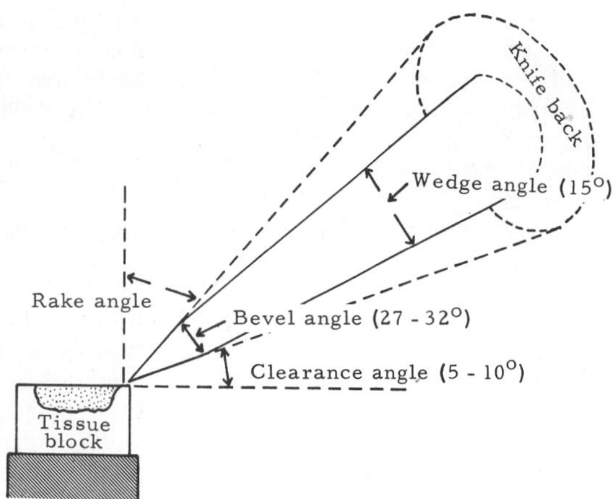

Figure 32–8 Setting the microtome knife.

one should never be used on another. Care should be taken that the back is put on evenly and symmetrically, otherwise the cutting facets will be unequal; normally, each should be 0.1 to 0.6 mm. Theoretically, facets of unequal length or depth are an advantage, but in practice this is not desirable, because the cant (slope or inclination) of the knife must then be adapted to whichever facet is presented to the block. Knives must be inclined relative to the cutting plane so that there is 5 to 10 degrees clearance between the cutting facet presenting to the block and the surface of the block. If there is not such clearance the cutting facet will wedge or compress the block as the latter slides under the knife; in this manner, no section may be obtained at all for two or three strokes; then the block suddenly expands and a very thick section is obtained.

Missed sections or alternately thin and thick sections are most commonly the result of neglecting to allow a proper angle or clearance between the block surface and the cutting facet. Normally (always in rotary microtomes), the plane (axis) of the knife edge is at right angles to the plane of cutting (line of movement of the block). For most tissues this is satisfactory; however, for large tissues, for hard tissue blocks, and for celloidin work it is advantageous to incline the axis of the knife edge so that it is oblique (30 to 45 degrees); this gives a slicing cut with less wedging.

CUTTING AND THE CUTTING EDGE

The actual mechanism by which sections are cut is not fully understood. However, it appears that the wax and wax-impregnated tissue in the block are compressed in front of the cutting edge, which then "wedges" off the section by a combination of tearing and crushing at submicroscopic levels. Therefore, the cutting edge must be thinner than the material (section) to be cut. Actually, the cutting edge is not a true edge in the theoretical sense; it is, in fact, a tiny part of the circumference of a minute circle of radius 0.1 to 0.35 μm. A good cutting edge demands that the knife be made of good quality steel; if too soft, it does not maintain the edge; if too highly tempered (hard), it is likely to "nick" against hard objects or even on honing. A good edge should cut good sections from a good paraffin wax block at 2 to 3μm thickness, and such an edge will show no serrations when examined under the microscope at × 100 magnifications. It will also comply with von Mohl's criterion; i.e., with a strong nearby source of light the cutting edge will show only a slight reflection as a very narrow, continuous straight line. Such an edge will split a hair that is drawn across it or will cut the hairs of the back of the hand against only their own resistance. However, hair cutting is not recommended, as it may damage the edge. The final test of sharpness is, as already stated, the ability to obtain good quality sections at 4 μm thickness from good quality blocks.

SHARPENING OF MICROTOME KNIVES

The degree of sharpness is proportional to the fineness of the abrasive used in sharpening. The final sharpening materials used must have a grain size smaller than the permissible serrations remaining in the edge. Sharpening may be carried out either by hand or by machine.

Hand Sharpening

This may be done in one of two ways: (1) by hones, (2) by plate glass and abrasives. A hone is a natural stone or hard grinding surface for sharpening a knife or other cutting tools. Good-quality hones are expensive, but only the best quality should be used. The finer the grain in a hone, the harder the hone. Carborundum hones are available in a wide variety of fineness. Arkansas stone is a stone of medium fineness, whereas the yellow Belgian and Belgian black vein (blue-green) are the finest available (in that order). It is convenient to purchase a combination hone, e.g., Belgian yellow and black vein mounted back to back, with a surface size 3 to 4 by 12 to 14 inches. Hones are also called oilstones because oil is commonly used as a lubricant. Many oils may be used; a light machine oil, e.g., 3-in-1, is probably best, although a neutral soap solution is just as good. Liquid paraffin (mineral oil), vegetable oils, and xylene may be used, but xylene tends to evaporate too rapidly, and natural oils become messy.

Procedure. The hone is first wiped clean with a soft cloth; occasionally, it should be wiped with a soft cloth moistened in xylene so as to remove loose particles of stone and metal. The hone is then covered with a thin film of

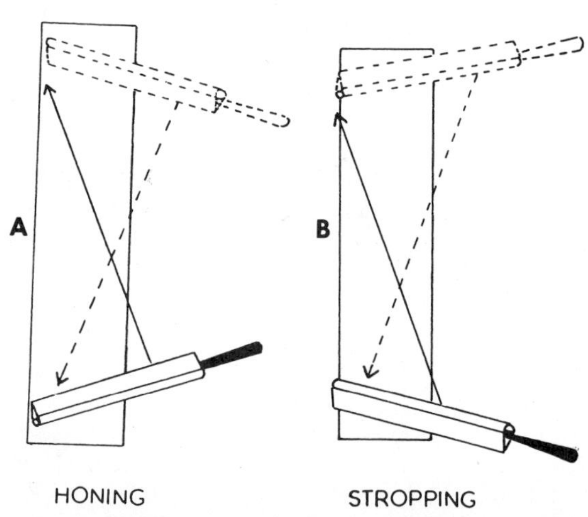

Figure 32–9 *A*, Honing. *B*, Stropping.

lubricant; the knife is fitted with its own back and laid obliquely on the stone, edge forward. Gentle, even pressure is made on the knife with the thumbs or forefingers, and the knife is drawn obliquely forward on the stone in an easy, steady motion, "heel" (handle end) first, so that when the other end of the stone is reached the "toe" is on the stone. The knife is then rotated, *on* its back, so that the other cutting facet rests on the stone, and the knife is drawn toward the operator, again from heel to toe. Such sequence forms a double stroke, and about 20 to 30 such strokes on the medium-grain stone and an equal number on the fine-grain stone usually suffice. The knife edge is then wiped clean with a rag moistened in xylene. The edge may then be inspected under the microscope, but the experienced honer will know at a glance as well as by the feel of the knife on the hone whether it is ready for stropping. Occasional small nicks in the knife edge may be left, as they will gradually be honed out, and the knife can be set in the microtome so that the nicks can be avoided. Large nicks demand regrinding of the edge, and this is best done at the factory. Excessive honing is harmful, as is excessive pressure; both may turn the edge or make the edge round. Too little pressure on the blade will lead to inadequate honing, and a jerky motion may lead to nicking. The knife edge must be pressed against the hone surface with a continuous, even, gentle pressure.

Plate Glass Honing

This is excellent. A piece of plate glass 1/4 to 3/8 inch thick, about 14 inches long and 1 to 2 inches wider than the length of the knife blade is used. Abrasive powder is used in conjunction with this; for grinding and removing nicks, using Corundum 303 or 304. This should be followed by levigated alumina or by Corundum 305s, both of which are sufficient for ordinary sharpening. Diamantine is used for the final polishing. The abrasives are made up as suspensions in water, the plate glass being thoroughly cleaned after each one. Since the plate glass is wider than the length of the knife blade, the latter does not have to be held obliquely but is pushed and pulled forward and backward at right angles to the transverse axis of the plate. For grinding, the average size of the abrasive particles should be 20 μm (not larger than 40 μm); for polishing, the average particle size should be 4 μm or less (and not larger than 8 μm).

Automatic Hones

These are rapidly becoming indispensable, but only those employing a flat plate glass hone can be recommended. Broadly speaking, these are of two types: a large circular glass plate, against the upper surface of which the knife facet is held by a clamping arm; and those (e.g., American Optical Company's model) employing a relatively small rectangular frosted glass plate which vibrates at high frequency and over which the knife, held by clamps on the end of a motor-driven shaft, is stroked. Because of the smaller hone's greater flatness, precision, ease of dressing, economical replacement, overall efficiency, and ease of operation, it enjoys wide popularity. It enables one to dispense entirely with stropping—provided a few simple rules are adhered to: (1) never use the same glass plate for knives of different lengths; (2) always center the knife precisely; (3) use one surface of the glass hone plate for coarse, the other for fine honing, and mark them accordingly; (4) use the proper oil-base abrasive for each type of honing, and wash both knife and plate well after each phase; and (5) follow the manufacturer's instructions.

Undoubtedly, the best automatic knife sharpeners are those using a large circular glass plate. Of these, the Fanz has deservedly enjoyed wide popularity, but the Shandon-Elliott* Autosharp III is currently highly favored and has many features to recommend it. Of the manual knife-sharpening devices, the most scientific and by far the best is undoubtedly that described by Bell.† The equipment includes a large circular bronze lapping plate, which has parallel grooves to prevent accumulation of debris on the honing surface. Knives are held at the right inclination by means of a special steel block that locks onto the knife back and rests on the lapping plate by means of tungsten carbide foot pads that are on self-aligning bearings. The facet angles are controlled by adjustable screws, and the correct angle for each facet of any knife is determined by a single optical device.

Factory Grinding of Microtome Knives

After repeated sharpening of wedge knives the cutting edge gradually retreats into thicker metal, with consequent widening of the bevel angle. When this angle becomes much greater than 35 degrees the knife should be returned so that both its wedge surfaces may be ground down and the correct bevel angle restored.

Stropping

Theoretically a perfectly honed knife does not require stropping; however, in practice, some stropping is still required after all but the best plate glass automatic sharpeners. Strops should be of the best quality shell-horse leather made from the rump or thick part of the horse hide. The leather or stop surface must be of good size, e.g., 3 to 4 by 18 inches and should be mounted on a solid wooden block. Strops not so supported sag in the middle and will turn or round the knife edge. It is convenient to have two qualities of strop mounted on the same block: one of pure fine leather, the other impregnated with a fine abrasive (diamond dust or fine carborundum paste), this second or coarser strop often serving to touch up a knife when there is not time or real need for honing. In all cases, the final finishing is done on the fine unimpregnated strop. To strop, the knife is first fitted with its appropriate knife-back, then laid obliquely on the strop and pushed backward and drawn forward (toe to heel), its back edge always leading, i.e., the opposite to honing. About 40 to 120 double strokes are usually required, but this has to be determined by experience. Before and after use, the strop must be wiped with a soft cloth so as to remove all particles. Occasionally, it is necessary to wipe with a cloth just moistened with xylene, but care must be exercised here, as xylene will remove the oil (castor oil) with which the strop is impregnated. From time to time the strop can be reoiled (about once a year). Some

---

*Shandon Southern Instruments Inc., Sewickley, Pa. 15143.
†P. T. Lawson, Sydney, Australia.

workers dust fine alumina on the strop to prevent the smooth leather from pulling out particles from the knife edge. Excessive stropping will turn the edge and may "burn" it, i.e., produce localized dark areas. This results from heat destroying the temper, and such areas have to be honed out. The knife edge must be wiped clean after each "series" of stropping, and before changing from coarse to fine strop, so as not to carry over any particles. Finally, when stropping is completed to satisfaction, the knife edge is oiled or greased to prevent rusting. The knife is then placed in its suspension box; knives must never by rested on their sides since this is bound to damage the edge.

ROUTINE PARAFFIN SECTION CUTTING

Preparation of the Block and Equipment

The numbered block is secured in place in the microtome object clamp. Special microtome clamps are available for unmounted (e.g., Peel-A-Way) blocks, for those mounted on fiber blocks, and for specific embedding systems, e.g., Tissue-Tek, TIMS. Experience and practice will teach how one should best orientate the blocks, but in general, when a tissue varies in consistency, e.g., skin, it is best to have the soft part of the tissue strike the knife edge first. The object holder is adjusted so that the top of the wax block just touches the knife edge. If the tissue has not been embedded in a flat plane it may be necessary to tilt the object holder so that the whole of the top surface of the block is in the plane of cutting.

By means of the coarse adjustment the microtome feed is then advanced some 10 to 15 μm between each stroke until the whole plane of the tissue is being cut. It is convenient to perform this trimming down with one end of the knife that is awaiting honing. As each block is trimmed down for sectioning it may be removed from the object holder and placed face down on a tray of ice cubes or, better, on a refrigerated plate. When all the blocks have been trimmed the knife is moved so that a fresh and sharp portion of its edge is in position for cutting. Alternatively, a block is recooled by holding an ice cube on its face, moving the knife, and cutting sections without having removed the block. The thumb screws of the knife clamp are tightened by finger pressure (no tools should ever be used), and if necessary the clearance angle of the knife is checked.

A series of glass slides is numbered with a diamond pencil, the numbers corresponding to those on the blocks to be cut and the slides being arranged in the same order as the blocks. There may be less chance of confusion if etched slides are used and numbered with pencil as each block is cut, a permanent label-number being applied after staining and mounting.

The slides are cleaned with a fine cloth and the numbered surface of each slide smeared with a very thin coat of adhesive mixture, which is spread with the pad of the index finger.

Adhesive Mixtures for Coating Slides

Although these are unnecessary for routine staining, provided that slides are clean and grease-free, they are essential for methods entailing significant exposure of sections to acids and especially alkalis (ammoniacal silver solutions). They are advisable for complex or prolonged sequences and for certain tissues such as nervous system and bone. They are all protein solutions and, since proteins retain many stains, the amount of concentration of the solution used to coat the slide must be kept to a minimum. They are all prone to contamination by organisms which could cause confusion, e.g., in Gram and PAS stains; thymol and the use of a glass rod applicator fixed in the stopper of the container help prevent this. It should be remembered that these adhesive mixtures cannot be used if protein histochemical investigations are contemplated. Lillie believes that these agents act mainly by reducing surface tension and thus producing closer capillary adhesion of the sections to the slide.

Mayer's Egg Albumen-Glycerol

Whites of fresh eggs	50 mL
Glycerol	50 mL

Mix well and filter through several layers of gauze. Add about 100 mg thymol to prevent mold growth. Some workers prefer to dilute the Mayer formula by adding 50 mL distilled water.

Gelatin in Floating-Out Bath

Adding 15 to 30 mL of 1% aqueous gelatin to the water in the floating-out bath and mixing well is a most convenient alternative to direct coating of slides.

Gelatin—Chrome Alum

This solution can be added to the water bath. It is made by placing 1 g of gelatin in 15 mL of cold water until it softens. 85 mL of boiling water is then added, and solution of the gelatin is assisted by gentle heat with a hot plate if necessary. Finally, 0.1 g of chrome alum is added to this solution, and the solution is mixed.

For use, 10 mL of the solution is added to the water bath and mixed well.

If desired, slides for use in frozen sections may be dipped into this solution diluted 1:3 with water and then air dried. The slides are kept available for use with the cryostat.

Floating-out Bath

It is convenient to have such a bath close by the microtome. A circular, thermostatically controlled bath 10 to 12 inches in diameter and 3 to 4 inches in depth is desirable; the inside surface should be black, thus enabling easier visualization of sections. The thermostat should be set at 45°C, i.e., about 10° below the melting point of the wax used for blocking out. The bath should be filled to within 1/2 to 1 cm from the top with water at approximately the required temperature and then plugged into the electrical outlet. The bath must be disconnected, emptied, and wiped dry and clean after use. Should a scum appear on the surface of the water before or during cutting, it may be removed by momentarily and gently resting a large sheet of filter or other suitable absorbent paper on the surface of the water and then pulling the paper off, raising the edge held in the fingers as little as possible above the water surface. It should be mentioned here that some workers prefer not to use a water bath, but place the sections on the slide, add 1 or 2 mL of water from a Pasteur pipette, and then place the slide on a warm plate (45 to 50°C) until the section has flattened out.

Section Cutting

Make sure that the microtome is set for the desired thickness of cut, which for routine work is normally 4 to 6 μm. The block is removed from the ice, wiped dry, and clamped firmly in the clamp or chuck of the microtome. The object holder is moved manually until the surface of the wax just touches the knife edge, cutting then being commenced with regular even strokes (there must be no jerking motion). Experience will be the best guide here, but generally a hard tissue, e.g., cervix or thyroid, is best cut with a firm, relatively quick stroke, whereas soft tissues are best cut with slow, gentle motion. Nervous tissue and lymph nodes should be cut slowly with a very even stroke. Breathing on the knife and block may help with such tissues. The ideal block is one with as little disparity as possible between the consistency or hardness of the tissue and that of the wax. It is not convenient to use waxes of different melting points for different tissues in a busy routine laboratory, but compensation may be made by varying the degree of cooling of the blocks; the harder the tissue, the harder (and therefore the cooler) the block should be so that the resistance between the knife edge, wax, and tissue will be as uniform as possible. However, if cooling, either by ice or cold water, is too prolonged, the wax may tend to retract so that the tissue protrudes and thus cannot be cut.

Wax solidifies or sets in crystalline form. The smaller these crystals, the better they support the tissue and the better are the sections obtained. In all these aspects Paraplast offers a distinct advantage over paraffin wax.

Cutting of Ribbon Sections

It is important that the upper and lower surfaces of the block to be cut be parallel in order that straight "ribbons" of sections be obtained. The first section is raised carefully with the index finger or a pencil camel's-hair brush. As the knife strikes the block to start cutting the next section, locally generated heat and pressure weld the edge of section number 2 to the back edge of section number 1. This continues with succeeding sections so that a ribbon of sections is formed. This may be supported by the moistened tip of an index finger under the first section (some prefer to use a camel's-hair brush, spatula, or flat-bladed forceps). A practiced section cutter can, by finger support, easily secure ribbons 9 to 12 inches long. Once cut, the ribbons are laid out in serial order on a sheet of cardboard or black x-ray wrapping paper, with each end of the ribbon secured by pressing the wax border onto the paper with the back of a scalpel blade.

For mounting, the ribbons are cut into convenient lengths (2 inches), the adhesion to the cardboard or paper at the line of cutting being freed by passing the scalpel blade obliquely under the line of adhesion. They are then placed on numbered slides, the serial order being maintained. A few mL of water are added to each slide, which is then placed on a hot plate until such time as the sections have flattened out (5 to 10 minutes). Any excess water is drained off, and the slides are stood at an angle of about 40 to 85 degrees to drain.

For routine sections, however, ribbons of two to six suitable sections are taken by the moistened tip of the index finger adhering to the edge of the first section, and the section ribbon is floated onto the surface of the water in the floating-out bath. With the aid of two dissecting needles such sections as are not required are flicked off smartly (the needle points must be clean and polished; otherwise they will adhere to and may destroy the ribbon). When the sections chosen have flattened out (1/2 to 2 minutes) the appropriately numbered slide is immersed nearly vertically in the water bath. The surface of the slide coated with adhesive is then gently approximated to the end of the section or ribbon. The slide is gently raised in an even motion and, as it touches the edge of the section, the section will adhere to it as the slide is drawn upward. The slide is then stood to drain at an angle of about 60 to 85 degrees for approximately 2 to 5 minutes.

Drying Sections on Slides

After draining, the sections must be fixed to the slides. This may be done in several ways: (1) in a wax oven at 56 to 60°C for 2 hours; (2) in an incubator at 37°C overnight; (3) on a hot plate at 45 to 55°C for 30 to 45 minutes, preferably inverted, the slide ends resting on tracklike supports 3 to 4 mm above the plate surface; (4) for 20 to 30 minutes at 50 to 55°C in a blower-type electric slide dryer; (5) by mounting the sections in 0.1 to 0.25% aqueous floating-out gelatin solution or onto albumenized slides, draining excess fluid, and, while still moist, placing them in a covered Coplin jar containing 2 to 3 mL 40% formaldehyde in the incubator at 37°C for 4 to 18 hours; and (6) in urgency, by carefully holding the slide, section upward, above a Bunsen flame until the wax just melts. In the case of nervous tissue, best results are obtained by overnight incubation at 37°C; the sections tend to crack at higher temperatures or if dried off rapidly.

DIFFICULTIES ENCOUNTERED IN SECTION CUTTING

Difficulties Deriving from Improper Fixation

Incomplete or inadequate fixation tends to produce a soft, mushy tissue block and sections that crumble and "feather" when cut. This occurs most frequently in the case of excessively mucinous tissues, e.g., pseudomucinous cystadenomas of the ovary, in which the fixative does not readily penetrate the viscous mucus. Fixation in buffered neutral formalin, using thin blocks, prior washing with normal saline to remove excess blood or mucus, and adequate fixation time will generally overcome this difficulty. On the other hand, prolonged fixation in fixatives such as Zenker's or Helly's produces hard, brittle blocks and may lead to discontinuous or fragmented sections. Such hard blocks may cause the knife to "ring" or "chatter," i.e., vibrate, and so produce in the section lines or scores that run parallel to the knife edge, or alternate thin and thick sections. If the block is excessively hard, the tissue may even tear or jump out of the block during sectioning. Very hard blocks may cut more easily if the entire block is soaked overnight in Mollifex (B.D.H.*).

Difficulties Deriving from Faulty Dehydration, Clearing, and Embedding

If the tissue has been insufficiently dehydrated, the clearing agent turns milky when the tissue is transferred into it. In such circumstances clearing, and therefore also wax impregnation, cannot proceed to completion and the resultant block will tend to be soft or even mushy. Sectioning such blocks is extremely difficult, and the sections tend to fray and crumble. If inadequate dehydration is detected during clearing, it can be remedied by returning the tissue for further treatment in absolute alcohol. Old blocks may require similar reprocessing.

Insufficient clearing causes the tissue to appear opaque or cloudy, and section cutting may be difficult or impossible. If the tissue has already been blocked, it will have to be returned to the wax bath until the wax is completely molten and the tissue then returned to the clearing agent for further treatment. Actually, in such cases, if possible, it is generally more satisfactory to select another block of tissue and to start from the beginning. At the other extreme, prolonged treatment with certain clearing agents, e.g., xylene, will cause the tissue to become excessively hard and brittle and may also lead to inordinate shrinkage.

Insufficient impregnation with wax will produce a "moist" block that tends to crumble and that smells of the clearing agent. Prolonged wax impregnation, on the other hand, will give a tissue block that is hard and unduly shrunken.

Difficulties Derived from the Tissue

Certain tissues, e.g., blood clot, cervix, and thyroid, tend to become very hard in routine processing. The block should be well cooled before cutting, which should be effected with a firm, sharp stroke. Hardness becomes less of a problem with such tissues if chloroform is used for clearing. Tetrahydrofuran, used instead of traditional dehydrating and clearing agents, may give better results. Fatty tissues, e.g., subcutaneous tissues, breast, and lipomas, tend to give soft blocks and shredded sections. This is owing mainly to inadequate removal of the fat. For tissues of this nature the selected blocks should be thin (2 mm), and wax impregnation in the vacuum bath is of great help. Brain and lymph nodes become very hard and brittle if xylene is used for dealcoholization. In their case chloroform is best, and vacuum impregnation helps with lymph nodes. Soft tissues are compressed by setting and cooling of the wax block (10 to 12% shrinkage). When sections of such tissues are cut they are compressed even further. On being floated out, these sections have a natural tendency to expand more than do sections of firmer tissues. The outer rim of wax should therefore be split with a dissecting needle (without damaging the tissue) or creases and wrinkles will result.

*B.D.H. Chemicals, Toronto, Ont. M8Z 1K5, or Gallard-Schlesinger Chemical Manufacturing Corp., Carle Place, N.Y. 11514.

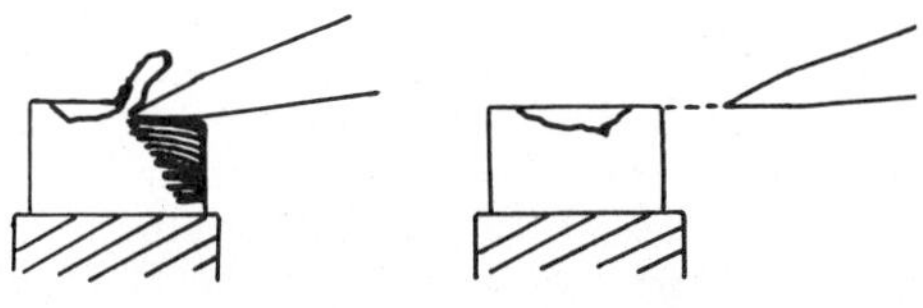

Figure 32–10 Wedging, caused by too small a clearance angle.

Difficulties Related to the Knife or Microtome

If the knife is not held securely in the microtome it will tend to jump, especially on striking hard tissues. Also, if the knife setting is such as to give excessive tilt, i.e., too great a clearance angle, the knife will be prone to vibrate, and "chattering" is likely to occur. This causes bands of unequal thickness parallel to the knife edge in the sections. If the tilt of the knife is very great, then scraping tends to replace cutting and it may be impossible to obtain a section. Provided the knife is correctly set and adequately clamped, the heavier the knife the less the tendency to vibration.

Inadequate clearance angle leads to block compression, so that a sequence of no section followed by a thick section, or alternate thin and thick sections, results. Sections of unequal or irregular thickness may also result from inadequate tightening of the block holder (object clamp).

A blunt knife will not cut good sections even though everything else is perfect. When the width of the cut section is much less than that of the block, the knife

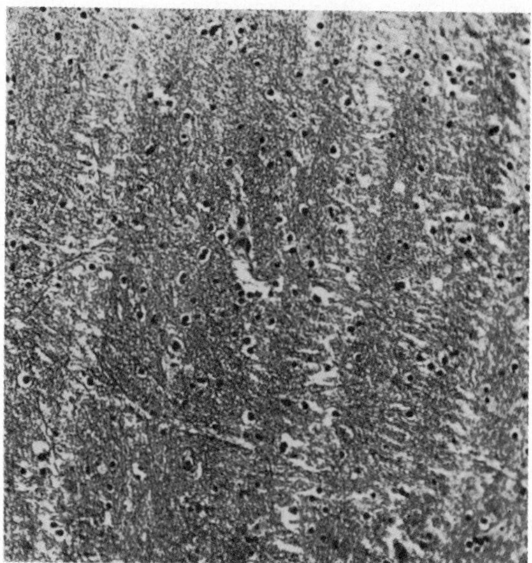

Figure 32–11 Scoring in brain section. The scores are in the line of cutting and may result from (1) minute nicks in the knife edge, (2) dust granules on the knife edge, or (3) hard granules, e.g., calcium or mercury salt deposits, in the tissue (or wax). Hematoxylin-eosin × 180.

has probably lost its bevel. Serrations or minute nicks in, or wax adhering to the back of, the knife edge will score or scratch the sections in the direction of the cutting stroke. Similar scratches may be caused by particles of dirt in the wax, or by minute spicules of calcium or silica in the tissue. If the knife edge is not really sharp, "ribboning" will be difficult. A blunt edge produces greater distortion and compression of the tissue section and enhances any tendency to wrinkles and folds.

Other causes of difficulties in cutting good sections may lie in the wax, the thickness setting of the microtome, or the type of cutting stroke used. If the wax is too hard (high melting point), ribboning may be difficult, and folds and wrinkles are very apt to occur in the case of softer tissues. If sections are cut too thick (more than 8 μm), they tend to roll up or fracture. Very thin sections (less than 4½ μm) must be cut with a gentle, even stroke, especially if the tissue is a cellular one with relatively little supporting stroma, e.g., lymph nodes. Hard tissues are best cut with a firm, sharp stroke. Ribbon formation may be prevented by the section's being lifted from the knife on the upstroke (rotary microtome) or backstroke (sliding microtome with fixed knife). This may be caused by the knife or wax block's being too warm or by the knife tilt's being too small.

Trouble may also be experienced from static electricity, especially during the winter months, when the atmosphere is very dry. The statically charged sections are extremely difficult to manipulate. This problem may be reduced by increasing the humidity of the atmosphere and by grounding (earthing) the microtome to a water pipe.

DISTORTION IN SECTIONS

This is the name given to any change in the form (shape) of the tissue in the section from that of the tissue in the block. It is occasionally also applied when the section thickness differs from the setting of the microtome. Because of the compressible nature of wax and of most tissues and because of the wedge-cutting action of the knife, sections are almost invariably a little wider and shorter than the surface dimensions of the block. On floating out, some of this distortion is corrected: but in the case of very soft and compressible tissues (e.g., fat, skin, and endometrium), the expansion on warm water may lead to folds and wrinkles unless the outer rim of wax is broken at points of stress by a sharp nick with the polished point of a mounting needle. In the case of hard tissues, on the other hand, folds may occur during cutting because the softer wax surrounding the tissue yields and distorts more than the tissue itself. Such folds may be eliminated by gentle needling in the water bath, though it is better to avoid them altogether by cooling the block so as to harden the wax.

FROZEN SECTIONING

Advantages of Frozen and Cryostat Sections

1. For certain staining procedures, e.g., the demonstration of fat by the oil red O method and for certain silver impregnation methods, as well as for certain methods in the central nervous system, frozen sections are essential.

2. Frozen or cryostat sections are indispensable for rapid diagnosis during operations.

3. All enzymes are destroyed at temperatures above 56°C, and although some, e.g., phosphatases, may be demonstrated in paraffin sections, all are best shown in cryostat or frozen sections of fresh tissue. The same applies for a number of histochemical methods.

Disadvantages

1. It is almost impossible to obtain serial sections.

2. Because of the lack of an embedding mass, structural details tend to be somewhat distorted during cutting and handling.

3. Staining of frozen sections of unfixed tissue is rarely as satisfactory as that obtained with properly fixed material.

4. Freezing artifact may be produced by inappropriate techniques. These include: the presence of ice crystals in the tissues, nuclear ballooning and vacuolation, and separation of a mucosal or other epithelial surface.

THE CRYOSTAT

The major advance made by the cryostat and its major advantage over freezing microtomes is that it maintains the tissue block, knife, and section at the same temperature. It does this by housing the entire operation in an insulated, thermostatically controlled, refrigerated cabinet. Modern cryostats are caster-mounted cabinet models of the open-top type, permitting easy access and visiblity through the hinged, double-thickness plastic cover. The rust-proof microtome is usually mounted at a 45-degree angle in the stainless steel cabinet, which is equipped with an antifogging air-circulating system, a drain for defrosting and sterilizing, and a shelf with spaces for four to six metal block carriers. Temperature control range varies from +10 to −30°C. Most use 120 mm wedge knives, the tilt of which can be adjusted. Some provide a razor blade attachment, but we have not found this to be satisfactory. Of the many models on the market, we have had sufficient experience with only three, viz., the A.O. Cryo-Cut,* I.E.C.'s model CTD,† and Ames Lab-Tek cryostat, all of which are excellent and are recommended. All three have superb rotary microtomes (A.O. Spencer and Minot type, respectively). They are equipped with antiroll devices, i.e., a plastic plate which, when in position, is separated from the knife surface by elevated shoulders (0.0635 mm high in A.O. Cryo-Cut), thus permitting the section to slide under the plate.

OPERATION AND MAINTENANCE OF CRYOSTAT

The cryostat should be left on at all times, since several hours are required to attain operating temperature from a room temperature start. It should be defrosted during the weekend, when the inside of the

*American Optical Co., Buffalo, N.Y. 14215.

†Damon Corp./IEC Division, Needham Heights, Mass. 02194.

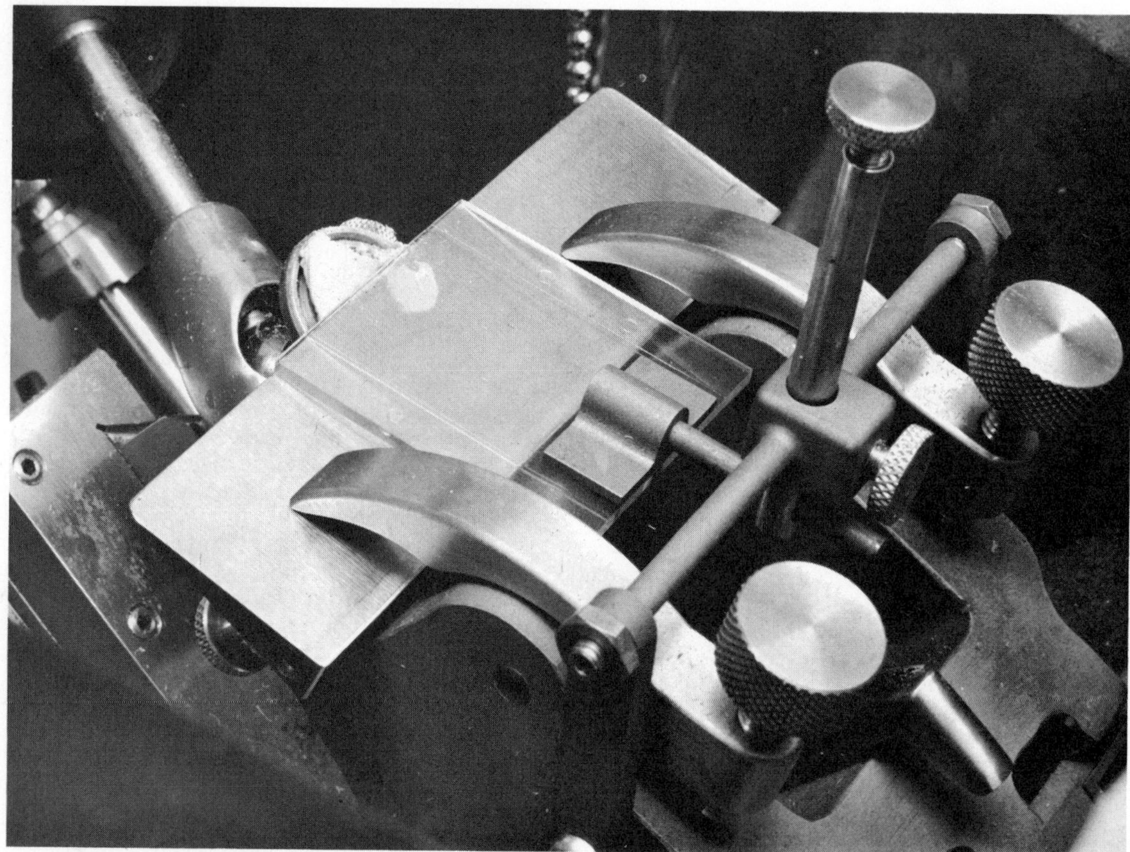

Figure 32–12 Close-up view of the antiroll device on the microtome of the I. E. C. cryostat. (Courtesy of International Equipment Company, Needham Heights, Mass. 02194.)

cabinet should be washed and dried, and the microtome cleaned and oiled with special low-temperature oil. Since a knife will require almost an hour to come down to operating temperature, one should always be kept in the cabinet—either in its box or in the holder (the A.O. model has a place for a spare knife). For good cryostat sectioning a faultlessly sharp knife is just as essential as for paraffin sectioning. Some problem arises from the fact that knives kept in the cabinet tend to rust. This can be minimized by purchasing best-quality knives and by cleaning them thoroughly with xylene followed by alcohol after each use: some workers advocate coating them with a light coating of silicone, using an aerosol spray. To ensure that the sections will glide smoothly and freely on its surface, the knife face must be kept scrupulously clean and dry; the same applies to the undersurface and edge of the antiroll plate. Also, one must not forget to clean the undersurface of the knife, where tissue and mounting compound tend to build up and may interfere with cutting by compressing the tissue. Cleaning is effected by soft paper tissue, either dry or moistened with absolute alcohol.

Operating Temperature and Type of Tissue

Because of differences in composition, cellularity, connective tissue, and fat content, the optimum temperature for cryostat sectioning varies with the tissue. In this regard animal tissue may be classed in three groups: (1) brain, lymph nodes, liver, spleen, kidney, testis, uterine curettings, soft cellular tumors, and thyroid section best at −5 to −15°C; (2) muscle, connective tissue, pancreas, uterus and cervix, skin (without fat), nonfatty breast tissue, ovary, prostate, tongue, and gut section best at −15 to −25°C; (3) fatty tissue, including skin with fatty subcutis, fatty breast, and omental tissues cut best at about −35°C.

Obviously, since any cryostat requires considerable time to attain temperatures that differ by more than ±5°C from its setting, it is impossible to cater to the tissue variations listed (unless one has three cryostats). However, these difficulties can be largely overcome by attention to three apsects:

Optimum Working Temperature of Cryostat. This is −18 to −20°C.

Cryostat Mounting Media. In ascending order of merit these are: water, 20 to 30% bovine albumin, and von Apathy's gum syrup; but best of all are formulas consisting of synthetic water-soluble glycols and resins. Especially recommended is Lab Tek's O.C.T. (optimal cutting temperature) compound,* marketed in convenient 8-oz plastic dispensers in three temperature ranges corresponding to those just outlined.

Carbon Dioxide Freezing of Fatty Tissues. Blocks of tissues of the third group may be quick-frozen in the

*Lab-Tek Products, Division of Miles Laboratories, Inc., Naperville, Ill. 60540.

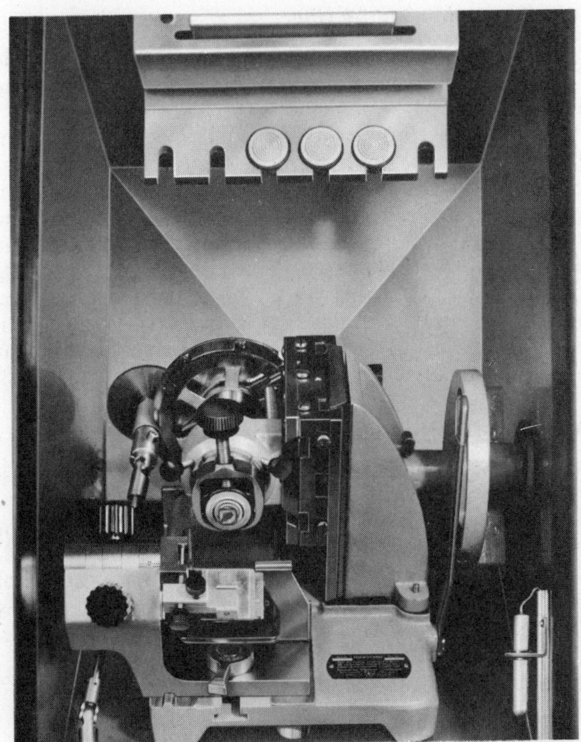

Figure 32–13 Detail of A. O. Cryo-Cut in cabinet. (Courtesy of American Optical Company, Buffalo, N.Y. 14240.

special CO_2-freezing chamber before being placed in the cryostat. Quick-freezing spray cans of fluorinated hydrocarbons, e.g., I.E.C.'s Cryokwik (fluorocarbon 22)* are a distinct advantage for freezing blocks of any type tissue rapidly.

Repeated episodes of severe palpitation in those exposed to fluorocarbons in pathology departments have been reported. It has been recommended that greater care be exercised in using such substances, especially in poorly ventilated places, and that inhalation of the fluorocarbon vapors be avoided.

Cryostat Sectioning Procedure

A suitable block of fresh tissue is selected and trimmed with a sharp scalpel so that its sides are parallel. Preferably, the block should be 2 to 4 mm thick so as to minimize the risk of the metal object disc's striking the knife edge; however, thinner blocks may be elevated by using a thicker base of O.C.T. compound. Within limits, the size of the block governs the thickness at which sections can be cut. Small fragments of tissue, e.g., curettings, are placed on a thick base of O.C.T. compound. The blocks are then surrounded and covered with a matrix of O.C.T. compound and placed in the quick-freeze shelf of the cryostat, where they will become adequately cooled and frozen in 1 to 3 minutes. This process may be expedited by (1) using cold object holders from the cryostat cabinet and (2) swinging the heat-exchanging metal block into position on the tissue.

When the tissue is adequately frozen the object disc is inserted into the microtome object clamp, the tilt and angle being so oriented that the face of the block (and of the object disc) is in the plane of sectioning and the block edge is parallel to that of the knife. Make sure the microtome advance feed mechanism is returned to its starting position. Release the knife-holder clamp and move the assembly until the knife edge just touches the block. Ensure that all clamps are tightened (manually). Using the quick or manual advance, trim the block until the desired full section is obtained. Now, set the section thickness control and automatic advance mechanism and make sure that the surfaces of the knife and the edge and undersurface of the antiroll plate are absolutely clean; if not, wipe them with fine tissue. Position the antiroll plate so that its edge is parallel to and even with the knife edge (in some makes it is advantageous to have it a fraction of a millimeter ahead of the knife edge; experience is the best guide). At this point it is advantageous to close the cabinet for a minute or two to allow temperatures to equilibrate, using this time to get slides and stains ready.

It must be realized that the cryostat cuts individual sections; it does not ribbon. Sections of most tissues are best cut with a slow, even motion; some, e.g., harder tissues, cut better with a firm, fast stroke. With correct adjustments, clean surfaces, and skilled technique, the section will glide smoothly and flat beneath the antiroll plate. Some workers like to use a camel's hair brush to start the section and to keep it flat as it glides out on the knife surface. Sectioning may be difficult in hot, humid weather.

Mounting Cryostat Sections

Once the section has been cut the cabinet is opened and the antiroll plate is flipped back. A clean slide is then carefully lowered onto the section. In practice, one edge of the glass slide is rested on the knife surface about 1 inch beyond the section and the other end is lowered gently until it is about ½ to 1 mm from the knife face, and the section will automatically transfer from the cold knife to the relatively warm slide. Never press the slide down on the section. A frost mark will remain where the section rested on the knife. This should be wiped away with soft tissue. The antiroll plate is repositioned and another section may be cut. Sections may also be picked up on coverglasses, which may be held by hand, by forceps, or by suction bulb.

Fixing Cryostat Sections to Slides

In the case of sections of fresh, unfixed tissue no adhesive is necessary; all that is required is a few seconds' waving in air, or *better,* fixing immediately in formol-alcohol (15 mL of 40% formaldehyde plus 85 mL of 95% ethanol; optionally, 5 mL glacial acetic acid may be added). Sections of formalin or otherwise fixed tissue, however, may not adhere and may therefore detach during staining. Some people prefer to wash such fixed tissue for several hours in running tap water before sectioning, the sections being picked up on clean slides coated with albumen or Zwemer's chrome-glycerin jelly (dissolve 0.2 g chrome alum in 30 mL distilled water; dissolve 3 g powdered gelatin in 50 mL distilled water; mix and add 20 mL glycerin; mix the two solutions and

*Damon Corp./IEC Division, Needham Heights, Mass. 02194.

adjust pH to 7.4 if necessary with $NaHCO_3$). The mounted sections are placed in a covered Coplin jar containing 1 to 5 mL of 40% formaldehyde for 1 to 5 minutes: this causes irreversible gelling of the gelatin. We have not usually found this to be necessary.

Fixed Tissue for Cryostat Examination

Since the major use of the cryostat is for rapid surgical diagnosis, time may be saved by using unfixed tissue. The latter will also adhere easily to the glass slide without need for any adhesive mixture. Unfixed frozen tissues also preserve their enzymes and other substances that may be studied by histochemical techniques.

However, fixed tissues may be used. The tissue block, selected by the pathologist, may be immersed in boiling 10% buffered formalin for 1 to 2 minutes before freezing and sectioning for rapid surgical diagnosis. Fixation artifact (such as shrinkage) may occur, and the consistency of the block may become less than optimal because of the additional water from the fixative fluid. Special fixatives, such as 10% formol calcium at 4°C, may be used in histochemistry and for lipid demonstration.

Tissues that have been fixed or stored in alcohol should be washed in water for 12 to 24 hours before sectioning, since the alcohol tends to inhibit freezing. Mercuric chloride fixative must be removed by alcoholic iodine and water, whereas potassium dichromate must be rinsed from the tissues with water before subjecting the material to the cryostat.

Staining of Cryostat Sections

There are numerous methods of staining frozen sections, but for rapid surgical diagnosis two methods are widely used: hematoxylin-eosin and polychrome methylene blue. There are numerous modifications of these methods, and those reproduced here are merely a selection from these.

Hematoxylin-Eosin

Sections are allowed to dry in air for ½ to 1 minute.

1. Fix air-dried sections in pure acetone for 15 to 20 seconds or in formol-alcohol for ½ to 1 minute.
2. Place in absolute ethanol, 5 to 10 seconds.
3. *Optimal:* Place in a second bath of absolute ethanol, followed by two changes of xylene (until clear); then return through two changes of 100% ethanol.
4. Place in 90% ethanol for 5 seconds.
5. Place in distilled water until no longer "greasy" or cloudy.
6. Place in Harris's hematoxylin for 1 to 2 minutes.
7. Place in distilled water, with agitation, for 5 to 10 seconds.
8. Dip in 0.5% sodium borate until blue.
9. Place in 70% ethanol for 5 seconds.
10. Place in 1% alcoholic eosin for 5 to 25 seconds.
11. Wash in water for 10 to 30 seconds.
12. Dehydrate through graded alcohols.
13. Clear in three changes of xylene and mount in Clarite, Permount, or H.S.R.

Note. Reagents for this rapid hematoxylin-eosin are conveniently set up in sequence in a series of Coplin jars on a tray.

Polychrome Methylene Blue

Methylene blue is one of the few utterly indispensable stains. It usually contains some azures or methylene violet. The zinc-free chloride is the form used.

The polychroming involves the oxidation of the methylene blue so that methyl groups are lost, leaving lower homologues of the dye (azures) and deaminized oxidation products (thiazoles). The resulting mixture of methylene blue, azures, and thiazoles is known as polychrome methylene blue (Bernthsen's methylene violet) and has a violet color. It stains nuclei blue; cartilage matrix, mucin, mast cell granules, and connective tissues generally are stained a reddish violet, i.e., somewhat similar to, but more polychromatic than, thionine.

Methods of Polychroming Methylene Blue

Polychroming occurs naturally in alkaline solutions, and the process is accelerated at pH levels above 8.0 and also by heat. Under these conditions it is not necessary to add oxidizers. The normal aging of methylene blue, either as a dry powder or in methyl alcohol solution, leads to oxidation and polychroming, but this is extremely slow. Acids generally retard polychroming.

Löffler's Polychrome Methylene Blue

Saturated solution of methylene blue in alcohol	30 mL
1:10,000 KOH (1 mL of 1% aqueous KOH to 99 mL distilled water)	100 mL

This is placed in bottles, which are only half filled. These are shaken from time to time, and the caps are removed for an hour or so occasionally. Under these conditions polychroming will be effected in about 1 year. The process may be expedited by placing the bottles in the incubator at 37°C or 58° to 60°C. The solution is also available commerically. For rapid diagnosis, frozen sections are stained with polychrome methylene blue for ½ to 1 minute and are then rinsed and mounted in an aqueous mountant or blotted dry, cleared in xylol, and mounted in H.S.R.

Comments on Cryostat Sections and Applications

The cryostat has become indispensable to the modern hospital laboratory. It has removed much of the guesswork and "art" from frozen section diagnosis and has elevated it to the level of an almost precise science—so much so that the hematoxylin-eosin–stained cryostat quick section should be kept and filed as a permanent record. Of course, it is strongly recommended that representative paraffin blocks and sections also be prepared, though it is recognized that some institutions use cryostat sections routinely for surgical and autopsy material.

The cryostat is also recommended for any technique requiring cold sectioning of unfixed (or fixed) material, e.g., for fats and lipids, and for some special methods for the nervous system. Even more indispensable is its use for such procedures as fluorescent antigen-antibody techniques, most enzyme and histochemical investigations, microincineration, autoradiography, and freeze-drying. Indeed, some research model cryostats are equipped with freeze-drying attachments.

MOUNTING STAINED SECTIONS

If an unmounted stained section is examined under the microscope, very little detail can be made out because of the great difference in the refractive index of the glass slide, the tissue components, and air. For the best results with stained tissue sections they must be impregnated by a transparent medium having a refractive index close to that of glass. Stained elements will then be visible and distinguishable by their color and differences in color tone. Mounting medium is also necessary to protect the stained section from physical injury and from bleaching or deterioration of the stain as a result of oxidation. The best mounting medium will have a refractive index close to that of glass (1.518), will be freely miscible with xylene and toluene, will be nonreactive and will not change in pH or color, will set without distortion or shrinkage of tissue sections, will set hard without granularity or cracking, and will not leach out any stain or cause any loss of staining over long periods. Such mounting media fall into the permanent category; there are also a number of temporary or semipermanent mounting media.

PERMANENT MOUNTING MEDIA

These are resins, either natural or synthetic.

Canada Balsam

Until 1939 this was the medium of choice. It is an oleoresin collected from blisters in the bark of the balsam fir, which is a native tree of the eastern half of Canada. It is transparent, almost colorless in thin layers, adheres firmly to glass, and sets to a hard consistency without granulation. A minor disadvantage is that Canada balsam darkens slightly with age, but a major disadvantage is that it slowly becomes acid because it oxidizes xylene to toluic and phthalic acids. This acidity causes gradual fading of many stains. Many attempts have been made to avoid this, but none has been successful; hence, Canada balsam has been superseded by more stable synthetic resins.

D.P.X. of Kirkpatrick and Lendrum

This is made of the resin "Distrene 80" plasticized by the addition of tricresylphosphate or dibutylphthalate. It is a good mounting medium, though H.S.R. (Harleco Synthetic Resin) Clarite or Permount is preferred, since D.P.X. shrinks somewhat on drying. Its refractive index is 1.52.

Clarite (also Clarite X)

This is one of the most widely used mounting media in North America. It is a synthetic resin with a refractive index of 1.544; it is soluble in and used as a 60% solution in xylene. Permount (made by Fisher Scientific) appears to be similar, if not the same.

Other synthetic mounting media recommended are H.S.R. (Harleco Synthetic Resin), Clearmount (Gurr), and Malinol.* Thin plastic sections stained for light microscopy may be mounted in Malinol or a similar mountant or in the plastic formula used for the parent block's embedment.

*Chroma Gesellschaft Schmid Co., Stuttgart-Untertürkheim, W. Germany.

TECHNIQUE OF PERMANENT MOUNTING

Since all the resins used for this purpose are soluble in xylene, it follows that the stained sections must be brought up to xylene, i.e., dehydrated and then cleared. This is usually done by passing through two changes of 95% ethyl alcohol, then one or two changes of 100% ethyl alcohol, and finally through two or three changes of xylene. Ethyl alcohol should be used with care for dehydrating sections stained by thiazine dyes, e.g., methylene blue, thionine, and toluidine blue. Alcohol may convert the metachromatic staining of dyes such as thionine, toluidine blue, methyl violet, and crystal violet to orthochromatic. An alternative to the use of alcohol is to blot sections dry and then clear in xylol. This procedure may need to be repeated to get the section properly clear.

When the sections are placed in the final bath of xylene, a series of suitable-sized coverglasses (coverslips) are selected, cleaned with a fine cloth (if necessary, after washing in alcohol), and placed on a sheet of white paper or large sheet of white blotting paper. Coverglasses may be round, square, or rectangular; 22 × 22, 22 × 30, 22 × 40, and 22 × 50 mm are popular sizes, and are sold in 1-oz packages in three thicknesses, the most commonly used being No. 1 (about 0.125 mm in thickness). The slide carrying the section to be mounted is taken from the xylene bath with forceps; the ends are first cleaned so that the diamond-inscribed number is seen and the front of the slide (side on which section is attached) can be identified. The back of the slide is then wiped dry with a clean, dry, fine cloth, and the excess xylene is wiped off the front to within 2 or 3 mm of the margin of the section. With a small glass rod a streak of mounting medium is placed down the center of a suitably sized coverglass. The slide is then placed lengthwise on its edge, touching the edge of the coverglass and gradually inclined, section side downward, onto the coverglass until the section touches the streak of mounting medium; the slide is then inverted. As this happens the mounting medium quickly spreads through the whole area of the section, which is still moist with xylene, and to the edges of the coverglass.

Only experience will teach one how much mounting medium to place on the coverglass: If too much is used, it will ooze out at the sides of the coverglass and should be carefully wiped away with the fingernail covered by a fine cloth dipped in xylene. If too little (or too diluted) mounting medium is used, as the medium sets it will draw away from the edges of the coverglass and the section must be remounted, removing the coverglass by soaking in xylene. Occasionally one may notice cloudy areas in the mounted section; these are caused by moisture. If this occurs, it means that dehydration has not been adequate. The coverglass must be soaked off in xylene and the slide dehydrated in two baths of absolute alcohol, passed through two baths of xylene, and remounted. The causes of such inadequate dehydration may be too rapid passage through the alcohols, water contamination of the absolute alcohol, splashing, breathing on the slide, or a very moist atmosphere. The absolute alcohol should be tested for water content by taking some copper sulfate, powdering it, heating it on a sand bath until white (anhydrous), and adding a little of it to the alcohol, which, if contaminated with water, will cause the anhydrous copper sulfate to become blue. Some workers keep a layer of copper sulfate powder (anhydrous) on the bottom of the absolute alcohol baths; this not only serves as an indicator but also absorbs a considerable amount of the moisture, thus prolonging the useful life of the alcohol. However, with a good source of supply this should not be necessary, especially if the alcohols are downgraded, say once each week; i.e., the first 100% (from the water side) becomes the 95%, and new alcohol is placed in the last 100% bath next to the xylene, and so forth. If a section has not been properly dehydrated, a milky cloudiness will appear in it when it is placed in the first xylene bath.

Another difficulty that dogs the beginner is the inclusion of air bubbles in the mounted section. This should not happen if the proper amount of xylene is on the section, if the streak of mountant on the coverglass is in line with the axis in which the slide is inclined down onto it, and if the slide is lowered gently and evenly onto the coverglass. It may be mentioned that some workers prefer to put the mounting medium on the xylene-moist section; this may be found easier by some. Should many bubbles be included it is better to remount the section; if only one or two are present they may be teased out by gentle pressure on the coverglass, with the point of a mounting needle.

Once the sections are mounted they are ready for microscopic examination but must be handled with care so that the coverglasses are not moved. If time allows setting of the mouting medium may be hastened by placing the slides on the hot plate (50°C) or in the wax oven for up to 2 hours. Before filing, the mounting medium must be thoroughly dried and hardened by placing the slides in a 37 to 60°C oven for 24 hours or by leaving them at room temperature for 2 to 3 days.

SEMIPERMANENT AND TEMPORARY MOUNTS

For some preparations it is imperative not to use the permanent xylene-resin mounting media, because xylene dissolves out the essential staining: an example is fat stains (neutral fats stained in frozen sections by oil red O, Sudan IV, and so forth). These may be mounted in one of the following:

Water

This has a low refractive index, is moderately transparent and, therefore, affords good visibility, but it is the least permanent, drying off very quickly, and does not permit oil immersion objectives to be used.

Glycerin (Glycerol)

This has a refractive index of 1.46, and is very suitable as a temporary mounting medium, lasting for months if care is taken in handling and if sealed; it also has a preservative action. Slight dilution with water (moist section) aids visibility. The edges may be sealed as described on this and the next page.

Mineral Oil (Liquid Paraffin)

This is a useful temporary mounting medium for Romanowsky-stained smears, which should be well dried before mounting.

Glycerin Jelly (Glycerol Gelatin), R.I. 1.4 to 1.47

This sets quite hard and will keep for years, especially if sealed. Many formulae are available, but that given by Baker is quite good; soak 5 g of fine gelatin for 1 hour at room temperature in 25 mL of distilled water, cover, and place in the paraffin wax oven, stirring occasionally until all the gelatin is dissolved. Meanwhile, mix 35 mL of glycerol, 40 mL of distilled water, and 0.25 mL of cresol (or 10 mg of thimerosal—Merthiolate) and place in the paraffin oven. When all the gelatin has dissolved, mix the two fluids. If necessary, filter through muslin in the oven and place in convenient-sized bottles (5 mL screw-cap) in which it is allowed to set and can be reheated at 55 to 60°C to melt when required for use.

Von Apathy's Gum Syrup Medium, R.I. 1.52

This is prepared as follows: Dissolve 50 g gum arabic (gum acacia) and 50 g of cane sugar in 50 mL (or 100 mL if a less viscid solution is required) of distilled water, with frequent shaking, in a water bath at 60°C, and add 50 mg of thymol (or 15 mg of thimerosal) as a preservative. While warm, place in a vacuum chamber to remove air bubbles. To prevent "bleeding" of metachromatic staining of amyloid by methyl or crystal violet, add 30 to 50 g of potassium acetate or 10 g of sodium chloride.

This is an excellent mounting medium since it sets as hard as do resins, and there is no need to seal the coverglasses.

Farrant's Medium, R.I. 1.43

Dissolve 50 g gum acacia in 50 mL distilled water with frequent shaking in the water bath at 55 to 60°C. When dissolved, add 25 mL glycerol, mix well, and filter through a fine-mesh cloth in the wax oven. It is not so good as von Apathy's gum syrup.

Levulose (Fructose) Syrup

This is a suitable temporary mounting medium because of its high refractive index (1.5), and because it does not leach metachromatic stains. To prepare, dissolve 30 g levulose in 20 mL of distilled water by placing in a stoppered bottle in the incubator (37°C) for 24 hours, with occasional shaking.

Water-miscible mounting media, e.g., of the polyethylene glycol group, may be used. Gurr's Aquamount is recommended.

Sealing Temporary and Semipermanent Mounts

Mounted preparations such as those for fat, metachromasia, and certain histochemical reactions may be protected and rendered more permanent by sealing (ringing) the cleaned and dried edges with one of several agents. These include paraffin wax, Kronig's (also called

Du Noyer's) mixture (8 parts powdered colophonium resin added slowly to 2 parts molten paraffin wax), nail varnish, or one of the many household plastic cements. A T-shaped metal applicator is advantageous for use with paraffin wax, and may be made from ⅛ inch thick brass sheet.

RESTAINING SECTIONS

Occasionally, it is necessary to restain sections because they have faded or because it is desired to use a different or additional (superimposed) stain. Also, if two or three pieces of tissue are on one slide, it may be desired to stain one by a technique different from that used for the others; in that case, the sections not to be stained should be mounted under suitably shaped coverglasses and the mountant allowed to set well before staining the uncovered section. Afterward the "partial" coverglass will be soaked off in xylene and a suitable coverglass chosen to cover the whole specimen. Before restaining old slides the coverglasses must first be removed by soaking in xylene for 24 hours, or they may be warmed gently over a bunsen burner; the coverglasses may then be gently pushed off with the point of a mounting needle. The sections are then taken down to 75% alcohol and placed in 1% acid alcohol until all the color has been removed. They are washed thoroughly in running tap water (if the tap water is acid, they should be placed in a weakly alkaline solution, e.g., Scott's tap water substitute, and then rinsed in distilled water) and are then ready for staining.

Alternatively, after hydration the sections are placed in 0.25% $KMnO_4$ for 5 minutes, then washed in water, and placed in 1% oxalic acid until white, followed by 5 minutes' washing in tap water and restaining.

Results with $KMnO_4$ and oxalic acid are superior to those obtained after acid alcohol decolorization without other treatment.

BROKEN SLIDES

If the slide has not been fragmented, and if the section is not too important, the pieces may be reassembled from xylene atop a clean xylene-moist slide on which a streak of Clarite has been placed. This will usually suffice for immediate examination, but a new section should be cut and stained. Occasionally, a very valuable slide becomes broken and a replacement is not available. If the section (or vital part thereof) has not been destroyed, it may with great care be transferred to another slide as follows:

Remove the coverslip by soaking in xylene. This may be expedited by placing in the incubator at 37°C. Leave in xylene until all mountant has been removed. Cover the whole slide with a mixture of 6 parts butyl acetate and 1 part Durofix. Harden off in the incubator at 37°C for 30 minutes. Using a sharp scalpel blade, cut the film around the section and place the slide in cold water until the film and section float off. Mount on a clean slide, drain, and place in the 37°C incubator until completely dry. Wash gently with butyl acetate, then wash well with xylene, and mount in Clarite.

PREPARATIONS OF BODY FLUIDS FOR MICROSCOPIC STUDY

Material from fluids of the body may be examined either by smear techniques or by the preparation of tissue blocks. Which of these procedures will be used will depend on the type of specimen and on the experience and expertise of the person who will examine the preparations.

Cervical and Vaginal Smears

These will be taken by the physician or cytotechnologist, and will be fixed immediately in Papanicolaou's fixative, which is equal parts 95% ethanol and ether. Because of the flammability and volatility of this mixture, most laboratories now use 95% ethanol alone. This fixative may also be used for smears of breast and prostatic secretions as well as other fluids. Fixation should be allowed to continue for 15 minutes; longer periods will not be deleterious. Smears may also be fixed by fixatives marketed in spray cans* that usually contain alcohol or ether-alcohol with a small proportion of polyethylene or propylene glycol as a coating agent.

Papanicolaou's Staining

Although the various stains used in Papanicolaou's technique may be made up as directed here, it is advisable for smaller laboratories to purchase them commercially.

Reagents

Harris' Hematoxylin. Prepare as on page 795, using ammonium aluminum sulfate; it may be used with or without glacial acetic acid. Filter into a dark bottle for storage. Filter the working solution regularly and replenish often by adding a small amount of fresh stock so as to maintain uniform staining results. Replace working solution every 1 to 3 weeks, depending on the number of slides being stained.

OG 6

Orange G—0.5 or 1.0% solution in 95% alcohol	100 mL
Phosphotungstic acid	0.015 g

EA 36†

Light green SF yellowish—0.14% in 95% alcohol	45 mL
Bismarck brown Y—0.5% in 95% alcohol	10 mL
Eosin yellowish (water and alcohol-soluble)—0.55% and 95% alcohol	45 mL
Phosphotungstic acid	0.2 g
Lithium carbonate, saturated aqueous solution	1 drop

Procedure

1. Transfer slides directly from alcohol-ether fixative, without drying, to 80% alcohol, and bring down through 70 and 50% alcohols to distilled water.

*Spraycyte, Clay Adams, Parsippany, N.J. 07054; Cyto Prep, Fisher Scientific Co., Pittsburg, Pa. 15219 and Don Mills, Ont. M3A 1A9; Pro-Fix, Scientific Products, Evanston, Ill. 60201.

†EA 50, Ortho Pharmaceutical Corp., Raritan, N.J. 08869, is a stain comparable to EA 36.

2. Stain in Harris' hematoxylin for 4 minutes.

3. Rinse briefly in distilled water. (All rinsing must be gentle—to prevent smears from being washed off slides.)

4. Dip in 0.25% HCl in 50% ethanol about six times (about 20 to 60 seconds).

5. Place in running tap water for 6 minutes.

6. Rinse in distilled water and run through 50%, 70%, and 80%, to 95% alcohol.

7. Stain in OG 6 for 1½ to 4 minutes.

8. Rinse in two changes of 95% alcohol.

9. Stain in EA 36 (or EA 50) for 1½ to 4 minutes.

10. Rinse in three changes of 95% alcohol. Dehydrate in absolute alcohol, followed by equal parts absolute alcohol and xylol; clear in xylol and mount.

Note. When variable times are given, choose that which gives optimal results and adhere to it routinely.

Sputum and Bronchopulmonary Specimens

Fresh early morning specimens of sputum may be delivered to the laboratory unfixed. Smears are made using applicator sticks, especially from blood-flecked areas or solid particles. Alternatively such areas may be flattened on slides by crushing them between two slides using a rotary motion and then moving the slides horizontally away from one another, producing a smeared imprint. Fixation is made in 95% ethanol, and such smears are stained by Papanicolaou's technique.

The patient may also be instructed to cough directly into Brasil's fixative. This will coagulate the specimen, as well as ensuring sterility and prompt fixation. The coagulated material can be processed along with other tissues and sections stained with hematoxylin and eosin (H & E). The fixative dyes the mucus a pale yellow, which assists embedding.

Pleural Fluid and Peritoneal Fluids

The fresh fluid is centrifuged, and from the button of material, smears can be made as described under Sputum. If desired, the specimen can be collected with 300 units of heparin added to each 100 mL of fluid to prevent clotting. Another technique is to add sufficient Brasil's fixative to the fluid shortly after collection and to allow protein to precipitate out. The supernatant fluid is poured off while the precipitate is centrifuged in polypropylene plastic centrifuge tubes. The resultant button of material is processed with other tissues, and sections can be stained with H & E or any special techniques desired.

Gastric Specimens

Gastric specimens are best obtained as brushings by the endoscopist. The smears thus obtained are fixed immediately in 95% ethanol and stained by Papanicolaou's method. Gastric aspirated material is often unsatisfactory for cytological study, since the cells (if present) are destroyed by gastric enzymes before they reach the slides. If aspirated material is to be examined it should be collected in bottles already one-third charged with 95% ethanol and cooled in ice. After fixation, suspicious areas of material are smeared on slides as described under sputum and bronchopulmonary specimens.

Spinal Fluids and Urine

These are usually fluids with few cells in a large amount of fluid that contains relatively little protein. A most elegant method for cytological examination of such fluids is the Millpore* filter technique.

Millipore Filter Technique for Cytology

Principle. Cells are filtered from a fluid through a porous membrane. They are subsequently fixed and stained, and the membrane is cleared and mounted on a slide. The cells on its surface are examined microscopically.

This is a very simple and useful technique for concentrating cells that are thinly dispersed in large volumes of fluid, e.g., urine for cytomegalic inclusions or for cancer cells. Practically no other method has such a high cell yield, and this aspect recommends its use for cerebrospinal and fluid samples. It may also be used for fluids of relatively high protein content, e.g., pleural and ascitic fluids, provided these are heparinized (1 to 3 units per mL) as soon as they are removed from patients. Citrate, oxalate, and EDTH are also satisfactory anticoagulants. Another virtue of the method is the even distribution of cells which it gives.

The filters used are of cellulose acetate and nitrate. For cytological purposes, type SM filter (pore size, 5.0 $\pm$ 1.2 μm) is used. Most popular is the regular 47 mm diameter filter, which has a filtering area of 9.6 cm^2 and can filter a relatively large volume of fluid without giving a crowded cell picture. This may be mounted whole on a 3 by 2 inch slide, using a 50 by 43 mm coverglass, or it may be cut in two and the halves mounted on two separate 3 by 1 inch slides. Rectangular filters (17 by 42 mm) are available and can be mounted on 3 by 1 inch slides; also, 25 and 13 mm round filters are supplied, but these are generally too small for all except very small samples, e.g., 5 mL of CSF or urine.

Specimens should be filtered as soon as possible after they are obtained from patients. If necessary, fluids of low protein content, such as urine, may be preserved for several hours by mixing with equal quantities of 50% ethanol. Addition of stronger preservatives will only lead to clogging of the filters with partly coagulated proteins. Filtration pressures should not exceed 100 mm Hg so as to avoid distortion of cells by their being partly pulled into the filter's pores. Millipore stresses that the important maneuver is to break the vacuum just as the last portion of the sample passes the filter surface. If the vacuum is not broken, air will be drawn through and will cause distortion and drying of cells. The Millipore data manual also recommends washing the filter immediately after specimen filtration by drawing 10 to 20 mL of 0.85% saline (prefiltered) through it. This washes through much if not most of the protein that has adhered to the filter. The specimen is then fixed by 95% ethanol. The cells may be stained by Papanicolaou's method or some other technique or modification. The filter with the stained cells is then dehydrated through graded alcohols and cleared in xylol. Finally it is immersed in Permount and then placed on a slide and

*Millipore, Bedford, Mass. 01730 and Mississauga, Ont. L4V 1M5.

coverslipped. The cells are seen against a filter background that is clear (transparent).

Procedure

1. Take a 47-mm SM Millipore filter and on its periphery write the serial accession number of the specimen in duplicate, using an indelible ballpoint pen.

2. Immerse the filter in 95% ethanol for 30 to 60 seconds to expand it.

3. Moisten the screen or fritted glass base of the filtration apparatus with 0.85% saline or Polysal and then center the preexpanded filter on it, numbered side upward. Now clamp the funnel portion to the base and filtration flask of the assembly.

4. Add 5 to 15 mL of Polysal to the funnel; then add specimen.

5. Apply vacuum (-100 mm Hg) until about 2 to 5 mL remains in the funnel (forming a thin layer of fluid on the filter). Then rinse the funnel well with 20 to 30 mL Polysal and continue vacuum filtration until the filter is just covered by a thin layer of fluid. Add 10 to 15 mL of 95% ethanol to the funnel and continue filtering to effect initial fixation of the material on the filter.

6. Apply filtration until only a very thin layer of fluid covers the filter. Then disconnect vacuum.

7. Remove the filter and place for at least 30 minutes in a Petri dish of 95% ethanol, numbered side up.

8. Other fluids, such as sputum and joint aspirates, may be treated so as to adapt them to filtration, and further information is obtainable from the Millipore Corporation (Exfoliative Cytology—Application Report AR–24).

Notes

1. The filter is numbered in duplicate, since it will be bisected for mounting.

2. To mark the filter use a pencil that will resist the processing to follow.

3. If the screen or fritted glass base is not premoistened the filter will cling to it and be difficult to center. The screen base is preferred to the fritted glass base as it permits more rapid filtration, does not become clogged, and is easier to clean.

4. Polysal* is superior to physiological saline. As with all fluids used in Millipore filtration, it is advisable to prefilter the saline or Polysal through a Millipore filter to remove particulate matter.

5. The volume of specimen per filter and the degree of its dilution depend on its protein and cell content. For clear fluids of low protein content, one may use up to 30 mL per filter; for very cellular, bloody, or high-protein fluids, not more than 5 mL per filter should be used, and this should be diluted with at least 30 mL of Polysal. Generally speaking, the only fluids that may be filtered without Polysal dilution (disregarding the 5 to 15 mL added initially to the funnel) are cerebrospinal fluid and urine. In the case of urine, it is advisable to test for protein (p. 209); if there is more than a trace of protein, dilute with Polysal. Ample dilution of protein-rich fluids aids in washing the protein through the filter pores and therefore ensures a clear background in the final stained preparation.

6. The filter must never be allowed to become dry, since this would ruin cytological detail. It must be emphasized that the filter still appears moist when its surface is dry and fluid is present only in its interstices.

*Cutter Laboratories, Berkeley, Calif. 94710, and Pointe Claire, Que. H9R 1G6.

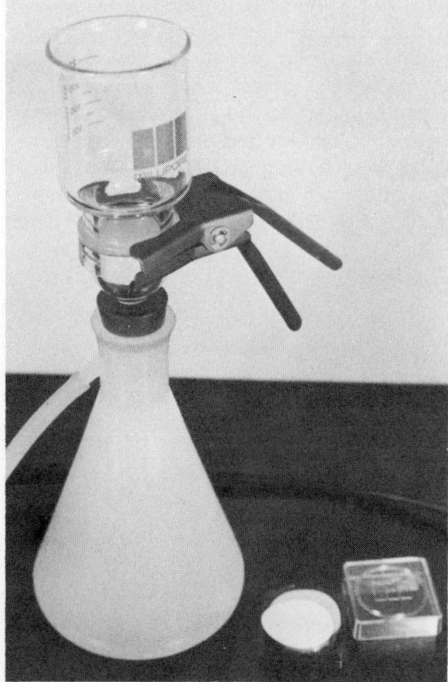

Figure 32–14 The apparatus necessary for Millipore filtration. The tube from the flask leads to a source of vacuum. To the right is a box of the filters. (Millipore, Bedford, Mass. 01730, and Mississauga, Ont. L4V 1M5.)

HANDLING AND EMBEDDING SMALL TISSUE FRAGMENTS

Minute fragments of tissue, e.g., bronchial biopsies, thin-needle biopsies, endoscopy fragments, and so forth may be lost through the perforations of tissue buttons. They may be wrapped in a small piece of cigarette or lens paper to prevent such an occurrence or may, subsequent to fixation, be embedded in 2% agar, which is solid at room temperature. The agar "block" may then be processed with other tissues.

A method for the processing of marrow fragments is described on p. 767. Another method that also may be used for marrow or similar small fragments, such as those from the needle biopsy of lung, is as follows (Bussolati, 1982).

Celloidin* flocks are soaked in absolute alcohol and then dissolved in ether to obtain a 10% solution in absolute alcohol-ether (1:1).

Celloidin bags are prepared by pouring this solution to the top of polypropylene plastic centrifuge tubes. The celloidin is then poured back into its jar and the tubes left draining upside down for a short while, after which a thin film of celloidin (20 to 50 μ thick) is left coating the inner aspect of the tube. The latter is filled with

*Chroma Gesellschaft Schmid Co., Stuttgart-Untertürkheim, W. Germany.

chloroform and stoppered. Immediately before use the chloroform is discarded and the material under study is placed inside the tube, which is then centrifuged. The supernatant is then discarded, and celloidin is peeled from the inner aspect of the tube to form a bag in which the sediment is already lodged. The excess of celloidin is discarded, and the bag with its content is dyed quickly in 1% alcoholic eosin before processing through paraffin. Staining subsequently may be with H & E or with other stains as required. The celloidin does not interfere with any processing or staining.

CHAPTER 32—REVIEW QUESTIONS

Review questions for Chapter 32 are included with those for Chapter 33 and will be found on p. 811.

STAINING PROCEDURES IN HISTOTECHNOLOGY

INTRODUCTION

If unstained sections of tissue are examined under the microscope with transmitted light, very little detail other then nuclear and cell boundaries can be identified. Dyeing or staining of the sections enables one to study and see the physical characteristics and relationships of the tissues and of their constituent cells. This is all the more possible since different tissues, and indeed different components of the cell, display differing affinities for most dyes or stains. These differences in staining are explicable on the basis of variations in physicochemical structure and composition of cells and tissues. However, histochemistry, the special branch of histology that attempts identification of cell and tissue components by virtue of specific chemical reactions, is of relatively recent development, and routine staining makes little pretense to such precise definition. Rather, its purpose is that of outlining the tissue and cellular components so that the trained pathologist or histologist may be able to identify tissue and to establish the presence or absence of disease processes. Such examination is facilitated if two contrasting stains are used, e.g., hematoxylin, which stains the nuclear detail, and eosin or phloxine, which bring into evidence the cytoplasmic detail of the cell and the tissue structure. Accordingly, the most commonly used routine staining method in histopathology is the hematoxylin-eosin sequence.

Before dealing with the technique of staining one should understand the different terms used in this aspect of histology.

STAINING AND IMPREGNATION

Cell and tissue components can be demonstrated not only by the use of stains but also by *impregnation*. These two methods differ in some respects. For example, in staining, the cells and tissue components combine with the active coloring agent so that no particulate dye is seen and the tissues remain relatively transparent, unless very deeply stained. Impregnation, on the other hand, makes use of the salts of heavy metals, which are precipitated with selectivity on certain cellular and tissue components. The impregnation method has its greatest application in tissue from the nervous system, but is also used for the demonstration of reticulin and, in the case of osmium tetroxide, for outlining fine intracellular structure. Broadly speaking, impregnation differs from staining in that it consists of an opaque particulate precipitate. However, this distinction is not absolute and, in the final analysis, impregnation displays many of the characteristics of true staining. Thus, osmium tetroxide combines with tissue components in an active chemical manner. Again, silver nitrate, which is the most commonly used agent for impregnation, can behave as a stain and can outline the tissue elements in a nonparticulate union.

Specific Staining

This is the basis of histochemistry, in which the identification of certain structures and chemical substances is accomplished by controlled, specific chemical reactions designed to give a final color (staining) at the site or location of the structure or substance in the cells or tissues. Such specific stains have little or no affinity for other tissue elements. Examples of specific staining are hemosiderin with Perls' Prussian blue reaction and polysaccharides with the periodic acid–Schiff technique. Specific demonstration of entities with relatively nonspecific stains may be achieved by the specific removal of an entity by chemical or enzymic methods, e.g., diastase for glycogen.

Direct Staining

This is the staining of tissue by means of simple solutions of dyes.

Indirect Staining

Here the action of the dye is intensified by some other agent, i.e., a mordant. By itself, the dye may stain weakly if at all. The mordant may be incorporated in the staining solution or may be used separately and, generally, has the effect of forming a link between the dye molecule and the tissue element.

Nature of Dye-Tissue Reactions

Most fall within the categories of chemical reactions or adsorption phenomena. The chemical reactions may be relatively nonspecific, e.g., staining of acidic nucleoproteins by basic dyes or of basic cytoplasmic constituents by acid dyes; group-specific, e.g., the PAS reaction; or highly specific, e.g., Perls' Prussian blue reaction for ferric iron. Adsorption involves the attraction and surface fixation of small molecules by large molecules, e.g., staining of dextrans by iodine. Probably, the majority of routine staining techniques represent a combination of chemical reactions and adsorption. A third principle involves differential solubilities and is the basis of staining lipids with alcoholic solutions of such dyes as oil red O and the Sudans, where the dye is more soluble in the fat than it is in the solvent in which it is employed (see also pp. 792 and 809).

COLOR

For the human eye the range of wavelengths in the visible spectrum lies between 400 and 750 nm. The naturally occurring mixture of all wavelengths between these limits gives white light. In the case of transparent and transilluminated objects such as a stained section, the color seen by the microscopist will be a combination of those components of the white light that remain after the selective absorption of light rays by the stained section. Thus, if blue (435 to 480 nm) is absorbed, the color seen will be yellow; if blue-green (490 to 500 nm) is absorbed, the color seen will be red (650 to 750 nm); if yellow (580 to 595 nm) is absorbed, the color seen will be blue.

The Chemical Basis of Color in Dyestuffs

This has been found to consist of certain atomic groupings known as *chromophores* (Gr. "color-bearers"), e.g., NO_2, N=O, N=N, C=C, C=O, C=N, C=S, and the quinonoid group or structure 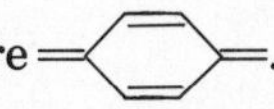 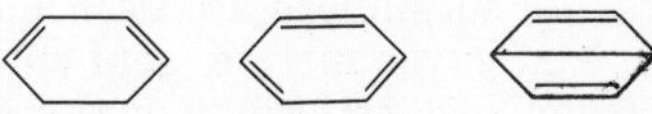. Such groupings introduce "resonance systems" into the molecule. Resonance systems result when a molecular formula can be written in several valid ways; thus:

The rapid change resulting from the presentation of alternate possible states involves the absorption of electromagnetic waves and the production of color. The formula above is that of benzene, which although not colored by white light shows color under ultraviolet. Many substances that could alternate their carbon bonds are colorless by ordinary light, but some molecular configurations are more likely to be colored. It is these systems that selectively absorb light rays and cause color to appear. The introduction of a *chromophoric* group into an uncolored molecule will cause it to be colored; it will then be a *chromogen*, which is colored, but not a dye. For a *chromogen* to be a dye it must be composed of an acid and a base, and therefore have salt-forming properties. This function is performed by a group known as *auxochromes* (Gr. "increasers"), which when attached to the dye molecule act as electron donors to the chromophore. The —OH and —NH_2 groups are the main auxochromes and, by virtue of their ability to dissociate and form compounds, they also serve to bind the dye to the tissues. Carboxyl (—COOH) and sulfonic groups (—SO_3H) may also be auxochromes.

Leuco Forms

Reduction of a colored dye yields a colorless or "leuco" form owing to hydrogenation of its chromophore, with the consequent loss of its resonance system. Schiff's reagent, which is colorless, is not a true leucobase, since it becomes colored on contact with an aldehyde and not by oxidation.

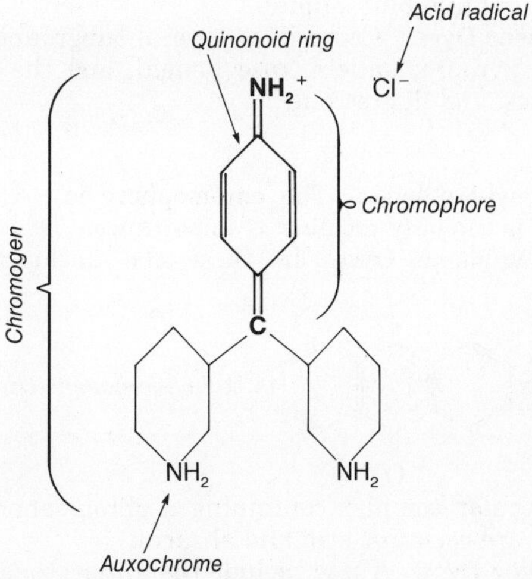

Figure 33–1 Basic fuchsin. The functions and nomenclature of parts of its molecule are illustrated.

Classification of Dyes

Dyes may be classified in a number of ways, e.g., natural or synthetic, or according to their reactions, tissue affinities, and main applications. Only four natural dyes are used extensively in histopathology. Hematoxylin is the most important; the three others are orcein, carmine, and saffron.

A few inorganic substances are used for staining or impregnation, e.g., silver nitrate, gold chloride, iodine, osmium tetroxide, and potassium permanganate, but, beyond tissue and the few natural dyes already mentioned, all staining agents employed in histological techniques are synthetic aromatic dyes made from coal tar derivatives. These synthetic dyestuffs may be classified in several groups.

Azo Dyes. This is the largest group, whose members are mono- and diazo dyes and are mainly cytoplasmic stains. Most are acid dyes, but a few are neutral or basic. Examples are: orange G, Ponceau de xylidine, chromotrope 2 R, Biebrich scarlet, azocarmine, Janus green, Bismarck brown, Congo red, and the Sudans. The chromophore is —N=N—.

Triphenylmethanes. These contain three aromatic nuclei and are quinonoid dyes in which the chromophore is =N—. They include aniline blue, crystal violet, fast green FCF, acid fuchsin, basic fuchsin, light green, patent blue, malachite green, gentian violet, methyl violet, pararosaniline, Victoria blue 4 R, and methyl green.

Thiazine Dyes. In these the chromophores are C—N=C and C—S=C. Members are methylene blue, thionine, toluidine blue, and the azures.

Azine Dyes. These have the chromophore C—N=C, but are also quinonoid dyes. They include neutral red, safranin, and azocarmine B.

Oxazine Dyes. These have the chromophore C—O=C and C—N=C. Examples are brilliant cresyl blue, celestine blue, cresyl violet (cresyl echt violet), and nile blue sulfate.

Xanthene Dyes. Comprising several subgroups, these include pyronin, gallein, rose Bengal, and the eosins, phloxines, and fluoresceins.

Diphenyl-Methanes. The chromophore is —C(=NH)—. Auramine is the only member of importance.

Anthraquinone Dyes. In these the anthraquinone complex is the *chromogen* (compound or molecular complex containing a chromophore). Examples are carminic acid and alizarin.

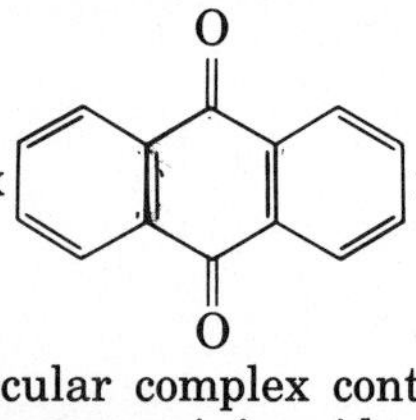

Acridine Dyes. These include the antiseptic acriflavine, but the only member widely used as a stain is acridine orange.

Direct Attachment of Stain to Tissues

In the tissues, there are electrically charged groups, especially the COOH and NH_2 groups of the amino acids. The ionization of these carboxyl and amino groups will depend partly on the pH. At an acid pH the amino groups are more ionized and at an alkaline pH, the carboxyl groups are ionized and the others suppressed. At the pH at which tissues are usually stained, the acid or alkali salt of the particular chromagen has an affinity for cell structures that are relatively alkali or acid, respectively. The process called *adsorption* is a phenomenon in which small particles in a medium are attracted by a larger structure. This phenomenon is affected by the pH of the reacting substances, and it appears that staining, as we know it, depends on both absorption and ionic affinity.

Hydrogen bonding occurs, it is believed, in nonaqueous solutions. Here, tissue hydrogen atoms between two electronegative atoms (oxygen and nitrogen) become attached to a dye. This is a minor method of dye attachment but may occur for example between Best's carmine and glycogen.

Other methods of coloring tissues, such as vital staining (in which a living organism takes up the coloring material) or phagocytosis (in which cells ingest the material) and injection of the colored material into vessels or channels need not concern us here. Subsequently we shall deal with both impregnation of tissues with metals and with histochemical staining, in which color-producing chemical reactions occur between fluid reagents and reactive cell components or contents.

Selective Solubility

Another mechanism of coloring is quite different from that described above. Here, the coloring agent is more soluble in certain tissue elements than in others. A good example of this phenomenon is the use of oil red O in the staining of neutral fat, in which the red material is dissolved unchanged by the fat and does not enter or color other tissue components.

Sulfonation of Dyes

Addition of the SO_3H group will convert a basic dye to an acid one, render an insoluble dye soluble in water, and bind the dye strongly to tissue proteins.

Basic Stains

In these the active or coloring substances is a base and is combined with a colorless acidic radical, e.g., basic fuchsin is the chloride salt of the base rosaniline. The acidic cell structures (chromatin, mucus, cartilage matrix, and so forth) have an affinity for basic dye ions and are therefore regarded as *basophilic*.

Acid Stains

In these it is the acidic radical that is the active, or coloring agent, the basic part being inactive, e.g., acid fuchsin consists of the sodium salt of a sulfonate of rosaniline. The basic cell structures (collagen, granules of eosinophil leukocytes, and so forth) have an affinity for the acidic dye ions and are regarded as *acidophilic*.

Neutral Dyes

These consist of mixtures of basic and acid dyes and, therefore, usually of large molecular complexes that are very sparingly soluble in water and usually must be dissolved in alcohol. Examples are the Romanowsky dyes used in hematology. Both acid and basic components retain their affinities for cell constituents of opposite reaction, and the whole compound dye stains neutrophilic structures.

STORAGE, IDENTIFICATION, AND MAINTENANCE OF DYES

Dyes are generally purchased in solid form and should be labeled with the date of receipt. They should be stored in a cool dark or shaded area in airtight bottles. In a solid form the dyes generally keep well, but if there is any suspicion that an old sample is inadequate then it should be subjected to quality control.

When stains are made up, distilled water should be used unless instructions specifically demand otherwise. An accurate balance and pure chemicals should be used in the formulation of dyes. When the latter are made, they should be kept in glass bottles with glass or plastic stoppers, and dark glass containers must be provided if necessary. The bottles are kept in a cool place and should be properly labeled. Filtering may be required before use.

Since the knowledge of dyes is very ancient, much of the nomenclature is confusing. This is especially so because dyes are used industrially as well as in biology. Many dyes are used that have several names, Brilliant crystal scarlet 6R, acid red 44, and crystal ponceau 6R are synonymous. However, they will all have one color index number, and to avoid confusion this number should be used to order dyes and should be present on the manufacturer's label along with the lot number. Should the stain not perform adequately, although it is of the correct color index, another lot number of the dye from another manufacturer should be tested. If the latter is satisfactory, the poor lot number of the dye should be brought to the attention of the supplier.

PROGRESSIVE AND REGRESSIVE STAINING

Staining with hematoxylin (and many other dyes also) may be of two types. In progressive staining, staining is continued until the desired intensity of coloring of the different tissue elements is attained.

In regressive staining the tissues are overstained and the excess dye is then removed selectively until the desired intensity is obtained.

METACHROMASIA

Most dyestuffs stain tissues orthochromatically, i.e., in shades of their own (the dyestuffs') color. Certain dyes, however, also stain certain tissues in a color or hue that is quite different from that of the stain itself.

Dyes Having Metachromatic Properties

These are all basic dyes of the aniline type and most actually belong to the thiazine group; the others are triphenylmethanes or azo dyes. They are:

Thionine	Crystal violet
New methylene blue	Methyl violet
Azure C	Safranine
Azure A	Azure B
Toluidine blue	

The ones most commonly employed are toluidine blue and thionine.

The property of metachromasia depends on (1) the dye and (2) the characteristics of the tissue components that unite with the dye to exhibit metachromasia. All metachromatic dyes are cationic, and their peculiar tinctorial properties almost certainly depend on their tendency to polymerize. Simply stated, the primary color of the dye is the result of the preponderance of the monomeric (single molecular) form in solution. Taking toluidine blue as an example, the color of a simple molecular solution is blue, and as dimers and trimers increase in number it becomes violet; finally, the full red metachromatic color is due to polymers of the basic dye molecule. It appears that all tissue components showing metachromasia are made up of large anionic molecules containing sulfate, phosphate, or carboxylic acid radicals in abundance. The acidic polysaccharides are the main group of substances of this nature and occur in the ground substance of cartilage (chondroitin sulfate) and in connective tissue mucin (acid mucopolysaccharides); heparin in mast cell granules is also an acid polysaccharide. Molecules of such substances, bearing SO_3H, PO_4, or COOH groups not more than 0.6 nm apart, exhibit metachromasia presumably because (1) these groups bind the basic dyes as salts and (2) these acidic groups are close enough to permit secondary bonding between the dye molecules so bound, i.e., polymerization of the bound dye. Water is essential for this union, which may be prevented by agents that interfere with the acidic radicals on the chromotropes. Though it may be preferable to employ frozen sections of fresh or rapidly fixed tissues, sections of formalin or formol-$HgCl_2$-fixed tissues are perfectly satisfactory.

Practical Considerations

In practice, metachromatic dyes are used in 0.1% (or less) concentration in 30% ethanol, or as 0.1 to 1% aqueous solutions. Care should be exercised not to overstain, as this may lead to the metachromatic being obscured by orthochromatic staining; less than one minute is adequate for most methods. Each batch of stain should be tested for polychromatic contaminants. Toluidine blue is one of the least objectionable in this regard, but other dyes, e.g., thionine, may contain impurities that stain in different colors, a phenomenon that may be mistaken for metachromasia.

Reversal and Induction of Metachromasia

Although true metachromasia—certainly that owing to ester sulfates—is probably not extracted or reversed by dehydration in alcohols, it is advisable to process a second section in parallel and to mount this in water or Apathy's syrup. Methylation abolishes metachromasia. As might be expected, sulfation induces metachromasia in tissue components that are not normally metachromatic, e.g., reticulin, basement membranes, and gastric and Brunner's gland mucins, and in thyroid and pituitary colloid.

PRINCIPLES OF HEMATOXYLIN STAINING

Hematoxylin is a natural dye that is extracted from the core or heartwood of the tree *Haematoxylon campechianum*. This tree was originally found in the state of Campeche in Mexico, where the native population was familiar with its properties as a dye. Nowadays, the tree is grown commercially, mainly in Jamaica. When they are about ten years old the trees are felled, the bark and sapwood (outer layers) are stripped off, and the heartwood is exported in logs about three feet long—hence the name "logwood." The logs are cut into fine chips for extraction, and the dye so obtained is used not only by microscopists but also in the dyeing of silks and wool. Indeed, for years its only use was in the textile industry until Waldeyer firmly established its use in histology in 1862.

The natural extract obtained from the logs (hematoxylon) is not an active dyestuff; it must first be oxidized to the active principle, i.e., hematein. In this process of oxidative conversion to hematein, hematoxylon loses two hydrogen atoms and assumes a quinonoid arrangement in one of its rings. Spontaneous oxidation occurs very slowly in watery or alcoholic solution, and it takes 3 to 4 months for this to be satisfactorily accomplished. This process of oxidation is known as "ripening," and it can be effected almost instantaneously by chemical oxidants such as mercuric oxide, sodium iodate, potassium permanganate, hydrogen peroxide, and calcium hypochlorite. During the process of oxidation compounds other than hematein are produced, and some of these are also active in staining, although hematein is the chief active ingredient. It should be understood that a ripened hematoxylin stain is a mixture of hematoxylin, hematein, active oxidation products of hematein and hematoxylon, and inactive ultraoxidation products. Excessive oxidation (over-ripening) leads to the production of a number of compounds, most of which are colorless and useless. *It is, therefore, essential that the correct amount of oxidant be used in making up hematoxylin stains* (naturally, the least amount of oxidant used, consistent with satisfactory staining, the longer will be the life of the stain):

Quantity of Hematoxylin	Type and Amount of Oxidant for Ripening	
1.0 g	Mercuric oxide (HgO)*	0.5 g
1.0 g	Sodium iodate ($NaIO_3 \cdot H_2O$)	0.05–0.15 g
1.0 g	Potassium permanganate ($KMnO_4$)	0.175 g
1.0 g	Hydrogen peroxide (H_2O_2), U.S.P.	2.0 mL
1.0 g	Potassium periodate (KIO_4)	0.05 g

*HgO: Either the red or yellow oxides.

For the reasons already given it is always preferable to use hematoxylin and not hematein in making up these stains, since solutions of commercial hematein become oxidized very easily and are unreliable in staining effect and lasting qualities.

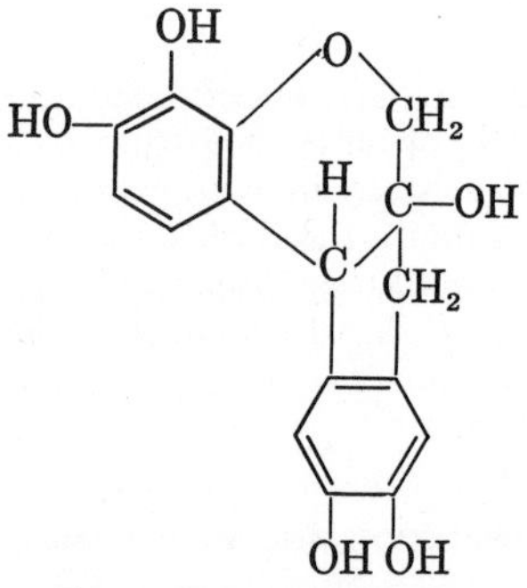

Figure 33–2 Hematoxylin.

MORDANTS AND HEMATEIN

Without a mordant hematein is almost useless, being a weak amber dye that stains an amber color. Mordants are substances that, by their physicochemical structure, aid in attaching a stain or dye to the tissues. They are essential to hematoxylin staining, for which the mordants used are always divalent or trivalent salts or hydroxides of metals. They probably combine as hydroxides with the dye by displacing a hydrogen atom from it, and their remaining valences serve to attach or bind the dye-mordant complex to the tissue components, especially to the phosphate groups of nucleic acids. The complex of stain and mordant is called a "lake." Salts of aluminum, iron, chromium, copper, molybdenum, and vanadium may all be used as mordants and, although simple salts such as sulfates and chlorides will do, the alum salts are most commonly used because they were more readily available in the earlier days and, therefore, have the sanction of tradition. Alums are double salts, i.e., one molecule of ammonium, sodium, or potassium sulfate crystallized with one molecule of the sulfate salt of a trivalent metal and 24 molecules of water. Potash alum (potassium aluminum sulfate, or simply "alum") is $K_2SO_4 \cdot Al_2(SO_4)_3 \cdot 24H_2O$. Iron alum (ferric ammonium sulfate) is $(NH_4)_2SO_4 \cdot Fe(SO_4)_3 \cdot 24H_2O$. Ammonium alum (aluminum ammonium sulfate) is $(NH_4)_2SO_4 \cdot Al_2(SO)_4)_3 \cdot 24H_2O$.

Aluminum salts give a blue lake, and increasing the amount of the aluminum salt increases the selectivity for nuclei, especially if acid is added or is used as a

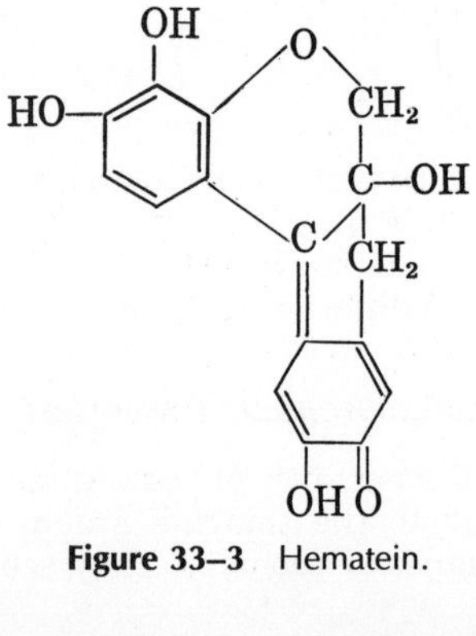

Figure 33–3 Hematein.

differentiating agent. The dye lake obtained when ferric salts are used as mordants is an intense blue-black one.

The use of mordants is not confined to hematoxylin stains and, although the salts listed are the most important mordants, they are not the only ones used in histology. Mordants do not have to be incorporated with the stain. Premordanting may be accomplished during fixation; e.g., mercurial or picric acid fixatives also act as mordants (premordants) for Mallory's phosphomolybdic and phosphotungstic acid methods for connective tissue. In some stains and staining methods a special mordant bath is incorporated in the technique, e.g., the ferric ammonium sulfate bath used in Heidenhain's iron hematoxylin.

Accentuators

These are chemical substances that heighten the color intensity, crispness, and selectivity of a stain. They differ from mordants in that they do not bind or link the dye to the tissue. Some appear to act as chemicophysical catalysts; others (e.g., aniline, and phenol) seem to work simply by reducing surface tension. Examples of accentuators are phenol in carbolthionine, aniline used with gentian violet, and potassium hydroxide used in Löffler's methylene blue. A rather special application of accentuators (here called "accelerators") is the use of certain hypnotic drugs such as barbital (Veronal), and chloral hydrate, in methods for the metallic impregnation of nerve fibers.

Differentiation

As mentioned already, staining with hematoxylins and with many other dyes may be (1) progressive or (2) regressive. In the latter method the excess stain is removed selectively until the right intensity is attained. The designation "selectively" derives from the fact that when the excess dye is removed it is cleared from certain cell constituents before others, or while other cell structures are still strongly stained. This process of selective removal of excess dye is called differentiation. However, in some staining techniques, e.g., with Romanowsky dyes, differentiation also implies the selective production of certain colors at specific pH values. The acid-alcohol bath in the routine Harris hematoxylin staining method is an example of simple differentiation used in a regressive staining technique. Generally, if the dye used is a basic one, differentiation is carried out by an acid solution, whereas an alkaline medium is used for differentiation after an acidic dye. However, for many dyes, both basic and acidic but especially the former, alcohol acts as a fairly efficient differentiator and probably acts by simply dissolving out the excess dye.

The fact that basic dyes stain chromatin rather selectively (union of basic dye with acidic nucleo-proteins) and that acid dyes stain the cytoplasm in a similarly selective fashion may make the use of differentiators seem superfluous to the beginner. However, the selectivity in these cases is not absolute, and basic dyes also stain the cytoplasm to some degree. Hence, in most cases differentiation is necessary. It is essential, though it is usually used after aluminum mordants because of the selectivity of these for nuclear staining.

Differentiators for mordant dyes may be divided into three classes: acids, oxidizers, and mordants.

Acid Differentiators

These act by combining with the metal, thus breaking the latter's union with the tissue or cell components. The acid chosen should be one that forms a soluble salt with the metal so that the latter is dissolved out. Examples are hydrochloric and acetic acids.

Oxidizing Differentiators

These act by oxidizing the dye to a colorless substance (leuco form). Components holding least dye will be bleached first. Examples are potassium ferricyanide, potassium permanganate, chromic acid, picric acid, and potassium dichromate. The last three are weak and slow differentiators.

Mordant Differentiators

The apparent paradox of a substance on the one hand binding a dye to the tissue, and on the other hand removing this same dye from its combination with the tissue, is explained in part by the phenomenon of mass action. When a section that has been stained by a mordant dye is placed in a solution of mordant, the latter is present in great excess and the dye gradually leaves the tissue to combine with the free mordant in solution. Also, mordants such as iron alum oxidize hematoxylin to a soluble colorless compound. Accordingly, the tissue components that contain the least dye will be decolorized first, and the structures containing most dye (nuclear chromatin) will still be deeply stained. This heavy staining of the chromatin results from the fact that the dye-mordant complexes are basic and unite preferentially with the acidic nuclear structures, especially if salts of aluminum are used as mordant.

Differentiators as Decolorizers

From the foregoing it follows that if a section that has been stained by a mordant dye is allowed to remain long enough in a differentiator, e.g., 1 to 2% acid alcohol, all the dye will be removed. Indeed, this is actually done as a preliminary step in the restaining of a faded slide. Accordingly, in routine staining, care must be taken that sections are not left too long in differentiators. The times stated under the various methods in this text are approximate; exact times must be established for each procedure by trial and error and by microscopic control.

Preparation of Alum Hematoxylins

Harris's Hematoxylin

In 1000 mL of distilled water in a large (3 to 4 liter) Erlenmeyer flask dissolve 100 g of ammonium or potassium alum by heating and shaking. Bring to 60°C; add a solution of 5 g of hematoxylin in 50 mL of absolute ethyl alcohol and bring rapidly to the boil. When it begins to boil remove from flame and add 2.5 g of mercuric oxide (red or yellow). Mix by swirling gently. The solution immediately becomes purple, and most workers suggest that the solution should then be immediately cooled by plunging the container into a sink filled with cold water. However, Lynch found that it was advantageous to continue heating, after addition of the mercuric oxide, for 1 to 3 minutes, sampling the color every half minute by streaking some on filter paper with a glass rod. The deep purple of the correctly ripened solution will soon be recognized and the formula should then be cooled rapidly. The oxidation or ripening here is artificial, being effected by the mercuric oxide. It will be found that it is convenient to add this rolled up loosely in a small (5 cm) circle of filter paper, thus preventing the mercuric oxide from sticking to the neck of the container. When cool, 20 to 40 mL of glacial acetic acid is added and the stain filtered before using. Since most of the alcohol is evaporated in the process of boiling, one may add 50 mL of ethyl alcohol to the final solution; it helps to prevent the growth of molds.

Harris's hematoxylin is a good regressive stain, easily made up and immediately ready for use. It is usually stable for about 6 months. The acid gives stability to the stain and improves nuclear staining. The staining time for Harris's hematoxylin varies between 4 and 30 minutes, depending on the batch of stain, its age, the nature of the tissue, and the depth of staining required. It is almost invariably used regressively. Best results are obtained if the formula is made up every 2 to 3 months. The precipitate that forms with age should be filtered off before use.

Mayer's Hemalum

One gram of hematoxylin is dissolved with vigorous shaking (in a stoppered flask or test tube) in 10 to 15 mL of absolute (or 90%) ethyl alcohol and is then added to 1000 mL of distilled water. Alternatively, the hematoxylin is dissolved overnight in the water or with the aid of gentle heat. This solution is ripened artificially and immediately by adding 0.05 to 0.15 g of sodium iodate ($NaIO_3$). Fifty grams of ammonium or potassium alum is then added and the solution is shaken until all the alum is dissolved. Citric acid, 1.0 g, is usually added at this stage; however, the addition of 20 mL glacial acetic acid seems to give better nuclear staining and a more stable solution. To the final solution, 50 mL of chloral hydrate may be added as a preservative. The life period of this stain is one of its greatest drawbacks; it keeps for only 3 to 6 months at the most.

Blueing

Alum (potassium aluminum sulfate) in watery solution tends to dissociate: the aluminum combines with the —OH of the water to form insoluble aluminum hydroxide, $Al(OH)_3$; the free hydrogen from the water tends to form sulfuric acid by uniting with the sulfate from the alum. However, if excess of acid (sulfuric or other acid) is present, the aluminum hydroxide cannot form. Under such circumstances, in an alum hematoxylin dye the insoluble dye lake cannot form because of lack of hydroxyl ions. Hence acid solutions of alum hematoxylin are reddish in color, whereas the aluminum lake of hematein is blue. In the blueing of sections that have been stained by an alum hematoxylin the alkaline solution used for blueing neutralizes the free acid and makes hydroxyl groups available so that the insoluble blue aluminum-hematein-tissue lake is formed. Accordingly, for blueing of alum-hematoxylin–stained sections warm (40 to 50°C) tap water is commonly used, since it is generally sufficiently alkaline. However, in many areas the tap water is acid and is unsuitable. In such regions lithium carbonate (1% w/v in water), bicarbonate (0.2 to 0.5% w/v in tap water), potassium or sodium acetate may be used. Alternatively, Scott's tap water substitute may be employed: sodium or potassium bicarbonate, 2 to 3.5 g, and magnesium sulfate, 20 g, dissolved separately, then combined and made up to 1000 mL with distilled water. (A few crystals of thymol or 5 to 10 mL of commercial formaldehyde [40%] solution are added to prevent the growth of molds.) The use of ammonia (0.5 to 1% in 80% alcohol) is deprecated by many because it may be "hard" on delicate tissues and will loosen sections from the slides. One per cent aqueous lithium carbonate and 1% alcoholic ammonia are good blueing agents following acid differentiations, but Scott's tap water substitute is preferable. If the acid is not completely neutralized, the stain is liable to fade rather rapidly. Also, blueing with ammonia, lithium carbonate, or Scott's tap water substitute has the added advantage of rapidity (about 15, 30, and 60 seconds, respectively, as against 5 to 15 minutes required for warm tap water). Lithium carbonate has a tendency to form crystalline deposits unless the slides are agitated in it and well washed afterwards.

Eosins, Eosin Staining, and Substitutes

Eosins are acid xanthene or phthalein dyes. The common members of this group of commercial dyes are eosin Y, eosin B, phloxine, and erythrosin (halogenated with iodine instead of the bromine of eosin). Eosin itself derives its name from its dawnlike color, and the "Y" stands for yellowish, which is its predominant shade of red. Eosin is most commonly used as a background or contrast stain because it gives a pleasing and useful contrast to nuclear stains such as hematoxylin.

The most frequently used of the eosins is eosin Y (solubility 44% w/v in water and 2% w/v in ethanol). Stock aqueous solutions are generally made up in 1% w/v concentration; a large crystal of thymol or 0.25 mL of 40% formaldehyde is added to each 100 mL of stock to prevent the growth of molds. The aqueous stain is usually used as the 1% solution for ¼ to 3 minutes, depending on the tissue, type of fixative (slightly longer time required after formalin than after Zenker), and intensity of color desired. The alcoholic solution (1% w/v) is made by dissolving 1 g in 20 mL distilled water and adding 80 mL of absolute or 95% ethanol. This may be diluted for use with 80% ethanol to give 0.25% or 0.5%, or it may be used undiluted. Addition of 0.2 mL

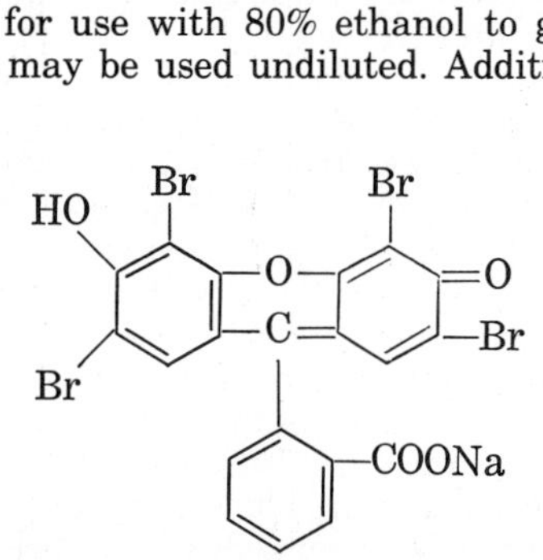

HO Br Br O O Br Br C COONa

Figure 33–4 Eosin (tetrabromofluorescein). In eosin Y the—OH is replaced by NaO—. In enthyl eosin the—OH is replaced by KO—, and the NaOOC by $H_5C_2 \cdot OOC$.

of glacial acetic acid, *or* 0.25 g tannic acid, to each 100 mL aqueous solution (up to 0.5 mL glacial acetic per 100 mL of alcoholic solution) makes eosin staining more intense and selective.

Eosin is the most widely employed cytoplasmic counterstain in hematoxylin techniques, but several substitutes are available, e.g., phloxine, erythrosin, azophloxin, Biebrich scarlet, and orange G—all in concentrations and modes similar to eosin.

Microscopic Control of Staining

From the outset, every student should develop the habit of controlling even the simplest staining procedures by microscopic examination during or after each step.

Hematoxylin Staining in Practice

The section when cut and mounted on the slide must first be drained and then thoroughly dried. The process of drying ensures the evaporation of all moisture between the section and slide, so that the section is brought completely into contact with the slide surface at all points and is thus firmly attached to it by surface tension and capillary attraction. If drying is not thoroughly accomplished, the section (or part of it) is likely to become detached during staining, most likely after the use of the acid differentiator, and especially in the case of bone and nervous tissue.

Since all stains are used in solution, usually aqueous, occasionally alcoholic, the section must be so treated that all parts of it are in the same phase as, and in contact with, the solvent medium of the stain. In the case of paraffin sections the wax must first be removed by xylene (two baths, each of 3 to 5 minutes). The xylene is, in turn, removed by passing through two baths of absolute alcohol (each of 2 minutes). The sections are then brought through "down-graded" alcohol baths: one bath of 95% alcohol for 2 minutes, followed by 2 minutes in 75 to 80% alcohol. If the stain to be employed is in alcohol solution, the sections are transferred directly into it from the alcohol baths. However, since most routine stains are in aqueous solutions the section must be taken from the 75 or 80% alcohol and placed in running tap water or in distilled water for about 1 minute before staining is begun.

Routine Hematoxylin-Eosin Stain

Procedure

1. The sections are arranged in a suitable bottomless, glass slide carrier, one slide to each slot. Immerse in the first xylene bath for 3 minutes.

2. Transfer to second xylene bath for 2 to 3 minutes. Excess solution should always be drained off by tilting the slide carrier and scraping it on the edge of the trough.

3. Immerse in the first bath of absolute ethyl alcohol for 2 minutes. If a second bath of absolute alcohol is included the sections may be passed through it very quickly, or it may be skipped altogether when bringing sections down to water.

4. Immerse in a bath of 95% ethyl alcohol for 1 or 2 minutes. (If a mercurial fixative has been used, the mercury must be removed in a 0.5% solution of iodine in 80 to 95% alcohol. Following this, the section should be rinsed in water and the iodine removed by placing for 1 to 5 minutes in 3% sodium thiosulfate solution [$Na_2S_2O_3 \cdot 5H_2O$], after which the section must be washed well by placing in running water for 3 to 5 minutes. Alternatively, mercury deposits may be removed after the sections are hydrated—by immersing in Gram's or Lugol's iodine for 5 minutes, followed by sodium thiosulfate and washing. Sections of mercurial fixed tissues are then ready for staining.)

5. Rinse in running water for about 1 minute, and then briefly in distilled water.

6. Stain 4 to 8 minutes in alum hematoxylin (e.g., Harris's).

7. Differentiate (after a quick rinse in water) by dipping three or four times (about 3 to 10 seconds) in 1% acid alcohol (1 mL conc HCl to 99 mL of 80% ethyl alcohol).

8. Rinse in water.

9. Blue by placing in Scott's tap water substitute *or* 1% aqueous lithium carbonate until the sections appear blue (about 30 seconds for the lithium and 1 minute for Scott's tap water substitute).

10. Rinse well in water.

11. Stain in acidified 1% aqueous eosin Y for ¼ to 2 minutes, depending on intensity desired; *or* rinse briefly in 80% ethanol and then stain for ½ to 3 minutes in acidified 0.5 or 1.0% eosin Y in 80% ethanol.

12. If aqueous eosin has been used, rinse briefly in water. If alcoholic eosin has been used, washing in running tap water for ½ to 2 minutes differentiates the eosin staining.

13. Dehydrate by passing through three or four baths of absolute ethanol with agitation; 10 to 20 seconds in each bath will suffice.

14. Pass through two or three baths of xylene, about 15 to 20 seconds in each.

15. Mount in Permount, Clarite, Malinol, or other suitable mountant.

Results. Using Harris's hematoxylin: Nuclei—blue. Bone and calcium—similar to nuclei but more brown and less intense. Erythrocytes, muscle, and eosinophil granules—bright red. Cytoplasm, proteins in edema fluid, and so forth—pale pink.

Preparation of Iron Hematoxylins

In contrast to the blue ammonium lake of hematein, the ferric lake is a deep blue-black or black. Ferric salts oxidize or ripen hematoxylin quickly, so that ripening, either artificial or natural, is not of great importance with iron hematoxylin stains. In mixtures of hematoxylin and ferric salts the insoluble lake gradually precipitates out, so that premixed stains are not very stable. For this reason, in the study of cytological detail, e.g., chromosomes, spindles, chromatin, mitochondria, and Golgi apparatus, cytologists usually use these in a "sequence" fashion; i.e., the sections, having been brought to water, are mordanted with a water solution of ferric salt and then stained with a simple aqueous solution of hematoxylin to a black color, after which they are differentiated with acid solution or with ferric salt solution to the degree of staining desired in the different components. This procedure, however, is a laborious one for routine work, in which one of the combined solution methods is usually employed. If acid or excess of mordant is present, these dyes behave like basic dyes, and progressive methods of staining may then be employed. Iron hematoxylins have found their greatest use in the study of fine cellular detail and are invaluable for this because they give very sharp, crisp staining; differentiation can be finely and accurately controlled; they give excellent results for photography; and the staining is most stable.

Solutions prepared with correct or optimal amounts of iron salts are used for dense, regressive staining (e.g., myelin methods). Addition of acid or of excess of ferric salt gives a stain that is more selective for nuclei. Lillie gives the optimal amount of iron as 0.5 g metallic iron (4.32 g iron alum, 2.419 g $FeCl_3 \cdot 6H_2O$, or 3.9 mL of U.S.P. solution or iron chloride) for each 1 g of hematoxylin, and states that doubling the amount of ferric iron in the mixed solution prevents overstaining.

Weigert's Iron Hematoxylin

Stock solution A is 1% w/v hematoxylin in ethanol. The working stain is made by taking 1 vol of solution A and *adding to it* 1 vol of solution B (95 mL distilled water, 4 mL of 29% aqueous $FeCl_3$, and 1 mL of conc. HCl). The stain is stable for not longer than 2 to 3 weeks, during which time its color changes from a deep blue-black-violet, through violet, purple, and brown, to yellowish brown. When turning brown it should be discarded. Sections stained 2 to 6 minutes are washed in tap water and should require no differentiation. However, it may be used regressively by staining for 12 to 30 minutes, followed by washing and differentiation in 0.5% to 1% acid alcohol. Nuclear staining is very sharp, black or blue-black, and fades much more slowly than alum hematoxylins; it also resists picric acid and is therefore very useful in conjunction with van Gieson, which combination is suitable for demonstrating connective tissue elements or *Entamoeba histolytica* in sections.

Procedure

1. **Sections are dewaxed and hydrated.**
2. **Stain 5 to 20 minutes in Weigert's iron hematoxylin.**
3. **Rinse in tap water and examine microscopically.**
4. **Differentiate if necessary in 0.5 or 1.0% HCl in 70% ethanol. Differentiation should not be completed if one plans to counterstain with van Gieson, since the picric acid component will complete the differentiation.**
5. **Wash at least 5 minutes in running tap water.**
6. **Counterstain to suit, e.g., 3 to 5 minutes in van Gieson's picrofuchsin.**
7. **Dehydrate, clear and mount.**

Results. Nuclei are stained blue-black, black, or brownish black; with van Gieson as a counterstain, collagen will be red to crimson, and muscle, fibrin, and red blood cells will be yellow.

CARBOHYDRATE STAINING AND IDENTIFICATION

Carbohydrates are the most important sources of energy for the cells of the body, and for this purpose they are mobilized as monosaccharides. For storage, however, they are polymerized by enzymatic action into polysaccharides. Polysaccharides are also used extensively in various types and chemical combinations—often with peptides, proteins, or lipids—in the formation of the different "cements" of the body (e.g., ground substances of tissues) or in the elaboration of many secretions (e.g., the mucins of mucus and the polysaccharide component of many hormones). Because of their extreme solubility the monosaccharides and disaccharides are lost easily during fixation and are difficult to demonstrate in tissues. The histological and histochemical study of the polysaccharides, however, has contributed greatly to our understanding of tissue structure.

The staining and identification of the various types of polysaccharides are beyond the scope of this work, which will deal only with two varieties: glycogen that is stored normally in the liver, heart, and striated muscle but that may be stored abnormally in disease and neutral mucopolysaccharide, which is the mucus secreted by gastrointestinal tract glands and in the respiratory lining cells. These mucins consist of hexosamines, whereas glycogen is made up of polysaccharides of glucose. Both are stained by the periodic acid–Schiff (PAS) technique.

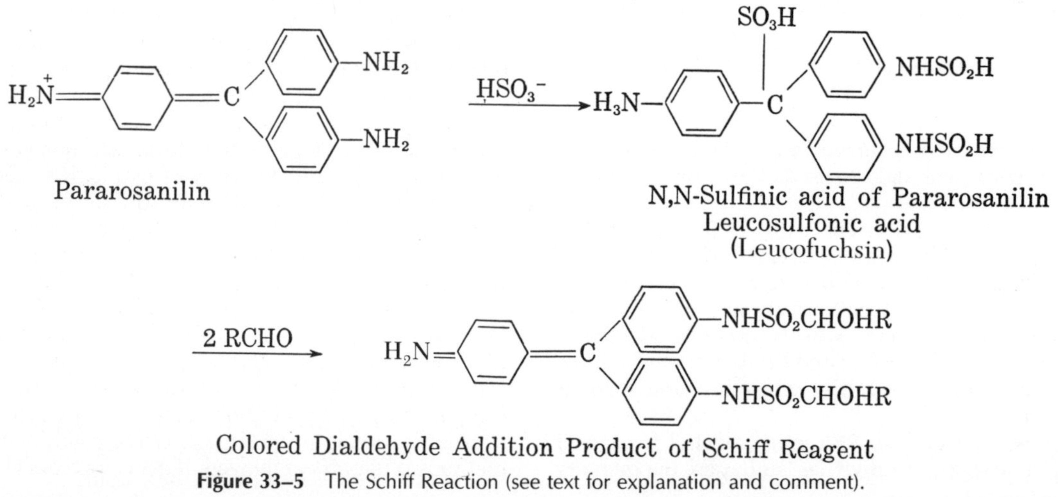

Pararosanilin

HSO_3^- →

N,N-Sulfinic acid of Pararosanilin
Leucosulfonic acid
(Leucofuchsin)

2 RCHO →

Colored Dialdehyde Addition Product of Schiff Reagent

Figure 33–5 The Schiff Reaction (see text for explanation and comment).

Schiff Reagent and Feulgen-Schiff Reaction: Theoretical Basis

Basic fuchsin is a mixture of three dyes of triamino triphenyl methane type, viz., rosanilin, pararosanilin, and magenta II. More than a century ago, H. Schiff (1866) showed that aldehydes restore the magenta color to fuchsin that has been decolorized (leucofuchsin) by sulfur dioxide. Leucofuchsin is colorless because its chromophoric double bond, and therefore its quinonoid structure (resonance system), has been destroyed (Fig. 33–5). Reoxidation, e.g., slowly by exposure to air and light, will restore the double bond and the color.

The quinonoid structure is also restored by aldehydes, but in this case the aldehydic compound is added to the "fuchsin-sulfurous acid compound" and the shade of reddish purple color resulting will be modified slightly by the nature of the additive compound.

The PAS Reaction

In 1928 Malaprade introduced periodic acid (HIO_4) for the chemical estimation of polyalcohols. In 1946 McManus first applied the periodic acid–Schiff reaction in histology. Periodic acid oxidizes compounds having free hydroxyl groups: when the OH groups are next to each other (vicinal), e.g., 1,2-glycols (CHOH · CHOH), the bond between the neighboring carbon atoms that carry the OH groups is broken and a dialdehyde structure is produced. Similarly, periodic acid attacks 1-hydroxy-2-amino substituted alcohols $\left(\begin{array}{ccc} OH & & NH_2 \\ | & & | \\ -C & - & C- \\ | & & | \\ H & & H \end{array}\right)$ and 1-hydroxy-2-alkylamino groups $\left(\begin{array}{ccc} & & R \\ & & | \\ OH & & N-H \\ | & & | \\ -C & - & C- \\ | & & | \\ H & & H \end{array}\right)$. In the case of 1-hydroxy-2-ketogroups $\left(\begin{array}{ccc} HO & & O \\ | & & \| \\ -C & - & C- \\ | & & \\ H & & \end{array}\right)$ the oxidation products are one aldehyde (HCHO) and one carboxyl (COOH) group; in the alpha diketones two carboxyl groups result, and subsequent application of Schiff's reagent gives no color. Obviously, the dialdehydic configuration resulting from the HIO_4 oxidation of glucose will react strongly with Schiff's reagent, and the same applies for galactose, mannose, the methylpentose fucose, and the hexasamines. As a general rule, the intensity of the PAS reaction is proportional to the content of these sugars in the reacting material. Thus, the 1-3 linkage between glucuronic acid and *N*-acetyl-glucosamine in hyaluronic acid prevents oxidation that would produce aldehyde groups; as a result hyaluronic acid is PAS-negative.

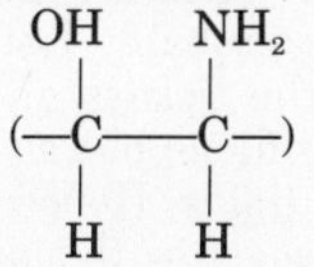

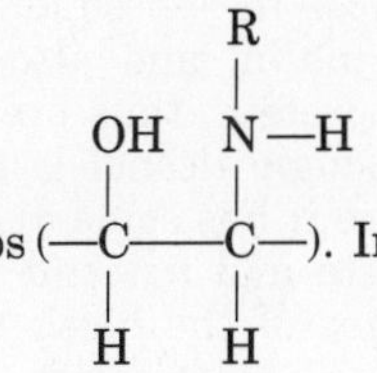

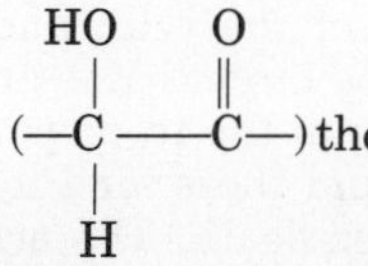

PAS-Positive Substances

Many substances other than glycogen and mucus are PAS positive. They include cartilaginous matrix, the granules of megakaryocytes, phospholipids, colloid of the thyroid gland, and other substances.

THE PAS TECHNIQUE IN PRACTICE

Fixation

Most fixatives except those containing osmic or chromic acids, chromates, and permanganate may be used. The usual fixation time in Zenker's and Helly's fluids, however, gives reasonably satisfactory results, though there is some reduction in the intensity of the reaction owing to chromate oxidation. Routine fixation and decalcification of bone causes considerable loss of PAS positivity.

Choice of Oxidant: Time and Temperature of Oxidation

Many oxidants have been used, e.g., chromic acid, potassium permanganate, lead tetraacetate, sodium bismuthate, manganese triacetate and tetraacetate, osmic acid, and hydrogen peroxide. None of these is as good as periodic acid, which is the most specific for 1,2-glycol, 1-OH-2-amino, 1-OH-2-alkylamino, and 1-OH-2-keto groups; it does not further oxidize the aldehydes formed, and the HIO_3 that results is inert toward them.

Periodic acid ($HIO_4 \cdot 2H_2O$) is generally employed as a 0.5 to 1.0% aqueous solution for 2 to 10 (usually 5) minutes at room temperature, but variations from 0.2 to 2.5% concentration seem to make little difference. The main reactive groups appear to be all oxidized to aldehydes in 5 minutes. Oxidation beyond 10 minutes increases tissue basophilia and methylene blue staining—probably by conversion of sulfhydryl groups to sulfonic acids. Even with the standard 5-minute oxidation the effect of this tissue acidification is seen in the increased affinity of the nuclei, for example, for hematoxylin counterstain. Prolonging the oxidation time may be advantageous in the case of glycolipids, phospholipids, and unsaturated lipids, but if used, a control section should be subjected to the usual 5 minute oxidation.

Temperatures above 25°C markedly accelerate the reaction and should not be used, since aldehydes and other groups, e.g., sulfhydryl and disulfide, are then also likely to be oxidized.

Methods of Preparing Schiff Reagent

Barger and Delamater Method. Dissolve 1 g basic fuchsin in 400 mL boiling distilled water. Cool to 50°C and filter. Add 1 mL thionyl chloride ($SOCl_2$) to the filtrate; stopper, shake, and then let stand in the dark for 12 hours. Now add 2 g activated charcoal, shake for 1 minute, and filter into a brown stock bottle. Store at 0 to 4°C. Before use, allow the aliquot required to reach room temperature. In this reagent the thionyl chloride reacts with water to release sulfur dioxide:

$$SOCl_2 + H_2O \rightarrow SO_2 + 2\,HCl$$

Barger and Delamater's is one of the most stable Schiff reagents—possibly too stable for tests such as the performic acid–Schiff for unsaturated lipids.

De Tomasi-Coleman Method. Dissolve 1 g basic fuchsin in 200 mL of boiling distilled water, shaking for 5 minutes. Cool to 50°C and filter. To the warm filtrate add 20 mL of 1 M HCl (98.3 mL HCl, sp gr 1.16, made to 1000 mL with distilled water, *or* 83.5 mL conc HCl, sp gr 1.19, made similarly to 1000 mL). Cool to 25°C and add 1 g anhydrous sodium or potassium metabisulfite ($Na_2S_2O_5$, $K_2S_2O_5$). Let stand in the dark for 16 to 24 hours, when the solution will be orange or straw-colored. Now add 2 g activated charcoal, shake for 1 minute, and filter into a brown stock bottle. Store in the dark at 0 to 4°C. Before use, allow the aliquot required to reach room temperature.

Itikawa and Ogura Method. With shaking, dissolve 1 g basic fuchsin in 200 mL boiling distilled water. Cool and filter. Bubble SO_2 gas slowly through the solution through a fritted glass filter, with occasional shaking. When the solution becomes a clear, transparent red, turn off the gas, stopper the flask, and let stand overnight in the dark at room temperature. The pink fluid is then decolorized by adding 1 g activated charcoal, shaking for 1 minute, and filtering into a brown stock bottle. Store in the dark at 0 to 4°C.

Life of Schiff Reagents: Testing For Potency

Of the 3 Schiff reagents given, the first two are the more stable and may last up to 6 months. However, it is preferable to make up fresh reagent every month, especially in the case of the Itikawa and Ogura method. Generally, when the reagent begins to become colored it should be discarded. Apart from running control sections in parallel, the reactivity of the Schiff reagent may be tested by adding a few drops to 3 to 5 mL of 40% formaldehyde on a watchglass: active Schiff reagent will lead to the rapid development of a reddish purple color; delayed development of a deep bluish purple indicates that the reagent is going off.

Sulfurous Acid (Sulfite) Rinse

This is optional: Culling regarded it as superfluous and replaced it with a 10-minute wash in running tap water. The purpose of the rinse is to remove excess leucofuchsin, which might become recolorized (on oxidation) and produce false positive staining of some structures. The sulfite rinse must be prepared fresh each day as follows (enough for three Coplin jars):

10% Sodium or potassium metabisulfite ($Na_2S_2O_5$)	7.5 to 9.0 mL
1 M Hydrochloric acid	7.5 mL
Distilled water	150 mL

The PAS Procedure (McManus)

1. Dewax and hydrate paraffin sections, removing mercury precipitate if indicated. Treat a positive control section in parallel.

2. Oxidize for 5 minutes in 0.5% aqueous periodic acid.

3. Rinse in tap and then in distilled water.

4. Place in Schiff's reagent for 15 minutes (10 minutes for frozen sections). Some use longer times in Schiff's reagent, e.g., 10 to 30 minutes, or 30 to 40 minutes.

5. Rinse for 2 minutes in each of three changes of freshly made sulfite rinse.

6. Wash 5 to 10 minutes in running tap water.

7. Optional: counterstain with Harris's hematoxylin for 1 to 3 minutes, *or* in light green (0.1% in 0.1% acetic acid) for 5 to 20 seconds. Light green is especially useful when searching for fungi.

8. If hematoxylin has been used as a counterstain, differentiate by means of three to five quick dips in 1% acid alcohol, wash in tap water, and blue in Scott's tap water substitute; then wash 5 minutes in running tap water.

9. Dehydrate, clear, and mount in Clarite or Permount.

Results. With hematoxylin counterstain, nuclei are blue. PAS-positive materials are magenta (purple-red).

GLYCOGEN

Glycogen is a polymer of glucose and, depending on the complexity and length of the polymer chain, there are many different types of glycogen present in the body tissues. It is manufactured and stored especially in the liver cells but is also found normally, although in lesser concentrations, in other tissues of the body, e.g., muscles, parathyroids, and cartilage. It is very soluble in water and insoluble in alcohol. Hence, *theoretically,* watery or aqueous fixatives are unsuitable, and alcoholic fixatives are *theoretically* the best. In practice, however, this is not entirely so, for many reasons: (1) The short-chain, or simple, glycogens are probably lost, no matter what method is used. (2) In the tissues glycogen appears to be present or located not alone but as part of a complex mixture of proteins and lipids. Hence, any good protein fixative will coat the glycogen with a protein membrane, which prevents glycogen loss in subsequent manipulations. (3) In addition, formalin, and also picric acid, tends to bind glycogen to protein, thus preventing any considerable loss. (4) Although alcohol is theoretically the best fixative, in practice it has some disadvantages. Alcohol is slow to penetrate and fix, and with it only the glycogen on the surface of the block may be preserved. Also, alcohol causes polarization of glycogen (streaming to one corner of the cell), and it tends to cause glycogen to appear as large coarse granules.

In the tissues, especially in the liver, powerful glycogenolytic enzymes exist, and these tend to break down glycogen very rapidly after death. The action of these enzymes is slowed by cooling. Hence, no matter what fixative is used, thin slices (2 mm or less in thickness) should be taken as soon after death as possible and should be placed immediately in fixative at 4°C. In glycogen storage disease, abnormally stable glycogens are stored in excess in the liver or the heart (e.g., von Gierke's and Pompe's diseases). Unfortunately, this in vivo stability does not hold true in histopathology.

Fixatives for Glycogen

One should remember that glycogen is soluble in all aqueous media but that it is insoluble in concentrations of alcohol greater than 70%. For routine demonstration of glycogen the best fixatives are formol-calcium, Brasil's, Gendre's, acetic acid–alcohol–formalin (5:85:10), Bouin's, and ethanol—more or less in this order. From the fixative the tissue blocks should go directly into absolute ethanol. If minimal loss of glycogen is desired, it is advisable to float the sections onto 75% ethanol when cutting, and also to mount them on slides from this. Celloidinization of the mounted sections offers some advantage but is not necessary with well-fixed tissues.

In staining, the sections should not be fully hydrated but should be taken directly from 70 or 80% ethanol into the staining solution or reagent. The latter is usually aqueous, and it is here that the advantage of those alcoholic fixatives containing picric acid or formalin over pure alcohol is manifest. Although alcohol precipitates glycogen well, it does not seem to enmesh it by, or fix it to, proteins, the way picric acid especially and also formalin do. Cryostat sections of fresh tissue are best handled similarly, e.g., fixed for 10 to 30 minutes in one of the agents listed, followed by 5 to 10 minutes in absolute ethanol, brought down to 80 or 70% alcohol, and stained.

If sufficient material is available for two blocks, one may be fixed for 18 to 72 hours in Lillie's 1% periodic acid in 10% formalin; subsequent oxidation of sections is unnecessary; a diastase control is impossible but may be carried out in the sections from the second block fixed in one of the usual fixatives.

STAINING OF GLYCOGEN

Two sections of the material under investigation should always be prepared, and one of these should be used as a control. This control slide, after it is brought to water, should be subjected to diastase digestion.

Diastase Digestion of Glycogen

Hydrated sections are treated for 30 minutes at room temperature with a 1% solution of malt diastase (buffering is unnecessary). Commercial malt diastase contains many enzymes besides alpha-amylase, and it removes substances other than glycogen, e.g., RNA. However, this is of no consequence when one is staining only for glycogen. If malt diastase is not available, the section should be treated with one's own saliva, the ptyalin of which digests glycogen. Common fixatives appear to have no inhibitory effect on diastase action; neither do they affect the nucleases or hyaluronidases.

RETICULIN (RETICULUM) AND COLLAGEN

Reticulin consists of a fibrillary extracellular scaffolding found throughout the tissues of the body; in this framework the parenchymal and special cells are held and their nutrient capillaries and so forth are carried. The fibrils of reticulin are delicate and isotropic, stain black on impregnation with silver, and are either unstained or a faint pinkish color with van Gieson's stain.

Collagen forms a coarser extracellular framework or scaffolding; its fibers are the coarse connective tissue fibers. They are doubly refractile and stain red with van Gieson's stain and yellow, lavender, or brown on silver impregnation.

Many believe that reticulin and collagen are basically similar and that reticulin precedes collagen and may be regarded as procollagen.

General Considerations of Silver Impregnation Methods

Many methods of silver impregnation of reticulin exist. They depend on the local reduction and selective precipitation of silver by the aldehydic groups of the carbohydrate of the reticulin. Of these, one method of Foot and the methods of Bielschowsky-Maresch, Perdrau da Fano, Wilder, Gomori, and Lillie all depend on silver oxide or hydroxide in ammoniacal solution. The del Rio-Hortega, Foot, and Laidlaw variants use ammoniacal solutions of silver carbonate. Most are prepared by producing a precipitate from silver nitrate with sodium, potassium, or ammonium hydroxide or with lithium or sodium carbonate. The type of reaction involved in the preparation of the silver solution may be exemplified by Laidlaw's method:

$$2\,AgNO_3 + Li_2CO_3 = Ag_2CO_3\downarrow + 2\,LiNO_3$$

The lithium nitrate is then removed by washing and the precipitated silver carbonate is dissolved with ammonia water:

$$Ag_2CO_3 + 4\,NH_3 = [Ag(NH_3)_2]_2CO_3$$

(ammonium silver carbonate)

The essential reactions in the impregnation are believed to be as follows:

1. The aldehydic groups of reticulum reduce the colorless silver complex (mixed solution and colloid) to a dark brown lower oxide, which is precipitated in particulate form on the reticulin fibers.

2. This silver oxide is reduced to black metallic silver by formalin. Sodium sulfite and hydroquinone will also accomplish this, but formalin is used in the majority of methods.

3. The unreduced silver is removed by solution in sodium thiosulfate (hypo). Various refinements are employed in different methods:

a. Many methods recommend some form of presilvering. All of these pretreatments involve oxidation: $KMnO_4$ has been used by some workers. Others have used acidified $KMnO_4$, 4% chromic acid, and 0.5% periodic acid or 10% phosphomolybdic acid. Many of the aminosilver methods employ "sensitizers," e.g., uranium or silver nitrate, ferric chloride, or iron alum. Some of these act as oxidants.

b. Toning with yellow gold chloride. This is a very valuable step. If the sections are untoned after silver impregnation, the background will be yellowish because of colloidal metallic silver. Toning removes this silver and replaces it with gold chloride. This, in turn, is reduced to metallic gold by metabisulfite. The formula for the reaction is:

$$3Ag\downarrow + AuCl_3 \rightarrow Au\downarrow + 3AgCl$$

Toning gives a very pale gray background, which is better for photography and which also improves subsequent counterstaining. The metallic gold is also more stable than the precipitated silver.

As regards fixation of tissues for silver impregnation, most methods specify formalin, but other fixatives may be employed. If mercurial fixatives are used, the iodine-thiosulfate sequence must be used after the sections are brought to water, to remove mercury deposits. Frozen sections may be used with all methods, and some workers prefer this. However, most use paraffin sections. The high alkalinity of the silver solutions tends to detach the sections from the slides. This may be overcome by: (1) Fixing the section well to an albumenized slide by thorough drying. (2) Celloidinizing the mounted sections. This is done, after removal of the wax, by transferring the slide from absolute alcohol into 1% celloidin (parlodion), where it is allowed to soak for 5 minutes. The excess celloidin is then drained off, and the celloidin film is hardened by immersing for 5 minutes in 80% alcohol followed by water. (3) Carrying out steps of the procedure by floating the paraffin section on the solutions, the section being mounted on completion of the staining procedures, drained dry, "baked" by placing in the paraffin oven for 10 minutes, cleared in xylene, and mounted.

Silver impregnations are notoriously capricious. Scrupulous techniques will ensure consistent results. In particular, all glassware used, especially before and for the silver bath and for the preparation of the silver solutions, must be thoroughly washed with 10% nitric acid and then rinsed in several changes of distilled water. The forceps used for slide manipulation during processing should be nonmetallic, i.e., plastic, until after the sodium thiosulfate stage. This will prevent the nonspecific precipitation of silver on the slide. Whenever indicated in the particular method, washing of the sections with distilled water must be thorough, especially before impregnation. In particular, dust must be avoided, since it (and not light) is the greatest single factor in the deterioration and precipitation of silver solutions. Improper procedure will lead to precipitate formation in almost any method. Splashing, or the use of glass rods without careful washing between solutions, must be avoided. Glass-distilled water should be used.

Explosive Hazards of Ammoniacal Silver Solutions

In the preparation of the commonly used silver impregnation solutions, various chemical reactions occur. These are outlined as follows:

1. $AgNO_3 + NaOH \rightarrow AgOH + NaNO_3$
2. $2\ AgOH = Ag_2O + H_2O$
3. $Ag_2O = 2\ Ag^+ + O^{--}$
4. $2\ NH_3 + Ag^+ \rightarrow [Ag(NH_3)_2]^+$

The hydrated silver oxide precipitate formed by the addition of aqueous NaOH to $AgNO_3$ solutions dissolves on addition of ammonia, with formation of the complex argentammonium ion $[Ag(NH_3)_2]^+$ and consequent shifting of the equilibrium of reaction 3 toward the right. With aging or exposure of ammoniacal silver solutions to air or light, shiny black crystals of explosive silver compounds, e.g., "fulminating silver," silver nitride (Ag_3N), and silver azide (AgN_3) are formed. If formaldehyde vapor is present or alcohol is included in the solutions, a further hazard emerges in the formation of silver fulminate (CNOAg). To avoid these very real dangers (violent explosions may occur while removing a stopper, throwing a solution down a sink, or even when holding it up to the light), it is recommended (1) that all ammoniacal silver solutions be prepared fresh just before use, (2) that "well-silvered" glassware never be used, and (3) that any unused solutions be inactivated by adding excess of sodium chloride solution or of dilute hydrochloric acid.

Of the many silver reticulin methods available, Gomori's is recommended for ease and reproducibility.

Gomori's Silver Impregnation Stain for Reticulin

We regard this as the most reliable method for reticulin; it works equally well for beginners and experts.

Preparation of Silver Solution. To 20 mL of 10% silver nitrate solution add 4 to 5 mL of 10% potassium hydroxide. Mark the fluid level on the flask and pour off the supernatant. Wash the precipitated silver with distilled water once or twice until the water is quite clear, and fill up to the fluid level with fresh distilled water; this step will result in a cleaner background. Then, with continuous shaking, add 28% ammonia water, drop by drop, until the precipitate is all dissolved. Now carefully add 10% silver nitrate solution, drop by drop, until the precipitate that forms easily disappears on shaking. Make the solution up to twice its volume with distilled water; i.e., add an equal volume of distilled water. If stored in a well-stoppered bottle in the dark, the solution may be used for 2 days.

Procedure

1. Bring paraffin sections of formalin-fixed material down to water.

2. Oxidize in 0.5% aqueous potassium permanganate for 1 to 2 minutes.

3. Rinse in tap water for 2 minutes.

4. Place in 2% aqueous potassium metabisulfite for 1 minute, or until colorless.

5. Wash in tap water for 2 to 5 minutes.

6. Place in 2% aqueous ferric ammonium sulfate for 1 minute to sensitize.

7. Wash in tap water for 2 minutes and then for 30 seconds in each of two changes of distilled water.

8. Allow impregnation in the silver solution for 1 minute.

9. Rinse in distilled water for 20 seconds.

10. Reduce for 3 minutes in 20% formalin (formaldehyde 10 mL, distilled water 40 mL).

11. Wash in tap water for 3 minutes.

12. Tone in 0.2% gold chloride solution for 10 minutes.

13. Rinse in distilled water.

14. Place in 2% aqueous potassium metabisulfite for 1 minute to reduce toning.

15. Fix in 2% aqueous sodium thiosulfate (hypo) for 1 minute.

16. Wash in tap water for 2 minutes.

17. Dehydrate, clear, and mount.

Results. Reticulin fibers—black.

STAINING OF COLLAGEN

Collagen and most reticulin stain selectively with acid aniline dyes (aniline blue, acid fuchsin, methyl blue, indigo carmine) from fairly strong acid solutions. The acid most used is picric acid, which, in addition to providing acidity and acting as a counterstain for muscle and cytoplasm, also appears to form a complex with the dyes mentioned. This complex seems to have a special affinity for collagen. These considerations form the basis of such stains for collagen as van Gieson's (picrofuchsin). Other methods have used phosphomolybdic or phosphotungstic acid with aniline dyestuffs in sequence (Mallory, Heidenhain and Masson).

Weigert–van Gieson Stain

van Gieson's Stain

Saturated aqueous picric acid	100 mL
1% acid fuchsin	10 mL

This may be kept as a stock solution, but a freshly prepared solution of 10 mL saturated aqueous picric acid and 1.5 mL of 1% acid fuchsin may give better staining quality.

Procedure

1. Bring sections to water.
2. Stain with Weigert's hematoxylin (p. 798) for 20 minutes.
3. Wash in tap water.
4. Differentiate in 1% acid alcohol.
5. Blue in tap water.
6. Counterstain in van Gieson's stain for 3–5 minutes.
7. Rinse rapidly in distilled water. Do *not* use tap water at this stage.
8. Differentiate by dipping in 95% ethanol saturated with picric acid.
9. Dehydrate rapidly in two changes of ethanol, clear in xylene, and mount.

Result. Cell nuclei—black. Collagen—red. Muscle fibers, red blood cells, fibrin—yellow.

Masson's Trichrome Stain

Bouin's (or Zenker's) fixation is best. Sections of formalin-fixed material should be premordanted in Bouin's fluid for 1 hour at 56°C or overnight at room temperature. Sections should be secured firmly to the slides.

Procedures

1. Bring paraffin sections to water and wash until the yellow color is gone, or remove mercury deposits with iodine-thiosulfate sequence, as indicated.
2. Stain nuclei for 10 to 30 minutes in Weigert's iron hematoxylin (p. 798).
3. Differentiate to a pure nuclear stain with 1% acid alcohol; wash in running tap water for 10 minutes until blue.
4. Rinse in distilled water and stain for 15 minutes in Biebrich scarlet-acid fuchsin (90 mL of 1% aqueous Biebrich scarlet, 10 mL of 1% aqueous acid fuchsin, and 1 mL glacial acetic acid), *or* for 5 minutes in a mixture of 2 parts 1% Ponceau de xylidine in 1% acetic acid plus 1 part 1% acid fuchsin in 1% acetic acid.
5. Rinse in distilled water.
6. Mordant for 10 to 15 minutes in a solution of 2.5 g phosphomolybdic acid, 2.5 g phosphotungstic acid, and 100 mL distilled water, if aniline blue is to be used. If light green is to be the counterstain, place for 5 to 15 minutes in 5% aqueous phosphotungstic acid. Discard acid solutions after use.
7. Drain and stain for 5 to 10 minutes in 2.5% aniline blue in 2.0% acetic acid, *or* for 1 to 3 minutes in 2% light green in 1% acetic acid.
8. Rinse or drain and differentiate for 1 to 3 minutes in 1% acetic acid.
9. Dehydrate, clear, and mount.

Results. Muscle, cytoplasm, and keratin—red. Nuclei—black. Collagen and mucus—blue (or green).

ELASTIC FIBERS

Elastic tissue is present in the skin, in ligaments, and in the elastic laminae of blood vessels, and it is very abundant in the lung, and especially so in the wall of the aorta. In these sites it serves the function implied by its name and often exists as a fenestrated membrane. The wrinkled skin of old age is largely a result of atrophy of elastic fibers. Elastic fibers are made up of fine, intertwining corkscrew filaments, which are very insoluble in organic and inorganic solvents (as distinct from collagen, which is soluble in 2% acetic acid) and are resistant to most enzymes (except elastase of the pancreas). Elastic tissue is isotropic and gives a yellowish (blue if unstained) fluorescence in ultraviolet light. Most of the staining methods employed for its demonstration are empiric. In the presence of ferric salts (oxidizers) elastic fibers stain with basic fuchsin, with or without resorcin. From acidic solutions the fibers are stained selectively by the weak acid orcein. Elastic fibers of the skin are much more easily stained than those in the walls of arteries, probably because of physicochemical differences.

Although rarely required, elastase, either from cultures of *Pseudomonas aeruginosa* or from pancreas, may be used for the specific identification of elastin. However, a simpler and cheaper method is to expose sections to pepsin for brief periods sufficient to digest the elastic fibers while leaving the collagen fibers undamaged.

Gomori's Aldehyde-Fuchsin Method for Elastic Fibers

Solutions Required

1. Basic fuchsin

Basic fuchsin	0.5 g
60–70% ethanol	100 mL
Paraldehyde (U.S.P)	1 mL
Concentrated HCl	1.5 mL

Dissolve the fuchsin in the alcohol and add the paraldehyde and hydrochloric acid. Shake well and leave at room temperature for 24 to 48 hours, until it is deep purple and ready for use. It should be stored in the refrigerator, where it will keep its staining properties for 2 to 3 months.

2. *Lugol's Iodine*

Iodine	1 g
KI	2 g
Distilled water	to 100 mL

Dissolve the KI in 4 to 5 mL of water and the iodine in this solution. Then make up to 100 mL.

3. *Light Green*

Light green SF	0.2 g
Orange G	1.0 g

Chromotrope 2R (may omit)	0.5 g
Phosphotungstic acid	0.5 g
Glacial acetic acid	1.0 mL
Distilled water	to 100 mL

Method. Formalin or Bouin's fixed tissues are preferred.

1. **Dewax and hydrate paraffin section.**
2. **Treat in Lugol's iodine for 30 minutes.**
3. **Bleach in 5% sodium thiosulfate for 2 minutes.**
4. **Wash in running tap water for 3 minutes.**
5. **Rinse in 90% ethanol.**
6. **Stain in aldehyde-fuchsin for 5 to 10 minutes (the stain is progressive).**
7. **Rinse in 90% ethanol.**
8. **Counterstain in light green.**
9. **Dehydrate, clear, and mount.**

Results. Elastic tissue—deep purple. Collagen—green. Other structures that take on the deep purple color include the granules of mast cells, beta cells of the pancreatic islets, gastric chief cells, and suprisingly, HBsAg, which is the surface antigen and the marker of hepatitis B virus in the tissues.

Verhoeff's Elastic Method

1. **Hydrate paraffin sections (use any fixative). The iodine-thiosulfate sequence is not essential as the mercury deposits are removed by the stain, but it is advantageous as a mordant.**
2. **Stain in Verhoeff's solution until the sections are black (15 to 45 minutes).** ***Verhoeff's solution:*** **to 30 mL of stock 5% alcoholic hematoxylin add 12 mL of 10% aqueous $FeCl_3$; mix, and then add 12 mL of a solution of 2 g iodine and 4 g KI in 100 mL distilled water; mix.** ***Note:*** **The ingredients must be added in the order given.**
3. **Differentiate in 2% aqueous $FeCl_3$ with agitation for a few minutes, checking by rinsing in distilled water and examining under the low power of the microscope—until only elastic fibers and nuclei are black and other tissues are gray. Should the section be overdifferentiated, it may be returned to Verhoeff's solution for further staining.**
4. **Rinse in water and then in 95% ethanol to remove iodine.**
5. **Wash for 5 minutes in water.**
6. **Counterstain 1 to 2 minutes with van Gieson.**
7. **Differentiate in 95% ethanol, dehydrate, clear, and mount.**

Results. Elastic fibers—black. Nuclei—gray to black. Collagen—red. Cytoplasm and muscle—yellow.

PIGMENTS IN TISSUES

CLASSIFICATION

Artifacts

These result from methods used in processing the tissues.

Formalin Pigment. Dark brown pigment (acid formaldehyde hematein) produced by the interaction of acidic formaldehyde solutions and blood. Remove by treating sections with alcoholic-picric acid (see p. 761).

Mercurial Deposits. Gray-black granular deposits resulting from the use of mercurial fixatives. Remove by treating sections with alcoholic iodine, followed by sodium thiosulfate.

Chrome Deposits

These are brownish black granules that are the result of alcohol treatment following chrome fixation; such pigment *cannot be removed.* Chrome-fixed tissues must be washed in running water for 12 to 18 hours immediately following fixation. This washing removes excess chromate from the tissue which can then safely be dehydrated in alcohol.

Endogenous and Exogenous Pigments

The endogenous pigments that will be considered here are hemosiderins and melanins. Other such pigments—as well as exogenous pigments such as carbon dust pigment, which is often present in lungs—will not be described.

HEMOSIDERINS

When hemoglobin is released from the red cells it is broken down by cells (mainly histiocytes) into iron-free hematoidin and iron-containing hemosiderin. The latter consists of ferric hydroxide ($Fe[OH]_3$) bound to protein (ferritin). It takes 2 to 3 days from the time of release of hemoglobin from the red cells before hemosiderin first appears. Normally a little hemosiderin is found in the bone marrow and in the spleen. It is seen in excess in the tissues in such conditions as hemosiderosis and hemochromatosis and in the bone marrow in pernicious anemia. Hemosiderin is a granular, yellowish brown or golden pigment. It is insoluble in alkalis but is soluble in acids. After fixation in formaldehyde solutions it is

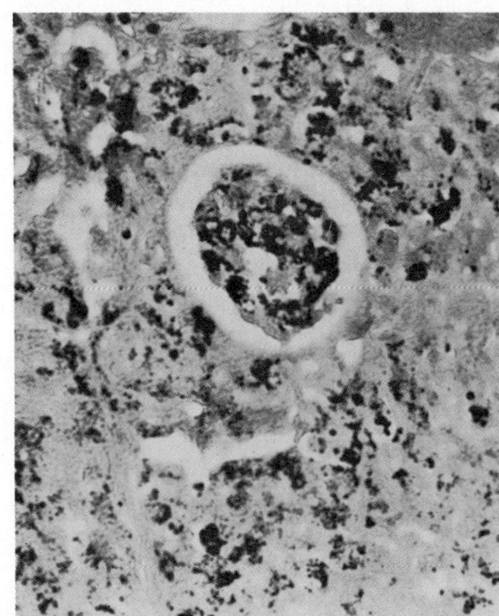

Figure 33–6 Pancreas from a patient with hemochromatosis. Stained for iron by the Gomori technique. × 300.

slowly dissolved by dilute acids; hence, formol-saline fixation may, if the formalin is not buffered, lead to complete loss of all but the grosser deposits of hemosiderin. Buffered neutral formalin should always be used as fixative. For further details on the deleterious effects of acids and Versene in the decalcification process of hemosiderin and on their avoidance see p. 765. There are several reactions by which hemosiderin (iron) may be demonstrated, but Perls' Prussian blue reaction (Gomori's method) is the best. It is important to use iron-free reagents and equipment to avoid any possibility of contamination.

Gomori's Application of Perls' Prussian Blue Reaction for Hemosiderin

This depends on the combination of inorganic iron with potassium ferrocyanide in acid solution to form ferric ferrocyanide (Prussian blue):

$$4FeCl_3 + 3\ K_4Fe(CN)_6 \rightarrow Fe_4\ (Fe(CN)_6)_3 + 12\ KCl.$$

Procedure

1. Bring paraffin sections down to water.
2. Place in freshly made 10% aqueous potassium ferrocyanide (note volume of ferrocyanide solution used).
3. After 5 minutes add 10% solution of HCl (must be free of iron) in an amount equal to half the volume of ferrocyanide used. Mix by stirring with a clean glass rod. Then leave for 20 minutes.
4. Wash well in distilled water.
5. A variety of counterstains may be used, viz., (a) 0.1% nuclear fast red in 5% aluminum sulfate for 2 to 5 minutes; (b) 0.5% aqueous eosin for 20 to 60 seconds; (c) 1% aqueous neutral red for 20 to 60 seconds; (d) 0.1% safranine for 10 to 30 seconds; (e) 0.5% phloxine and 0.5% tartrazine for 5 minutes; (f) van Gieson's stain for 1 to 3 minutes.

Results. Ferric iron—blue. Other tissues—shades of red or pink, depending on the counterstain used.

Melanins

These are granular, yellow, brown, or black pigments that are believed to be formed from tyrosine and related compounds by the action of tyrosinase (dopa oxidase). They appear to be combined firmly with proteins and are extremely difficult to extract. They are insoluble in organic solvents and indeed in any solvent other than those that destroy the tissues. They are, however, soluble in 1 M sodium hydroxide. Melanins are slowly bleached by strong oxidizing agents, e.g., hydrogen peroxide, peracetic acid, potassium permanganate, ferric chloride, potassium chlorate and HCl, and ascorbic acid. Melanins also reduce solutions of ammoniacal silver nitrate to black metallic silver. Normally, melanins occur in the skin, hair, choroid and iris of the eye, meninges, and substantia nigra of the brain. The importance of their identification in routine histopathology lies in the fact that some melanomas have only minute traces of melanin, and the demonstration of this may be decisive in the recognition of these malignant tumors. Melanin is increased in the skin and other tissues in Addison's disease (acquired adrenal insufficiency) and in hemochromatosis.

Masson-Fontana Ammoniacal Silver Reaction for Melanin

Procedure

1. To 20 mL of 10% aqueous silver nitrate add strong (28%) ammonia water drop by drop until the dark brown precipitate that forms is *almost* all redissolved (about 2 mL of ammonia will be required). Add 20 mL distilled water and allow the solution to settle for 18 to 24 hours. Place the supernatant in a dark brown bottle, where it will keep for 1 to 3 months. (*Note dangers associated with such solutions, p. 802.*) Filter before use.
2. Bring paraffin sections down to water.
3. Treat with Gram's iodine solution for 10 minutes. Wash well in three changes of distilled water.
4. Place the sections in the silver solution in the dark for 18 to 24 hours.
5. Rinse in distilled water. Toning in 0.1 to 0.2% gold chloride for 3 to 7 minutes, followed by rinsing in distilled water, is done at this stage.
6. Fix in 5% sodium thiosulfate for 1 to 2 minutes. Then wash 3 minutes in running tap water.
7. Counterstain with 0.5% safranine for 15 to 45 seconds.
8. Rinse in water.
9. Dehydrate rapidly in alcohol, clear in xylene, and mount.

Results. Melanin and argentaffin cell granules—black. In this test melanin granules are argentaffin; i.e., they reduce ammoniacal silver solution to metallic silver. Besides being argentaffin, melanin granules are also argyrophilic; i.e., they are colored black by silver impregnation methods using a reducing agent.

STAINING OF BACTERIA

For general purposes of staining, bacteria fall into two broad divisions, gram-positive and gram-negative. The classification "acid- and/or alcohol-fast" is also used for identifying bacilli of the mycobacteria class. Many bacteria, e.g., staphylococci, streptococci, and streptobacilli, are shown by ordinary hematoxylin-eosin staining, appearing as light brown to brown black bodies; i.e., they take up the hematoxylin. This staining is enhanced after periodic acid oxidation, e.g., when hematoxylin is used as a counterstain in the PAS technique.

Gram's Stain for Tissues

The dyes that may be used in Gram staining are: crystal, methyl, ethyl, and Hoffman's violets, brilliant green, malachite green, basic fuchsin, and Victoria blue R. All of these form precipitates with iodine, and all but the last are triphenylmethanes. Methyl violet is a mixture of tetra-, penta-, and hexamethyl pararosaniline. The designation R is applied to those methyl violets having a reddish shade and B to those having a bluish shade, 10 B being the bluest. As indicated in Figure 33–7, crystal violet is hexamethyl pararosaniline; it is easily prepared in pure form and hence is the one most widely used, especially when a deep blue-violet shade is desired. Gentian violet is an ill-defined mixture of methyl violets with or without dextrin; it is not a certifiable stain and should not be used.

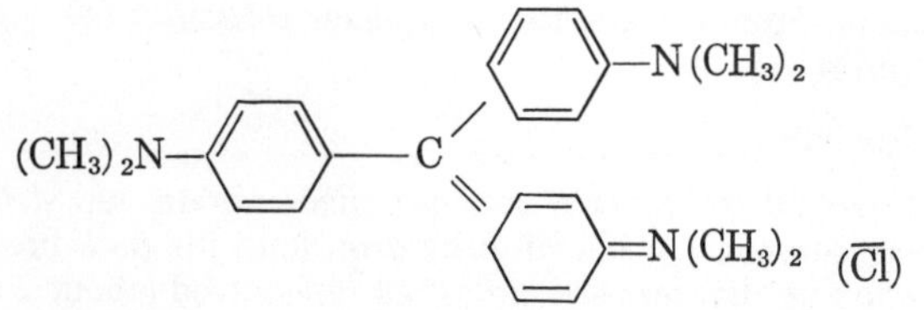

$(CH_3)_2N$—C$_6H_4$—C(—C$_6H_4$—$N(CH_3)_2$)=C$_6H_4$=$N(CH_3)_2$ $(\overline{Cl})$

Figure 33–7 Hexamethyl pararosaniline (crystal violet).

Brown and Brenn Technique for Gram Stain

Formalin fixation is preferred. Paraffin sections are cut at 4 to 6 μm.

Procedure

1. Hydrate paraffin sections; remove mercury deposits with iodine-thiosulfate sequence if indicated.

2. Place slides on staining rack and flood with a freshly prepared mixture of 1 mL of 1% aqueous crystal violet and 5 drops (0.25 mL) of 5% aqueous sodium bicarbonate. Leave 1 minute.

3. Rinse in water.

4. Flood for 1 minute with Gram's iodine (KI, 2 g; I_2, 1 g dissolved in 300 mL of distilled water).

5. Rinse in water; blot completely dry with filter paper, but do not allow to dry further in the atmosphere (see precautions).

6. Decolorize with a mixture of equal parts ether and acetone (or briefly with acetone alone) from a dropping bottle until no more blue color runs off.

7. Stain 1 minute with 0.1% basic fuchsin (0.1 mL of saturated basic fuchsin in 100 mL distilled water; saturated basic fuchsin = 0.25 g in 100 mL distilled water).

8. Wash in water; blot gently but not completely dry.

9. Dip briefly in acetone.

10. Differentiate immediately in 0.1% picric acid in acetone until the sections are yellowish pink.

11. Rinse quickly in acetone, and then in a mixture of equal parts acetone and xylene.

12. Clear in three or four changes of xylene; mount in Permount.

Results. Gram-positive bacteria—blue; gram-negative bacteria—red; nuclei—red; other tissue elements—yellow.

Precautions. Complete drying at any time after the crystal violet staining leads to the formation of a new compound that is difficult to differentiate with ether-acetone. Drying after the basic fuchsin leads to an insoluble compound resistant to picric acid in acetone. The picric acid must be anhydrous (dried in vacuum desiccator over calcium chloride); and the picric acid–acetone solution must be yellow; if any greenish tint is present, it must be discarded.

Theories of Gram Staining

See p. 347.

DEMONSTRATION OF ACID-FAST ORGANISMS IN TISSUES

Certain bacteria, e.g., *Mycobacterium tuberculosis* and leprosy bacillus, are relatively resistant to staining, but when stained by a strong stain with the aid of heat they resist decolorization by acid. This property is due to the structural incorporation of lipids in the organism. Other bacteria that are commonly found in butter, milk, tap water, grass, and manure, and the smegma bacillus are also acid-fast but are decolorized by alcohol. *M. tuberculosis* is both alcohol- and acid-fast, and the leprosy bacillus is similar but is less easily stained and more easily decolorized. Certain species of *Nocardia,* e.g., *N. asteroides* and *N. brasiliensis* are acid-fast, but *N. madurae, N. pelletieri,* and *N. paraguayensis* are not and are actually now regarded as members of the *Streptomyces* genus.

Of the methods to be described, the Ziehl-Neelsen is the traditional one; it is reliable, but can be improved by dewaxing sections in one of the oil mixtures. The Wade-Fite-Faraco and Wade-Fite methods employ this and are preferred for *M. leprae.* Fluorescent staining offers rapid and easy identification of acid-fast organisms at low magnification (× 180 to 350) but the preparation is not permanent. Although some workers use up to 3% HCl in 70% alcohol for decolorization, 1% is adequate.

Ziehl-Neelsen Stain for Acid- and Alcohol-Fast Bacteria in Tissues

Fixation. Buffered neutral formalin and mercuric fixatives are satisfactory.

Preserving Acid Fastness. Especially in the case of Hansen's bacillus *(M. leprae),* but also with old tubercle bacilli, acid fastness may be lost in processing. Faraco first guarded against this by placing olive oil or mineral lubricating oil on the section after dewaxing with xylene, heating for a few minutes, and blotting to opacity before staining. Fite et al. removed the wax with 2 parts xylene + 1 part cottonseed oil. Wade improved on the method by dewaxing for 1 to 2 minutes in a 1:2 mixture of paraffin oil and aviation gasoline *or* of paraffin oil and rectified turpentine, and showed also that imbedding in Carbowax safeguarded acid fastness, which could be restored to a considerable degree by soaking the sections in a heavy grade of paraffin oil for up to 3 to 6 hours.

Carbolfuchsin Solution

Basic fuchsin	1 g
Absolute ethyl alcohol	10 mL
Carbolic acid	5 mL
Distilled water	100 mL

Dissolve the basic fuchsin in the alcohol and the phenol in the water; mix the two solutions. Filter before use.

Procedure

1. Bring paraffin sections to water.

2. Stain in carbolfuchsin at 37°C for 1 hour, or at 56°C (in wax oven) for 30 minutes, or overnight at room temperature.

3. Rinse well in tap water.

4. Decolorize with 3% HCl in 70% alcohol (1% aqueous H_2SO_4 for non–alcohol-fast bacilli).

5. Wash in water and counterstain in 1% methylene blue 10 to 30 seconds (pale blue color desired).

6. Rinse in water.

7. Dehydrate in two changes each of 95% and absolute alcohol.

8. Clear in xylene and mount in Clarite or Permount.

Results. Tubercle bacilli—bright red. Tissue—blue. Caseous material—very pale grayish blue. *Note:* Red blood cells should show a very slight reddish tint and are a good index against overdecolorization.

Rapid Ziehl-Neelsen Method (Culling, 1974)

1. Hydrate sections; place face up on staining rack and cover with rectangular piece of filter paper (prevents precipitate).

2. Flood with carbolfuchsin solution, heat to steaming, and leave for 10 minutes.

3. Wash in water.

4. Decolorize as in step 4 of the regular method until sections are pale pink (1 to 5 minutes).

5. Wash and counterstain as in step 5 of the regular method.

6. Wash in water, dehydrate, clear, and mount.

Wade-Fite-Faraco Stain for Acid-Fast Bacilli

This method is suitable for delicate organisms such as *M. leprae.*

Procedure

1. Deparaffinize by immersing for 1 to 2 minutes in a mixture of 1 part paraffin oil (light or heavy grade) and 2 parts aviation gasoline *or* of 1 part paraffin oil and 2 parts rectified turpentine. Some use equal parts xylene and peanut oil, but this is not Wade's method.

2. Drain, wipe excess oil from edges, and blot to opacity; place in water until ready to stain.

3. Stain in Ziehl-Neelsen carbolfuchsin for 20 to 30 minutes at room temperature.

4. Rinse in water and decolorize in 1% HCl in 70% ethanol until sections are faint pink (about 1 to 2 minutes). *Note:* If *M. leprae* is being stained, only aqueous 0.5 to 1% H_2SO_4 should be used—for ½ to 1 minute.

5. Wash in water and counterstain 10 to 20 seconds with 0.1 to 0.5% methylene blue.

6. Rinse in tap water, wipe edges clean, blot, and then allow to dry in the air. When thoroughly dry, mount directly in synthetic mounting medium such as Permount or Clarite.

Results. Acid-fast bacilli—red on light blue background.

Wade-Fite Stain for Acid-Fast Bacilli

Fixation. Zenker or formalin fixation is used.

Procedure

1. Dewax paraffin sections with a mixture of 2 parts rectified turpentine and 1 part heavy paraffin oil—2½ minutes in each of two changes. Removal of mercury deposits is not necessary.

2. Drain, wipe oil from edges, and blot to opacity; place in water for a few minutes.

3. Stain 6 to 24 hours (longer times, e.g., 18 to 24 hours, for old or poorly preserved bacilli) at room temperature in carbol–new fuchsin (0.5 g new fuchsin dissolved in 10 mL alcohol and mixed with a solution of 5 mL melted phenol crystals in 100 mL distilled water).

4. Wash in water; then place for 5 minutes in *reagent-grade* 37 to 40% formaldehyde. This causes the bacilli to assume a permanent blue color that is owing to fuchsin-aldehyde reaction.

5. Wash in water.

6. Decolorize for 1 minute in 5% aqueous H_2SO_4.

7. Wash in running tap water for 5 minutes.

8. Place in 1% $KMnO_4$ for 3 minutes.

9. Wash in tap water.

10. Bleach ½ to 1 minute in 2% oxalic acid.

11. Wash 5 to 10 minutes in running tap water.

12. Stain 3 minutes in dilute van Gieson (acid fuchsin, 0.01 g, + 1 g picric acid in 100 mL distilled water).

13. Without washing, dehydrate rapidly through 95% and absolute alcohols; clear in xylene and mount.

Results. Acid-fast bacilli—deep blue to blue-black; collagen—red; other elements—yellow.

STAINING OF FUNGI

A number of stains may be used to demonstrate these organisms, but they may have disadvantages. H and E may be used, but some of the fungi do not take up hematoxylin; only a few of the fungi are acid-fast; the PAS techniques have few disadvantages, but the Gram stain is little used, since the organism has relatively little affinity for the stain.

Gomori's Methenamine–Silver Nitrate Method

Principle. Aldehydogenic groups are uncovered by chromic acid oxidation and subsequently reduce methenamine–silver nitrate in alkaline solution. The method is specific for aldehydes if certain phenols and uric acid can be ruled out. It is an extremely good method for demonstrating fungi in tissue. The usual precautions when using silver impregnation methods apply here.

Stock Silver Nitrate–Methenamine Complex

Add 5 mL of 5% $AgNO_3$ to 100 mL of 3% methenamine (hexamethylenetetramine). The initial heavy white precipitate easily disappears on shaking, and the crystal clear solution will keep for several months in the refrigerator and about 2 weeks at room temperature.

Procedure

1. Deparaffinize sections; celloidinize if glycogen is being sought.

2. Oxidize the hydrated sections 1 to 1½ hours in 5% chromic acid (or in 1% periodic acid for 10 to 15 minutes).

3. Wash in running tap water for 10 minutes.

4. Treat 1 minute with 1 to 2% sodium bisulfite to remove the last traces of chromic acid.

5. Wash 5 minutes in running tap water; rinse in distilled water.

6. Incubate in working silver-methenamine solution (25 mL each of stock silver nitrate–methenamine and distilled water, + 1 to 2 mL of 5% borax—$Na_2B_4O_7 \cdot 10H_2O$) for 1 to 3 hours at 37 to 45°C, or for ½ to 1 hour at 58 to 60°C (Grocott) until sections turn yellowish brown. Using wax-coated or plastic forceps, rinse sections in distilled water and examine every 15 minutes after the first half. The end point is reached when glycogen, mucin, basement membranes, or fungi are dark brown to brownish black.

7. Rinse in three or more changes of distilled water.

8. Tone 2 to 5 minutes in 0.1% gold chloride.

9. Rinse well for 3 to 5 minutes in 2 to 3% sodium thiosulfate to remove unreacted silver. Then wash well in tap water.

10. Counterstain as desired, e.g., ½ to 1 minute in dilute light green (0.2 g light green S F in 100 mL distilled water + 0.2 mL acetic acid; dilute 10 mL of this to 60 mL with distilled water for use.

11. Dehydrate; remove celloidin film if indicated, with alcohol-ether or acetone; clear in xylene and mount.

Results. Glycogen, mucin, fungi, basement membranes, reticulin, and elastin—brownish black to black. The preparations are especially suited for black and white photography.

Grocott's Adaptation of Gomori's Methenamine-Silver for Fungi

Grocott showed that Gomori's method was well suited to the demonstration of fungi in sections. He used 1 hour's incubation in methenamine-silver at 45 to 50°C, but otherwise his technique is that of Gomori.

FIXATION AND PRESERVATION OF LIPIDS

There is no really good fixative for lipids. Formalin fixes only a minority of lipids, e.g., those already more or less firmly bound to proteins. It is inert toward simple lipids and allows appreciable diffusion loss of phospholipids. Addition of calcium, cobalt, or cadmium ions prevents phospholipids from dissolving or leaching out in formalin by forming temporary intermolecular linkage complexes between these lipids and large molecules such as proteins and mucopolysaccharides. However, these temporary linkages do not alter the solubility of phospholipids in subsequent fluid phases, and they may therefore be lost even during washing in water for more than 2 to 4 hours; they will certainly be lost in routine dehydration and embedding unless chromated. In addition, prolonged fixation in formalin (and aldehydes generally) alters the chemical and physical state of many lipids other than neutral fats.

Chromate fixatives oxidize phospholipids, rendering them nonextractable by alcohols, toluene, xylene, or chloroform in paraffin embedding. Osmium tetroxide is reduced by fatty acids and unsaturated lipids, and forms strongly bound, nonextractable additive compounds with these and other lipids, coloring them black and rendering them electron dense so that they are visualized with the electron microscope. Polyethylene glycols (carbowaxes), used in lieu of the usual dehydration and embedding, are sometimes used as a method of preserving lipids in tissues. Cryostat sections of fresh unfixed tissue involve the least loss of lipids.

Demonstration of Fat (Neutral Fat)

Demonstration of neutral fat in tissues is called for in a variety of circumstances.

Neutral fats are dissolved out by fat solvents such as benzene, xylene, toluene, and alcohol and are, therefore, not demonstrable in routine paraffin sections. Prior treatment of the tissue with potassium dichromate or osmic acid will render the fats insoluble in, and nonextractable by, the solvents mentioned. The use of Carbowax embedding excludes fat solvents and offers an elegant means of studying fats in thin sections. However, the Carbowax technique has not received wide application, so that in most centers neutral fats and fat embolism are still best demonstrated by means of frozen sections of fixed or unfixed tissue. The stains used belong to a group that is more soluble in fat than in alcohols, and they are employed in saturated solutions so that their take-up by fat is facilitated.

In staining for neutral lipids by any of the differential solubility transfer dye methods, e.g., oil red O or the Sudans, it is better to use free-floating sections. If one uses mounted sections, especially cryostat sections of fresh tissue, the staining of fat tends to be incomplete, superficial, capricious, and to lack crispness.

Supersaturated Isopropanol Oil Red O Method for Neutral Fats (Lillie)

Prepare a stock saturated solution of the disazo dye, oil red O (xylene-azo-xylene-azo-beta-naphthol) by dissolving 250 to 500 mg in 100 mL of 99% isopropyl alcohol. For use, dilute in the proportion of 6 mL of stock to 4 mL of distilled water. Mix, allow to stand for 5 to 10 minutes, and then filter. This working dilution should be used within 2 to 4 hours. Such saturated staining solutions must be kept in air-tight staining vessels to avoid precipitation of the dye (because of evaporation of the solvent).

Procedure

1. Cut frozen sections at 10 to 40 μm. (Fat, e.g., emboli, may be lost from thin sections of certain tissues, e.g., lung, which is best cut at 25 to 35 μm, and brain, which is best cut at 15 to 25 μm. Actually, for scanty fat emboli, brain tissue is best embedded in gelatin; indeed, it is far more rewarding to section the choroid plexus when looking for scanty fat emboli in the nervous system.)

2. Wash well in distilled water and stain in oil red O for 10 minutes.

3. Rinse in tap water. On being placed in water the sections unfold very nicely, and if diagnosis only is required, e.g., of fat embolism, they may be mounted with ease at this stage and examined.

4. Counterstain 1 to 3 minutes in Mayer's hemalum. (Alternatively, both fat and nuclear staining may be accomplished simultaneously by dissolving 0.1 to 0.3 g pinacyanole in 100 mL of the stock saturated isopropanol solution of oil red O.)

5. Blue in tap water to which a few drops of saturated sodium carbonate have been added (or in 1% disodium phosphate).

6. Transfer to a fresh water bath. Float onto a clean slide. Drain but do not allow to dry. Mount in glycerin jelly, Farrant's medium, or von Apathy's gum syrup.

Results. Neutral fats—bright red; nuclei—blue; other tissues—pale brown.

Oil red O (xylene-azo-xylene-azo-beta-naphthol; M.W. 408.48)

Sudan black B (Solvent black 3; M.W. 456.53)

Figure 33–8 Structural formulas of oil red O and Sudan black B. Sudan III has the same formula as oil red O but lacks all four methyl groups; Sudan IV lacks the two methyl groups marked with asterisks in the oil red O formula.

Notes on Oil-Soluble Dye Staining of Fats

Sudan III was the first of these dyes to be introduced (1896). It was followed in 1901 by Sudan IV (Scharlach R or scarlet red). As will be seen from Figure 33–8 (legend), both these dyes are very closely related to oil red O. The latter was recommended for use as a fat stain in 1926, but did not become widely used until Lillie and Ashburn popularized it in 1943 by advocating its use as a 50 to 60% fresh aqueous dilution of a saturated 99% isopropanol stock solution. Hence *sudanophilia* has come to mean stainability with fat- or oil-soluble dyes regardless of the dye used, and the term also implies a fatty nature for the substances so staining. Sudan black B (Fig. 33–8) is also a diazo dye (two azo groups), and is the most sensitive lipid stain known, being actually too sensitive as a general fat stain. All of these dyes are insoluble in water and stain fats by being more soluble in them than in the aqueous-alcoholic or acetone-alcoholic phase in which they are applied.

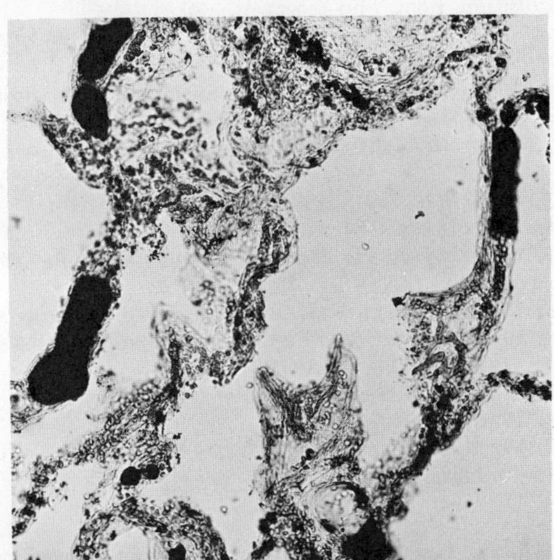

Figure 33–9 Fat emboli in lung resulting from fractures of the long bones. Frozen section stained by oil red O and lightly counterstained with Mayer's hemalum × 180.

Valid objections exist to the use of acetone and ethanol as vehicles for these dyes in that these solvents remove a significant portion of the lipids. As a result, small fat droplets are likely to be dissolved out and escape detection. Isopropyl alcohol is less objectionable in this regard. Propylene or ethylene glycol is even less objectionable (Culling, 1974).

Specificity of Oil-Soluble Dyes. Although based only on simple physical differential solubility, staining with these dyes is regarded as specific for lipids, especially for simple lipids (neutral fats). However, cholesterol and its esters, and also tristearin and carotenoids, do not take these dyes, or do so very weakly, at room temperature. Oil red O stains neutral fats and some lipofuscins well.

Nuclear Staining. Because of its simplicity, Mayer's hemalum is recommended in the routine method.

Precipitates with Oil-Soluble Dyes. Precipitates commonly form during staining with saturated aqueous-alcoholic solutions of these dyes. The tendency can be minimized by staining in airtight containers, using only freshly made and filtered working dilution of the stain, and by not staining for longer than 10 minutes (5 to 7 minutes is usually adequate). The sections should be agitated in the stain and rinsed well in distilled water after staining. Some workers recommend a quick rinse in 50 to 60% ethanol before the water rinse.

THE CENTRAL NERVOUS SYSTEM (CNS)

In the simplest analogy the nervous system may be likened to the most complex electronic "brain" that man is capable of assembling. It has millions of transistor units (nerve cells), which are interconnected in a most complex but orderly manner. The nerve cell sends out its physicochemically generated and propagated message as an electric impulse along its efferent fiber (axon). The same cell receives impulses or messages from other cells by means of short-branched processes (dendrites), which relay the message from the axons of other cells.

Obviously, since the messages are relayed as electric impulses, the conducting fibers or axons must be insulated from each other. This insulation is effected by means of a white fatty substance (myelin), which surrounds each fiber in a manner similar to the insulating plastic or rubber tube that covers household electrical wiring. Parts of the brain and most peripheral nerves consist mainly of insulated conducting circuits (myelinated fibers), and the abundance of myelin gives to these areas and structures a white appearance (white matter). Some nerves, e.g., sympathetic and parasympathetic fibers, are nonmyelinated (nonmedullated). Areas of the brain where nerve cells abound have a gray color (gray matter); examples are the cortex or rind of the brain and certain nuclear masses, e.g., basal ganglia.

Supporting Structures of Nervous System (Neuroglia)

The nerve cells (neurons) and their dendrites and myelinated axons are supported by various specialized cells and fibers known as *neuroglia,* which are the specialized connective tissue of the CNS. Throughout the whole nervous system fine capillary blood vessels serve as a nutrient framework and are covered by prolongations of the very fine leptomeninges, which enclose a microscopic space (Virchow-Robin space) around the tiny blood vessels.

Microglia are small phagocytic cells with nuclei of irregular outlines. They are probably derived from the pia mater that surrounds the capillaries and brain cortex. Collectively, three types of "supporting" cell—astrocytes, oligodendroglia, and microglia—are called *neuroglia,* but, as just stated, the microglia differ from the other two in being mesenchymal in origin. Astrocytes and oligodendroglia, like all other nervous structures (with the exception of the meninges, blood vessels, and microglia), are ectodermal in origin. In the gray matter microglia tend to occur as perineural satellites, though they are less abundant here than the oligodendroglia. Microglia are the scavenger or "macrophage" cells of the brain. When injured brain tissue undergoes degeneration the microglia increase in number and size in the affected area, and their cytoplasm becomes swollen and clear; they are then known as "gitter cells" or "compound granular corpuscles."

Fixation of Nervous System Tissues

This has already been described in the discussion of fixatives. Undoubtedly, the best general fixative for nervous tissue is formol-saline but buffered formalin gives excellent results. Formalin fixation renders cephalin and sphingomyelin insoluble even in hot alcohol and ether. A minimum of 48 hours should be allowed for fixation of the embalmed brain and 1 week for the unembalmed brain. The spinal cord is best fixed by suspension for 2 to 4 days (after opening the covering dura mater) in a tall cylinder of fixative.

Pathological Changes in the Central Nervous System

The responses to disease or injury occur in the cells and in the axons. The cells lose their Nissl's granules, and the nucleus moves from its central location to the periphery of the cytoplasm, which becomes increasingly eosinophilic and shrinks. If the axon is myelinated, the response of myelin to injury or disease is to degenerate and finally to be lost. A number of diseases, e.g., multiple sclerosis, have as the basis of their pathology a demyelinating process.

There are a large number of histological and histochemical methods to demonstrate changes in the nervous system; for these, larger works must be consulted. Simple hematoxylin and eosin stains will often give sufficient information for diagnosis, although the myelin sheath will not be seen. Luxol fast blue–cresyl echt violet will stain the cells in the nervous system and will show the myelin sheaths.

Luxol fast blue combines with lipoprotein of the myelin (simple lipids will have been dissolved during the processing of paraffin sections), and the cresyl echt violet stains the cells.

Luxol Fast Blue–Cresyl echt Violet (Kluver and Barrera)

Solutions Required

1. *Luxol fast blue* — 1 g
   Luxol fast blue MBSN (solvent blue 38)
   95% ethanol — 1 L

To the solution add:
   10% acetic acid — 5 mL

Filter before use.

2. *Cresyl echt violet*
   Cresyl violet* — 0.25% aqueous solution

Before use, add 5 drops of 10% acetic acid to 30 mL of the solution, heat, and filter.

Method

1. Dewax the formalin-fixed paraffin sections and rinse in several changes of 95% ethanol.

2. Stain overnight (16 to 24 hours) in Luxol fast blue at 57 to 60°C.

3. Rinse in 95% ethanol to remove excess stain.

4. Wash in distilled water.

5. Quickly immerse in 0.05% lithium carbonate (10 to 20 seconds).

6. Differentiate carefully in 70% ethanol until gray and white matter can be identified. Do not overdifferentiate.

7. Wash in distilled water.

8. Immerse in cresyl echt violet for 5 minutes.

9. Wash in 95% ethanol.

10. Wash in ethanol to which has been added 3 drops of neutral balsam.

---

*Matheson, Coleman, and Bell, Norwood, Ohio 45212.

11. Repeat step 10 in a second jar containing ethanol with 3 drops of neutral balsam.

12. Clear in xylene and mount.

Results. Normal myelin—blue to green-blue. Cells—pink to violet.

CHAPTERS 32 AND 33—REVIEW QUESTIONS

1. Define *fixation*. Give the requirements of an ideal fixative. Explain autolysis and putrifaction. Give the advantages and disadvantages of fixatives based on formaldehyde, on alcohol, and on mercuric chloride.

2. Describe the action of nitric acid and EDTA in decalcification. Explain the methods of testing whether decalcification is complete. What is the consequence of using these agents on subsequent staining for hemosiderin, and how may you avoid them?

3. Give the purposes of dehydration, clearing, wax impregnation, embedding, and frozen sectioning.

4. Explain the following terms in relation to dyes and dyeing:

Color index	Selective solubility
Progressive staining	Chromagen
Auxochromes	Mordants
Metachromasia	Argentaffin
Resonance system	Accentuators

5. Describe a method for demonstrating neutral fat, melanin, and reticulin. Explain the principle involved in each reaction.

6. Describe a PAS (periodic acid–Schiff) technique to show carbohydrate. Explain the principle involved in the technical steps. Comment on the use of a diastase control. Name three substances other than mucus and glycogen that are PAS positive.

REFERENCES FOR HISTOTECHNOLOGY SECTION

Baker, JR. Principles of Biological Microtechnique. London, Methuen & Co., Ltd., 1958.

Bussolati, G. A celloidin bag for the histological preparation of cytologic material. J Clin Pathol 1982; *35*:574–576.

Clark, G, ed. Staining procedures used by the biological stain commission, 3rd ed. Baltimore, Williams & Wilkins Co., 1960.

Conn, HJ. Biological Stains, 6th ed. Geneva, NY, Biotech, 1953.

Conn, HJ, Darrow, MA, and Emmel, VM. Staining Procedures, 2nd ed. Baltimore, Williams & Wilkins, 1960.

Culling, CFA. Handbook of Histopathological and Histochemical Techniques, 3rd ed. Reading, Mass., Butterworths, 1974.

Drury, RAB, and Wallington, EA. Carleton's Histological Technique, 4th ed. New York, Oxford University Press, 1967.

Lillie, RD, and Fullmer, HM. Histopathologic Technic and Practical Histochemistry, 4th ed. New York, McGraw-Hill Book Co., 1976.

Luna, LG, ed. Manual of Histological Staining Methods, 3rd ed. New York, McGraw-Hill Book Co., 1968.

Sheehan, DC, and Hrapchak, BB, eds. Theory and Practice of Histotechnology, 2nd ed. St. Louis, CV Mosby Co., 1980.

Silverton, RE, and Anderson, MJ. Handbook of Medical Laboratory Formulae. London, Butterworths, 1961.

APPENDICES

APPENDIX A. CONVERSION FACTORS

The term *millimicron,* used to describe the wavelength of radiant energy, is more correctly replaced by the term *nanometer,* abbreviated nm. (One nanometer = 10^{-9} meter.) The term *micromicrogram,* used as a unit for expressing such things as the hemoglobin content of a single red cell, should be replaced by the term *picogram.*

Conversion Factors

Inches to centimeters	× 2.54
Yards to meters	× 0.91
Gallons (U.S.) to liters	× 3.78
Gallons (British) to liters	× 4.54
Fluid ounces (U.S.) to milliliters	× 29.6
Fluid ounces (British) to milliliters	× 28.4
Ounces to grams	× 28.35
Pounds to kilograms	× 0.45
Centimeters to inches	× 0.39
Meters to yards	× 1.09
Liters to gallons (U.S.)	× 0.26
Liters to gallons (British)	× 0.22
Milliliters to fluid ounces (U.S.)	× 0.034
Milliliters to fluid ounces (British)	× 0.035
Grams to ounces	× 0.035
Kilograms to pounds	× 2.2
Millimicrons (nanometers) to angstroms	× 10

Apothecaries' Weights—Equivalents

1 grain = 65 milligrams
1 ounce = 29.57 grams or milliliters
1 dram = 60 grains = 3.7 grams or milliliters

SI System Equivalents

Present Common Usage	SI Equivalent
μ or micron	μm (micrometer; 10^{-6} meter)
μ^3 or cubic micron	fl (femtoliter; 10^{-15} liter)
μμg or micromicrogram	pg (picogram; 10^{-12} gram)
mcg or microgram	μg (microgram; 10^{-6} gram)
Å or Angstrom	nm × 10 (Å ÷ 10 = nm)
mμ or millimicron	nm (10^{-9} meter, nanometer)
calorie	4.1868 J (J = joule)
Calorie (kilocalorie)	4186.8 J or 4.1868 kJ (kilojoules)
mm Hg (millimeters of mercury)	kPa (kilopascals) = mm Hg × 0.133
mOsm (milliosmoles)	mmol/kg (millimol per kg): numerical value unchanged
volumes per cent (gases)	mmol/L (millimol per liter) = vols% × 0.446

Pressure Conversions

1 mm water	9.806 N/m²
1 mm Hg	133.322 N/m²
1 torr	133.322 N/m²
1 inch water gauge	249.089 N/m²
1 lb/sq in	6.895 kN/m²
1 kg/cm²	98.066 kN/m²
1 bar	100 kN/m²
1 atmosphere	101.325 kN/m²

mm water × 9.806 = Pa
mm Hg × 133.322 = Pa
torr × 133.322 = Pa
inches water × 249.089 = Pa
lb/sq inch × 6.895 = kPa
kg/cm² × 98.066 = kPa
bar × 100 = kPa
atmospheres × 101.325 = kPa
N/m² = pascal: symbol Pa, 1000 pascals = 1 kilopascal, symbol kPa

The most convenient working unit is the kilopascal, symbol kPa, and an approximate conversion is

$$\frac{\text{mm Hg} \times 2}{15} = \text{kPa}.$$

$$\text{Thus } 760 \text{ mm Hg} = \frac{760 \times 2}{15} = 101.3 \text{ kPa}.$$

To convert standard temperature and pressure—STP, 0°C at 760 mm Hg—to SI units, in theory the temperature should be converted to the thermodynamic temperature in kelvins (symbol K) when K = degrees Celsius plus 273.15. In practice this change is made in calculations by adding 273.15 to the stated temperature in degrees Celsius. The conversion to SI units of the pressure is made by the relationship 760 mm Hg = 101.3 kPa. Thus STP in SI units = 273.15° K at 101.3 kPa. (One might speculate that the choice of a standard pressure of 750 mm Hg instead of 760 mm Hg would simplify the system, since this would be 100 kPa in SI units.)

Wavelength and Wave Number

For radiation in the visible and ultraviolet regions of the spectrum, the usual and most convenient unit is the nanometer (nm, 10^{-9}m). In the infrared region, designation by wavelength would involve numbers ranging from about 1000 to 100,000 nm. It is customary and more convenient to describe infrared radiation in terms of wave number, which is the number of waves per unit length, usually per cm. Thus 1000 nm becomes 10,000 cm^{-1}; 50,000 nm becomes 200 cm^{-1}. The formula for conversion is:

$$\frac{\text{Number of nanometers in 1 cm} = 10^7}{\text{Wavelength in nanometers}} =$$

Number of waves per cm.

The symbol for wave number is the Greek letter nu—ν Useful tables of conversions from the present usage to SI unit convention, for use in many of the reports issued by hospital laboratories, may be found in the text *SI Units in Medicine—An Introduction to the International System of Units with Conversion Tables and Normal Ranges*, by Lippert, H., and Lehmann, H. P., published by Urban & Schwarzenberg, Baltimore, 1978.

APPENDIX B. ATOMIC WEIGHTS

Before 1961, atomic weights (more correctly, atomic masses) calculated by reference to naturally occurring oxygen as the standard, with a value of 16.0, differed slightly from the values found when the predominant isotope of oxygen, ^{16}O, was used. This was due to the presence of three isotopes in natural oxygen—^{16}O, ^{17}O, and ^{18}O. By a decision of the International Union of Pure and Applied Chemistry in 1961, the table of atomic weights is now based on the isotope carbon-12 (^{12}C) to which is assigned the exact atomic weight of 12. The table included here uses the values calculated on this basis. It will be noted that the atomic weight of natural carbon has the value 12.01; this is the weighted mean of the two predominant carbon isotopes—^{12}C, which forms 98.89% of natural carbon, and ^{13}C, which forms 1.11%. (The isotope of carbon used for dating purposes—^{14}C—forms only a minute proportion of natural carbon, and is detectable only by reason of its radioactivity.)

Element	Symbol	Atomic Weight (to Two Decimal Places)	Valence
Aluminum	Al	26.98	3
Antimony	Sb	121.75	3,5
Argon	Ar	39.95	0
Arsenic	As	74.92	3,5
Barium	Ba	137.34	2
Beryllium	Be	9.01	2
Bismuth	Bi	208.98	3,5
Boron	B	10.81	3
Bromine	Br	79.91	1,3,5,7
Cadmium	Cd	112.40	2
Calcium	Ca	40.08	2
Carbon	C	12.01	2,4
Cerium	Ce	140.12	3,4
Cesium	Cs	132.90	1
Chlorine	Cl	35.45	1,3,5,7
Chromium	Cr	52.00	2,3,6
Cobalt	Co	58.93	2,3
Copper	Cu	63.54	1,2
Dysprosium	Dy	162.50	3
Erbium	Er	167.26	3
Europium	Eu	151.96	2,3
Fluorine	F	19.00	1
Gadolinium	Gd	157.25	3
Gallium	Ga	69.72	2,3
Germanium	Ge	72.59	2,4
Gold	Au	196.97	1,3
Hafnium	Hf	178.49	4
Helium	He	4.00	0
Holmium	Ho	164.93	3
Hydrogen	H	1.01	1
Indium	In	114.82	1,3
Iodine	I	126.90	1,3,5,7
Iridium	Ir	192.20	3,4
Iron	Fe	55.85	2,3,6
Krypton	Kr	83.80	0
Lanthanum	La	138.91	3

Element	Symbol	Atomic Weight (to Two Decimal Places)	Valence
Lead	Pb	207.19	2,4
Lithium	Li	6.94	1
Lutetium	Lu	174.97	3
Magnesium	Mg	24.31	2
Manganese	Mn	54.94	2,3,4,6,7
Mercury	Hg	200.59	1,2
Molybdenum	Mo	95.94	2,3,4,5,6
Neodymium	Nd	144.24	3
Neon	Ne	20.18	0
Nickel	Ni	58.71	2,3
Niobium	Nb	92.91	3,5
Nitrogen	N	14.01	3,5
Osmium	Os	190.20	2,3,4,6,8
Oxygen	O	16.00	2
Palladium	Pd	106.40	2,4
Phosphorus	P	30.97	3,5
Platinum	Pt	195.09	2,4
Potassium	K	39.10	1
Praseodymium	Pr	140.91	3,4,5
Rhenium	Re	186.20	3,4,5,6,7
Rhodium	Rh	102.91	1,2,3,4
Rubidium	Rb	85.47	1
Ruthenium	Ru	101.07	3,4,6,8
Samarium	Sm	150.35	2,3
Scandium	Sc	44.96	3
Selenium	Se	78.96	2,4,6
Silicon	Si	28.09	4
Silver	Ag	107.87	1
Sodium	Na	22.99	1
Strontium	Sr	87.62	2
Sulfur	S	32.06	2,4,6
Tantalum	Ta	180.95	3,5
Tellurium	Te	127.60	2,4,6
Terbium	Tb	158.92	3
Thallium	Tl	204.37	1,3
Thorium	Th	232.04	4

Element	Symbol	Atomic Weight (to Two Decimal Places)	Valence
Thulium	Tm	168.93	3
Tin	Sn	118.69	2,4
Titanium	Ti	47.90	2,3,4
Tungsten	W	183.85	2,4,5,6
Uranium	U	238.03	3,4,6
Vanadium	V	50.94	2,3,4,5
Xenon	Xe	131.30	0
Ytterbium	Yb	173.04	3
Yttrium	X	88.91	3
Zinc	Zn	65.37	2
Zirconium	Zr	91.22	2,4

APPENDIX C. IMPORTANT RADIOACTIVE ELEMENTS

In addition to the 274 known stable isotopes of the elements, there are at least 1300 or more radioactive isotopes. The short list here includes only those of interest because they are used in diagnosis and treatment, or because of their historical importance.

Element	Atomic Number Z	Mass Number A	Half-Life
Antimony	51	122	67 hr
		124	60 days
Arsenic	33	74	17.5 days
		76	26.8 hr
Beryllium	3	7	53 days
Bismuth	83	210	5 days
Bromine	35	82	35.7 hr
Calcium	20	45	164 days
(with scandium 47)		47	4.7 days
Carbon	6	11	20.4 min
		14	5730 years
Cerium	58	141	33 days
Chlorine	17	38	37.3 min
Chromium	24	51	27.8 days
Cobalt	27	57	270 days
		58	72 days
		60	5.2 yr
Copper	29	64	12.8 hr
Gold	79	198	2.69 days
		199	3.15 days
Hydrogen (tritium)	1	3	12.26 yr
Iodine	53	125	60 days
		130	12.6 hr
		131	8.1 days
		132	2.33 hr
Iron	26	55	2.94 yr
		59	45 days
Magnesium	12	28	21.2 hr
(with aluminum 28)			
Manganese	25	52	5.8 days
		54	320 days
Mercury	80	197	2.7 days
		203	47.9 days
Nickel	28	56	6.4 days
		63	125 yr
Phosphorus	15	32	14.3 days
Potassium	19	42	12.5 hr
Radium	88	228	1620 yr
Radon	86	222	3.83 days
Rubidium	37	86	18.6 days
Selenium	34	75	127 days
Silver	47	111	7.5 days
Sodium	11	22	2.6 yr
		24	15 hr
Strontium	38	85	65 days
		89	54 days
(with yttrium 90)		90	28 yr
Sulfur	16	35	87 days
Technetium	43	93	2.7 hr
Tellurium	52	121	17 days
Thallium	81	204	4.1 yr
Thorium	90	232	1.39×10^{10} yr
Tin	50	113	115 days
(with indium 113m)			
Tungsten	74	185	74 days
Vanadium	23	48	16 days
Xenon	54	133	5.27 days
Zinc	30	65	245 days

APPENDIX D. MEASUREMENT OF TEMPERATURE

The accepted temperature scale for scientific purposes is the Celsius (centigrade) system, which is based on two defined points:

1. *The Triple-Point State of Water:* The temperature at which water exists simultaneously as a liquid, a solid, and a gas. It occurs at a pressure of 611 N/m² and corresponds to 273.15°K or 0°C.

2. *The Steam Point:* The equilibrium temperature between water and water vapor, commonly referred to as the boiling point of water—designated as 100 degrees Celsius (100°C), determined at 760 mm pressure.

For certain calculations in clinical chemistry, such as those involving the gas laws, the absolute, or Kelvin, temperature scale is used. The zero point on this scale is defined from thermodynamic considerations, but corresponds to the theoretic temperature at which all kinetic energy of the molecules of a perfect gas has ceased. 0 degrees Kelvin (0°K) corresponds to −273.15°C; thus, for practical purposes, degrees K = degrees C + 273.15.

The Fahrenheit Scale: The defined points are the same as for the Celsius scale, but are allotted different numerical values: the triple point is 32°F and the steam point 212°F, so that one Fahrenheit degree equals 100/180 or 5/9 of a Celsius degree. The two scales may be interconverted by the following expressions:

$$(°C \times 1.8) + 32 = °F \text{ or } (°C \times 9/5) + 32 = °F.$$
$$(°F - 32) \times 0.55 = °C \text{ or } (F° - 32) \times 5/9 = °C.$$

The Rankine scale, in which absolute temperatures are measured using Fahrenheit units, and the Réaumer scale, which divides the span between the triple point and the steam point into 80°R, are now little used.

APPENDIX E. INDICATORS

In the following list of indicators, those most widely used in medical laboratory technology are marked with an asterisk.

Indicator	pH Range(s)	Color Change Over the Range
Methyl violet	0.2–1.8	Colorless to blue
	2.0–3.2	Blue to violet
Metacresol purple	1.2–2.8	Red to yellow
	7.6–9.2	Yellow to purple
Thymol blue	1.2–2.8	Red to yellow
	8.0–9.6	Yellow to blue
*Topfer's reagent (dimethyl yellow)	2.9–4.0	Red to yellow
*Bromphenol blue	3.0–4.6	Yellow to blue
Congo red	3.0–5.0	Blue to red
*Methyl orange	3.1–4.4	Red to yellow
*Bromcresol green	3.8–5.4	Yellow to blue
Methyl red	4.2–6.3	Red to yellow
Litmus	4.5–8.3	Red to blue
Chlorphenol red	5.1–6.7	Yellow to red
*Bromcresol purple	5.2–6.8	Yellow to purple
*Bromthymol blue	6.0–7.6	Yellow to blue
*Neutral red	6.8–8.0	Red to yellow
*Phenol red	6.8–8.4	Yellow to red
Cresol red	7.2–8.8	Yellow to red
*Phenolphthalein	8.3–10.0	Colorless to red
Thymolphthalein	9.3–10.5	Colorless to blue
Alizarin yellow GG	10.0–12.0	Yellow to lilac
Tropeolin 0	11.1–12.7	Yellow to orange
1,3,5-Trinitrobenzene	12.0–14.3	Colorless to orange

Preparation of Indicator Solutions

For volumetric titrations, the commonly used indicators are available commercially in convenient plastic dropping bottles, as dilute (0.1 to 0.5%) aqueous or alcoholic solutions. If the sulfonephthalein group of indicators is used for pH determination—e.g., for adjustment of bacteriological media—conversion to the salt form of the indicator is accomplished by the following procedure.

Mix 0.1 g of the indicator in a mortar with the volume of 0.01 M sodium hydroxide shown here and dilute the solution up to 250 mL with distilled water that has been boiled and cooled to remove carbon dioxide.

Bromcresol green	14.3 mL
Bromcresol purple	18.5 mL
Bromphenol blue	14.9 mL
Bromthymol blue	16.0 mL
Chlorphenol red	23.6 mL
Cresol red	26.2 mL
Metacresol purple	26.2 mL
Phenol red	28.2 mL
Thymol blue	21.5 mL

The Use of Indicators in Acid-Base Titrations

When titrating:

1. Strong acid with strong base—use an indicator that changes color at an alkaline pH, e.g., phenolphthalein.
2. Strong base with strong acid—use an indicator that changes color at an acid pH, e.g., methyl orange.
3. Weak acid with strong base—use an indicator that changes color at an alkaline pH, e.g., phenolphthalein.
4. Weak base with strong acid—use an indicator that changes color at an acid pH, e.g., methyl orange.

When titrating strong acids with strong bases, and vice versa, the rate of change of pH as the equivalence point is approached is so great that the choice of indicator is not very critical; the indicator will be completely converted from one form to the other by a very small addition of titrant. But for titrations involving weak acids and weak bases, the indicator must be selected by reference to its equivalence point and the degree of hydrolysis of the salts produced during titration. For example, an indicator changing color in the acid pH range would be useless for titrations of weak acids with strong bases because the indicator would change color before the neutral point was reached.

APPENDIX F. HYDROGEN ION CONCENTRATION AND PREPARATION OF STANDARD SOLUTIONS AND BUFFERS

HYDROGEN ION CONCENTRATION AND pH

Pure water is ionized to a small degree; some of the water molecules are split into hydrogen ions (H^+) and hydroxyl ions (OH^-). At 24°C the concentration of hydrogen ions in pure water is 10^{-7} gram molecules per liter, i.e., 1/10,000,000 g per liter. The symbol used to denote hydrogen ion concentration is C_H. The number of hydroxyl ions (OH^-) in pure water will, of course, be equal to the number of hydrogen ions. The dissociation constant of water is the product of the hydrogen and hydroxyl ion concentrations:

$$K_W = [H^+] \times [OH^-]$$

The hydrogen ion concentration varies slightly with temperature, e.g., at 18°C $C_H = 10^{-7.07}$, and at 24°C $C_H = 10^{-7}$. The dissociation constant will, therefore, also vary slightly, e.g.:

$$\text{at 18°C } K_W = 10^{-7.07} \times 10^{-7.07} = 10^{-14.14}$$
$$\text{at 24°C } K_W = 10^{-7} \times 10^{-7} = 10^{-14}.$$

For practical purposes, however, K_W is taken as 10^{-14}. The dissociation constant of water, K_W, holds for all aqueous solutions.

Neutral Solution. A neutral solution is one in which hydrogen ions and hydroxyl ions are equal, as in pure water.

Acid Solution. This is one in which the hydrogen ion concentration is greater than the hydroxyl ion concentration.

Alkaline Solution. In an alkaline solution the hydroxyl ion concentration is greater than the hydrogen ion concentration.

pH

When dealing with solutions in terms of acidity or alkalinity, it is usual to refer only to the hydrogen ion concentration. (The hydroxyl ion concentration can easily be calculated from the K_W formula.) Since hydrogen ion concentrations are very small numbers, and therefore cumbersome, the Sorensen notation, called pH, is used. This is the logarithm, to base 10, of the reciprocal of the hydrogen ion concentration, i.e.,

$$pH = \log 1/C_H.$$

To convert C_H to pH:

EXAMPLE. $C_H = 2 \times 10^{-6}$ g ions per liter

$$pH = \log \frac{1}{2 \times 10^{-6}} = \log \frac{10^6}{2}$$
$$= 6.0 - 0.301 = 5.699.$$

To convert C_{OH} to pOH:

EXAMPLE. $C_{OH} = 5 \times 10^{-8}$ g ions per liter

$$pOH = \log \frac{1}{5 \times 10^{-8}} = \log \frac{10^8}{5}$$
$$= 8.0 - 0.699 = 7.301.$$

To calculate pOH when pH is known:

From $K_W = [H] \times [OH] = 10^{-14}$

$$pH + pOH = 14.$$

EXAMPLE. pH $= 6.0$
pOH $= 14 - 6 = 8.$

Calculation of pH of an Acid Solution

In a solution containing a weak acid, its conjugate base, and the hydronium ions derived from dissociation of the acid, if it is assumed that the concentration of water undergoes a negligible change (and this assumption is largely true for most solutions of this type in common use), the dissociation constant of the acid—K_a—can be derived from the formula:

$$K_a = \frac{[H_3O^+][A^-]}{[HA]},$$

when $[H_3O^+]$ is the concentration of hydronium ion in moles per liter, $[A^-]$ is that of the conjugate base, and [HA] that of the undissociated acid. The value obtained reflects the strength of the acid; it is more conveniently expressed in an exponential form analogous to the pH notation: $pK_a = \log \frac{1}{K_a}$ ·A strong acid has a low pK_a value; an acid with a pK_a value greater than 7.0 will hardly redden litmus paper. If the pK_a of a weak acid is known from tables, and provided that the calculated hydronium concentration from the expression

$$[H_3O^+] = \sqrt{K_a \times \text{Concentration of acid in moles per liter } C_a}$$

is not greater than $0.05 \times [C_a]$, the pH can be found from the expression:

$$pH = -\log(K_aC_a)^{1/2} \text{ or } pH = \tfrac{1}{2}pK_a - \tfrac{1}{2}\log C_a.$$

If the hydronium ion concentration is found to be greater than the limit $0.05 \times C_a$, the more accurate formula must be used:

$$[H_3O^+] = \frac{-K_a \pm (K_a^2 + 4\,C_aK_a)^{1/2}}{2}.$$

The hydronium ion concentration now being known, the pH is determined from the usual relationship:

$$pH = -\log [H_3O^+] \text{ or } pH = \log \frac{1}{[H_3O^+]}.$$

For example, to find the pH of a 0.2 molar solution of acetic acid: K_a for acetic acid = 1.75×10^{-5}; pK_a = 4.76; C_a = 0.2 moles per liter.

$[H_3O] = \sqrt{K_aC_a} = \sqrt{1.75 \times 10^{-5} \times 0.2} = \sqrt{0.35 \times 10^{-5}}$ = 0.00187 mole per liter. This value is less than $0.05 \times C_a$ ($0.05 \times 0.2 = 0.01$). Therefore:

$$\begin{aligned} pH &= \tfrac{1}{2}pK_a - \tfrac{1}{2}\log C_a \\ &= \frac{4.76}{2} - \tfrac{1}{2}(\bar{2} + 1.3010) \\ &= 2.38 - (\bar{1} + 0.6505) \\ &= 2.38 + 1 - 0.6505 \\ &= 2.73. \end{aligned}$$

PREPARATION OF STANDARD SOLUTIONS

Primary Standards

Substances that are stable, can be accurately weighed, and are available in pure form are primary standards, e.g., constant-boiling hydrochloric acid, sodium carbonate, sodium oxalate, and potassium hydrogen phthalate. Accurately prepared solutions of these substances do not require standardization and can be used to standardize solutions of other substances.

STANDARD HYDROCHLORIC ACID

Constant Boiling Method

When hydrochloric acid is distilled, ultimately the undistilled portion reaches a state of constant composition, and from then on the distillate has the same concentration as that of the undistilled portion.

This method was described by Hulett and Bonner (1909).

Procedure. Dilute concentrated hydrochloric acid with an equal volume of distilled water; bring the specific gravity of the solution to 1.096 with the addition of more acid or water.

Using an all glass still, distill off three-quarters of the solution at the rate of 3 to 4 mL per minute. The remaining solution will have the concentration listed in the following table, depending on the barometric pressure.

Barometric Pressure at the Time of Distillation	Hydrochloric Acid Concentration by Weight	Amount Required, by Weight, to Make 1 Liter of 0.1 M Hydrochloric Acid
730 mm	20.293 g /100 g	17.956 g
740 mm	20.269 g /100 g	17.977 g
750 mm	20.245 g /100 g	17.998 g
760 mm	20.221 g /100 g	18.019 g
770 mm	20.197 g /100 g	18.041 g
780 mm	20.173 g /100 g	18.062 g

Distill all but the last 50 mL of the remaining solution into a clean, dry flask. Use the distillate to prepare standard solutions. Stored in a polyethylene or waxed glass bottle, this solution keeps indefinitely.

0.1 M Hydrochloric Acid Solution

Place about 16 mL of constant boiling hydrochloric acid solution in a weighed beaker of 50 or 100 mL capacity and add or remove acid until the desired weight (obtained from the preceding table) is achieved. Pour the acid into a liter volumetric flask, wash in with 2 or 3 lots of distilled water, and then make the volume up to 1 liter with distilled water. This solution does not require standardization, and is regarded as a primary standard against which other solutions may be standardized.

Note. Concentrated hydrochloric acid, specific gravity 1.18, is about 10 times molar; therefore, an approximately molar solution may be prepared by diluting the concentrated acid 1 in 10.

STANDARD SODIUM HYDROXIDE SOLUTIONS

Removal of Sodium Carbonate

Dissolve 100 g of pure sodium hydroxide pellets or sticks in 1 dL of distilled water. Cap the flask and leave overnight at room temperature. The carbonate will settle out as an insoluble precipitate. Filter the solution through a sintered glass filter, applying gentle suction if necessary.

1.0 N (1.0 M) Sodium Hydroxide Solution

Dilute 50 mL of the carbonate-free sodium hydroxide solution (see the preceding paragraph) to 1 liter with freshly boiled and cooled distilled water in a liter volumetric flask. Standardize against 1.0 M hydrochloric acid.

Calculation of Normality

For example, 20 mL of a 1.0 N (1.0 M) solution of hydrochloric acid required 19.5 mL of a sodium hydroxide solution for complete neutralization. Normality of the hydroxide solution:

$$\frac{1.0 \text{ N} \times 20 \text{ mL}}{19.5 \text{ mL}} = 1.025 \text{ N}$$

If it is desired to dilute the hydroxide solution to exactly 1.0 N, the amount of hydroxide to be diluted to 1 liter is calculated as follows:

$$\frac{1000 \text{ mL} \times 1.0 \text{ N}}{\text{normality of solution}} = \frac{1000 \text{ mL} \times 1.0 \text{ N}}{1.025 \text{ N}} = 975.6 \text{ mL}$$

Note. All dilutions must be made with freshly boiled and cooled distilled water. The normality of the solution must be checked by titration after dilution. At least 3 titrations of each solution should be made and the mean value taken. Phenolphthalein is a suitable indicator for these titrations; the acids are titrated with the hydroxide solutions when using this indicator.

0.1 N (0.1 M) Sodium Thiosulfate

1. $2\ Na_2S_2O_3 + I_2 = 2\ NaI + Na_2S_4O_6$.
2. $I_2 + H_2O = 2\ HI + O$.

From equation 1 it is seen that two molecules of thiosulfate react with one molecule of iodine; therefore, one molecule of thiosulfate will react with one atom of iodine. In equation 2, one atom of iodine is seen to replace one equivalent of oxygen; the equivalent weight of iodine is then the same as its atomic weight. From this it follows that the equivalent weight of sodium thiosulfate is the same as its molecular weight.

Dissolve 25 g of crystalline sodium thiosulfate in 1 liter of distilled water.

Standardization

1. Make an accurate 0.1 N potassium iodate solution by dissolving 3.567 g of pure dry potassium iodate (KIO_3) in a liter flask with distilled water; make the volume up to 1 liter with distilled water.
2. Prepare an approximately 10% w/v solution of potassium iodide (KI) in distilled water.
3. Mix about 1 g of soluble starch with a little cold distilled water and pour it slowly, with constant stirring, into 200 mL of boiling distilled water. Continue heating until the starch is in solution.
4. In a 200-mL beaker or flask, place 20 mL of the 0.1 N potassium iodate solution, 10 mL of potassium iodide solution, and 20 mL of 1.0 N hydrochloric acid. The solution in the flask will become amber as a result of liberated iodine:

$$KIO_3 + 5\ KI + 6\ HCl = 3\ I_2 + 6\ KCl + 3\ H_2O$$

5. Titrate this solution with the approximately 0.1 N thiosulfate solution until almost all the amber color has been discharged. Add 1.0 mL of the starch solution; a blue color will result. Continue the titration until the blue color is just discharged. Repeat the titration twice more, and take the mean of the titration values.

Normality of the sodium thiosulfate solution is calculated as follows:

$$\frac{20\ \text{mL} \times 0.1\ \text{N}}{\text{mL of thiosulfate used in titration}}$$

If the solution is not exactly 0.1 N, calculate the factor by which titration values obtained with this solution may be multiplied to convert them to terms of 0.1 N:

$$\text{Factor} = \frac{\text{Normality of thiosulfate}}{0.1}$$

0.1 N Iodine Solution

Dissolve 24 g of pure potassium iodide in about 100 mL of distilled water in a liter volumetric flask. Add 13.5 g of pure sublimed iodine and dissolve completely. Make the volume up to 1 liter with distilled water. Standardize against 0.1 N sodium thiosulfate solution.

Standard Potassium Permanganate Solution

One gram molecule of potassium permanganate (158 g) yields 5 gram equivalents of oxygen in acid solution; therefore, 158/5 = 31.6 g of potassium permanganate will yield 1 gram equivalent of oxygen.

0.1 N Potassium Permanganate Solution

Dissolve 3.16 g of pure potassium permanganate in, and make the volume up to 1 liter with distilled water. Store in a brown glass bottle. The normality of this solution may be checked against 0.1 N oxalic acid solution as follows: Place 20 mL of 0.1 N oxalic acid solution in a conical flask, add 10 mL of approximately normal sulfuric acid, heat to about 80°C, and then titrate with the potassium permanganate solution to the first appearance of a persistent pale pink color. A blank solution consisting of 20 mL of distilled water and 10 mL of normal sulfuric acid is titrated to the same end point and the titer subtracted from the first titration.

1.0 N Oxalic Acid Solution

Dissolve 63.035 g of pure crystalline oxalic acid $(COOH)_2 \cdot H_2O$ in and make the volume up to 1 liter with distilled water. Dilute volumetrically 1 in 10 for 0.1 N oxalic acid.

PREPARATION OF BUFFER SOLUTIONS

The suitability of a buffer solution for a particular procedure depends on:

(i) Buffer capacity: the total capacity of the buffer to minimize the effect of added strong acid or base. This in turn depends on the concentration of the buffer constituents, and the difference between the buffer pH and the pK_a of its acid component. The buffer has its highest buffering ability when its $pH = pK_a$.

(ii) Buffer efficiency: the smaller the change in pH for a given addition of strong acid or base, the greater is the efficiency of the buffer. In most cases the buffer efficiency is close to its maximum value in the range $pK_a \pm 0.5$, although many buffers are effective in the range $pH = pK_a \pm 1.0$.

(iii) Particularly in enzyme applications, the chemical composition of the buffer must be compatible with the reaction in which it is used. In some instances—for example, the amino alcohol buffers used in some alkaline phosphatase assay methods—the type of buffer has a significant enhancing effect on enzymatic activity. In critical enzyme work the buffer constituents must be free of any trace metals which might inhibit the reaction, and in general only highest purity reagent chemicals should be used. In some instances when a buffer of low capacity is used, the distilled water used in its preparation must be boiled to remove dissolved carbon dioxide.

Storage of Buffers

Wherever possible, buffers should be prepared and stored in concentrated form, and kept either refrigerated or with a suitable preservative. For nonenzymatic procedures, a trace of sodium azide (about 0.01% w/v) will inhibit mold growth in phosphate buffers. The problem with refrigeration of concentrated buffers is crystallization of a constituent salt; the form of such crystals often makes them slow to redissolve. The alternative is to keep preweighed vials of the salt component(s) of a buffer to facilitate rapid preparation when required. Except for use in fluorometric methods, in which interference may occur from plasticizers extracted from some plastics, buffers should be stored in polypropylene bottles, or good-quality polyethylene.

"Zwitterion" Buffers

In recent years the traditional buffers, using phosphates, acetates, TRIS, and so forth, have been supplemented by some new groups of compounds such as the amino alcohols and the ethane and propanesulfonic acids. For biochemical and tissue culture purposes they have some important advantages—compatibility with enzymes, and freedom from heavy metal contamination. In addition they are simple to use. Select a buffer substance from the list with a pK_a value close to the desired value of pH required and below it. Prepare a solution of it in a smaller volume than stipulated by the required molarity, and titrate with a suitable base to the exact pH desired, using a pH meter and stirring constantly. Finally make up to the required volume. By this means small amounts of buffer can be prepared quickly and accurately for special or occasional requirements. The use of the more exotic and expensive compounds is confined largely to tissue culture work, but recent alkaline phosphatase assay methods employ the amino alcohols.

Formulating a Buffer

For convenience, the tables give the volumes of stock solutions that are combined to yield a buffer of a required pH. The following examples illustrate the procedure for arriving at these volumes.

The weak acid/salt pair used and the molarity will be governed by the use to which the buffer will be put; generally speaking, it is more convenient to make the buffer as a relatively concentrated solution from which working solutions may be prepared by dilution. It is also convenient to prepare the acid and salt solutions in equimolar concentrations, since this simplifies the calculations.

To prepare a buffer of pH 5.4 with a final molarity of 0.1 M, use acetic acid and sodium acetate solutions, each 0.2 molar.

$$pH = pK_a + \log \frac{[salt]}{[acid]}$$

$$5.4 = 4.76 + \log x$$
$$\text{Log } x = 5.4 - 4.76 = 0.64$$
$$x = \text{antilog } 0.64 = 4.37$$

Since both acid and salt solutions are 0.2 molar, the ratio of their volumes will be the same as the ratio of their concentrations. Therefore 4.37 volumes of salt solution will be required for each volume of acid. That is, the mixture will contain $\frac{4.37}{5.37}$ parts of salt solution and $\frac{1.0}{5.37}$ parts of acid solution. To finish up with a 0.1

BUFFERS ARRANGED BY pK_a AND EFFECTIVE BUFFER RANGE*

Abbreviated Name	Chemical Name	pK_a	Range
	Citric acid (pK_a1)	3.2	
	Citric acid (pK_a2)	4.8	3.0– 6.0
	Citric acid (pK_a3) trisodium	5.4	
	Succinic acid (pK_a1)	4.2	3.8– 6.0
	Succinic acid (pK_a2)	5.6	
MES	2(Morpholino)ethanesulfonic acid	6.1	5.8– 6.5
	Maleic acid	6.2	5.2– 7.2
ADA	*N*–(2–Acetamido)iminodiacetic acid	6.6	6.2– 7.2
PIPES	Piperazine–*N,N'*–bis(2–ethanesulfonic acid)	6.8	6.4– 7.2
ACES	N–(2–Acetamido)–2–aminoethanesulfonic acid	6.9	6.4– 7.4
BES	*N,N*–Bis(2–hydroxyethyl)–2–aminoethane sulfonic acid	7.1	6.6– 7.6
MOPS	3–(*N*-Morpholino)propanesulfonic acid	7.2	6.5– 7.9
TES	*N*–Tris(hydroxymethyl)methyl–2–amino–ethanesulfonic acid	7.5	7.0– 8.0
HEPES	*N*–2–Hydroxyethylpiperazine–*N'*–2–ethanesulfonic acid	7.5	7.0– 8.0
EPPS	*N*–2–Hydroxyethylpiperazine–*N'*–3–propanesulfonic acid	8.0	7.6– 8.6
TRIS	Tris(hydroxymethyl)aminomethane	8.3	7.3– 9.3
TRICINE	*N*–Tris(hydroxymethyl)methylglycine	8.2	7.6– 8.8
BICINE	*N,N*–Bis(2–hydroxyethyl)glycine	8.3	7.8– 8.8
	Glycylglycine	8.3	7.3– 9.3
	2–Amino–2–ethyl–1,3–propanediol	9.4	8.6–10.2
	2–Amino–2–methyl–1,3–propanediol	9.4	8.6–10.2
CHES	2–(Cyclohexylamino)ethanesulfonic acid	9.6	9.0–10.1
AMP	2–Amino–2–methyl–1–propanol	9.6	8.6–10.6
CAPS	3–(Cyclohexylamino)–1,1–propane-sulfonic acid	10.4	9.7–11.1

***Table is reproduced by permission of P–L Biochemicals, Inc., Milwaukee, Wis., 53205, from their reference guide, 1973 edition, p. 123.**

M solution, the mixture must have a final volume of twice the total volumes of acid and salt solution. For a final volume of 200 mL the sum of acid and salt solutions must be 100 mL, and of this amount $\frac{4.37}{5.37} \times 100$ mL = 81.4 mL will be 0.2 M sodium acetate solution, and $\frac{1.0}{5.37} \times 100$ mL = 18.6 mL will be 0.2 M acetic acid. When mixed and made up to 200 mL, the solution will have a pH of 5.4 and a molarity of 0.1.

When using polyprotic acids such as phosphoric, the pK_a which corresponds to the particular state of ionization must be used. For example, to prepare a phosphate buffer of pH 7.0, the dissociation of the $H_2PO_4^-$ ion has a pK_a of 7.19, which is close to the required buffer pH, and will therefore be the most efficient.

$$pH = pK_a + \log \frac{[salt]}{[acid]}$$

In this example, the salt is the $HPO_4^=$ ion and the acid the $H_2PO_4^-$ ion.

$$7.0 = 7.19 + \log \underline{x}$$
$$\log x = -0.19 = \bar{1} + 0.81 \text{ by the usual logarithmic transformation}$$
$$x = \text{antilog } \bar{1}.81 = 0.646$$

Thus the ratio of salt to acid is 0.646/1.0; in each 100 mL of mixture, $\frac{0.646}{1.646} \times 100 = 39.25$ mL of 0.2 M monohydrogen phosphate plus $\frac{1.0}{1.646} \times 100 = 60.75$ mL of dihydrogen phosphate, 0.2 M. The final molarity will be 0.2 M, and from this buffers of other molarities can be made by suitable dilution.

Buffers for Histochemical and Enzyme Studies

HCl-KCl Buffer—pH Range 1.0 to 2.2

Stock Solution A. Dissolve 14.91 g potassium chloride (KCl) in 1 liter distilled water, making a 0.2 M solution.

Stock Solution B. 0.2 M hydrochloric acid (HCl), checked by titration.

mL of Solution B	Final pH
97.0	1.0
78.0	1.1
64.5	1.2
51.0	1.3
41.5	1.4
33.3	1.5
26.3	1.6
20.6	1.7
16.6	1.8
13.2	1.9
10.6	2.0
8.4	2.1
6.7	2.2

Mix 50.0 mL of solution A with the volume of solution B as shown in the table, and make up to a final total volume of 200 mL to obtain the pH values shown.

Glycine-HCl Buffer—pH Range 2.2 to 3.6

Stock Solution A. Dissolve 15.01 g glycine (NH_2CH_2COOH) in 1 liter distilled water, making a 0.2 M solution.

Stock Solution B. 0.2 M hydrochloric acid (HCl).

Mix 50.0 mL of solution A with the volume of solution B as shown in the table, and make up to a final total volume of 200 mL to obtain the pH values shown.

mL of Solution B	Final pH
44.0	2.2
32.4	2.4
24.2	2.6
16.8	2.8
11.4	3.0
8.2	3.2
6.4	3.4
5.0	3.6

Phthalate-HCl Buffer—pH Range 2.2 to 3.8

Stock Solution A. Dissolve 40.85 g potassium acid phthalate (potassium biphthalate—$HOOCC_6H_4COOK$) in 1 liter distilled water, making a 0.2 M solution.

Stock Solution B. 0.2 M hydrochloric acid (HCl).

Mix 50.0 mL of solution A with the volume of solution B as shown in the table, and make up to a final total volume of 200 mL to obtain the pH values shown.

mL Solution B	Final pH
46.7	2.2
39.6	2.4
33.0	2.6
26.4	2.8
20.3	3.0
14.7	3.2
9.9	3.4
6.0	3.6
2.63	3.8

Acetate Buffer—pH Range 3.5 to 5.6

Stock Solution A. Dilute 11.55 mL glacial acetic acid ($CH_3 \cdot COOH$) up to 1 liter with distilled water, making a 0.2 M solution.

Stock Solution B. Dissolve 16.41 g anhydrous sodium acetate ($CH_3 \cdot COONa$) or 27.22 g $CH_3 \cdot COONa \cdot 3H_2O$ in 1 liter distilled water, making a 0.2 M solution.

Mix the volumes of the stock solutions as shown in the table and dilute to a final volume of 100 mL to obtain the pH values shown.

mL of Solution A	mL of Solution B	Final pH
46.3	3.7	3.6
44.0	6.0	3.8
41.0	9.0	4.0
36.8	13.2	4.2
30.5	19.5	4.4
25.5	24.5	4.6
20.0	30.0	4.8
14.8	35.2	5.0
10.5	39.5	5.2
8.8	41.2	5.4
4.8	45.2	5.6

Phthalate–Sodium Hydroxide Buffer—pH Range 4.2 to 6.0

Stock Solution A. Dissolve 40.85 g potassium acid phthalate ($HOOCC_6H_4COOK$) in 1 liter distilled water, making a 0.2 M solution.

Stock Solution B. 0.2 M sodium hydroxide (NaOH).

Mix 50.0 mL of solution A with the volume of solution B as shown in the table, and make up to a final total volume of 200 mL to obtain the pH values shown.

mL of Solution B	Final pH
3.7	4.2
7.5	4.4
12.2	4.6
17.7	4.8
23.9	5.0
30.0	5.2
35.5	5.4
39.8	5.6
43.0	5.8
45.5	6.0

Phosphate Buffer—pH Range 5.7 to 8.0

Sock Solution A. Dissolve 27.6 g of monobasic sodium phosphate ($NaH_2PO_4 \cdot H_2O$) in 1 liter of distilled water, making a 0.2 M solution.

Stock Solution B. Disssolve 28.39 g of dibasic sodium phosphate (Na_2HPO_4 *or* 53.62 g $Na_2HPO_4 \cdot 7H_2O$) in 1 liter of distilled water, making a 0.2 M solution.

Mix the volumes of the stock solutions as shown in the table and dilute to a final volume of 200 mL to obtain the pH values shown.

mL of Solution A	mL of Solution B	Final pH
93.5	6.5	5.7
92.0	8.0	5.8
90.0	10.0	5.9
87.7	12.3	6.0
85.0	15.0	6.1
81.5	18.5	6.2
77.5	22.5	6.3
73.5	26.5	6.4
68.5	31.5	6.5
62.5	37.5	6.6
56.5	43.5	6.7
51.0	49.0	6.8
45.0	55.0	6.9
39.0	61.0	7.0
33.0	67.0	7.1
28.0	72.0	7.2
23.0	77.0	7.3
19.0	81.0	7.4
16.0	84.0	7.5
13.0	87.0	7.6
10.5	90.5	7.7
8.5	91.5	7.8
7.0	93.0	7.9
5.3	94.7	8.0

Barbital Buffer—pH Range 6.8 to 9.2

Stock Solution A. Dissolve 41.2 g sodium diethylbarbiturate (sodium barbital) in 1 liter distilled water, making a 0.2 M solution.

Stock Solution B. 0.2 M hydrochloric acid (HCl).

Mix 50.0 mL of solution A with the volume of solution B as shown in the table, and make up to a final total volume of 200 mL to obtain the pH values shown.

mL of Solution B	Final pH
45.0	6.8
43.0	7.0
39.0	7.2
32.5	7.4
27.5	7.6
22.5	7.8
17.5	8.0
12.7	8.2
9.0	8.4
6.0	8.6
4.0	8.8
2.5	9.0
1.5	9.2

Tris Buffer—pH Range 7.2 to 9.0

Stock Solution A. Dissolve 24.2 g tris (hydroxymethyl) aminomethane (tris, THAM; $C_4H_{11}NO_3$) in 1 liter of distilled water, making a 0.2 M solution.

Stock Solution B. 0.2 M hydrochloric acid (HCl).

Mix 50.0 mL of solution A with the volume of solution B as shown in the table, and make up to a final total volume of 200 mL to obtain the pH values shown.

mL of Solution B	Final pH
44.2	7.2
41.4	7.4
38.4	7.6
32.5	7.8
26.8	8.0
21.9	8.2
16.5	8.4
12.2	8.6
8.1	8.8
5.0	9.0

Barbital–Sodium Barbital Buffer—pH Range 7.0 to 8.9

Stock Solution A. Dissolve 8.24 g pure sodium diethyl barbiturate (sodium barbital, sodium Veronal) in, and make up to 1 liter with, distilled water, making a 0.04 M solution.

Stock Solution B. Dissolve 7.36 g pure diethyl barbituric acid (barbital, barbitone, Veronal) in, and make up to 1 liter with distilled water, making a 0.04 M solution.

Solution is effected by gentle heat plus constant stirring; a combined hot plate and magnetic mixer is useful.

Mix the volumes of solution A and solution B shown in the table to obtain the pH values indicated. The pH values are for a temperature of 25°C; subtract 0.1 to obtain the pH values at 37°C.

mL of Solution A	mL of Solution B	Final pH
10.0	90.0	7.0
12.5	87.5	7.1
15.5	84.5	7.2
19.0	81.0	7.3
22.5	77.5	7.4
26.0	74.0	7.5
30.0	70.0	7.6
34.5	65.5	7.7
39.5	60.5	7.8
44.5	55.5	7.9
50.0	50.0	8.0
57.5	42.5	8.1
65.0	35.0	8.2
72.0	28.0	8.3
76.5	23.5	8.4
80.0	20.0	8.5
83.0	17.0	8.6
85.5	14.5	8.7
88.0	12.0	8.8
90.0	10.0	8.9

Boric Acid–Borate Buffer pH Range 7.6 to 9.2

Stock Solution A. Dissolve 12.36 g pure boric acid (H_3BO_3) in, and make up to 1 liter with, distilled water, making a 0.2 M solution.

Stock Solution B. Dissolve 19.07 g borax (sodium tetraborate, $Na_2B_4O_7 \cdot 10H_2O$) in, and make up to 1 liter with, distilled water. This solution is 0.05 M with respect to borax, and 0.2 M with respect to sodium borate.

Mix 50.0 mL of solution A with the volume of solution B as shown in the table, and make up to a final total volume of 200 mL to obtain the pH values shown.

mL of Solution B	Final pH
2.0	7.6
3.1	7.8
4.9	8.0
7.3	8.2
11.5	8.4
17.5	8.6
22.5	8.7
30.0	8.8
42.5	8.9
59.0	9.0
83.0	9.1
115.0	9.2

Glycine-Sodium Hydroxide Buffer—pH Range 8.6 to 10.6

Stock Solution A. Dissolve 15.01 g pure glycine (aminoacetic acid, NH_2CH_2COOH) in, and make up to 1 liter with, distilled water, forming a 0.2 M solution.

Stock Solution B. 0.2 M sodium hydroxide (NaOH).

Mix 50.0 mL of solution A with the volume of solution B as shown in the table, and make up to a final total volume of 200 mL to obtain the pH values shown.

mL of Solution B	Final pH
4.0	8.6
6.0	8.8
8.8	9.0
12.0	9.2
16.8	9.4
22.4	9.6
27.2	9.8
32.0	10.0
38.6	10.2
42.6	10.4
45.5	10.6

Sodium Carbonate–Bicarbonate Buffer—pH Range 9.2 to 10.7

Stock Solution A. Dissolve 21.2 g pure anhydrous sodium carbonate (Na_2CO_3) in, and make up to 1 liter with, distilled water, making a 0.2 M solution.

Stock Solution B. Dissolve 16.8 g pure sodium bicarbonate ($NaHCO_3$) in, and make up to 1 liter with, distilled water, making a 0.2 M solution.

Mix the volumes of solution A and solution B shown in the table, and dilute to final total volume of 200 mL to obtain the pH values shown.

mL of Solution A	mL of Solution B	Final pH
4.0	46.0	9.2
7.5	42.5	9.3
9.5	40.5	9.4
13.0	37.0	9.5
16.0	34.0	9.6
19.5	30.5	9.7
22.0	28.0	9.8
25.0	25.0	9.9
27.5	22.5	10.0
30.0	20.0	10.1
33.0	17.0	10.2
35.5	14.5	10.3
38.5	11.5	10.4
40.5	9.5	10.5
42.5	7.5	10.6
45.0	5.0	10.7

Glycine–Sodium Hydroxide–Sodium Chloride Buffer—pH Range 8.4 to 12.8

Stock Solution A. Dissolve 7.505 g pure glycine (aminoacetic acid, NH_2CH_2COOH) and 5.85 g pure sodium chloride (NaCl) in, and make up to 1 liter with, distilled water, making a 0.1 M solution of both solutes.

Stock Solution B. 0.1 M sodium hydroxide (NaOH).

Mix the volumes of solution A and solution B shown in the table to obtain the pH values shown at 25°C.

mL of Solution A	mL of Solution B	Final pH
95.0	5.0	8.4
90.0	10.0	8.7
80.0	20.0	9.1
70.0	30.0	9.5
60.0	40.0	9.9
55.0	45.0	10.3
51.0	49.0	10.8
50.0	50.0	11.1
49.0	51.0	11.4
45.0	55.0	11.8
40.0	60.0	12.2
30.0	70.0	12.4
20.0	80.0	12.6
10.0	90.0	12.8

Walpole's Sodium Acetate–HCl Buffer—pH Range 0.65 to 5.2

Stock Solution A. Dissolve 82.04 g anhydrous sodium acetate ($CH_3{\cdot}COONa$) in, and make up to 1 liter with, distilled water, making a 1.0 M solution.

Stock Solution B. 1.0 M hydrochloric acid (HCl), checked by titration.

Mix 100 mL of solution A with the volume of solution B as shown in the table below, and make up to a final total volume of 500 mL with distilled water to obtain the pH values shown.

mL of Solution B	Final pH
200	0.65
160	0.91
140	1.09
130	1.24
120	1.42
110	1.71
105	1.99
102	2.32
99.5	2.72
97	3.09
95	3.29
92.5	3.5
85	3.79
80	3.95
70	4.19
50	4.58
40	4.76
30	4.92
20	5.2

Gomori's Tris-Maleic Acid Buffer—pH Range 5.08 to 8.45

Stock Solution A. Dissolve 116.0 g maleic acid (HOOC·CH-CH·COOH) in, and make up to 1 liter with, distilled water, making a 1.0 M solution.

Stock Solution B. Dissolve 121.0 g tris (hydroxymethyl) aminomethane $NH_2{\cdot}C(CH_2OH)_3$ in, and make up to 1 liter with, distilled water, making a 1.0 M solution.

Stock Solution C. 0.5 M sodium hydroxide (NaOH).

Mix the indicated volumes of these stock solutions shown in the table below to obtain the given pH values.

Michaelis' Veronal Acetate Buffer—pH Range 2.62 to 9.16

Stock Solution A. Sodium acetate ($C_2H_3NaO_2{\cdot}3H_2O$), 19.428 g (11.704 g of anhydrous salt), and 29.428 g Veronal (sodium diethylbarbiturate) dissolved in and made to 1000 mL with CO_2-free distilled water.

Stock Solution B, 0.1 N HCl. 8.4 mL concentrated hydrochloric acid added to distilled water and made to 1000 mL with same.

To obtain buffer of a certain pH, mix the quantities of the various ingredients as set out opposite that pH value in the table on the following page.

mL of Solution A	mL of Solution B	mL of Solution C	mL distilled water	pH
5	5	1	39	5.08
5	5	2	38	5.30
5	5	3	37	5.52
5	5	4	36	5.70
5	5	5	35	5.88
5	5	6	34	6.05
5	5	7	33	6.27
5	5	8	32	6.50
5	5	9	31	6.86
5	5	10	30	7.20
5	5	11	29	7.50
5	5	12	28	7.75
5	5	13	27	7.97
5	5	14	26	8.15
5	5	15	25	8.30
5	5	16	24	8.45

REFERENCE SOLUTIONS FOR pH METERS

pH 4.01 at 38°C

Dry pure potassium hydrogen phthalate (potassium biphthalate, acid potassium phthalate; $HOOCC_6H_4COOK$) for 4 to 6 hours at 105 to 110°C: cool in desiccator before weighing. Dissolve 1.021 g in, and make up to 100 mL with, distilled water. Bring to 38°C before use. pH at 25°C—4.01.

pH 6.85 at 38°C

Dry pure potassium dihydrogen phosphate (potassium phosphate monobasic; KH_2PO_4) and disodium hydrogen phosphate (sodium phosphate dibasic; Na_2HPO_4) as for pH 4.01 buffer. Dissolve 0.340 g KH_2PO_4 plus 0.355 g Na_2HPO_4 in, and make up to 100 mL with, distilled water. Bring to 38°C before use. pH at 25°C—6.86. This solution can be kept for up to 3 months if transferred to small ampules, sealed, and deep-frozen.

pH 7.381 at 38°C

Dry KH_2PO_4 and Na_2HPO_4 as for the pH 6.85 buffer. Dissolve 0.1179 g KH_2PO_4 and 0.4303 g Na_2HPO_4 in, and make up to 100 mL with, distilled water. This solution will keep if sealed in small ampules and frozen.

pH 9.18 at 25°C

Dissolve 0.381 g pure sodium tetraborate ($Na_2B_4O_7 \cdot 10H_2O$) in, and make up to 100 mL with distilled water. This solution keeps well in the refrigerator.

For the best accuracy the reference solutions should only be made in small amounts, and if stored frozen they should be discarded after they are opened.

PREPARATION OF APPROXIMATELY NORMAL SOLUTIONS

For some histological and chemical purposes, when volumetric accuracy is not required approximately nor-

pH	Stock Solution A (mL)	Stock Solution B (mL)	CO_2-Free Distilled Water
2.62	5.0	16.0	2.0
3.20	5.0	15.0	3.0
3.62	5.0	14.0	4.0
3.88	5.0	13.0	5.0
4.13	5.0	12.0	6.0
4.33	5.0	11.0	7.0
4.66	5.0	10.0	8.0
4.93	5.0	9.0	9.0
5.32	5.0	8.0	10.0
6.12	5.0	7.0	11.0
6.75	5.0	6.5	11.5
6.99	5.0	6.0	12.0
7.25	5.0	5.5	12.5
7.42	5.0	5.0	13.0
7.66	5.0	4.0	14.0
8.18	5.0	2.0	16.0
9.16	5.0	0.25	17.75

mal solutions of acids and bases may be made by dissolving in, or diluting up to, 1 liter the following quantities of the reagent-grade acids and bases.

Acetic acid (glacial)	58.0 mL
Ammonium hydroxide, sp gr 0.89 to 0.90	68.0 mL
Boric acid	20.7 g
Citric acid	70.0 g
Formic acid, 90%	43.0 mL
Hydrochloric acid, concentrated	83.0 mL
Lactic acid, 88%	85.0 mL
Nitric acid, concentrated	65.0 mL
Perchloric acid, 70 to 72%	86.0 mL
Phosphoric acid, ortho	23.0 mL
Potassium hydroxide	56.0 g
Sodium carbonate (anhydrous)	53.0 g
Sodium hydroxide	40.0 g
Sulfuric acid, concentrated	28.0 mL

IONIC STRENGTH OF SOLUTIONS

Ionic strength is a concept used to relate activity coefficients of solutions of electrolytes, and is calculated as follows:

$$\text{Ionic strength } \mu = \frac{1}{2}\sum cZ^2$$

where c is the molarity and Z the charge on the ion.

EXAMPLE 1. Calculate the ionic strength of a 0.1 M solution of sodium chloride.

Sodium = 0.1 M; charge = 1

Chloride = 0.1 M; charge = 1

$$\therefore \mu = \frac{1}{2}(0.1 \times 1^2 + 0.1 \times 1^2) = 0.1$$

EXAMPLE 2. Calculate the ionic strength of 0.1 M solution of sodium sulfate (Na_2SO_4).

Sodium = 0.1 × 2 = 0.2 M; charge = 1

Sulfate ion = 0.1 M; charge = 2

$$\therefore \mu = \frac{1}{2}(0.2 \times 1^2 + 0.1 \times 2^2)$$

$$\therefore \mu = \frac{1}{2}(0.2 + 0.4) = 0.3$$

EXAMPLE 3. Calculate the ionic strength of a buffer solution which is 0.01 M for disodium hydrogen phosphate and 0.005 M for sodium dihydrogen phosphate.

Sodium = (0.01 × 2 + 0.005) = 0.025 M;
charge = 1
Hydrogen = (0.01 + 0.005 × 2) = 0.02 M;
charge = 1
Phosphate = (0.01 + 0.005) = 0.015 M;
charge = 3

$$\therefore \mu = \frac{1}{2}(0.025 \times 1^2 + 0.02 \times 1^2 + 0.015 \times 3^2)$$

$$\mu = \frac{1}{2}(0.025 + 0.02 + 0.135) = 0.09$$

SOLUBILITY PRODUCT

The solubility concept applies to saturated solutions of slightly soluble electrolytes. The electrolytes are assumed to be completely ionized and in equilibrium with the undissolved salt, e.g.,

$$AgCl \rightleftharpoons Ag^+ + Cl^-.$$

Since the amount of undissolved solid does not affect the number of ions in solution, the solubility product is the product of the ions in solution.

$$K_{sp} = (Ag^+)(Cl^-)$$

EXAMPLE 1. A solution of silver chloride contains 1.3×10^{-5} g ions of both silver and chloride per liter of solution when in equilibrium with undissolved silver chloride.

Calculate the solubility product of silver chloride.

$$K_{sp} = (1.3 \times 10^{-5})(1.3 \times 10^{-5}) = 1.69 \times 10^{-10}$$

The solubility product varies with temperature, but unless otherwise stated the values given in tables are for 25°C.

If the product of the ions in solution is not greater than the solubility product, precipitation will not occur.

EXAMPLE 2. A solution contains 10^{-6} g ions of chloride per liter. Calculate the concentration of silver ions necessary to initiate precipitation of silver chloride.

$$(Ag^+)(Cl^-) = 1.8 \times 10^{-10}$$

$$(Ag^+) = \frac{1.8 \times 10^{-10}}{(Cl^-)} = \frac{1.8 \times 10^{-10}}{1.0 \times 10^{-6}}$$

$$= 1.8 \times 10^{-4} \text{ g ions/liter.}$$

APPENDIX G. TABLE OF SOLUBILITIES

The following abbreviated list contains only those compounds of laboratory interest.

For solubilities of organic compounds, see *Handbook of Chemistry and Physics,* and *Documenta Geigy Scientific Tables,* 7th ed., Montreal, Geigy Pharmaceuticals, 1970.

Table of Solubilities

Compound	Formula Weight	Grams Soluble in 100 mL Water	Temperature °C
Ammonium acetate. $NH_4C_2H_3O_2$	77.08	148	4
Ammonium carbonate $(NH_4)_2CO_3$	96.09	100	15
Ammonium chloride NH_4Cl	53.50	29.7	0
Ammonium molybdate $(NH_4)_2MoO_4$	196.03	sol with decomposition	
Ammonium nitrate NH_4NO_3	80.05	118.3	0
Ammonium oxalate	142.12	2.54	0
$(NH_4)_2C_2O_2 \cdot H_2O$		4.0	16.8
Antimony trichloride	228.13	601.6	0
$SbCl_3$			
Barium chloride	208.27	31.0	0
$BaCl_2$			
$BaCl_2 \cdot 2H_2O$	244.31	35.7	20
Barium hydroxide	315.51	5.6	15
$Ba(OH)_2 \cdot 8H_2O$			
Boric acid (boracic acid)	61.84	1.95	0
H_3BO_3		5.15	21
Bromine	159.83	4.17	0
Br_2		3.58	20
Cadmium chloride	183.32	140.0	20
$CdCl_2$			
$CdCl_2 \cdot 2\frac{1}{2}H_2O$	228.36	168.0	20
Calcium acetate	158.17	37.4	0
$Ca(C_2H_3O_2)_2$			
$Ca(C_2H_3O_2)_2 \cdot H_2O$	176.18	43.6	0
$Ca(C_2H_3O_2)_2 \cdot 2H_2O$	194.20	34.7	20
Calcium D-gluconate	448.39	3.3	15
$Ca(C_6H_{11}O_7)_2 \cdot H_2O$			
Calcium orthophosphate	310.20	0.002	
$Ca_3(PO_4)_2$			
Copper acetate (cupric)	199.64	7.2	
$Cu(C_2H_3O_2)_2 \cdot H_2O$			
Copper chloride (cupric)	134.45	70.6	0
$CuCl_2$			
$CuCl_2 \cdot 2H_2O$	170.49	110.4	0
Copper sulfate (cupric)	159.61	14.3	0
$CuSO_4$			
$CuSO_4 \cdot 5H_2O$	249.69	31.6	0
Ferric chloride	162.22	74.4	0
$FeCl_3$			
$FeCl_3 \cdot 6H_2O$	270.32	91.9	20
Ferric citrate	299.00	soluble	
$FeC_6H_5O_7 \cdot 3H_2O$			
Ferric nitrate	349.97	soluble	
$Fe(NO_3)_3 \cdot 6H_2O$			
$Fe(NO_3)_3 \cdot 9H_2O$	404.02	soluble	
Ferrous sulfate	278.03	15.65	
$FeSO_4 \cdot 7H_2O$			
Gold chloride (auric)	303.57	68	
$AuCl_3$			
Lead acetate	379.35	45.61	15
$Pb(C_2H_3O_2) \cdot 3H_2O$			
Lead acetate, basic	608.56	very soluble	
$Pb_2OH(C_2H_3O_2)_3$			
Lead nitrate	331.23	56.5	20
$Pb(NO_3)_2$			
Lithium chloride	42.40	45.4	25
$LiCl$			
Lithium nitrate	68.95	52.2	
$LiNO_3$			
Lithium carbonate	73.89	1.33	20
Li_2CO_3			

Table continued on following page

Table of Solubilities *(Continued)*

Compound	Formula Weight	Grams Soluble in 100 mL Water	Temperature °C
Magnesium chloride $MgCl_2 \cdot 6H_2O$	203.33	167	
Magnesium nitrate $Mg(NO_3)_2 \cdot 6H_2O$	256.43	42.33	18
Manganese chloride $MnCl_2 \cdot 4H_2O$	197.91	151	8
Mercuric chloride $HgCl_2$	271.52	6.9	20
Mercuric nitrate $HgNO_3 \cdot H_2O$	342.64	soluble	
Molybdic acid H_2MoO_4	161.97	slightly soluble	
$H_2MoO_4 \cdot H_2O$	179.98	0.133	18
Osmium tetroxide OsO_4	254.20	6.23	25
Potassium Compounds			
Acetate $KC_2H_3O_2$	98.14	253	20
Bromate $KBrO_3$	167.01	13.3	40
Bromide KBr	119.01	53.48	0
Carbonate, anhydrous K_2CO_3	138.20	112.0	20
$K_2CO_3 \cdot 1\frac{1}{2}H_2O$	165.24	129.4	
Chlorate $KClO_3$	122.55	7.1	20
Chloride KCl	74.55	34.7	20
Cyanide KCN	65.11	very soluble	
Dichromate $K_2Cr_2O_7$	294.21	4.9	0
Ferricyanide $K_3Fe(CN)_6$	329.25	33.0	4
Ferrocyanide $K_4Fe(CN)_6 \cdot 3H_2O$	422.39	27.8	12
Fluoride KF	58.10	92.3	18
Hydrogen carbonate (bicarbonate, $KHCO_3$)	100.11	22.4	
Hydrogen phosphate, mono-H K_2HPO_4	174.18	167	20
Hydrogen phosphate, di-H KH_2PO_4	136.09	33.0	25
Hydrogen phthalate $KHC_8H_4O_4$	204.22	10	25
Hydrogen sulfate (bisulfate) $KHSO_4$	136.17	36.3	0
Hydroxide KOH	56.10	107	15
Hypochlorite KClO	90.55	very soluble	
Iodate KIO_3	214.02	4.74	0
Iodide KI	166.02	127.5	0
Metaperiodate KIO_4	230.02	0.66	13
Nitrate KNO_3	101.10	31.6	20
Nitrite KNO_2	85.10	313	25
Oxalate $K_2C_2O_4 \cdot H_2O$	184.23	33	16
Permanganate $KMnO_4$	158.03	6.38	20

Table continued on opposite page

Table of Solubilities *(Continued)*

Compound	Formula Weight	Grams Soluble in 100 mL Water	Temperature °C
Persulfate $K_2S_2O_8$	270.32	5.3	20
Phosphate K_3PO_4	212.27	90	20
Pyrophosphate $K_4P_2O_7 \cdot 3H_2O$	384.39	soluble	
Sulfate K_2SO_4	174.26	12	25
Tartrate, D- $K_2C_4H_4O_6 \cdot \frac{1}{2}H_2O$	235.27	150	14
Tellurite K_2TeO_3	253.80	very soluble	
Thiocyanate KSCN	97.18	217	20
Silver nitrate $AgNO_3$	169.89	122	0
Sodium Compounds			
Acetate $NaC_2H_3O_2$	82.04	119	0
$NaC_2H_3O_2 \cdot 3H_2O$	136.09	76.2	0
Azide NaN_3	65.02	41.7	17
Barbital $NaC_8H_{11}N_2O_3$	206.18	20	25
Benzoate $NaC_7H_5O_2$	144.11	66	20
Borohydride $NaBH_4$	37.85	decomposes	
Bromate $NaBrO_3$	150.91	27.5	0
Bromide NaBr	102.91	116	50
Carbonate Na_2CO_3	106.00	7.1	0
$Na_2CO_3 \cdot H_2O$	124.02	33	
Chlorate $NaClO_4$	106.45	79	0
Chloride NaCl	58.45	35.7	0
Chromate Na_2CrO_4	162.00	87.3	30
Citrate $Na_3C_6H_5O_7 \cdot 2H_2O$	294.12	72	25
Cyanide NaCN	49.02	soluble	
Ferricyanide $Na_3Fe(CN)_6 \cdot H_2O$	298.97	18.9	0
Ferrocyanide $Na_4Fe(CN)_6 \cdot 10H_2O$	484.11	31.85	20
Fluoride NaF	42.00	4.22	18
Formate $NaCHO_2$	68.02	97.2	20
Hydrogen carbonate (bicarbonate) $NaHCO_3$	84.02	6.9	0
Hydrogen phosphate (monobasic, dihydrogen) $NaH_2PO_4 \cdot H_2O$	138.01	110.3	20
Hydrogen phosphate (dibasic, monohydrogen) $Na_2HPO_4 \cdot 7H_2O$	268.09	104	40
Hydrogen sulfate (bisulfate) $NaHSO_4 \cdot H_2O$	138.09	67, decomposes	
Hydrosulfite (dithionite) $Na_2S_2O_4 \cdot 2H_2O$	210.16	25.4	20
Hydroxide NaOH	40.01	42	0
		347	100
Iodate $NaIO_3$	197.92	2.5	0

Table continued on following page

Table of Solubilities *(Continued)*

Compound	Formula Weight	Grams Soluble in 100 mL Water	Temperature °C
Iodide NaI	149.92	158.7	0
Molybdate $Na_2MoO_4 \cdot 2H_2O$	241.98	56.2	0
Nitrate $NaNO_3$	85.01	73	0
Nitrite $NaNO_2$	69.01	81.5	15
Nitroprusside $Na_2(NO)Fe(CN)_5 \cdot 2H_2O$	297.97	40	16
Oxalate $Na_2C_2O_4$	134.01	3.7	20
Pentobarbital $NaC_{11}H_{17}N_2O_3$	248.26	soluble	
Perchlorate $NaClO_4 \cdot H_2O$	140.47	209	15
Phenobarbital $NaC_{12}H_{11}N_2O_3$	254.22	very soluble	
Phosphate (tribasic) $Na_3PO_4 \cdot 12H_2O$	380.16	25.8	20
Pyrophosphate $Na_4P_2O_7 \cdot 10H_2O$	446.11	5.41	0
Pyrosulfite (metabisulfite) $Na_2S_2O_5$	190.13	54	20
Salicylate $NaC_7H_5O_3$	160.11	111	15
Sulfate, rhombic	142.06	4.76	0
monoclinic Na_2SO_4	142.06	48.8	40
Sulfate (Glauber's salt) $Na_2SO_4 \cdot 10H_2O$	322.22	92.7	30
Sulfite Na_2SO_3	126.06	12.54	0
Tetraborate, borax $Na_2B_4O_7 \cdot 10H_2O$	381.43	1.6	10
Thiosulfate, hypo $Na_2S_2O_3 \cdot 5H_2O$	248.21	79.4	0
Tungstate $Na_2WO_4 \cdot 2H_2O$	329.95	82.5	20
Stannous chloride $SnCl_2 \cdot 2H_2O$	225.65	118.7, decomposes	
Uranyl nitrate $UO_2(NO_3)_2 \cdot 6H_2O$	502.18	170.3	0
Zinc acetate $Zn(C_2H_3O_2)_2 \cdot 2H_2O$	219.50	31.1	20
Zinc chloride $ZnCl_2$	136.29	432	25

Reference

Handbook of Chemistry and Physics. 48th ed., Cleveland, The Chemical Rubber Co., 1967.

APPENDIX H. BLOOD GLUCOSE ESTIMATION (Dubowski, 1962)

Principle

See paragraph 2, p. 126.

Procedure

1. Using a positive-displacement, piston type pipettor, add 0.1 mL of whole blood, serum, or plasma to 1.9 mL of 3.0% w/v trichloracetic acid in a 100 by 13 mm test tube. Mix well, allow to stand for at least five minutes, and centrifuge for 10 minutes at 2500 rpm.

2. Set up three 150 by 16 mm tubes, marked Test, Blank, and Standard.

3. Transfer accurately 1.0 mL of clear supernatant from step 1 into the Test tube. Into the Blank tube pipette 1.0 mL of distilled water. Into the Standard tube pipette 1.0 mL of working standard solution.

4. Using a suitable automatic dispensing device, add to all tubes 5.0 mL of o-toluidine reagent.

5. Mix by careful lateral shaking; cap tubes with aluminum caps. Heat in a boiling water bath for exactly 10 minutes

6. Cool in cold tap water for at least 4 minutes.

7. Read the absorbance of Test and Standard at 630 nm in the spectrophotometer, setting zero absorbance with the Blank. (See Note 2 below.)

Calculation

$$\frac{\text{Absorbance of Test}}{\text{Absorbance of Standard}} \times 200 = \text{mg glucose per dL}$$

$$\text{Mg glucose per dL} \times 0.056 = \text{mmol/L}$$

Normal Values

See p. 127.

Reagents

3.0% w/v Trichloroacetic Acid. Dissolve 30.0 g pure trichloroacetic acid in distilled water and make up to one liter. Mix well.

o-Toluidine Reagent. This is most conveniently obtained commercially. The original reagent is made by dissolving 1.5 g of pure thiourea in 200 mL glacial acetic acid, using gentle heat if necessary. Transfer to a one liter volumetric flask, washing in with glacial acetic acid. Add 60.0 mL pure o-toluidine (use the grade identified as "from nitrate"), mix, make up to one liter with glacial acetic acid, mix well. Keep in a brown glass bottle in the refrigerator.

Stock Glucose Standard Solution. 1.0 g of pure, dry, anhydrous glucose dissolved in, and made up to 100 mL with, a saturated solution of benzoic acid.

Working Glucose Standard. Dilute volumetrically 1.0 mL of stock to 100 mL with a saturated solution of benzoic acid. Make weekly to minimize changes due to evaporation.

Notes

1. For CSF use 0.4 mL of CSF plus 1.6 mL trichloroacetic acid: divide the final result by four.
2. To minimize the chance of accidents with the strongly acid reagent, use high-grade test tubes in step 2 and use the same tubes for the absorbance readings. A flow-through type cuvette may be used, but very thorough flushing will be essential.
3. Unacceptably high blanks may be due to the use of poor grades of o-toluidine.
4. Results under 40 mg/dL may be unreliable; repeat the assay using a 0.2 mL sample, dividing the final result by two.
5. If interference from galactose is suspected or possible, use the specific hexokinase method given on p. 127. Interference from xylose after oral administration of that carbohydrate in the investigation of malabsorption will show as a brown color instead of emerald green. Administration to the patient of one of the dextran plasma volume expanders will cause severe turbidity in the final reaction: use the specific hexokinase method.

References

Dubowski KM. An o-toluidine method for body-fluid glucose determination. Clin Chem 1962; *8*:215–235.

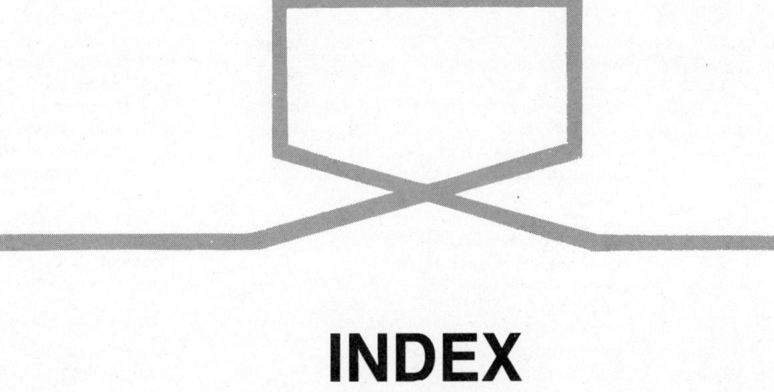

INDEX

Page numbers in *italics* refer to illustrations; numbers followed by T indicate tables

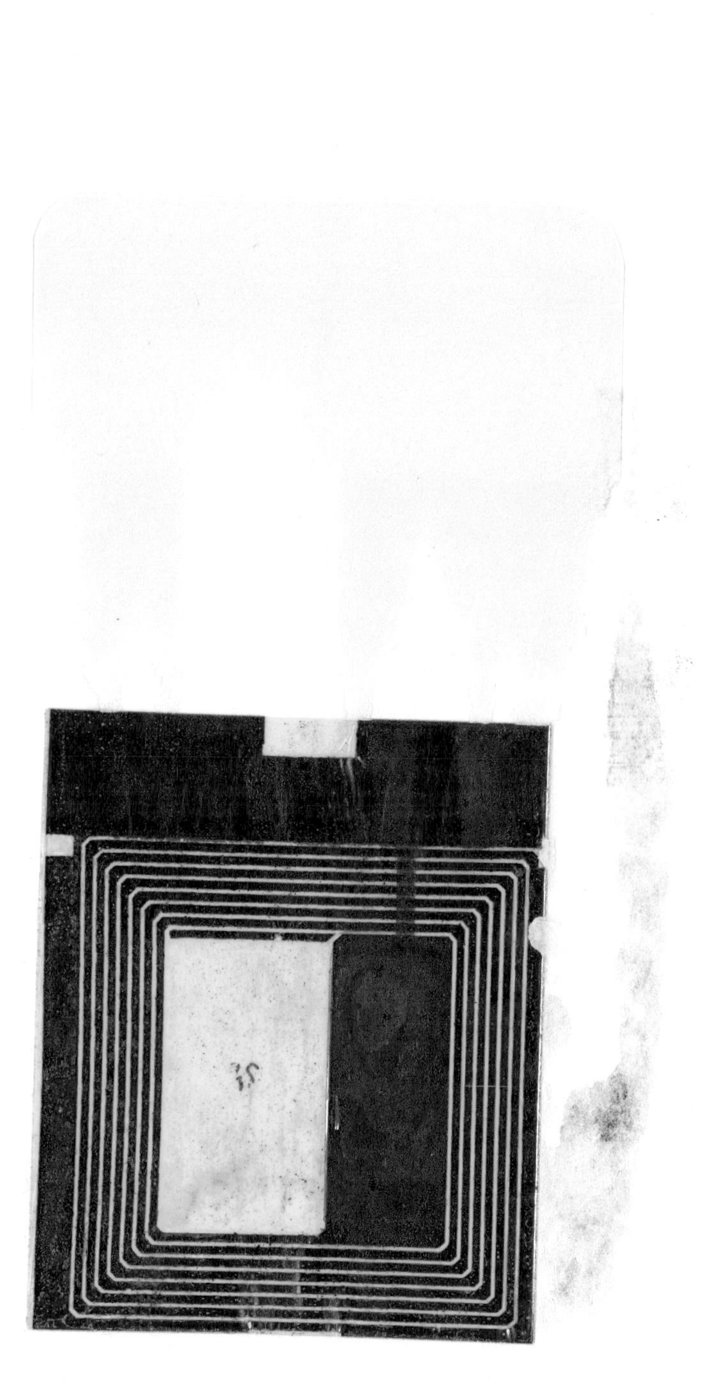

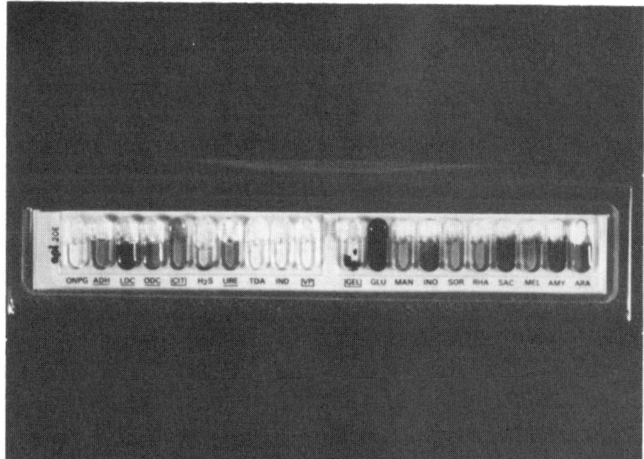

API 20E strip inoculated and incubated with *S. typhi*.

Immunoplate for IgA estimation.

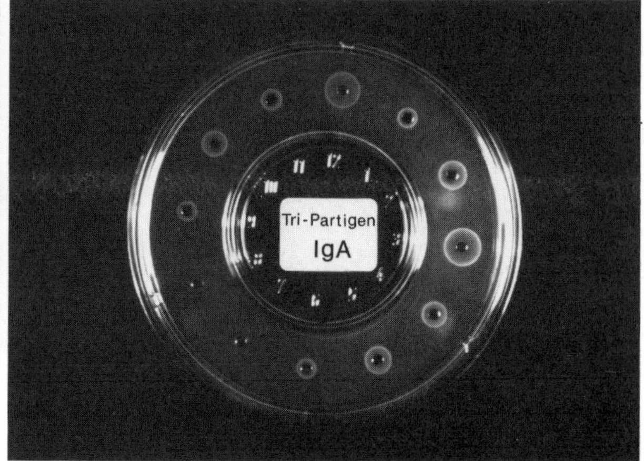

Schistosoma mansoni ova in rectal wall.

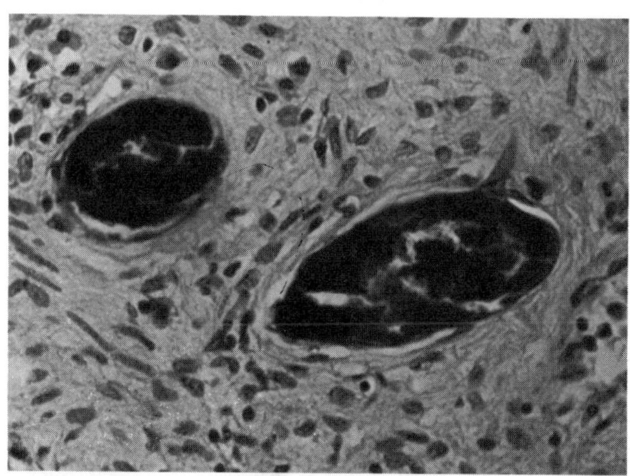

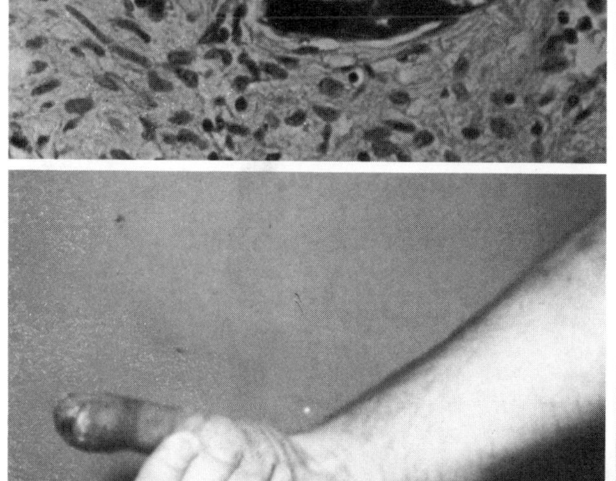

Inflammation and ulceration of thumb due to sporotrichosis.

Tuberculous pus stained by Ziehl-Neelsen technique.

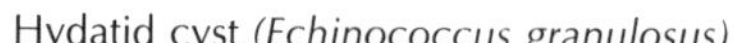

Hydatid cyst *(Echinococcus granulosus)*.

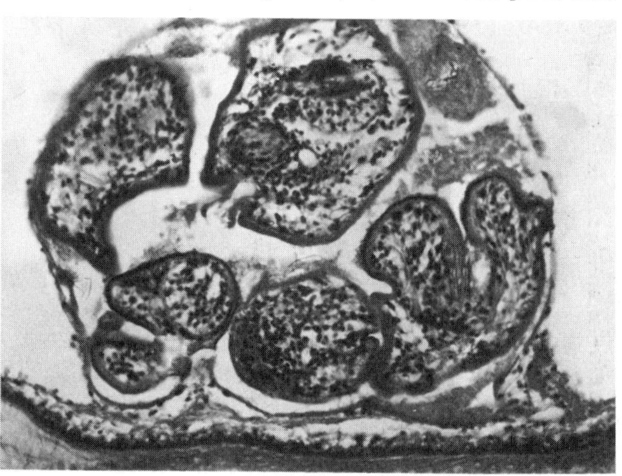